Sloane's
Medical
Word
Book

Sloane's Medical Word Book

A spelling and vocabulary guide
to medical transcription

---

fourth edition
ELLEN DRAKE, CMT

W.B. SAUNDERS COMPANY
A Harcourt Health Sciences Company
Philadelphia   London   New York   St. Louis   Sydney   Toronto

W.B. SAUNDERS COMPANY
A Harcourt Health Sciences Company

The Curtis Center
Independence Square West
Philadelphia, Pennsylvania 19106

www.wbsaunders.com

Library of Congress Cataloging-in-Publication Data

Drake, Ellen
   Sloane's medical word book / Ellen Drake.—4th ed.

     p. cm.

   Rev. ed. of: Medical word book / Sheila B. Sloane. 3rd. ed. 1991.

   ISBN 0-7216-7626-X
   1. Medicine–Terminology. I. Sloane, Sheila B. Medical word book. II. Title.

R123 .S57 2001
610'.1'4–dc21

2001020706

Acquisitions Editor: Maureen Pfeifer

Production Editor: Edna Dick

Production Manager: Pete Faber

Book Designer: Ellen Zanolle

Sloane's Medical Word Book   ISBN 0–7216–7626–X

Printed in the United States of America.

Last digit is the print number: 9   8   7   6   5   4   3   2   1

*Dedicated to
the memory of
Sheila B. Sloane*

Preface

It was an honor for me to be requested by Sheila Sloane herself to complete this update of *The Medical Word Book.* I had met Sheila a couple of times at medical transcription meetings, and she made a point of encouraging me and complimenting me on my own book, the *Saunders Pharmaceutical Word Book.* I felt I should have been salaaming at *her* feet!

To me, Sheila was an icon in our profession because she was one of the first, if not *the* first, to recognize our need for quick-reference books. Her many books have contributed immeasurably to the quality of transcribed medical reports, not to mention their role in the greater ease with which we MTs do our work. *The Medical Word Book* is no doubt the most popular and treasured of Sheila's books. Although my personal contact with Sheila was limited, my respect and admiration for her were immense. I will miss her greatly, and I'm certain many others will also.

In this fourth edition of *The Medical Word Book,* I have tried to remain true to Sheila's original and ongoing purpose:

> . . . to introduce the newcomer and the seasoned [medical] transcriptionist to the available information and to provide, collected in one place, the essentials necessary to make their task of transcribing medical reports an easier one. The transcriptionist new to the profession is relieved of the responsibility of guessing whether a disease entity, an instrument, or the like is listed in one particular specialty rather than another. If a word applies to several specialties, it is listed in [all] the appropriate section[s]. In this respect, repetition of terms has not been avoided; rather, it has been sought out.

> For example, "sarcoidosis" appears in the [*Cardiology, Internal Medicine, Obstetrics and Gynecology, Oncology and Hematology, Orthopedics and Sports Medicine,* and *Pulmonary Medicine*] sections, thus making it unnecessary to flip pages back and forth between sections to find the proper spelling.

> As in the past, no attempt has been made to make this a complete listing of medical terms. Such an undertaking would be overwhelming and cumbersome. The attempt here is to give the reader a listing of commonly used uncommon medical terms to ease the burden of searching through many books.

I have continued to include individual terms in multiple sections when they apply to more than one specialty. All surgical hardware is listed in *General Surgical Terms.* Surgical terms that apply only to a particular specialty are listed in that specialty. I have expanded the use of phonetic spellings to aid in locating difficult-to-spell terms, including some eponyms. Occasionally, I have included clues for use of individual terms to help readers distinguish, for example, between nouns and adjectives (e.g., mucous and mucus), common nouns and eponyms (e.g., Green, Angle, Bar), homonyms (e.g., principal and principle), anatomy and pathogen (e.g., pediculus and *Pediculus*), or anatomy and surgical term (e.g., suture). Note that explanatory notes are enclosed in brackets after the terms. In addition, I have added about 200 nonmedical terms that are frequently used in medical reports as well as about 90 of the most frequently misspelled English words. Most of these appear in General Medical Terms, a few in relevant specialty sections.

Irregularly formed plurals, followed by the notation "plural of . . ." in parentheses, are included as individual entries and also in parentheses following the singular form of a term. The exception to this is if the plural entry would appear immediately before or after the singular entry. Common units of measure are followed by the appropriate abbreviation (e.g., milligrams [mg], centimeters [cm], etc.) and can be found in **Part One** in the section most relevant to that term.

I have cross-referenced variant spellings for eponyms to the preferred or most widely used spelling. The entry for the preferred spelling often includes the variant spelling in parentheses. Any subentries that apply to that eponym will be under the more common spelling. Occasionally, two spellings for an eponym seemed equally common, and you will find subentries under both spellings. When there were two or more spellings for a single common noun or noneponymic term, I have tried to include only the most frequently used spelling (i.e., the one with the definition in *Dorland's Illustrated Medical Dictionary,* 29th ed.).

In keeping with widely accepted style for medical reporting, I have dropped the possessive forms of eponyms as well as periods from uppercase abbreviations. You will find the use of hyphens much less frequent and the spaces removed from abbreviations that include an ampersand symbol (e.g., D&C). When special characters (e.g., μ [Greek letter mu], superscripts, subscripts, etc.) are part of an abbreviation or term, I have tried to include in brackets an acceptable alternative for those unable to transcribe special characters because of font or printer limitations. Please consult your supervisor or institution's approved style manual for any questions relating to style.

I have made some changes to the overall structure of the book as well. The three major parts (**General Terms, Specialties,** and **Guide to Terminology**) have been retained. However, I have moved the *Anatomy Plates* section from **Part One: General Terms** to **Part Three: Guide to Terminology.** Also, I have omitted the section *Drugs and Chemistry.* The rapid changes in pharmaceuticals make it impractical to include a listing of drugs in a book that is updated only every 4 to 5 years.When *The Medical Word Book* was first published, there were no good, up-to-date pharmaceutical references for our field. Today there are—the best of which is the *Saunders Pharmaceutical Word Book,* which is updated annually and available from this same publisher. I did retain and add a substantial number of drug-related terms (200 drug classes have been added, for example) and include those terms in *General Medical Terms*. Chemistry terms have been moved to *Laboratory, Pathology, and Chemistry Terms*.

An entirely new section in **Part Two: Specialties** is *Oncology and Hematology*. The *Dentistry* section, omitted from the third edition, has been restored and updated in this edition. In addition, I have moved *Allergy* from *Dermatology* to the *Infectious Diseases and Immunology* (formerly *Immunology*) section and separated *Psychiatry* from *Neurology*. In many cases the specialties have been expanded and the titles changed. Please review the **Contents** page before using the book to refamiliarize yourself with its organization.

As noted above, this book is not comprehensive. It would take a large, single volume to do justice to each specialty. However, I hope that readers will find that this edition lives up to the purpose and standards set by Sheila Sloane.

I would like to thank Maureen Pfeifer, Acquisitions Editor; the editorial and production staff at W.B. Saunders, particularly Pete Faber and Edna Dick; as well as Sheila's family for their patience and support while I have been working on this revision. The work has not been without setbacks, and I know their patience has been tried many times. I would also like to thank Susan Dooley and the Medical Transcription Class at Seminole Community College in Sanford, Florida for help in verifying many terms.

As with my other books, I welcome readers' feedback. If you have comments, corrections, or questions, you may e-mail me at the address below or send them to me via U.S. mail in care of Sloane's Medical Word Book, W.B. Saunders Company, The Curtis Center, Independence Square West, Philadelphia, PA 19106-3399. To order additional copies, individuals can call 800-545-2522; schools call 800-782-4479, 8 AM to 7 PM, central time.

Author's e-mail address: Ellen Drake, CMT
MedicalWordBook@Saunders.net   Peachtree City, GA

Contents

Part Three
Guide to Terminology

Appendix

Sloane's
Medical
Word
Book

Part One

General Terms

General Medical Terms
Includes Emergency Medicine and Drug-Related Terminology

A$_2$ [A2]—aortic second sound
AA—Alcoholics Anonymous
AAFP—American Academy of
    Family Practice
        American Association of
        Family Physicians
AAGP—American Academy of
    General Practice
AAL—anterior axillary line
AAO3, AAOx3—awake, alert, and
    oriented times three [to time,
    place, and person]
Aaron
      sign
AAS—acute abdominal series
abapical
abate
abatement
abaxial
ABC—airway breathing circulation
    [protocol]
ABD, Abd, abd—abdomen, abdom-
    inal
abdomen
abdominal
        a. cavity
        a. crisis
        a. reflexes
abdominoanterior
abdominoposterior
abduct
abduction
abductor
abenteric
aberrancy
abeyance
abiatrophy

ability
      general a.
abionergy
abiotrophic
abiotrophy
abirritant
abirritation
abirritative
ablate
ablation
abluent
abluminal
ablution
abmortal
ABN, Abn, abn—abnormal, abnor-
      mality
abnerval
abnormal
abnormality (abnormalities)
abnormity
ABO
      blood groups
aborad [adv.]
aboral [adj.]
abortifacients [a class of drugs]
abortive
abouchement
ABP—arterial blood pressure
ABR—absolute bed rest
abrachius
abradant
abrade
abrasion
      dicing a.
      marginal a.
abrasive

abscess
>apical a.
>caseous a.
>cheesy a.
>chronic a.
>circumscribed a.
>deep a.
>diffuse a.
>dry a.
>encapsulated a.
>encysted a.
>gas a.
>glandular a.
>gravitation a., gravity a.
>gummatous a.
>helminthic a.
>hematogenous a.
>hemorrhagic a.
>hot a.
>hypostatic a.
>idiopathic a.
>marginal a.
>migrating a.
>miliary a.
>milk a.
>mother a.
>mural a.
>peritoneal a.
>phlegmonous a.
>primary a.
>pyemic a.
>pyogenic a.
>recrudescent a.
>residual a.
>satellite a.
>secondary a.
>septicemic a.
>serous a.
>shirt-stud a.
>stellate a.
>stercoraceous a., stercoral a.
>sterile a.
>stitch a.
>strumous a.
>subacute a.
>subaponeurotic a.
>subdiaphragmatic a.
>subfascial a.

abscess (continued)
>subpectoral a.
>subscapular a.
>sudoriparous a.
>sympathetic a.
>traumatic a.
>tuberculous a.
>tympanitic a.
>verminous a.
>walled-off a.
>wandering a.
>warm a.

absinthe
absorb
absorbent
absorption
>percutaneous a.

abstergent
abstinence
abstract
abstraction
absurdity (absurdities)
abundance
abuse
>alcohol a.
>chemical a.
>child a.
>drug a.
>elder a.
>ethanol a.
>inhalant a.
>mixed drug a.
>physical a.
>polydrug a.
>polypharmacy a.
>polysubstance a.
>psychoactive substance a.
>sexual a.
>spousal a., spouse a.
>substance a.
>tobacco a.

abut
a.c.—before meals (L. ante cibum)
ACA—adenocarcinoma
acanthoid
acanthopelvis
acanthopelyx

a capite ad calcem (L. from the
    head to the heel)
acaudal
acaudate
ACC—ambulatory care center
accede
accelerant
accelerated
acceleration
accelerator
    thromboplastin generation a.
accentuation
    presystolic a.
access
accessiflexor
accessorius
accessory
    a. muscles of respiration
    a. nerve
    a. sign
accident
    cardiovascular a.
    car versus pedestrian a.
    cerebrovascular a. (CVA)
    motor vehicle a. (MVA)
acclimate, acclimated
accommodate
accommodation
accommodative
accomplice
accrementition
accretion
accuracy
ACE—angiotensin-converting
    enzyme
ACEIs—ACE inhibitors [a class of
    drugs]
acenesthesia
acentric
ACEP—American College of
    Emergency Physicians
acerate
acerbity
acerola
acervuline
acetaminophen poisoning
acetanilid
    a. poisoning

acetic
acetify
acetin
acetonitrile
acetous
acetum
acetylcholinesterase (AChE) inhibi-
    tors [a class of drugs]
acetylsalicylic acid poisoning
ACF—acute care facility
ache
AChE (acetylcholinesterase) inhibi-
    tors [a class of drugs]
achievement
    a. scores
achroodextrin
acicular
aciculate
aciculum
acid
    acetylsalicylic a. (ASA)
    alpha-lipoic a. (ALA)
    boric a.
    citric a.
    muriatic a.
    salicylic a.
    saturated fatty a. (SFA)
    sulfuric a.
    tannic a.
    trichloroacetic a.
    unsaturated fatty a.
acidic
acidification
acidity
acid-proof
acid rain
acies
ackee, akee
ACLF—adult congregate living
    facility
ACLS—advanced cardiac life support
acme
acolous
aconite
acoustic
acoustics
acquired
acquisition

acrid
acrimony
acritical
acrocephalous
acrocinesis
acrocinetic
acromelia
acromelic
acromphalus
acronarcotic
acroteric
acrotic
acrotism
acrylic acid
actinolyte
action
    cumulative a.
activate
activated charcoal
activator
    plasminogen a.
    single-chain urokinase-type
      plasminogen (scu-PA) a.
      (prourokinase)
    tissue plasminogen a. (t-PA,
      tPA, TPA)
    urinary plasminogen a., u-
      plasminogen a. (urokinase)
active
activity
    a.'s of daily living (ADL,
      ADLs)
aculeate
acupuncture
acus
acute
acute on chronic
    a.o.c. illness
    a.o.c. symptoms
ACVD—acute cardiovascular disease
    arteriosclerotic cardiovascu-
      lar disease
acyanotic
acyclic
AD—admitting diagnosis
    advance directive
    right ear (L. auris dextra)
adaptability

adaptation
    physiologic a.
    sensory a.
adaxial
additive
ADDU—alcohol and drug depen-
    dency unit
adduct
adduction
adenalgia
adenectopia
adenic
adeniform
adenine
    a. arabinoside
adenitis
adenization
adenocarcinoma
adenodynia
adenogenous
adenoma
adenomatoid
adenomyomatous
adenoneural
adenosine
    a. deaminase
    a. diphosphate (ADP)
    a. kinase
    a. monophosphate (AMP)
    a. triphosphate (ATP)
adenous
adenoviral
adeps
    a. praeparatus
adequacy
adhere
adherent
adhesiveness
adiathermancy
adient
adipofibroma
adipogenic
adipogenous
adipoid
adipometer
adiposalgia
adipose
adipositis

adjacent
adjunct
adjunctive
adjustment
    a. disorder
adjuvant
    double-emulsion a.
    Freund a.
    oil emulsion a.
    solubilized water-in-oil a.
    a. therapy
    water-in-oil-in-water emul-
      sion a.
ADL, ADLs—activities of daily liv-
    ing
ad lib—as desired, at pleasure (L.
    ad libitum)
adm, admit—admission
admedial
admedian
admittance
admixture
ad nauseam
adnerval
adneural
adolescence
adolescent
ADR—adverse drug reaction
adrenal cortical steroids, adrenocor-
    tical steroids [a class of drugs]
adrenaline
adrenergic
    a. agonists [a class of drugs]
adrenogenic
adsorb
adsorbate
adsorbent
adsorption
adsternal
adterminal
adtorsion
adult
adulterant
adulteration
advance
adventitia
adventitious
    a. sounds

adverse effects
adversive
advocate
    patient a.
AED—antiepileptic drug
aerate
aerated
aeration
aeremia
aerial
aeroembolism
aeromedicine
aeropathy
aerophagia
aerosol
aerosolization
aesculapian
Aesculapius, staff of
AF—Asian female
afebrile
affect [verb: influence]
affect [noun: state of mind]
    apathetic a.
    bland a.
    blunted a.
    congruent a.
    constricted a.
    depressed a., depressive a.
    euphoric a.
    flat a.
    impaired a.
    inappropriate a.
    labile a.
    restricted a.
affection
affective
afflux
aforementioned
aftercare
afterdamp
aftereffect
aftermath
aftertaste
afunction
against medical advice (AMA)
age
    anatomical a.
    bone a.

age (continued)
>   childbearing a.
>   chronological a.
>   a. of consent
>   developmental a.
>   emotional a.
>   functional a.
>   mental a.
>   physical a., physiologic a.
>   skeletal a.

agent
>   adrenergic blocking a.
>   chemotherapeutic a.
>   myoneural blocking a.
>   neuromuscular blocking a.
>   virus-inactivating a.

Agent Orange
agerasia
ageusic
aggregate
aggregated
aggressive
>   a. manner
>   a. treatment

aging
agitated
agminated
agmination
agnogenic
agnosic
agonal
agonist
>   cholinergic a.'s [a class of
>   drugs]
>   muscarinic a.'s [a class of
>   drugs]
>   narcotic a.'s [a class of drugs]
>   narcotic a.-antagonists [a
>   class of drugs]
>   prostaglandin a.'s [a class of
>   drugs]

agony
agrypnotic
ague
"ah-boosh-maw" Phonetic for
>   abouchement.
aid
>   first a.

aid (continued)
>   pharmaceutic a., pharmaceu-
>   tical a.
>   prosthetic speech a.
>   speech a.

aide
>   nurse's a.

AIDS—acquired immunodeficiency
>   syndrome

ailment
air
>   ambient a.
>   a. cushion
>   a. embolism
>   vitiated a.

airborne
airsickness
airway
>   anatomical a.
>   artificial a.
>   esophageal obturator a.
>   lower a.
>   nasopharyngeal a.
>   oropharyngeal a.
>   upper a.

akee, ackee
akinetic
ALA—alpha-lipoic acid
alanine (Ala, A)
alar
alate
albeit
albidus
Albuminar-5
albuminoid
albuminous
alcohol
>   grain a.
>   a. intoxication
>   wood a.

alcoholic
Alco-Sensor
alga (algae)
>   blue-green a.

algesia
algesic
algicide
algogenesia

align
alimentary
alimentation
aliquot
alkalinity
alkalinization
alkalinize
alkaloid
alkalosis
    altitude a.
"alk. phos." Slang for alkaline phosphatase.
alkylamines [a class of drugs]
alkylate
alkylation
alkylator
allantoid
allergenic extracts [a class of drugs]
alliance
    therapeutic a.
    working a.
allopathic
allopathy
alloploid
allowance
    recommended daily a. (RDA)
allude, alluded
allusion
allylamines [a class of drugs]
almond
    bitter a.
aloe
alpha
    a.-tocopherol
ALS—advanced life support
alter
alterative
alternation
altricious
aluminum (Al)
    a. acetate
    a. hydroxide
    a. nicotinate
    a. phosphate
    a. sulfate
alveolate
alvus

a.m.—before noon (L. ante meridiem)
AM—Asian male
AMA—against medical advice
amacrinal
amacrine
amalgamation
amaranth
amaroid
amatol
ambidexterity
ambidextrism
ambidextrous
ambient
ambiguity
ambiguous
ambilateral
ambilevosity
ambilevous
ambisinister
ambisinistrous
ambivalence
ambivalent
Ambu bag
ambulance
ambulant
ambulation
ambulatory
ambustion
amebicides [a class of drugs]
ameliorate, ameliorated
amelioration
amenable
amerism
ameristic
AMI—acute myocardial infarction
p-aminobenzoic acid (PABA) [p-,
   para-]
aminoglycosides [a class of drugs]
aminoketones [a class of drugs]
aminopenicillins [a class of drugs]
21-aminosteroids [a class of drugs]
ammoniacal
amobarbital
amok, amuck
amorphous
"amp" Slang for ampicillin.

"amp and gent" Slang for ampicillin and gentamicin.
amperage
amphetamine
    a. aspartate
    a. sulfate
amphetamines [a class of drugs]
amphitheater
ampule
amuck, amok
anabolic steroids [a class of drugs]
anabolism
anacatharsis
analeptics [a class of drugs]
analgesia
analgesics [a class of drugs]
analog [electronic]
analogous
analogue [anatomical, chemical]
analogy
analysis
anaphrodisiacs [a class of drugs]
anaphylactoid
anasarca
anatomic, anatomical
anatomicity
ancillary
    a. measures
    a. therapy
androgens [a class of drugs]
anemia
anemic
anergy
anesthesia
    See in *General Surgical Terms.*
anesthesiologist
anesthesiology
anesthetics [a class of drugs]
anesthetist
aneurysm
aneurysmatic
angina
anginal
angioma
    spider a.
angiomatoid
angiomatosis

angiotensin
    a. II
    a. III
    a. amide
    a.-converting enzyme (ACE)
    a.-converting enzyme inhibitors (ACEIs) [a class of drugs]
    a. II receptor antagonists (AIIRAs) [a class of drugs]
angle
angor
    a. animi
    a. nocturnus
    a. ocularis
    a. pectoris
Angström
    reciprocal
    unit
angulated
anhidrosis
anhidrotics [a class of drugs]
anicteric
aniline
    a. fuchsin
    a. gentian violet
    a. red
anima
    a. mundi
animation
annectent
annihilation
annular
anodynes [a class of drugs]
anomalous
anomaly
    developmental a.
anonymous
anophelicide
anophelifuge
anopheline
anophelism
anorectic
anorectics [a class of drugs]
anorexiants [a class of drugs]
anorexigenics [a class of drugs]
anoxemia
ansate

Ansbacher unit
antacids [a class of drugs]
antagonist
    histamine H_1 a.'s [a class of drugs]
    histamine H_2 a.'s [a class of drugs]
    5-HT_3 (hydroxytryptamine) receptor a.'s [a class of drugs]
    leukotriene receptor a.'s [a class of drugs]
antecedent
anteflexion
antegrade
anterior
anteriorly
anteroexternal
anterograde
anteroinferior
anterointernal
anterolateral
anteromedial
anteromedian
anteroposterior
anteroposteriorly
anterosuperior
anterosuperiorly
anteroventral
anteversion
anteverted
antexed
anthelmintics [a class of drugs]
anthorisma
anthracene
anthracic
anthracotherapy
anthracyclines [a class of drugs]
anthropokinetics
anthropology
    social a.
anthropomorphic
anthropomorphism
anthroponosis
anthropopathy
anthroposcopy
antiadrenergics [a class of drugs]
antiandrogens [a class of drugs]

antianxiety
antibiotics [a class of drugs]
    aminoglycoside a.
    bactericidal a.
    bacteriostatic a.
    broad-spectrum a.
    carbapenem a.
    cephalosporin a.
    fluoroquinolone a.
    glycopeptide a.
    β-lactam a. [beta-]
    lincosamide a.
    macrolide a.
    oral a.
    polyene a.
    sulfonamide a.
    tetracycline a.
    topical a.
antibromics [a class of drugs]
anticholinergic
anticholinergics [a class of drugs]
anticoagulants [a class of drugs]
anticoagulated
anticonvulsants [a class of drugs]
antidepressants [a class of drugs]
antidiuretic
    a. hormone
antidiuretics [a class of drugs]
antidopaminergics [a class of drugs]
antidotes [a class of drugs]
antiemetics [a class of drugs]
antiepileptic drugs (AEDs) [a class of drugs]
antiestrogens [a class of drugs]
antihistamines [a class of drugs]
antihydrotics [a class of drugs]
antihyperlipidemic agents [a class of drugs]
antilipemics [a class of drugs]
antilithics [a class of drugs]
antimuscarinics [a class of drugs]
antinauseants [a class of drugs]
antineoplastics [a class of drugs]
antineoplastons [a class of drugs]
antiperiodics [a class of drugs]
antiphlogistics [a class of drugs]
antipyretics [a class of drugs]
antisense drugs [a class of drugs]

antisepsis
antiseptics [a class of drugs]
antispasmodics [a class of drugs]
antitoxins [a class of drugs]
antituberculous agents [a class of drugs]
antitussives [a class of drugs]
antivenins [a class of drugs]
antivirals [a class of drugs]
anulus (anuli) [compare: annulus]
AOB—alcohol on breath
A&P—auscultation and percussion
APACHE—acute physiology and chronic health evaluation
apathetic
apathy
APC—acetylsalicylic acid, phenacetin, caffeine
    aspirin, phenacetin, caffeine
APC-C—aspirin, phenacetin, caffeine with codeine
APE—aminophylline, phenobarbital, ephedrine
aperture
apex (apices, apexes)
aphagia
    a. algera
aphasic
apical
apices (plural of apex)
apogee
apparatus
appearance
    angry a.
    shocklike a., shocky a.
    toxic a.
appendices (plural of appendix)
appendicitis
    acute a.
    a. by contiguity
    chronic a.
    fulminating a.
    gangrenous a.
    a. granulosa
    helminthic a.
    a. larvata
    myxoglobulosis a.
    necropurulent a.

appendicitis (continued)
    nonobstructive a.
    a. obliterans
    perforating a.
    perforative a.
    stercoral a.
    subperitoneal a.
    suppurative a.
    syncongestive a.
    verminous a.
apperception
apperceptive
appraisal
    health risk a.
approximal
approximate
"appy" Slang for appendectomy.
apron
    abdominal a.
apyretic
apyrexia
apyrexial
apyrogenetic
apyrogenic
aqua (aquae)
aquatic
AR—artificial respiration
AIIRAs—angiotensin II receptor antagonists [a class of drugs]
arboroid
ARC—American Red Cross
arcate
arch
    U-shaped a.
archaic
archetype
arciform
arctation
arcual
arcuate
arcuation
ARD—acute respiratory disease
    acute respiratory distress
area (areae, areas)
    body surface a. (BSA)
    genital a.'s
    triangular a.
areolar

areolate
ARF—acute renal failure
    acute respiratory failure
armadillo
armamentarium
armpit
aromatase
    a. inhibitors
arrested
arrhythmic
arthritis (arthritides)
articulate
articulation
articulo
    a. mortis
artifact
artificial sweeteners
    aspartame
    Equal
    saccharine
    Splenda
    stevia
    sucralose
    Sweet and Low
AS—left ear (L. auris sinistra)
ascending
ascertain, ascertained
ascertainment
ascorbic acid
asepsis
aseptic
aspartame
aspect
    dorsal a.
    ventral a.
asphyxia
    autoerotic a.
    sexual a.
asphyxiant
asphyxiate, asphyxiated
asphyxiation
aspirate
aspirating
aspiration
aspirator
assault
    felonious a.
assaultive

assessment
assimilation
association
assumption
    a. of care
    a. of risk
asterixis
asteroid
asthenic
astringents [a class of drugs]
asymmetric, asymmetrical
asymmetry
asymptomatic
asynchronism
atelectasis
atelectatic
athlete
atonia
atonic
atonicity
atony
atopic
atopy
ATPase (adenosine triphosphatase)
    inhibitors [a class of drugs]
atraumatic
atretic
atrium (atria)
    a. of infection
atrophied
atrophy
attenuant
attenuate, attenuated
atypia
AU—each ear (L. auris utraque)
    [not: auris uterque]
augmentation
aura
auris (aures)
    a. dextra (AD) (L. right ear)
    a. sinistra (AS) (L. left ear)
    a. utraque (AU) (L. each ear)
auscultation
autogenesis
autogenous
autonomy
autopsy
autosome

auxiliary
avascular
avulsion
    scalp a.
A&W—alive and well
axilla (axillae)
axillary
axis (axes)
azaspirones [a class of drugs]
azoles [a class of drugs]
background
bacterium (bacteria)
    See specific bacteria in *Lab-
      oratory, Pathology, and
      Chemistry Terms.*
Bair-Hugger Convective Warming
  Unit
baldness
    male pattern b.
ballooning
ballotable
balsamics; balsams
banana
    b. bag
    b. spider
bandage
    See also *dressing.*
    See in *General Surgical
      Terms.*
    b. shears
Band-Aid
bandeau
banding
barba (barbae)
barberry
barbiturates [a class of drugs]
bare, bared
bariatrics
barley
barrel
    b. chest
barrel hoop
    b.h. sign
barrier
    architectural b.
basal
    b. body temperature
bases (plural of basis)

basically
basilad
basilar
basilateral, basolateral
basilic
basin
    kidney b.
basis (bases)
basolateral, basilateral
bastion
BAT—blunt abdominal trauma
battalion
battery
    b. of tests
beanbag
bed
    Gatch b.
bedbug
bedpan
bedrest, bed rest
bedridden
bedsore
bedwetting
beetle
    blister b.
behavior
belching
belly
bellyache
bellybutton
beneficence
beneficial
beneficiary
benefit
    indemnity b.
    maximum hospital b.
    maximum medical b.
    service b.
benefited
benign
benzimidazoles, substituted [a class
  of drugs]
benzisoxazoles [a class of drugs]
benzodiazepines [a class of drugs]
benzothiazepines [a class of drugs]
benzylamines [a class of drugs]
bergamot, scarlet
beseech, beseeched

beta
    b. blockers [a class of drugs]
    b.-lactams [a class of drugs]
BHAPs—bisheteroarylpiperazines
    [a class of drugs]
BI—burn index
bibasilar
    b. rales
bibulous
bicameral
bicarbonate
    b. of soda, sodium b.
bicaudal
bicaudate [pref: bicaudal]
bicephalus
bicorporate
b.i.d.—twice a day (L. bis in die)
biduous
bifid
biforate
bifurcate
bigeminal
bigonial
bilateral
bilious
biliousness
binaural
    b. stethoscope
bind
bioavailability
biocidal
biocompatibility
biocompatible
bioflavonoid
biohazard
biologic, biological
biology
biomedicine
biophysics
biophysiology
biorhythm
biparietal
biperforate
birthing
    b. center
bisaxillary
bischloromethyl ether

bisheteroarylpiperazines (BHAPs)
    [a class of drugs]
bisphosphonates [a class of drugs]
bitter
bizarre
blacksnake
Blakemore-Sengstaken
    tube
blanket
    hypothermic b.
blast
    b. chest
    b. effect
    lung b.
BLB—Boothby-Lovelace-Bulbulian
BLB mask
blennogenic
blockade
blockage
blocker
    beta b.'s (β-blockers) [a
       class of drugs]
    H_1 b.'s [a class of drugs]
    H_2 b.'s [a class of drugs]
    selective serotonin 5-HT_3
       (hydroxytryptamine) b.'s
       [a class of drugs]
    slow-channel b.'s [a class of
       drugs]
    starch b.
blood
    b. bank
    banked b.
    whole b.
blood-brain barrier
blood plasma
blood volume expanders [a class of
    drugs]
blotchy
BLS—basic life support
BM—bone marrow
    bowel movement
BMR—basal metabolic rate
board
    back b.
    spine b.
    transfer b.
board certified, board-certified

board eligible, board-eligible
body (bodies)
boggy
bolus
BOM—bilateral otitis media
Boothby
    mask
"boo-ton-year" Phonetic for bouton-
    nière.
"boo-yaw," "boo-yawn" Phonetic
    for bouillon.
borborygmus (borborygmi)
borderline
bosselated
bouillon
bout
boutonnière
bowel
    b. movement (BM)
    b. obstruction
    b. sounds
boxing
BP—blood pressure
BPH—benign prostatic hyperplasia
    benign prostatic hypertrophy
bracelet
bradykinesia
bradykinetic
brain-dead
brash
    water b.
BRAT—bananas, rice cereal, apple-
    sauce, toast [diet]
breadth
breast
breast-fed
breast-feed, breast-feeds
breast-feeding
breath
Breathalyzer
breathiness
breathing
    labored b.
    mouth-to-mouth b.
    shallow b.
breathless
breathlessness
brewer's yeast

bridou
broad-spectrum antibiotics [a class
    of drugs]
bromide
bronchitis
"broo-ee" Phonetic for bruit.
BRP—bathroom privileges
"bru-ee" Phonetic for bruit.
bruise
bruit
    See in *Cardiology* and *Pul-
    monary Medicine* sections.
bruxism
"brwe" Phonetic for bruit.
BS—blood sugar
    bowel sounds
B/S—breath sounds
BSA—body surface area
BSE—bilateral, symmetrical, and
    equal
BSF—basal skull fracture
BSS—balanced salt solution
    buffered saline solution
BU—burn unit
buccal
    b. mucosa
    b. smear
buckling
BUE—both upper extremities
bulbar
bulboid
bulbous
bulk-producing laxatives [a class of
    drugs]
bumps
    goose b.
BUN—blood urea nitrogen
BUO—bleeding of undetermined
    origin
burn
    brush b.
    chemical b.
    first-degree b.
    flash b.
    fourth-degree b.
    full-thickness b.
    high-tension b.
    immersion b.

burn (continued)
    partial-thickness b.
    powder b.
    radiation b.
    respiratory b.
    second-degree b.
    thermal b.
    third-degree b.
burnisher
burnishing
burn-out
burst
buttock
button
    belly b. [pref: bellybutton]
buttonhole
butyrophenones [a class of drugs]
BW—birthweight
bystander
c̄—with (L. cum)
C—Celsius
CA—chronological age
Ca, CA—cancer
    carcinoma
cachectic
cachet
cacoethic
CAD—coronary artery disease
cadaver
cadaveric
cadaverous
caduceus
café coronary
caffeinated
caffeine
CAHD—coronary arteriosclerotic
    heart disease
    coronary atherosclerotic
      heart disease
Cal, Kcal—kilocalorie
calcium (Ca)
    c. alginate
    c. antagonists [a class of
      drugs]
    c. carbonate
    c. channel blockers [a class
      of drugs]
    cyclamate c.

calcium (Ca) (continued)
    docusate c.
    c. edetate sodium
Caldwell
    protection
calendar
callous [adj.]
calorie
CAM—Caucasian adult male
Cammann
    stethoscope
canker sore
cap.—capsule (L. capsula)
capacious
capitation
CAPS—caffeine, alcohol, pepper,
    spicy foods
CAPS-free diet
capsaicin
Capsicum, capsicum
carbacephems [a class of drugs]
carbonaceous
carbon dioxide (CO_2)
carbonic anhydrase inhibitors [a
    class of drugs]
carbuncle
carbuncular
carbunculoid
carbunculosis
carcinogenesis
carcinomatoid
carcinomatous
cardiac glycosides [a class of drugs]
cardiac risk factors (CRFs)
cardiomegaly
cardiomyopathy
cardioprotective agents [a class of
    drugs]
cardiovascular
care
    acute c.
    ambulatory c.
    continuity of c.
    custodial c.
    extended c.
    home health c.
    skilled nursing c.
    tertiary c.

carnivorous
carnosity
caroticoclinoid
carotidynia
carpal
carrot
cartilaginification
cartilaginiform
cartilaginous
cascade
case history
caseous
cast room
catabolism
catamnesis
catastrophe
category
"cath" Slang for catheter, catheterization, catheterize.
catharsis
Caucasian
caudad [adv.]
caudae
caudal [adj.]
caudalis
caudalward
caudate
causalgia
causation
 legal c.
causative
cause
 contributory c. of death
 underlying c. of death
caustic
caustics [a class of drugs]
cauterants [a class of drugs]
cauterization
CBC—complete blood count
cc, cm³ [cm3], cu cm—cubic centimeter(s)
CC—clinical course
 current complaints
CC, C/C—chief complaint
CCU—coronary care unit
 critical care unit
C/D, C/d—cigarettes per day

CDC—Centers for Disease Control and Prevention
CDP—comprehensive discharge planning
CDU—chemical dependency unit
cecal
Celsius (C)
 thermometer
censorship
center
 birthing c.
 burn c.
 poison control c.
Centers for Disease Control and Prevention (CDC)
centigrade thermometer
centimeter (cm)
centimeters squared (cm², sq cm)
centrad
central
 c. nervous system (CNS)
centralis
centration
centraxonial
centric
centrilobular
Centruroides
 C. suffusus
cephalad [adv.]
cephalalgia
cephalic
cephalosporins [a class of drugs]
cephamycins [a class of drugs]
cereal
cerebrospinant
cerebrovascular
 c. accident (CVA)
cervical
CF—Caucasian female
CG—choking gas (phosgene)
challenge
 fluid c.
chamber
 decompression c.
channel
character
characteristic

charcoal
    activated c.
chart
    flow c.
chelating agents [a class of drugs]
chem—chemistry [panel, profile]
chem-6 [chem-7, chem-12, chem-
    12/60, etc.]
"chemo" Slang for chemotherapy.
chemistry (chemistries)
    blood c. studies
    clinical c.
    histological c.
chemopharmacodynamics
chemoprophylaxis
chemoresistance
chemoresistant
chemosensitive
chemotherapeutics
chemotherapy
"chemstick" Slang.
chest
    barrel c.
    emphysematous c.
    fissured c.
    hourglass c.
    pendelluft c.
    rachitic c.
    stove-in c.
CHF—congestive heart failure
CIII—closed head injury
chlordane
chlorophyll
chocolate
cholesterol
cholesterolemia
cholinergic
    c. agonists [a class of drugs]
cholinesterase inhibitors [a class of
    drugs]
chromosome
chronic
chyliform
chyloid
chylous
chymotrypsin
cicatrices (plural of cicatrix)
cicatricial

cicatrix (cicatrices)
cicatrization
CICU—cardiac intensive care unit
    coronary intensive care unit
cig—cigarettes
CIL—center for independent living
cin–. See also words beginning
    sin–, syn–.
cinnamon
circadian
    c. rhythm
circinate
circuitous
circular
circulation
circumferential
circumflex
    c. artery
circumscribed
circumstantiality
cirrhotic
CIS—carcinoma in situ
citric acid
classification
    Karnofsky status c. [score
        0–100]
CLD—chronic lung disease
clinical
Clonopin [now: Klonopin]
clubbing
clysis
cm—centimeter
cm^2 [cm2], sq cm—square centimeter
cm^3 [cm3], cc, cu cm—cubic cen-
    timeter(s)
CM—costal margin
cm H_2O [cm H2O]—centimeter(s)
    of water
CMO—comfort measures only
CN—cranial nerve
CNS—central nervous system
CO—carbon monoxide
CO_2 [CO2]—carbon dioxide
coagulants [a class of drugs]
coalesce
coalescence
coapt
coarctate

coarse
coarsening
cocaine
        c. HCl
coccyx
COD—cause of death
        condition on discharge
Coe-Pak dressing
coffee
        c. enema
coffee-grounds
        c-g. vomit, c.-g. vomitus
cognizant
coherent
coincidence
colic
colicky pain
collarbone, collar bone
colony-stimulating factors [a class
        of drugs]
colorblind, color-blind
comatose
Combitube
comitant
commensurate
comminuted
commitment
comparable
compatible
compendium (compendia)
        drug c.
compensation
compensatory
competence
competent
competitive
complaint
complexion
compress
compression
COMT inhibitors [a class of drugs]
concavity
concede
concentric
concomitant
        c. condition
        c. disease
        c. medical problem

concomitantly
concrescence
concretion
concussion
confidentiality
confluent
Conform dressing
congenital
congested
congestion
conglomerate
congruence
congruent
congruous
conical
coniotomy
consanguineous
consanguinity
conscious
consciousness
consensus
conservative
constellation
        c. of symptoms
constipated
constitution
constitutional
consultant
consultation
contagious
contamination
contiguity
contiguous
contour
contouring
contraindication
contusion
convalescence
convalescent
conventional (typical) antipsychot-
        ics [a class of drugs]
convexity
convoluted
convulsion
cornucopia
coronal
coronary
        café c.

coronary artery disease (CAD)
coronary heart disease (CHD)
coroner
corpora (plural of corpus)
corporeal
corporic
corps ["kor"]
     medical c.
corpse ["korps"]
corpulency
corpuscle
corpuscular
correlation
corticosteroids [a class of drugs]
cortisol
coryza
costal
     c. margin
costovertebral
     c. angle (CVA)
     c. angle tenderness (CVAT)
coumarins [a class of drugs]
counterirritants [a class of drugs]
course
     convalescent c., c. of conva-
       lescence
     downhill c.
     treatment c.
coursing
COX-2 (cyclooxygenase-2) inhibi-
    tors [a class of drugs]
CPR—cardiopulmonary resuscitation
CPS—clinical performance score
cranberry juice
cranial [adj.]
crank amphetamine
CRC—crisis resolution center
crease
crepitant
crepitation
crepitus
crescendo
crescent
crescentic
CRF—cardiac risk factor(s)
crisis (crises)
criterion (criteria)
critical

cross-tolerance
croupette
crustacean
crustal
cryotherapy
cryptic
cryptogenetic
cryptogenic
cryptomere
cryptopyic
cryptotoxic
crypt
C&S—culture and sensitivity
CSA—criminal sexual assault
CSF—cerebrospinal fluid
     colony-stimulating factor
CSIU—cardiac surgery intermedi-
    ate unit
CTAP—clear to auscultation and
    percussion
CTx—chemotherapy
CTZ—chlorothiazide
CU—convalescent unit
cubic centimeters (cm^3 [cm3], cc,
    cu cm)
cu cm, cm^3 [cm3], cc—cubic cen-
    timeter(s)
cue [signal, hint, suggestion]
     verbal c.'s
cuff
culprit
cu mm, mm^3 [mm3]—cubic millime-
    ter(s)
cuneate
curiosity
curious
curriculum (curricula)
cutaneous
CV—cardiovascular
CVA—cerebrovascular accident
     costovertebral angle
CVD—cardiovascular disease
     cerebrovascular disease
CVIU—cardiovascular intermediate
    unit
CVR—cardiovascular-respiratory
    [system]

CVS—cardiovascular surgery
    cardiovascular system
CW—chest wall
cyanosis
cyanotic
cyclamate calcium
cyclooxygenase-2 (COX-2) inhibi-
    tors [a class of drugs]
cyclopean
cycloplegics [a class of drugs]
cystoid
cytoid
cytoprotective agents [a class of
    drugs]
DAT—diphtheria antitoxin
data (plural of datum)
database
datum (data)
DB—date of birth
DBP—diastolic blood pressure
DC—direct current
    discharge
    discontinue
DC, D.C.—Doctor of Chiropractic
DD—differential diagnosis
D&D—Drake and Drake [medical
    reference books]
DDS, D.D.S.—Doctor of Dental
    Surgery
dead time
deaf
deaf-mute
deaf-mutism
dealt
dearth
    d. of evidence
    d. of findings
    d. of symptoms
debilitate
debilitation
debility
débouchement
débride
deceleration
decontamination
decrement
decrepitate
decrepitation

decrudescence
decrustation
decubation
decubitus
deem, deemed
defecation
defervescence
defervescent
deficit
definitely
definition
definitive
definitively
degenerative
dehydration
deleterious
    d. effects
delineate
delinquency
delinquent
    juvenile d.
delirious
delitescence
deltoid
demise
demulcents [a class of drugs]
dendritic
denervation
denudation
deodorants
dependency
dependent
depressants [a class of drugs]
deprivation
DermaBond [topical adhesive]
dermis
DES—diethylstilbestrol
DES daughter
descending
desiccant
desiccate
desiccative
despair
despairing
desperate [hopeless, despairing]
desperation
deter
detergent

deterioration
deterrent
detumescence
deviation
dextran
dextroposition
dextrose
dg—decigram
DG, Dx—diagnosis
DHE—dihydroergotamine
diagnose
diagnosis
    biological d.
    clinical d.
    cytohistologic d.
    cytologic d.
    differential d.
    d. ex juvantibus
    niveau d.
    pathologic d.
    provocative d.
    roentgen d.
    serum d.
diagnostic
diagnostician
dial-a-flow IV line
diaphoresis
diaphoretic
diaphoretics [a class of drugs]
diarrhea
diathermy
diathesis
dibenzodiazepines [a class of drugs]
dibenzothiazepines [a class of drugs]
dibenzoxazepines [a class of drugs]
dichotomy
diet
    Atkins d.
    CAPS-free d.
    high-protein d.
    low-carbohydrate d.
    paleolithic d.
    reducing d.
dietary
dietetic
diethylstilbestrol (DES)
dieting
    yo-yo d.

dietitian
"diff" Slang for differential.
differential
    d. stethoscope
differentiate
diffuse
"dig" Slang for digitalis, digoxin.
digestion
digestive
digit
digitalis
    d. effect
digitalis glycosides [a class of drugs]
digitation
digitize
dihydroindolones [a class of drugs]
dihydropyridines [a class of drugs]
"dij" Phonetic for "dig"; slang for
    digitalis, digoxin.
dilemma
dilution
dimension
diminution
dimpling
diphenylalkylamines [a class of
    drugs]
diphenylbutylpiperidines [a class of
    drugs]
dire
    d. consequences
    d. straits
dis–. See also words beginning dys–.
discharge
disciform ["disiform"]
disciplinary
disclosing
discoid
discoloration
discontinuity
discord
discordance
discordant
discrepancy
discrete
    d. disease
    d. masses
    d. nodule
    d. organ enlargement

discrimination
discutient
disease
>See also in medical specialty sections.
>congenital d.
>end-stage renal d. (ESRD)
>nosocomial d.
>occupational d.
>psychosomatic d.

disesthesia
"disiform" Phonetic for disciform.
disinfect
disinfectant
disintegration
disk
>floppy d.

diskiform
dislocated
disorganization
disorientation
disparate [distinct, different]
disposition
dissipate
dissociative
dissolution
dissonance
distad
distal
distalis
distally
distention
distraught
diuresis (diureses)
diuretics [a class of drugs]
diurnal
divergent
diverticula (plural of diverticulum)
diverticulae [incorrect spelling/pronunciation of diverticula]
diverticuli [incorrect spelling/pronunciation of diverticula]
diverticulum (diverticula)
divulsion
dizziness
DJD—degenerative joint disease
DKA—diabetic ketoacidosis
dL, dl—deciliter

DMARD—disease-modifying antirheumatic drug
DMD, D.M.D.—Doctor of Dental Medicine
DNR—do not resuscitate
DO, D.O.—Doctor of Osteopathy
DOA—dead on arrival
DOB—date of birth
DOD—date of death
DOE—dyspnea on exertion
doffing
Döhle
>inclusion bodies

donning
donor
"doosh" Phonetic for douche.
dopaminergics [a class of drugs]
dorsad [adv.]
dorsal [adj.]
dorsum
dose
>loading d.

dotage
double-blind
>d.-b. clinical trial
>d.-b. experiment
>d.-b. study
>d.-b. test

douche
>Betadine d.

doughy
>d. abdomen
>d. consistency

DP—diastolic pressure
DPM, D.P.M.—Doctor of Podiatric Medicine
DPT—diphtheria, pertussis, tetanus
DPT vaccine
Dr.—doctor
drainage
>d. tube

dressing
>See in *General Surgical Terms.*
>Coe-Pak d.
>Conform d.

DRGs—diagnosis related groups
droplet

DT, DTs—delirium tremens
DTP—diphtheria and tetanus (tox-
    oids) pertussis (vaccine)
DTRs—deep tendon reflexes
D/W—dextrose in water
D5W, D$_5$W, D5/W—5% dextrose in
    water
Dx, DG—diagnosis
DXM—dexamethasone
dys–. See also words beginning dis–.
dysbarism
dyschezia
dysesthesia
dyslipidosis
dyspepsia
dyspneic
dysponderal
dyspragia
dyssymmetry
dystonia
dystonic
dysuria
EBBS—equal bilateral breath sounds
ebrietas
ebriety
ECC—edema, clubbing, cyanosis
eccentric
ecchymosed
ecchymosis (ecchymoses)
        multiple e.'s
        old e.
        scattered e.'s
ecchymotic
ECF—extended care facility
ECG—electrocardiogram
        electrocardiography
eclampsia
écouvillon
écouvillonage
ecstasy
ectad
ectal
ectoentad
ectopic
edematous
edentulism
edentulous

EDTA—ethylenediaminetetra-acetic
    acid
        ethylenediaminetetra-acetate
EENT—eyes, ears, nose, and throat
effect [noun: result, outcome]
        additive e.
        adverse e.
        blast e.
        contrast e.
        cumulative e.
        deleterious e.'s
        digitalis e.
        placebo e.
        side e.'s
        untoward e.'s
effect [verb: to produce, to bring
    about]
        to e. a cure
effectiveness
effector
effect [noun: result, outcome]
        untoward e.'s
efferent
efficacious
efficacy
efflux
effraction
effusion
egophony
egress
EH—essential hypertension
EKG [pref: ECG]—electrocardio-
    gram
        electrocardiography
elaboration
elastica
elasticity
elective
electric, electrical
electrocardiogram (ECG)
electrocardiography (ECG)
electrocution
electrolytic
electronic
        e. stethoscope
electronics
electropathology
electropyrexia

electrothanasia
electrotherapy
elicit
elicited
ellipsis
elongation
elucidate
elude, eluded
EM—ejection murmur
emaciated
emanate
embarrass
embarrassment
    e. of choices
    e. of riches
embed, embedding
embryo
embryonic
emerge, emerged
emergency
emetics [a class of drugs]
emetocathartic
eminent [distinguished, prominent, outstanding]
emollient laxatives [a class of drugs]
emollients [a class of drugs]
empathize
empiric, cmpirical
empiricism
EMS—emergency medical service
EMT—emergency medical technician
en bloc
encapsulated
encased
encompass, encompassed, encompassing
endemic
endocardium
endocrine
endogenous
endomorph
endomorphic
endomorphy
endoplasm
endothelin-1 receptor antagonists [a class of drugs]
end point

end-stage renal disease (ESRD)
enema
    coffee e.
engender, engendered
engorged
engorgement
enigmatic, enigmatical
en plaque
"en-sed" Phonetic for NSAID (nonsteroidal anti-inflammatory drug).
ENT—ear, nose, and throat
entad
ental
entirety
entropy
enucleate
environment
environmental
eparsalgia
"epi" Slang for epinephrine.
epicentral
epicostal
epidemic
epidermiologic, epidemiological
epidemiologist
epidemiology
epidermic
epigastric
epigastrium
epinephrine
epiphenomenon
episode
epistasis
epistatic
epistaxis
episternal
episternum
epithet
eponym
eponymic, eponymous
"eppy" Slang for epinephrine.
equivocal
ER—emergency room
erosion
erosive
erratic
eructation

erudite
eruption
erythrism
erythristic
eschar
escharotic
eschew
"eskar" Phonetic for eschar.
estrogens [a class of drugs]
ET—endotracheal
et al.—and others (L. et alii)
ethanol
ethanolamines [a class of drugs]
ether
ethylene glycol
etiologic, etiological
etiology
ETKM—every test known to man
ETOH, EtOH—ethyl alcohol
eucrasia
euphoretics, euphoriants, euphora-
    gens [a class of drugs]
euphoria
eupnea
eupneic
euthanasia
euthyroid
evacuation
eval—evaluation
evanescent
eversion
evert
everted
evisceration
Ewald
        tube
exacerbate
exacerbation
        abrupt e.
        sudden e.
        explained e.
exam—examination
exceed
excise
excitable
excrement
excrescence
excretion

exenteration
exhaustion
exhilarated
existence
exogenous
exophytic
exp, expir—expiration
        expired
expectancy
expectant
expectorants [a class of drugs]
expediency
expedient
expedite
expeditious
expeditiously
experiment
        double-blind e.
expiration
expire
exsanguinate
exsanguination
extraocular
extrapolate
extravasation
extremital
extrinsic
extubate
extubation
exuberance
exuberant
        e. tumor
exudate
F—Fahrenheit
facial
facies (facies)
        f. hepatica
facilitation
facility
        acute care f. (ACF)
        adult congregate living f.
            (ACLF)
        extended care f. (ECF)
        intermediate care f. (ICF)
        skilled nursing f. (SNF)
FACP—Fellow of the American
    College of Physicians

FACS—Fellow of the American College of Surgeons
factitious
factor
        cardiac risk f.'s (CRFs)
Fahrenheit (F)
        thermometer
"fahr-ma–" Phonetic for words beginning pharma–.
"fal–" Phonetic for words beginning phal–.
falces
falciform
familial
fascia (fasciae)
fascial
fascicle
fasciculation
fasciculus
fastigium
fatigability
fatigue
faveolate
FB—foreign body
F&D—fixed and dilated
FDA—Food and Drug Administration
Fe—iron
febrile
feces [grammatically plural; no singular form]
feeblemindedness
felony
female
feminine
femininity
feminism
fenestrated
"fenil–" Phonetic for words beginning phenyl–.
"fenomenon" Phonetic for phenomenon.
Fermi vaccine
fervescence
fetid
FFP—fresh frozen plasma
FH—family history
"fib" Slang for fibrillation.

5150 hold
filament
filamentous
filial
filterable
fimbrial
fimbriated
fimbriation
fimbriatum
fingerbreadth (fingerbreadths)
fissural
fistula (fistulas, fistulae)
5-HT$_3$ (hydroxytryptamine) receptor antagonists [a class of drugs]
"fizeo–" Phonetic for words beginning physio–.
flaccid
flank
"flatlined" Slang for expired.
flatness
flattening
flatulence
flatus
flaunt [show off]
"flebitis" Phonetic for phlebitis.
"flebo–" Phonetic for words beginning phlebo–.
"flegmatik" Phonetic for phlegmatic.
flesh
        goosebump f.
        proud f.
flexibility
flight
        f. into disease
flocculus
floppy disk
florid
        f. infection
flout [scorn]
fluctuant
fluoride
fluoroquinolones [a class of drugs]
fluoroscope
focus (foci)
foliaceous
folic acid
folinic acid
follicle

follow-up care
footprint
forego
foreign body (FB)
      retained f.b. (RFB)
forensic
formative
forme (formes)
      f. fruste, formes frustes
      f. tardive
former and latter
formic acid
formula
      Berkow f.
      chemical f.
formulary
formulate
formulation
fossette
fossulate
foveola (foveolae)
      f. coccygea
FP—family practice
fragmentation
fraught
frenetic, frenetical
frenzy, frenzied
friable
frontal
frustration
FU—follow-up
fulgurate
fulguration
fulminant
fumigation
functional
funduscopy
fungus (fungi)
      See specific fungi in *Labo-*
      ratory, Pathology, and
      Chemistry Terms.
FUO—fever of undetermined origin
      fever of unknown origin
furor
furuncle
fusible
fusiform
FW—fragment wound

fx—fracture
g—gram(s)
GABA—γ-aminobutyric acid
      [gamma-]
gait and station
galactagogues [a class of drugs]
gallstone-solubilizing agents [a
      class of drugs]
ganglionic
gangrenous
garrulous
gaseous
gastric acid inhibitors [a class of
      drugs]
gastrogavage
gastrointestinal (GI)
Gatch
      bed
gauge
GB—gallbladder
GC—gonococcus
GCS—Glasgow Coma Scale
gefilte fish
geminate
genera (plural of genus)
general
generalization
generalize
generation
generic
genesis
gene-splicing
geneticist
genetics
geniculum (genicula)
genitalia [grammatically plural; no
      singular form]
genitorectal
genu
genus (genera)
geographic, geographical
geometric, geometrical
geriatric
geriatrician
geriatrics
germicides
GI—gastrointestinal
gibberish

GIS—gastrointestinal system
glacial
glare
Glasgow
    Coma Scale (GCS)
    sign
glassy
glaze
gleaned
global
globose
globule
glucagon
glucocorticoids [a class of drugs]
glycerin
glycine
glycopeptides [a class of drugs]
glycoprotein (GP) IIb/IIIa receptor
    antagonists [a class of drugs]
glycosaminoglycans [a class of
    drugs]
glycosides, cardiac [a class of drugs]
GM—general medicine
gonadotropin-releasing hormone
    (Gn-RH)
        g.-r.h. analogues [a class of
        drugs]
gonadotropins [a class of drugs]
GP—general practice
        general practitioner
GP (glycoprotein) IIb/IIIa inhibitors
    [a class of drugs]
gr.—grain(s)
gracile
granulate
granulation
grass [street slang for marijuana]
gratification
grave
        g. condition
        g. illness
gravida (0, 1, 2, etc.) [number of
    pregnancies]
grotesque, grotesquely
grumous
GS—general surgery
GSW—gunshot wound
gt.—drop (L. gutta)

gtt.—drops (L. guttae)
GTT—glucose tolerance test
GU—genitourinary
guaiac
guardian ad litem
guarding
guideline
GUS—genitourinary system
gyn, GYN—gynecology
gyration
gyrose
H_1 blockers [a class of drugs]
H_2 blockers [a class of drugs]
habit
habitat
habitual
habitus
Haldane
halitosis
hallucination
        See in *Psychiatry* section.
hallucinogen
handedness
handicap
handicapped
handpiece
handprint
handshaking
harassment
hardness
harm's way
Hb, Hgb—hemoglobin
HBO—hyperbaric oxygen
HC—hospital course
Hct, hct—hematocrit
HCTZ—hydrochlorothiazide
HDCV—human diploid cell
        (rabies) vaccine
HDL—high-density lipoprotein
headache
        cluster h.
        exertional h.
        meningeal h.
        migraine h.
        muscle contraction h.
        postconcussional h.
        tension h.
        thunderclap h.

headache (continued)
    traumatic h.
    vascular h.
healing
    faith h.
hedgehog proteins [a class of drugs]
HEENT—head, eyes, ears, nose,
    and throat
helicine
helicoid
heliosis
helminthic
hematinics [a class of drugs]
hematochezia
hematogenous
hematologic, hematological
hematology
hematoma
hematopoietics [a class of drugs]
hcmc
hemiparesis
hemiplegia
hemoglobin (Hb, Hgb)
hemoptysis
hemorrhage
    critical h.
hemorrhagic
    h. shock
hemostasis
hemostatics [a class of drugs]
hence
henceforth
heparin
    low-molecular-weight h.'s [a
        class of drugs]
hepatomegaly
hepatorenal
hepatosplenomegaly
hereditary
heredity
heretofore
hermetically
heroin
hertz (Hz)
heterogenic
heterotopia
heterotopic
HF—heart failure

Hg—mercury
Hgb, Hb—hemoglobin
hiccup
high-risk
"hipo–" Phonetic for words begin-
    ning hypo–.
"hipocrasy" Phonetic for hypocrisy.
hippocratic
    h. oath
hirci (plural of hircus)
hircismus
hircus (hirci)
hirsute
histamine
    h. diphosphate
    h. phosphate
histamine H$_1$ antagonists [a class of
    drugs]
histamine H$_2$ antagonists [a class of
    drugs]
histology
history
    case h.
    family h. (FH)
    incongruous h.
    marital h. (MH)
    medical h. (MH)
    occupational h. (OH)
    past h. (PH)
    past surgical h. (PSH)
    h. and physical examination
        (HPE)
    h. of present illness (HPI)
    social h. (SH)
    surgical h. (SH)
HIV protease inhibitors [a class of
    drugs]
HMG-CoA (3-hydroxy-3-methylglu-
    taryl–coenzyme A) reductase
    inhibitors [a class of drugs]
HMO—health maintenance organi-
    zation
h/o, H/O—history of
H$_2$O$_2$ [H2O2]—hydrogen peroxide
holism
holistic
homicidal
homicide

homogeneous
homogeneously
homogenous
homolateral
homologous
hook-up
horizontal
hormone
hospital
hospitalist
hostility
hot
    h. appendix
hot line, hotline
H&P—history and physical
HPE—history and physical examination
HPI—history of present illness
HPV—*Haemophilus pertussis* vaccine
HR—heart rate
h.s.—at bedtime (L. hora somni)
HSA—human serum albumin
HSV—herpes simplex virus
HT, htn—hypertension
HVM—high-velocity missile
Hx—history
hyalinization
hydantoins [a class of drugs]
hydration
hydrocholeretics [a class of drugs]
3-hydroxy-3-methylglutaryl–coenzyme A (HMG-CoA) reductase inhibitors [a class of drugs]
5-hydroxytryptamine$_3$ (5-HT$_3$) receptor antagonists [a class of drugs]
hygiene
hygienic
hypalgesia
hypasthenia
hyperactive
hyperactivity
hyperacute
hypercupremia
hypercupriuria
hyperdynamia
hyperelastic

hyperemization
hyperevolutism
hyperfunction
hyperfunctioning
hypergenesis
hypergenetic
hyperglycemia
Hypericum
    H. perforatum
hyperkalemia
hyperkinesia
hyperkinesis
hyperkinetic
hyperlethal
hypermedication
hypermimia
hypermnesia
hypermnesic
hypernomic
hypernormal
hyperocclusion
hyperosmotic laxatives [a class of drugs]
hyperplasia
hyperplastic
hyperresonance
hyperresonant
hypersensibility
hypersensitive
hyperthermia
hypertonicity
hypertoxic
hypertoxicity
hypertrophic
hyperventilation
hypervolemia
hypervolemic
hypnopedia
hypnotics [a class of drugs]
hypochlorite
    sodium h.
hypochondriac
hypocrisy
hypodermic
    h. needle
hypofunction
hypogastric
hypoglycemia

hypohydration
hypointense
hypolethal
hypopexia
hypoplasia
hypostypsis
hypostyptic
hypothermal
hypothermia
hypothermic
hypothesis (hypotheses)
hypotonia
hypotonic
hypotoxicity
hypotrophy
hypoxemia
hypoxemic
hypoxia
hypoxic
hysteric, hysterical
hysterics
iatrogenic
IC—intensive care
    intermediate care
ICC—intensive coronary care
ICCU—intensive coronary care unit
ICD—International Classification of
    Diseases
ICF—intermediate care facility
ichorous
ichthyoid
ichthyosiform
ICM—intercostal margin
ictal
icteric
icterus
ictus
ICU—intensive care unit
ID—identification
    Infectious Disease [service]
    infectious disease(s)
idealization
ideology
idiogenesis
idiologism
idiopathic
idiopathy
idioreflex

idiosyncrasy
idiosyncratic
idiot *
    i.-savant
"ikthe–" Phonetic for words begin-
    ning ichthy–.
"iktus" Phonetic for ictus.
ileac [pertaining to ileus or ileum
    (bowel)]
ileal [pertaining to ileum (bowel)]
ileum [bowel]
iliac [hip bone]
ilium (ilia) [hip bone]
illness
    acute on chronic i.
    grave i.
    refractory i.
illumination
illusion
IM—internal medicine
    intramuscular
imagery
imbed [pref: embed]
imbricated
IMHP—1-iodomercuri-2-hydroxy-
    propane
imitate
immature
immediate
immediately
imminent [about to occur, impending]
immobility
immunologic, immunological
immunosuppressants [a class of
    drugs]
immunotherapy
impalpable
impatency
impatent
imperforate
impermeable
impingement
implantation
impoverishment
impression
inactivity
inadequacy
inadequate

in articulo mortis
incarcerated
incarceration
incidence
incipient
incisive
incoherent
incompatibility
incompetence
incompetent
incongruent
incongruous
    i. findings
    i. history
incontinence
incontinent
incorrigible
incubation
incumbent
incurable
indanediones [a class of drugs]
independent
indifferent
indigenous
indigestion
indiscernible
indiscrete
indisposition
indistinct
indium (In)
indolent
indolones [a class of drugs]
induced
inebriation
inebriety
inert
inexorable
in extremis
infancy
infanticide
infantile
infarct
infarction
inferior
inferolateral
inferomedian
inferoposterior
infestation

infirm
infirmity
inflammation
inflammatory
inflation
inflexion
infusion
ingenious
ingestion
ingravescent
ingress
inguinal
inhalation
inherent
inhibitor
    acetylcholinesterase (AChE)
      inhibitors [a class of drugs]
    ATPase (adenosine triphos-
      phatase) i.'s [a class of
      drugs]
    carbonic anhydrase i.'s [a
      class of drugs]
    cholinesterase i.'s [a class of
      drugs]
    COMT i.'s [a class of drugs]
    COX-2 (cyclooxygenase-2)
      i.'s [a class of drugs]
    gastric acid i.'s [a class of
      drugs]
    GP (glycoprotein) IIb/IIIa
      i.'s [a class of drugs]
    HIV protease i.'s [a class of
      drugs]
    HMG-CoA (3-hydroxy-3-
      methylglutaryl–coenzyme
      A) reductase i.'s [a class
      of drugs]
    leukotriene receptor i.'s [a
      class of drugs]
    matrix metalloproteinase
      (MMP) i.'s [a class of
      drugs]
    MMP i.'s [a class of drugs]
    monoamine oxidase i.'s
      (MAOIs) [a class of drugs]
    non-nucleoside reverse
      transcriptase i.'s (NNR-
      TIs) [a class of drugs]

inhibitor (continued)
  phosphodiesterase III (PDE
   III) i.'s [a class of drugs]
  protease i.'s [a class of drugs]
  proton pump i.'s [a class of
   drugs]
  reverse transcriptase (RT)
   i.'s [a class of drugs]
  selective serotonin reuptake
   i.'s (SSRIs) [a class of
   drugs]
  thymidylate synthase (TS)
   i.'s [a class of drugs]
  topoisomerase I i.'s [a class
   of drugs]
inhibitory
inhomogeneous
initial
injury
innate
innominate
inoculate
inoculation
inoperable
inotropes [a class of drugs]
insalubrious
insanitary
inscription
insidious
in situ
insomnia
inspiration
inspiratory
  post-tussive i. rhonchi
  i. rhonchi
inspissated
instillation
instinctive
insufflation
insular
insulate
insulation
insulator
insulin
insult
integration
integument
integumentary

intensity
intensive
intention
intercede
intercostal
intercourse
interim
International Classification of Diseases (ICD)
international unit(s) (IU)
interpretation
interrogation
intersection
interstitial
intestine
intima
intolerance
in toto
intoxication
  alcohol i.
  substance i.
intractable
intramuscular
intrathecal
intravenous
intravitam
intrinsic
introflexion
introversion
intubate
intubation
  i. tube
invaginate
in vivo
involuntary
involutional
I&O—in and out (surgery)
  intake and output
iodine (I)
  Lugol i.
  povidone-i.
  radioactive i. (iodine I 131)
IOU—intensive therapy observation
  unit
ipsilateral
IPU—inpatient unit
IQ—intelligence quotient
irascibility

irradiation
irreducible
irregular
irreversible
irritability
irritable
irritant
    i. laxatives [a class of drugs]
irritation
irritative
"is-mus" Phonetic for isthmus.
isolate
isolateral
isolation
isotonia
isotonic
isotope
    radioactive i.
isthmic
IT—intrathecal
IU—international unit(s)
IV—intravenous
IV cocktail
IVC—intravenous cholangiogram
IVH—intraventricular hemorrhage
jactitation
Janeway
    sphygmomanometer
jaundice
JCAHO—Joint Commission on
    Accreditation of Healthcare
    Organizations
"jibberish" Phonetic for gibberish.
joule
judgment
judicious
jugate
jugular
jugulation
juncture
juxtaposition
JV—jugular vein
    jugular venous
JVP—jugular venous pressure
    jugular venous pulse
K—potassium
"kahk–," "kak–" Phonetic for words
    beginning cac–, cach–.

kaliuretic
katzenjammer [a hangover or
    depression]
Kcal, Cal—kilocalorie
KCl—potassium chloride
"kemo–" Phonetic for words begin-
    ning chemo–.
keratolytics [a class of drugs]
kg—kilogram(s)
kilogram
kinetic
kininase
    k. II inhibitors [a class of
      drugs]
KLS—kidneys, liver, spleen
"kolee–" Phonetic for words begin-
    ning chole–, choli–, coli–.
KUB—kidney, ureter, bladder [x-ray]
KVO—keep vein open [IV line]
kyphosis
lab—laboratory
labile
lability
labored breathing
laborious
lacerate, lacerated
β-lactams [beta-] [a class of drugs]
lactiferous
lactivorous
lactovegetarian
lactovegetarianism
lactulose
laden
lambdoid, lambdoidal
laminated
lamination
lana (lanae)
lancinating pain
laparotomy
larvaceous
larvate
laser
lassitude
latency
latent
laterad
lateral
laterality

lateralization
lateritious
lateroabdominal
laterodeviation
laterodorsal
latex
lathyrism
lathyritic
lathyrogen
lathyrogenic
latrodectism
latter
laxatives [a class of drugs]
      bulk-producing l.
      emollient l.
      hyperosmotic l.
      stimulant l.
      stool-softening l.
      surfactant l.
lazaroids [a class of drugs]
LBM—lean body mass
LC—living children
LCM—left costal margin
lead (Pb) ["led"]
Leff
      stethoscope
lentigo (lentigines)
      senile lentigines
leprostatics [a class of drugs]
lethal
lethargic
lethargy
leukotriene receptor antagonists
    (LTRAs) [a class of drugs]
leukotriene receptor inhibitors [a
    class of drugs]
lhistory
      past medical h. (PMH)
liaison
license
licentiate
licentious
limb
lime
limes ["li-meez"] [limit, boundary]
lime solution
lincosamides [a class of drugs]
lindane

linguistic deficit
lipoma
lipotropics [a class of drugs]
liquefacient
liquefaction
liquefy
liquescent
liquiform
liquor (liquors, liquores)
liquorice
litholytics [a class of drugs]
LLE—left lower extremity
LLQ—left lower quadrant
LMD—local medical doctor
loading dose
lobular
lobulization
local
localized
locular
loculate
loculated
loculation
loculus (loculi)
locum
locus (loci)
longitudinal
loop
      l. diuretics [a class of drugs]
LOQ—lower outer quadrant
loquacious
low-molecular-weight heparins [a
    class of drugs]
LP—lumbar puncture
LPN—licensed practical nurse
LR—lactated Ringer
LRQ—lower right quadrant
LRS—lactated Ringer solution
LSB—left sternal border
LSD—lysergic acid diethylamide
LTRAs—leukotriene receptor
    antagonists [a class of drugs]
lucid
lucidity
LUE—left upper extremity
lugubrious
lumbar
luminal

LUQ—left upper quadrant
LW—lacerating wound
L&W, L/W—living and well
lymphangiogram
lymphatic
lymphs—lymphocytes
lyse
lysergic acid diethylamide (LSD)
lysine
lysis
μ—micro- [prefix; alphabetized as m]
maceration
macrolides [a class of drugs]
maim
mal
      m. rouge
malabsorption
malacia
maladjustment
malady
malaise
malar
malformation
malfunction
malign
malignancy
malignant
malingerer
malingering
malleable
malnutrition
malposition
malpractice
malt
malum
mamelon
mammiform
mammillated
mammillation
mammilliform
mammose
mandate, mandated
mandible
maneuver
      See also in *General Surgical*
        Terms.
      Heimlich m.
      Valsalva m.

manifest
manifestation
manipulation
mannerism
mannitol
manual
MAO—monoamine oxidase
MAOI, MAOIs—monoamine oxidase
      inhibitor(s) [a class of drugs]
marasmus
marbleization
marcid
margin
      m. of safety
marginal
marihuana, marijuana
marital
marking pen
marsupialization
masculine
masculinization
masculinize
masculinizing
MASH—Mobile Army Surgical
      Hospital
MAST—military antishock trousers
matrix (matrices)
matrix metalloproteinase (MMP)
      inhibitors [a class of drugs]
mature, matured
max—maximum
maxima (plural of maximum)
maximal
maximum (maxima)
mazel tov
mcg, μg—microgram(s)
MCH—mean corpuscular hemoglo-
      bin
MCHC—mean corpuscular hemo-
      globin concentration
MCL—midclavicular line
MCV—mean corpuscular volume
MD, M.D.—medical doctor (L.
      Medicinae Doctor)
MDA—methylenedioxyamphetamine
MDMA—methylenedioxymetham-
      phetamine
MDR—minimum daily requirement

measurement
    skinfold m.'s
mediad
medial
medialis
median
medianus
mediate
mediator
medicable
medicate
medication
    conservative m.
    sublingual m.
medicinal
medicine
    adolescent m.
    aerospace m.
    aviation m.
    behavioral m.
    clinical m.
    community m.
    emergency m.
    environmental m.
    experimental m.
    family m.
    fetal-maternal m.
    folk m.
    geriatric m.
    holistic m.
    hyperbaric m.
    industrial m.
    internal m.
    manipulative m.
    neonatal m.
    nuclear m.
    occupational m.
    oral m.
    osteopathic m.
    patent m.
    perinatal m.
    physical m.
    preclinical m.
    preventive m.
    proprietary m.
    rehabilitation m.
    social m.
    socialized m.

medicine (continued)
    space m.
    sports m.
    tropical m.
    veterinary m.
medicochirurgic
medicolegal
mediocre
mediolateral
medius
meds—medications
    medicines
medusa
"meelu" Phonetic for milieu.
melancholic
melanemesis
melanotic [pertaining to melanin]
melenic [pertaining to melena,
    blood in the stool]
mellitum (mellita)
"melyuh" Phonetic for milieu.
membraniform
membranoid
membranous
mentoanterior
mentoposterior
mentotransverse
mep—meperidine
mEq—milliequivalent(s)
6-mercaptopurine
mercurial
mercury (Hg)
    millimeters of m. (mm Hg)
meridian
meridional
meritorious
meromelia
mescaline
mesentery
mesion
metabolic
metabolism
metastasize
metastatic
method
    See in *General Surgical
      Terms.*
MFB—metallic foreign body

MFWs—multiple fragment wounds
μg, mcg—microgram(s)
mg—milligram(s)
mg/L—milligrams per liter
MH—marital history
    medical history
MHB—maximum hospital benefit
mication
microaerosol
microdosage
microdose
microfilm
microgram(s) (μg, mcg)
microinjection
micronize, micronized
micronutrient
microscopic, microscopical
microtrauma
microwave
MICU—medical intensive care unit
"middle-shmertz" Phonetic for mit-
    telschmerz.
migrate
migration
migratory
milieu
    m. extérieur
    m. intérieur
milk of magnesia (MOM)
millennium
milliequivalent(s) (mEq)
milligram(s) (mg)
    m.'s per liter (mg/L)
milliliter(s) (mL, ml)
millimeter(s) (mm)
    m.'s of mercury (mm Hg)
    square m. (mm^2, sq mm)
    m.'s of water (mm H$_2$O)
mineralocorticoids [a class of drugs]
minimal
minuscule
minute [small]
minute (M, min)
miotics [a class of drugs]
misanthropy
mischievous
mitotic
    m. inhibitors [a class of drugs]

mittelschmerz [pain with ovulation]
μL, μl—microliter(s)
mL, ml—milliliter(s)
mm—millimeter(s)
mm^2 [mm2], sq mm—square mil-
    limeter(s)
mm^3 [mm3], cu mm—cubic mil-
    limeter(s)
mm Hg—millimeters of mercury
mm H$_2$O [mm H2O]—millimeters
    of water
MMP—matrix metalloproteinase
MMP inhibitors [a class of drugs]
MO—mineral oil
moccasin
    cottonmouth water m.
modality (modalities)
modeling
MOM—milk of magnesia
monoamine oxidase (MAO)
monoamine oxidase inhibitors
    (MAOIs) [a class of drugs]
monobactams [a class of drugs]
monogamous
monogamy
monomorphous
monos—monocytes
monosyllabic
monstrosity
moot
    m. point
    m. question
morbid
morbidity
morcel
morcellated
morcellation
moribund
morphology
mortal
mortality
mosquito (mosquitoes)
motile
motility
mottled
MS—mental status
    morphine sulfate
MSG—monosodium glutamate

MSL—midsternal line
mucilaginous
mucolytics [a class of drugs]
mucopurulent
mucopus
mucoraceous
mucosanguineous
mucous [adj.]
mucronate
mucroniform
mucus [noun]
muffle
multicystic
multifactorial
multifocal
multiform
multilobar
multilobular
multilocular
multinodular
multiple
multisystem
    m. disease
multivitamin (MV)
mummying
Münchausen
    by proxy syndrome
    syndrome
mural
muscarine
muscarinic
    m. agonists [a class of drugs]
muscle
    See also in *Orthopedics and*
       Sports Medicine section.
    accessory m.'s of respiration
    extraocular m.'s (EOMs)
    inspiratory m.
muscular
muscularity
mushroom
mustard
    white m.
    yellow m.
mutilate
mutilation
myalgia
mydriatics [a class of drugs]

"my-nute" Phonetic for minute
    [small].
"mytotic" Phonetic for mitotic.
Na—sodium
N/A, NA—not applicable
    not available
NaCl—sodium chloride
NAD—no active disease
    no acute distress
    no apparent distress
    no appreciable disease
nail bed
narcostimulant
narcotic
narcotic agonist-antagonists [a
    class of drugs]
narcotics; narcotic agonists [a class
    of drugs]
narcotize
nare [incorrect term for naris, sin-
    gular of nares]
nares (plural of naris)
naris (nares)
National Formulary (NF)
natis (nates)
natriuretic
nausea
nauseated
nauseous
NC—noncontributory
N/C—no complaints
ND—no disease
nebulization
NEC—not elsewhere classified, not
    elsewhere classifiable
necessary
necropurulent
    n. appendicitis
NED—no evidence of disease
neoadjuvant
    n. therapy
neologism
neoplastic
NER—no evidence of recurrence
NERD—no evidence of recurrent
    disease
nervous
    n. breakdown

nervous (continued)
    central n. system
    peripheral n. system
nervousness
nettle
neural
neurasthenia
neuro—neurologic
neurologic, neurological
neurologist
neurology
    clinical n.
neuromimetic
neurovascular
nevertheless
nexus
NF—National Formulary
NIA—no information available
niche
NICU—neonatal intensive care unit
    neurological intensive care
      unit
nidus (nidi)
nitrates [a class of drugs]
nitrosoureas [a class of drugs]
NK—not known
NKA—no known allergies
NKDA—no known drug allergies
NM—neuromuscular
    nuclear medicine
NNRTIs—non-nucleoside reverse
    transcriptase inhibitors [a class
    of drugs]
NO—nitric oxide
No.—number
nocturia
nocturnal
nocuous
nodular
nodularity
nodulated
nodulation
nomen (nomina)
    nomina generalia
nomenclature
noncompliance, noncompliant
nonetheless
nonfunctioning

noninfectious
nonlymphocytic
non-nucleoside reverse transcriptase
    inhibitors (NNRTIs) [a class
    of drugs]
nonpermissive
nonplused, nonplussed
nonspecific
nonsteroidal anti-inflammatory drugs
    (NSAIDs) [a class of drugs]
nonsurgical
nonviable
norlupinanes [a class of drugs]
normoactive
normotensive
normothermia
normotonia
normotopia
normotrophic
NOS—not otherwise specified
nosocomial
notching
noticeable
    n. improvement
novel (atypical) antipsychotics [a
    class of drugs]
Novocain [anesthetic agent]
noxa (noxae)
NP—nasopharyngeal
    nasopharynx
    nurse practioner
n.p.o., NPO—nothing by mouth (L.
    nil per os)
NS—normal saline
NSA—no significant abnormality
NSAIA—nonsteroidal anti-inflam-
    matory agent
NSAID, NSAIDs—nonsteroidal
    anti-inflammatory drug(s) [a
    class of drugs]
NSR—normal sinus rhythm
NTP—normal temperature and
    pressure
nucha
nucleoplasm
nutrition
nux
    n. vomica

Nv—naked vision
N&V—nausea and vomiting
NVD—nausea, vomiting, diarrhea
NWB—nonweightbearing, non-weightbearing, non–weight-bearing, no weightbearing
O₂ [O2]—oxygen
OA—osteoarthritis
oasis (oases)
OB—obstetrics
obese
obesity
    exogenous o.
obfuscation
OBG, OB-GYN—obstetrics and gynecology
obliteration
obsolescence
obsolete
obstetric, obstetrical
obstipation
obtund
obtundation
obtundent
obturation
obtuse
occasion
occipital
occiput
occult
occurrence
oculus (oculi)
    o. dexter (OD) [L. right eye]
    o. sinister (OS) [L. left eye]
    o. uterque (OU) [L. each eye]
OD—overdose
    right eye (L. oculus dexter)
OH—occupational history
OJ—orange juice
oleaginous
oleander
olei (genitive of oleum)
oleum (olea)
oligodipsia
OM—otitis media
omnivorous
OMPA—otitis media, purulent, acute
omphalic

omphalus
oneiroid
OP—operation
OP, OPT—outpatient
O&P—ova and parasites
opaque
OPD—outpatient department
operable
operation
    See in *General Surgical Terms.*
opiate
opioid
opium
    crude o.
OPS—outpatient service
OPT—outpatient treatment
OPT, OP—outpatient
optic, optical
optimal
optimum
OR—operating room
orbicular
organomegaly
oriented
    alert and o. (AO)
    o. to time, place, and person (OTPP)
    o. to time, place, person, and situation [or circumstance]
    o. times three, o. x3
orificial
ORS—orthopedic surgery
orth, ortho—orthopedics
orthopedics
orthopedist
orthopnea
    three-pillow o.
    two-pillow o.
orthostatic
    o. hypotension
orthotopic
os (ossa) [bone]
    See in *Orthopedics and Sports Medicine* section.
OS—left eye (L. oculus sinister)
oscillator
oscitate

oscitation
osculum
OSHA—Occupational Safety and
  Health Administration
osmotic diuretics [a class of drugs]
ossiform
ossify
ossifying
osteal [bony, osseous]
osteoid
osteolysis
osteopath
osteopathic
osteopathy
ostia (plural of ostium)
ostial [pertaining to opening, aperture, orifice]
ostium (ostia)
ostraceous
ostreotoxism
OT—occupational therapy
OTC—over-the-counter
OU—each eye (L. oculus uterque)
OURQ—outer upper right quadrant
OV—office visit
oval
overcorrection
overdosage
overdose (OD)
overflow
overgrowth
overhang
overlap
overlay
overload
overprotection
overreaching
overriding
overstress
overt
overtone
overweight
oxazolidinediones [a class of drugs]
oxidize
oximeter
    finger o.
    pulse o.

oximetry
    finger o.
    pulse o.
oxygen (O)
    molecular o. (O_2) [O2])
oxytocics [a class of drugs]
oxytocin
P—pulse
P_1—pulmonic first sound
P_2—pulmonic second sound
PA, P.A.—physician's assistant
P&A—percussion and auscultation
PAB—*p*-aminobenzoate [p-, para-]
PABA—*p*-aminobenzoic acid [p-,
  para-]
PAC—phenacetin, aspirin, caffeine
    premature atrial contraction
pagetoid
pain
    bearing-down p.
    lancinating p.
palliate
palliative
pallor
palpable
palpate
palpation
palpebrate
palpebration
palpitation
panel
    urine drug p. (UDP)
panhidrosis
panhyperemia
Papanicolaou (Pap)
    smear
    stain
    test
papyraceous
para
para (0, 1, 2, etc.) [number of deliv-
  eries]
para
    p.-aminobenzoic acid (PABA)
paracenesthesia
paracentral
paradoxic, paradoxical
parallel

paralytic
paramedian
paranoid
paranormal
paraphernalia
paraprofessional
parapsychology
parasite
    See specific parasites in
    Laboratory, Pathology,
    and Chemistry Terms.
parasympathetic
parasympathomimetics [a class of
    drugs]
parenchymal
parenteral
paresis
paresthesia
parietal
pari passu
paroxysm
paroxysmal
parried
parry
particulate
PASA—*p*-aminosalicylic acid [p-,
    para-]
PAS-C—*p*-aminosalicylic acid,
    crystallized [p-, para-]
PASG—pneumatic antishock garment
passive
pasteurizer
PAT—paroxysmal atrial tachycardia
path—pathology
pathogen
    See specific pathogens in
    Laboratory, Pathology,
    and Chemistry Terms.
pathologic, pathological
pathology
pathosis
pattern
    rugal p.
patulous
paucity
    p. of findings
    p. of speech
PBZ—pyribenzamine

p.c.—after meals (L. post cibum)
PC—phosphatidyl choline
PCA—patient-controlled analgesia
PCM—protein-calorie malnutrition
PCP—phencyclidine
    phenylcyclohexyl piperidine
    [now: phencyclidine]
PD—pediatrics
    pulmonary disease
PDE III (phosphodiesterase III)
    inhibitors [a class of drugs]
PDR—*Physicians' Desk Reference*
PE—phenylephrine
    physical evaluation
    physical examination
peau
    p. d'orange (Fr. orange peel
    skin)
pectinate
ped, peds pediatrics
pedal
pediculicides
pedicure
peduncular
pedunculated
peeling
pelvic
    p. inflammatory disease (PID)
pendelluft
    p. chest
pendulous
penems [a class of drugs]
penicilliary
penicillinase-resistant penicillins [a
    class of drugs]
penicillins [a class of drugs]
percussible
perennial
perfusion
peripheral
    p. vasodilators [a class of
    drugs]
peripherally
periphery
peritoneum
PERL—pupils equal, react to light
PERLA—pupils equal, react to
    light and accommodation

permeability
permeation
pernicious
per os (p.o.) (L. by mouth)
perplexed
per rectum
PERRLA—pupils equal, round, react
      to light and accommodation
per se (L. of, in, or by itself)
persecuted
persecutory
perseverance
perspiration
per tubam
perusal
perversion
pervert
pessimism
pest
pesticide
pestiferous
pestilence
pestilential
pestle
"petekeah" Phonetic for petechia.
petrous
PFT—pulmonary function test
pg—picogram(s)
PH—past history
phalliform
phalloid
phanerogenic
pharmaceutical
pharmacist
phenolphthalein
phenol red
phenolsulfonphthalein
phenomenology
phenomenon (phenomena)
      anaphylactoid p.
phenothiazines [a class of drugs]
phenylbutylpiperadines [a class of
      drugs]
phenyltriazines [a class of drugs]
phlebitis
phleboclysis
      drip p.
      slow p.

phleboid
phlebotomy
phlegmatic
phonetic
phonetics
phosphatidylcholine (PC)
phosphodiesterase III (PDE III)
      inhibitors [a class of drugs]
phosphorous [adj.]
phosphorus (P) [noun]
phosphuretic
Physalia
physaliform
physaliphorous
physician
physiognomy
physiognosis
physiologic, physiological
physiologicoanatomical
physiology
physiopathologic
physiopathology
physique
PI—present illness
pica
picogram(s) (pg)
PICU—pediatric intensive care unit
      pulmonary intensive care unit
pièce de résistance
piecemeal
piggyback
piggybacking
pigmentation
pigmented
"piknic" Phonetic for pyknic.
piliform
pill
pillet
pillion
pilula (pilulae)
pilular
pilule
piperidines [a class of drugs]
pizzeria
placebo
plasma expanders [a class of drugs]
plasma protein fractions [a class of
      drugs]

platelet
plethora
       p. of complaints
       p. of problems
plethoric
plexiform
plicate
PM—after death (L. post mortem)
       physical medicine
       preventive medicine
p.m., PM—afternoon, evening,
     nighttime
       after noon (L. post meridian)
PMH—past medical history
PMI—point of maximal impulse
       point of maximal intensity
PMR—physical medicine and reha-
     bilitation
PND—paroxysmal nocturnal dyspnea
       postnasal drip, postnasal
        drainage
pneumatized
p.o.—by mouth (L. per os)
POC—point of care
       postoperative care
       postoperative course
poculiform
POD—postoperative day
podium (podia)
podophyllotoxins [a class of drugs]
"po do rahnj" Phonetic for peau
     d'orange.
poinsettia
poison
         corrosive p.
         narcotic p.'s
         puffer p.
poison control center (PCC)
poisonous
pokeweed
polarity
polarization
polarize
Polaroid
pole
         apical p.
         cephalic p.
         negative p.

pole (continued)
         positive p.
         twin p.'s
police officer
polio—poliomyelitis
polishing
poll, polled
pollution
polychlorinated biphenyl (PCB)
polydipsia
polyenes [a class of drugs]
polygamy
polyleptic
polymerization
polypharmaceutic
polypharmacy
polypiform
polyunsaturated
polyuria
POMR—problem-oriented medical
     record
"poo-drahzh" Phonetic for poudrage.
POP—plaster of Paris
POR—problem-oriented record
porcelain
porcelaneous
porous
Portuguese man-o'-war
position
     See in *General Surgical*
      Terms.
postanoxic
posterior
posteriorly
posteroinferior
posterolateral
posteromedial
postictal
postmortem
postnatal
postop—postoperative
postprandial
potassium (K)
         p. acetate
         p. chloride
         p. gluconate
         p. hydroxide
         p. iodide

potassium (K) (continued)
    p. perchlorate
    p. permanganate
    p. phosphate
potassium-sparing diuretics [a class
    of drugs]
potency
poudrage
poultice
p.p.—after meals (L. post prandium)
PP—postprandial
    private practice
PPB—positive-pressure breathing
PPD—purified protein derivative
    (of tuberculin)
PPD-S—purified protein deriva-
    tive–standard
PPO—preferred provider organiza-
    tion
prandial
PRCs—packed red cells
preagonal
precarious
precede
precipitate
precipitately
precipitous
precipitously
precocious
precocity
precursor
predilection
predisposition
prejudice
premonitory
preop—preoperative
prescription
presentation
       See in *Obstetrics & Gyne-*
         cology section.
preventive
primary
principal [primary, main]
    p. aspect
    p. reason
    p. symptom
principle [rule]

privilege
    admitting p.'s
    bathroom p.'s
    conversion p.
    staff p.'s
p.r.n., prn, PRN—as necessary (L.
    pro re nata)
procedure
proceed
prodroma (plural of prodromon)
prodromal
prodromata [incorrect term for pro-
    droma, plural of prodromon]
prodrome
prodromon (prodroma) [singular
    form rarely used]
pro-drugs
Professional Standards Review
    Organization (PSRO)
professor
profound
    p. anemia
    p. debility
    p. hematuria
profundus
progeny
progeria
progesterone
progestins [a class of drugs]
prognosis
proliferation
promontory
prone
prophylactic
propositus (propositi)
proprioceptive
prosody
prostaglandin (PG)
    p. agonists [a class of drugs]
prostaglandins [a class of drugs]
prostate
prosthetics
prostration
protease inhibitors [a class of drugs]
proton pump inhibitors [a class of
    drugs]
protuberant
    p. abdomen

proud flesh
provisional
provocative
proximal
proximalis
proximally
PRRE—pupils round, regular, and
    equal
pruritus
PS—plastic surgery
PSH—past surgical history
psoas
       p. sign
psoralens [a class of drugs]
psy, psych—psychiatry, psychiatric
psychiatric
psychiatrist
psychiatry
psychic
psychogenic
psychologic, psychological
psychologist
psychology
psyllium
       p. hydrophilic mucilloid
       p. seed
pt—patient
PT—prothrombin time
PTA—post-traumatic amnesia
    prior to admission
    prior to arrival
PTD—permanent and total disability
pterins [a class of drugs]
ptosis
PTT—partial thromboplastin time
puberty
pubescence
pubescent
publicly
puerile
pulicicide
pulley
pulmonary
       p. toilet
pulpless
pulpy
pulsatile
pulsion

pultaceous
pulverization
pulverulent
pulvinate
pulvis
punctate
pura (plural of pus)
purgatives [a class of drugs]
puris (genitive of pus)
purulent
puruloid
pus (pura)
    anchovy sauce p.
    blue p.
    burrowing p.
    cheesy p.
    curdy p.
    green p.
    ichorous p.
    laudable p., p. laudandum
    p. tube
"pussy" Slang for pustular, puslike.
pustular
pustule
putative
putrid
PVP—polyvinylpyrrolidone [now:
    povidone]
Px—physical examination
    prognosis
pyemesis
pyknic
pyogenesis
pyogenic
pyramidal
pyrazolopyrimidines [a class of
    drugs]
pyrethrins
pyretic
pyrexia (pyrexiae)
pyrexial
pyrosis
q.—every (L. quaque)
Q—query [sometimes used for
    questionable diagnosis]
q.a.m.—every morning (L. quaque
    ante meridiem)
q.d.—every day (L. quaque die)

q.h.—every hour (L. quaque hora)
q.2h.—every two hours
q.3h.—every three hours
q.4h.—every four hours
q.h.s.—every hour of sleep
q.i.d.—four times a day (L. quater in die)
q.o.d.—every other day [coined expression, not Latin]
quadrant
qualitative
quandary
quantal
quantitate
quantitative
quantization
quantize, quantized
quantum (quanta)
quarantine
querulous
queue [line]
quiescent
quinolizidines [a class of drugs]
quinolones [a class of drugs]
R—respiration
RA—rheumatoid arthritis
raccoon eyes
radialis
radiate
radical [adj.]
radicle [noun: branch of nerve or vessel]
radiologic, radiological
"rah-mo-lees-maw" Phonetic for ramollissement.
"rahpor" Phonetic for rapport.
"rakoma" Phonetic for rhacoma.
rale
>   See in *Pulmonary Medicine* section.
>   bibasilar r.'s
Rally pack
ramal
ramification
ramify
ramollissement
ramose
rampart

ramus (rami)
rapport
rarefaction
ratio
>   body-weight r.
>   risk r.
>   risk-benefit r.
rationalization
RBC—red blood cell(s)
RCM—right costal margin
RCU—respiratory care unit
RDA—recommended daily allowance
RDS—respiratory distress syndrome
rebound
recalcitrant
>   r. disease
>   r. hemorrhage
>   r. patient
recapitulation
recede
receive
recidivation
reciprocal
recommend
recommendation
recrudescence
recrudescent
>   r. pain
rectus
recumbent
recuperation
recurred
recurrence
recurrent
red herring
red tide
reducible
redundant
reentry
reflex
>   See also in *Neurology and Pain Management* section.
>   deep tendon r.'s (DTRs)
>   light r.
>   red r.
refractory
>   r. illness

refractory (continued)
    r. period
regimen
regio (regiones)
region
    core r.
    focal r.
    hypochondriac r.
    hypogastric r.
    inguinal r.
    lateral abdominal r.
    pelvic r.
    sternocleidomastoid r.
    submental r.
    temporal r.
    umbilical r.
regional
region of interest
"regma" Phonetic for rhegma.
regurgitant
rehab—rehabilitation
rehabilitation
rehydration
rejoinder
"reksis" Phonetic for rhexis.
relapse
remediable
    surgically r.
remedial
remedy
reminiscent
remittent
renown
"rentgen" Phonetic for roentgen.
reoccurrence [incorrect word for
    recurrence]
repertoire
repetition
residual
residue
resilience
resinoid
resinous
resistance
    drug r.
    multidrug r., multiple drug. r.
    natural r.
resorption

respiration
    See also in the *Pulmonary*
      Medicine section.
    absent r.
    accelerated r.
    forced r.
    labored r.
    mouth-to-mouth r.
    spontaneous r.'s
respiratory
    r. acidosis
    r. arrest
    r. distress
    r. distress syndrome (RDS)
    r. system
    r. tract
restaurateur
restiform
restitutio
    r. integrum
restitution
restoration
resuscitation
retching
retention
"retic" Slang for reticulocyte (count).
retinoids [a class of drugs]
retrocedent
retrograde
retroperitoneal
retropulsion
retroversion
reverse transcriptase (RT) inhibitors
    [a class of drugs]
reversion
RFB—retained foreign body
Rh—Rhesus
Rh
    antibody
    blood group
    factor
    immunization
    incompatibility
    isoantigen
rhacoma
rhagades [grammatically plural; no
    singular form]
rhagadiform

rhegma
rhexis
rhizoid
rhonchal, rhonchial
rhonchus (rhonchi)
      audible rhonchi
      bibasilar rhonchi
      bilateral rhonchi
      coarse rhonchi
      diffuse rhonchi
      expiratory rhonchi
      faint rhonchi
      few rhonchi
      harsh rhonchi
      high-pitched rhonchi
      humming rhonchi
      inspiratory rhonchi
      low-pitched rhonchi
      marked rhonchi
      musical rhonchi
      occasional rhonchi
      post-tussive inspiratory
        rhonchi
      rare rhonchi
      scattered rhonchi
      sibilant rhonchi
      sonorous rhonchi
      upper respiratory rhonchi
      whistling rhonchi
rhythm
      circadian r.
rhythmic, rhythmical
rhythmicity
rictus
rigidity
      nuchal r.
rigor
      r. mortis
rigors
"rith-ing" Phonetic for writhing.
"rithm" Phonetic for rhythm.
rivalry
"rizo–" Phonetic for words begin-
    ning rhizo–.
RLE—right lower extremity
RLQ—right lower quadrant
RLS—Ringer lactated solution
RN, R.N.—registered nurse

RO, R/O—rule out
roentgen (R)
roentgenologic, roentgenological
ROMI—rule out myocardial infarc-
    tion
"romied" Slang for myocardial
    infarction ruled out.
"rongk–" Phonetic for words begin-
    ning rhonch–.
ROS—review of systems
rostra (plural of rostrum)
rostrad
rostrate
rostriform
rostrum (rostrums, rostra)
rotexion
RPG—retrograde pyelogram
RR—recovery room
      respiratory rate
R&R—rest and recuperation
RR&E—round, regular, and equal
RR-HPO—rapid
      recompression–high-pressure
      oxygen
RSR—regular sinus rhythm
RT (reverse transcriptase) inhibitors
    [a class of drugs]
rub
      friction r.
      pericardial r.
      pleural r.
      pleuritic r.
      pleuropericardial r.
rubedo
rubefacients
ruber
ruberous
rubescent
rubiginose, rubiginous
rubor
ruborous
rubric
rubrous
ructus
rudimentary
RUE—right upper extremity
rufous

rugal pattern
rugate
rugose, rugous
rugosity
rule
    r. of nines
runoff
rupture
    traumatic r.
RUQ—right upper quadrant
℞ [R_x, Rx]—prescription
    take (L. recipe)
    therapy
    treatment
S_1–S_4 [S1–S4]—heart sounds (first
    through fourth)
sacciform
saccular
sacculation
saccule
sacculiform
sacral
sacrifice
sacrilegious
sacroiliac
sagacious
sagacity
sagittal
SAH—subarachnoid hemorrhage
salicylates [a class of drugs]
salient
    s. findings
saline
    s. laxatives
    s. solution
saliva
salivary
salivation
salubrious
saluretic
salutary
salvo
sanative
sanatorium
sang-froid
sanguine
sanguineous

sarcoma (sarcomas, sarcomata)
    See in *Oncology and Hema-*
        tology section.
sardonic
satellite
satiate, satiated
satiety
saturated
save, save that
SBP—systolic blood pressure
scabicides [a class of drugs]
scalariform
scale
    Celsius s.
    centigrade s.
    Fahrenheit s.
    Glasgow Coma S.
scalene
scalloped
scalloping
scanning
scaphoid
scarification
scarify
scavenger
SCBA—self-contained breathing
    apparatus
scenario
schizoid
sciatica
sclerogenous
sclerogummatous
scleroid
sclerose
sclerosed
sclerosis
sclerotic
sclerous
scop—scopolamine
"scopes" See under full name.
    stethoscope
screen
    urine drug s. (UDS)
SCU—special care unit
scurrile
scurrilous
scyphoid
scythropasmus

SD—sudden death
SDS—sudden death syndrome
secede
second (s, sec.)
    inverse s.
    reciprocal s.
secretion
sectioning
sed rate—sedimentation rate
sedate
sedation
sedatives [a class of drugs]
    general s.
sedentary
segmented neutrophils (segs, segmenteds)
segs—segmented neutrophils
seizure
selective estrogen receptor modulators (SERMs) [a class of drugs]
selective serotonin 5-HT$_3$ (hydroxytryptamine) blockers [a class of drugs]
selective serotonin reuptake inhibitors (SSRIs) [a class of drugs]
self-care
self-limited, self-limiting
semilunar
senescence
senility
sensorium
    general s.
separation
sequela (sequelae)
sequestral
serendipitous
serendipity
serial
serially
seriatim
SERMs—selective estrogen receptor modulators [a class of drugs]
serology
    diagnostic s.
seroma
seropurulent
seropus
serosa

serosanguineous
serous
serpiginous
serrated
"ser-sin-ate" Phonetic for circinate.
serum (serums, sera)
    anticrotalus s.
    antirabies s.
    antisnakebite s.
    antitetanic s. (ATS)
    North American antisnakebite s.
    Sclavo s.
    truth s.
sessile
seta (setae)
setaceous
sexuality
SH—social history
    surgical history
shagreen
shears
    bandage s.
Sherman unit
shivering
shock
    anaphylactic s.
    electric s.
    hemorrhagic s.
    hypoglycemic s.
    hypovolemic s.
shrapnel
SI—self-inflicted
sialagogues [a class of drugs]
sibling
sick bay
SICU—surgical intensive care unit
side effect
sig—let it be labeled (L. signetur)
sign
    Aaron s.
    accessory s.
    antecedent s.
    assident s.
    auscultatory s.'s
    Ballance s.
    Burton s.
    commemorative s.

sign (continued)
    Cope s.
    Corrigan s.
    Federici s.
    Gubler s.
    Horn s.
    Kernig s.
    Klemm s.
    McBurney s.
    objective s.'s
    obturator s.
    physical s.'s
    psoas s.
    Robertson s.
    Rovsing s.
    soft s.'s
    subjective s.'s
    vital s.'s
signa (S)
signature
significance
    statistical s.
significant
"sike–" Phonetic for words beginning psych–.
silhouette
"sil-oo-et" Phonetic for silhouette.
silver (Ag)
    s. nitrate
Simon
    position
sin–. See also words beginning cin–, syn–.
single-blind [clinical trial]
singultation
singultous [adj.]
singultus [noun]
sinister
sinistrad
sinusal
sinusoidal
sinusoidalization
"sithropazmus" Phonetic for scythropasmus.
SIW—self-inflicted wound
SK—streptokinase
skeleton
skeletonized

skew
"sklero–" Phonetic for words beginning sclero–.
sleeplessness
sleeptalking
sleepwalking
slough
sloughing
slow-channel blockers [a class of drugs]
"sluff" Phonetic for slough.
"sluffing" Phonetic for sloughing.
slurry
SMA—sequential multiple analyzer [SMA 6/60, SMA 12/60, SMA 20/60]
SMAC ["smack"]—sequential multiple analyzer plus computer [SMAC 7, SMAC 12, SMAC 20]
SNF ["sniff"]—skilled nursing facility
SOAP—Subjective, Objective, Assessment, Plan [format for medical reports]
SOB—shortness of breath
sociology
sodium (Na)
    s. amobarbital
    s. ampicillin
    s. ascorbate
    s. bicarbonate
    s. bromide
    s. butabarbital
    s. carbonate
    s. channel
    s. chloride (Cl [NaCl])
    s. citrate
    s. folate
    s. glutamate
    s. hydroxide
    s. iodide
    s. lauryl sulfate
    s. methicillin
    monohydrated s. carbonate
    s. nitrite
    s. nitroprusside
    s. oxacillin

sodium (Na) (continued)
    s. penicillin G
    s. pentobarbital
    s. phenobarbital
    s. phenytoin
    s. propionate
    s. salicylate
    s. secobarbital
    s. warfarin
solanine
solanism
solanoid
Solanum carolinense
solarium
soluble
Soma
somatic
somnolence
sonorous
"soo-chee," "soo-shee" Phonetic for
    sushi.
"soo-fl," "soo-flay" Phonetic for
    souffle.
SOP—standard operating procedure
sophomore
sorbefacient
souffle
sound
        vesicular breath s.'s
        white s.
souvenir
S/P, SP—status post
spasmodic
spatial
specialist
        clinical nurse s., nurse s.
specialization
specialize
specialty
specific
specimen
spectral
spermicides [a class of drugs]
Sphaeroides
        S. maculatus
sphenoid
spheroid
sphincteral

sphincteralgia
sphygmomanometer
spider
        banana s.
spinate
spontaneous
sporadic
spurious
        s. findings (on laboratory
          tests)
SPWB—Saunders Pharmaceutical
    Word Book
squamate
square millimeter(s) (mm^2, sq mm)
SR—systems review
SSRIs—selective serotonin reuptake
    inhibitors [a class of drugs]
stab [German word for band, imma-
    ture neutrophil]
stability
stabilization
stable
stab wound
stamina
standardize
standby
stat, STAT—immediately (L. statim)
statins [a class of drugs]
status
        mental s.
        nutrition s.
        s. post [event]
        s. praesens
steatorrhea
steatosis
stellate
stenosed
stenosing
stenosis (stenoses)
stenotic
stercoral
stercus (stercora)
stereoscopic
sterile, sterilely
sterility
sterilize
Steri-Strip

stethoscope
    binaural s.
    Cammann s.
    differential s.
    electronic s.
    Leff s.
stigma (stigmas, stigmata)
stimulant laxatives [a class of drugs]
stimulants [a class of drugs]
stimulation
stimulus (stimuli)
STK—streptokinase
stool-softening laxatives [a class of drugs]
streptogramins [a class of drugs]
striatal
striated
stroke
    exertional heat s.
    heat s.
    lightning s.
    sun s. [pref: sunstroke]
study
    double-blind s.
stupor
    benign s.
    Cairns s.
    catatonic s.
    depressive s.
stuporous
styptics
subacute
subconscious
subcostal
subcostalis (subcostales)
subcu, subq—subcutaneous
subcutaneous
subcuticular
subjective
sublimate
subluxation
subside
subsidence
substituted benzimidazoles [a class of drugs]
subtle
subtly
succagogue

succedaneous
succedaneum
succeed
succenturiate
succession
succinimides [a class of drugs]
succulence
succus (succi)
    s. cerasi
sudorifics [a class of drugs]
suicide
suit
    antiblackout s.
    anti-G s.
    antishock s.
suite ["sweet"]
    operating s.
sulciform
sulfamates [a class of drugs]
sulfonamides [a class of drugs]
sulfonylureas [a class of drugs]
sunstroke
superficial
superficialis
supersede
supination
supine
suppression
suppuration
suppurative
surfactant laxatives [a class of drugs]
surfeit
surgery
    ambulatory s.
    conservative s.
    cosmetic s.
    day s.
    elective s.
    exploratory s.
    general s.
    in-and-out s.
    major s.
    minor s.
    palliative s.
    radical s.
    rapid in-and-out (RIO) s.
surprise
surprisingly

surrogate
surveillance
susceptible
sushi
"sut-el" Phonetic for subtle.
"sut-lee" Phonetic for subtly.
suture [material]
    See in *General Surgical Terms.*
suture [technique]
    See in *General Surgical Terms.*
"sweet" Phonetic for suite.
sweetener
    artificial s. [q.v. for specific kinds]
swelling
    fugitive s.
symbiosis
symmetric, symmetrical
sympatholytics [a class of drugs]
sympathomimetics [a class of drugs]
symptom
    accessory s.
    acute on chronic s.'s
    assident s.
    cardinal s.
    characteristic s.
    concomitant s.
    consecutive s.
    constitutional s.
    deficiency s.
    delayed s.
    direct s.
    equivocal s.
    factitious s.
    fundamental s.
    general s.
    guiding s.
    indirect s.
    induced s.
    local s.
    localizing s.'s
    negative s.
    objective s.
    pathognomonic s.
    precursor s.
    premonitory s.

symptom (continued)
    presenting s.
    prodromal s.
    rational s.
    reflex s.
    signal s.
    static s.
    subjective s.
    sympathetic s.
    systemic s.
symptomatic
symptomatology
syn–. See also words beginning cin–, sin–.
syncopal
syndrome
    See in medical specialty sections.
synergetic
synkinesis
T—temperature
tab—tablet
"tabeez" Phonetic for tabes.
tabella (tabellae)
tabescent
tabular
tachypnea
tactile
taeniacides [a class of drugs]
"takipneah" Phonetic for tachypnea.
talcum
tamponade
    nasal t.
    postnasal balloon t.
taper
TAT—tetanus antitoxin
    turn-around time
tattoo
taut
    t. skin
taxanes, taxoids [a class of drugs]
TBSA—total body surface area
TCIE—transient cerebral ischemic episode
TD—tetanus-diphtheria [vaccine—pediatric initial dose]
Td—tetanus-diphtheria [vaccine—adult booster dose]

TDE—tetrachlorodiphenylethane
(pesticide)
TDI—toluene-diisocyanate
Te—tetanus
tease, teased
technique
See in *General Surgical Terms.*
temperature (T, temp)
body t.
core t.
maximum t.
minimum t.
normal t.
temporal
tenable
tenacious
tenacity
tenuous
t. situation
teratoid
terminad
terminal
grapelike t.'s
terminalization
termination
terminology
tessellated
test
See also in *Laboratory, Pathology, and Chemistry Terms.*
double-blind t.
screening t.
testimony
expert t.
testis (testes)
testosterone
t. cypionate
t. propionate
tetracyclics [a class of drugs]
tetracyclines [a class of drugs]
texture
THC—tetrahydrocannabinol
theraccines [a class of drugs]
therapeutic
therapist

therapy
multiple t.
thermometer
axilla t.
Celsius t.
centigrade t.
clinical t.
Fahrenheit t.
infrared tympanic t.
oral t.
rectal t.
tympanic t.
thiazides [a class of drugs]
thiazolidinediones [a class of drugs]
thienamycins [a class of drugs]
thienobenzodiazepines [a class of drugs]
thioxanthenes [a class of drugs]
thoraces (plural of thorax)
thoracic
thoracodorsal
thorax (thoraces)
amazon t.
barrel-shaped t.
cholesterol t.
Peyrot t.
pyriform t.
three-pillow orthopnea
threshold
t. of discomfort
pain t.
throbbing
thrombin
thrombolytics [a class of drugs]
thymidylate synthase (TS) inhibitors [a class of drugs]
thyromegaly
TIA—transient ischemic attack
t.i.d.—three times a day (L. ter in die)
TIE—transient ischemic episode
tigroid
time (T)
dead t.
tincture of t.
turn-around time (TAT)
tinctura (tincturae)
tincturation

tincture
    t. of time
tinnitus
tiqueur
tissue
    t. plasminogen activator (t-PA, tPA, TPA)
titration
TM—tympanic membrane
tocolytics [a class of drugs]
α-tocopherol [alpha-]
toilet
tolerance
    drug t.
tomogram
tonicity
tonus
toothache
toothed
toothpick
topical
topographic, topographical
topography
topoisomerase I inhibitors [a class of drugs]
TOPS—Take Off Pounds Sensibly [program]
torpid
torpidity
torpor
torsion
tortuous
tortured
    t. expression
"tosis" Phonetic for ptosis.
toxemia
toxic
toxicity
toxoids [a class of drugs]
t-PA, tPA, TPA—tissue plasminogen activator
TPN—total parenteral nutrition
TPPN—total peripheral parenteral nutrition
TPR—temperature, pulse, respiration
TPT—typhoid-paratyphoid
TPT vaccine

track
    needle t.'s
tragedy
trajector
tranquilizer
transaminase
transference
transillumination
transition
translucent
transmigration
transmissible
transmission
transudate
transverse
trauma (traumas, traumata)
traumatherapy
traumatic
traumatism
traumatize
treatment
    conservative t.
    drug t.
    empiric t.
    expectant t.
    palliative t.
    preventive t., prophylactic t.
    protracted t.
    radical t.
    surgical t.
    symptomatic t.
tremor
tremulous
trial
    double-blind t.
tricyclics [a class of drugs]
trigeminy
triiodothyronine
triple-blind [clinical trial]
troche
trochiscus (trochischi)
trochlear
truly
truncate
trypsin
L-tryptophan
TS—thoracic surgery
tsp.—teaspoon(s), teaspoonful

tubercular
tuberculin
    Old t. (OT)
    purified protein derivative
      (PPD) t.
    Seibert t.
tuberculosis (TB)
tuberculostatic
tubuliform
tumefacient
tumefaction
tumentia
tumescence
tumescent
tumid
tumor
    benign t.
tunicate
tunnel
turbid
turbidity
turgescence
turgescent
turgid
tussive
twinge
twitch
two-pillow orthopnea
Tx—treatment
tympanic
tympanitic
typhoid-paratyphoid (TPT) vaccine
"u–" Phonetic for words beginning
    eu–.
U—unit
UA—urinalysis
ubiquitous
UCD, UChD—usual childhood dis-
    eases
UDP—urine drug panel
UDS—urine drug screen
UE—upper extremity
"ufor–" Phonetic for words begin-
    ning euphor–.
UG—urogenital
UGI—upper gastrointestinal
UIQ—upper inner quadrant
UK—urokinase

"ukraseah" Phonetic for eucrasia.
ulcerate
ulcerating
ulceration
ulcerative
ULN—upper limit of normal
ULQ—upper left quadrant
umbilical
umbilicus
unarousable
unbeknownst
uncia (unciae)
uncompensated
unconditioned
unconscious
unconsciousness
unction
unctuous
undernutrition
undifferentiated
undulating
undulation
"ungk-shun" Phonetic for unction.
unguent
unguenta (plural of unguentum)
unguenti (genitive of unguentum)
unguentum (unguenta)
unicentral
unilateral
unit
    See also in *Laboratory,*
      Pathology, and Chemistry
      Terms.
    alcohol and drug dependen-
      cy u. (ADDU)
    antitoxic u.
    burn u.
    cardiac care u. (CCU)
    cardiology intensive care u.
      (CICU)
    coronary care u. (CCU)
    coronary intensive care u.
      (CICU)
    critical care u. (CCU)
    intensive care u. (ICU)
    intensive coronary care u.
      (ICCU)
    international u. of penicillin

unit (continued)
> international u. of vitamin A
> international u. of vitamin D
> medical intensive care u.
> (MICU)
> u. of penicillin
> pulmonary intensive care u.
> (PICU)
> respiratory care u. (RCU)
> SI (Système International) u.
> special care u. (SCU)
> Steenbock u. of vitamin D
> surgical intensive care u.
> (SICU)
> USP (United States Pharma-
> copeia) u.
> u. of vasopressin
> vitamin A u.
> u. of vitamin B_1 [B1]
> vitamin D u.

United States Adopted Names
(USAN) Council
United States Pharmacopeia (USP)
unnecessary
unresponsive
"unsi–" Phonetic for words beginning unci–.
untenable
untoward
> u. effects

UOQ—upper outer quadrant
"up-nee-a" Phonetic for eupnea.
UR—upper respiratory [tract]
URI—upper respiratory infection
urinalysis
urine
> u. drug panel (UDP)
> u. drug screen (UDS)

urokinase
urologic, urological
URQ—upper right quadrant
URTI—upper respiratory tract
infection
"uthanazea" Phonetic for euthanasia.
"uthiroid" Phonetic for euthyroid.
UTI—urinary tract infection
UV—ultraviolet
uva (uvae)

uviform
UVL—ultraviolet light
VA, V.A.—Veterans Administration
Veterans Affairs
vaccinate
vaccines [a class of drugs]
vacillate
vaginate
vallate
vapor (vapores, vapors)
vaporization
vaporize
variability
variable
variant
vascular serotonin 5-HT_1 [5-HT1]
receptor agonists [a class of
drugs]
vasiform
vasoconstrictors [a class of drugs]
vasodilators [a class of drugs]
vasopressin
vasopressors [a class of drugs]
"veez-a-vee" Phonetic for vis-à-vis.
velamentous
venation
ventral
ventralis
ventromedial
vermicides [a class of drugs]
vermicular
vermiculation
vermiculous
vermiform
vermifugal
vermifuges
vertebra (vertebrae)
> See in *Orthopedics and*
> *Sports Medicine* section.

vertebral
vertical
vertiginous
vertigo
vesicants
vestige
vestigial
viability

viable
>   v. alternative
vial
vicious
vinca alkaloids [a class of drugs]
viral
virile
virulent
virus
>   See specific viruses in *Laboratory, Pathology, and Chemistry Terms.*
vis (vires)
>   v. conservatrix
>   v. formativa
>   v. a fronte
>   v. in situ
>   v. medicatrix naturae
>   v. a tergo
>   v. vitae, v. vitalis
vis-à-vis [opposite to, compared with, in relation to]
viscera (plural of viscus)
visceromegaly
visceroptosis
viscid
viscose [noun or adj.]
viscosity
>   absolute v.
viscous [adj.]
viscus (viscera)
vit—vitamin
vital
vitality
vitamin
vitamin B$_{12}$ [B12]
vitiate
vitiation
voces (plural of vox)
vocis (genitive of vox)
voix
>   v. de Polichinelle
volar
volatile
volenti non fit injuria
volvulate
vomica

vomit
>   coffee-grounds v.
vomiting
vomitus
>   coffee-grounds v.
>   v. cruentus
vox (voces)
VR—vocational rehabilitation
vs—against (L. versus)
VS—vital signs
VSS—vital signs stable
vulnera (plural of vulnus)
vulnerability
vulnerable
vulnerant
vulneraries [a class of drugs]
vulnerary
vulnerate
vulnus (vulnera)
vulsellum
"vwah" Phonetic for voix.
wakefulness
waxed and waned
>   fever w.a.w.
>   symptoms w.a.w.
WD—well-developed
WDWN—well-developed, well-nourished
weight
>   apothecaries' w.
>   avoirdupois w.
>   troy w.
well-developed
well-nourished
WF—white female
wheal
wheeze
whelk
whereupon
wherewithal
WHO—World Health Organization
whorl
wintergreen
wizened
>   w. appearance
WM—white male
WMF—white middle-aged female
WMM—white middle-aged male

WN—well-nourished
WNF—well-nourished female
WNL—within normal limits
WNM—well-nourished male
w/o, wo—without
World Health Organization (WHO)
wound
writhing
    w. in pain
x—times
xanthic
xanthines, xanthine derivatives [a
    class of drugs]
xanthous
xiphoid

y/o, Y/O—-year-old
    years old
YOB—year of birth
"yoo–" Phonetic for words begin-
    ning eu–.
"yoop-nee-a" Phonetic for eupnea.
yo-yo dieting
"zifoid" Phonetic for xiphoid.
zigzag
    z. laceration
zonal
zonary
zone
    comfort z.
zoning
zoster

General Surgical Terms

Abbe
    rings
Abbé-Zeiss
Abbott-Miller
    tube
Abbott-Rawson
    tube
abdominal
    a. incision
    a. retractor
    a. splenectomy
abdominoscopy
abdominothoracic
    a. incision
Abelson
    adenotome
    cannula
Abernethy
    fascia
    operation
ab externo
    a.e. incision
abrader
    Howard a.
Abraham
    cannula
Abrams
    needle
Abramson
    catheter
abscess
    axillary a.
    blind a.
abscise
absorbable
    a. dressing
    a. surgical suture
    a. suture
absorptive lenses
accordion drain
Ace-Fischer external fixator

acetabular
    a. cup
Acland
    clip
ACMI
    bronchoscope
    gastroscope
    laparoscope
    Martin endoscopy forceps
    proctoscope
    telescope
    valve
Acmistat
    catheter
Acmi-Valentine
    tube
acorn-tip catheter
acromionizer
activator
    bow a.
    functional a.
    monoblock a.
    Schwarz a.
Acufex
    forceps
    instrument
    punch
acusection
acusector
Acutrol
    suture
Adair
    forceps
    tenaculum
Adams
    clasp
    forceps
    position
    saw
Adams-DeWeese device

adapter, adaptor
    House a.
    McReynolds a.
    Ralks a.
Adaptic
    gauze dressing
adenectomy
adenoid
    a. curet
    a. forceps
adenomatome
adenopathy
    axillary a.
adenotome
    Abelson a.
    Kelley a.
    Kelly a.
    LaForce a.
    LaForce-Grieshaber a.
    Shambaugh a.
    Sluder a.
adhesiectomy
adhesion
    anomalous mesenteric a.'s
    attic a.
    banjo-string a.
    filmy a.'s
    primary a.
    secondary a.
    serologic a.
adhesiotomy
adhesive
    a. dressing
adjuster
    Negus ligature a.
Adler
    punch
adrenalectomize
adrenalectomy
adrenalorrhaphy
adrenalotomy
Adson
    bur
    cannula
    chisel
    clip
    conductor
    drill

Adson (continued)
    elevator
    forceps
    hook
    knife
    needle
    retractor
    rongeur
    scissors
    tube
Aebli
    scissors
AED—automatic external defibrillator
aerocystoscope
aerogel
Aeroplast
    dressing
aerourethroscope
Agnew
    keratome
    splint
Agnew-Verhoeff
    incision
Agrikola
    retractor
AICD—automatic implantable cardioverter-defibrillator
Ainsworth punch
airplane splint
Åkerlund
    diaphragm
alar
    a. incision
Albee
    fracture table
    osteotome
    saw
Albers-Schönberg
    bone
Albert
    bronchoscope
    suture
Albert-Andrews
    laryngoscope
Alcock
    catheter
    lithotrite

Alcock-Hendrickson lithotrite
Alcock-Timberlake obturator
Alcon
    suture
Alexander
    chisel
    gouge
    incision
    osteotome
    periosteotome
Alexander-Farabeuf
    elevator
    periosteotome
Alfred M. Large
    vena cava clamp
Alger brush
Allarton
    operation
Allen
    clamp
    implant
    orbital implant
    root pliers
    trocar
Allingham
    rectal speculum
Allis
    clamp
    forceps
Allis-Ochsner
    forceps
Allison
    retractor
    suture
allograft
    cadaveric a.
    living related a.
    living unrelated a.
alloplast
allotriolith
alloy
    amalgam a.
    dental a.
    solid solution a.
Allport
    retractor
    searcher

Alm
    retractor
Alpar implant
alternating
    a. suture
Alyea
    clamp
AMBI
    hip screw
    nail
amblyoscope
Amico
    drill
    extractor
    nail nipper
    skin lifter
amnioscope
amniotome
    Baylor a.
    Beacham a.
Amoils
    cryoextractor
    cryoprobe
    retractor
Amplatz
    cardiac catheter
    coronary catheter
amputating saw
amputation
    Farabeuf a.
    major a.
Amsler
    needle
anal
    a. speculum
anastomosis (anastomoses)
    antiperistaltic a.
    Brackin a.
    Clado a.
    a. clamp
    Coffey a.
    end-to-end a.
    end-to-side a.
    Furniss a.
    genicular a.
    Haight a.
    intestinal a.
    isoperistaltic a.

anastomosis (anastomoses) (contin-
    ued)
        side-to-end a.
        side-to-side a.
        sutureless a.
        triple a.
anastomotic
    a. operation
anchoring suture
Anderson
    appliance
    splint
Andresen
    appliance
Andrews
    applicator
    gouge
    retractor
Andrews-Hartmann
    forceps
Andrews-Pynchon
    suction tube
Anel
    probe
aneurysm
    a. needle
Angelchik antireflux prosthesis
angiocatheter
    Ependorf a.
angiocheiloscope
angioscope
angle
    a. suture
Angle [eponym]
    splint
angle-former
angular
    a. incision
ankylotome
annulorrhaphy
anomaloscope
    Nagel a.
anorthoscope
anoscope
    See also *colonoscope, procto-
       scope,* and *sigmoidoscope.*
    Bacon a.
    Bodenheimer a.

anoscope (continued)
    Boehm a.
    Brinkerhoff a.
    Buie-Hirschman a.
    Fansler a.
    Goldbacher a.
    Hirschman a.
    Ives a.
    Muer a.
    Otis a.
    Pratt a.
    Pruitt a.
    rotating a.
    Sims a.
    speculum a.
    Welch-Allyn a.
anosigmoidoscopy
Anson-McVay
    operation
Anthony
    tube
antroscope
antrum (antra)
    pyloric a.
    a. pyloricum
    a. of Willis
anvil
    Bunnell a.
AOA splint [All Orthopedic Appli-
    ances]
aortic
    a. flush pigtail catheter
    a. prosthesis
    trileaflet a. prosthesis
AO soft lens
aponeurosis (aponeuroses)
    a. of external oblique muscle
apoplexy
    splenic a.
apparatus
    hyoid a.
    Knipping a.
    Krogh a.
appendix (appendices)
    cecal a.
    ensiform a.
    pelvic a.
    a. vermiformis

appendotome
appliance
See also *brace, prosthesis,*
and *splint.*
crown of thorns a.
Crozat a.
functional a.
Hawley a.
light round-wire a.
multibanded a.
occlusal overlay a.
pin and tube a.
regulating a.
retaining a.
Roger Anderson pin fixation
a.
speech a.
applicator
Andrews a.
Brown a.
Dean a.
Ernst a.
Fletcher-Suit a.
Gifford a.
Holinger a.
Lathbury a.
Lejeune a.
Plummer-Vinson radium a.
Pynchon a.
Roberts a.
sandwich-mold a.
surface a.
Appolito
operation
suture
apposition
a. suture
approximation
a. suture
approximator
rib a.
skin-edge a.
Aquaflex lens
Arbuckle
probe
arch
prepancreatic a.

arch bar
Erich a.b.
Jelanko a.b.
Winter a.b.
Arco pacemaker
arcuate
a. incision
a. suture
ARD—anorectal dressing
areolar
a. incision
Argyle
catheter
chest tube
endotracheal tube
Argyle-Salem
sump tube
Argyll Robertson
suture
Arlt (von Arlt)
scoop
suture
Armsby
operation
Army-Navy
retractor
Arruga
expressor
forceps
implant
operation
protector
trephine
arterial
a. catheter
artery
appendicular a.
calcareous a.
epigastric a.
hepatic a.
intramural a.
sternocleidomastoid a.
suprascapular a.
temporal a.
thoracoacromial a.
arthroscope
arthrotome

articulator
ASAS—American Society of
     Abdominal Surgeons
Asch
     forceps
     splint
Ashcath
     hemodialysis catheter
Ashhurst splint
Ashley
     breast prosthesis
aspheric
     a. lens
aspirating
     a. needle
aspirator
     blue-tip a.
     Broyles a.
     Dieulafoy a.
     Gottschalk a.
     red-tip a.
     Thorek a.
     vacuum a.
     yellow-tip a.
astigmatoscope
astigmoscope
Atkins-Cannard
     tracheotomy tube
Atkins-Tucker
     laryngoscope
Atlee
     clamp
     dilator
atomizer
     Devilbiss a.
Atraloc
     suture
atraumatic
     a. needle
     a. suture
Atricor pacemaker
Auchincloss
     operation
audiometer
Aufranc-Turner
     cup
     hip prosthesis

Aufricht
     elevator
     rasp
     retractor
     speculum
Aufricht-Lipsett
     rasp
aught [zero, transcribe 0; used to indi-
     cate size of suture or instrument]
Augustine nail
aural
     a. speculum
auriscope
auscultoscope
Austin
     knife
     retractor
Austin Moore
     femoral head remover
     hip prosthesis
     inside-outside calipers
     mortising chisel
     rasp
     straight-stem endoprosthesis
autechoscope
Autoclip
autofundoscope
autofundoscopy
autologous
     a. fat graft
automatic
     a. rotating tourniquet
automatic implantable cardioverter-
     defibrillator (AICD)
autoscopy
autotransplantation
     pancreatic a.
Auvard
     cranioclast
     weighted vaginal speculum
Auvard-Remine
     speculum
Auvray
     incision
avascularization
Avitene
     hemostat

awl
    Carroll a.
    curved a.
    Rochester a.
    Wangensteen a.
    Wilson a.
Ayerst
    knife
Ayre
    brush
    cervical spatula
    cone knife
    tube
Babcock
    clamp
    forceps
    needle
    suture
back-and-forth suture
backcut incision
Backhaus
    forceps
    towel clamp
Bacon
    anoscope
    forceps
Badgley
    plate
bag
    Pilcher hemostatic b.
Baggish
    hysteroscope
Bagolini lenses
Bahn
    spud
Bahnson
    clamp
Bailey
    catheter
    clamp
    leukotome
    rib contractor
Bailey-Glover-O'Neill
    knife
Bailey-Morse
    knife
Bailey-Williamson
    forceps

Bainbridge
    anastomosis clamp
    hemostatic forceps
Baker
    jejunostomy tube
    self-sumping tube
Bakes
    bile duct dilator
    dilator
    probe
Balfour
    bladder blade
    retractor
    retractor with fenestrated
      blade
    self-retaining retractor
Balkan
    frame
    splint
ball
    b.-valve prosthesis
Ballantine
    clamp
    hemilaminectomy retractor
    hysterectomy forceps
    uterine curet
Ballenger
    curet
    elevator
    forceps
    swivel knife
Ballenger-Sluder
    tonsillectome
balloon
    ACS b.
    b. biliary catheter
    b. catheter
    b. defecation
    b. dilatation, b. dilation
    Fogarty b.
    Garren b.
    Grüntzig (Gruentzig) b.
    Grüntzig-type b.
    Honan b.
    Hunter b.
    Hunter-Sessions b.
    image data intra-aortic
      counter-pulsation b.

balloon (continued)
    intranasal b.
    pilot b.
    pneumatic b. dilator
Baloser
    hysteroscope
banana
    b. blade
bandage
    See also *dressing.*
    Ace b.
    adhesive b.
    barrel b.
    Barton b.
    capeline b.
    Champ elastic b.
    circular b.
    compression b.
    cotton elastic b.
    cotton-wool b.
    cravat b.
    crepe b.
    crucial b.
    Curad plastic b.
    demigauntlet b.
    E cotton b.
    elastic b.
    Elasticon b.
    Elastomull b.
    Elastoplast b.
    Esmarch b.
    figure-of-eight b.
    fixation b.
    Flexilite b.
    four-tailed b.
    Fricke b.
    gauntlet b.
    gauze b.
    Gibney b.
    hammock b.
    Hueter b.
    Hydron Burn B.
    immobilizing b.
    Kerlix b.
    Kling b.
    many-tailed b.
    Marlex b.
    Martin b.

bandage (continued)
    oblique b.
    plaster b.
    POP (plaster of Paris) b.
    pressure b.
    reversed b.
    roller b.
    Sayre b.
    Scultetus b.
    Seutin b.
    b. shears
    spica b.
    spiral b.
    stockinette b.
    Surgiflex b.
    suspensory b.
    T b.
    Theden b.
    Thillaye b.
    triangular b.
    Velpeau b.
    Y b.
Band-Aid
    dressing
Bane
    forceps
banjo curet
Bankhart
    retractor
bar
    Erich arch b.
    House b.
    Jelanko arch b.
    Mercier b.
    metatarsal b.
    Passavant b.
    sublingual b.
    thyroid b.
    Winter arch b.
Bard
    catheter
Bardex
    catheter
Bardic
    cannula
Bard-Parker
    blade
    dermatome

Bard-Parker (continued)
   knife
Barkan
   knife
Barker
   Vacu-tome dermatome
Barlow
   forceps
Barnes
   bag
   cervical dilator
   common duct dilator
   dilator
   trocar
Barnes-Crile
   forceps
Barnhill
   curet
baroscope
Barr
   anal speculum
   bolt
   crypt hook
   fistula hook
   fistula probe
   rectal hook
   rectal probe
   rectal speculum
   self-retaining rectal retractor
Barraquer
   brush
   ciliary forceps
   corneal forceps
   erysiphake
   irrigator spatula
   keratoplasty knife
   microkeratome
   needle holder
   scissors
   speculum
   trephine
Barraquer-Colibri
   speculum
Barraquer-DeWecker
   scissors
Barraya
   forceps

barrel
   b. dressing
Barrett
   forceps
   tenaculum
Barrett-Adson
   retractor
Barrett-Allen
   forceps
Barsky
   elevator
Barton
   bandage
   forceps
   tongs
   traction handle
Barton-Cone
   tongs
baseball
   b. suture
baseball lens
basilar
   b. suture
Basile hip screw
basket
   Browne b.
   Councill b.
   Dormia b.
   Ferguson b.
   Howard b.
   Johnson b.
   Mitchell b.
   stone b.
Bassini
   operation
bastard suture
basting stitch
   Parker-Kerr b.s.
Bateman
   prosthesis
bath
   sitz b.
Battle
   incision
Battle-Jalaguier-Kammerer
   incision
Baumrucker
   resectoscope

Baylor
    amniotome
    splint
    sump
Baynton
    bandage
    operation
bayonet
    b. forceps
    b. incision
    b. saw
BB—breast biopsy
BDE—bile duct exploration
Beacham
    amniotome
Beall
    mitral valve
    mitral valve prosthesis
Beardsley
    aortic dilator
    cecostomy trocar
    empyema tube
    esophageal retractor
    intestinal clamp
Beaupre
    forceps
Beaver
    blade
    handle
    keratome
    knife
Beaver-DeBakey
    blade
Bechtol
    hip prosthesis
Beck
    clamp
    gastrostomy scoop
    knife
    rasp
Beckman
    adenoid curet
    goiter retractor
    nasal speculum
    retractor
    self-retaining retractor
Beckman-Adson
    laminectomy retractor

Beckman-Colver
    nasal speculum
Beckman-Eaton
    laminectomy retractor
Beck-Mueller
    tonsillectome
Beck-Schenck
    tonsillectome
Béclard
    hernia
    suture
bed
    air-fluidized b.
    circle b.
    CircOlectric b.
    Clinitron b.
    Gatch b.
    rocking b.
    Roto-Rest b.
    Sanders oscillating b.
Beebe
    forceps
Beer
    canaliculus knife
    cataract knife
    ciliary forceps
Begg
    appliance
    straight-wire combination
        bracket
Belfield
    wire retractor
Bell
    erysiphake
    suture
Bellocq
    cannula
    sound
    tube
Bellows cryoextractor
Bellucci
    scissors
Belmas
    operation
belonoskiascopy
Benaron
    forceps

Benedict
>gastroscope
>retractor

Benedict-Roth
>spirometer

Bengolea
>forceps

Béniqué
>catheter
>dilator
>sound

Bennett
>elevator
>forceps
>retractor

Berbridge
>scissors

Berens
>dilator
>forceps
>implant
>keratome
>lid everter
>muscle clamp
>punch
>retractor
>scissors
>scoop
>spatula
>speculum

Berens-Rosa implant

Berger. See *Buerger.*

Bergmann
>incision

Bergmann-Israel
>incision

Berke
>double-end lid everter
>ptosis clamp
>ptosis forceps

Berlind-Auvard
>speculum

Berman locator

Berna
>infant abdominal retractor

Bernard
>operation

Bernay
>sponge
>tracheal retractor
>uterine gauze packer

Berne
>forceps
>rasp

Bernstein
>gastroscope

Berry
>uterine-elevating forceps

Best
>clamp
>common duct stone forceps
>direct forward-vision tele-
>>scope
>gallstone forceps
>intestinal forceps

Betadine

Bethune
>lung tourniquet
>periosteal elevator
>phrenic retractor
>rib cutter
>rib shears

Bevan
>gallbladder forceps
>hemostatic forceps
>incision

Beyea
>operation

Beyer
>forceps
>rongeur

Bier
>block anesthesia
>method
>passive hyperemia

Bigelow
>lithotrite

bilabe

biliary
>b. prosthesis

Billeau
>ear wax curet

Billroth
>forceps
>ovarian retractor

Billroth (continued)
  uterine tumor forceps
Bill traction handle
binangle, binangled
  b. chisel
binder
  Velcro b.
Binkhorst
  implant
  lens
Binkhorst-Fyodorov lens
binocular
  b. ophthalmoscope
binophthalmoscope
binoscope
biologic, biological
  b. dressing
biomicroscope
biopsy
    aspiration b.
    cervical punch b.
    b. needle
    open b.
    surface b.
    wound b.
bioptome
    Stanford b.
biospectroscopy
biparietal
    b. suture
Bircher
    operation
Birch-Hirschfeld
    lamp
bird's nest filter
Birtcher
    cautery
    Hyfrecator cautery wire
Bishop
    sphygmoscope
    tendon tucker
Bishop-Black tendon tucker
Bishop-DeWitt tendon tucker
Bishop-Harmon
    anterior chamber irrigating
      cannula
    bladebreaker
    forceps

Bishop-Harmon (continued)
    Superblade
Bishop-Peter tendon tucker
bistoury
    b. blade
    Brophy b.
    Jackson b.
biteblock, bite-block, bite block
bite gauge, bitegage, bite-gage
bitelock, bite-lock, bite lock
biterminal
bitoric contact lens
bivalve, bivalved
    b. incision
    b. speculum
Bizzarri-Guiffrida
    laryngoscope
Björk-Shiley
    aortic valve prosthesis
    convexoconcave 60-degree
      valve prosthesis
    floating-disk prosthesis
BL—blood loss
black braided suture
black silk suture
Black-Wylie
    obstetric dilator
bladder
    b. blade
blade
    Bard-Parker b.
    Beaver b.
    Beaver-DeBakey b.
    bistoury b.
    bladder b.
    Cooley-Pontius b.
    DeBakey b.
    Foregger b.
    Macintosh fiberoptic laryn-
      goscope b.
    McPherson-Wheeler b.
bladebreaker
    b. knife
Blair
    cleft palate knife
    Gigli-saw guide
    modification of Gellhorn
      pessary

Blair (continued)
    nasal chisel
    palate hook
    serrefine
    stiletto
Blair-Brown
    knife
Blake
    disk
    ear forceps
    embolus forceps
    forceps
    gallstone forceps
    uterine curet
Blakemore
    esophageal tube
    nasogastric tube
Blakemore-Sengstaken
    tube
Blakesley
    forceps
Blanchard
    cryptotome
    hemorrhoidal forceps
    pile clamp
blanket
    b. suture
Blasucci
    curved-tip ureteral catheter
    pigtail ureteral catheter
Bledsoe
    brace
block
    anesthetic b.
    Bier b.
    bite b. [also: biteblock, bite-
      block]
    regional b.
Blom-Singer
    valve
    voice prosthesis
blood flow probe
Bloodgood
    disease
bloodless
    b. operation
Blot
    perforator

Blount
    osteotome
    plate
    retractor
    stapler
blunt probe
Boari
    button
Bobb
    operation
Bodenheimer
    anoscope
Boehm
    anoscope
    proctoscope
    sigmoidoscope
Bogue
    operation
Böhler
    clamp
    splint
Böhler-Braun splint
Bohlman pin
Boies
    forceps
bolster suture
bolt
    Webb b.
    Wilson b.
bolus
    b. dressing
Bonaccolto
    forceps
    scleral ring
Bond [eponym]
    forceps
    splint
bone
    b. clamp
    b.-cutting forceps
    b. forceps
    b.-nibbling forceps
Bonn
    forceps
Bonner position
Bonta
    knife

"boo-she-ron" Phonetic for
    Boucheron.
"boo-shoo" Phonetic for Bouchut.
boot
    air b.
    gelatin compression b.
    Gibney b.
    Jobst b.
    pneumatic b.
    Unna b.
    Unna paste b.
Boros
    esophagoscope
Bose
    operation
    tracheostomy hook
Bosher
    knife
Boston
    brace
Bosworth
    coracoclavicular screw
    nasal snare
Böttcher (Boettcher)
    forceps
    hook
    scissors
Boucheron
    speculum
Bouchut
    laryngeal tube
bougie
    b. à boule
    acorn-tipped b.
    common duct b.
    coudé b.
    Gruber b.
    Hurst b.
    Jackson b.
    Le Fort b.
    olive-tip b., olive-tipped b.
    Otis b.
    Phillips b.
    Plummer b.
    polyvinyl b.
    Ruschelit b.
    soluble b.
    Trousseau b.

bougie (continued)
    tunneled b.
    wax-tipped b.
    whistle b.
bougienage
bovied
Bovie unit
Bowen
    osteotome
Bowen-Grover
    meniscotome
Bowlby splint
Bowman
    eye knife
    iris needle
    iris scissors
    lacrimal dilator
    lacrimal probe
    needle
    strabismus scissors
Boyce position
Boyd
    implant
Boyes-Goodfellow
    hook
Boynton
    needle holder
Boys-Allis
    forceps
Bozeman
    forceps
    position
    speculum
    suture
Bozeman-Fritsch
    catheter
Braasch
    catheter
    cystoscope
    forceps
brace
    See also *appliance, prosthe-*
       sis, and *splint.*
    Bledsoe b.
    Boston b.
    chair-back b.
    clam-shell b.
    drop foot b.

brace (continued)
    49'er knee b.
    Goldthwait b.
    Hudson b.
    ischial weightbearing
      (weight-bearing) b.
    Klenzak b.
    Knight b.
    Knight-Taylor b.
    Kydex b.
    Lenox Hill b.
    long leg b.
    LSU reciprocation-gait
      orthosis b.
    Lyman-Smith b.
    Milwaukee b.
    Moe b.
    Roylan tibia fracture b.
    Seton hip b.
    SMo (stainless steel and
      molybdenum) b.
    SOMI (sternal occipital
      mandibular immobilizer) b.
    Taylor b.
    toe drop b.
    UBC (University of British
      Columbia) b.
    weightbearing (weight-bear-
      ing) b.
Bracken
    forceps
Brackett
    probe
Brackin
    incision
Bradford
    forceps
    frame
Bradshaw-O'Neill
    clamp
braided
    black b. suture
    b. suture
    white b. suture
Brant aluminum splint
Brantley-Turner
    retractor

brassiere
    b.-type dressing
Braun
    cranioclast
    hook
    scissors
    tenaculum
Braun-Jardine-DeLee
    hook
Braunwald
    prosthesis
Brawley
    retractor
bregmatomastoid suture
Brenner
    operation
Brewer
    speculum
Brewster
    retractor
bridge
bridgework
bridle
    b. suture
Brinkerhoff
    anoscope
    rectal speculum
Bristow
    periosteal elevator
broach
    b. holder
    root-canal b.
Brock
    incision
    knife
    punch
Brockenbrough
    catheter
Brodny
    clamp
bronchofiberscope
bronchoscope
    ACMI b.
    Albert b.
    Broyles b.
    Bruening b.
    Chevalier Jackson b.
    coagulation b.

bronchoscope (continued)
    costophrenic b.
    Davis b.
    double-channel irrigating b.
    Emerson b.
    fiberoptic b.
    Foregger b.
    Haslinger b.
    Holinger b.
    Holinger-Jackson b.
    hook-on b.
    Jackson b.
    Jesberg b.
    Kernan-Jackson b.
    Michelson b.
    Moersch b.
    Negus b.
    Overholt-Jackson b.
    Pilling b.
    Riecker b.
    Safar b.
    Storz b.
    telescope b.
    Tucker b.
    ventilation b.
    Waterman b.
    Yankauer b.
bronchotome
Bronson-Turz
    retractor
Brooks
    scissors
Brophy
    bistoury
    forceps
    knife
    plate
Broviac
    catheter
Brown
    applicator
    dermatome
    forceps
    graft
    knife
    needle
    retractor
    snare

Brown (continued)
    splint
    tendon sheath syndrome
    tonsillectome
Brown-Adson
    forceps
Brown-Buerger
    cystoscope
Brown-Dohlman implant
Browne
    basket
Brown-McHardy
    dilator
Broyles
    aspirator
    bronchoscope
    dilator
    esophagoscope
    forceps
    laryngoscope
    nasopharyngoscope
    telescope
    tube
Bruening
    bronchoscope
    esophagoscope
    forceps
    otoscope
    snare
Brun
    curet
Brunner
    dissector
    forceps
Brunton
    otoscope
brush
    Ayre b.
    Barraquer b.
    electrical b.
    Haidinger b
Bryant
    operation
BSS—black silk suture
Buck
    curet
    hook
    knife

Buck (continued)
    splint
Buckstein insufflator
Bucy
    knife
    retractor
Bucy-Frazier
    cannula
buddy splint
Buerger-McCarthy
    forceps
Bugbee electrode
Buie
    clamp
    forceps
    irrigator
    position
    probe
    procedure
    rectal suction tube
    scissors
    sigmoidoscope
    technique
Buie-Hirschman
    anoscope
    clamp
Buic-Smith
    retractor
    speculum
bulky dressing
bulldog clamp
Buller
    bandage
    shield
bullet probe
Bumm
    curet
Bumpus
    forceps
    resectoscope
bunching suture
Bunge
    spoon
Bunim
    forceps
Bunnell
    anvil
    drill

Bunnell (continued)
    needle
    probe
    splints
    suture
bur
    Adson b.
    Burwell b.
    D'Errico b.
    diamond b.
    Hall b.
    b.-hole incision
    Hudson b.
    Jordan-Day b.
    Lempert b.
    McKenzie b.
    round b.
    Wullstein b.
Burch
    calipers
    pick
Burch-Greenwood tendon tucker
Burford rib spreader
buried suture
Burnham
    scissors
burr [pref: bur]
Burwell
    bur
Butcher
    saw
Butterfield
    cystoscope
butterfly
    b. bandage
    b. drain
    b. dressing
    b. needle
button
    Boari b.
    Chlumsky b.
    Jaboulay b.
    Lardennois b.
    Moore tracheostomy b.
    Murphy b.
    Panje voice b.
    peritoneal b.
    polyethylene collar b.

button (continued)
    b. suture
    Villard b.
buttonhole
    b. incision
    b. operation
    b. suture
butyroscope
Buxton
    clamp
Byford
    retractor
bypass
    axillo-axillary b.
    axillofemoral b.
    carotid-subclavian b.
    extra-anatomic b.
    ileojejunal b.
    infrapopliteal b.
    in situ b.
    obturator b.
    subclavian-subclavian b.
cable
    c. wire suture
CAD prosthesis
cage
    Faraday c.
caged-ball
Cairns
    forceps
Calhoun
    needle
Calhoun-Merz
    needle
calibrated
    c. probe
calipers
    Austin Moore inside-outside
      c.
    Burch c.
    Castroviejo c.
    Green c.
    Jameson c.
    Ladd c.
    Lange skinfold c.
    Machemer c.
    Oscher c.
    Stahl c.

calipers (continued)
    Thorpe c.
    ultrasonic c.
    Vernier c.
    walking c.
Callisen
    operation
caloriscope
Calot
    triangle
Caltagirone
    knife
camera
Cameron-Haight
    elevator
Camino
    intracranial catheter
Campbell
    catheter
    elevator
    forceps
    osteotome
    retractor
    sound
    trocar
canal
    crural c.
canalicular
    c. scissors
Canfield
    knife
Cannon
    Bio-Flek nasal splint
    endarterectomy loop
cannula
    Abelson c.
    Abraham c.
    Adson c.
    Bardic c.
    Bellocq c.
    Bishop-Harmon c.
    Bucy-Frazier c.
    Castroviejo c.
    Coakley c.
    Concorde suction c.
    Cone c.
    Cooper c.
    Day c.

cannula (continued)
    Flexicath c.
    Floyd c.
    Frazier c.
    Goldstein c.
    Goodfellow c.
    Haynes c.
    Holman-Mathieu c.
    Hudgins c.
    infusion c.
    Ingals c.
    irrigation c.
    Jarcho c.
    Kahn c.
    Kanavel brain-exploring c.
    Karman c.
    Kos c.
    Krause c.
    Lifemed c.
    Mayo c.
    Mercedes tip c.
    Moncrieff irrigating c.
    Morris c.
    Neal c.
    Packo pars plana c.
    Padgett shark-mouth c.
    Paterson laryngeal c.
    perfusion c.
    Polystan c.
    Portnoy c.
    Pritchard c.
    Randolph c.
    Rockey c.
    Roper c.
    Rubin c.
    Sachs c.
    Scheie c.
    c. scissors
    Scott c.
    Seletz c.
    Silastic coronary artery c.
    Soresi c.
    Tenner c.
    Tulevech c.
    USCI c.
    Veirs c.
    venous c.
    ventricular c.

cannula (continued)
    Veress c.
Cantlie
    cannula
Cantor
    tube
Capetown
    aortic prosthetic valve
    aortic valve prosthesis
capitonnage
    c. suture
capsule
    c. forceps
capsulotome
    Darling c.
Carabelli
    aspirator
    endobronchial tube
    lumen finder
Carbo-Jet [bone-cleaning device]
carcinolysis
cardiac
    c. tube
cardiovalvulotome
cardiovascular
    c. suture
cardioverter
    automatic implantable c.-
        defibrillator (AICD)
Carlens
    catheter
    mediastinoscope
    tube
Carmack
    ear curet
Carmalt
    arterial forceps
    clamp
    hemostatic forceps
    hysterectomy forceps
    splinter forceps
    thoracic forceps
Carman
    rectal tube
Carmichael crown
Carmody
    forceps

Carpenter
    dissector
    knife
Carpentier
    heart valve
Carpentier-Edwards valve
Carrel
    clamp
    mosquito forceps
    operation
    tube
Carrel-Girard screw
carrier
    Deschamps c.
    Lahey c.
    ligature c.
    Mayo c.
    Wangensteen c.
Carroll
    awl
    bone-holding forceps
    bone hook
    finger goniometer
    forearm tendon stripper
    hook curet
    osteotome
    periosteal elevator
    self-retaining spring retractor
    tendon-passing forceps
    tendon-pulling forceps
    tendon retriever
Carroll-Legg
    osteotome
Carroll-Smith-Petersen
    osteotome
Carson
    catheter
Carter
    clamp
    introducer
    retractor
    thoracosplenectomy
cartilage
    c. forceps
Cartwright
    prosthesis
Casselberry
    position

Cassidy-Brophy
    forceps
Castallo
    retractor
Castaneda
    forceps
Castelli
    tube
Castroviejo
    calipers
    cannula
    dilator
    forceps
    holder
    keratome
    knife
    needle
    needle holder
    punch
    retractor
    scissors
    spatula
    speculum
    trephine
Castroviejo-Arruga
    forceps
Castroviejo-Kalt
    needle holder
cataract
    c. needle
catgut
    carbolized c.
    chromic c. suture
    c. suture
"cath" Slang for catheter, catheterization, catheterize.
cathematic catheter
catheter
    Abramson c.
    Acmistat c.
    acorn-tip c.
    Alcock c.
    Amplatz cardiac c.
    Amplatz coronary c.
    aortic flush pigtail c.
    Argyle c.
    arterial c.
    Ashcath hemodialysis c.

catheter (continued)
    Bailey c.
    balloon c.
    Bard c.
    Bardex c.
    Blasucci curved-tip ureteral c.
    Blasucci pigtail ureteral c.
    Bozeman-Fritsch c.
    Braasch c.
    Brockenbrough c.
    Broviac c.
    Camino intracranial c.
    Campbell c.
    Carlens c.
    Carson c.
    cathematic c.
    central venous pressure
      (CVP) c.
    c. clip
    coaxial counterflow single-
      needle blood access c.
    coudé c.
    Councill c.
    Cournand c.
    Coxeter c.
    CVP (central venous pres-
      sure) c.
    de Pezzer c.
    double-J stent c.
    double-lumen c.
    Edwards c.
    filiform c.
    flexible c.
    Fogarty c.
    Foley c.
    Foley-Alcock c.
    French polyethylene c.
    French-Robinson c.
    Fritsch c.
    Furniss c.
    Goodale-Lubin c.
    Gouley c.
    Grollman pigtail c.
    Groshong c.
    Grüntzig (Gruentzig) bal-
      loon-tip c.
    headhunter c.
    Hickman c.

catheter (continued)
    indwelling c.
    Ingram trocar c.
    intracardiac c.
    Intracath c.
    intraluminal c.
    intraperitoneal c.
    Itard c.
    Jackson-Pratt c.
    Karman c.
    KISS (kidney internal
      splint/stent) c.
    Lane c.
    latex c.
    Le Fort c.
    Lehman c.
    Lloyd c.
    Malecot c.
    McIver nephrostomy c.
    Metras c.
    mushroom c.
    nasogastric c.
    nasotracheal c.
    Nélaton c.
    NIH (National Institutes of
      Health) c.
    Nutricath c.
    Nycore pigtail c.
    olive-tip c.
    opaque c.
    oropharyngeal c.
    Owen c.
    Pezzer c.
    Phillips c.
    pigtail c.
    pigtail angiographic c.
    polyethylene c.
    radiopaque c.
    red Robinson c.
    red rubber c.
    retention c.
    retrograde c.
    return flow hemostatic c.
    Ring-McLean c.
    self-retaining c.
    sheathed c.
    sidewinder c.
    Silastic mushroom c.

catheter (continued)
 Simmons c.
 Sones coronary c.
 spiral-tip c.
 split-sheath c.
 subclavian c.
 Swan-Ganz c.
 Teflon c.
 Tenckhoff peritoneal c.
 Texas c.
 thermodilution c.
 Thompson c.
 Tiemann c.
 trocar c.
 umbilical c.
 ureteral c.
 venous c.
 ventricular c.
 Virden c.
 von Sonnenberg c.
 Weber c.
 whip c.
 whistle-tip c.
 Winer c.
 Wishard c.
 Wurd c.
 Yankauer c.
 Zavod c.
Cattell
 operation
 tube
Caulk punch
cauterization
 c. by points
 cold c.
cautery
 bicap c.
 Corrigan c.
cavascope
cavernoscope
Cavitron
 aspiration unit
 dissector
 ultrasonic aspirator (CUSA)
cavity
 peritoneal c.
cavum (cava)
 c. peritonei

C-clamp
CD—cadaver donor
 consanguineous donor
Cecil-Culp repair
cecostomy
 Beardsley c. trocar
cecum
 hepatic c.
 mobile c.
Celestin
 tube
celiectomy
celioscopy
cellophane
 c. dressing
cell saver
 c.s. transfusion
celluloid
 c. suture
cement
 black copper c.
 c. dressing
 oxyphosphate c.
centesis
central venous pressure (CVP) catheter
cephalotome
ceramic
 c. head of hip prosthesis
cerebroscope
cerecloth
cereolus (cereoli)
cervical
 c. incision
 c. punch biopsy clamp
cervitome
 Milex c.
CGS—catgut suture
Chaffin-Pratt
 tube
chain
 c. suture
chair-back brace
chalazion (chalazia)
 c. forceps
Chamberlen
 forceps

Chandler
    elevator
    forceps
    retractor
    splint
Chaoul
Chaput
    operation
Charles
    operation
Charnley
    total hip prosthesis
Charnley-Mueller
    hip prosthesis
Charrière
    bone saw
Chaussier
    tube
cheiloangioscopy
cheiroscope
Chelsea-Eaton
    speculum
chemosterilization
Cherney
    incision
Chernez
    incision
Cherry
    osteotome
    retractor
    tongs
Cherry-Kerrison
    forceps
chest
    c. tube
Chevalier Jackson
    bronchoscope
    esophagoscope
    gastroscope
    laryngoscope
    speculum
    tube
chevron
    c.-shaped incision
Cheyne
    operation
Chiazzi
    operation

Chiba
    needle
Chiene
    incision
Child
    operation
Child-Phillips
    needle
chisel
    Adson c.
    Alexander c.
    binangle c., binangled c.
    Converse c.
    Derlacki c.
    Derlacki-Shambaugh c.
    Fomon c.
    Freer c.
    guarded c.
    Hajek c.
    House c.
    Killian c.
    Moore c.
    Sewall c.
    Shambaugh-Derlacki c.
    Sheehan c.
    Troutman c.
Chlumsky button
cholangiogastrostomy
cholecystenteroanastomosis
cholecystenterorrhaphy
cholecystenterostomy
choledochectomy
choledochocholedochorrhaphy
choledochocholedochostomy
choledochoenterostomy
choledochogastrostomy
choledochohepatostomy
choledochoileostomy
choledochojejunostomy
choledochoplasty
choledochoscope
chromatoscope
chromatoscopy
chromic
    c. catgut suture
    gut c. suture
chromocholoscopy
chromocystoscopy

chronoscope
CHS—compression hip screw
Cibis
    ski needle
cicatrectomy
cicatricotomy
Cicherelli
    forceps
cigarette drain
ciliariscope
CircOlectric bed
circular
    c. incision
    c. suture
circulus (circuli)
    c. articuli vasculosus
circumareolar
    c. incision
circumcision, circumcisional
    c. incision
    c. suture
circumferential
    c. incision
circumlimbal
    c. incision
circumscribed
    c. clamp
circumscribing
    c. incision
cirsectomy
cirsodesis
cirsotome
cirsotomy
Citelli
    rongeur
Citelli-Meltzer
    atticus punch
Clagett
    operation
clamp
    Alfred M. Large vena cava c.
    Allen c.
    Allis c.
    Alyea c.
    anastomosis c.
    Atlee c.
    Babcock c.
    Backhaus towel c.

clamp (continued)
    Bahnson c.
    Bailey c.
    Bainbridge anastomosis c.
    Ballantine c.
    Beardsley intestinal c.
    Beck c.
    Berens muscle c.
    Berke ptosis c.
    Best c.
    Blanchard pile c.
    Böhler c.
    bone c.
    Bradshaw-O'Neill c.
    Brodny c.
    Buie c.
    Buie-Hirschman c.
    bulldog c.
    Buxton c.
    C c.
    Carmalt c.
    Carrel c.
    Carter c.
    cervical punch biopsy c.
    circumscribed c.
    Cooley c.
    Cope c.
    cord c.
    Cottle c.
    Craford c.
    Crile c.
    crushing c.
    Crutchfield c.
    Cunningham c.
    Daniel c.
    Davidson c.
    Davis c.
    DeBakey c.
    DeMartel-Wolfson c.
    Dennis c.
    Derra c.
    Diethrich shunt c.
    Dixon-Thomas-Smith c.
    Doyen c.
    Eastman c.
    Edwards c.
    Fehland c.
    fenestrated c.

clamp (continued)
>Forrester c.
>Foss c.
>Friedrich-Petz c.
>Furniss c.
>Furniss-Clute c.
>Furniss-McClure-Hinton c.
>Gandy c.
>Gant c.
>Glassman c.
>Glover c.
>Goldblatt c.
>Gomco c.
>Gross c.
>Guyon c.
>Guyon-Péan c.
>Halsted c.
>Hayes c.
>Heaney c.
>hemostatic c.
>Herbert-Adams c.
>Herff c.
>Herrick c.
>Hey Groves c.
>c. holder
>Hopkins c.
>Hudson c.
>Hufnagel c.
>Hume c.
>Humphries c.
>Hunt c.
>Hurwitz c.
>Hyams c.
>Jackson c.
>Jacobson c.
>Jarvis c.
>Javid bypass c.
>Jesberg c.
>Johns Hopkins c.
>Joseph c.
>Juevenell c.
>Kane c.
>Kantor c.
>Kantrowicz c.
>Kapp-Beck c.
>Kelly c.
>Kinsella-Buie c.
>Kocher c.

clamp (continued)
>Lahey c.
>Lambotte c.
>Lane c.
>Lee c.
>Lees c.
>lever-compression c.
>Liddle aorta c.
>Linton c.
>Lockwood c.
>Lowman c.
>MacDonald c.
>Martel c.
>Mastin c.
>Mattox c.
>Mayo c.
>McDonald c.
>microvascular c.
>Mikulicz c.
>Moreno c.
>mosquito c.
>Moynihan c.
>Mueller c.
>Nichols c.
>Noon AV fistula c.
>Nussbaum c.
>occlusion c.
>Ochsner c.
>Ockerblad c.
>Parker c.
>Payr c.
>Péan c.
>pedicle c.
>Pemberton c.
>penile c.
>Pennington c.
>Phillips c.
>Poppen c.
>Poppen-Blalock c.
>Potts c.
>Potts-Niedner c.
>Potts-Smith c.
>Price-Thomas c.
>Ralks c.
>Rankin c.
>Ranzewski c.
>Reich c.
>Reich-Nechtow c.

clamp (continued)
    Rienhoff c.
    Rockey c.
    Roosevelt c.
    rubber-shod c.
    Rubin c.
    Rumel c.
    Salibi c.
    Sarot c.
    Satinsky c.
    Schoemaker c.
    Scudder c.
    Sehrt c.
    Selverstone c.
    serrefine c.
    Shoemaker c.
    splenectomy c.
    Stevenson c.
    Stille c.
    Stockman c.
    Stone c.
    Stone-Holcombe c.
    Tatum c.
    c. technique
    Thomson c.
    towel c.
    Trendelenburg-Crafoord c.
    vascular c.
    Verbrugge c.
    von Petz c.
    Walther c.
    Walther-Crenshaw c.
    Wangensteen c.
    Watts c.
    W. Dean McDonald c.
    Wertheim c.
    Wertheim-Cullen c.
    Wertheim-Reverdin c.
    Wester c.
    Willett c.
    Williams c.
    Wilman c.
    Wilson c.
    Wolfson c.
    Yellen c.
    Young c.
    Zachary-Cope-DeMartel c.
    Zipser c.

clam-shell brace
clasp
    Adams c.
    ball c.
Clayton
    osteotome
cleft palate
    c.p. prosthesis
Clerf
    laryngoscope
    saw
Cleveland procedure
Clinitron bed
clinoscope
clip
    Acland c.
    Adson c.
    catheter c.
    Cushing c.
    dura c.
    Halberg c.
    Heifitz c.
    Hulka c.
    Mayfield c.
    McKenzie c.
    Michel c.
    Olivecrona c.
    Paterson long-shank brain c.
    Raney c.
    Schütz c.
    Schwartz c.
    Scoville c.
    Scoville-Lewis c.
    skin c.
    Smith c.
    Sugar c.
    tantalum c.
    towel c.
    Weck c.
    Yasargil c.
Cloquet
    canal
    fascia
    ganglion
    hernia
    ligament
    node
    pseudoganglion

Cloquet (continued)
    septum
closure
    delayed primary c.
    Smead-Jones c.
Cloward
    osteotome
    retractor
Cloward-Hoen
    retractor
Clute
    incision
coagulation
    c. bronchoscope
    infrared c.
coagulator
Coakley
    cannula
    curet
    forceps
    speculum
    suture
    trocar
coaptation
    c. suture
coaxial counterflow single-needle
    blood access catheter
Cobb
    elevator
    osteotome
cobbler's suture
cobra retractor
cocoon dressing
Codman
    incision
Coe-Pak dressing
Coffey
    incision
Cohen
    forceps
coil
    Gianturco wool-tufted wire c.
    Margulles c.
cold punch resectoscope
Cole
    retractor
Colibri
    forceps

collagen
    c. suture
collar
    c. dressing
    c. incision
Collin
    forceps
    osteoclast
    speculum
Collings electrode
collodion
    c. dressing
colohepatopexy
cololysis
colonoscope
    See also *anoscope, procto-*
      scope, and *sigmoidoscope.*
    fiberoptic c.
colopexostomy
colopexotomy
color-contrast microscope
colpomicroscope
colposcope
Colver
    forceps
    knife
Comberg lens
commissure
    c. laryngoscope
common duct bougie
Communitrach
    tube
comparascope
comparison microscope
compound
    c. dressing
    c. suture
compression
    c. dressing
    fluffy c. dressing
conchoscope
conchotome
Concorde
    suction cannula
conductor
    Adson c.
    Bailey c.
    Davis c.

conductor (continued)
    Kanavel c.
Cone [eponym]
    cannula
    needle
    retractor
confirmatory incision
Conform dressing
conjunctival
    c. incision
Connell
    suture
constriction
    duodenopyloric c.
contactoscope
continuous
    c. suture
contour
    c. retractor
contracture
    Dupuytren c.
    Volkmann c.
Converse [eponym]
    chisel
    osteotome
    speculum
convex lens
convexoconcave
Conzett goniometer
Cook
    speculum
Cooley
    clamp
    dilator
    forceps
    prosthesis
    retractor
    scissors
Cooley-Pontius
    blade
Cooper
    cannula
    operation
Cope
    clamp
    needle
Copeland
    retinoscope

Coppridge
    forceps
coquille plano lens
Corbett
    forceps
cord
    c. clamp
Cordes
    forceps
Cordes-New
    forceps
Corey
    forceps
corneal
    c. microscope
corneoscleral
    c. incision
    c. scissors
Corner [eponym]
    tampon
Cornet
    forceps
Corning
    anesthesia
    method
Cornish
    wool dressing
Corrigan
    cautery
cortical
    c. incision
Corwin
    hemostat
Coryllos
    raspatory
    retractor
costophrenic
    c. bronchoscope
costotome
    Tudor-Edwards c.
Cotrel cast
Cotting
    operation
Cottle
    clamp
    elevator
    forceps
    knife

Cottle (continued)
    osteotome
    rasp
    retractor
    saw
    scissors
    speculum
    tenaculum
Cottle-Arruga
    forceps
Cottle-Jansen
    forceps
Cottle-Kazanjian
    forceps
Cottle-Neivert
    retractor
cottonoid patty
cotton-wool
    c.-w. bandage
coudé
    c. bougie
    c. catheter
Councill
    basket
    catheter
    stone dislodger
Cournand
    catheter
    needle
Courvoisier
    incision
Coxeter
    catheter
Crafoord
    clamp
    forceps
    scissors
Craig
    forceps
    needle
    scissors
Cramer splint
Crane
    mallet
    osteotome
craniotome
craniotomy
    c. scissors

Crawford
    retractor
Crawford-Adams
    acetabular cup
Crawford-Cooley
    tunneler
Creech technique
Crenshaw
    forceps
crescent
    c. incision
crib
    Jackson c.
Crile
    clamp
    forceps
    knife
    retractor
Crile-Matas
    operation
Cripps
    obturator
    operation
crocodile forceps
Cronin
    prosthesis
Crookes lens
cross-clamp
crosshatch incision
Crowe-Davis mouth gag
crown
    c. saw
Crozat
    appliance
    clasp
crucial
    c. incision
cruciate
    c. incision
cruciform
    c. suture
crushing clamp
Crutchfield
    clamp
    drill
    tongs
Crutchfield-Raney
    tongs

Cruveilhier
    fascia
    ulcer
Cryer
    elevator
cryocautery
cryoscope
cryoscopy
cryostat
cryptotome
    Blanchard c.
cuffed tube
culdoscope
    Decker c.
Cunningham
    clamp
Curdy
    sclerotome
curet, curette
    adenoid c.
    Ballenger c.
    banjo c.
    Barnhill c.
    Beckmann c.
    Billeau ear wax c.
    Brun c.
    Buck c.
    Bumm c.
    Carmack ear c.
    Coakley c.
    Delstanche c.
    Derlacki c.
    Faulkner c.
    Fox c.
    Freimuth c.
    Gifford c.
    Goldman c.
    Gottstein c.
    Govons c.
    Gracey c.
    Green c.
    Greene c.
    Gross c.
    Gusberg c.
    Halle c.
    Hannon c.
    Hartmann c.
    Hayden c.

curet, curette (continued)
    Heaney c.
    Heath c.
    Hibbs c.
    Holden c.
    Holtz c.
    Hotz c.
    House c.
    Hunter c.
    Ingersoll c.
    Jones c.
    Kelly c.
    Kelly-Gray c.
    Kevorkian c.
    Kushner-Tandatnick c.
    Lempert c.
    Lounsbury c.
    McCaskey c.
    Meyerding c.
    Meyhoeffer c.
    Middleton c.
    Mosher c.
    Moult c.
    Myles c.
    Novak c.
    Piffard c.
    Pratt c.
    Randall c.
    Raney c.
    Récamier c.
    Reich-Nechtow c.
    Richards c.
    Ridpath c.
    Rosenmüller c.
    Schaeffer c.
    serrated c.
    Shapleigh c.
    Shea c.
    Sims c.
    Skeele c.
    Skene c.
    Spratt c.
    St. Clair-Thompson c.
    Stubbs c.
    Tabb c.
    Thomas c.
    Vogel c.
    Volkmann c.

curet, curette (continued)
  Walsh c.
  Weisman c.
  Whiting c.
  Yankauer c.
curetted
curioscopy
Curry
  needle
  splint
Curtis
  forceps
curved incision
curvilinear
  c. incision
CUSA—Cavitron ultrasonic aspirator
Cusco
  speculum
Cushing
  clip
  depressor
  drill
  forceps
  needle
  operation
  periosteal elevator
  retractor
  spatula
  spoon
  suture
cushioning suture
cutaneous
  c. suture
  c. suture of palate
cuticular
  c. suture
Cutter-SCDK
  prosthesis
Cutter-Smeloff
  cardiac valve prosthesis
cutting loops
cutting needle
CVC—central venous catheter
CVP (central venous pressure) catheter
cycloscope
cyclotome

cyst
  Baker c.
  branchial c.
  echinococcus c.
  involution c.
  sacrococcygeal c.
cystauchenotomy
cysticolithectomy
cysticolithotripsy
cysticorrhaphy
cysticotomy
cystidolaparotomy
cystis
  c. fellea
cystitome [instrument for incising cornea]
cystodiaphanoscopy
cystoscope
  Braasch c.
  Brown-Buerger c.
  Butterfield c.
  fiberoptic c.
  Kelly c.
  Lowsley-Peterson c.
  McCarthy c.
  McCarthy-Campbell c.
  McCarthy-Peterson c.
  National c.
  Nesbit c.
  Ravich c.
  Storz c.
  Wappler c.
cystotome
  See also *cystitome*.
  Graefe (von Graefe) c.
  Wheeler c.
cystourethroscope
cytoscopy
Czerny
  operation
  suture
Czerny-Lembert
  suture
Dacron
  prosthesis
  suture
dactyloscopy

Dakin
    antiseptic solution
    fluid
Dallas
    operation
D'Allesandro
    serial suture-holding forceps
Dandy
    hemostat
    hook
    scissors
Daniel
    clamp
Daniels
    tonsillectome
Darling
    capsulotome
Darrach
    procedure
D'Assumpcao
    rhytidoplasty marker
David
    speculum
Davidoff (Davidov)
    retractor
Davidson
    clamp
    retractor
Daviel
    scoop
    spoon
Davis
    bronchoscope
    clamp
    conductor
    crown
    forceps
    gag
    knife needle
    needle
    retractor
    spatula
    splint
    stone dislodger
Davis-Crowe mouth gag
Day
    cannula

"day-zhar-dahz" Phonetic for Des-
    jardins.
De Alvarez
    forceps
Dean
    applicator
    forceps
    knife
    periosteotome
    scissors
Deaver
    incision
    retractor
    scissors
DeBakey
    blade
    clamp
    forceps
    prosthesis
    scissors
    tunneler
DeBakey-Bahnson
    forceps
DeBakey-Bainbridge
    forceps
DeBakey-Balfour
    retractor
DeBakey-Cooley
    dilator
    forceps
    retractor
DeBakey-Metzenbaum
    scissors
Debove
    tube
débridement
    tangential d.
débrider
Decker
    culdoscope
declinator
decompression
    d. incision
    d. operation
Dedo
    laryngoscope
Dedo-Pilling
    laryngoscope

Dees
>   needle
defibrillator
>   automatic implantable cardioverter-d. (AICD)
deformity
>   Akerlund d.
dehiscence
>   wound d.
"dehisens" Phonetic for dehiscence.
dekalon suture
Deknatel
>   suture
delayed
>   d. primary suture
>   d. suture
DeLee
>   forceps
>   maneuver
>   retractor
>   suction
>   tenaculum
Delstanche
>   curet
deltopectoral
>   d. incision
DeMartel-Wolfson
>   clamp
Denans
>   operation
Denhardt
>   mouth gag
Denhardt-Dingman mouth gag
Denis Browne
>   clubfoot splint
>   needle
>   pouch
Dennis
>   clamp
>   forceps
Denoff splint
dental
>   prosthesis
Denver shunt
Depage
>   position
DePalma
>   prosthesis

Depaul
>   tube
dependent
>   d. drainage
de Pezzer
>   catheter
depilatory forceps
DePuy
>   orthopedic implant
>   prosthesis
Derf
>   needle holder
Derlacki
>   chisel
>   curet
>   knife
Derlacki-Shambaugh
>   chisel
dermabrader
dermal
>   d. suture
Dermalene
>   suture
Dermalon
>   suture
dermatome
>   Bard-Parker d.
>   Barker Vacu-tome d.
>   Brown d.
>   drum d.
>   Hall d.
>   Hood d.
>   Meek-Wall d.
>   Padgett d.
>   Reese d.
>   Stryker d.
Derra
>   clamp
>   dilator
>   knife
D'Errico
>   bur
>   drill
>   forceps
>   retractor
D'Errico-Adson
>   retractor

Desault
  apparatus
  bandage
descensus
  d. ventriculi
Deschamps
  carrier
  needle
Desjardins
  forceps
  probe
  scoop
Desmarres
  forceps
  knife
  lid elevator
  retractor
device
DeVilbiss
  atomizer
  forceps
  irrigator
  nebulizer
  rongeur
  speculum
  trephine
DeVilbiss-Stacey
  speculum
DeWecker
  scissors
DeWecker-Pritikin
  scissors
Dewey
  forceps
Dexon
  mesh
  suture
Deyerle
  drill
diamond bur
diaphanoscope
diaphanoscopy
Dick
  dilator
diechoscope
Diethrich
  shunt clamp

Dieulafoy
  aspirator
  ulcer
dilating urethrotome
dilation
  digital d.
dilator
  Atlee d.
  Bakes d.
  Barnes d.
  Beardsley aortic d.
  Berens d.
  Black-Wylie obstetric d.
  Brown-McHardy d.
  Broyles d.
  Castroviejo d.
  Cooley d.
  DeBakey-Cooley d.
  Derra d.
  Dick d.
  Einhorn d.
  esophageal d.
  Ferris d.
  French d. Nos. 8 to 36
  Gohrbrand d.
  Goodell d.
  Guyon d.
  Hank d.
  Hank-Bradley d.
  Heath d.
  Hegar d.
  Hurtig d.
  Jackson d.
  Jackson-Mosher d.
  Jackson-Trousseau d.
  Jolly d.
  Jones d.
  Kelly d.
  Kollmann d.
  Kron d.
  Laborde d.
  Leader-Kollmann d.
  Maloney d.
  Mantz d.
  Mixter d.
  Mosher d.
  Muldoon d.
  Murphy d.

dilator (continued)
    Negus hydrostatic d.
    Nettleship-Wilder d.
    Ottenheimer d.
    Palmer d.
    Patton d.
    Plummer d.
    Plummer-Vinson d.
    pneumatic balloon d.
    Pratt d.
    Ramstedt d.
    Reich-Nechtow d.
    Savary-Gilliard d.
    Sippy d.
    Starlinger d.
    Steele d.
    tracheal d.
    Trousseau d.
    Trousseau-Jackson d.
    Tubbs d.
    Tucker d.
    Van Buren d.
    Wales d.
    Walther d.
    Wylie d.
    Young d.
Dimitry
    erysiphake
Dimitry-Bell erysiphake
Dimitry-Thomas erysiphake
Dingman
    elevator
    forceps
    osteotome
    retractor
diploscope
direct
    d. ophthalmoscope
director
    Larry d.
    Pratt d.
discission
    d. needle
discoid
    d. aortic prosthesis
discoidectomy (pref: diskectomy)
disk valve prosthesis
disposable sigmoidoscope

dissecting
    d. forceps
    d. microscope
dissection
    blunt d.
    radical neck d.
    sharp d.
    supraomohyoid neck d.
dissector
    Brunner d.
    Fisher d.
    Green d.
    Holinger d.
    Hurd d.
    Kocher d.
    Lewin d.
    Lynch d.
    McWhinnie d.
    Oldberg d.
    Pierce d.
    Roger d.
    Sheldon-Pudenz d.
    Walker d.
    Wangensteen d.
diverticularization
Dixon-Thomas-Smith
    clamp
Dobbhoff
    feeding tube
docking needle
Dohlman
    operation
Donaldson
    tube
Dorian
    rib stripper
Dormia
    basket
    stone dislodger
dorsal [adj.]
    d. lithotomy position
dorsolateral
    d. incision
Dott
    mouth gag
double-action forceps
double-armed suture, doubly armed
    suture

double-button suture
double-channel irrigating bronchoscope
double-J stent catheter
double-lumen catheter
double-Y incision
Douglas
  knife
Dowell
  operation
Downing
  knife
Doyen
  clamp
  elevator
  forceps
  gag
  retractor
  scissors
drain
  accordion d.
  butterfly d.
  cigarette d.
  Hemovac d.
  latex d.
  Malecot d.
  Penrose d.
  Pezzer d.
  polyethylene d.
  polyvinyl d.
  quarantine d.
  Redivac d.
  rubber dam d.
  stab wound d.
  suction d.
  sump d.
  whistle-tip d.
drainage
  Roux-Y d.
  d. tube
drainage system
  closed water-seal d.s.
  continuous suction d.s.
  Glover d.s.
  Monaldi d.s.
  postural d.s.
  Redivac d.s.
  Snyder Surgivac d.s.

drainage system (continued)
  sump d.s.
  Surgivac suction d.s.
  three-bottle d.s.
  tidal d.s.
  two-bottle d.s.
  vacuum d.s.
  waterseal d.s.
  water-seal d.s.
dressing
  See also *bandage.*
  absorbable d.
  Adaptic gauze d.
  adhesive d.
  Aeroplast d.
  Band-Aid d.
  barrel d.
  biologic d., biological d.
  bolus d.
  brassiere-type d.
  bulky d.
  butterfly d.
  cellophane d.
  cement d.
  cocoon d.
  Coe-Pak d.
  collar d.
  collodion d.
  compound d.
  compression d.
  Conform d.
  Cornish wool d.
  dry pressure d.
  felt d.
  fine mesh d.
  fluff d.
  fluffy compression d.
  foam rubber d.
  four-tailed d.
  Fricke scrotal d.
  Gelfilm d.
  Gelfoam d.
  Gelocast d.
  impregnated d.
  iodoform d.
  Lister d.
  Lubafax d.
  many-tailed d.

dressing (continued)
>Mersilene gauze d.
>mustache d.
>Nu-gauze d.
>occlusive d.
>paraffin d.
>patch d.
>petrolatum gauze d.
>plastic d.
>pressure d.
>propylene d.
>Ray-Tec d.
>sheepskin d.
>stent d.
>stockinette d.
>Styrofoam d.
>surgical gauze d.
>Surgicel gauze d.
>Telfa d.
>tulle gras d.
>Vaseline gauze d.
>Velcro d.
>Velroc d.
>Vioform d.
>Wangensteen d.
>wet-to-dry d.
>Xeroform gauze d.

drill
>Adson d.
>Amico d.
>Bunnell d.
>Cloward d.
>Crutchfield d.
>Cushing d.
>D'Errico d.
>Deyerle d.
>Hall d.
>Hall air d.
>Hall surgical d.
>Hudson d.
>intramedullary d.
>Jordan-Day d.
>Lentulo spiral d.
>McKenzie d.
>mirror d.
>Ralks d.
>Raney d.
>Shea d.

drill (continued)
>Smedberg d.
>Spirec d.
>Stille d.
>Stryker d.
>Vitallium d.

drop foot brace

drum
>d. dermatome
>d. probe

Drummond-Morison
>operation

dry pressure dressing

duckbill, duck-billed
>d. speculum

duct
>alveolar d.
>common hepatic d.
>efferent d.
>excretory d.
>lactiferous d.
>mammary d.
>papillary d.
>parotid d.
>prostatic d.
>salivary d.
>d. of Santorini
>semicircular d.
>d. of Wirsung

Dudley
>hook

Dudley-Smith
>speculum

Dührssen
>incision

Duke
>trocar

Dulox
>suture

Dunhill
>hemostat

Duplay
>hook
>speculum
>tenaculum

Duplay-Lynch
>speculum

Dupuytren
    enterotome
dura
    d. clip
dural
    d. forceps
    d. hook
Dur-A-Sil
Durham
    trocar
    tube
Duromedics
    prosthesis
Duval
    intestinal forceps
    lung-grasping forceps
Duval-Crile
    forceps
Duvergier
    suture
dye laser
dynamometer
dynamoscope
Eagleton
    operation
Earle
    probe
Eastman
    clamp
    retractor
Eaton
    speculum
Eber
    forceps
echinococcotomy
echoscope
ectocolostomy
ectokelostomy
ectomy
ectoscopy
Edebohls
    incision
Eder
    forceps
    gastroscope
    laparoscope
Eder-Chamberlin
    gastroscope

Eder-Hufford
    esophagoscope
    gastroscope
Eder-Palmer
    gastroscope
edge-to-edge suture
Edwards
    catheter
    clamp
    hook
    prosthesis
effect [verb: to produce, to bring
   about]
    to e. closure of an incision
Eicher
    prosthesis
Einhorn
    dilator
Ekehorn
    operation
elastic
    e. suture
electric
    e. probe
electrobioscopy
electrocoagulation
electrode
    ureteral meatotomy e.
electrodermatome
electrodesiccation
electrodiaphake
electrodiaphane
electrodiaphanoscope
electrodiaphanoscopy
electrodynamometer
electroencephaloscope
electroexcision
electrogastroenterostomy
electrohemostasis
electroresection
electroscission
electroscope
electrosection
electrosurgery
electrosurgical needle
electrotherm
electrotome
    Stern-McCarthy e.

electrotomy
elevator
    Adson e.
    Ballenger e.
    Barsky e.
    Bennett e.
    Cameron-Haight e.
    Campbell e.
    Chandler e.
    Cobb e.
    Cottle e.
    Cryer e.
    Cushing periosteal e.
    Desmarres lid e.
    Dingman e.
    Doyen e.
    Farabeuf e.
    Frazier c.
    Freer e.
    Hajek-Ballenger e.
    Hamrick e.
    Hedblom e.
    Hibbs e.
    House e.
    Hurd e.
    Jackson e.
    joker e.
    Killian e.
    Lamont e.
    Lane e.
    Langenbeck (von Langenbeck) e.
    Lempert e.
    Love-Adson e.
    MacKenty e.
    Matson e.
    McIndoe e.
    Overholt e.
    palatal e.
    Pennington e.
    periosteal e.
    Phemister e.
    Pierce e.
    Proctor e.
    Ralks e.
    Ray-Parsons-Sunday e.
    Rochester e.
    Sédillot e.

elevator (continued)
    Shambaugh e.
    Shambaugh-Derlacki e.
    Soonawalla uterine e.
    Sunday e.
    Veau e.
    Woodson e.
Elliot
    position
    trephine
Elliott
    forceps
    plate
elliptic, elliptical
    e. incision
Ellis
    needle holder
Ellsner
    gastroscope
Elsberg
    incision
Elschnig
    forceps
    knife
    retractor
    spatula
    spoon
Elschnig-O'Brien
    forceps
embryoscope
Emerson
    bronchoscope
    pump
    stripper
Emmet
    hook
    retractor
    scissors
    suture
empyema
    e. tube
encephaloscope
encephalotome
end
    e. tracheostome
endarterectomy
    Cannon e. loop

endaural
 e. incision
endobronchial
 e. tube
endocardial
 e. tube
endodiascope
end-on mattress suture
endoscope
 Kelly e.
 Rockey e.
endoskeletal prosthesis
endothyropexy
endotoscope
endotracheal (ET)
 e. tube
end-to-end anastomosis
end-to-side anastomosis
Engelmann
 splint
Engen extension orthosis
enterohepatopexy
enterotome
 Dupuytren e.
entoptoscope
epauxesiectomy
epigastrocele
epigastrorrhaphy
epineural
 e. suture
epiplocele
epiploectomy
epiploic
epiploitis
epiplomerocele
epiplomphalocele
epiplosarcomphalocele
epiploscheocele
epithesis
Epstein
 osteotome
Equen-Neuffer
 knife
Equisetene
 suture
Erich
 arch bar
 forceps

Ernst
 applicator
erysiphake
 Barraquer e.
 Bell e.
 Dimitry e.
 Dimitry-Bell e.
 Dimitry-Thomas e.
 Harrington e.
 Kara e.
 L'Esperance e.
 Maumenee e.
 Nugent-Green-Dimitry e.
 Post-Harrington e.
 Sakler e.
 Searcy e.
 Viers e.
Esmarch
 bandage
 scissors
 tourniquet
 tube
eso—esophagoscopy
esophageal
 e. dilator
 e. speculum
 e. tube
esophagocardiomyotomy
esophagoscope
 Boros e.
 Broyles e.
 Bruening e.
 Chevalier Jackson e.
 Eder-Hufford e.
 fiberoptic e.
 full-lumen e.
 Haslinger e.
 Holinger e.
 Jackson e.
 Jesberg e.
 Lell e.
 Moersch e.
 Mosher e.
 Moure e.
 Negus e.
 optical e.
 oval e.
 Roberts e.

esophagoscope (continued)
    Schindler e.
    Tucker e.
    Yankauer e.
esophagotome
Ethibond
    suture
Ethicon
    suture
Ethiflex
    suture
Ethilon
    suture
eupatheoscope
euthyscope
Evans
    forceps
everting
    e. interrupted suture
    e. suture
Eves tonsillar snare
Ewald
    tube
excavator
    dental e.
    hatchet e.
    Schuknecht whirlybird e.
    spoon e.
excision
    wound e.
exoskeletal prosthesis
exploratory
    e. incision
    e. operation
exteriorize
external
    e. stripper
extractor
    Saalfield e.
eye
    e. speculum
eyed probe
fallostomy
Fansler
    anoscope
    proctoscope
    speculum
fantascope

Farabeuf
    elevator
    forceps
    saw
    triangle
Farabeuf-Lambotte
    forceps
far-and-near suture
Farr
    retractor
Farrington
    forceps
Farrior
    speculum
Farris
    forceps
fascia (fasciae)
    Cloquet f.
    cribriform f.
    external oblique f.
    infundibuliform f.
    f. of insertion
    pectineal f.
    prepubic f.
    psoas f.
    subcutaneous f.
    f. subscapularis
    f. of Toldt
    transverse f.
    f. of Treitz
fasciatome
    Luck f.
Faulkner
    curet
Fauvel
    forceps
FB—fingerbreadth
Federoff
    splenectomy
feeding
    f. prosthesis
    f. tube
Fehland
    clamp
Feilchenfeld
    forceps
Feleky instrument
Fell-O'Dwyer apparatus

felt dressing
fenestrated
    f. clamp
fenestrater
Fenger
    probe
Ferguson
    basket
    forceps
    scissors
    scoop
Ferguson-Moon
    retractor
Fergusson
    speculum
Ferris
    dilator
    forceps
    scoop
Ferris-Robb
    knife
Ferris-Smith
    forceps
    retractor
    technique
Ferris-Smith-Kerrison
    forceps
Ferris-Smith-Sewall
    retractor
fetoscope
fibercolonoscope
fibergastroscope
fiber-illuminated
fiberoptic
    f. bronchoscope
    f. colonoscope
    f. cystoscope
    f. esophagoscope
    f. gastroscope
    f. laryngoscope
    f. probe
    f. sigmoidoscope
    f. tube
fiberscope
    gastric f.
    Hirschowitz gastroduodenal f.
    Olympus f.

fibrin
    f. sponge
fibrinopurulent
fibrinoscopy
fibromyotomy
Ficoll-Hypaque technique
figure-of-eight suture
filiform
    f. catheter
    f. and follower
filter
    bird's nest f.
    Kimray-Greenfield f.
    Mobin-Uddin umbrella f.
fine mesh dressing
fine-needle
Fink
    laryngoscope
    retractor
    tendon tucker
Finochietto
    forceps
    rib spreader
    stirrup
Fischer
    needle
Fish
    forceps
Fisher
    dissector
    knife
    spud
fishmouth
    f. incision
fistulatome
Fitzgerald
    forceps
fixation
    f. forceps
    f. hook
    f. suture
Flagg
    laryngoscope
flank
    f. incision
    lateral f. incision
Flannery
    speculum

flap
    cellulocutaneous f.
    island f.
    musculocutaneous f.
    sliding f.
    surgical f.
    tensor fasciae latae muscle f.
Flaxedil
    suture
Fleming
    knife
Fletcher
    knife
Fletcher-Suit
    applicator
Fletcher-Van Doren
    forceps
flexed incision
flexible
    f. catheter
    f. gastroscope
flexible shaft retractor
Flexicath
    cannula
Flexitone
    suture
Flexon
    suture
flexure
    duodenojejunal f.
    fluctuant
    hepatic f.
    iliac f.
    sigmoid f.
floating-disk prosthesis
Floyd
    cannula
    needle
fluffy compression dressing
fluoroscope
flying spot microscope
Flynt
    needle
foam rubber dressing
Fogarty
    catheter
Foley
    catheter

Foley (continued)
    forceps
Foley-Alcock
    catheter
follower
    filiform and f.
Foltz valve
Fomon
    chisel
    knife
    periosteotome
    rasp
    scissors
fontactoscope
Fontan
    procedure
forceps
    ACMI f.
    ACMI Martin endoscopy f.
    Acufex f.
    Adair f.
    Adams f.
    adenoid f.
    Adson f.
    Allis f.
    Allis-Ochsner f.
    Andrews-Hartmann f.
    Arruga f.
    Asch f.
    Babcock f.
    Backhaus f.
    Bacon f.
    Bailey-Williamson f.
    Bainbridge hemostatic f.
    Ballantine hysterectomy f.
    Ballenger f.
    Bane f.
    Barlow f.
    Barnes-Crile f.
    Barraquer ciliary f.
    Barraquer corneal f.
    Barraya f.
    Barrett f.
    Barrett-Allen f.
    Barton f.
    bayonet f.
    Beaupre f.
    Beebe f.

forceps (continued)
    Beer ciliary f.
    Benaron f.
    Bengolea f.
    Bennett f.
    Berens f.
    Berke ptosis f.
    Berne f.
    Berry uterine-elevating f.
    Best common duct stone f.
    Best gallstone f.
    Best intestinal f.
    Bevan gallbladder f.
    Bevan hemostatic f.
    Beyer f.
    Billroth f.
    Billroth uterine tumor f.
    Bishop-Harmon f.
    Blake f.
    Blake ear f.
    Blake embolus f.
    Blake gallstone f.
    Blakesley f.
    Blanchard hemorrhoidal f.
    Boies f.
    Bonaccolto f.
    Bond f.
    bone f.
    bone-cutting f.
    bone-nibbling f.
    Bonn f.
    Böttcher (Boettcher) f.
    Boys-Allis f.
    Bozeman f.
    Braasch f.
    Bracken f.
    Bradford f.
    Brophy f.
    Brown f.
    Brown-Adson f.
    Broyles f.
    Bruening f.
    Brunner f.
    Buerger-McCarthy f.
    Buie f.
    Bumpus f.
    Bunim f.
    Cairns f.

forceps (continued)
    Campbell f.
    capsule f.
    Carmalt arterial f.
    Carmalt hemostatic f.
    Carmalt hysterectomy f.
    Carmalt splinter f.
    Carmalt thoracic f.
    Carmody f.
    Carrel mosquito f.
    Carroll bone-holding f.
    Carroll tendon-passing f.
    Carroll tendon-pulling f.
    cartilage f.
    Cassidy-Brophy f.
    Castaneda f.
    Castroviejo f.
    Castroviejo-Arruga f.
    chalazion f.
    Chamberlen f.
    Chandler f.
    Cherry-Kerrison f.
    Cicherelli f.
    Coakley f.
    Cohen f.
    Colibri f.
    Collin f.
    Colver f.
    Cooley f.
    Coppridge f.
    Corbett f.
    Cordes f.
    Cordes-New f.
    Corey f.
    Cornet f.
    Cottle f.
    Cottle-Arruga f.
    Cottle-Jansen f.
    Cottle-Kazanjian f.
    Crafoord f.
    Craig f.
    Crenshaw f.
    Crile f.
    crocodile f.
    Curtis f.
    Cushing f.
    D'Allesandro serial suture-
        holding f.

forceps (continued)
Davis f.
De Alvarez f.
Dean f.
DeBakey f.
DeBakey-Bahnson f.
DeBakey-Bainbridge f.
DeBakey-Cooley f.
DeLee f.
Dennis f.
depilatory f.
D'Errico f.
Desjardins f.
Desmarres f.
DeVilbiss f.
Dewey f.
Dingman f.
dissecting f.
double-action f.
Doyen f.
dural f.
Duval-Crile f.
Eber f.
Eder f.
Elliott f.
Elschnig f.
Elschnig-O'Brien f.
Erich f.
Evans f.
Farabeuf f.
Farabeuf-Lambotte f.
Farrington f.
Farris f.
Fauvel f.
Feilchenfeld f.
Ferguson f.
Ferris f.
Ferris-Smith f.
Ferris-Smith-Kerrison f.
Finochietto f.
Fish f.
Fitzgerald f.
fixation f.
Fletcher-Van Doren f.
Foerster f.
Foley f.
Förster iris f.
Foss f.

forceps (continued)
Foster-Ballenger f.
Fränkel f.
Frankfeldt f.
Fricke arterial f.
Fuchs f.
Fulpit f.
Garrigue f.
Gaylor f.
Gellhorn f.
Gelpi-Lowrie f.
Gerald f.
Gifford f.
Glassman f.
Glassman-Allis f.
Glenner f.
Glover f.
Goldman-Kazanjian f.
Goodhill f.
Gordon f.
gouge f.
Graefe (von Graefe) f.
Gray f.
Green f.
Gruenwald f.
Gruenwald-Bryant f.
Guggenheim f.
Gutglass f.
Haig Ferguson f.
Hajek-Koffler f.
Hale f.
Halsted f.
Harken f.
Harrington f.
Harrington-Mayo f.
Harris f.
Hartmann f.
Hartmann-Citelli f.
Hartmann-Gruenwald f.
Hawkins cervical biopsy f.
Hawks-Dennen f.
Healy f.
Heaney f.
Heaney-Ballantine f.
Heaney-Kanter f.
Heaney-Rezek f.
Heath f.
Heise f.

forceps (continued)
    Hendren f.
    Henrotin f.
    Hess f.
    Hess-Barraquer f.
    Hess-Horwitz f.
    Hibbs f.
    Hirschman f.
    Hodge f.
    Hoffmann f.
    Holinger f.
    Holth f.
    Horsley bone-cutting f.
    House f.
    Howard f.
    Hoxworth f.
    Hudson f.
    Hunt f.
    Hurd f.
    Imperatori f.
    inlet f.
    insertion f.
    Iowa f.
    Jackson f.
    Jacobs f.
    Jacobson f.
    Jameson f.
    Jansen f.
    Jansen-Middleton f.
    Jansen-Struycken f.
    Jarcho f.
    Johns Hopkins f.
    Johnson f.
    Jones f.
    Judd f.
    Judd-Allis f.
    Judd-DeMartel f.
    Juers-Lempert f.
    Julian f.
    Jurasz f.
    Kahler f.
    Kalt f.
    Katzin-Barraquer f.
    Kazanjian f.
    Kelly f.
    Kelman f.
    Kennedy f.
    Kern f.

forceps (continued)
    Kerrison f.
    Kielland (Kjelland) f.
    Kielland-Luikart f.
    Killian f.
    Kirby f.
    Kittner f.
    Knapp f.
    Knight f.
    Knight-Sluder f.
    Kocher f.
    Koeberlé f.
    Koffler f.
    Koffler-Lillie f.
    Kolb f.
    Krause f.
    Kronfeld f.
    Kuhnt f.
    Kulvin-Kalt f.
    Laborde f.
    Lahey f.
    Lahey-Péan f.
    Lambert f.
    Lambotte f.
    Lane f.
    Laufe f.
    Laufe-Barton-Kielland f.
    Laufe-Piper f.
    Lebsche f.
    Leksell f.
    Leland-Jones f.
    Lempert f.
    Leriche f.
    Levret f.
    Lewin f.
    Lewis f.
    Lewkowitz f.
    Leyro-Diaz f.
    Lillie f.
    lion-jawed f.
    Lister f.
    Liston-Stille f.
    Littauer f.
    Littauer-Liston f.
    lock f.
    Lockwood f.
    Long f.
    Long Island f.

forceps (continued)
>> Love-Kerrison f.
>> Lovelace f.
>> Lowenberg f.
>> Lower f.
>> Lowsley f.
>> Luc f.
>> Lucae f.
>> Luer f.
>> Luikart f.
>> Luikart-Simpson f.
>> Lutz f.
>> Lynch f.
>> Maier f.
>> Mann f.
>> Marshik f.
>> Martin f.
>> Maryan f.
>> Mathieu f.
>> Mayo f.
>> Mayo-Blake f.
>> Mayo-Ochsner f.
>> Mayo-Robson f.
>> Mayo-Russian f.
>> McCarthy f.
>> McCarthy-Alcock f.
>> McCullough f.
>> McHenry f.
>> McKay f.
>> McKenzie f.
>> McLane f.
>> McLane-Tucker f.
>> McLane-Tucker-Luikart f.
>> McNealy-Glassman-Bab-
cock f.
>> McNealy-Glassman-Mixter f.
>> McPherson f.
>> Metzenbaum f.
>> Millin f.
>> Mitchell-Diamond f.
>> Mixter f.
>> Moersch f.
>> Moritz-Schmidt f.
>> mosquito f.
>> Mount-Mayfield f.
>> mouse-tooth f.
>> Moynihan f.
>> Mundie f.

forceps (continued)
>> Museholdt f.
>> Myerson f.
>> Myles f.
>> Negus ligature f.
>> Nelson f.
>> Neubauer f.
>> New f.
>> Newman f.
>> Noble f.
>> nonfenestrated f.
>> Noyes f.
>> Nugent f.
>> O'Brien f.
>> obstetric f.
>> Ochsner f.
>> Ochsner-Dixon f.
>> O'Hanlon f.
>> Oldberg f.
>> O'Shaughnessy f.
>> Ostrom f.
>> outlet f.
>> Overstreet f.
>> ovum f.
>> Palmer f.
>> Pang f.
>> Parker-Kerr f.
>> Paterson brain clip f.
>> Paterson laryngeal f.
>> Patterson bronchoscopic f.
>> Péan f.
>> Pennington f.
>> Percy f.
>> Perritt f.
>> Phaneuf f.
>> Piper f.
>> Pitha f.
>> placental f.
>> Pley f.
>> polyp f.
>> Porter f.
>> Potts-Smith f.
>> Poutasse f.
>> Pratt-Smith f.
>> Price-Thomas f.
>> Prince f.
>> Providence f.
>> punch f.

forceps (continued)

Quevedo f.
Randall stone f.
Raney f.
Rankin f.
Ratliff-Blake f.
rat-tooth f.
Ray f.
Reese f.
Reiner-Knight f.
rib-cutting f.
Rienhoff f.
ring f.
Robb f.
Roberts f.
Robertson f.
Rochester f.
Rochester-Carmalt f.
Rochester-Ewald f.
Rochester-Mixter f.
Rochester-Ochsner f.
Rochester-Péan f.
Rochester-Rankin f.
Rockey f.
Roeder f.
Rolf f.
root-splitting f.
Rowland f.
Rumel f.
Ruskin f.
Russell f.
Russian f.
Sam Roberts f.
Sanders f.
Sarot f.
Satinsky f.
Sauer f.
Sauerbruch f.
Sawtell f.
Scheinmann f.
Schlesinger f.
Schoenberg f.
Schroeder f.
Schubert f.
Schutz f.
Schwartz f.
Schweigger f.
Schweizer f.

forceps (continued)

Scoville f.
Scudder f.
Segond f.
Seiffert f.
Selman f.
Semb f.
Semken f.
Senn f.
Sewall f.
Shaaf f.
Shallcross f.
Shearer f.
Simpson f.
Simpson-Luikart f.
Singley f.
sinus f.
Skene f.
Skillern f.
Smart f.
Smith f.
Smithwick f.
Somers f.
Spence f.
Spence-Adson f.
Spencer Wells f.
Spero f.
sponge f., sponge-holding f.
spring f.
Spurling f.
Staude f.
Staude-Moore f.
Steinmann f.
Stevens f.
Stevenson f.
Stille f.
Stille-Liston f.
Stille-Luer f.
stone f.
Strassmann f.
Struempel f.
Struempel ear alligator f.
Struempel ear punch f.
Struyken f.
Suker iris f.
suture-holding f.
Sweet f.
Takahashi f.

forceps (continued)
Tarnier f.
Teale f.
Thoms f.
Thoms-Allis f.
Thoms-Gaylor f.
Thorek-Mixter f.
Thorpe f.
Tischler f.
tissue f.
Tivnen f.
Tobold f.
Tobold-Fauvel f.
f. tourniquet
towel f.
tubular f.
Tucker-McLean f.
Tuttle f.
Tydings f.
Tydings-Lakeside f.
uterine f.
Van Buren f.
Vanderbilt f.
Van Doren f.
Verhoeff f.
Virtus f.
von Mondak f.
vulsellum f.
Waldeau f.
Walsham f.
Walter f.
Walther f.
Walton f.
Walton-Schubert f.
Wangensteen f.
Washam f.
Watson-Williams f.
Watze f.
Weil f.
Weingartner f.
Weisenbach f.
Weisman f.
Welch-Allyn f.
Wertheim f.
Wertheim-Cullen f.
White f.
White-Lillie f.
White-Oslay f.

forceps (continued)
Wilde f.
Willett f.
Williams f.
Wittner f.
Wullstein f.
Wullstein-House f.
Yankauer f.
Yankauer-Little f.
Yeoman f.
Young f.
Zenker f.
Ziegler f.
Zollinger f.
fore-and-aft suture
Foregger
bronchoscope
laryngoscope
Foroblique
McCarthy F. panendoscope
Forrester
clamp
Förster (Foerster)
forceps
iris forceps
photometer
49'er knee brace
Foss
clamp
forceps
retractor
Foster-Ballenger
forceps
four-tailed dressing
Fowler
incision
sound
Fowler-Weir
incision
Fox
curet
scissors
splint
Fraenkel. See *Fränkel.*
fraise
frame
Bradford f.
Foster f.

frame (continued)
 Hibbs f.
 Stryker f.
 Whitman f.
Francke
 needle
Fränkel (Fraenkel)
 forceps
 speculum
Frankfeldt
 forceps
 needle
 sigmoidoscope
 snare
Franklin-Silverman
 needle
Franz
 retractor
Frazier
 cannula
 elevator
 hook retractor
 osteotome
 retractor
 suction tube
 tube
Frederick
 needle
free ligature suture
Freer
 chisel
 elevator
 knife
freezing microtome
Freiberg
 knife
Freimuth
 curet
Frejka
 pillow splint
French
 catheter
 dilator Nos. 8 to 36
 polyethylene catheter
 S-shaped retractor
French-McCarthy
 panendoscope

French-Robinson
 catheter
Fricke
 arterial forceps
 bandage
 scrotal dressing
Friedenwald
 ophthalmoscope
Friedman
 retractor
Friedrich-Petz
 clamp
Friesner
 knife
Fritsch
 catheter
frog, frogleg
 f. splint
Frost [eponym]
 suture
Fuchs
 forceps
full-lumen esophagoscope
Fulpit
 forceps
fundoplication
 Nissen f.
funduscope
fundusectomy
Furniss
 anastomosis
 catheter
 clamp
 incision
Furniss-Clute
 clamp
Furniss-McClure-Hinton
 clamp
furrier's suture
fusion
 f. tubes
Futura splint
Gabriel
 proctoscope
Gabriel Tucker
 tube
gag
 McIvor g.

Gaillard-Arlt
   suture
galactoscope
gallbladder
      Courvoisier g.
Gallie
      operation
      transplant
Galt
      trephine
Gambee
      suture
Gamgee
      tissue
Gandhi
      knife
Gandy
      clamp
ganglionostomy
Gant
      clamp
gantry
Gardner
      needle
Garfield-Holinger
      laryngoscope
Gariel pessary
Garrigue
      forceps
      speculum
gas-permeable lens
gasserectomy
Gass scleral punch
gastric
      g. fiberscope
gastrocamera
gastrofiberscope
gastroscope
      ACMI g.
      Benedict g.
      Bernstein g.
      Chevalier Jackson g.
      Eder g.
      Eder-Chamberlin g.
      Eder-Hufford g.
      Eder-Palmer g.
      Ellsner g.
      fiberoptic g.

gastroscope (continued)
      flexible g.
      Herman-Taylor g.
      Hirschowitz g.
      Housset-Debray g.
      Janeway g.
      Kelling g.
      Schindler g.
      Wolf-Schindler g.
gastrostomy
      Beck g. scoop
gastrotome
Gatch
      bed
Gatellier
      incision
gauze
      antiseptic g.
      iodoform g.
      Kling g.
      ribbon g.
      g. sponge
      tulle gras g.
      Xeroform g.
Gaylor
      forceps
GDC—Guglielmi detachable coil
Gehrung pessary
Geissler
      tube
gelatin
      absorbable g. sponge
      g. sponge
Gelfilm
      dressing
Gel Flex lens
Gelfoam
      cookie
      dressing
      packing
Gellhorn
      forceps
Gelocast
      dressing
Gelpi
      retractor
Gelpi-Lowrie
      forceps

Gély
    suture
generator
Geomedic
    prosthesis
geometric
    g. prosthesis
Gerald
    forceps
Gerzog
    speculum
ghost
    g. ophthalmoscope
Gibbon
    stent
Gibney
    bandage
Gibson
    incision
    suture
Gibson-Balfour
    retractor
Giertz-Shoemaker
    rib shears
Gifford
    applicator
    curet
    forceps
    retractor
Gigli
    wire saw
Giliberty
    prosthesis
Gill
    knife
Gillies
    hook
Gillies-Dingman
    hook
Gilmer splint
Girdner
    electric probe
Glassman
    clamp
    forceps
Glassman-Allis
    forceps

Glenner
    forceps
    retractor
Glisson
    sling
Glover [eponym]
    clamp
    drainage system
    forceps
glover's suture
Gluck
    incision
    rib shears
Goelet
    retractor
Gohrbrand
    dilator
gold (Au)
Goldbacher
    anoscope
    needle
    proctoscope
    speculum
Goldberg
    MPC mediastinoscope
Goldblatt
    clamp
Goldman
    curet
Goldman-Kazanjian
    forceps
Goldmann applanation tonometer
Goldstein
    cannula
    retractor
Goldthwait
    brace
Gomco
    clamp
goniometer
    Carroll finger g.
    Conzett g.
    finger g.
    universal g.
goniometry
gonioscope
Good [eponym]
    rasp

Goodale-Lubin
    catheter
Goodell
    dilator
Goodfellow
    cannula
Goodhill
    forceps
Goodyear
    knife
Gordon
    forceps
    splint
Gosset
    retractor
Gott
    prosthesis
Gottschalk
    saw
Gottstein
    curet
gouge
        Alexander g.
        Andrews g.
        Cobb g.
        Derlacki g.
        g. forceps
        Hibbs g.
        Holmes g.
        Meyerding g.
        Moore g.
        Todd g.
        Troutman g.
Gould
    suture
Gouley
    catheter
Govons
    curet
Gracey
    curet
Gradle
    retractor
Graefe (von Graefe)
    cystotome
    forceps
    hook
    knife

Graefe (von Graefe) (continued)
    needle
graft
    See also *prosthesis* and *valve*.
    bifurcation g.
    fascial g.
    fiber glass g.
    Marlex g.
    tantalum mesh g.
    Teflon g.
grafting
Graham
    hook
Graham-Roscie
    operation
Graves
    speculum
Gray [eponym]
    forceps
Green [cponym]
    calipers
    curet
    dissector
    forceps
    hook
    knife
    needle holder
    retractor
Greene
    curet
Greenfield
    filter
Greenhow
    incision
Greiling
    tube
gridiron incision
Grieshaber
    keratome
    needle
    needle holder
    retractor
Groenholm
    retractor
Grollman
    pigtail catheter
Grondahl-Finney
    operation

groove
    g. suture
Groshong
    catheter
Gross
    clamp
    curet
    retractor
    spoon
Gross-Pomeranz-Watkins
    retractor
Gruber
    bougie
    speculum
    suture
    test
Gruenwald
    forceps
Gruenwald-Bryant
    forceps
Grüntzig (Gruentzig)
    balloon-tip catheter
guarded
    g. chisel
Gudebrod
    suture
Guedel
    laryngoscope
Guepar
    prosthesis
Guggenheim
    forceps
guide
    Blair Gigli-saw g.
guidewire, guide wire
Guild-Pratt
    speculum
guillotine
    g. incision
    Sluder g.
    Sluder-Sauer g.
    Sluder tonsillar g.
    tonsil g.
Guisez
    tube
Gundelach punch
Gusberg
    curet

Gussenbauer
    operation
    suture
Gusto
    speculum
gut
    g. chromic suture
    ribbon g. suture
    silkworm g. suture
    tiger g. suture
Gutglass
    forceps
Guttmann
    retractor
    speculum
Guyon
    clamp
    dilator
Guyon-Péan
    clamp
guy suture
Guyton-Friedenwald
    suture
Guyton-Maumenee
    speculum
Guyton-Park
    speculum
Hagedorn
    needle
Hahn
    operation
Haidinger brushes
Haig Ferguson
    forceps
Haight
    retractor
Hajek
    chisel
    retractor
Hajek-Ballenger
    elevator
Hajek-Koffler
    forceps
Hajek-Skillern punch
Halberg
    clip
Hale
    forceps

Hall
    air drill
    bur
    dermatome
    surgical drill
    drill
    neurotome
Halle
    curet
    speculum
Halle-Tieck
    speculum
Hallux
    h. malleus
    h. valgus
    h. varus
Halsey
    needle holder
Halsted
    clamp
    forceps
    hemostat
    incision
    operation
    suture
Hamby
    retractor
Hamm electrode
Hamrick
    elevator
Hancock
    M.O. bioprosthesis, M.O. II
        bioprosthesis
    II tissue valve
Handley
    incision
    lymphangioplasty
    operation
"Haney" Phonetic for Heaney.
Hank
    dilator
Hank-Bradlcy
    dilator
Hannon
    curet
Hansen-Street
    nail
    pin

haploscope
Hardy-Duddy
    speculum
harelip
    h. suture
Harken
    forceps
    prosthesis
Harmon
    incision
Harrington
    erysiphake
    forceps
    instrumentation
    retractor
    rod
Harrington-Mayo
    forceps
Harrington-Pemberton
    retractor
Harris
    forceps
    segregator
    separator
    suture
    tube
Harrison
    knife
    scissors
Hartmann
    curet
    dewaxer speculum
    forceps
    fossa
    point
    pouch
    procedure
    punch
Hartmann-Citelli
    forceps
Hartmann-Gruenwald
    forceps
Hartmann-Herzfeld
    rongeur
Hartstein
    retractor
Haslinger
    bronchoscope

Haslinger (continued)
    esophagoscope
    laryngoscope
    retractor
    tracheobronchoesophago-
      scope
Hawkins
    cervical biopsy forceps
Hawks-Dennen
    forceps
Hawley
    appliance
    retainer
Hayden
    curet
Hayes
    clamp
Hayes Martin
    incision
Haynes
    cannula
hayrake splint
headhunter catheter
headrest
    Light-Veley h.
    Shambaugh h.
Healy
    forceps
Heaney
    clamp
    curet
    forceps
    needle holder
    retractor
Heaney-Ballantine
    forceps
Heaney-Kanter
    forceps
Heaney-Rezek
    forceps
Heaney-Simon
    retractor
heart valve prosthesis
heat
    h. probe
Heath
    curet
    dilator

Heath (continued)
    forceps
Heaton
    operation
Hedblom
    elevator
    retractor
Heermann
    incision
Heffernan
    speculum
Hegar
    dilator
    sign
Heifitz
    clip
Heineke
    operation
Heise
    forceps
helical suture
Helmont
    speculum
HEMA—hydroxyethyl methacrylate
hematoma
    retroperitoneal h.
hematospectroscope
hematospectroscopy
hemicorporectomy
hemilaminectomy
    Ballantine h. retractor
hemithyroidectomy
hemitransfixion incision
hemocryoscopy
hemorrhoid
    combined h.
    external h.
    internal h.
    lingual h.
    mixed h.
    mucocutaneous h.
    prolapsed h.
    strangulated h.
    thrombosed h.
hemostat
    Avitene h.
    Corwin h.
    Dandy h.

hemostat (continued)
    Dunhill h.
    Halsted h.
    Kolodny h.
    Maingot h.
hemostatic
    h. clamp
    return flow h. catheter
    h. sutures
Hemovac
    drain
Hendren
    forceps
Henke triangle
Henner
    retractor
Henrotin
    forceps
    speculum
Henry
    incision
    operation
    splenectomy
hepatectomize
hepaticocholangiocholecystoen-
    terostomy
hepaticocholangiojejunostomy
hepatolithectomy
hepatopexy
hepatoscopy
Herbert-Adams
    clamp
Herff
    clamp
Herman-Taylor
    gastroscope
hernia
    abdominal h.
    acquired h.
    h. adiposa
    amniotic h.
    Barth h.
    Béclard h.
    Birkett h.
    cecal h.
    Cloquet h.
    Cooper h.
    crural h.

hernia (continued)
    diverticular h.
    duodenojejunal h.
    encysted h.
    epigastric h.
    extrasaccular h.
    femoral h.
    foraminal h.
    funicular h.
    gastroesophageal h.
    Gibbon h.
    gluteal h.
    Goyrand h.
    Gruber h.
    Grynfelt h.
    Hesselbach h.
    Hey h.
    Holthouse h.
    incisional h.
    indirect h.
    infantile h.
    inguinocrural h.
    inguinofemoral h.
    inguinoproperitoneal h.
    inguinosuperficial h.
    h. in recto
    intermuscular h.
    interparietal h.
    intersigmoid h.
    interstitial h.
    irreducible h.
    ischiatic h.
    ischiorectal h.
    Krönlein h.
    Küster h.
    labial h.
    Laugier h.
    levator h.
    linea alba h.
    Littré h.
    Littré-Richter h.
    lumbar h.
    Maydl h.
    mesenteric h.
    mesocolic h.
    mucosal h.
    oblique h.
    obturator h.

hernia (continued)
 omental h.
 ovarian h.
 pantaloon h.
 paraesophageal h.
 paraperitoneal h.
 parasaccular h.
 paraumbilical h.
 h. par glissement
 parietal h.
 pectineal h.
 perineal h.
 Petit h.
 properitoneal h.
 pudendal h.
 pulsion h.
 rectal h.
 reducible h.
 retrograde h.
 retroperitoneal h.
 Richter h.
 Rieux h.
 Rokitansky h.
 sciatic h.
 scrotal h.
 sliding h.
 strangulated h.
 subpubic h.
 synovial h.
 thyroidal h.
 tonsillar h.
 Treitz h.
 tunicary h.
 uterine h.
 vaginal h.
 vaginolabial h.
 Velpeau h.
 ventral h.
 vesical h.
 voluminous h.
 Von Bergman h.
 W h.
hernioappendectomy
hernioenterotomy
herniolaparotomy
herniopuncture
herniotome
herniotomy

Herrick
 clamp
Hess
 forceps
 spoon
Hess-Barraquer
 forceps
Hess-Horwitz
 forceps
heteroautoplasty
heteroscope
Hey
 skull saw
Heyer
 valve
Heyer-Schulte
 prosthesis
Hey Groves
 operation
hiatopexy
Hibbs
 curet
 elevator
 forceps
 frame
 gouge
 osteotome
 retractor
Hickman
 catheter
Higgins
 incision
Hildreth cautery
Hill-Ferguson
 retractor
Hillis
 retractor
Himmelstein
 valvulotome
Hinkle-James
 rectal speculum
Hippel. See *von Hippel.*
Hirschman
 anoscope
 forceps
 proctoscope
Hirschman-Martin
 proctoscope

Hirschowitz
    gastroduodenal fiberscope
    gastroscope
Hirst-Emmett
    forceps
histotome
Hochenegg
    operation
hockey-stick incision
Hodge
    forceps
    pessary
    plane
Hodgen
    apparatus
    splint
hoe
    Hough h.
Hoen
    plate
    skull plate
Hoffmann
    forceps
    punch
    rongeur
Hoguet
    maneuver
    operation
Hohmann
    retractor
Hoke
    osteotome
Holden
    curet
holder
    broach h.
    Castroviejo h.
    clamp h.
    needle h.
    rubber dam clamp h.
    sponge h.
hole saw
Holinger
    applicator
    bronchoscope
    dissector
    esophagoscope
    forceps

Holinger (continued)
    laryngoscope
    telescope
    tube
Holinger-Jackson
    bronchoscope
Holman-Mathieu
    cannula
Holmes
    gouge
    nasopharyngoscope
Holter shunt
Holth
    forceps
Holtz
    curet
homoplasty
Hood [eponym]
    dermatome
Hood and Kirklin
    incision
hook
    Adson h.
    Barr crypt h.
    Barr fistula h.
    Barr rectal h.
    Blair palate h.
    Boettcher h.
    Bose tracheostomy h.
    Boyes-Goodfellow h.
    Braun h.
    Braun-Jardine-DeLee h.
    Buck h.
    Carroll bone h.
    Carroll h. curet
    Dandy h.
    Dudley h.
    Duplay h.
    dural h.
    Edwards h.
    Emmet h.
    fixation h.
    Frazier h. retractor
    Gillies h.
    Gillies-Dingman h.
    Graefe (von Graefe) h.
    Graham h.
    Green h.

hook (continued)
- House h.
- Jameson h.
- Kelly h.
- Kimball h.
- Kirby h.
- Lillie h.
- Linton h.
- Mayo h.
- New h.
- Newman h.
- Nugent h.
- O'Connor h.
- Pratt h.
- Rosser h.
- Schuknecht h.
- Schwartz h.
- Shambaugh h.
- Shea h.
- Smith h.
- Stevens h.
- Stewart h.
- tracheostomy h.
- Tyrell h.
- Welch-Allyn h.
- Wiener h.

hook-on bronchoscope

Hopkins
- clamp
- operation

Hopp
- laryngoscope

horizontal
- h. incision
- h. mattress suture

horsehair suture

Horsley
- bone-cutting forceps
- test
- wax

hot-tip, hot-tipped
- h.-t. laser probe
- h.-t. probe

Hotz
- curet

Hough
- hoe

Hourin
- needle

House
- chisel
- curet
- elevator
- forceps
- hook
- knife
- needle
- prosthesis
- scissors
- tube

House-Barbara
- needle

House-Rosen
- needle

House-Urban
- retractor

Housset-Debray
- gastroscope

Howard
- abrader
- basket
- forceps
- method

Howard-Dolman
- apparatus

Hoxworth
- forceps

Hruby lens

Hudgins
- cannula

Hudson
- brace
- bur
- clamp
- drill
- forceps

Hueter
- bandage

Huey
- scissors

Huffman-Graves
- speculum

Hufnagel
- clamp
- knife

Hufnagel (continued)
    prosthesis
Hulka
    clip
Hume
    clamp
Humphries
    clamp
Hunt
    clamp
    forceps
    operation
Hunter
    curet
Hurd
    dissector
    elevator
    forceps
Hurst
    bougie
Hurtig
    dilator
Hurwitz
    clamp
    trocar
Hutchins
    needle
Hyams
    clamp
    scleral knife
hydrodiascope
Hydroflex
    penile prosthesis
hydrophilic lens
hydrotomy
hypodermatomy
hypodermic
    h. needle
hypodermoclysis
hypopharyngoscope
hysterectomy
    Ballantine h. forceps
    Carmalt h. forceps
    h. and radiation (H&R)
hysterocolposcope
hysteroscope
    Baggish h.
    Baloser h.

hysteroscope (continued)
    Storz h.
hysterostat
hysterotome
ICLH apparatus
I&D—irrigation and débridement
Iglesias
    resectoscope
iliocolotomy
Ilizarov leg-lengthening procedure
imbricated
    i. suture
Immergut
    tube
immersion
    i. microscopy
Imperatori
    forceps
implant
    sponge i.
    wire mesh i.
implanted suture
impregnated
    i. dressing
incised
incision
    abdominal i.
    abdominothoracic i.
    ab externo i.
    Agnew-Verhoeff i.
    alar i.
    Alexander i.
    angular i.
    arcuate i.
    areolar i.
    Auvray i.
    backcut i.
    Battle i.
    Battle-Jalaguier-Kammerer i.
    bayonet i.
    Bergmann i.
    Bergmann-Israel i.
    Bevan i.
    bivalve i., bivalved i.
    Brackin i.
    Brock i.
    bur-hole i.
    buttonhole i.

incision (continued)
    cervical i.
    Cherney i.
    Chernez i.
    chevron-shaped i.
    Chiene i.
    circular i.
    circumareolar i.
    circumcisional i.
    circumferential i.
    circumlimbal i.
    circumscribing i.
    Clute i.
    Codman i.
    Coffey i.
    collar i.
    confirmatory i.
    conjunctival i.
    corneoscleral i.
    cortical i.
    Courvoisier i.
    crescent i.
    crosshatch i.
    crucial i.
    cruciate i.
    curved i.
    curvilinear i.
    Deaver i.
    decompression i.
    deltopectoral i.
    dorsolateral i.
    double-Y i.
    Dührssen i.
    dural i.
    Edebohls i.
    elliptical i.
    Elsberg i.
    endaural i.
    exploratory i.
    Fergusson i.
    fishmouth i.
    flank i.
    flexed i.
    Fowler i.
    Fowler-Weir i.
    Furniss i.
    Gatellier i.
    Gibson i.

incision (continued)
    Gluck i.
    Greenhow i.
    gridiron i.
    guillotine i.
    Halsted i.
    Handley i.
    Harmon i.
    Hayes Martin i.
    Heermann i.
    hemitransfixion i.
    Henry i.
    Higgins i.
    hockey-stick i.
    Hood and Kirklin i.
    horizontal i.
    inframammary i.
    infraumbilical i.
    inguinal i.
    intercartilaginous i.
    intracapsular i.
    Jackson i.
    J-shaped i.
    Kammerer i.
    Kehr i.
    Kocher i.
    Küstner i.
    lamellar i.
    Lamm i.
    lateral flank i.
    lateral rectus i.
    lazy H i.
    lazy S i.
    lazy Z i.
    Lempert i.
    Lilienthal i.
    limbal i.
    linear i.
    Linton i.
    longitudinal i.
    Lynch i.
    MacFee i.
    Mackenrodt i.
    Mason i.
    mastoid i.
    Maylard i.
    Mayo-Robson i.
    McArthur i.

incision (continued)
McBurney i.
McLaughlin i.
McVay i.
meatal i.
median i.
Meyer hockey-stick i.
midline i.
Mikulicz i.
Morison i.
muscle-splitting i.
Nagamatsu i.
oblique i.
Ollier i.
Orr i.
paracostal i.
parainguinal i.
paramedian i.
paramuscular i.
parapatellar i.
pararectus i.
parasagittal i.
parascapular i.
paraumbilical i.
paravaginal i.
Parker i.
Péan i.
perianal i.
periareolar i.
perilimbal i.
periscapular i.
peritoneal i.
Perthes i.
Pfannenstiel i.
Phemister i.
popliteal i.
postauricular i.
posterior i.
posterolateral i.
proximal i.
racquet i.
radial i.
rectus muscle–splitting i.
recumbent i.
relief i.
retroauricular i.
rim i.
Robertson i.

incision (continued)
Rockey-Davis i.
Rodman i.
Rollet i.
Rosen i.
Roux-en-Y jejunal loop i.
Ruddy i.
saber-cut i.
salmon backcut i.
Sanders i.
Schobinger i.
Schuchardt i.
scratch-type i.
semicircular i.
semiflexed i.
semilunar i.
serpentine i.
Shambaugh i.
shelving i.
shoulder-strap i.
Simon i.
Singleton i.
Sloan i.
spiral i.
stab wound i.
stellate i.
sternal-splitting i.
Stewart i.
Strömbeck i.
subcostal i.
subinguinal i.
submammary i.
subtrochanteric i.
subumbilical i.
supracervical i.
suprapubic i.
supraumbilical i.
temporal i.
Thomas-Warren i.
thoracoabdominal i.
Timbrall-Fisher i.
transection i.
transmeatal i.
transrectus i.
transverse i.
trap-door i.
T-shaped i.
U-shaped i.

incision (continued)
    vertical i.
    Vischer i.
    V-shaped i.
    Warren i.
    Watson-Jones i.
    Weber-Fergusson i.
    wedge i.
    Whipple i.
    Wilde i.
    W-shaped i.
    Y i., Y-type i.
    Yorke-Mason i.
    Z-flap i.
    Z-shaped i.
incisional
indigo carmine
indirect
    i. ophthalmoscope
indwelling
    i. catheter
inframammary
    i. incision
infraumbilical
    i. incision
infusion
    i. cannula
Ingals
    cannula
    speculum
Ingersoll
    curet
Ingram
    trocar catheter
inguinal
    i. incision
inlet
    i. forceps
inoscopy
insertion
    i. forceps
insufflator
    Buckstein i.
    Kidde tubal i.
    Weber i.
integrating microscope
intercartilaginous
    i. incision

interlocking
    i. sutures
internal
    i. stripper
interrupted
    i. suture
interval
    i. operation
intestinal
    i. tube
intracapsular
    i. incision
intracardiac
    i. catheter
Intracath
    catheter
intradermal
    i. mattress suture
    i. suture
intradermic suture
intraluminal
    i. catheter
    i. stripper
intramedullary
    i. drill
intraperitoneal
    i. catheter
intratracheal
introducer
    Carter i.
    Littleford-Spector i.
intubation
    i. tube
invaginating suture
inverted, inverting
    i. suture
iodoform
    i. dressing
    i. gauze packing
IOL—intraocular lens
Ionescu-Shiley
    prosthesis
ionoscope
Iowa
    forceps
iridectomy
    laser i.

iris
 i. scissors
irrigation
 i. cannula
irrigator
 Buie i.
 Rollet i.
Irvine
 scissors
 syndrome
ischial
 i. weightbearing (weight-
  bearing) brace
isograft
isolator
isoscope
Israel
 retractor
Itard
 catheter
Ivalon
 implant
 suture
Iverson dermabrader
Ives
 anoscope
Ivy
 loop wiring
 wire
Jaboulay
 button
 operation
Jackson
 appliance
 bistoury
 bougie
 bronchoscope
 clamp
 dilator
 elevator
 esophagoscope
 forceps
 incision
 laryngoscope
 retractor
 safety triangle
 scalpel
 scissors

Jackson (continued)
 tenaculum
 tube
Jackson-Babcock
 operation
Jackson-Mosher
 dilator
Jackson-Pratt
 catheter
 tube
Jackson-Trousseau
 dilator
Jacobaeus
 thoracoscope
Jacobs
 forceps
 uterine tenaculum
Jacobson
 clamp
 forceps
 retractor
 scissors
 spatula
Jacobs-Palmer
 laparoscope
Jaeger
 keratome
Jako
 laryngoscope
Jameson
 calipers
 forceps
 hook
Jamshidi
 needle
Janeway
 gastroscope
Jansen
 forceps
 retractor
Jansen-Middleton
 forceps
Jansen-Newhart
 probe
Jansen-Struycken
 forceps
Jarcho
 cannula

Jarcho (continued)
    forceps
Jarvis
    clamp
Javid
    bypass clamp
Javid shunt
jejunostomy
    Baker j. tube
Jelanko arch bar
Jelk
    operation
Jenckel method
Jennings mouth gag
Jesberg
    bronchoscope
    clamp
    esophagoscope
Jewett
    extractor
    nail
    plate
Jobert
    suture
Johns Hopkins
    clamp
    forceps
Johnson
    basket
    calculation
    forceps
    needle holder
    stone dislodger
    tube
joker elevator
Jolly
    dilator
Jonas-Graves
    speculum
Jones
    curet
    dilator
    forceps
    scissors
Jonge position
Jordan-Day
    bur
    drill

Jorgenson
    scissors
Joseph
    clamp
    knife
    periosteotome
    saw
    scissors
Joseph-Maltz
    saw
J-shaped incision
Judd
    forceps
    retractor
Judd-Allis
    forceps
Judd-DeMartel
    forceps
Judd-Masson
    retractor
Judet
    prosthesis
Juers-Lempert
    forceps
Juevenell
    clamp
Julian
    forceps
Jurasz
    forceps
Jutte
    tube
Kader-Senn
    operation
Kahler
    forceps
Kahn
    cannula
    tenaculum
Kahn-Graves
    speculum
Kalt
    forceps
    needle holder
    suture
Kammerer
    incision

Kanavel
    apparatus
    brain-exploring cannula
    conductor
    splint
Kane
    clamp
kangaroo tendon suture
Kantor
    clamp
Kantrowicz
    clamp
Kaplan
    needle
Kapp-Beck
    clamp
Kara erysiphake
Karman
    cannula
    catheter
Katzin
    scissors
Katzin-Barraquer
    forceps
Kay-Shiley
    prosthesis
Kay Suzuki
    prosthesis
Kazanjian
    forceps
    line
    splint
keel
    McNaught k.
Keeley
    stripper
Kehr
    incision
Keith
    needle
Keitzer
    urethrotome
Keller-Blake
Kelley adenotome
Kelling
    gastroscope
Kelly
    adenotome

Kelly (continued)
    clamp
    curet
    cystoscope
    dilator
    endoscope
    forceps
    hook
    proctoscope
    retractor
    scissors
    sigmoidoscope
    speculum
    sphincteroscope
    suture
    tube
Kelly-Gray
    curet
Kelman
    forceps
kelotomy
Kennedy
    bar
    forceps
keratoiridoscope
keratome
    Agnew k.
    Beaver k.
    Berens k.
    Castroviejo k.
    Grieshaber k.
    Jaeger k.
    Kirby k.
keratoplasty
    Barraquer k. knife
keratoscope
Kern
    forceps
Kernan-Jackson
    bronchoscope
Kerrison
    forceps
    punch
    retractor
    rongeur
Kessel plate
Kestenbach-Anderson procedure

Kevorkian
    curet
Keyes
    biopsy punch
    dermal punch
    lithotrite
Kezerian
    osteotome
Kidde tubal insufflator
kidney
    k. internal splint/stent
        (KISS) catheter
Kielland (Kjelland)
    forceps
Kielland-Luikart
    forceps
Killian
    chisel
    elevator
    forceps
    knife
    nasal speculum
    rectal speculum
    tube
Killian-King
    retractor
Kimball
    hook
Kimpton-Brown
    tube
kinescope
kinetoscope
King
    retractor
Kingsley
    appliance plate
    splint
Kinsella-Buie
    clamp
Kirby
    forceps
    hook
    keratome
    knife
    retractor
    scissors
    spoon

Kirkland
    knife
Kirschner
    apparatus
    splint
    suture
    wire
    wire splint
KISS—kidney internal splint/stent
    [catheter]
Kistner
    tube
Kittner
    forceps
Klatskin
    needle
KleenSpec
    sigmoidoscope
Klemme
    retractor
Klenzak
    brace
Kloehn headgear
Knapp
    forceps
    knife
    needle
    retractor
    scissors
    scoop
    spatula
    speculum
    spoon
knife
    Adson k.
    Austin k.
    Ayerst k.
    Bailey-Glover-O'Neill k.
    Bailey-Morse k.
    Ballenger swivel k.
    Bard-Parker k.
    Barkan k.
    Barraquer keratoplasty k.
    Beaver k.
    Beck k.
    bladebreaker k.
    Blair-Brown k.
    Blair cleft palate k.

knife (continued)
- Bonta k.
- Bosher k.
- Brock k.
- Brophy k.
- Brown k.
- Buck k.
- Bucy k.
- Caltagirone k.
- Canfield k.
- Carpenter k.
- Castroviejo k.
- Colver k.
- Cottle k.
- Crile k.
- Dean k.
- Derlacki k.
- Derra k.
- Desmarres k.
- Douglas k.
- Downing k.
- Elschnig k.
- Equen-Neuffer k.
- Ferris-Robb k.
- Fisher k.
- Fleming k.
- Fletcher k.
- Fomon k.
- Freer k.
- Freiberg k.
- Friesner k.
- Gandhi k.
- Gill k.
- Goodyear k.
- Graefe (von Graefe) k.
- Green k.
- Harrison k.
- House k.
- Hufnagel k.
- Hyams scleral k.
- Joseph k.
- Killian k.
- Kirby k.
- Kirkland k.
- Knapp k.
- Lancaster k.
- Lebsche k.
- Leland k.

knife (continued)
- Lempert k.
- lenticular k.
- Liston k.
- Lothrop k.
- Löwe-Breck k.
- Lundsgaard k.
- Lynch k.
- MacKenty k.
- Maltz k.
- McHugh k.
- McPherson-Wheeler k.
- McPherson-Ziegler k.
- McReynolds k.
- meniscectomy k.
- k. needle
- Niedner k.
- Nunez-Nunez k.
- Pace k.
- Parker k.
- Robertson k.
- Rochester k.
- Rosen k.
- Scheie k.
- Schuknecht k.
- Seiler k.
- Sellor k.
- Sexton k.
- Shambaugh-Lempert k.
- Shea k.
- Sheehy k.
- Smillie k.
- Smith-Green k.
- Thiersch k.
- Tobold k.
- Tooke k.
- Tydings k.
- Virchow k.
- Weber k.
- Wheeler k.
- Wullstein k.
- Ziegler k.

knife needle
- Davis k.n.

Knight
- brace
- forceps
- scissors

Knight-Sluder
    forceps
Knight-Taylor
    brace
knitted vascular prosthesis
Knowles
    scissors
Kocher
    clamp
    dissector
    forceps
    incision
    retractor
    ulcer
Kocher-Crotti
    retractor
Koeberlé
    forceps
Koffler
    forceps
Koffler-Lillie
    forceps
Kolb
    forceps
Kollmann
    dilator
Kolodny
    hemostat
Kondoleon
    operation
Kos
    cannula
Kowalzig
    operation
Kramer
    speculum
Kraske
    position
Kratz lens
Krause
    cannula
    forceps
    snare
Kreuscher
    scissors
Kron
    bile duct probe
    dilator

Kronecker
    needle
Kronfeld
    forceps
    retractor
Krupin valve
Kruse brush
kryoscopy
Kuhn
    tube
Kuhnt
    forceps
Kulvin-Kalt
    forceps
Kurten
    stripper
Kushner-Tandatnick
    curet
Küstner
    incision
Kydex
    brace
Kyle
    speculum
kymoscope
Laborde
    dilator
    forceps
lace
    l. suture
lacrimal
    l. probe
lacrimotome
lactoscope
Ladd
    calipers
LaForce
    adenotome
    spud
    tonsillectome
LaForce-Grieshaber
    adenotome
Lagrange
    scissors
Lahey
    carrier
    clamp
    forceps

Lahey (continued)
    operation
    retractor
    tenaculum
Lahey-Péan
    forceps
Laing plate
Lambert
    forceps
Lambotte
    clamp
    forceps
    osteotome
Lambotte-Henderson
    osteotome
lamellar
    l. incision
laminectomy
    Beckman-Adson l. retractor
Lamm
    incision
Lamont
    elevator
    saw
Lancaster
    knife
    speculum
Lane
    catheter
    clamp
    elevator
    forceps
    mouth gag
    operation
Lange
    skinfold calipers
    speculum
Langenbeck (von Langenbeck)
    elevator
    saw
Lanz
    tube
laparocystidotomy
laparoenterotomy
laparogastroscopy
laparogastrostomy
laparogastrotomy
laparohepatotomy

laparoileotomy
laparorrhaphy
laparoscope
    ACMI l.
    Eder l.
    Jacobs-Palmer l.
    Lent l.
    Wolf l.
laparotome
laparotrachelotomy
laparotyphlotomy
Lapides
    needle holder
Lardennois button
LaRocca
    tube
Larry
    rectal director
    rectal probe
laryngendoscope
laryngoscope
    Albert-Andrews l.
    Atkins-Tucker l.
    Bizzarri-Guiffrida l.
    Broyles l.
    Chevalier Jackson l.
    Clerf l.
    commissure l.
    Dedo l.
    Dedo-Pilling l.
    fiberoptic l.
    Fink l.
    Flagg l.
    Foregger l.
    Garfield-Holinger l.
    Guedel l.
    Haslinger l.
    Holinger l.
    Hopp l.
    Jackson l.
    Jako l.
    Lewy l.
    Lundy l.
    Lynch l.
    MacIntosh l.
    Magill l.
    Miller l.
    reverse-bevel l.

laryngoscope (continued)
    Roberts l.
    rotating l.
    Rusch l.
    Sanders l.
    self-retaining l.
    Siker l.
    slotted l.
    suspension l.
    Tucker l.
    Welch-Allyn l.
    Wis-Foregger l.
    Wis-Hipple l.
    Yankauer l.
laryngostomy
    l. tube
laryngostroboscope
laryngotomy
    l. tube
laser
    argon l.
    carbon dioxide l.
    dye l.
    helium-neon l.
    Hruby l.
    ion l.
    l. iridectomy
    krypton l.
    neodymium:yttrium-alumi-
       num-garnet (Nd:YAG) l.
    l. photocoagulation
    ruby l.
    Sharplan 733 CO_2 [CO2] l.
    Visulas Nd:YAG l.
    xenon arc l.
LASER—light amplification by
    stimulated emission of radia-
    tion [now: laser]
lateral
    l. flank incision
    l. rectus incision
latex
    l. catheter
    l. drain
Lathbury
    applicator
Latrobe
    retractor

Laufe
    forceps
Laufe-Barton-Kielland
    forceps
Laufe-Piper
    forceps
Laugier hernia
Lawson
    operation
Lawson-Thorton plate
lazy H incision
lazy S incision
lazy Z incision
Leader-Kollmann
    dilator
Lebsche
    forceps
    knife
    shears
Le Dentu
    suture
Le Dran
    suture
Lee
    bronchus clamp
    wedge resection clamp
Le Fort
    bougie
    catheter
    sound
    suture
Legg
    osteotome
Legueu
    retractor
Lehman
    catheter
Leinbach
    osteotome
Lejeune
    applicator
    scissors
Leksell
    forceps
    rongeur
Leland
    knife

Leland-Jones
>forceps
Lell
>esophagoscope
Lembert
>suture
Lempert
>bur
>curet
>elevator
>forceps
>incision
>knife
>perforator
>retractor
>rugine
Lempert-Colver
>endaural speculum
Lempka
>stripper
Lennarson
>tube
Lenox Hill
>brace
lens
>l. sutures
Lent
>laparoscope
lenticular
>l. knife
Lentulo
>spiral drill
Lepley-Ernst
>tube
leptoscope
Leriche
>forceps
Lermoyez
>punch
L'Esperance erysiphake
Lester Martin procedure
leukoscope
leukotome
>Bailey l.
>Love l.
Levant
>stone dislodger

levator (levatores)
>l. resection
LeVeen
>peritoneal shunt
lever-compression clamp
Levin
>tube
Levret
>forceps
Lewin
>dissector
>forceps
Lewin-Stern splint
Lewis
>forceps
>rasp
>scoop
>tube
Lewkowitz
>forceps
Lewy
>laryngoscope
Lewy-Rubin
>needle
Leyro-Diaz
>forceps
Lichtwicz
>trocar
lid
>l. speculum
Liddle
>aorta clamp
Lieb and Guerry
>cataract implant lens
Lieberman
>proctoscope
>sigmoidoscope
Lifemed
>cannula
ligament
>Cooper l.
>gastrocolic l.
>gastrolienal l.
>gastrophrenic l.
>Gimbernat l.
>hepatogastric l.
>Hesselbach l.
>lienorenal l.

ligament (continued)
    pancreaticosplenic l.
    pectineal l.
    phrenicocolic l.
    phrenicolienal l.
    phrenicosplenic l.
    Poupart l.
    splenocolic l.
    splenorenal l.
    l. of Treitz
ligamentopexy
ligation
    high saphenous vein l.
    l. suture
ligature
    free l. suture
    McGraw elastic l.
    l. needle
    suture l.
light
Light-Veley headrest
Lilienthal
    incision
    probe
Lillehei-Kaster
    prosthesis
Lillie
    forceps
    hook
    scissors
    speculum
limbal
    l. incision
Limberg flap
Lincoff
    sponge
Lindeman-Silverstein
    tube
Lindner
    spatula
line
    iliopectineal l.
    median l.
    pectinate l.
    pectineal l.
    semilunar l. of Spieghel
    Spieghel l.
    spigelian l.

line (continued)
    Spigelius l.
linear
    l. incision
linguotrite
Linton
    clamp
    hook
    incision
    operation
    procedure
    retractor
    tube
lion-jawed forceps
lip
    l. adhesion operation
Lippman
    prosthesis
Lister
    dressing
    forceps
    scissors
Lister-Burch
    speculum
Liston
    knife
    scissors
    shears
Liston-Stille
    forceps
lithoscope
lithotome
lithotomy
    dorsal l. position
    l. position
lithotresis
lithotripsy
lithotriptor
    Dornier gallstone l.
lithotriptoscope
lithotrite
    Alcock l.
    Alcock-Hendrickson l.
    Bigelow l.
    cystoscopic l.
    electrohydraulic l.
    Hendrickson l.
    Keyes l.

lithotrite (continued)
    Löwenstein l.
    Lowsley l.
    Reliquet l.
    Thompson l.
Littauer
    forceps
    scissors
Littauer-Liston
    forceps
Little [eponym]
    intraocular lens (IOL) implant
    retractor
Littleford-Spector
    introducer
Littre
    hernia
    suture
Litwak
    scissors
Lloyd
    catheter
locator
lock
    bite l. [also: bitelock, bite-lock]
    l. forceps
locking
    l. suture
lock-stitch suture
Lockwood
    clamp
    forceps
Löffler
    suture
logoscope
Lombard-Boies rongeur
Long
    forceps
Long Island
    forceps
longitudinal
    l. incision
long leg brace
loop
    Cannon endarterectomy l.
    cutting l.
    l.-on mucosa suture

loop (continued)
    Silastic l.'s
    l. suture
loopful
Lord
    operation
Lore-Lawrence
    tube
Loreta
    operation
Loring
    ophthalmoscope
Lotheissen
    operation
Lothrop
    knife
    retractor
Lounsbury
    curet
loupe [magnifying lens]
Love
    leukotome
    retractor
Love-Adson
    elevator
Love-Gruenwald
    forceps
    rongeur
Love-Kerrison
    forceps
Lovelace
    forceps
Löwe-Breck
Lowe-Breck
    knife
Löwenberg
    forceps
Löwenstein
    lithotrite
Lower [eponym]
    forceps
Lowman
    clamp
Lowsley
    forceps
Lowsley-Peterson
    cystoscope
LSU reciprocation-gait orthosis brace

Lubafax
    dressing
Luc
    forceps
Lucae
    forceps
    mallet
Lucas
    chisel
    curet
    gouge
Luck
    fasciatome
Luer
    forceps
    retractor
    syringe
    tube
Luer-Korte
    scoop
Luhr maxillofacial system
Luikart
    forceps
Luikart-Bill traction handle
Luikart-Simpson
    forceps
Lukens
    retractor
    trap
lumbar puncture needle
luminoscope
Lundsgaard
    knife
Lundsgaard-Burch
    sclerotome
Lundy
    laryngoscope
Luongo
    retractor
Lutz
    forceps
Lyman-Smith
    brace
lymphadenectomy
lymphadenocele
lymphadenotomy
lymphangiectomy

lymphangioplasty
    Handley l.
lymphaticostomy
lymphotome
Lynch
    dissector
    forceps
    incision
    knife
    laryngoscope
    operation
    scissors
Lyster
    tube
Lytle splint
MA—Miller-Abbott (tube)
MacDonald
    clamp
MacFee
    incision
Machemer
    calipers
MacIntosh
    fiberoptic laryngoscope blade
    laryngoscope
    prosthesis
Mack
    tonsillectome
Mackenrodt
    incision
MacKenty
    elevator
    knife
    tube
Mackenzie
    See *McKenzie.*
Mackid
    operation
Maclay
    scissors
Madden technique
Magill
    laryngoscope
Magovern
    prosthesis
Mahoney
    speculum

Maier
    forceps
Maingot
    hemostat
Mair
    operation
Maisonneuve
    urethrotome
major
    m. operation
    m. surgery
malacotomy
Malecot
    catheter
    drain
Malis coagulator
mallet
    Crane m.
    Lucae m.
    Meyerding m.
    Rush m.
malleus
    m. shears
Malm-Himmelstein
    valvulotome
Maloney
    dilator
Maltz
    knife
    rasp
    saw
Maltz-Lipsett
    rasp
mammectomy
Mancini plates
Mann
    forceps
manner
    in a m. after Tom Jones
manoptoscope
manoscopy
Mantz
    dilator
many-tailed dressing
Maquet technique
Marcy
    operation

margin
    falciform m. of fascia lata
    falciform m. of saphenus
        hiatus
    falciform m. of white line of
        pelvic fascia
marker
    D'Assumpcao rhytidoplasty
        m.
Marlex
    atraumatic tenaculum
    bandage
    graft
    mesh
    suture
Marshall
    surgical sucker
Marshik
    forceps
Martel
    clamp
Martin
    forceps
    needle
    pelvimeter
    retractor
    speculum
    tube
Martin and Davy
    speculum
Martius
    fat pad graft
Marwedel
    operation
Maryan
    forceps
mask
    tracheostomy m.
    Venturi m.
Mason
    incision
Mason-Allen splint
Mason-Auvard
    speculum
Massiot
    polytome
Masson-Judd
    retractor

Mastin
    clamp
mastoid
    m. incision
Matchett-Brown
    prosthesis
Mathews
    speculum
Mathieu
    forceps
Matson
    elevator
Mattox
    clamp
mattress
    end-on m. suture
    horizontal m. suture
    intradermal m. suture
    right-angle m. suture
    m. suture
    vertical m. suture
Maumenee erysiphake
Maumenee-Park
    speculum
Maunsell
    suture
maxillofacial
    m. prosthesis
Maydl
    hernia
Mayer
    pessary
    speculum
Mayfield
    clip
    osteotome
Maylard
    incision
Mayo
    cannula
    carrier
    clamp
    forceps
    hook
    linen suture
    needle
    probe
    retractor

Mayo (continued)
    scissors
    scoop
    stripper
Mayo-Blake
    forceps
Mayo-Collins
    retractor
Mayo-Harrington
    scissors
Mayo-Lovelace
    retractor
Mayo-Noble
    scissors
Mayo-Ochsner
    forceps
Mayo-Robson
    forceps
    incision
    operation
    position
    scoop
Mayo-Russian
    forceps
Mayo-Sims
    scissors
McArthur
    incision
    method
    operation
McAtee screw
McBurney
    incision
    operation
    point
McCarthy
    cystoscope
    forceps
    Foroblique panendoscope
    resectoscope
    telescope
McCarthy-Alcock
    forceps
McCarthy-Campbell
    cystoscope
McCarthy-Peterson
    cystoscope

McCaskey
    curet
McClure
    scissors
McCrea sound
McCullough
    forceps
McCurdy
    needle
McDonald
    clamp
McDonald, W. Dean
    clamp
McEvedy
    operation
McGannon
    retractor
McGoon technique
McGraw elastic ligature
McGuire
    scissors
McHenry
    forceps
McHugh
    knife
    speculum
McIndoe
    elevator
McIntire aspiration-irrigation system
McIver
    nephrostomy catheter
McIvor mouth gag
McKay
    forceps
McKee-Farrar
    acetabular cup
    prosthesis
McKeever
    prosthesis
McKenzie
    bur
    clip
    drill
    forceps
McLane
    forceps
McLane-Tucker
    forceps

McLane-Tucker-Luikart
    forceps
McLaughlin
    incision
McLean
    scissors
McNealy-Glassman-Babcock
    forceps
McNealy-Glassman-Mixter
    forceps
McPherson
    forceps
    needle holder
    scissors
    spatula
    speculum
McPherson-Castroviejo
    scissors
McPherson-Vannas
    scissors
McPherson-Wheeler
    blade
    knife
McPherson-Ziegler
    knife
McReynolds
    knife
McVay
    incision
McWhinnie
    dissector
meatal
    m. incision
meatometer
meatoscope
meatotome
median
    m. incision
mediastinoscope
    Carlens m.
    Goldberg MPC m.
MediPort vascular access device
Medrafil
    wire suture
Medtronic-Hall valve
Meek-Wall
    dermatome

Meigs
    suture
Meller
    retractor
Mellinger
    speculum
Meltzer
    nasopharyngoscope
membrane
    Cargile m.
    serous m.
membranous
    m. adhesions
Menge
    pessary
Menghini
    needle
meniscectomy
    m. knife
meniscotome
    Bowen-Grover m.
meniscus lens
Mercedes
    tip cannula
Mercurio position
Mermingas
    operation
Mersilene
    gauze dressing
    suture
mesh
    Dexon m.
    fine m. dressing
    Marlex m.
    steel m. suture
    tantalum m.
    Teflon m.
    Vitallium m.
    wire m.
meshwork
    trabecular m.
mesocolon
    ascending m.
    descending m.
    sigmoid m.
    transverse m.
metalloscopy

method
    See also *maneuver, operation, procedure, surgery,* and *technique.*
    Jenckel m.
    Torkildsen shunt m.
    Wardill four-flap m.
    Wardill two-flap m.
Metras
    catheter
metronoscope
metroscope
Metzenbaum
    forceps
    scissors
Metzenbaum-Lipsett
    scissors
Meyer
    hockey-stick incision
    operation
    retractor
    stripper
Meyerding
    curet
    osteotome
    retractor
Meyhoeffer
    curet
Michel
    clip
    trephine
Michelson
    bronchoscope
microdermatome
microdissection
microelectrode
microgonioscope
microinjector
microneedle
microphthalmoscope
micropolariscope
microprobe
microscope
    corneal m.
    dissecting m.
    ocular m.
    Omni operating m.
    operating m.

microscope (continued)
    optical m.
    slit lamp m.
    surgical m.
    Wild operating m.
    Zeiss m.
microscopy
    immersion m.
    television m.
microspectroscope
microsuture
microsyringe
microtome
    freezing m.
    rocking m.
    rotary m.
    sliding m.
    Stadie-Riggs m.
microvascular clamp
Middleton
    curet
midline
    m. incision
Mikulicz (von Mikulicz)
    clamp
    incision
    pack
    resection
Miles
    operation
Milex
    cervitome
Millen technique
Miller
    laryngoscope
    scissors
    speculum
Miller-Abbott (MA)
    tube
Millin
    forceps
    tube
Millin-Bacon
    retractor
    spreader
milliner's needle
Milwaukee
    brace

Miner
    osteotome
Minnesota
    tube
minor
    m. operation
    m. surgery
mirror
    m. drill
Mitchell
    basket
Mitchell-Diamond
    forceps
mitral
    m. prosthesis
Mixter
    dilator
    forceps
MMK operation
modular prosthesis
Moe
    brace
    plate
Moersch
    bronchoscope
    esophagoscope
    forceps
molecular
    m. hybridization probe
Moltz-Storz
    tonsillectome
Monaldi
    drainage system
Moncrieff
    irrigating cannula
Monks
    malar elevator
monofilament
    nylon m. suture
    m. suture
Monro
    line
Montague
    proctoscope
    sigmoidoscope
Montgomery
    tracheocannula
    T tube

moon boot
Moore
    chisel
    extractor
    gouge
    nail
    osteotome
    pin
    prosthesis
    reamer
    scoop
    tracheostomy button
Moorehead
    retractor
Moorhead
    foreign body locator
Morch
    tube
Moreno
    clamp
Morison
    incision
    method
Moritz-Schmidt
    forceps
Morris
    cannula
Morse
    scissors
Mosher
    curet
    dilator
    esophagoscope
    speculum
    tube
mosquito
    m. clamp
    m. forceps
Moult
    curet
Mount-Mayfield
    forceps
Moure
    esophagoscope
Moure-Coryllos
    rib shears
mouse-tooth forceps

mouth gag
    Crowe-Davis m.g., Davis-
      Crowe m.g.
    Denhardt m.g.
    Denhardt-Dingman m.g.
    McIvor m.g.
mouth prop
Moynihan
    clamp
    forceps
    operation
    position
    probe
    scoop
mucotome
Mueller
    cautery
    clamp
    needle
    prosthesis
    retractor
    speculum
Mueller-Frazier
    tube
Mueller-Pool
    tube
Mueller-Pynchon
    tube
Mueller-Yankauer
    tube
Muer
    anoscope
Muldoon
    dilator
multifilament suture
multistrand suture
multitoothed forceps
Mundie
    forceps
Munster
    prosthesis
Murdock-Wiener
    speculum
Murphy
    button
    dilator
    needle
    retractor

Murphy (continued)
    treatment
muscle-splitting incision
Museholdt
    forceps
mushroom
    m. catheter
    Silastic m. catheter
mustache dressing
myelotome
Myerson
    forceps
    saw
Myles
    curet
    forceps
    speculum
    tonsillectome
myoelectric prosthesis
myoscope
myotome
myringoscope
myringotomy
    Venturi m. tube
Nabatoff
    stripper
Nachlas
    tube
Nagamatsu
    incision
nail
    Augustine n.
    Hansen-Street n.
    Harrington n.
    Jewett n.
    Kuntscher n.
    Lottes n.
    Massie n.
    Moore n.
    Neufeld n.
    Pugh n.
    Schneider n.
    Smillie n.
    Smith-Petersen n.
    Thornton n.
    Venable-Stuck n.
    Zickel n. fixation
nail nipper

nasal
    n. speculum
nasoendoscope
nasoendoscopy
nasogastric
    n. catheter
    n. tube
nasopharyngeal
    n. speculum
    n. tube
nasopharyngolaryngoscope
nasopharyngoscope
    Broyles n.
    Holmes n.
    Meltzer n.
nasoscope
nasotracheal
    n. catheter
    n. tube
National
    cystoscope
Neal
    cannula
near-and-far suture
needle
    Abrams n.
    Adson n.
    Amsler n.
    aneurysm n.
    aspirating n.
    atraumatic n.
    Babcock n.
    biopsy n.
    Bowman iris n.
    Brown n.
    Bunnell n.
    butterfly n.
    Calhoun n.
    Calhoun-Merz n.
    cataract n.
    Chiba n.
    Child-Phillips n.
    Cibis ski n.
    coaxial counterflow single-n.
      blood access catheter
    Cone n.
    Cope n.
    Cournand n.

needle (continued)
    Craig n.
    Curry n.
    Cushing n.
    cutting n.
    Davis n.
    Davis knife n.
    Dees n.
    Denis Browne n.
    Deschamps n.
    discission n.
    docking n.
    electrosurgical n.
    fascia n.
    fine n.
    Fischer n.
    Floyd n.
    Flynt n.
    Frankfeldt n.
    Franklin-Silverman n.
    Frederick n.
    Gardner n.
    Goldbacher n.
    Graefe (von Graefe) n.
    Grieshaber n.
    Hagedorn n.
    Hourin n.
    House n.
    House-Barbara n.
    House-Rosen n.
    Hutchins n.
    hypodermic n.
    Jamshidi n.
    Kaplan n.
    Keith n.
    Klatskin n.
    Knapp n.
    knife n.
    Kronecker n.
    Lewy-Rubin n.
    ligature n.
    lumbar puncture n.
    Martin n.
    Mayo n.
    McCurdy n.
    Menghini n.
    milliner's n.
    Mueller n.

needle (continued)
    Murphy n.
    New n.
    Parhad-Poppen n.
    Pereyra n.
    pop-off n.
    radium n.
    Retter n.
    Reverdin n.
    Rochester n.
    Rosen n.
    Sachs n.
    Sanders-Brown-Shaw n.
    Seldinger n.
    Shambaugh n.
    Sheldon-Spatz n.
    Shirodkar n.
    side-cutting spatulated n.
    Silverman n.
    skinny n.
    Smiley-Williams arteriography n.
    spinal n.
    Stocker n.
    stop n.
    swaged n.
    Travenol n.
    Tru-Cut n.
    Tuohy n.
    Turkel n.
    Updegraff n.
    Veenema-Gusberg n.
    ventriculopuncture n.
    Veress n.
    Vicat n.
    Vim-Silverman n.
    Voorhees n.
    Ward-French n.
    Weeks n.
    Wood n.
needle holder
    Barraquer n.h.
    Boynton n.h.
    Castroviejo n.h.
    Castroviejo-Kalt n.h.
    Derf n.h.
    Ellis n.h.
    Green n.h.

needle holder (continued)
  Grieshaber n.h.
  Halsey n.h.
  Heaney n.h.
  Johnson n.h.
  Kalt n.h.
  Lapides n.h.
  McPherson n.h.
  Paton n.h.
  Stratte n.h.
  Young n.h.
  Young-Millin n.h.
Neer
  prosthesis
Negus
  bronchoscope
  esophagoscope
  hydrostatic dilator
  ligature forceps
  tube
Neil-Moore electrode
Neivert
  retractor
Nélaton
  catheter
Nelson
  forceps
  scissors
nephroscope
nephrostomy
  n. tube
nerve
  n. suture
Nesbit
  cystoscope
  resectoscope
Nettleship-Wilder
  dilator
Neubauer
  forceps
Neurolon
  suture
neuropacemaker
neurotome
  Hall n.
Neville
  prosthesis

New [eponym]
  forceps
  hook
  needle
  scissors
  tube
New-Lambotte
  osteotome
Newman
  forceps
  hook
  proctoscope
Nichols
  clamp
Niebauer
  prosthesis
Niedner
  knife
NIH (National Institutes of Health)
  catheter
nipple
  invaginated n.
Noble
  forceps
nonabsorbable, unabsorbable
  n. surgical suture
  n. suture
nonadherent
nonencapsulated
nonfenestrated forceps
nonviable
  n. tissue
nonweightbearing, non-weightbearing
Noon
  AV fistula clamp
noose suture
Northbent
  scissors
Norwood snare
nose
  telescope n.
Nott
  speculum
Novak
  curet
novoscope
Noyes
  forceps

Noyes-Shambaugh
    scissors
Nu-gauze
    dressing
Nugent
    forceps
    hook
Nugent-Gradle
    scissors
Nugent-Green-Dimitry
    erysiphake
Nunez-Nunez
    knife
Nussbaum
    clamp
Nutricath
    catheter
Nuttall
    operation
Nycore
    pigtail catheter
nylon
    n. monofilament suture
0 [zero]—suture size
O'Beirne
    sphincter
    tube
Ober-Barr procedure
Oberst
    operation
oblique
    external o. muscle
    o. incision
    internal o. muscle
obliteration
    percutaneous transhepatic o.
        of varices
O'Brien
    forceps
observation tube
obstetric, obstetrical
    o. forceps
obturator
    Cripps o.
occlusion
    o. clamp
occlusive dressing

Ochsner
    clamp
    forceps
    probe
    scissors
    trocar
    tube
Ochsner-Dixon
    forceps
Ockerblad
    clamp
OCL—Ortho Casting Lab
OCL splint
O'Connor
    hook
ocular
    o. microscope
    o. prosthesis
oculometroscope
odontoscope
odontoscopy
off-loading splint
Ogilvie
    operation
O'Hanlon
    forceps
Oldberg
    dissector
    forceps
    retractor
oligonucleotide
olive
    o. ring
    o. wire
Olivecrona
    clip
olive-tip, olive-tipped
    o.t. bougie
    o.t. catheter
Ollier
    incision
Olympus
    fiberscope
omentectomy
omentopexy
omentoplasty
omentorrhaphy
omentosplenopexy

omentotomy
omentum (omenta)
    colic o.
    gastric o.
    gastrocolic o.
    gastrohepatic o.
    gastrosplenic o.
    greater o.
    lesser o.
    o. majus
    o. minus
    pancreaticosplenic o.
    splenogastric o.
Ommaya reservoir
Omni
    operating microscope
Omnicarbon valve
Omniscience valve
omphalectomy
omphalotomy
oncotomy
opaque
    o. catheter
open
    o. operation
operating microscope
operation
    Abernethy o.
    Allarton o.
    anastomotic o.
    Anson-McVay o.
    Appolito o.
    Armsby o.
    Auchincloss o.
    Bassini o.
    Baynton o.
    Belmas o.
    Bernard o.
    Beyea o.
    Bircher o.
    bloodless o.
    Bobb o.
    Bogue o.
    Bose o.
    Brenner o.
    Bryant o.
    buttonhole o.
    Callisen o.

operation (continued)
    Carrel o.
    Cattell o.
    Chaput o.
    Charles o.
    Cheyne o.
    Chiazzi o.
    Child o.
    Clagett o.
    Cooper o.
    Cotting o.
    Crile-Matas o.
    Cripps o.
    Cushing o.
    Czerny o.
    Dallas o.
    decompression o.
    Denans o.
    Dohlman o.
    Dowell o.
    Drummond-Morison o.
    Eagleton o.
    Ekehorn o.
    exploratory o.
    Franke tabes o.
    Gallie o.
    Graham-Roscie o.
    Grondahl-Finney o.
    Gussenbauer o.
    Hahn o.
    Halsted o.
    Handley o.
    Heaton o.
    Heineke o.
    Henry o.
    Hey Groves o.
    Hochenegg o.
    Hoguet o.
    Hopkins o.
    Hunt o.
    interval o.
    Jaboulay o.
    Jackson-Babcock o.
    Jelk o.
    Kader-Senn o.
    Kondoleon o.
    Kowalzig o.
    Lahey o.

operation (continued)
  Lane o.
  Lawson o.
  Linton o.
  lip adhesion o.
  Lord o.
  Loreta o.
  Lotheissen o.
  Lynch o.
  Mackid o.
  Mair o.
  major o.
  Marcy o.
  Marwedel o.
  Mayo-Robson o.
  McArthur o.
  McBurney o.
  McEvedy o.
  Mermingas o.
  Meyer o.
  Miles o.
  minor o.
  Moynihan o.
  Nuttall o.
  Oberst o.
  Ogilvie o.
  open o.
  Owen o.
  Patey o.
  Peet o.
  Physick o.
  Pirogoff o.
  Pollock o.
  Portmann interposition o.
  Poth o.
  radical o.
  Rashkind o.
  reconstructive o.
  Rehn-Delorme o.
  Ripstein o.
  Roux-en-Y o.
  Scarpa o.
  Schlatter o.
  Senn o.
  seton o.
  Smith-Gibson o.
  Sotteau o.
  State o.

operation (continued)
  subcutaneous o.
  Tanner o.
  Tansini o.
  Taussig o.
  Taussig-Morton o.
  Thomas o.
  Thomson o.
  Travel o.
  Trendelenburg o.
  Treves o.
  Turner o.
  van Buren .o
  Vermale o.
  Verneuil o.
  Watson o.
  Waugh o.
  Weve o.
  Whipple o.
  Whitehead o.
  Winiwarter o.
  Wise o.
  Witzel o.
  Wützer o.
  Wyllys-Andrews o.
  Zieman o.
  Zimmerman o.
ophthalmofunduscope
ophthalmoleukoscope
ophthalmometroscope
ophthalmoscope
  binocular o.
  direct o.
  Friedenwald o.
  ghost o.
  indirect o.
  Loring o.
optical
  o. esophagoscope
  o. microscope
oral
  o. panendoscope
orbitostat
oropharyngeal
  o. catheter
orotracheal tube
Orr
  incision

Orr-Loygue technique
orthodiascope
orthoradioscopy
orthoscope
orthosis (orthoses)
    See also *appliance, brace,*
       prosthesis, and *splint.*
    Toronto Legg-Perthes o.
orthostereoscope
orthotopic
    o. transplantation
Oscher
    calipers
O'Shaughnessy
    forceps
osmoscope
osteoclast
osteotome
    Albee o.
    Alexander o.
    Blount o.
    Bowen o.
    Campbell o.
    Carroll o.
    Carroll-Legg o.
    Carroll-Smith-Petersen o.
    Cherry o.
    Clayton o.
    Cloward o.
    Cobb o.
    Converse o.
    Cottle o.
    Crane o.
    Dingman o.
    Epstein o.
    Frazier o.
    Hibbs o.
    Hoke o.
    Kezerian o.
    Lambotte o.
    Lambotte-Henderson o.
    Legg o.
    Leinbach o.
    Mayfield o.
    Meyerding o.
    Miner o.
    Moore o.
    New-Lambotte o.

osteotome (continued)
    Rowland o.
    Sheehan o.
    Silver o.
    Smith-Petersen o.
    Stille o.
osteotribe, osteotrite
Ostrom
    forceps
O'Sullivan
    retractor
O'Sullivan-O'Connor
    retractor
    speculum
"ot" Phonetic for aught. [zero, tran-
    scribe 0; used to indicate size
    of suture or instrument]
Otis
    anoscope
    bougie
    urethrotome
otolith apparatus
otomicroscope
otoscope
    Bruening o.
    Brunton o.
    pneumatic o.
    Siegle o.
    Toynbee o.
    Welch-Allyn o.
Ottenheimer
    dilator
"ought" Phonetic for aught. [zero,
    transcribe 0; used to indicate
    size of suture or instrument]
outlet
    o. forceps
oval
    o. esophagoscope
over-and-over suture
Overholt
    elevator
Overholt-Jackson
    bronchoscope
overlapping sutures
Overstreet
    forceps
overtube

ovum (ova)
    o. forceps
Owen
    catheter
    position
    operation
Oxycel pack
oxygenator
    bubble o.
    disk o.
    film o.
    membrane o.
    pump-o.
    rotating-disk o.
    screen o.
Pace
    knife
pacemaker
    p. catheter
pack
    Mikulicz p.
packing
    denture p.
    Gelfoam p.
    iodoform gauze p.
    vaginal p.
Packo
    pars plana cannula
Padgett
    See also *Paget.*
    dermatome
    shark-mouth cannula
Pagenstecher
    linen thread suture
Paget
    See also *Padgett.*
palatal
    p. elevator
palate
    p. retractor
Palfyn
    suture
Palmer
    dilator
    forceps
Pancoast
    suture
pancreaticoduodenostomy

pancreaticoenterostomy
pancreaticogastrostomy
pancreaticojejunostomy
pancreatoduodenectomy
pancreatoduodenostomy
pancreatoenterostomy
pancreatolithectomy
pancreatolithotomy
pancreolithotomy
panelectroscope
panendoscope
    French-McCarthy p.
    McCarthy Foroblique p.
    oral p.
Pang
    forceps
Panje
    voice button
    voice prosthesis
panniculectomy
Panzer
    scissors
Paparella
    tube
papillectomy
papillotome
PAR—postanesthesia room
paracentesis
    abdominal p.
    p. abdominis
    p. tunicae vaginalis
    p. tympani
    p. vesicae
parachlorophenol (PCP)
paracostal
    p. incision
paraffin
    p. dressing
parainguinal
    p. incision
paramedian
    p. incision
paramuscular
    p. incision
pararectus
    p. incision
parasagittal
    p. incision

parascapular
    p. incision
paraumbilical
    p. incision
Paré
    suture
Parhad-Poppen
    needle
Park
    speculum
Parker
    clamp
    incision
    knife
    retractor
    tube
Parker-Kerr
    basting stitch
    forceps
    suture
paste
    Unna p.
patch
    p. dressing
patency
Paterson
    See also *Patterson*.
    brain clip forceps
    laryngeal cannula
    laryngeal forceps
    long-shank brain clip
Patey
    operation
Paton
    needle holder
Patterson
    See also *Paterson*.
    bronchoscopic forceps
    empyema forceps
    specimen forceps
    trocar
Patton
    dilator
Paul-Mixter
    tube
Payr
    clamp
PE—polyethylene

Péan
    clamp
    forceps
    incision
    position
peanut sponge
Pederson
    speculum
pediatric
    p. speculum
pedicle
    p. clamp
Peet
    operation
peg-and-socket suture
pelvimeter
    Martin p.
pelviscope
Pemberton
    clamp
penile
    p. clamp
    Hydroflex p. prosthesis
    p. prosthesis
Pennington
    clamp
    elevator
    forceps
    speculum
Penrose
    drain
Percy
    cautery
    forceps
Pereyra
    needle
perforator
    Blot p.
    Lempert p.
    Royce p.
    Smellie p.
    Wellaminski p.
perfusion
    p. cannula
perianal
    p. incision
periareolar
    p. incision

pericostal suture
perilimbal
    p. incision
periodontal
    p. disease
    p. probe
periodontoscope
periosteal
    p. elevator
    p. retractor
periosteotome
    Alexander p.
    Alexander-Farabeuf p.
    Dean p.
    Fomon p.
    Joseph p.
periscapular
    p. incision
peritoneal
    p. incision
peritoneocentesis
peritoneoclysis
peritoneoplasty
peritoneoscope
    Wolf p.
peritoneoscopy
peritoneotomy
peritonization
peritonize
Per-Lee
    tube
Perritt
    forceps
Perthes
    incision
pessary
    Mayer p.
    Menge p.
Petersen
    bag
Petit
    hernia
    suture
petrolatum
    p. gauze dressing
Pezzer
    catheter
    drain

Pfannenstiel
    incision
phacoidoscope
phacoscope
Phaneuf
    forceps
pharyngoscope
Pheifer-Young
    retractor
Phelps-Gocht osteoclast
Phemister
    elevator
    incision
phenakistoscope
Phillips
    bougie
    catheter
    clamp
phonacoscope
phonacoscopy
phonendoscope
phonendoskiascope
phonoscope
phonoscopy
phonoselectoscope
phoriascope
phoroscope
phosphoroscope
photocoagulator
    Zeiss p.
photofluoroscope
photofluoroscopy
photogastroscope
photomicroscope
photomicroscopy
photoscope
photoscopy
photostethoscope
Physick
    operation
pick
    apical p.
    Burch p.
    crane p.
    Rhein p.'s
    root p.
Picot
    speculum

Pierce
    dissector
    elevator
    retractor
Pietrie cast
Piffard
    curet
pigtail
    p. angiographic catheter
    aortic flush p. catheter
    p. catheter
Pilcher
    hemostatic bag
Pilling
    bronchoscope
    tube
pillow
piloting trocar
pin
    Bohlman p.
    Compere p.
    Ender p.
    friction-retained p.
    Hagie p.
    Hansen-Street p.
    Hatcher p.
    incisal guide p.
    Knowles p.
    Kuntscher p.
    Moore p.
    Pischel p.
    retention p.
    Rush p.
    self-threading p.
    Steinmann p.
    Street p.
    p. suture
    Turner p.
    von Saal p.
    Zimmer p.
pinchcock mechanism
Piper
    forceps
Pirogoff
    operation
Pitha
    forceps
pituitectomy

placental
    p. forceps
plain
    p. catgut suture
    p. suture
plasma
    p. scalpel
plastic
    p. dressing
    p. suture
plate
    bone p.
    compression p.
    Deyerle p.
    Eggers p.
    Elliott p.
    Hoen p.
    Hoen skull p.
    Jewett p.
    jumping the bite p.
    Kessel p.
    Kingsley p.
    Laing p.
    Lane p.'s
    Lawson-Thornton p.
    McLaughlin p.
    Moe p.
    Sherman p.
    Thornton p.
    Wilson p.
    Wright p.
pleurotome
Pley
    forceps
plicating suture, plication suture
pliers
    Allen root p.
Plummer
    bougie
    dilator
Plummer-Vinson
    dilator
    radium applicator
pneoscope
pneumascope
pneumatic
    p. balloon dilator
    p. otoscope

pneumatic (continued)
    p. prosthesis
    p. tourniquet
pneumatoscope
pocket
    p. probe
PODx—preoperative diagnosis
point
    Hartmann p.
    McBurney p.
polariscope
polariscopy
Polisar-Lyons
    tube
Politzer
    speculum
Pollock
    operation
poloxamer
Polydek
    suture
polyester
    p. suture
polyethylene
    p. catheter
    p. drain
    p. suture
polyfilament suture
polyglactin 910
polyglycolic acid
polyp
    p. forceps
polypotome
polypropylene suture
polyscope
Polystan
    cannula
polytome
    Massiot p.
polyvinyl
    p. bougie
    p. drain
Ponka technique
Pool [eponym]
    tube
popliteal
    p. incision
pop-off needle

Poppen
    clamp
Poppen-Blalock
    clamp
"port-a-gwe" Phonetic for porte-
    aiguille.
portal
    intestinal p.
porte-aiguille
portepolisher, porte-polisher
Porter
    forceps
Portmann
    interposition operation
Portnoy
    cannula
portoenterostomy
position
    Adams p.
    Albert p.
    anatomical p.
    arm-extension p.
    Bonner p.
    Boyce p.
    Bozeman p.
    Buie p.
    Casselberry p.
    coiled p.
    decortical p.
    Depage p.
    dorsal p.
    dorsal elevated p.
    dorsal inertia p.
    dorsal lithotomy p.
    dorsal recumbent p.
    dorsal rigid p.
    dorsodecubitus p.
    dorsorecumbent p.
    dorsosacral p.
    dorsosupine p.
    Duncan p.
    Edebohls p.
    Elliot p.
    emprosthotonos p.
    fetal p.
    Fowler p.
    Fuchs p.
    genucubital p.

position (continued)
    genufacial p.
    genupectoral p.
    head dependent p.
    hinge p.
    horizontal p.
    hornpipe p.
    jackknife p.
    Jones p.
    Jonge p.
    kidney p.
    knee-chest p.
    knee-elbow p.
    kneeling-squatting p.
    Kraske p.
    lateral decubitus p.
    lateral prone p.
    lateral recumbent p.
    leapfrog p.
    lithotomy p.
    Mayo-Robson p.
    Mercurio p.
    Moynihan p.
    neck extension p.
    Noble p.
    opisthotonos p.
    orthopnea p., orthopneic p.
    orthotonos p.
    Owen p.
    Péan p.
    Proetz p.
    Robson p.
    Rose p.
    Samuel p.
    Scultetus p.
    semiprone p.
    semireclining p.
    shoe-and-stocking p.
    Simon p.
    Sims p.
    Stern p.
    upright p.
    Valentine p.
    Walcher p.
    Waters-Waldron p.
    Wolfenden p.
postauricular
    p. incision

posterior
    p. incision
posterolateral
    p. incision
Post-Harrington erysiphake
postural
    p. drainage system
Potain
    trocar
Poth
    operation
Potts
    clamp
    procedure
    rib shears
    scissors
Potts-Niedner
    clamp
Potts-Smith
    clamp
    forceps
    scissors
pouch
    Willis p.
Poupart
    ligament
    shelving edge
Poutasse
    forceps
Pratt
    anoscope
    curet
    dilator
    director
    hook
    probe
    scissors
    sound
    speculum
Pratt-Smith
    forceps
prep—prepare
prepped and draped
presection suture
pressure
    p. dressing
    dry p. dressing
pressure ring

Price-Thomas
    clamp
    forceps
primary
    p. suture
Prince
    forceps
    scissors
Pritchard
    cannula
Pritikin punch
probe
    Anel p.
    Arbuckle p.
    Bakes p.
    Barr fistula p.
    Barr rectal p.
    blood flow p.
    blunt p.
    Bowman lacrimal p.
    Brackett p.
    Buie p.
    bullet p.
    Bunnell p.
    calibrated p.
    Desjardins p.
    drum p.
    Earle p.
    electric p.
    eyed p.
    Fenger p.
    Girdner electric p.
    heat p.
    hot-tip p.
    Jansen-Newhart p.
    Kron bile duct p.
    lacrimal p.
    Larry rectal p.
    Lilienthal p.
    Mayo p.
    molecular hybridization p.
    Moynihan p.
    nuclear p.
    Ochsner p.
    oligonucleotide p.
    periodontal p., pocket p.
    Pratt p.
    priapus p.

probe (continued)
    root canal p.
    Rosen p.
    scissors p.
    Spencer p.
    syringe p.
    telephonic p.
    Theobald p.
    ultrasound p.
    uterine p.
    vertebrated p.
    Welch-Allyn p.
    WHO (World Health Organization) periodontal p.
    Williams p.
    Yankauer p.
    Ziegler p.
procedure
    See also *method, maneuver, operation, surgery,* and *technique.*
    Buie p.
    Mikulicz p.
    Rashkind o.
proctococcypexy
proctocolonoscopy
proctocolpoplasty
proctocystotome
Proctor
    elevator
    retractor
proctoscope
    See also *anoscope, colonoscope,* and *sigmoidoscope.*
    ACMI p.
    Boehm p.
    Fansler p.
    Gabriel p.
    Goldbacher p.
    Hirschman p.
    Hirschman-Martin p.
    Kelly p.
    Lieberman p.
    Montague p.
    Newman p.
    Pruitt p.
    Strauss p.
    Turell p.

proctoscope (continued)
>Tuttle p.
>Vernon-David p.
>Welch-Allyn p.
>Yeoman p.

proctoscopic
>p. speculum

proctosigmoidoscope

proctotome

Proetz position

prolapse
>rectal p.

prolapsus
>p. ani
>p. recti

Prolene
>suture

propylene
>p. dressing

prosthesis (prostheses)
>See also *appliance, brace,*
>and *splint.*
>Alvarez p.
>Angelchik antireflux p.
>aortic p.
>Ashley breast p.
>Aufranc-Turner p.
>Austin Moore p.
>Bateman p.
>Beall mitral valve p.
>Bechtol hip p.
>biliary p.
>Björk-Shiley aortic valve p.
>Björk-Shiley convexocon-
>cave 60-degree valve p.
>Björk-Shiley floating-disk p.
>Blom-Singer voice p.
>Braunwald p.
>CAD (computer-assisted
>design) p.
>caged-ball p.
>Capetown aortic valve p.
>Cartwright p.
>Charnley-Mueller hip p.
>Charnley total hip p.
>cleft palate p.
>Cooley p.
>Cronin p.

prosthesis (prostheses) (continued)
>Cutter-SCDK p.
>Cutter-Smeloff cardiac valve
>p.
>Dacron p.
>DeBakey p.
>dental p.
>DePalma p.
>DePuy p.
>discoid aortic p.
>disk-valve p.
>Duromedics p.
>Edwards p.
>Eicher p.
>endoskeletal p.
>exoskeletal p.
>feeding p.
>Geomedic p.
>geometric p.
>Giliberty p.
>Gott p.
>Guepar p.
>Harken p.
>heart valve p.
>Heyer-Schulte p.
>House p.
>Hufnagel p.
>Hydroflex penile p.
>Ionescu-Shiley p.
>Judet p.
>Kay-Shiley p.
>Kay-Suzuki p.
>knitted vascular p.
>Lillehei-Kaster p.
>Lippman p.
>MacIntosh p.
>Magovern p.
>Matchett-Brown p.
>maxillofacial p.
>McKee-Farrar p.
>McKeever p.
>mitral p.
>modular p.
>Moore p.
>Mueller p.
>Munster p.
>myoelectric p.
>Neer p.

prosthesis (prostheses) (continued)
    Neville p.
    Niebauer p.
    ocular p.
    Panje voice p.
    pneumatic p.
    SACH (solid-ankle, cush-
      ioned-heel) foot p.
    SE (Starr-Edwards) p.
    semirigid p.
    Sheehy-House p.
    Shier p.
    Silastic testicular p.
    Smeloff-Cutter p.
    Smith-Petersen p.
    speech-aid p.
    Starr-Edwards p.
    Swanson p.
    Syme p.
    Teflon p.
    Thompson p.
    tilting-disk p.
    total ossicular replacement
      p. (TORP)
    Townley p.
    tracheoesophageal fistula
      voice button p.
    trileaflet aortic p.
    Vanghetti p.
    Vitallium p.
    Wada p.
    Walldius p.
    Weavenit p.
    Wesolowski p.
    woven vascular p.
    Zimaloy p.
    Zimmer p.
prosthetics
protractor
    Robinson p.
Providence
    forceps
proximal
    p. incision
Pruitt
    anoscope
    proctoscope

Pryor-Péan
    retractor
psauoscopy
pseudocyst
    pancreatic p.
PTBD—percutaneous transhepatic
    biliary drainage
PTBD catheter
pubioplasty
pubiotomy
Pudenz
    reservoir
    shunt
    tube
    valve
Pudenz-Heyer valve
Puestow-Gillesby procedure
Puestow procedure
pulley
    p. suture
pull-out wire suture
pulsator
pump
punch
    Adler p.
    Ainsworth p.
    Berens p.
    Brock p.
    Castroviejo p.
    cervical p. biopsy clamp
    Citelli-Meltzer atticus p.
    Deyerle p.
    p. forceps
    Gundelach p.
    Hajek-Skillern p.
    Hartmann p.
    Hoffmann p.
    Holth p.
    Kerrison p.
    Keyes biopsy p.
    Keyes dermal p.
    Lermoyez p.
    Meltzer p.
    Mosher p.
    Myles p.
    Pritikin p.
    rubber dam p.
    Rubin-Holth p.

punch (continued)
    Schmeden p.
    Spencer p.
    sphenoidal p.
    Spies p.
    Takahashi p.
    Wagner p.
    Walton p.
    Watson-Williams p.
    Wilde p.
    Yankauer p.
puncture
    exploratory p.
    splenic p.
pupilloscope
Purcell
    retractor
pursestring suture
Putti
    rasp
pylorectomy
pylorodilator
Pynchon
    applicator
    speculum
    tube
pyramid
    p. of thyroid
quarantine
    q. drain
Quevedo
    forceps
quilt suture, quilted suture
racquet incision
radial
    r. incision
radical [adj.]
    r. operation
radiopaque
    r. catheter
radioscope
rake retractor
Ralks
    clamp
    drill
    elevator
Ramdohr
    suture

Ramirez shunt
Rammstedt (pref: Ramstedt)
Ramsden eyepiece
Ramses diaphragm
Ramstedt
    dilator
Randall
    curet
    stone forceps
Randolph
    cannula
Raney
    clip
    curet
    drill
    forceps
Raney-Crutchfield
    tongs
Rankin
    clamp
    forceps
    retractor
Ranzewski
    clamp
Rashkind
    procedure
    operation
rasp
    Aufricht r.
    Aufricht-Lipsett r.
    Beck r.
    Berne r.
    Cottle r.
    Fomon r.
    Good r.
    Lewis r.
    Maltz r.
    Maltz-Lipsett r.
    Putti r.
    Wiener-Pierce r.
raspatory
    Coryllos r.
    Kirmisson r.
Ratliff-Blake
    forceps
rat-tooth forceps
Ravich
    cystoscope

Ray [eponym]
    forceps
    speculum
Ray-Parsons-Sunday
    elevator
Ray-Tec
    dressing
Rebuck skin window technique
Récamier
    curet
receiver
reconstructive
    r. operation
rectal
    r. speculum
    r. trocar
    r. tube
rectoromanoscope
rectoscope
rectosigmoidoscopy
rectus
    lateral r. incision
    r. muscle–splitting incision
recumbent
    r. incision
Redivac
    drain
    drainage system
red Robinson
    catheter
red rubber catheter
Reese
    dermatome
    forceps
reflecting microscope
Regaud and Lacassagne technique
region
    inframammary r.
    mammary r.
    subphrenic r.
    supraomental r.
Rehfuss
    tube
Rehn-Delorme
    operation
Reich
    clamp

Reich-Nechtow
    clamp
    curet
    dilator
Reiner-Beck snare
Reiner-Knight
    forceps
reinforcing suture
relaxation
    r. suture
relief
    r. incision
resection
    levator r.
    Mikulicz r.
    root r.
    wedge r.
resectoscope
    Baumrucker r.
    Bumpus r.
    cold punch r.
    Iglesias r.
    McCarthy r.
    Nesbit r.
    Stern-McCarthy r.
    Thompson r.
resectoscopy
reservoir
    Kock r.
    Ommaya r.
    Pecquet r.
    Pudenz r.
    Rickham r.
    Rickham-Salmon r.
respirator
    BABYbird r.
    Bird r.
    cabinet r.
    cuirass r.
    demand r.
    Drinker r.
    Engström r.
    negative-pressure r.
retention
    r. catheter
    r. suture
retinaculum (retinacula)
retinascope

retinophotoscopy
retinoscope
    Copeland r.
retractor
    abdominal r.
    Adson r.
    Agrikola r.
    Allison r.
    Allport r.
    Alm r.
    Amoils r.
    Andrews r.
    Army-Navy r.
    Aufricht r.
    Austin r.
    Balfour r.
    Balfour self-retaining r.
    Balfour r. with fenestrated
      blade
    Ballantine hemilaminectomy
      r.
    Bankhart r.
    Barrett-Adson r.
    Barr self-retaining rectal r.
    Beardsley esophageal r.
    Beckman r.
    Beckman-Adson laminecto-
      my r.
    Beckman-Eaton laminecto-
      my r.
    Beckman goiter r.
    Beckman self-retaining r.
    Belfield wire r.
    Benedict r.
    Bennett r.
    Berens r.
    Berna infant abdominal r.
    Bernay tracheal r.
    Bethune phrenic r.
    Billroth ovarian r.
    Blount r.
    Brantley-Turner r.
    Brawley r.
    Brewster r.
    Bronson-Turz r.
    Brown r.
    Bucy r.
    Buie-Smith r.

retractor (continued)
    Byford r.
    Campbell r.
    Carroll self-retaining spring r.
    Carter r.
    Castallo r.
    Castroviejo r.
    Chandler r.
    Cherry r.
    Cloward r.
    Cloward-Hoen r.
    cobra r.
    Cole r.
    Cone r.
    contour r.
    Cooley r.
    Coryllos r.
    Cottle r.
    Cottle-Neivert r.
    Crawford r.
    Crile r.
    Cushing r.
    Davidoff (Davidov) r.
    Davidson r.
    Davis r.
    Deaver r.
    DeBakey-Balfour r.
    DeBakey-Cooley r.
    DeLee r.
    D'Errico r.
    D'Errico-Adson r.
    Desmarres r.
    Dingman r.
    Doyen r.
    Eastman r.
    Elschnig r.
    Emmet r.
    Farr r.
    Ferguson-Moon r.
    Ferris-Smith r.
    Ferris-Smith-Sewall r.
    Fink r.
    flexible shaft r.
    Foss r.
    Franz r.
    Frazier r.
    Frazier hook r.
    French S-shaped r.

retractor (continued)

    Friedman r.
    Gelpi r.
    Gibson-Balfour r.
    Gifford r.
    Glenner r.
    Goelet r.
    Goldstein r.
    Gosset r.
    Gradle r.
    Green r.
    Grieshaber r.
    Groenholm r.
    Gross r.
    Gross-Pomeranz-Watkins r.
    Guttmann r.
    Haight r.
    Hajek r.
    Hamby r.
    Harrington r.
    Harrington-Pemberton r.
    Hartstein r.
    Haslinger r.
    Heaney r.
    Heaney-Simon r.
    Hedblom r.
    Henner r.
    Hibbs r.
    Hill-Ferguson r.
    Hillis r.
    Hohmann r.
    House-Urban r.
    Israel r.
    Jackson r.
    Jacobson r.
    Jansen r.
    Judd r.
    Judd-Masson r.
    Kelly r.
    Kerrison r.
    Killian-King r.
    King r.
    Kirby r.
    Klemme r.
    Knapp r.
    Kocher r.
    Kocher-Crotti r.
    Krasky r.

retractor (continued)

    Kronfeld r.
    Lahey r.
    Latrobe r.
    Legueu r.
    Lempert r.
    Linton r.
    Little r.
    Lothrop r.
    Love r.
    Luer r.
    Lukens r.
    Luongo r.
    Martin r.
    Masson-Judd r.
    Mayo r.
    Mayo-Collins r.
    Mayo-Lovelace r.
    McGannon r.
    Meller r.
    Meyer r.
    Meyerding r.
    Millin-Bacon r.
    Moorehead r.
    Mueller r.
    Murphy r.
    Neivert r.
    Oldberg r.
    O'Sullivan r.
    O'Sullivan-O'Connor r.
    palate r.
    Parker r.
    periosteal r.
    Pheifer-Young r.
    Pierce r.
    Proctor r.
    Pryor-Péan r.
    Purcell r.
    rake r.
    Rankin r.
    rib r.
    Richardson r.
    Richardson-Eastman r.
    Rigby r.
    Rizzo r.
    Rizzuti r.
    Robinson r.
    Rochester-Ferguson r.

retractor (continued)
    Rollet r.
    Ross r.
    Roux r.
    Sachs r.
    Sauerbruch r.
    Schuknecht r.
    Scoville r.
    self-retaining r.
    Semb r.
    Senn r.
    Senn-Dingman r.
    Shambaugh r.
    Sheldon r.
    Shurly r.
    Sims r.
    Sims-Kelly r.
    Sistrunk r.
    Sloan r.
    Sluder r.
    Smith-Buie r.
    Snitman r.
    Stevenson r.
    Sweet r.
    Taylor r.
    Theis r.
    tonsil pillar r.
    Tower r.
    Tuffier r.
    Tuffier-Raney r.
    Ullrich r.
    Veenema r.
    vein r.
    Volkmann r.
    Walker r.
    Walter-Deaver r.
    Webster r.
    Weinberg r.
    Weitlaner r.
    Wesson r.
    White-Proud r.
    Wolfson r.
    Wullstein r.
    Yasargil r.
    Young r.
retroauricular
    r. incision

retrograde
    r. catheter
retromammary
Retter
    needle
return
    r. flow hemostatic catheter
Reuter
    tube
Reverdin
    needle
reverse-bevel laryngoscope
Rhein
    picks
rheoscope
rhinoscope
rhytidoplasty
    D'Assumpcao r. marker
rib
    r. retractor
ribbon
    r. gut suture
rib contractor
rib cutter
    Bethune r.c.
rib-cutting forceps
rib shears
    Bethune r.s.
    Giertz-Shoemaker r.s.
    Gluck r.s.
    Moure-Coryllos r.s.
    Potts r.s.
    Sauerbruch r.s.
    Shoemaker r.s.
rib spreader
    Finochietto r.s.
rib stripper
    Dorian r.s.
Richards
    curet
Richardson
    retractor
    suture
Richardson-Eastman
    retractor
Richards screw
Richter
    hernia

Richter (continued)
    suture
Rickham reservoir
Rickham-Salmon reservoir
Ridpath
    curet
Riecker
    bronchoscope
Rienhoff
    clamp
    forceps
Rieux hernia
Rigal
    suture
Rigby
    retractor
right-angle
    r.-a. mattress suture
    r.-a. telescope
rim
    r. incision
ring
    Abbe r.
    Flieringa r.
    r. forceps
    inguinal r.
    inguinal r., deep
    inguinal r., external
    inguinal r., internal
    inguinal r., superficial
Ring-McLean
    catheter
Ripstein
    operation
Risdon
    wire
Risser cast
Ritchie
    tenaculum
Rives
    splenectomy
Rizzo
    retractor
Rizzoli
    osteoclast
Rizzuti
    retractor
RM—radical mastectomy

RO—Ritter-Oleson [technique]
Robb
    forceps
Roberts
    applicator
    esophagoscope
    forceps
    laryngoscope
Robertshaw
    tube
Robertson
    forceps
    incision
    knife
Robinson
    catheter, red
    protractor
    retractor
    stone dislodger
Robson position
Rochester
    awl
    connector
    elevator
    forceps
    knife
    needle
Rochester-Carmalt
    forceps
Rochester-Ewald
    forceps
Rochester-Ferguson
    retractor
    scissors
Rochester-Mixter
    forceps
Rochester-Ochsner
    forceps
Rochester-Péan
    forceps
Rochester-Rankin
    forceps
Rockey
    cannula
    clamp
    endoscope
    forceps

Rockey-Davis
    incision
rocking microtome
Rodman
    incision
Roeder
    forceps
roentgenoscope
roentgenoscopy
Roger
    dissector
Rolf
    forceps
Rollet
    incision
    irrigator
    retractor
romanoscope
Rommel cautery
Rommel-Hildreth cautery
rongeur
    Beyer r.
    Cloward r.
    Converse r.
    DeVilbiss r.
    duckbill r.
    gooseneck r.
    Hartmann r.
    Hartmann-Herzfeld r.
    Hoffmann r.
    Husks r.
    Ivy r.
    Kerrison r.
    Leksell r.
    Lombard-Boies r.
    Love-Gruenwald r.
    Rowland r.
    Ruskin r.
    Schlesinger r.
    Spurling r.
    Stille-Luer r.
    Struempel f.
    Tobey r.
    Whiting r.
Roosevelt
    clamp
root canal
    r.c. probe

Roper
    cannula
Rosen
    incision
    knife
    needle
    probe
    tube
Rosenmüller
    curet
Rosenthal
    speculum
Roser
    mouth gag
Ross
    retractor
Rosser
    hook
rotating
    r. anoscope
    automatic r. tourniquet
    r. laryngoscope
round bur
Roux
    retractor
Roux-en-Y
    jejunal loop incision
Rowland
    forceps
    osteotome
Royce
    perforator
Roylan
    tibia fracture brace
rubber
    r. suture
rubber dam
    r.d. clamp holder
    r.d. drain
rubber-shod clamp
Rubin
    cannula
    clamp
    tube
Rubin-Holth punch
Ruddy
    incision

rugine
Lempert r.
rule
M'Naghten r.
Rumel
clamp
forceps
tourniquet
running continuous suture
rupture
incidental r.
Rusch
laryngoscope
Ruschelit
bougie
Rush
mallet
pin
reamer
rod
Ruskin
forceps
Russell
forceps
Russian
forceps
Ryerson
tenotome
Ryle
tube
saber-cut incision
sac
hernial s.
serous s.
saccharascope
sacculotomy
SACH—solid-ankle, cushioned-heel
(foot prosthesis)
Sachs
cannula
guard
needle
retractor
spatula
suction tube
Saenger
suture

Safar
bronchoscope
Sakler erysiphake
Salibi
clamp
salpingoscope
Salter
line
Salvatore-Maloney
tracheotome
Sam Roberts
forceps
Samuel position
Sanders
forceps
incision
laryngoscope
oscillating bed
Sanders-Brown-Shaw
needle
sandwich
s.-mold applicator
Santorini duct
saphenectomy
Sarot
clamp
forceps
Satinsky
clamp
forceps
scissors
Satterlee
saw
saucerization
Sauer
forceps
speculum
tonsillectome
Sauerbruch
forceps
prosthesis
retractor
rib shears
Sauer-Sluder
tonsillectome
Savary-Gilliard
dilator

saw
> Adams s.
> Albee s.
> amputating s.
> bayonet s.
> Blair Gigli-s. guide
> Butcher s.
> Charrière bone s.
> Clerf s.
> Cottle s.
> crown s.
> Farabeuf s.
> Gigli wire s.
> Gottschalk s.
> Hey skull s.
> hole s.
> Joseph s.
> Joseph-Maltz s.
> Lamont s.
> Langenbeck (von Langen-
>   beck) s.
> Maltz s.
> Myerson s.
> Satterlee s.
> separating s.
> Shrady s.
> Slaughter s.
> Stille-Gigli s.
> Stryker s.
> Woakcs s.

Sawtell
> forceps

scale
> French s.

scalenectomy

scalenotomy

scaler
> chisel s.
> deep s.
> double-ended s.
> hoe s.
> sickle s.
> superficial s.
> ultrasonic s.
> watch-spring s.

scalp
> s. tourniquet

scalpel
> Jackson s.
> plasma s.

scanning

scapulary

scarifier

Scarpa
> operation

scatoscopy

Schaefer
> fixation forceps
> sponge holder

Schaeffer
> curet
> ethmoid curet
> mastoid curet

"schafer" Phonetic for Schaefer,
>   Schaeffer, Schäfer, Schäffer,
>   Shaeffer, and Shaffer.

Schall
> tube

Schamberg
> extractor

Scheie
> cannula
> knife

Scheinmann
> forceps

Schindler
> esophagoscope
> gastroscope

schistosomiasis
> intestinal s.
> Manson s.

Schlange sign

Schlatter
> operation

Schlesinger
> forceps

schlieren microscope

Schmeden punch

Schobinger
> incision

Schoemaker
> clamp

Schoenberg
> forceps

Schroeder
    forceps
    scissors
    tenaculum
Schubert
    forceps
Schuchardt
    incision
Schuknecht
    hook
    knife
    retractor
    speculum
Schüller position
Schutz
    clip
    forceps
Schwartz
    clip
    forceps
    hook
Schweigger
    forceps
Schweizer
    forceps
scialyscope
scintillation
    s. probe
scissors
    Adson s.
    Aebli s.
    Barraquer s.
    Barraquer-DeWecker s.
    Bellucci s.
    Berbridge s.
    Berens s.
    Boettcher s.
    Braun s.
    Brooks s.
    Buie s.
    Burnham s.
    canalicular s.
    cannula s.
    Castroviejo s.
    Cooley s.
    corneoscleral s.
    Cottle s.
    Crafoord s.

scissors (continued)
    Craig s.
    craniotomy s.
    Dandy s.
    Dean s.
    Deaver s.
    DeBakey s.
    DeBakey-Metzenbaum s.
    DeWecker s.
    DeWecker-Pritikin s.
    Doyen s.
    Emmet s.
    Esmarch s.
    Ferguson s.
    Fomon s.
    Fox s.
    Harrison s.
    House s.
    Huey s.
    iris s.
    Irvine s.
    Jackson s.
    Jacobson s.
    Jones s.
    Jorgenson s.
    Joseph s.
    Katzin s.
    Kelly s.
    Kirby s.
    Knapp s.
    Knight s.
    Knowles s.
    Kreuscher s.
    Lagrange s.
    Lejeune s.
    Lillie s.
    Lister s.
    Liston s.
    Littauer s.
    Litwak s.
    Lynch s.
    Maclay s.
    Mayo s.
    Mayo-Harrington s.
    Mayo-Noble s.
    Mayo-Sims s.
    McClure s.
    McGuire s.

scissors (continued)
    McLean s.
    McPherson s.
    McPherson-Castroviejo s.
    McPherson-Vannas s.
    Metzenbaum s.
    Metzenbaum-Lipsett s.
    Miller s.
    Morse s.
    Nelson s.
    New s.
    Northbent s.
    Noyes-Shambaugh s.
    Nugent-Gradle s.
    Ochsner s.
    Panzer s.
    Potts s.
    Potts-Smith s.
    Pratt s.
    Prince s.
    s. probe
    Rochester-Ferguson s.
    Satinsky s.
    Schroeder s.
    Seiler s.
    Shortbent s.
    Sims s.
    Sistrunk s.
    Smart s.
    Spencer s.
    Stevens s.
    Stevenson s.
    stitch s.
    Strully s.
    Sweet s.
    Taylor s.
    Thorek s.
    Thorek-Feldman s.
    Thorpe s.
    Thorpe-Castroviejo s.
    Thorpe-Westcott s.
    Toennis s.
    umbilical s.
    Vannas s.
    Verhoeff s.
    Vezien s.
    Waldmann s.
    Walker s.

scissors (continued)
    Westcott s.
    Wester s.
    Wilmer s.
scleroscope
scleroticotomy
sclerotome
    Curdy s.
    Lundsgaard-Burch s.
scoop
    Arlt s.
    Beck gastrostomy s.
    Berens s.
    Daviel s.
    Desjardins s.
    Ferguson s.
    Ferris s.
    Knapp s.
    Lewis s.
    Luer-Korte s.
    Mayo s.
    Mayo-Robson s.
    Moore s.
    Moynihan s.
    Mules s.
    Wilder s.
"scopes" See under full name.
    amnioscope
    angioscope
    anoscope
    antroscope
    arthroscope
    bronchofiberscope
    bronchoscope
    choledochoscope
    colonoscope
    colposcope
    culdoscope
    cystoscope
    cystourethroscope
    dynamoscope
    endoscope
    esophagoscope
    fibercolonoscope
    fibergastroscope
    fiberscope
    gastroscope
    hypopharyngoscope

"scopes" See under full name. (continued)
    hysterocolposcope
    hysteroscope
    laparoscope
    laryngoscope
    laryngostroboscope
    lithoscope
    lithotriptoscope
    meatoscope
    mediastinoscope
    metroscope
    myoscope
    nasoendoscope
    nasopharyngoscope
    nasoscope
    nephroscope
    panendoscope
    peritoneoscope
    pharyngoscope
    photogastroscope
    pneumatoscope
    proctoscope
    proctosigmoidoscope
    rectoscope
    resectoscope
    romanoscope
    saccharascope
    salpingoscope
    sigmoidoscope
    sphincteroscope
    stereocolposcope
    telescope
    thoracoscope
    tonsilloscope
    tracheobronchoesophago-
        scope
    tracheoscope
    ureterocystoscope
    urethroscope
    uteroscope
    vaginoscope
    ventriculoscope
scotoscopy
Scott
    cannula
    speculum

Scoville
    clip
    forceps
    retractor
Scoville-Lewis
    clip
scratch-type incision
screw
    Basile s.
    Bosworth s.
    Collison s.
    Coventry s.
    dentin s.
    Eggers s.
    expansion s.
    Kristiansen s.
    Leinbach s.
    McAtee s.
    McLaughlin s.
    Richards hip s.
    Sherman s.
    Thornton s.
    Vitallium s.
    Zimmer s.
Scudder
    clamp
    forceps
Scultetus
    bandage [also: scultetus]
    position
SE—Starr-Edwards (prosthesis)
searcher
    Allport s.
    Allport-Babcock s.
Searcy
    erysiphake
    tonsillectome
secondary
    s. suture
second intention
section
    transverse s.
sectioning
    surgical s.
Sédillot
    elevator
Segond
    forceps

Segond (continued)
    spatula
Sehrt
    clamp
Seiffert
    forceps
Seiler
    knife
    scissors
Seldinger
    needle
Seletz
    cannula
self-retaining
    s.-r. catheter
    s.-r. laryngoscope
    s.-r. retractor
Sellor
    knife
Sclman
    forceps
Selverstone
    clamp
Semb
    forceps
    retractor
semicircular incision
semiflexed incision
semilunar
    s. incision
semirigid prosthesis
Semken
    forceps
Sengstaken
    tube
Sengstaken-Blakemore
    tube
Senn
    forceps
    operation
    retractor
Senn-Dingman
    retractor
Senturia
    speculum
separating saw
separator
    Horsley s.

separator (continued)
    House s.
    Remy s.
    Rosen s.
septotome
serioscopy
"ser-kloth" Phonetic for cerecloth.
seromuscular
    s. suture
seroserosal silk suture
seroserous
    s. suture
serpentine
    s. incision
serrated
    s. curet
serrefine
    s. clamp
seton
    s. opcration
Seton [eponym]
    hip brace
Sewall
    chisel
    forceps
Sexton
    knife
Shaaf
    forceps
Shaeffer
    rigid orthosis
"shafer" Phonetic for Schaefer,
    Schaeffer, Schäfer, Schäffer,
    Shaeffer, and Shaffer.
Shaffer
    modification of Barkan knife
Shallcross
    forceps
Shambaugh
    adenotome
    elevator
    hook
    incision
    needle
    retractor
Shambaugh-Derlacki
    chisel
    elevator

Shambaugh-Lempert
    knife
Shapleigh
    curet
sharp spoon
sharp-toothed tenaculum
Shaw
    stripper
Shea
    curet
    drill
    hook
    knife
    tube
Shearer
    forceps
Shearing lens
shears
    bandage s.
    Lebsche s.
    Liston s.
    malleus s.
sheath
    peel-away s.
    rectus s.
    s. of rectus abdominis muscle
sheathed
    s. catheter
Sheehan
    chisel
    osteotome
Sheehy
    knife
    tube
Sheehy-House
    prosthesis
sheepskin dressing
Sheets lens
Sheldon
    retractor
Sheldon-Pudenz
    dissector
Sheldon-Spatz
    needle
shelving
    s. incision
Shenstone
    tourniquet

Shepard
    tube
Sherman plate
Shier
    prosthesis
Shiley
    tube
Shiner
    tube
Shirodkar
    needle
Shoemaker
    clamp
    rib shears
Shortbent
    scissors
shotted suture
shoulder-strap incision
Shrady
    saw
shunt
    Denver s.
    Javid s.
    LeVeen peritoneovenous s.
    mesocaval s.
    peritoneovenous s.
    PFTE (polyfluorotetraethyl-
        ene) s.
    Pudenz s.
    Quinton-Scribner s.
    reversed s.
    Scribner s.
    splenorenal s.
    splenorenal s., distal
    Stookey-Scarff s.
    Thomas appliqué s.
    ventriculojugular s.
    Warren s.
Shurly
    retractor
side-cutting spatulated needle
sideroscope
sidewinder catheter
Siegle
    otoscope
    pneumatic ear speculum
Sierra-Sheldon
    tracheotome

sigmoidopexy
sigmoidoscope
    See also *anoscope, colono-*
       scope, and *proctoscope.*
    Boehm s.
    Buie s.
    disposable s.
    fiberoptic s.
    Frankfeldt s.
    Kelly s.
    KleenSpec s.
    Lieberman s.
    Montague s.
    Solow s.
    Turell s.
    Tuttle s.
    Vernon-David s.
    Welch-Allyn s.
    Yeoman s.
sigmoidosigmoidostomy
Siker
    laryngoscope
Silastic
    coronary artery cannula
    cup
    implant
    mushroom catheter
    patch
    testicular prosthesis
    ventriculoperitoneal shunt
silk
    s.-braided suture
    seroserosal s. suture
    s. suture
    white s. suture
silkworm gut suture
Silver [eponym]
    osteotome
Silverman
    needle
silver wire
    s.w. suture
Simcoe lens
Simmonds
    speculum
Simmons
    catheter

Simon
    incision
    suture
simple
    s. suture
Simpson
    forceps
Simpson-Luikart
    forceps
Sims
    anoscope
    curet
    position
    retractor
    scissors
    speculum
    suture
Sims-Kelly
    retractor
single-armed suture
Singleton
    incision
single-tooth, single-toothed
    s.-t. forceps
    s.-t. tenaculum
Singley
    forceps
Sinskey lens
sinus (sinus, sinuses)
    s. of Bochdalek
    s. forceps
    sacrococcygeal s.
siphon
Sippy
    dilator
Sistrunk
    retractor
    scissors
Skeele
    curet
Skene
    curet
    forceps
skenoscope
skiaporescopy
skiascope
Skillern
    forceps

skin
  s. clip
skin lifter
  Amico s.l.
skinny needle
skull
  s. tongs
Slaughter
  saw
slide
  microscope s.
sliding microtome
sling
  Glisson s.
  s. suture
slit lamp
  s.l. microscope
Sloan
  incision
  retractor
slotted laryngoscope
Sluder
  adenotome
  guillotine
  guillotine tonsillectomy
  retractor
  tonsillectome
Sluder-Demarest
  tonsillectome
Sluder-Jansen mouth gag
Sluder-Sauer
  tonsillar guillotine
  tonsillectome
Smart
  forceps
  scissors
Smead-Jones closure
Smedberg
  drill
Smellie
  perforator
Smeloff-Cutter
  prosthesis
Smiley-Williams
  needle
Smillie
  knife
  meniscotome

Smith
  clip
  dislocation
  expressor
  forceps
  hook
  pessary
Smith-Buie
  retractor
Smith-Gibson
  operation
Smith-Green
  knife
Smith-Hodge pessary
Smith-Petersen
  osteotome
  prosthesis
Smith-Peterson
  incision
Smithwick
  forceps
SMo (stainless steel and molybdenum) brace
SMR (submucous resection) speculum
snare
  Eves tonsillar s.
  Frankfeldt s.
  Norwood s.
SNB—scalene node biopsy
Snitman
  retractor
Snyder
  Surgivac drainage system
  Surgivac suction tube
Solow
  sigmoidoscope
soluble
  s. bougie
somatoscopy
Somers
  forceps
SOMI—sternal occipital mandibular immobilizer
SOMI brace
Sones
  coronary catheter

Sonnenschein
   speculum
sonofluoroscope
sonoscope
Soonawalla
   uterine elevator
Soresi
   cannula
Sotteau
   operation
sound
   Campbell s.
   Davis s.
   Dittel s.
   esophageal s.
   Fowler s.
   Guyon s.
   Jewett s.
   lacrimal s.
   Le Fort s.
   McCrea s.
   Otis s.
   Pratt s.
   Simpson s.
   Sims s.
   urethral s.
   uterine s.
   Van Buren s.
   Walther s.
Southey
   trocar
Southey-Leech
   tube
Souttar
   tube
SPA—suprapubic aspiration
space
   axillary s.
   extraperitoneal s.
   peritoneal s.
   pleuroperitoneal s.
   retropubic s.
   subphrenic s.
   subumbilical s.
spatula
   Berens s.
   Castroviejo s.
   Cushing s.

spatula (continued)
   Davis s.
   Elschnig s.
   Jacobson s.
   Knapp s.
   Lindner s.
   McPherson s.
   Sachs s.
   Segond s.
   Tauber s.
   tongue s.
   Wheeler s.
   Woodson s.
speaking tube
speculum (specula, speculums)
   Allingham rectal s.
   anal s.
   s. anoscope
   Aufricht s.
   aural s.
   Auvard-Remine s.
   Auvard weighted s.
   Barr anal s.
   Barraquer s.
   Barraquer-Colibri s.
   Barr rectal s.
   Beckman-Colver nasal s.
   Beckman nasal s.
   Berens s.
   Berlind-Auvard s.
   bivalve s., bivalved s.
   Boucheron s.
   Bozeman s.
   Brewer s.
   Brinkerhoff rectal s.
   Buie-Smith s.
   Castroviejo s.
   Chelsea-Eaton s.
   Chevalier Jackson s.
   Coakley s.
   Collin s.
   Converse s.
   Cook s.
   Cottle s.
   Cusco s.
   David s.
   DeVilbiss s.
   DeVilbiss-Stacey s.

speculum (specula, speculums)
  (continued)
    duckbill s., duck-billed s.
    Dudley-Smith s.
    Duplay s.
    Duplay-Lynch s.
    Eaton s.
    esophageal s.
    eye s.
    Fansler s.
    Farrior s.
    Fergusson s.
    Flannery s.
    Fränkel s.
    Garrigue s.
    Gerzog s.
    Goldbacher s.
    Graves s.
    Gruber s.
    Guild-Pratt s.
    Gusto s.
    Guttmann s.
    Guyton-Maumenee s.
    Guyton-Park s.
    Halle s.
    Halle-Tieck s.
    Hardy-Duddy s.
    Hartmann dewaxer s.
    Heffernan s.
    Helmont s.
    Henrotin s.
    Hinkle-James rectal s.
    Huffman-Graves s.
    Ingals s.
    Jonas-Graves s.
    Kahn-Graves s.
    Kelly s.
    Killian nasal s.
    Killian rectal s.
    Knapp s.
    Kramer s.
    Kyle s.
    Lancaster s.
    Lange s.
    Lempert-Colver endaural s.
    lid s.
    Lillie s.
    Lister-Burch s.

speculum (specula, speculums)
  (continued)
    Mahoney s.
    Martin s.
    Martin and Davy s.
    Mason-Auvard s.
    Mathews s.
    Maumenee-Park s.
    Mayer s.
    McHugh s.
    McPherson s.
    Mellinger s.
    Miller s.
    Mosher s.
    Mueller s.
    Murdock-Wiener s.
    Myles s.
    nasal s.
    nasopharyngeal s.
    Nott s.
    O'Sullivan-O'Connor s.
    Park s.
    Pederson s.
    pediatric s.
    Pennington s.
    Picot s.
    Politzer s.
    Pratt s.
    proctoscopic s.
    Pynchon s.
    Ray s.
    rectal s.
    Rosenthal s.
    Sauer s.
    Schuknecht s.
    Scott s.
    Senturia s.
    Siegle pneumatic ear s.
    Simmonds s.
    Sims s.
    SMR s.
    Sonnenschein s.
    stop eye s.
    Thudichum nasal s.
    Toynbee s.
    Tröltsch s.
    urethral s.
    vaginal s.

speculum (specula, speculums)
   (continued)
     van Helmont s.
     Vernon-David s.
     Vienna s.
     Weeks s.
     weighted s.
     Weisman-Graves s.
     Welch-Allyn s.
     Wiener s.
     Williams s.
     wire s.
     wire bivalve s.
     Yankauer s.
speech-aid prosthesis
Spence
     forceps
Spence-Adson
     forceps
Spencer
     probe
     scissors
Spencer Wells
     forceps
Spero
     forceps
sphincter
     O'Beirne s.
     ostial s.
     physiologic s.
     segmental s.
sphincteroscope
     Kelly s.
sphincterotome
sphygmomanometer
sphygmoscope
sphygmoscopy
Spieghel line
Spies punch
spinal
     s. needle
spiral
     s. incision
     s. suture
     s.-tip catheter
Spirec
     drill
spiroscope

spiroscopy
splanchnoscopy
splanchnotomy
splenectomize
splenectomy
     abdominal s.
     s. clamp
     Federoff s.
     Henry s.
     Rives s.
     subcapsular s.
splenorenal
splenorrhaphy
splenotomy
splint
     See also *appliance, brace,*
       and *prosthesis.*
     Engelmann s.
     Gilmer s.
     Gordon s.
     Keller-Blake s.
     Thomas knee s.
     Valentine s.
split-sheath catheter
sponge
     absorbable gelatin s.
     Bernay s.
     fibrin s.
     s. forceps, s.-holding forceps
     gauze s.
     gelatin s.
     s. holder
     s. implant
     Lincoff s.
     peanut s.
     s. stick
     Weck s.
     Weck-cel s.
spoon
     Bunge s.
     Cushing s.
     Daviel s.
     Elschnig s.
     s. excavator
     Gross s.
     Hess s.
     Kirby s.
     Knapp s.

spoon (continued)
    sharp s.
    Volkmann s.
Spratt
    curet
spreader
    gutta-percha s.
    Millin-Bacon s.
    root canal filling s.
    Turek s.
    Wiltberger s.
spring
    s. forceps
Spurling
    forceps
    rongeur
SSU—sterile supply unit
stab wound
    s.w. drain
    s.w. incision
Stader splint
Stadie-Riggs
    microtome
stage
    microscope s.
Stahl
    calipers
stainless steel suture
Stanford
    bioptome
Staple
    bronchoscope
stapler
    Blount s.
    TA-55 s.
staple suture
Starlinger
    dilator
Starr-Edwards
    prosthesis
State [eponym]
    operation
Staude
    forceps
Staude-Moore
    forceps
Staunton

stay
    s. suture
St. Clair-Thompson
    curet
steel
    s. mesh suture
    stainless s. suture
Steele
    dilator
Steinmann
    extension
    forceps
    pin
stellate
    s. incision
stellectomy
stenoses (plural of stenosis)
stent
    s. dressing
stereocolposcope
stereomonoscope
stereophantoscope
stereophoroscope
stereoscope
stereostroboscope
sternal
    s.-splitting incision
Stern-McCarthy
    electrotome
    resectoscope
Stern position
stethendoscope
stethopolyscope
stethoscope
stethoscopy
Stevens
    forceps
    hook
    scissors
Stevenson
    clamp
    forceps
    retractor
    scissors
Stewart
    hook
    incision

stick
  sponge s.
  s.-tie suture
Stille
  clamp
  drill
  forceps
  osteotome
Stille-Gigli
  saw
Stille-Liston
  forceps
Stille-Luer
  forceps
  rongeur
stirrup
  Finochietto s.
stitch
  s. scissors
St. Jude valve
Stocker
  needle
stockinette
  s. dressing
stocking
Stockman
  clamp
stomach
  dumping s.
  s. tube
stomatoscope
stone
  s. basket
  s. forceps
Stone [eponym]
  clamp
  forceps
stone dislodger
  Councill s.d.
  Davis s.d.
  Dormia s.d.
  Johnson s.d.
  Levant s.d.
  Robinson s.d.
  woven loop s.d.
Stone-Holcombe
  clamp

stop
  s. eye speculum
  s. needle
Storz
  bronchoscope
  cystoscope
  hysteroscope
  magnet
Storz-Beck snare
straight tenaculum
Strassman
  forceps
  uterine forceps
Stratte
  needle holder
Strauss
  proctoscope
streak
  s. retinoscope
stripper
  Carroll forearm tendon s.
  Emerson s.
  external s.
  internal s.
  intraluminal s.
  Keeley s.
  Kurten s.
  Lempka s.
  Mayo s.
  Meyer s.
  Nabatoff s.
  Shaw s.
  thrombus s.
  vein s.
  Webb s.
  Wilson s.
  Wylie s.
stroboscope
strobostereoscope
Strömbeck
  incision
Struempel (Strümpel)
  ear alligator forceps
  ear punch forceps
  rongeur
Strully
  scissors

struma
      Riedel s.
Strümpel. See *Struempel*.
Struyken
      forceps
Stryker
      dermatome
      drill
      frame
      saw
Stubbs
      curet
stump
      invaginated s.
Sturmdorf
      suture
Stutsman snare
stylet
Styrofoam
      dressing
subcapsular
      s. splenectomy
subclavian
      s. catheter
subcostal
      s. incision
subcutaneous
      s. operation
subcuticular
      s. suture
subinguinal
      s. incision
subjectoscope
submammary
      s. incision
subtrochanteric
      s. incision
subumbilical
      s. incision
sucker
      Marshall surgical s.
suction
      s. drain
      s. tube
      Wangensteen s.
suction tube
      Adson s.t.
      Andrews-Pynchon s.t.

suction tube (continued)
      Buie rectal s.t.
      Frazier s.t.
      Sachs s.t.
Sugar [eponym]
      clip
sugar-tong splint
Sugiura procedure
suit
      body exhaust s.
Suker
      iris forceps
sump
      s. drain
      s. drainage system
      s. tube
sump tube
      Argyle-Salem s.t.
Sunday [eponym]
      elevator
Superblade
superficial
      s. suture
supermicroscope
support
      s. suture
supracervical
      s. incision
Supramid
      suture
suprapubic
      s. incision
supraumbilical
      s. incision
surface
      s. applicator
surgical
      s. microscope
      s. suture
Surgicel
      gauze dressing
Surgilene
      suture
Surgilon
      suture
Surgilope
      suture

Surgivac
  drainage system, Snyder
  suction drainage system
suspension
  s. laryngoscope
suturation
suture [material]
  See also *suture [technique]*.
  0 s. [size zero]
  00 s., 2-0 s.
  000 s., 3-0 s.
  4-0 s. [sizes 5-0 through 11-0]
  #1 s. [sizes 2, 3, etc.]
  absorbable s.
  absorbable surgical s.
  Acutrol s.
  Alcon s.
  Atraloc s.
  black braided s.
  black silk s.
  braided s.
  cardiovascular s.
  catgut s.
  celluloid s.
  chromic catgut s.
  collagen s.
  Dacron s.
  dekalon s.
  Deknatel s.
  Dermalene s.
  Dermalon s.
  Dexon s.
  Dulox s.
  elastic s.
  Equisetene s.
  Ethibond s.
  Ethicon s.
  Ethiflex s.
  Ethilon s.
  Flaxedil s.
  Flexitone s.
  Flexon s.
  gut chromic s.
  horsehair s.
  Marlex s.
  Mayo linen s.
  Medrafil wire s.
  Mersilene s.

suture [material] (continued)
  monofilament s.
  multifilament s.
  multistrand s.
  Neurolon s.
  nonabsorbable s.
  nonabsorbable surgical s.
  nylon monofilament s.
  Pagenstecher linen thread s.
  plain s.
  plain catgut s.
  Polydek s.
  polyester s.
  polyethylene s.
  polyfilament s.
  polypropylene s.
  Prolene s.
  ribbon gut s.
  rubber s.
  silk s.
  silk-braided s.
  silkworm gut s.
  silver wire s.
  stainless steel s.
  staple s.
  steel mesh s.
  Supramid s.
  Surgilene s.
  Surgilon s.
  Surgilope s.
  tantalum wire s.
  Tevdek s.
  Thermo-flex s.
  Ti-Cron s., Tycron s.
  tiger gut s.
  unabsorbable s.
  Vicryl s.
  Viro-Tec s.
  white braided s.
  white silk s.
  wire s.
  Zytor s.
suture [technique]
  See also *suture [material]*.
  Albert s.
  Allison s.
  alternating s.
  anchoring s.

suture [technique] (continued)
   angle s.
   Appolito s.
   apposition s.
   approximation s.
   arcuate s.
   Argyll Robertson s.
   Arlt s.
   atraumatic s.
   Axenfeld s.
   Babcock s.
   back-and-forth s.
   Barraquer s.
   baseball s.
   basilar s.
   bastard s.
   Béclard s.
   Bell s.
   biparietal s.
   blanket s.
   bolster s.
   Bozeman s.
   bregmatomastoid s.
   bridle s.
   bunching s.
   Bunnell s.
   buried s.
   button s.
   buttonhole s.
   cable wire s.
   capitonnage s.
   Carrel s.
   chain s.
   circular s.
   circumcision s.
   Coakley s.
   coaptation s.
   cobbler's s.
   compound s.
   Connell s.
   continuous s.
   cruciform s.
   Cushing s.
   cushioning s.
   cutaneous s.
   cutaneous s. of palate
   cuticular s.
   Czerny s.

suture [technique] (continued)
   Czerny-Lembert s.
   delayed s.
   delayed primary s.
   dermal s.
   double-armed s., doubly
     armed s.
   double-button s.
   Dupuytren s.
   edge-to-edge s.
   Emmet s.
   end-on mattress s.
   epineural s.
   everting s.
   everting interrupted s.
   far-and-near s.
   figure-of-eight s.
   fixation s.
   fore-and-aft s.
   free ligature s.
   Frost s.
   furrier's s.
   Gaillard-Arlt s.
   Gambee s.
   Gély s.
   Gibson s.
   glover's s.
   Gould s.
   groove s.
   Gruber s.
   Gudebrod s.
   Gussenbauer s.
   guy s.
   Guyton-Friedenwald s.
   Halsted s.
   harelip s.
   Harris s.
   helical s.
   hemostatic s.'s
   horizontal mattress s.
   imbricated s.
   implanted s.
   interlocking s.
   interrupted s.
   intradermal s.
   intradermal mattress s.
   intradermic s.
   invaginating s.

suture [technique] (continued)
  inverted s., inverting s.
  Ivalon s.
  Jobert s.
  Kalt s.
  kangaroo tendon s.
  Kelly s.
  Kirschner s.
  lace s.
  Le Dentu s.
  Le Dran s.
  Le Fort s.
  Lembert s.
  lens s.'s
  ligation s.
  s. ligature
  Littré s.
  locking s.
  lock-stitch s.
  Löffler s.
  loop s.
  loop-on mucosa s.
  mattress s.
  mattress s., end-on
  mattress s., horizontal
  mattress s., intradermal
  mattress s., right-angle
  mattress s., vertical
  Maunsell s.
  Meigs s.
  near-and-far s.
  nerve s.
  noose s.
  over-and-over s.
  overlapping s.'s
  Palfyn s.
  Pancoast s.
  Paré s.
  Parker-Kerr s.
  peg-and-socket s.
  pericostal s.
  Petit s.
  pin s.
  plastic s.
  plicating s., plication s.
  presection s.
  primary s.
  pulley s.

suture [technique] (continued)
  pull-out wire s.
  pursestring s.
  quilt s., quilted s.
  Ramdohr s.
  reinforcing s.
  relaxation s.
  retention s.
  Richardson s.
  Richter s.
  Rigal s.
  right-angle mattress s.
  running continuous s.
  Saenger s.
  secondary s.
  seromuscular s.
  seroserosal silk s.
  seroserous s.
  shotted s.
  Simon s.
  simple s.
  Sims s.
  single-armed s.
  sling s.
  spiral s.
  stay s.
  stick-tie s.
  Sturmdorf s.
  subcuticular s.
  superficial s.
  support s.
  surgical s.
  Taylor s.
  tendon s.
  tension s.
  Thiersch s.
  through-and-through s.
  Tom Jones s.
  tongue-and-groove s.
  traction s.
  transfixing s., transfixion s.
  twisted s.
  uninterrupted s.
  Verhoeff s.
  vertical mattress s.
  whipstitch s.
  Wolfler s.
  Wysler s.

suture [technique] (continued)
    Y-s.
    Z-s.
suture-holding forceps
suture ligature
swaged
    s. needle
Swan-Ganz
    catheter
Swanson
    prosthesis
Sweet
    forceps
    retractor
    scissors
Syme
    prosthesis
symphysiotome
synechotome
Syner-G
synoptiscope
syringe
    probe s.
syringectomy
syringotome
syringotomy
Tabb
    curet
tachistoscope
tachistoscopy
Taillefer valve
Takahashi
    forceps
tampon
    Dührssen t.
    Genupak t.
    nasal t.
    Trendelenburg t.
    t. tube
    vaginal t.
Tanner
    operation
    procedure
Tansini
    operation
tantalum (Ta)
    t. clip
    t. mesh

tantalum (Ta) (continued)
    t. plate
    t. ring
    t. sheet
    t. wire
    t. wire suture
Tarnier
    forceps
TA-55 stapler
Tatum
    clamp
Tauber
    spatula
Taussig
    operation
Taussig-Morton
    operation
Taylor
    apparatus
    brace
    retractor
    scissors
    splint
    suture
T bandage
Teale
    forceps
    gorget
technique
    See also *method, maneuver,*
       operation, procedure, and
       surgery.
    Buie t.
    clamp t.
    La Roque t.
    Lotheissen-McVay t.
    Madden t.
    Ponka t.
    vest-over-pants t.
    Yasargil t.
Teflon
    catheter
    graft
    membrane
    mesh
    prosthesis
    tube
telephonic probe

telescope
    t. bronchoscope
    Broyles t.
    Holinger t.
    McCarthy t.
    right-angle t.
    Vest t.
telesthetoscope
television microscopy
Telfa
    dressing
temporal
    t. incision
tenaculum
    Adair t.
    Barrett t.
    Braun t.
    Cottle t.
    DeLee t.
    Duplay t.
    Jackson t.
    Jacobs t.
    Kahn t.
    Lahey t.
    Marlex atraumatic t.
    Ritchie t.
    Schroeder t.
    sharp-toothed t.
    straight t.
Tenckhoff
    peritoneal catheter
tendon
    conjoined t.
    kangaroo t. suture
    t. suture
    t. tucker
tendon-passing forceps
tendon-pulling forceps
tendon tucker
    Bishop t.t.
    Bishop-Black t.t.
    Bishop-DeWitt t.t.
    Bishop-Peter t.t.
    Burch-Greenwood t.t.
    Fink t.t.
tenectomy
Tenner
    cannula

tenomyoplasty
tenotome
    Ryerson t.
tension
    t. suture
tensor
    t. fasciae latae
Terrier valve
test
    scleroscope t.
Tevdek
    suture
Texas
    catheter
Theis
    retractor
Theobald
    probe
therapy
    sparing t.
    surgical maggot t.
thermocauterectomy
thermodilution
    t. catheter
Thermo-flex
    suture
thermoscope
Thiersch
    knife
    suture
Thomas
    curet
    operation
Thomas-Warren
    incision
Thompson
    catheter
    prosthesis
    resectoscope
Thoms
    forceps
    pelvimeter
Thoms-Allis
    forceps
Thoms-Gaylor
    forceps
Thomson
    clamp

Thomson (continued)
    operation
thoracoabdominal
    t. incision
thoracoscope
thoracostomy
    t. tube
Thorek
    aspirator
    scissors
Thorek-Feldman
    scissors
Thorek-Mixter
    forceps
Thornwald
    perforator
Thorpe
    calipers
    forceps
    scissors
Thorpe-Castroviejo
    scissors
Thorpe-Westcott
    scissors
thread
    celluloid t.
    Pagenstecher linen t. suture
three-bottle drainage system
thrombus (thrombi)
    t. stripper
through-and-through suture
Thudichum
    speculum
thyrohyal
thyroidea
    t. accessoria
    t. ima
thyroidectomize
thyrotomy
Ti-Cron, Tycron
    suture
tidal drainage system
Tiemann
    catheter
tiger gut suture
tilting-disk prosthesis
Timberlake obturator

Timbrall-Fisher
    incision
time (T)
    decimal reduction t. (D)
    thermal death t.
tincture
    benzethonium chloride t.
    benzoin t., compound
    iodine t.
    iodine t., strong
Tischler
    forceps
Tissot spirometer
tissue
    t. expander
    t. forceps
    Gamgee t.
Tivnen
    forceps
Tobey
    rongeur
Tobold
    forceps
    knife
Tobold-Fauvel
    forceps
Tobruk splint
Todd
    gouge
toe
    t. drop brace
Toennis
    scissors
Toldt
    ligament
Tom Jones
    closure
    suture
tongs
    Barton t.
    Barton-Cone t.
    Cherry t.
    Crutchfield t.
    Crutchfield-Raney t.
    Raney-Crutchfield t.
    skull t.
tongue
    t. spatula

tongue-and-groove suture
tonoscope
tonsil
    t. pillar retractor
    t. snare
tonsillectome
    Ballenger-Sluder t.
    Beck-Mueller t.
    Beck-Schenck t.
    Brown t.
    Daniels t.
    LaForce t.
    Mack t.
    Moltz-Storz t.
    Myles t.
    Sauer t.
    Sauer-Sluder t.
    Searcy t.
    Sluder t.
    Sluder-Demarest t.
    Sluder-Sauer t.
    Tydings t.
    Van Osdel t.
    Whiting t.
tonsilloscope
tonsillotome
Tooke
    knife
toric
    t. lens
TORP—total ossicular replacement
   prosthesis
tourniquet
    automatic rotating t.
    Bethune lung t.
    Esmarch t.
    forceps t.
    pneumatic t.
    Rumel t.
    scalp t.
    Shenstone t.
    windlass t.
towel clamp
    Backhaus t.c.
towel clip
towel forceps
Tower
    retractor

Townley
    prosthesis
Toynbee
    otoscope
    speculum
TQ—tourniquet
trabecular
    t. meshwork
tracheal
    t. dilator
    t. tube
tracheobronchoesophagoscope
    Haslinger t.
tracheocannula
tracheoesophageal
    t. fistula voice button pros-
       thesis
tracheoscope
tracheostome
    end t.
tracheostomy
    Bose t. hook
    t. hook
    t. mask
    Moore t. button
    t. tube
tracheotome
    Salvatore-Maloney t.
    Sierra-Sheldon t.
tracheotomy
    t. tube
traction
    t. suture
traction handle
tractor
    prostatic t.
    Syms t.
    urethral t.
    Young t.
transduodenal
transection
    t. incision
transfixing suture
transfixion
    t. suture
transmeatal
    t. incision

transplant
    Gallie t.
transplantation
    allogeneic t.
    heterotopic t.
    homotopic t.
    liver t.
    orthotopic t.
    orthotopic liver t.
    syngeneic t.
    syngenesioplastic t.
transrectus
    t. incision
transverse
    t. incision
transversostomy
trap-door incision
Travel [eponym]
    operation
Travenol
    needle
treatment
    Murphy t.
Trendelenburg
    operation
    tampon
Trendelenburg-Crafoord
    clamp
trephine
    Arruga t.
    Barraquer t.
    Castroviejo t.
    DeVilbiss t.
    Elliot t.
    Galt t.
    Grieshaber t.
    Michel t.
    Paufique t.
    Turkel t.
trephiner
Treves
    operation
triangle
    Calot t., t. of Calot
    Henke t.
    Hesselbach t.
trichinoscope
trichoscopy

Tri-Flow incentive spirometry
trigonectomy
trileaflet aortic prosthesis
trinocular microscope
trocar
    Allen t.
    Barnes t.
    Beardsley cecostomy t.
    Campbell t.
    t. catheter
    Coakley t.
    Duke t.
    Durham t.
    Hurwitz t.
    Ingram t. catheter
    Lichtwicz t.
    Ochsner t.
    Patterson t.
    piloting t.
    Potain t.
    rectal t.
    Southey t.
Tröltsch
    speculum
troposcope
Trousseau
    bougie
    dilator
Trousseau-Jackson
    dilator
Troutman
    chisel
Tru-Cut
    needle
T-shaped incision
T tube, T-tube
Tubbs
    dilator
tube
    Abbott-Miller t.
    Abbott-Rawson t.
    Acmi-Valentine t.
    Adson suction t.
    Andrews-Pynchon suction t.
    Anthony t.
    Argyle chest t.
    Argyle endotracheal t.
    Argyle-Salem sump t.

tube (continued)
- Atkins-Cannard tracheotomy t.
- Ayre t.
- Baker jejunostomy t.
- Baker self-sumping t.
- Beardsley empyema t.
- Bellocq t.
- Blakemore esophageal t.
- Blakemore nasogastric t.
- Blakemore-Sengstaken t.
- Bouchut laryngeal t.
- Broyles t.
- Buie rectal suction t.
- Cantor t.
- Carabelli endobronchial t.
- cardiac t.
- Carlens t.
- Carman rectal t.
- Carrel t.
- Castelli t.
- Cattell t.
- Celestin t.
- Chaffin-Pratt t.
- Chaussier t.
- chest t.
- Chevalier Jackson t.
- Communitrach t.
- cuffed t.
- Debove t.
- Depaul t.
- Dobbhoff feeding t.
- Donaldson t.
- drainage t.
- Durham t.
- empyema t.
- endobronchial t.
- endocardial t.
- endotracheal t.
- Esmarch t.
- esophageal t.
- Ewald t.
- feeding t.
- fiberoptic t.
- Frazier t.
- Frazier suction t.
- fusion t.'s
- Gabriel Tucker t.

tube (continued)
- Greiling t.
- Guisez t.
- Harris t.
- Holinger t.
- House t.
- Immergut t.
- intestinal t.
- intratracheal t. (IT)
- intubation t.
- Jackson t.
- Jackson-Pratt t.
- Johnson t.
- Jutte t.
- Kelly t.
- Killian t.
- Kistner t.
- Kuhn t.
- Lanz t.
- LaRocca t.
- laryngostomy t.
- laryngotomy t.
- Lennarson t.
- Lepley-Ernst t.
- Levin t.
- Lewis t.
- Lindeman-Silverstein t.
- Linton t.
- Lore-Lawrence t.
- Luer t.
- Lyster t.
- MacKenty t.
- Martin t.
- Miller-Abbott (MA) t.
- Millin t.
- Minnesota t.
- Montgomery T t.
- Morch t.
- Mosher t.
- Mueller-Frazier t.
- Mueller-Pool t.
- Mueller-Pynchon t.
- Mueller-Yankauer t.
- Nachlas t.
- nasogastric t.
- nasopharyngeal t.
- nasotracheal t.
- Negus t.

tube (continued)
  nephrostomy t.
  New t.
  O'Beirne t.
  observation t.
  Ochsner t.
  orotracheal t.
  Paparella t.
  Parker t.
  Paul-Mixter t.
  Per-Lee t.
  Pilling t.
  pin and t. appliance
  Polisar-Lyons t.
  Pool t.
  Pudenz t.
  Pynchon t.
  rectal t.
  Rehfuss t.
  Reuter t.
  Robertshaw t.
  Rosen t.
  Rubin t.
  Ryle t.
  Sachs suction t.
  Schall t.
  Sengstaken t.
  Sengstaken-Blakemore t.
  Shea t.
  Sheehy t.
  Shepard t.
  Shiley t.
  Shiner t.
  Southey-Leech t.
  Souttar t.
  speaking t.
  stomach t.
  suction t.
  sump t.
  T t.
  tampon t.
  Teflon t.
  thoracostomy t.
  tracheal t.
  tracheostomy t.
  tracheotomy t.
  Tucker t.
  tympanostomy t.

tube (continued)
  U t.
  Valentine t.
  ventilation t.
  Venturi myringotomy t.
  vertical t.
  Voltolini t.
  Wangensteen t.
  Welch-Allyn t.
  Yankauer t.
tubectomy
tuber (tubers, tubera)
  t. omentale
tubular
  t. forceps
tucker
  Bishop-Black tendon t.
  Bishop-DeWitt tendon t.
  Bishop-Peter tendon t.
  Bishop tendon t.
  Burch-Greenwood t.
  Burch-Greenwood tendon t.
  Fink tendon t.
Tucker [eponym]
  bronchoscope
  dilator
  esophagoscope
  laryngoscope
  tube
Tucker-McLean
  forceps
Tudor-Edwards
  costotome
Tuffier-Raney
  retractor
Tulevech
  cannula
tulle gras
  t.g. dressing
  t.g. gauze
Tulpius valve
tumorectomy
tunneled bougie
tunneler
  Crawford-Cooley t.
  DeBakey t.
Tuohy
  needle

Turek spinous process spreader
Turell
    proctoscope
    sigmoidoscope
Turkel
    needle
Turner
    operation
    pin
Tuttle
    forceps
    proctoscope
    sigmoidoscope
twisted suture
two-bottle drainage system
Tycron, Ti-Cron
    suture
Tydings
    forceps
    knife
    tonsillectome
Tydings-Lakeside
    forceps
tylectomy
tympanostomy
    t. tube
typoscope
Tyrrell
    hook
UBC—University of British
   Columbia
UBC brace
ulcer
    Allingham u.
    Cruveilhier u.
    Cushing u.
    Dieulafoy u.
    follicular u.
    gastroduodenal u.
    gastrojejunal u.
    Kocher u.
    Mann-Williamson u.
    marginal u.
    perforating u.
Ullrich
    retractor
ultramicroscope
ultramicroscopy

ultrasonic
    u. calipers
ultrasound
    u. probe
umbilectomy
umbilical
    u. catheter
    u. scissors
umbrascopy
umbrella
    Mobin-Uddin u.
unabsorbable, nonabsorbable
    n. surgical suture
    n. suture
uncipressure
underwater
    u. seal drainage system
uninterrupted suture
unit
    Bovie u.
Unna
    extractor
    paste
    paste boot
Updegraff
    needle
ureteral
    u. catheter
ureterocystoscope
ureterorenoscope
urethral
    u. speculum
urethroscope
urethrotome
    dilating u.
    Keitzer u.
    Maisonneuve u.
    Otis u.
USCI—United States Catheter and
   Instrument [Company]
USCI cannula
U-shaped incision
uterine
    u. forceps
    u. probe
uteroscope
uvulotome

vacuum
    v. drainage system
vagectomy
vaginal
    v. speculum
vaginoscope
Valentine
    position
    splint
    tube
valve
    See also *graft* and *prosthesis.*
    artificial v.
    ball-type v.
    Björk-Shiley v.
    Blom-Singer v.
    caged-ball v.
    cardiac v., artificial
    Carpentier-Edwards v.
    Duromedics v.
    Hancock v.
    heart v., artificial
    Houston v.'s
    Ionescu v.
    Ionescu-Shiley v.
    Kerckring (Kerkring) v.'s
    Lillehei-Kaster v.
    Medtronic-Hall v.
    Omnicarbon v.
    Omniscience v.
    pop-off v.
    porcine v.
    pressure-limiting v.
    Pudenz v.
    Pudenz-Heyer v.
    speaking v.
    Starr-Edwards v.
    St. Jude v.
    tilting-disk v.
valved
valvula (valvulae)
    v. ileocolica
    v. pylori
valvulotome
    Himmelstein v.
    Malm-Himmelstein v.
van Buren
    dilator

van Buren (continued)
    forceps
    operation
    sound
Vanderbilt
    forceps
Van Doren
    forceps
Vanghetti
    prosthesis
van Helmont
    speculum
Vannas
    scissors
Van Osdel
    tonsillectome
vaporizer
    anesthetic v.
varicotomy
vascular
    v. clamp
    knitted v. prosthesis
Vaseline
    gauze dressing
vasoligature
Vater
    papilla
Veau
    elevator
vectorscope
Veenema
    retractor
Veenema-Gusberg
    needle
vein
    femoral v.
    v. retractor
    v. stripper
Veirs
    cannula
Velcro
    binder
    dressing
Velpeau
    bandage
    hernia
Velroc
    dressing

velum (vela)
    artificial v.
Venable-Stuck nail
venoperitoneostomy
venous
    v. cannula
    v. catheter
ventilation
    v. bronchoscope
    v. tube
ventricular
    v. cannula
    v. catheter
ventriculopuncture
    v. needle
ventriculoscope
ventroscopy
ventrotomy
Venturi
    myringotomy tube
Verbrugge
    clamp
Veress
    cannula
    needle
verge
    anal v.
Verhoeff
    forceps
    scissors
    suture
Vermale
    operation
Verneuil
    operation
Vernier [eponym]
    calipers
Vernon-David
    proctoscope
    sigmoidoscope
    speculum
vertebrated
    v. probe
vertical
    v. incision
    v. mattress suture
    v. tube

Vest [eponym]
    telescope
vest-over-pants technique
Vezien
    scissors
Vicat
    needle
Vicryl
    suture
videomicroscopy
Vi-drape
Vienna
    speculum
Viers erysiphake
Villard button
villusectomy
Vim-Silverman
    needle
Vioform
    dressing
Virchow
    knife
Virden
    catheter
Viro-Tec
    suture
Virtus
    forceps
VISC—vitreous infusion suction
    cutter
viscerad
viscerotome
viscerotomy
Vischer
    incision
visuoscope
visuscope
Vitallium
    drill
    implant
    mesh
    prosthesis
"Vo" Phonetic for Veau.
Vogel
    curet
Volkmann
    curet
    retractor

Volkmann (continued)
    splint
    spoon
Voltolini
    tube
von Arlt. See *Arlt.*
von Bergmann
    hernia
    operation
von Graefe. See *Graefe.*
von Hippel (Hippel)
    trephine
von Langenbeck. See *Langenbeck.*
von Mikulicz. See *Mikulicz.*
von Mondak
    forceps
von Petz
    clamp
von Saal
    pin
von Sonnenberg
    catheter
von Zenker. See *Zenker.*
Voorhees
    bag
    needle
V-shaped incision
vulsella, vulsellum
vulsellum
    v. forceps
Wada
    prosthesis
Wadsworth-Todd cautery
Wagner punch
Wahl sign
Walcher position
Waldeau
    forceps
Waldmann
    scissors
Wales
    dilator
Walker
    dissector
    retractor
    scissors
walking
    w. calipers

Walldius
    prosthesis
Walsh
    curet
Walsham
    forceps
Walter
    forceps
    spud
Walter-Deaver
    retractor
Walther
    clamp
    dilator
    forceps
Walther-Crenshaw
    clamp
Walton
    forceps
    punch
Walton-Schubert
    forceps
Wangensteen
    apparatus
    awl
    carrier
    clamp
    dissector
    drainage
    dressing
    forceps
    suction
    tube
Wappler
    cystoscope
Ward-French
    needle
Warren
    incision
Washam
    forceps
Waterman
    bronchoscope
water-seal drainage system
Waters-Waldron position
Watson
    operation

Watson-Jones
 incision
Watson-Williams
 forceps
Watts
 clamp
Watze
 forceps
Waugh
 operation
wax-tipped bougie
W. Dean McDonald
 clamp
Weavenit
 prosthesis
Webb
 bolt
 stripper
Weber
 catheter
 insufflator
 knife
Weber-Fergusson
 incision
Webster
 retractor
Weck
 clip
Weck-cel sponge
wedge
 w. incision
Weeks
 needle
 speculum
weightbearing, weight-bearing
 w. brace
weighted speculum
Weil
 forceps
Weinberg
 retractor
Weingartner
 forceps
Weisenbach
 forceps
Weisman
 curet
 forceps

Weisman-Graves
 speculum
Weitlaner
 retractor
Welch-Allyn
 anoscope
 forceps
 hook
 laryngoscope
 otoscope
 probe
 proctoscope
 sigmoidoscope
 speculum
 tube
Wellaminski
 perforator
"Werd" Phonetic for Wurd.
Wertheim
 clamp
 forceps
 splint
Wertheim-Cullen
 clamp
 forceps
Wertheim-Reverdin
 clamp
Wesolowski
 prosthesis
Wesson
 retractor
Westcott
 scissors
Wester
 clamp
 scissors
wet-to-dry dressing
Weve
 operation
Wheeler
 cystotome
 knife
 spatula
whip catheter
Whipple
 incision
 operation
whipstitch suture

whirligig apparatus
whistle
    w. bougie
whistle-tip
    w.-t. catheter
    w.-t. drain
white
    w. braided suture
    w. silk suture
White [eponym]
    forceps
Whitehead
    operation
White-Lillie
    forceps
White-Oslay
    forceps
White-Proud
    retractor
Whiting
    curet
    tonsillectome
whitlow
    melanotic w.
WHO periodontal probe
Wiener
    hook
    speculum
Wiener-Pierce
    rasp
Wigby-Taylor position
Wild
    operating microscope
Wilde
    forceps
    incision
Wilde-Bruening snare
Wilder
    scoop
Willett
    clamp
    forceps
Williams
    clamp
    forceps
    probe
    speculum

Willis
    antrum
Wilman
    clamp
Wilmer
    scissors
Wilson
    awl
    bolt
    clamp
    leads
    plate
    rib spreader
    stripper
    wrench
Wiltberger spreader
windlass
    w. tourniquet
Winer
    catheter
Winiwarter
    operation
Winslow
    foramen
    pancreas
Winter arch bar
wire
    alignment w.
    alveolar w.
    arch w.
    arch w., ideal
    w. bivalve speculum
    cable w. suture
    continuous loop w.
    guide w., guidewire
    interdental w.
    intraoral w.
    Ivy w.
    Kirschner w.
    ligature w.
    Medrafil w. suture
    w. mesh
    orthodontic w.
    pull-out w. suture
    Risdon w.
    silver w. suture
    w. speculum
    w. suture

wire (continued)
  tantalum w. suture
  twin w.
Wise
 operation
Wis-Foregger
 laryngoscope
Wishard
 catheter
Wis-Hipple
 laryngoscope
Wittner
 forceps
Witzel
 operation
Woakes
 saw
Wolf
 laparoscope
 peritoneoscope
Wolfenden position
Wölfler
 sign
 suture
Wolf-Schindler
 gastroscope
Wolfson
 clamp
 retractor
Wolkowitsch sign
Wood [cponym]
 needle
Woodson
 elevator
 spatula
"Word" Phonetic for Wurd.
woven loop stone dislodger
woven vascular prosthesis
Wright
 plate
 snare
W-shaped incision
Wullstein
 bur
 forceps
 knife
 retractor

Wullstein-House
 forceps
Wurd
 catheter
Wützer
 operation
Wylie
 dilator
 stripper
Wyllys-Andrews
 operation
Wysler
 suture
xenograft
 Hancock porcine x.
Xeroform
 gauze dressing
xyster
YAG—yttrium-aluminum-garnet
YAG laser
Yankauer
 bronchoscope
 catheter
 curet
 esophagoscope
 forceps
 laryngoscope
 probe
 speculum
 tube
Yankauer-Little
 forceps
Yasargil
 clip
 retractor
Yellen
 clamp
Yeoman
 forceps
 proctoscope
 sigmoidoscope
Y incision, Y-type incision
Yorke-Mason
 incision
Young
 clamp
 dilator
 forceps

Young (continued)
    needle holder
    retractor
Young-Millin
    needle holder
Y suture
Y-type incision, Y incision
Zachary-Cope-DeMartel
    clamp
Zancolli
    procedure
Zanelli position
Zavod
    catheter
Zeiss
    microscope
Zenker
    forceps
zeoscope
zero [suture size: 0, 00, 2-0, etc.]
Z-flap
    incision
Ziegler
    forceps
    knife

Ziegler (continued)
    probe
Zieman
    operation
zigzag
    z. incision
Zimaloy
    prosthesis
Zimmer
    prosthesis
Zimmerman
    operation
Zipser
    clamp
"zister" Phonetic for xyster.
zoescope
Zollinger
    forceps
Z-shaped incision
Z suture
Zwanck pessary
Zweifel-DeLee cranioclast
Zytor
    suture

Laboratory, Pathology, and Chemistry Terms

a—[as a subscript] symbol for arterial blood
A—adenine
    adenosine
    [as a subscript] symbol for alveolar gas
A_{1c} [A1C]—hemoglobin A_{1c} [glycosylated hemoglobin]
A-a, $(A-a)O_2$, $P(A-a)O_2$—alveolar-arterial [oxygen gradient]
AABB—American Association of Blood Banks
AAP—American Association of Pathologists
AAPB—American Association of Pathologists and Bacteriologists
AAV—adeno-associated virus
Ab—antibody
abbau
Abbé-Zeiss
Abbe-Zeiss
    apparatus
    counting cell
ABC—aspiration biopsy cytology
abequose
aberration
    chromosome a.
    heterosomal a.
    intrachromosomal a.
ABG, ABGs—arterial blood gas(es)
abiuret
abiuretic
ABO
    antibodies
    antigens
    blood groups
    compatibility
    incompatibility
    typing

Abrams
    test
abscess
    sterile a.
absorptiometer
absorption
    fat a.
    intestinal a.
    iron a.
    percutaneous a.
    protein a.
absorptivity
Acanthamoeba
    A. astronyxis
    A. castellani
    A. culbertsoni
    A. hatchetti
    A. polyphaga
    A. rhisodes
Acanthia lectularia
acanthocyte
acanthocytosis
acari (plural of acarus)
acarologist
Acarus
    A. hordei
    A. rhyzoglypticus hyacinthi
accelerator
    serum prothrombin conversion a. (SPCA)
    serum thrombotic a.
    thromboplastin generation a.
accelerin
accolé
acellular
acephalocyst
acetanilid
    a. poisoning
acetas

acetate
acetoacetic acid
acetoacetyl-CoA (coenzyme A)
acetoacetyl-CoA (coenzyme A)
    reductase
acetoacetyl-CoA (coenzyme A) thi-
    olase
acetoacetyl coenzyme A
Acetobacter
    A. aceti
acetoin
acetolysis
acetonation
acetonitrile
acetonumerator
aceto-orcein
acetosoluble
acetous
acetylcholine
    a. receptor antibody
        (AChRab)
acetyl-CoA acetyltransferase
acetyl-CoA acyltransferase
acetyl-CoA carboxylase
acetyl-CoA: α-glucosaminide-*N*-
    acetyltransferase
acetyl-CoA synthetase
N-acetylgalactosamine-4-sulfatase
N-acetylgalactosamine-6-sulfatase
α-*N*-acetylgalactosaminidase [alpha-]
β-*N*-acetylgalactosaminidase [beta-]
N-acetylglucosamine-6-sulfatase
α-*N*-acetylglucosaminidase [alpha-]
N-acetylglucosaminylphosphotrans-
    ferase
N-acetyl-β-hexosaminidase
acetylization
acetylsulfadiazine
acetylsulfaguanidine
acetylsulfathiazole
acetyltransferase
ACF—acid-fast culture
Achatina
AChRab—acetylcholine receptor
    antibody
achromasia
achromat
achromatin

achromatinic
achromatize
achromatolysis
achromatophil
achromatophilia
achromatopia
achromatopic
achromatous
achromia
    central a.
achromophilous
achrooamyloid
Achúcarro stain
acid
    acetic a.
    acetoacetic a.
    acetylacetic a.
    acetylsalicylic a. (ASA)
    amino a.
    aminobenzoic a.
    aminocaproic a.
    aminolevulinic a. (ALA)
    argininosuccinic a.
    ascorbic a.
    chloracetic a., chloroacetic a.
    chloranilic a.
    citric a.
    deoxyribonucleic a. (DNA)
    diacetic a.
    ethacrynic a.
    folic a.
    formic a.
    formiminoglutamic a.
    glucuronic a.
    glutamic a.
    glycolic a.
    hippuric a.
    homogentisic a.
    homovanillic a.
    hydrochloric a.
    5-hydroxyindoleacetic a.
    lactic a.
    linoleic a.
    linolenic a.
    linolic a.
    lysergic a.
    muriatic a.
    nalidixic a.

acid (continued)
    nicotinic a.
    nitric a.
    oleic a.
    oxalic a.
    pantothenic a.
    pentanoic a.
    perchloric a.
    phenylpyruvic a.
    phosphoric a.
    pyruvic a.
    ribonucleic a. (RNA)
    salicylic a.
    sodium *p*-aminohippuric
      (PAH) a. [*p*-, para-]
    stearic a.
    succinic a.
    sulfosalicylic a.
    sulfuric a.
    tannic a.
    teichoic a.
    titratable a.
    tricarboxylic a.
    trichloroacetic a.
    uric a.
    valproic a.
    vanillylmandelic a.
    xanthurenic a.
acidalbumin
Acidaminococcus
acid-forming
acidimeter
acidophilia
acidophilus [*Lactobacillus acido-*
    philus]
acidosis
    carbon dioxide a.
acidulated
aciduria
    glutamic a.
    glycolic a.
    L-glyceric a.
    xanthurenic a.
Acinetobacter
    A. calcoaceticus
acipenserin
ackee, akee
aconitine

acoustic
    a. microscope
Acremoniella
acroblast
acrolein
acrosomal
acrosome
acrylate
acrylic acid
acrylonitrile
ACT—activated coagulation time
ACTH—adrenocorticotropic hor-
    mone
ACTH-RF—ACTH-releasing factor
ACTH stimulation test
Actinobacillus
    A. actinomycetemcomitans
    A. lignieresii
    A. mallei
    A. pseudomallei
Actinomadura
    A. madurae
    A. pelletierii
Actinomyces
    A. israelii
    A. muris
    A. naeslundii
actinomycete
    nocardioform a.
actinomycetin
actinophage
action
    a. spectrum
activated coagulation time (ACT)
activated partial thromboplastin
    time (APTT, aPTT)
activity
    leukemia-associated inhibi-
      tory a. (LIA)
    nonsuppressible insulin-like a.
    plasma renin a.
actodigin
actomyosin
acyl carrier protein
acyl-CoA [coenzyme A]
acyl-CoA dehydrogenase
acyl-CoA desaturase
acyl-CoA synthetase

acyl coenzyme A
acyl enzyme
acylsphingosine deacylase
acyltransferase
adamantoblast
Adamkiewicz
    test
Addis
    count
    test
addisin
adelomorphic
adelomorphous
adendritic
adenine deaminase
adenoblast
adenocyte
adenopituicyte
adenosine
    a. deaminase
    a. diphosphate (ADP)
    a. kinase
    a. monophosphate (AMP)
    a. triphosphate (ATP)
adenosinetriphosphatase (ATPase)
adenylate
adenylate cyclase
adenylate deaminase
adenylate kinase
adenyl cyclase
adenylic acid
adenylic acid deaminase
adenylosuccinase
adenylosuccinate lyase
adenylpyrophosphate
adenylyl, adenyl
adenylyl transferase
ADH—antidiuretic hormone
adherence
    bacterial a.
    immune a.
adiaspore
adipic acid
adipocellular
adipocere
adiposuria
Adler
    test

adrenocorticotropic hormone (ACTH)
adrenocorticotropin
adrenoreceptor
ADS—antidiuretic substance
Aedes
    A. aegypti
    A. albopictus
    A. cinereus
    A. flavescens
    A. leucocelaenus
    A. scutellaris pseudoscutel-
        laris
    A. sollicitans
    A. spencerii
    A. taeniorhynchus
AER—albumin excretion rate
aerobe
aerobic
Aerococcus
    A. viridans
aerogen
aerogenesis
Aeromonas
    A. hydrophila
    A. liquefaciens
    A. punctata
    A. salmonicida
    A. shigelloides
aerophil
aerophilic
aerosis
aerotonometer
AF—acid-fast
AFB—acid-fast bacilli
affinity
    antibody a. chromatography
    a. chromatography
    functional a.
    a. labeling
    selective a.
AFP—alpha-fetoprotein
AFS—acid-fast smear
aftergilding
AG—anion gap
    antiglobulin
Ag—antigen
agammaglobulinemia
    Bruton a.

agammaglobulinemia (continued)
  Swiss-type a.
Agamofilaria
agar
  See also *culture medium.*
  bacteriostasis a.
  bile-esculin a.
  bird seed a.
  bismuth sulfite a.
  blood a.
  Bordet-Gengou a.
  brain-heart infusion a.
  Brucella a.
  Campylobacter selective a.
  cetrimide a.
  charcoal yeast extract a.
  chocolate a.
  clostrisel a.
  Columbia blood a.
  corn meal a.
  Czapek-Dox a.
  deoxycholate-citrate a.
  deoxyribonuclease a.
  dextrose a.
  DNase a.
  egg-yolk a.
  Endo a.
  eosin-methylene blue
    (EMB) a.
  GC a.
  gelatin a.
  heart infusion a.
  Hektoen a.
  inhibitory mold a.
  Kligler iron a.
  Krumwiede triple sugar a.
  Levine EMB a.
  Löffler serum a.
  Löwenstein-Jensen a.
  lysine iron a.
  MacConkey a.
  Middlebrook a.
  modified TM a.
  Mueller-Hinton a.
  mycobiotic a.
  Mycoplasma a.
  neomycin assay a.
  nitrate a.

agar (continued)
  nutrient a.
  nystatin assay a.
  phenylalanine a.
  phenylethyl alcohol a.
  polymyxin test a.'s
  potato-blood a.
  potato dextrose a.
  Pseudomonas-selective a.
  rabbit blood a.
  Russell double-sugar a.
  Sabhi a.
  Sabouraud a.
  Sabouraud dextrose a.
  saccharose-mannitol a.
  Salmonella-Shigella a.
  Schaedler blood a.
  seed a.
  Simmons citrate a.
  standard methods a.
  streptomycin assay a. with
    yeast extract
  sulfite a.
  tellurite a.
  tellurite glycine a.
  Thayer-Martin (TM) a.
  thistle seed a.
  Trichophyton a.
  triple sugar iron a.
  tryptic soy a.
  urea a.
  Wilkins-Chilgren a.
  xylose-lysine-deoxycholate a.
  Zein a.
agar-agar
agaric acid
AGC—absolute granulocyte count
agent
  alkylating a.
  disclosing a.
agglutinable
agglutinant
agglutination
  acid a.
  alpha a.
  bacteriogenic a.
  beta a.
  cold a.

agglutination (continued)
    flagellar a.
    H a.
    immune a.
    intravascular a.
    latex a.
    macroscopic a.
    mediate a.
    microscopic a.
    O a.
    platelet a.
    Rh a.
    salt a.
    spontaneous a.
    T a.
    Vi a.
    warm a.
agglutinative
agglutinin
    alpha a.
    anti-A a.
    anti-B a.
    anti-M a.
    anti-N a.
    anti-P a.
    anti-Rh a.
    anti-S a.
    beta a.
    chief a.
    cold a.
    febrile a.
    flagellar a.
    group a.
    H a.
    immune a.
    latex a.
    leukocyte a.
    Mg a.
    natural a.
    O a.
    platelet a.
    Rh a.
    serum a.
    somatic a.
    warm a.
agglutinogenic
agglutinophilic

aggregate
    tubular a.
aggregated human IgG (AHuG)
aggregation
    cell a.
    platelet a.
aggregometer
aggregometry
aglandular
agminated
agmination
agranular
agyric
air
    alveolar a.
    residual a.
    tidal a.
akee, ackee
ALA—aminolevulinic acid
alanine aminotransferase
alanine transaminase
Albert
    diphtheria stain
albumin
    a. A
    acetosoluble a.
    acid a.
    alkali a.
    a. of Bence Jones
    caseiniform a.
    coagulated a.
    derived a.
    hematin a.
    normal human serum a.
    Patein a.
    radioiodinated serum a.
    serum a.
    a. tannate a.
    triphenyl a.
albuminate
albuminimeter
albuminimetry
albuminocholia
albuminocytological
albuminolysis
albuminoptysis
albuminoreaction
albuminous

Alcaligenes
    A. faecalis
alcohol dehydrogenase
Alco-Sensor
algal
alkalimeter
alkalimetry
alkaline
    a. phosphatase
alkalosis
"alk. phos." Slang for alkaline phos-
    phatase.
allele
allelic
allelism
allelochemics
Allodermanyssus
    A. sanguineus
Allomonas
allopregnanediol
allotoxin
Almén test
alpha
    a.-*N*-acetylgalactosaminidase
    a.-*N*-acetylglucosaminidase
    a. acid glycoprotein
    a.-adrenergic receptor
    a. amino acids
    a. amino nitrogen
    a.-amylose
    a. antichymotrypsin
    a. antiplasmin
    a.-1-antitrypsin
    a. band
    a.-beta variation
    a. cells
    a. chain
    a. decay
    a.-dextrinase
    a.-dinitrophenol
    a.-estradiol [now: estradiol
        17α (17-alpha)]
    a.-fetoprotein (AFP)
    a.-L-fucosidase
    a.-galactosidase A
    a. globulin
    a. globulin antibodies
    $a._2$ globulins

alpha (continued)
    1,4-a.-glucan branching
        enzyme
    a.-glucosidase
    a. 1,4-glucosidase
    a.-hemolytic streptococci
    17-a.-hydroxyprogesterone
        aldolase
    a.-L-iduronidase
    a.-keto acid dehydrogenase
    a.-ketoglutarate
    a.-ketoglutaric acid
    a.-lipoprotein
    a.-macroglobulin
    a.-2-macroglobulin
    a.-mannosidase
    a. melanocytic-stimulating
        hormone
    a.-methylacetoacetyl CoA
        thiolase
    a.-methyldopa
    a.-naphthol thiourea
    a. protease inhibitor
    a. receptors
    a. seromucoid
    a.-streptococci
    a.-thalassemia
    a.-trypsin
Alsberg
    angle
    triangle
alteplase
Altmann
    anilin-acid fuchsin stain
    fixative
    fluid
    granule
    liquid
    theory
Altmann-Gersh method
alum hematoxylin
alveus (alvei)
    a. hippocampi, a. of hip-
        pocampus
Alzheimer
    cell
    fibril
    stain

AMA—antimitochondrial antibody
amacrine
    a. cells
Amanita
    A. muscaria
    A. pantherina
    A. phalloides
    A. rubescens
    A. verna
    A. virosa
ambiguity
    ribosomal a.
amblychromasia
amblychromatic
ameba
ameloblast
ameloblastoma
    acanthomatous a.
    basal cell a.
    cystic a.
    extraosseous a.
    follicular a.
    granular cell a.
    malignant a.
    melanotic a.
    multicystic a.
    peripheral a.
    pigmented a.
    pituitary a.
    plexiform a.
    plexiform unicystic a.
    solid a.
    unicystic a.
amelogenin
American Type Culture Collection
    (ATCC)
Ames test
amianthoid
Amici
    disk
    line
    striae
amino acid
    a.a. residue
    aromatic a.a.
    a.a. sequence
    basic a.a.'s
    ketogenic a.a.

amino acid (continued)
    sulfur-containing a.a.'s
    uncoded a.a.
o-aminoazotoluene [o-, ortho-]
γ-aminobutyrate [gamma-]
γ-aminobutyric acid (GABA)
    [gamma-]
p-aminohippuric acid (PAH, PAHA)
    synthetase [p-, para-]
δ-aminolevulinic acid (ALA) [delta-]
aminopeptidase
    leucine a.
Ammon
    filaments
    fissure
    horn
ammonium
    a. oxalate crystal violet
    a. sulfate
amniocyte
Amoeba
    A. proteus
AMP—adenosine monophosphate
AMP, cyclic
AMP deaminase
amplification
    gene a.
    image a.
Amussat
    valve
    valvula
amylase
    pancreatic a.
    salivary a.
    serum a.
    urinary a.
amyloid
ANA—antinuclear antibody
anaerobe
    facultative a.
    obligate a.
analogue [anatomical, chemical]
analysis
    antigenic a.
    chemical a.
    gastric a.
    pentagastrin stimulated a.
    tubeless gastric a.

analyzer
    sequential multiple a. (SMA)
anamnesis
anatomy
    cross-sectional a.
ANC—absolute neutrophil count
Ancylostoma
    A. *braziliense*
    A. *caninum*
    A. *duodenale*
Andernach ossicles
Andersch
    ganglion
Anderson and Goldberger test
Andrade
    indicator
    syndrome
androgen
Angiostrongylus
    A. *cantonensis*
    A. *costaricensis*
angiotensin
    a. III
Anichkov (Anitschkow)
    cell
    myocyte
anion
    a. gap
anionic
anochromasia
anomaly
    Hegglin a.
    Huët-Pelger nuclear a.
    Jordan a.
    May-Hegglin a.
    Pelger-Huët a.
    Pelger-Huët nuclear a.
Anopheles
    A. *maculipennis*
anthranilic acid
anthropoid
anthropology
    forensic a.
    hematological a.
    pathologic a.
anthropometry
    forensic a.
anthropophilic

anthropozoophilic
antibody (antibodies)
    ABO a.
    a. affinity chromatography
    albumin-agglutinating a.
    anti-A a.
    anti-acetylcholine receptor
        (anti-AChR) a.
    anti-B a.
    anti-basement membrane a.
    anticardiolipin a.
    anticentromere a.
    anticytoplasmic a.
    antifibrin a.
    anti–glomerular basement
        membrane (anti-GBM) a.
    antikidney a.'s
    anti-La a.
    anti-M a.
    antimicrosomal a.
    antimitochondrial a.
    antinuclear a. (ANA)
    anti-P a.
    antireceptor a.
    anti-Rh (Rhesus) a.
    anti-Ro a.
    anti-S a.
    anti-Sm a.
    anti-smooth muscle a.
    anti-T-cell a.
    auto–anti-idiotypic a.
    autoimmune a.
    autologous a.
    basement membrane a.
    B-cell a.
    bivalent a.
    blocking a.
    combining-site a.
    complement-fixing a.
    coprecipitating a.
    cross-reacting a.
    cryptosporidiosis a.
    cytophilic a.
    cytotoxic a.
    a. deficiency syndrome
    a.-dependent cell–mediated
        cytotoxicity
    Donath-Landsteiner a.

antibody (antibodies) (continued)
    Duffy a.: FyFy
    Duffy blood a. type
    enhancing a.
    a. excess
    fluorescein-labeled a.
    H a.
    heat-labile a.
    hepatitis B core a. (HBcAb)
    hepatitis B e a. (HBeAb)
    hepatitis B surface a.
      (HBsAb)
    heteroclitic a.
    heterogenetic a.
    heteroligating a.
    heterophile a.
    homocytotropic a.
    humoral a.
    hybrid a.
    hybridoma a.
    IgM-RF (rheumatoid factor)
      a.
    immunosorbent a.
    inhibiting a.
    isoimmune a.
    isophil a.
    Kell blood a. type
    Kidd blood a. type
    Lewis a.: LeLe
    Lewis blood a. type
    Lutheran blood a. type
    maternal a.
    monoclonal a.
    neutralizing a.
    nonprecipitation a.
    nuclear a.
    O a.
    opsonizing a.
    Ortho-mune a.
    saline-agglutinating a.
    skin-sensitizing a.
    T a.
    Thomsen a.
    thyroglobulin a.
    thyroid microsomal a.'s
    treponema-immobilizing a.
    TSH-displacing a.
    univalent a.

antibody (antibodies) (continued)
    Vi a.
    warm-reactive a.
    Wassermann a.
    xenocytophilic a.
antigen (Ag)
    A a.
    ABO a.
    accessible a.
    allogeneic a.
    alpha a. of adenovirus
    alum-precipitated a.
    a.-antibody complex
    Australia a.
    autologous a.
    ayr a.
    ayw1 a. (ayw2, ayw3, ayw4)
    B a.
    bacterial a.
    beta a. of adenovirus
    a.-binding capacity
    C a.
    carbohydrate a.'s
    carcinoembryonic a. (CEA)
    chick embryo a.
    Chido-Rodgers a.
    common enterobacterial a.
    complement-fixing a.
    cross-reacting a.
    cryptic T a.
    cryptococcal a.
    Diego a.
    differentiation a.
    Duffy a.
    E a.
    endogenous a.
    epsilon a.
    erythrocyte a.
    a. excess
    exogenous a.
    F a.
    factor VIII a.
    fetal a.'s
    Forssman a.
    gamma a.
    group-specific a.
    H a.

antigen (Ag) (continued)
  hepatitis a., hepatitis-associated a. (HAA) [now: hepatitis B surface antigen]
  hepatitis B core a. (HBcAg)
  hepatitis B e a. (HBeAg)
  hepatitis B surface a. (HBsAg)
  heterogeneic a.
  heterophile a.
  Hikojima a.
  human leukocyte a. (HLA)
  I a.
  Ia a.
  idiotypic a.
  Inaba a.
  incomplete a.
  inhalant a.
  isophile a.
  Kell a.
  Kidd a.
  Kunin a.
  Kveim a.
  lens a.'s
  leukocyte common a.
  Ly a.
  lymphocyte function–associated a. 1 (LFA-1)
  lymphocyte function–associated a. 2 (LFA-2)
  lymphocyte function–associated a. 3 (LFA-3)
  NP a.
  O a.
  Ogawa a.
  oncofetal a.
  organ-specific a.
  Oz a.
  P54 a.
  PHA (phytohemagglutinin) a.
  plasma cell a.
  a.-presenting cell
  proliferating cell nuclear a.
  protective a.
  QA a.
  R a.
  Rh (Rhesus) factor a.
  S a.

antigen (Ag) (continued)
  SD a.
  skin-specific histocompatibility a.
  surface a.
  SV 40 T a.
  synthetic a.
  T a.
  T-cell a.
  Thomas a.
  Thomsen-Friedenreich a.
  thymus-dependent a.
  thymus-independent a.
  transplantation a.
  tumor-associated a.
  tumor-specific a.
  Vi a.
  viral capsid a.
  von Willebrand a.
  yolk sac a.
antihyaluronidase
  a. titer
anti-invasin
  a. I
  a. II
antilewisite
  British a. (BAL)
anti-Rho-D titer
antistreptolysin
  a. O
α_1-antitrypsin [alpha-1-]
AP—alkaline phosphatase
APH—adenohypophysial hormone
      anterior pituitary hormone
apo—apolipoprotein
apolipoprotein
  a. A-I
  a. B
  a. C-II
  a. D
  a. E (Apo-E)
apparatus
appearance
APTT, aPTT—activated partial thromboplastin time
Arachnia
  A. propionica

Arantius
    body (bodies)
    canal
    duct
    ligament
    nodules
arboroid
area (areae, areas)
    areae gastricae
Argas
    A. reflexus
argininosuccinicacidemia
Arias-Stella
    cells
    effect
    phenomenon
    reaction
Arizona
Armanni-Ebstein
    cell
    change
    lesion
Arneth
    classification
    count
    formula
    index
    stages
Arnold
    ganglion
    bundle
    canal
    tract
Arrhenius
    doctrine
    equation
    formula
    theory
ART—automated reagin test
arterial
    a. blood gas (ABG)
    a. oxygen saturation
Arthrographis
    A. langeroni
AS—antistreptolysin
Ascaris
    A. lumbricoides

ASCI—American Society for Clinical Investigation
ASCLT—American Society of Clinical Laboratory Technicians
ASCP—American Society of Clinical Pathologists
ASF—aniline, sulfur, formaldehyde
Askanazy cell
Asn—asparagine
Aspergillus
    A. auricularis
    A. barbae
    A. bouffardi
    A. clavatus
    A. concentricus
    A. flavus
    A. fumigatus
    A. giganteus
    A. glaucus
    A. gliocladium
    A. mucoroides
    A. nidulans
    A. niger
    A. ochraceus
    A. oryzae
    A. pictor
    A. repens
asphyxia
asphyxiation
assay
    biologic a.
    cancer antigen 125 (CA 125) a.
    CA15-3 RIA (radioimmunoassay)
    competitive protein-binding a.
    C-terminal a.
    D-dimer a.
    enzyme-linked immunosorbent a. (ELISA)
    estrogen receptor a. (ERA)
    factor III multimer a.
    glycosylated hemoglobin a.
    hemagglutination inhibition (HI, HAI) a.
    hemoglobin A_{1c} a. [A1C]
    immune a.

assay (continued)
    immune adherence hemag-
        glutination a. (IAHA)
    immunofluorescence a. (IFA)
    immunoradiometric a.
        (IRMA)
    Jerne plaque a.
    leukotactic a.
    microhemagglutination–*Tre-*
        ponema pallidum (MHΛ-
        TP)
    plaque-forming cell a.
    polyethylene glycol precipi-
        tation a.
    radioimmunoprecipitation a.
        (RIPA)
    Raji cell a.
    staphylococcal protein A
        binding a.
    Treponema pallidum hemag-
        glutination a. (TPHA)
Astra [chemistry profile: Astra-7,
    Astra-8]
astrocyte
    atypical a.
Astrup method
ATG—antithymocyte globulin
ATP—adenosine triphosphate
ATPase—adenosine triphosphatase
ATT—arginine tolerance test
Audouin microsporon
Auer
    bodies
    rods
Auerbach
    ganglion (ganglia)
    node
    plexus
aurococcus
Australia antigen (Au)
Australian X disease virus
autoagglutination
autoagglutinin
autoantibody
Automatic Clinical Analyzer
Automeris io
autoprothrombin
    a. IIa

autopsy
    forensic a.
    medicolegal a.
    psychological a.
autoradiography
    contact a.
    dip-coating a.
    film-stripping a.
    thick-layer a.
    two-emulsion a.
autosomal
    a. dominant
    a. recessive
Babès
    nodes
    nodules
    tubercles
Babès-Ernst
    bodies
    corpuscles
    granules
Babesia
    B. microti
bacillus (bacilli)
    acid-fast b.
    Battey b.
    Boas-Oppler b.
    Bordet-Gengou b.
    Calmette-Guérin b.
    Döderlein b.
    Ducrey b.
    enteric b.
    Escherich b.
    Flexner b.
    Friedländer b.
    Frisch b.
    Gärtner b.
    Ghon-Sachs b.
    glanders b.
    Hansen b.
    hay b.
    Hofmann b.
    influenza b.
    Klebs-Löffler b.
    Koch b.
    Koch-Weeks b.
    Morgan b.
    Newcastle-Manchester b.

bacillus (bacilli) (continued)
    paracolon b.
    Pfeiffer b.
    plague b.
    Preisz-Nocard b.
    rhinoscleroma b.
    Schmitz b.
    Shiga b.
    smegma b.
    Sonne-Duval b.
    Strong b.
    swine rotlauf b.
    tubercle b.
    typhoid b.
    Vincent b.
    Weeks b.
    Welch b.
    Whitmore b.
Bacillus
    B. anthracis
    B. cereus
    B. stearothermophilus
    B. subtilis
    B. tularense
bacteria (plural of bacterium)
bacteriform
bacteriologic, bacteriological
bacteriologist
bacterium (bacteria)
    gram-negative bacteria
    gram-positive bacteria
    lactic acid b.
Bacteroides
    B. corrodens
    B. fragilis
    B. funduliformis
    B. melaninogenicus
Bactigen
Baillarger
    bands
    lines
    striae
    stripes
Balantidium
    B. coli
Balbiani
    body
    nucleus

Balbiani (continued)
    ring
band
    MB b.
    MM b.
    Soret b.
Bang
    bacillus
    method
    test
Barcroft apparatus
Bargen streptococci
Barger method
Barr
    body
    chromatin body
Bartholin
    anus
Bartonella
    B. bacilliformis
base
    b. excess
basicaryoplastin
basichromatin
basichromiole
basicity
basicytoparaplastin
Basidiobolus
basilemma
basiparachromatin
basiparaplastin
Batson
    plexus
    system
Baumé
    law
    scale
Bayle
    granulations
BCAA—branched-chain amino acid
B cell [noun]
B-cell [adj.]
    B-c. antibody
    B-c. antigen receptors
beaker
Beale ganglion cell
Bekhterev (Bechterew)
    nucleus

belladonnine
Bence Jones
    albumin
    albumosuria
    body
    cylinders
    globulin
    protein
    protein method
    protein test
    proteinuria
    reaction
bench method
Benedict
    method
    test
Benedict-Roth
    apparatus
Bennet corpuscles
Bensley specific granules
bentonite
    b. flocculation test
benzanthracene
benzene
benzene hexachloride
benzenoid
benzin, benzine
benzopurpurine
benzo[a]pyrene
benzoquinone
benzoxiquine
benzoylecgonine
benzoylphenylcarbinol
Bergey classification
Bergmann
    cells
    cords
    fibers
Berkefeld filter
Bernard
    canal
    duct
Bernouilli
    law
    principle
    theorem
Bernstein
    test

Best
    carmine stain
beta
    b.-N-acetylgalactosaminidase
    b.-erythroidine
    b.-estradiol [now: estradiol
        17β]
    b.-galactosidase
    b. globulin
    b.-glucuronidase
    b. hCG (human chorionic
        gonadotropin)
    3-b.-hydroxy-delta-5-steroid
        dehydrogenase
    b.-lactamase negative
    b.-lactamase positive
    b.-lipotropin
    b.-methylcrotonylglycinuria
    b.-nicotyrine
    b. quick strep test
    b. ray microscope
    b.-sitosterolemia
Betz
    cell area
    cells
Bevan Lewis cells
Bezold (von Bezold)
    ganglion
Bial
    reagent
    test
Bianchi
    valve
bicarbonate
    b. of soda, sodium b.
    standard b.
Bichat
    canal
    fissure
    foramen
    membrane
Bielschowsky
    method
Bifidobacterium
    B. eriksonii
"big 7" Slang for a chemistry-7.
Bili-Labstix

bilirubin
    conjugated b.
    direct b.
    indirect b.
    unconjugated b.
binocular
    b. microscope
binuclear
binucleation
binucleolate
bioactive
bioassay
biochemorphic
biohazard
biologist
biotoxin
Bird
    formula
bisalbuminemia
bischloromethyl ether
biurate
Bizzozero
    cells
    corpuscles
    platelets
black B, Sudan
Blastocystis
    B. hominis
Blastomyces
    B. brasiliensis
    B. coccidioides
    B. dermatitidis
blastomycete
bleeding time
    Duke method b.t
    Ivy method b.t.
Blessig
    groove
Bloch
    method
    reaction
blood
    b. bank
    banked b.
    cord b.
    whole b.
blood groups
    ABO

blood plasma
blood serum
    Loeffler b.s., Löffler b.s.
    Lorrain Smith b.s.
blood type
BM—bone marrow
BMET—basic metabolic panel
    [also: profile]
BMP—basic metabolic panel [also:
    profile]
Boas
    test
Boas-Oppler
    bacillus
    lactobacillus
Bodian
    copper-Protargol stain
    method
Bodo
    B. caudatus
    B. saltans
    B. urinaria
body (bodies)
    Auer b.
    bacillary b.
    Barr b.
    Bollinger b.'s
    Cabot ring b.
    chromatin b.
    creola b.
    cytomegalic inclusion b.
    cytoplasmic inclusion b.
    Donovan b.
    embryoid b.
    fuchsin b.
    Gamna-Favre b.
    Gamna-Gandy b.
    glass b.
    Heinz b.
    Heinz-Ehrlich b.
    hematoxylin b.
    Howell b.
    Howell-Jolly b.
    inclusion b.
    Jolly b.
    ketone b.
    Leishman-Donovan b.
    Mallory b.

body (bodies) (continued)
    malpighian b.'s of kidney
    malpighian b.'s of spleen
    Negri b.
    Nissl b
    pacchionian b
    psammoma b.
    psittacosis inclusion b.
    reticulate b.
    tingible b.
    X chromatin b.
body snatching
Bollinger
    bodies
    granules
bone
bone marrow
"boo-shahr(z)" Phonetic for
    Bouchard.
"boo-shahr-dah(z)" Phonetic for
    Bouchardat.
"boo-yaw," "boo-yawn" Phonetic
    for bouillon.
Bordetella
    B. bronchiseptica
    B. parapertussis
    B. pertussis
Bordet-Gengou
    agar
    bacillus
    culture medium
    phenomenon
Born method
Borrelia
    B. anserina
    B. berbera
    B. buccalis
    B. burgdorferi
    B. carteri
    B. caucasica
    B. duttonii
    B. hermsii
    B. hispanica
    B. kochii
    B. parkeri
    B. persica
    B. recurrentis
    B. refringens

Borrelia (continued)
    B. turicatae
    B. venezuelensis
    B. vincentii
Bouchard
    coefficient
Bouchardat
    test
bouillon
Bouin
    fixative
    fluid
    solution
Bowman
    disks
BPH—benign prostatic hyperplasia
bradyzoite
branched-chain α-keto acid dehy-
    drogenase [alpha-]
brancher enzyme, branching enzyme
Branhamella
    B. catarrhalis
Brevibacterium
brightfield microscopy
BRM—biuret-reactive material
bromphenol
bromthymol
broth
    brain-heart infusion b.
    hippurate b.
    indole-nitrate b.
    Middlebrook b.
    Mueller-Hinton b.
    nutrient b.
    selenite b.
    thioglycolate (THIO) b.
    Todd-Hewitt b.
    Voges-Proskauer b.
Brucella
    B. abortus
    B. bronchiseptica
    B. canis
    B. melitensis
    B. suis
Brugia
    B. malayi
    B. microfilariae
BS—blood sugar

BSA—bismuth-sulfite agar
BSI—bound serum iron
BU—Bodansky unit
Büchner
    extract
    tuberculin
buffy coat, buffy-coated
    b.c. cells
    b.c. smear
BUN—blood urea nitrogen
Bunsen
    burner
    coefficient
Burdach
    bundle
    columns
    cuneate fasciculus
    fasciculus
    fissure
    fibers
    tract
buret, burette
burner
Burnett
    disinfecting fluid
    solution
BV—blood volume
C.—*Clostridium*
    Cryptococcus
C1–C9—complement components
    1–9 (C1q, C1r, C1s to C9q,
    C9r, C9s)
CA—cholic acid
    cold agglutinin
    corpora amylacea
Ca—calcium
Cabot
    ring bodies
CAD—cadaver
Cajal
    astrocyte
    cells
    interstitial nucleus
    stain
C_{alb}—albumin clearance
calcium (Ca)
    c. chloride
    c. ion(s)

Caldwell-Moloy
    classification
CALLA—common acute lym-
    phoblastic leukemia antigen
Calleja
    islands of C.
    islets
Calliphora
    C. vomitoria
Callison fluid
Calmette-Guérin bacillus
Calymmatobacterium
    C. granulomatis
C_{am}—amylase clearance
cAMP, cyclic AMP—cyclic adeno-
    sine monophosphate
3',5'-cAMP synthetase
Campylobacter
    C. cinaedi
    C. fennelliae
    C. fetus
    C. jejuni
    C. pyloris
canalicular
canaliculus (canaliculi)
    bile canaliculi, biliary
        canaliculi
    intercellular c.
    intercellular canaliculi of
        parietal cells
    pseudobile c.
    secretory c.
Candida
    C. albicans
    C. albidus
    C. guilliermondi
    C. krusei
    C. laurentii
    C. luteolus
    C. parakrusei
    C. parapsilosis
    C. pseudotropicalis
    C. stellatoidea
    C. tropicalis
    C. vulvovaginitis
cannabinol
Cannizzaro reaction

CAP—College of American Pathologists

capacity
  antigen-binding c.
  forced vital c. (FVC)
  total iron-binding c. (TIBC)

Capillaria
  C. hepatica
  C. philippinensis

capillarity

capillaroscopy

capillary (capillaries)
  c. microscope
  c. tube

capillus (capilli)

capsaicin

Capsicum, capsicum

capsule
  anthrax c.

carbolfuchsin
  Ziehl-Neelsen c.

carbon (C)
  c. 12
  c. 14
  c. dioxide
  c. monoxide

γ-carboxyglutamate [gamma-]

carboxyhemoglobin (HbCO)

carcinoembryonic antigen (CEA)

carcinogen

carcinoma (carcinomas, carcinomata)
  See in *Oncology and Hematology* section.

carcinomatoid

carcinomatous

Cardiobacterium
  C. hominis

Carpoglyphus
  C. passularum

Carrel-Lindberg pump

Carr-Price test

caseous

Casoni
  intradermal test
  reaction

cast
  blood c.
  epithelial c.

cast (continued)
  fat c.
  granular c.
  hyaline c.
  pigmented c.'s
  wax c., waxy c.

Castellanella
  C. castellani

Castellani
  test

cataphoresis

cataphoretic

catecholamines

catechol-*O*-methyl transferase (COMT)

cause
  contributory c. of death
  underlying c. of death

caustic

CBC—complete blood count

CBG—corticosteroid-binding globulin
  cortisol-binding globulin

cc, cm^3 [cm3], cu cm—cubic centimeter(s)

CC, C_{cr}—creatinine clearance

CCAT—conglutinating complement absorption test

CCK—cholecystokinin

C_{cr}, CC—creatinine clearance

CDC—chenodeoxycholate

CDCA—chenodeoxycholic acid

CEA—carcinoembryonic antigen

cell
  acanthoid c.
  agranular c.
  air c.'s of Mosher
  alpha c.
  amacrine c.
  anaplastic c.
  aneuploid c.
  anterior ethmoidal air c.'s
  anterior horn c.
  antigen-presenting c.
  argentaffin c.
  Armanni-Ebstein c.
  Aschoff c.
  Askanazy c.

cell (continued)

    atypical c.

    autologous lymphokine activated killer c.

    B c.

    band c.

    bank c.

    basal c.

    basilar c.

    basket c.

    basophilic c. of anterior lobe of hypophysis

    beta c.

    biochemical fuel c.

    bite c.

    Bizzozero c.

    blast c.

    bloated c.

    body c.

    bone marrow c.

    bristle c.'s

    brush bipolar c.

    buffy coat c., buffy-coated c.

    bulliform c.

    burr c.

    C c.

    cardiac failure c.'s

    centrifugal bipolar c.

    chromaffin c.

    ciliated c.

    clear c. of parathyroid gland

    cleaved follicular center c.

    clonogenic c.

    clue c.

    columnar c.

    comet c.

    companion c.

    cone bipolar c.

    conjunctival c.

    cornified c.

    crenated c.

    c. cycle

    cytomegalic c.

    cytotoxic c.

    daughter c.

    decidual c.

    deep c.

    delta c.

cell (continued)

    dendritic epidermal c.

    c. differentiation

    diffuse ganglion c.

    diploid c.

    displaced ganglion c.

    c. division

    dust c.

    EAC rosette-forming c.

    eating c.

    ectoblastic c.

    ectodermal c.

    electromotive force c.

    end c.

    endocervical c.

    endocrine c.

    endometrial c.

    endothelial c.

    enterochromaffin c.

    ependymal c.

    epithelial c.

    epithelioid c.

    E rosette-forming c.

    erythroid c.

    eta c.

    faggot c.

    c. of Fañanás

    Ferrata c.

    fixed c.

    flat bipolar c.

    follicular dendritic c.

    free c.

    fuchsinophil c.

    gamma c.

    ganglion c. of retina

    Gaucher c.

    gemistocytic c.

    generative c.

    germinal c.

    glandular c.

    glitter c.

    goblet c.

    Golgi c.

    granulosa c.

    guard c.

    haploid c.

    HEK (human embryo kidney) c.

cell (continued)
 HeLa c.
 HEL (human embryo lung) c.
 helper c.
 helper T c.'s
 hematopoietic stem c.
 hemopoietic c.
 hilar c.
 H-2 mouse c.
 homozygous typing c.
 horny c.
 Hortega c.
 hot c.
 Hürthle c.
 hybrid c.
 hyperchromatic c.
 immunocompetent c.
 immunologically competent
  c.
 inclusion c.
 inducer c.
 inner hair c.
 inner phalangeal c.
 intercalary c.
 internuncial c.
 interstitial c.
 intracytoplasmic inclusion c.
 islet c.
 K c.
 keratinized c.
 killer c.
 koilocytotic c.
 Kupffer c.
 Kurloff c.
 lacunar c.
 Langerhans c.
 Langhans c.
 LE c.
 Leclanché c.
 Leydig c.
 Lipschütz c.
 locomotive c.
 lupus erythematosus (LE) c.
 lutein c.
 luteum c.
 lymphoblastic plasma c.
 lymphoid c.
 lymphoreticular c.

cell (continued)
 M c.
 macroglial c.
 malpighian c.
 mast c.
 maturation B c.
 c.-mediated immunity
 mediator c.
 medullary interstitial c.
 medulloepithelial c.
 melanotropic c.
 Merkel c.
 Merkel-Ranvier c.'s
 mesothelial c.
 metallophil c.
 metaplastic c.
 Mexican hat c.
 microglial c.
 midget bipolar c.
 migratory c.
 Mikulicz c.'s
 monocytoid c.
 mononuclear c.
 monosomic c.
 monosynaptic bipolar c.
 mop bipolar c.
 motile c.
 mucous c.
 multipolar c.
 mural c.
 myeloid c.
 myogenic c.
 navicular c.
 nerve c.
 neurosecretory c.
 NK (natural killer) c.
 nonadherent c.
 noncleaved follicular center c.
 null c.
 oligodendroglial c.
 Opalski c.
 osteochondrogenic c.
 osteogenic c.
 outer hair c.
 outer phalangeal c.
 P c.
 packed c.
 Paget c.

cell (continued)

Paneth c.
parabasal c.
parafollicular c.
parent c.
Pelger-Huët c.
perineurial c.
peritoneal exudate c.
petrosal c.'s
phagocytic c.
phalangeal c. of Deiters
phantom c.
plaque-forming c.'s
plasma c.
pluripotent c.
polygonal c.
postmitotic c.
pre-B c.
precornified c.
pregranulosa c.
prickle c.
progenitor c.
pyknotic c.
pyroninophilic blast c.
red c.'s, red blood c.'s (RBCs)
Reed-Sternberg giant c.
regeneration c.
renal c.
renal tubular c.
reproductive c.
responder c.
reticuloendothelial c.
reticulum c.
sarcogenic c.
Schwann c.
serous c.
Sertoli c.
sickle c.
signet c.
sinusoidal endothelial c.
skein c.
smooth muscle c.
somatic c.
spindle-shaped c.
splenic c.
squamous c.
static balance receptor c.
stem c.

cell (continued)

stimulator c.
strap c.
stroma c.
superficial c.
suppressor c.
sympathetic formative c.
sympathotropic c.
syncytial c.
T c.
tadpole c.
tagged red c.'s
tailed red c.
tapetal c.
target c.
tart c.
T-cytotoxic c.
teardrop c.
theca c.
theca interna c.
theca-lutein c.
thymic epithelial c.
thymus-dependent c.
thymus-derived c.
thymus nurse c.
Tiselius electrophoresis c.
Touton giant c.
transducer c.
transitional c.
trisomic c.
T-suppressor c.
tube c.
Türk c.
Tzanck c.
umbrella c.
undifferentiated c.
unipolar c.
unit c.
van Hansemann c.'s
vegetative c.
veiled c.
Vero c.'s
vestibular hair c.'s
Walthard c.
white c.'s, white blood c.'s
  (WBCs)
zymogenic c.

cell body

Cellvibrio
    C. flavescens
    C. fulvus
    C. ochraceus
    C. vulgaris
centrifugal
centrifugalization
centrifugate
centrifugation
    cesium chloride gradient c.
    zonal c.
centrifuge
    c. microscope
centriole
Centruroides
    C. suffusus
CEP—counterelectrophoresis
Cephalosporium
    C. falciforme
    C. granulomatis
ceramidase
cerebronic acid
cerebroside
ceroid lipofuscin
cesarean section
    postmortem c.s.
CF—carbolfuchsin
    Christmas factor
    complement fixation, com-
        plement-fixing
CF antibody titer
CFA—complement-fixing antibody
CFT—complement fixation test
cfu—colony-forming unit(s)
CG—chorionic gonadotropin
    colloidal gold
cGMP, 3′,5′-GMP—cyclic guano-
    sine monophosphate
CGP—choline glycerophosphatide
    chorionic growth hormone
        prolactin
    circulating granulocyte pool
CGRP—calcitonin gene-related
    peptide
CGT—chorionic gonadotropin
CGTT—cortisone glucose tolerance
    test

chamber
    Petroff-Hauser counting c.
change
    fatty c.
Charcot-Leyden crystals
Charcot-Neumann crystals
Chauveau
    bacillus
    bacterium
CHE—cholinesterase
chem—chemistry [panel, profile]
chem-6 [chem-7, chem-12, chem-
    12/60, etc.]
chemistry (chemistries)
    blood c. studies
    clinical c.
    histological c.
Cheyletiella
    C. parasitovorax
Chievitz
    layer
    organ
Chilomastix
    C. mesnili
Chlamydia
    C. trachomatis
    C. oculogenitalis
    C. psittaci
Chlamydia sepsis
Chlamydiazyme test
chol—cholesterol
cholecystokinin (CCK)
Choleraesuis
    C. salmonella
Chol est—cholesterol esters
cholesterol
    c. acyltransferase
    c. esterase
choline
choline acetyltransferase
chorionic gonadotropin (CG)
    human c.g. (hCG)
chromatography
    affinity c.
    antibody affinity c.
    electric c.
    filter paper c.
    gas c. (GC)

chromatography (continued)
    gas-liquid c. (GLC)
    gas-solid c. (GSC)
    high-performance liquid c.
      (HPLC)
    high-pressure liquid c.
      (HPLC)
    instant thin-layer c. (ITLC)
    thin-layer c. (TLC)
    two-dimensional c.
chrome hematoxylin
Chromobacterium violaceum
chromomycosis
chromoscopy
    gastric c.
chromosomal
    c. markers
chromosome
    fragile X c.
    gametic c.
    Philadelphia c.
    X c.
    Y c.
Chrysops
    C. cecutiens
    C. dimidiata
    C. discalis
    C. silacea
CHS—cholinesterase
chylomicron
chymotrypsin
Ciaccio
    glands
    method
    stain
CIE, CIEP—counterimmunoelec-
    trophoresis
Cimex, cimex (cimices)
cin–. See also words beginning
    sin–, syn–.
C_{in}—insulin clearance
CIN—cervical intraepithelial neo-
    plasia
cirrhonosus
CIS—carcinoma in situ
Citrobacter
    Bethesda-Ballerup *C.*
    C. diversus

Citrobacter (continued)
    C. freundii
Civatte
    bodies
CK—creatine kinase
Cl—chloride
    chlorine
Cladosporium
    C. bantianum
    C. carrionii
    C. mansonii
    C. trichoides
    C. werneckii
Clara cells
Clark
    electrode
Clark-Collip method
Clarke
    column
    dorsal nucleus
    collateral bundle
classification
    See also *index.*
    Arneth c.
    bacterial c.
    Breslow c.
    Broders c.
    Caldwell-Moloy c.
    French-American-British
      (FAB) c.
    Griffith c.
    Kaufman-White c.
    Kennedy c.
    Lancefield c. (groups A −O)
    Landsteiner c.
    Lukes-Collins c. of non-
      Hodgkin lymphoma
    REAL (Revised European
      American Lymphoma) c.
    Runyon c.
    Rye histopathologic c. of
      Hodgkin disease
    Schilling c.
    Skinner c.
Claudius cell
clearance
    blood urea c.
    creatinine c.

clearance (continued)
    urea c.
cleavage
clinical
    c. microscopy
Clonorchis
    C. endemicus
    C. sinensis
Clostridium
    C. acetobutylicum
    C. aerofoetidum
    C. agni
    C. bifermentans
    C. botulinum
    C. butylicum
    C. chauvoei
    C. cochlearium'
    C. difficile
    C. fallax
    C. feseri
    C. haemolyticum
    C. histolyticum
    C. kluyveri
    C. multifermentans
    C. nigrificans
    C. novyi
    C. oedematiens
    C. ovitoxicus
    C. paludis
    C. parabotulinum
    C. parabotulinum equi
    C. pasteurianum
    C. pastorianum
    C. perfringens
    C. ramosum
    C. septicum
    C. sordellii
    C. sporogenes
    C. sticklandii
    C. tertium
    C. tetani
    C. tetanomorphum
    C. thermosaccharolyticum
    C. tyrosinogenes
    C. welchii
CLOtest
cm^3 [cm3], cc, cu cm—cubic centimeter(s)

CMET—comprehensive metabolic panel [also: profile]
CMP—complete metabolic panel [also: profile]
    comprehensive metabolic panel [also: profile]
    cytidine monophosphate
cnidarian
CO_2 [CO2]—carbon dioxide
CoA—coenzyme A
coarse
    c. gravel
    c. markings
    c. material
cocci (plural of coccus)
coccidial
coccidian
Coccidioides
    C. immitis
coccus (cocci)
    gram-negative cocci
    gram-positive cocci
    pyogenic cocci
COD—cause of death
COGTT—cortisone-primed oral glucose tolerance test
COIIb—carboxyhemoglobin
colonization
colony count
color-contrast microscope
comparison microscope
compatibility
    ABO c.
complement
    c. activation
    c. fixation
    normal c. of cells
    c. receptors [CR1, CR2, CR3, CR4, C1qR, C3aR, C5aR]
complex
    Ghon c.
compound
    c. microscope
COMT—catechol-*O*-methyl transferase
condensation
Congo red
    stain

Congo red (continued)
   test
Conidiobolus
   C. coronatus
contact
   c. autoradiography
contagium
   c. animatum
   c. vivum
conversion
   Mantoux c.
Coombs test
   direct
   indirect
Copromastix
   C. prowazeki
Copromonas
   C. subtilis
coracidia (plural of coracidium)
Cordylobia
   C. anthropophaga
Cori
   cycle
   ester
corpora (plural of corpus)
corps ["kor"]
   c. ronds
corpse ["korps"]
corpus (corpora)
   c. delicti
corpuscle
corpuscula (plural of corpusculum)
corpuscular
corpusculum (corpuscula)
Corynebacterium
   C. acnes
   C. belfantii
   C. diphtheriae
   C. enzymicum
   C. equi
   C. hemolyticum
   C. hofmannii
   C. infantisepticum
   C. minutissimum
   C. murisepticum
   C. mycetoides
   C. necrophorum
   C. ovis

Corynebacterium (continued)
   C. parvulum
   C. parvum
   C. pseudodiphtheriticum
   C. pseudotuberculosis
   C. pyogenes
   C. renale
   C. tenuis
   C. ulcerans
   C. vaginale
   C. xerosis
Coryneform, coryneform
count
   Addis c.
   Arneth c.
   reticulocyte c.
   Schilling blood c.
counter
   Coulter c.
Cowdry inclusion bodies (type A, type B)
Coxiella
   C. burnetii
coxsackievirus (group A, group B)
C/P—cholesterol-phospholipid ratio
C_{pah}—para-aminohippurate clearance
CPD—calcium pyrophosphate dihydrate (crystals)
CPK—creatine phosphokinase [now: creatine kinase (CK)]
CPK-MB
CPPD—calcium pyrophosphate dihydrate (crystals)
CPS—carbamoyl phosphate synthetase
C1q (to C9q) assay
CR1, C3b/C4b r., CD35; CR2, C3d/C3bi r. C3dg, CD21; CR3, C3bi r., CD11b/18; CR4, C3bi r., CD11c/18; C3aR (C3a r.); C5aR (C5a r.); C1qR (C1q r.) [various complement receptor designations]
Craigies
   tube
creatine
   c. kinase (CK)
   c. phosphate

creatine (continued)
    c. phosphokinase (CPK)
    [now: creatine kinase
    (CK)]
cresyl violet, cresylecht violet
CRF—corticotropin-releasing factor
CRH—corticotropin-releasing hormone
CRP—C-reactive protein
crust
    buffy c.
crusta (crustae)
    c. inflammatoria
    c. phlogistica
cryoprecipitability
cryoprecipitate
cryoprecipitation
cryostat
    Ames Lab-Tek c.
Cryptococcus
    C. albidus
    C. neoformans
cryptomere
cryptoplasmic
Cryptosporidium
    C. listeria
Cryptostroma
    C. corticale
crystal
    Charcot-Leyden c.
    Leyden c.'s
C&S—culture and sensitivity
CSF—cerebrospinal fluid
CSR—corrected sedimentation rate
CT—clotting time
    coagulation time
Ctenocephalides
    C. canis
CTH—ceramide trihexoside
CTL—cytotoxic T lymphocyte
C_u—urea clearance
cubic centimeters (cm^3 [cm3], cc,
   cu cm)
cubic millimeter(s) (cu mm, mm^3
   [mm3])
cu cm, cm^3 [cm3], cc—cubic cen-
   timeter(s)
cuffing

culture
    attenuated c.
    blood c.
    chorioallantoic c.
    direct c.
    flask c.
    hanging-block c.
    hanging-drop c.
    needle c.
    plate c.
    sensitized c.
    shake c.
    slant c.
    smear c.
    stab c.
    stock c.
    streak c.
    stroke c.
    thrust c.
    tissue c.
    tube c.
    type c.
culture medium
    Bordet-Gengou c.m.
    defined c. m.
    indicator c. m.
    N.N.N. (Novoy, McNeal,
      Nicolle) c. m.
    Thayer-Martin c.m.
cumulus (cumuli)
CV—corpuscular volume
    cresyl violet, cresylecht violet
CVS—clean-voided specimen
cyclase
    adenyl c.
    adenylate c.
cyclic
    c. adenosine monophosphate
      (cAMP)
    c. guanosine monophosphate
      (cGMP, 3',5'-GMP)
    c. nucleotides
cyclic AMP, cAMP—cyclic adenosine monophosphate
3',5'-cyclic AMP synthetase
cyclic GMP, cGMP—cyclic guanosine monophosphate
Cys—cysteine

Cys-Cys—cystine
cystathionine γ-lyase [gamma-]
cysticercosis
Cysticercus
    C. acanthrotrias
    C. bovis
    C. cellulosae
    C. fasciolaris
    C. ovis
    C. tenuicollis
cytologic, cytological
cytolysate
    blood c.
cytomegalovirus (CMV)
Cytospin
DAB—dimethylaminoazobenzene
DAG—diacylglycerol
DAP—dihydroxyacetone phosphate
DAPT—direct agglutination pregnancy test
darkfield
    d. microscope
    d. microscopy
DAT—differential agglutination titer
data (plural of datum)
database
datum (data)
Davidoff (Davidov) cells
DBA—dibenzanthracene
DBCL—dilute blood clot lysis (method)
DC—diphenylarsine cyanide
DCA—deoxycholate-citrate agar
    deoxycholic acid
DCHFB—dichlorohexafluorobutane
D_{co} [DCO]—diffusing capacity for carbon monoxide
DCTMA—desoxycorticosterone trimethylacetate
DCTPA—desoxycorticosterone triphenylacetate
DDD—dichlorodiphenyl-dichloroethane
D-dimer
DDT—dichlorodiphenyl-trichloroethane
Debove
    membrane

debris
    inflammatory cell d.
    purulent d.
    stonelike d.
definition
dehydrogenase
    isocitric d.
    lactate d. (LDH)
Delafield
    fluid
    hematoxylin
delta
    d.-aminolevulinic acid (ALA)
Demodex
    D. folliculorum
Dermacentor
    D. andersoni
    D. occidentalis
    D. variabilis
Dermanyssus
    D. avium et gallinae
Dermatobia
    D. hominis
Dermatophagoides
    D. pteronyssinus
    D. scheremetewskyi
Dermatophilus
    D. penetrans
dermatozoon (dermatozoa)
detergent
α-dextrinase [alpha-]
dextrose
DFA—direct fluorescent antibody [test]
DFDT—difluorodiphenyl-trichloroethane
DHEA—dehydroepiandrosterone
DHEAS—dehydroepiandrosterone sulfate
d'Herelle phenomenon
DHFR—dihydrofolate reductase
Dialister
    D. pneumosintes
Dicrocoelium
    D. dendriticum
Dientamoeba
    D. fragilis
"diff" Slang for differential.

differential
"difilo–" Phonetic for words begin-
    ning diphyllo–.
"dig" Slang for digitalis, digoxin.
"dij" Phonetic for "dig"; slang for
    digitalis, digoxin.
dimer
    D-d.
p-dimethylaminoazobenzene [p-,
    para-]
7,12-dimethylbenz[a]anthracene
    (DMBA)
DIP—diisopropyl phosphate
dip-coating autoradiography
Dipetalonema
    D. perstans
Diphyllobothrium
    D. latum
    D. parvum
    D. taenioides
Diplococcus
    D. pneumoniae
diplococcus (diplococci)
    d. of Morax-Axenfeld
    d. of Neisser
    Weichselbaum d.
Diplogonoporus
    D. brauni
    D. grandis
Dipylidium
    D. caninum
direct
    d. vision spectroscope
Dirofilaria
    D. immitis
    D. tenuis
dis–. See also words beginning dys–.
disc
    See also *disk.*
    embryonic d.
discharge
    d. tube
discrete
    d. lesion
    d. nodule
disease
    See in medical specialty sec-
    tions.

dish
    Petri d.
disk
disorder
    XXX d.
    XXXX d.
    XXXXY d.
    XXXY d.
    XXYY d.
dissecting
    d. microscope
DIT—diiodotyrosine
divisio (divisiones)
division
dL, dl—deciliter
DL—Donath-Landsteiner (test)
D_L [DL]—diffusing capacity of lung
D_LCO [DLCO]—diffusing capacity
    of lung for carbon monoxide
DMA—dimethyladenosine
DMAB—dimethylamino-benzalde-
    hyde
DMBA—dimethylbenzanthracene
DMPE—3,4-dimethoxyphenyleth-
    ylamine
DMSO—dimethylsulfoxide
D/N—dextrose-nitrogen [ratio]
DNA—deoxyribonucleic acid
DNA-directed DNA polymerase
DNA-directed RNA polymerase
DNA polymerase
DNase—deoxyribonuclease
DNB—dinitrobenzene
DNC—dinitrocarbanilide
DNFB—dinitrofluorobenzene
DNP—deoxyribonucleoprotein
DNPH—dinitrophenylhydrazine
DNPM—dinitrophenylmorphine
Dogiel corpuscles
Döhle
    inclusion bodies
Dolichos
    D. biflorus
Donath-Landsteiner
    antibody
    phenomenon
    syndrome
    test

Donovania
    D. granulomatis
dopamine β-hydroxylase [beta-]
dopamine β-monooxygenase [beta-]
Dorothy Reed cells
dose
dot
    See *macula* and *spot.*
Downey cell
Dracunculus
    D. medinensis
Drysdale corpuscles
DTM—dermatophyte test medium
Ducrey
    bacillus
    test
Duffy blood antibody type
DUMP—deoxyuridine monophosphate
Durham
    tube
Dutcher body
Dutton
    spirochete
dye
    aniline d.
dys–. See also words beginning dis–.
dyscrasia
    blood d.
    lymphatic d.
E.—Entamoeba
    Escherichia
EA—erythrocyte antibody
EAC—erythrocyte antibody complement
eating cell
EB—Epstein-Barr [virus]
EBNA—Epstein-Barr nuclear antigen [test]
EBV—Epstein-Barr virus
EC—*Escherichia coli*
ecchymosis (ecchymoses)
    cadaveric e.
ECF—eosinophil chemotactic factor
ECFA—eosinophil chemotactic factor of anaphylaxis
Echinococcus
    E. granulosus

Echinococcus (continued)
    E. multilocularis
ECHO—enteric cytopathogenic human orphan [now: echovirus]
echovirus (serotypes 1–7, 9, 11–18, 20–27, 29–34)
E. coli—Escherichia coli
ectozoon (ectozoa)
Edwardsiella
    E. tarda
EEC—enteropathogenic *Escherichia coli*
EFA, EFAs—essential fatty acid(s)
effect [noun: result, outcome]
    Arias-Stella e.
    Haldane e.
    Mierzejewski e.
    pressure e.
    Soret e.
EGF—epidermal growth factor
EGOT—erythrocyte glutamic-oxaloacetic transaminase
Ehrlich
    body
    reaction
    reagent
    test
    theory
    tumor
EID—electroimmunodiffusion
EIEC—enteroinvasive *Escherichia coli*
Eikenella
    E. corrodens
"ekinokokus" Phonetic for *Echinococcus.*
ELAM—endothelial leukocyte adhesion molecule
electric
    e. chromatography
electrode
    Clark e.
electrofocusing
electrolyte
    amphoteric e.
    colloidal e.
    protein e.
    serum e.'s

electrolytic
electromanometer
electromanometry
electron
    e. microscope
    e. microscopy
    e. multiplier tube
    scanning transmission e.
       microscopy
electron-dense
electron microscope
    scanning e.m.
electron-microscopical
electronograph
electropherogram
electrophoresis
    serum protein e.
electrophoretic
electrophoretically
electrophoretogram
electrophotometer
electrosynthesis
ELT—euglobulin lysis time
EM, EMC—electron microscopy
embed, embedding
EMB (eosin-methylene blue) agar
EMF—erythrocyte maturation factor
EMIT—enzyme-multiplied immu-
    noassay technique
Encephalitozoon
    E. cuniculi
    E. hellem
    E. intestinalis
Endo agar
Endolimax
    E. nana
Endomyces
    E. albicans
    E. capsulatus
    E. epidermatidis
    E. epidermidis
endothelin-1 receptor antagonists
endothelioid
Entamoeba
    E. buccalis
    E. buetschlii
    E. coli
    E. gingivalis

Entamoeba (continued)
    E. hartmanni
    E. histolytica
    E. kartulisi
    E. nana
    E. nipponica
    E. polecki
    E. tetragena
    E. tropicalis
    E. undulans
Enterobacter
    E. aerogenes
    E. agglomerans
    E. alvei
    E. cloacae
    E. gergoviae
    E. hafniae
    E. liquefaciens
    E. sakazakii
Enterobius
    E. vermicularis
Enteromonas
    E. hominis
Enterovirus, enterovirus
enterozoon (enterozoa)
entozoon (entozoa)
enzyme
    serum e.
EO—eosinophil
eos—eosinophils
eosinopenia
eosinophil
    polymorphonuclear e.
EPEC—enteropathogenic *Esche-*
    richia coli
Epidermophyton
    E. floccosum
    E. inguinale
    E. rubrum
epistasis
epistatic
epithelia (plural of epithelium)
epitheliitis
epithelioglandular
epitheliolysis
epitheliolytic
epithelium (epithelia)
    surface e.

epithelium (epithelia) (continued)
    visceral e.
epitype
epizoon (epizoa)
ERA—estrogen receptor assay
"erithro–" Phonetic for words
    beginning erythro–.
ERP—estrogen receptor protein
Erwinia
    E. amylovora
Erysipelothrix
    E. insidiosa
    E. rhusiopathiae
erythremia
erythroblast
erythroblastic
erythroblastosis
    e. fetalis
    e. neonatorum
erythroblastotic
erythrochromia
erythroclasis
erythroclast
erythroclastic
erythrocytapheresis
erythrocyte
    dichromatic e.
    reticulated e.
    e. transketolase
erythrocytic
erythrocytolysin
erythrocytolysis
erythrocytometer
erythrocytometry
erythrocytophagy
erythrocytorrhexis
erythrocytoschisis
erythrocytosis
    leukemic e.
    e. megalosplenica
erythrodegenerative
erythrogenesis
erythrogenic
erythroid
β-erythroidine [beta-]
erythrokinetics
erythron
erythroneocytosis

erythropenia
erythrophage
erythrophagocytosis
erythrophil
erythrophobic
erythropoiesis
erythropoietic
erythropoietin
erythropyknosis
Escherichia
    E. aerogenes
    E. alkalescens
    E. aurescens
    E. coli [virulent strain
      0157:h7]
    E. dispar
    E. dispar var. *ceylonensis*
    E. dispar var. *madampensis*
    E. freundii
    E. intermedia
ESF—erythropoietic-stimulating
    factor
"es-pep" Phonetic for SPEP (serum
    protein electrophoresis).
ESR—erythrocyte sedimentation rate
Essic cell band
β-estradiol [now: estradiol 17β (17-
    beta)]
α-estradiol [now: estradiol 17α [17-
    alpha]
estradiol
    e.-17α [e.-17-alpha]
    e.-17β [e.-17-beta]
ETEC—enterotoxic *Escherichia coli*
ETOH, EtOH—ethyl alcohol
Eubacterium
    E. alactolyticum
    E. lentum
    E. limosum
Euglena
    E. gracilis
Euproctis
    E. chrysorrhoea
Eurotium
    E. malignum
Eutrombicula
    E. alfreddugesi
exopeptidase

Exophiala
> *E. jeanselmei*
> *E. jeanselmi*
> *E. mycetoma*
> *E. werneckii*

exuberant
> e. infection
> e. tumor

FA—fluorescence assay
> fluorescent antibody

Fab—fragment, antigen-binding
FAB—French-American-British
> [classification]

Facb—fragment, antigen-and-com-
> plement-binding

FACS—fluorescence-activated cell
> sorter

factor
> f. I
> f. II
> f. III
> f. IV
> f. V
> f. VI
> f. XII
> f. VIII
> f. VIII:c
> f. VIII:CAg
> f. VIIIR:Ag
> f. VIII T
> f. IX
> f. X
> f. XI
> f. XII
> f. XIII
> activated clotting f.'s
> coagulation f.'s I–V, VII–XII
> colony-stimulating f. (CSF)
> Hageman f.
> platelet-activating f.
> rhesus (Rh) f.
> thyroid-stimulating hor-
>   mone–releasing f. (TSH-
>   RF)
> tissue plasminogen f.
> vascular permeability f.
> von Willebrand f.

FADF—fluorescent antibody dark-
> field [examination]

"fago–" Phonetic for words begin-
> ning phago–.

Fannia
> *F. canicularis*

Fasciola
> *F. gigantica*
> *F. hepatica*

Fasciolopsis
> *F. buski*

FAT—fluorescent antibody test
FBP—fibrinogen breakdown product
FBS—fasting blood sugar
FCA—ferritin-conjugated antibodies
FDP—fibrin degradation product
Fe—iron
FEF—forced expiratory flow
"feno–" Phonetic for words begin-
> ning pheno–.

"fenomenon" Phonetic for phenom-
> enon.

"fenotype" Phonetic for phenotype.
"feo–" Phonetic for words begin-
> ning pheo–.

fermentation
> mannitol f.
> f. tube

FET—forced expiratory time
α-fetoprotein (AFP) [alpha-]
FETS—forced expiratory time in
> seconds

FFP—fresh frozen plasma
FG—fibrinogen
FIA—fluoroimmunoassay
Fibrillenstruktur
fibrinolysin
> seminal f.

FIF—forced inspiratory flow
FIGLU—formiminoglutamic acid
filament
filamentous
filaria
> Bancroft f.
> Brug f.

filarial
filariform
"fi-lay" Phonetic for fillet.

fillet, filleted, filleting
film-stripping autoradiography
filter
    f. paper chromatography
filtrate
FiO$_2$ [FiO2]—fractional concentration of inspired oxygen
fixative
    Heidenhain Susa f.
    Zenker f.
"fizeo–" Phonetic for words beginning physio–.
flatworm
Flavobacterium
    F. meningosepticum
"flebektomee" Phonetic for phlebectomy.
"flebo–" Phonetic for words beginning phlebo–.
Flexner
    bacillus
    dysentery
    serum
flocculation
    cephalin f.
    Ramon f.
floccule
    toxoid-antitoxin f.
florid
    f. infection
fluid
    See also *liquid, liquor,* and *solution.*
    Zenker f.
fluke
    blood f.
fluorescence
    f. microscope
    f. microscopy
fluorescent
    f. antibody (FA)
    direct f. antibody (DFA) test
    indirect f. antibody (IFA)
    f. treponemal antibody (FTA)
fluorometry
p-fluorophenylalanine [p-, para-]
flying spot microscope

focus (foci)
    dysplastic f.
Fonsecaea
    F. compactum
    F. pedrosoi
forensic
form
    appliqué f.
    ring f.
formaldehyde dehydrogenase
formalin
formalinize
formatio (formationes)
formation
    coffin f.
    palisade f.
    rouleau f., f. of rouleaux
formic acid
formiminoglutamic acid (FIGLU)
formocortal
formol
formula
    See also *law* and *method.*
    Van Slyke f.
Forssman
    antibody
    antigen
    lipoid
    shock
"fos–" Phonetic for words beginning phos–.
FPM—filter paper microscopic (test)
fragility
    erythrocyte f.
    osmotic f.
    red cell f.
    f. test
fragmentography
    mass f.
Francisella
    F. tularensis
FRC—functional reserve capacity
    functional residual capacity
freeze-cleaving
freeze-drying
freeze-etching
freeze-fracturing
freeze-substitution

freezing microtome
Frei
    antigen
    test
Friedländer
    bacillus
    bacillus pneumonia
    disease
    pneumobacillus
    pneumonia
Frohn
    reagent
    test
FSF—fibrin-stabilizing factor
FSH—follicle-stimulating hormone
FSH/LH-RH—follicle-stimulating hormone and luteinizing hormone–releasing hormone
FSH-RF—follicle-stimulating hormone–releasing factor
FSH-RH—follicle-stimulating hormone–releasing hormone
FSPs—fibrin split products
FTA—fluorescent treponemal antibody
FTA-AB, FTA-ABS—fluorescent treponemal antibody absorption test
α-L-fucosidase [alpha-]
function
    liver f.
Fusobacterium
    F. gonidiaformans
    F. mortiferum
    F. naviforme
    F. nucleatum
    F. russii
    F. varium
FVC—forced vital capacity
FW—Felix-Weil (reaction)
FWR—Felix-Weil reaction
g—gram(s)
GABA—γ-aminobutyric acid [gamma-]
Gaffky
    scale
    table
galactitol

galactocerebroside
galactometer
α-galactosidase [alpha-]
α-galactosidase A [alpha-]
β-galactosidase [beta-]
galactoside
galactosyl
galacturonic acid
GALT—gastrointestinal-associated lymphoid tissue
    gut-associated lymphoid tissue
gamete
gametic
gametocyst
gametoid
gamma
    g.-aminobutyrate
    g.-aminobutyric acid (GABA)
    g.-carboxyglutamate
    g.-glutamyltransferase (GGT)
Gandy-Gamna
    nodules
    spleen
gangliosides
Ganser
    basal nucleus of G.
    commissure
    ganglion
    nucleus basalis of G.
Gardnerella
    G. vaginalis
gas
    g. chromatography (GC)
    g.-liquid chromatography (GLC)
    g.-solid chromatography (GSC)
gastric
    g. chromoscopy
Gaucher
    cells
    histiocyte
GBM—glomerular basement membrane
GC—gas chromatography
    gonococcus
    granular cast

GCSF—granulocyte colony-stimulating factor
G/E—granulocyte-erythroid [ratio]
Gegenbaur cell
gene
    autosomal g.
    g. bank
    chimeric g.
    g. code
    codominant g.
    dominant g.
    complementary g.
    g. complex
    lethal g.
    major g.
    g. mapping
    marker g.
    mutant g.
    recessive g.
    reciprocal g.
    regulator g., regulatory g.
    repressor g.
    sex-linked g.
    silent g.
    suicide g.
    supplementary g.
    tumor-suppressor g.
    X-linked g.
    Y-linked g.
genera (plural of genus)
generation time
genetic
    g. code
Gengou phenomenon
genotype
genus (genera)
Geotrichum
    G. candidum
Gerhardt
    test for acetoacetic acid
    test for urobilin in urine
GERL—Golgi endoplasmic reticulum lysosomes
germline, germ line
GG—gamma globulin
GGT—gamma-glutamyl transferase
GGTP—gamma-glutamyl transpeptidase

GH—growth hormone
GH-IH—growth hormone-inhibit-
  ing hormone
Ghon
    complex
    focus
    lesion
Ghon-Sachs
    bacillus
    complex
    focus
    primary lesion
    tubercle
GH-RF—growth hormone–releas-
  ing factor
GH-RH—growth hormone–releasing hormone
GH-RIH—growth hormone
  release–inhibiting hormone
giant cell
Giardia
    G. lamblia
Giemsa
    method
    stain
Gierke (von Gierke)
    cells
    corpuscles
GIP—gastric inhibitory polypeptide
Girard
    method
GITT—glucose-insulin tolerance test
glaze
GLC—gas-liquid chromatography
glioblast
glitter cell
globule
globulin
    alpha$_2$ g.
    beta g.
    gamma g.
    immune serum g.
    g. X
1,4α-glucan branching enzyme
  [-alpha-]
glucan-1,4α-glucosidase [-alpha-]
α-glucosidase [alpha-]
β-glucuronidase [beta-]

Gluge corpuscles
γ-glutamylcysteine synthetase
    [gamma-]
γ-glutamyltransferase (GGT)
    [gamma-]
Glyciphagus
    G. buski
    G. domesticus
GM-CSF—granulocyte-macrophage
    colony-stimulating factor
GMP—guanosine monophosphate
3′,5′-GMP, cGMP—cyclic guano-
    sine monophosphate
GN—gram-negative
G/N—glucose-nitrogen [ratio]
GNB—gram-negative bacilli
GNID—gram-negative intracellular
    diplococci
Gn-RH—gonadotropin-releasing
    hormone
Golgi cells
Gomori
    method
    stains
gonadotropin
    chorionic g.
Gongylonema
    G. pulchrum
Goodpasture
    stain
    syndrome
Gordon
    test
GOT—glutamic-oxaloacetic
    transaminase
GP—glycoprotein
G6PD, G6PDH—glucose-6-phos-
    phate dehydrogenase
GPT—glutamic-pyruvic transaminase
GPUT—galactose phosphate uridyl
    transferase
GR—glutathione reductase
Gram
    method
    solution
    stain
Grandry corpuscles
granulatio (granulationes)

granule
    Bensley specific g.'s
    Bollinger g.'s
gravity
    specific g.
GRF—gonadotropin-releasing factor
    growth hormone–releasing
      factor
GRH—growth hormone–releasing
    hormone
GRP—gastrin-releasing peptide
GSC—gas-solid chromatography
GSH—glutathione (reduced)
    growth-stimulating hormone
GSSG—glutathione (oxidized)
GT—glutamyl transpeptidase
GTH—gonadotropic hormone
GTP—glutamyl transpeptidase
    guanosine triphosphate
GTT—glucose tolerance test
Günzberg (Guenzberg) test
Gymnodinium
    G. breve
H.—Haemophilus
HA—hemagglutinating antibody
    hyaluronic acid
Haemonchus
    H. contortus
Haemophilus
    See also *hemophilus.*
    H. aegyptius
    H. aphrophilus
    H. bovis
    H. bronchisepticus
    H. ducreyi
    H. duplex
    H. haemolyticus
    H. hemoglobinophilus
    H. pertussis
    H. influenzae (type a, type b)
    H. parahaemolyticus
    H. parainfluenzae
    H. parapertussis
    H. paraphrophilus
    H. pertussis
    H. suis
    H. vaginalis

Hafnia
> *H. alvei*

HAI—hemagglutination inhibition
> hemagglutinin inhibition ·

Hamberger phenomenon

Hansen
> bacillus

hapten
> group A h.

Harris
> hematoxylin
> staining method

Hartmannella
> *H. hyalina*

HAT—hypoxanthine-aminopterin-
thymidine (medium)

HAV—hepatitis A virus

Haverhillia
> *H. moniliformis*
> *H. multiformis*

Hayem
> corpuscles
> solution

Hb, Hgb—hemoglobin

HbCO—carboxyhemoglobin

HBD, HBDH—hydroxybutyrate
dehydrogenase

HBLV—human B lymphotropic virus

HbO_2 [HBO2]—oxyhemoglobin

HBV—hepatitis B virus

HC—hyaline cast(s)

hCG—human chorionic gonadotropin

β-hCG [beta hCG]

HCO_3 [HCO3]—bicarbonate

hCS, hCSM—human chorionic
somatomammotropin

Hct, hct—hematocrit

HDL—high-density lipoprotein

H&E—hematoxylin and eosin [stain]

HEAT—human erythrocyte agglutination test

Heinz
> bodies
> granules

HEK—human embryo kidney (cell
culture)

Hektoen phenomenon

HEL—human embryo lung (cell
culture)

Helicobacter
> *H. cinaedi*
> *H. pylori*

helix (helices, helixes)
> α h. [alpha]

helper cell

Helvella
> *H. esculenta*

hemalum
> Mayer h.

hematoblast

hematocrit (Hct, hct)
> mean circulatory h.

hematologic, hematological

hematopoiesis
> extramedullary h.

hematoxylin
> Ehrlich h.
> h. and eosin (H&E) [stain]
> Harris h.
> Heidenhain iron h.
> Mayer h.
> Weigert iron h.

Hemispora stellata

hemizygosity

Hemoccult

hemochromogen

hemochromometry

hemocytoblast

hemocytometer

"hemofilus" Phonetic for *Haemophilus.*

hemoglobin (Hb, Hgb)
> sickle h.

hemolysin

hemolyze

"hemonkus" Phonetic for
> *Haemonchus.*

hemophilus
> See also *Haemophilus.*
> h. of Koch-Weeks
> h. of Morax-Axenfeld

hemorrhage
> petechial h.

hepatocuprein

Herbst corpuscles

Herellea
    H. vaginicola
Herpesvirus
    H. hominis
    H. papio
    H. simiae
    H. suis
Herter
    test
Heterodera
    H. marioni
Heterophyes
    H. heterophyes
    H. katsuradai
HF—Hageman factor
Hgb, Hb—hemoglobin
hGG—human gamma globulin
hGH—human growth hormone
HHb—hypohemoglobin, reduced hemoglobin, un-ionized hemoglobin
HI—hemagglutination inhibition
HIA—hemagglutination-inhibition antibody
5-HIAA—hydroxyindoleacetic acid
high-density lipoprotein (HDL)
"hipo–" Phonetic for words beginning hypo–.
Hirudo
    H. japonica
    H. medicinalis
His [eponym]
    isthmus
    space
histiocyte
histocompatibility
    h. complex
histodiagnosis
histodifferentiation
histofluorescence
histogram
histography
histologist
histolysis
histolytic
histometaplastic
histomorphology
histopathology

Histoplasma
    H. capsulatum
    H. duboisii
histospectroscopy
histotomy
HIT—hemagglutination-inhibition test
HIV—human immunodeficiency virus
HJ—Howell-Jolly
HJB—Howell-Jolly bodies
HL—histocompatibility locus
HLDH—heat-stable lactate dehydrogenase
hLH—human luteinizing hormone
HLV—herpes-like virus
HM—hydatidiform mole
HMG—hydroxymethylglutaryl
Hodgkin
    Rye classification of H. disease
Hofbauer cells
Hofmeister
    test
Holmgren-Golgi canals
Hormodendrum
    H. carrionii
    H. compactum
    H. pedrosoi
Howell
    bodies
HPAA—hydroxyphenylacetic acid
hpf—high-power field
HPF—heparin-precipitable fraction
hPFSH—human pituitary follicles-timulating hormone
hPG—human pituitary gonadotropin
HPLC—high-performance liquid chromatography
    high-pressure liquid chromatography
HPPA—hydroxyphenylpyruvic acid
HPS—hematoxylin-phloxine-saffron
HPV—human papillomavirus
HS—herpes simplex
HSA—human serum albumin
HT—histologic technician
HTP—hydroxytryptophan

HTV—herpes-type virus
HU—hydroxyurea
hyperemia unit
Huët-Pelger nuclear anomaly
human papillomavirus (HPV)
Hürthle
cell
HUS—hyaluronidase unit for semen
HV—herpesvirus
HVM—high-velocity missile
Hydatigera
H. infantis
hydrophobic
5-hydroxyindoleacetic acid (5-HIAA)
hydroxylase
11β-h. [11-beta-]
17α-h. [17-beta-]
21-h.
p-hydroxyphenylpyruvic acid
(PHPPA) [p-, para-]
17α-hydroxyprogesterone aldolase
[17-alpha-]
3β-hydroxy-δ5-steroid dehydrogenase [3-beta-, delta-5-]
Hylemyia
H. antiqua
H. brassicae
hymenolepiasis
Hymenolepis
H. diminuta
H. fraterna
H. murina
H. nana
hypercellular
hypercellularity
hyperchromatin
hyperchromatosis
hyperchromic
hypermetaplasia
hyperneocytosis
hyperplasia
benign prostatic h. (BPH)
cystic prostatic h.
Swiss-cheese h.
hyperplastic
hypersegmentation
hereditary h. of neutrophils

hypertrophy
benign prostatic h. (BPH)
hyphal
hypnotoxin
hypnozoite
hypobromous acid
hypocalcinuria
hypocellular
hypocellularity
hypochlorite
hypochlorous acid
Hypoderma
H. bovis
hypodermic
h. microscope
IADH—inappropriate antidiuretic
hormone
IAHA—immune adherence hemagglutination assay
IB—immune body
IBC—iron-binding capacity
ICAM-1—intercellular adhesion
molecule-1
ICG—indocyanine green
idioheteroagglutinin
idioheterolysin
idioisoagglutinin
IDL—intermediate-density lipoprotein
α-L-iduronidase [alpha-]
I/E—inspiratory-expiratory [ratio]
IEM—immune electron microscopy
IEOP—immunoelectro-osmophoresis
IEP—immunoelectrophoresis
IF—immunofluorescence
IFA—immunofluorescence assay
indirect fluorescent antibody
IFR—inspiratory flow rate
IFRA—indirect fluorescent rabies
antibody (test)
Ig—immunoglobulin [IgA, IgD,
IgE, IgG, IgM]
IGF-1—insulin-like growth factor-1
IHA—indirect hemagglutination
IIF—indirect immunofluorescence
"ikso–" Phonetic for words begin-
ning ixo–.
ill-defined

IMAA—iodinated macroaggregated albumin
imbed [pref: embed]
immune
    i. adherence
    i. complex
    i. response
    i. surveillance
    i. system
immunocatalysis
immunoelectrophoresis
    countercurrent i.
immunofluorescence
    direct i.
    indirect i.
    i. microscopy
immunoglobulin (Ig)
    i. A (IgA)
    i. D (IgD)
    i. E (IgE)
    i. G (IgG)
    i. M (IgM)
    thyroid-binding inhibitory i. (TBII)
    thyroid-stimulating i.
    thyrotropin-binding inhibitory i. (TBII)
    TSH-binding inhibitory i.
incompatibility
    ABO i.
index (indexes, indices)
    See also *classification.*
    acidophilic i.
    free thyroxin i. (FTI)
    hematopneic i.
    hemolytic i.
    icteric i.
    Krebs leukocyte i.
    maturation i.
    phagocytic i.
    pyknotic i.
    red blood cell indices, red cell indices
    sedimentation i.
indiscrete
indole
infrared
    i. microscope

infrared (continued)
    i. spectroscopy
inhibitor
    inter-alpha-trypsin i.
inspiratory
    i.-expiratory (I/E) phase ratio
    forced i. flow (FIF)
    i. flow
    i. flow rate (IFR)
    maximum i. flow (MIF)
    maximum i. pressure (MIP)
    peak i. flow (PIF)
    i. reserve capacity (IRC)
    i. reserve volume (IRV)
integrating microscope
in tela
interference
    i. microscope
intracytoplasmic inclusion cell
Iodamoeba
    I. buetschlii
    I. williamsi
iodine (I)
    Lugol i.
ion
    i. microscope
ions
IRC—inspiratory reserve capacity
IRV—inspiratory reserve volume
island
    i.'s of Langerhans
    i.'s of pancreas
isolate
isolation
Isoparorchis
    I. trisimilitubis
Isospora
    I. belli
    I. hominis
IST—insulin sensitivity test
ITT—insulin tolerance test
Ivy
    bleeding time test
    method
Ixodes
    I. bicornis
    I. cavipalpus
    I. dammini

Ixodes (continued)
  I. frequens
  I. pacificus
  I. persulcatus
  I. ricinus
  I. scapularis
Izar reagent
Jaffe
  reaction
  test
Jaksch (von Jaksch)
  test
Jansky classification
Jaworski
  bodies
  corpuscles
  test
Jenner stain
Joest bodies
Jung
  muscle
K—potassium
Kaes
  feltwork
  line
Kaes-Bekhterev
  band
  layer
  stripe
Kahler
  law
Kaiserling
  fixative
  method
  solution
Kaplan test
karyotype
Katayama
  test
KB—ketone body
KCl—potassium chloride
Kell blood antibody type
Kelvin
  scale
  thermometer
Kendall
  method
  rank correlation coefficient

Kendall (continued)
  tau
α-keto acid dehydrogenase [alpha-]
α-ketoglutaric acid [alpha-]
ketone bodies
Kidd blood antibody type
King
  unit
Klebsiella
  K. friedländeri
  K. pneumoniae
  K. oxytoca
  K. ozaenae
  K. pneumoniae
  K. rhinoscleromatis
Kligler agar
Koch
  bacillus
Koch-Weeks
  bacillus
  hemophilus
"kol–" Phonetic for words beginning chol–.
"kolee–" Phonetic for words beginning chole–, choli–, coli–.
Kovalevsky canal
Krause
  end bulbs
Krumwiede agar
Kuhne
  methylene blue
  spindle
  terminal plates
Kveim
  antigen
  test
Kyasanur Forest
  virus
LA—latex agglutination (test)
label
  radioactive l.
laboratory
labrocyte
lactaciduria
β-lactamase [beta-]
lactate
  l. dehydrogenase (LDH)

lactic
  l. acid
lactobacillus (lactobacilli)
  l. of Boas-Oppler
Lactobacillus
  L. acidophilus
  L. bifidus
  L. bulgaricus
lactoglobulin
  immune l.
Lafora
  bodies
lame foliacée ["lahm fol-yah-say"]
lamina (laminae)
  Rexed laminae
laminar
Lancefield classification
Landsteiner classification
Langer
  lines
Langhans cells
LAP—leucine aminopeptidase (test)
larva (larvae)
  l. currens
  cutaneous l. migrans
  l. migrans
  ocular l. migrans
  visceral l. migrans
larval
laser
  l. microscope
latent
latentiation
latex
Latrodectus
law
  See also *formula* and *method*.
  Avogadro l.
  Boyle l.
  Pascal l.
  Poiseuille l.
LCFA—long-chain fatty acid
LCT—long-chain triglyceride
LDH—lactate dehydrogenase
LDL—low-density lipoprotein
LDLP—low-density lipoprotein
Leclanché cell

leech
  American l.
  artificial l.
  medicinal l.
Legal
  test
Legionella
  L. bozemanii
  L. dumoffii
  L. feeleii
  L. gormanii
  L. longbeachae
  L. micdadei
  L. pittsburgensis
  L. pneumophila
  L. wadsworthii
Leishman-Donovan
  bodies
leishmania
Leishmania
  L. braziliensis
  L. donovani
  L. infantum
  L. tropica
  L. tropica mexicana
Lendrum inclusion body stain
lentivirus
Leptomitus
  L. epidermidis
  L. urophilus
  L. vaginae
Leptospira
  L. australis
  L. autumnalis
  L. biflexa
  L. canicola
  L. grippotyphosa
  L. hebdomidis
  L. hyos
  L. icterohaemorrhagiae
  L. interrogans
  L. icterohaemorrhagiae
  L. interrogans
  L. pomona
leptospirosis
  l. icterohemorrhagica
Leptotrichia
  L. buccalis

Leptotrichia (continued)
    L. placoides
Leptotrombidium
    L. akamushi
    L. deliense
lesion
    Armanni-Ebstein l.
    Bracht-Wächter l.
    Councilman l.
    diffuse l.
    Ebstein l.
    focal l.
    frondy l.
    gross l.
    histologic l.
    indiscriminate l.
    Kimmelstiel-Wilson l.
    local l.
    macroscopic l.
    mass l.
    molecular l.
    onionskin l.
    organic l.
    partial l.
    precancerous l.
    primary l.
    structural l.
    systemic l.
    total l.
    trophic l.
    tumor-like l.
"lesithin" Phonetic for lecithin.
leukapheresis
leukocyte
    granular l.'s (granulocytes)
    mononuclear l.
    Türk irritation l.
leukocythemia
leukocytic
leukocytosis
    absolute l.
    agonal l.
    basophilic l.
    eosinophilic l.
    lymphocytic l.
    neutrophilic l.
    l. of the newborn
    pathologic l.

leukocytosis (continued)
    physiologic l.
    pure l.
    relative l.
    terminal l.
    toxic l.
level
    barbiturate l.
    ethanol l.
    isoelectric l.
    lead l.
Levine
    EMB (eosin-ethylene blue)
      agar
Leyden
    crystals
Leydig cell
LFT—liver function test
LGV—lymphogranuloma venereum
LH—luteinizing hormone
LHRF—luteinizing
    hormone–releasing factor
LHRH—luteinizing
    hormone–releasing hormone
Liebermann-Burchard
    reaction
    test
Liebermeister
    furrows
    grooves
light
    l. microscope
    l. microscopy (LM)
Limnatis
    L. granulosa
    L. mysomelas
    L. nilotica
Limulus
    L. polyphemus
line
    See also *band, layer, streak,*
      and *stria.*
    Retzius l.'s
lineage
Linguatula
    L. rhinaria
    L. serrata
lipophage

lipophagic
lipoprotein
α-lipoprotein [alpha-]
lipoprotein
       high-density l. (HDL)
       intermediate-density l. (IDL)
       l. lipase (LPL)
       low-density l. (LDL)
       Lp(a) l.
       very low-density l. (VLDL)
β-lipotropin [beta-]
Lipschütz
       bodies
       cell
liquefacient
liquefaction
liquefy
liquid
       See also *fluid, liquor,* and
          solution.
       gas-l. chromatography (GLC)
       high-performance l. chro-
          matography (HPLC)
       high-pressure l. chromatog-
          raphy (HPLC)
liquiform
liquor (liquors, liquores)
       See also *fluid, liquid,* and
          solution.
       l. cerebrospinalis
       l. puris
Listeria
       L. monocytogenes
livor (livores)
       l. mortis
LM—light microscopy
Loa loa
Lobstein
       ganglion
loculus (loculi)
Loeffler
       agar
       blood serum
       culture medium
       stain
Loevit cell
Löffler
       See *Loeffler.*

low-density lipoprotein (LDL)
Löwenstein-Jensen agar
Loxosceles
       L. reclusa
LP—lipoprotein
LPE—lipoprotein electrophoresis
LPL—lipoprotein lipase
L/S—lecithin-sphingomyelin [ratio]
LSH—lutein-stimulating hormone
Lukes-Collins classification
"luko–" Phonetic for words begin-
       ning leuko–.
Luys segregator (separator)
Lyb antigens
lymphocyte
       atypical l.
       Downey-type l.
       plasmacytoid l.
lymphocytosis
       neutrophilic l.
       l.-promoting factor
lymphs—lymphocytes
lysis
Lyt antigens
μ—micro- [prefix; alphabetized as
       m]
Macracanthorhynchus
       M. hirudinaceus
Macrobdella
       M. decora
macrocythemia
       hyperchromatic m.
macroglobulin
Macromonas
       M. bipunctata
       M. mobilis
macroscopy
macula (maculae)
       maculae albidae
       maculae lacteae
       maculae tendineae
macular
macule
Madurella
       M. grisea
       M. mycetomi
MAI—*Mycobacterium avium-intra-*
       cellulare

Malassezia
    M. furfur
    M. macfadyani
    M. tropica
Malleomyces
    M. mallei
    M. pseudomallei
    M. whitmori
α-mannosidase [alpha-]
Mansonella
    M. ozzardi
    M. streptocerca
Mantoux
    conversion
    reaction
    skin test
    test
Marburg
    virus
marrow
    bone m.
Martinotti cells
mass
    m. fragmentography
    m. miniature radiography
      (MMR)
    m. radiography
    m. roentgenography
massa (massae)
MAST—multiple antigen stimulation test
mast cell
Maximow
Mayer
    hemalum
    hematoxylin
Mazzoni corpuscle
MB bands
MBP—myelin basic protein
MCBR—minimum concentration of bilirubin
McCarey-Kaufman (M-K) medium
MCFA—medium-chain fatty acid(s)
mcg, μg—microgram(s)
MCH—mean corpuscular hemoglobin
MCHC—mean corpuscular hemoglobin concentration

MCHg—mean corpuscular hemoglobin
M-CSF—macrophage colony-stimulating factor
MCT—medium-chain triglyceride [oil]
MCV—mean corpuscular volume
MDA—methylenedioxyamphetamine
MDMA—methylenedioxymethamphetamine
ME—medical examiner
M/E—myeloid-erythroid [ratio]
Meckel
    plane
media (plural of medium)
mediation
medicine
    forensic m.
medium (media, mediums)
    See also *culture medium.*
    active m.
    brain-heart infusion m.
    Bruns glucose m.
    clearing m.
    dispersion m.
    dispersive m.
    Löffler m.
    McCarey-Kaufman (M-K) m.
    mounting m.
    Novy, McNeal and Nicolle m.
    nutrient m.
    Sabouraud m.
    Stuart transport m.
    Thayer-Martin m.
    Wickersheimer m.
MEF—maximal expiratory flow
MEFR—maximum expiratory flow rate
MEFV—maximum expiratory flow volume
meg—megakaryocyte
megaloblast
melanin
melanoblast
melanocyte
Melanolestes
    M. picipes

membrane
    croupous m.
    diphtheritic m.
    false m.
    Volkmann m.
meningococci (plural of meningo-
    coccus)
meningococcus (meningococci)
meningocyte
mEq—milliequivalent(s)
Merkel
    cell
    cell carcinoma
Merkel-Ranvier
    cells
merotomy
"mersa" Phonetic for MRSA
    (methicillin-resistant *Staphylo-*
    coccus aureus).
metacercaria (metacercariae)
metHb—methemoglobin
methemoglobin (metHb)
method
    See also *technique.*
    See also *formula* and *law.*
    Bence Jones protein m.
    India ink m.
    Ivy m.
    Westergren m.
α-methylacetoacetyl CoA thiolase
    [alpha-]
β methylcrotonylglycinuria [beta-]
methylene blue
Mett (Mette)
    test tubes
μg, mcg—microgram(s)
mg—milligram(s)
mg%—milligrams percent
mg/L—milligrams per liter
MHA—microhemagglutination assay
MHB—methemoglobin
micaceous
micranatomy
microabsorption spectroscopy
microanatomy
micro-Astrup method
microbacteria
microbe

microbial
microbiologist
microbiology
microchemistry
microcyte
microelectrophoresis
microerythrocyte
microfilaria
    m. bancrofti
    m. diurna
    m. loa
    m. malaya
    sheathed m.
    m. streptocerca
    m. volvulus
microflora
microglia
microglial
microglobulin
microgram(s) (μg, mcg)
micrograph
    acoustic m.
    electron m.
micrography
microhematocrit
microhistology
microimmunofluorescent test
microinvasion
microinvasive
microlesion
micrometastasis
micrometer
Micromonospora
    M. inyoensis
    M. keratolyticum
    M. purpurea
micronodular
micropathology
micropipet
microplasia
Micropolyspora
    M. faeni
micropore
microprecipitation
microprobe
    laser m.
microscope
    acoustic m.

microscope (continued)
    beta ray m.
    binocular m.
    capillary m.
    centrifuge m.
    color-contrast m.
    comparison m.
    compound m.
    darkfield m.
    dissecting m.
    electron m.
    fluorescence m.
    flying spot m.
    hypodermic m.
    infrared m.
    integrating m.
    interference m.
    ion m.
    laser m.
    light m.
    opaque m.
    phase m., phase-contrast m.
    polarizing m.
    polarizing m., rectified
    projection x-ray m.
    reflecting m.
    Rheinberg m.
    schlieren m.
    simple m.
    stereoscopic m.
    stroboscopic m.
    trinocular m.
    ultra-m.
    ultrasonic m.
    ultraviolet m.
    x-ray m.
microscopic, microscopical
microscopy
    brightfield m.
    clinical m.
    darkfield m.
    electron m.
    fluorescence m.
    immune electron m. (IEM)
    immunofluorescence m.
    light m. (LM)
    phase-contrast m.
    scanning electron m. (SEM)

microscopy (continued)
    scanning transmission electron m.
    transmission electron m. (TEM)
microsection
microslide
microspectrophotometer
Microsporum
    M. audouinii
    M. canis
    M. ferrugineum
    M. furfur
    M. gypseum
    M. lanosum
microtome
    freezing m.
    rocking m.
    rotary m.
    sliding m.
    Stadie-Riggs m.
microtomization
microtomy
microvillus (microvilli)
microvivisection
"miel–" Phonetic for words beginning with myel–.
MIF—macrophage-inhibiting factor
MIFR—maximal inspiratory flow rate
Mikulicz (von Mikulicz) cells
milliequivalent(s) (mEq)
milligram(s) (mg)
    m.'s per liter (mg/L)
milligrams percent (mg%)
millikatal(s) (mkat)
milliliter(s) (mL, ml)
millimeter(s) (mm)
    cubic m. (c mm, cu mm, mm^3)
millimolar (mM)
millimole(s) (mmol)
milliosmole(s) (mOsm)
milliunit(s) (mU)
Mills-Reincke phenomenon
Mima
    M. polymorpha

minuscule
minute [small]
MIP—maximum inspiratory pressure
mitochondria (plural of mitochondrion)
mitochondrial
mitochondrion (mitochondria)
    giant m.
    m. of hemoflagellates
mitosis (mitoses)
mitotic
Miyagawanella
    M. illinii
    M. louisianae
    M. lymphogranulomatosis
    M. ornithosis
    M. pneumoniae
    M. psittaci
μL, μl—microliter(s)
mL, ml—milliliter(s)
M/L—monocyte-lymphocyte [ratio]
mm—millimeter(s)
mm^3 [mm3], cu mm—cubic millimeter(s)
MMEF—maximal midexpiratory flow
MMEFR—maximal midexpiratory flow rate
mmol—millimole(s)
mmol/L—millimoles per liter
MMR—mass miniature radiography
MNU—methylnitrosourea
modeling
molecule
    adhesion m.'s, cell adhesion m.'s (CAM)
    cell interaction (CI) m.'s
    intercellular adhesion m. 1 (ICAM-1)
    intercellular adhesion m. 2 (ICAM-2)
molluscum
    m. bodies
Monakow (von Monakow)
    bundle
    fascia
    striae

Monilia
    M. albicans
monomorphous
monos—monocytes
monosomic
Monosporium
    M. apiospermum
Morax-Axenfeld
    bacillus
    diplococcus
    hemophilus
Moraxella
    M. bovis
    M. lacunata
    M. liquefaciens
Morgagni
    humor
    liquor
morpio, morpion (morpiones)
Mosher
    air cells
mOsm—milliosmole(s)
mosquito (mosquitoes)
MOTT—mycobacteria other than tubercle (bacilli) [nontuberculous mycobacteria]
MOTT bacilli
MRF—mesencephalic reticular formation
MRSA—methicillin-resistant *Staphylococcus aureus*
MSH—melanocyte-stimulating hormone
MSVC—maximal sustained ventilatory capacity
MT—medical technologist
μU [microU]—microunit(s)
mucoprotein
Mucor
    M. corymbifer
    M. mucedo
    M. pusillus
    M. racemosus
    M. ramosus
    M. rhizopodiformis
Murray Valley
    virus

muscle
> See in *Orthopedics and Sports Medicine* section.

musculus (musculi)
> See in medical specialty sections.

MVP—mean platelet volume
mycobacterium (mycobacteria)
Mycobacterium
> *M. avium-intracellulare* (MAI)
> *M. balnei*
> · *M. berolinenis*
> *M. bovis*
> *M. butyricum*
> *M. chelonae*
> *M. flavescens*
> *M. fortuitum*
> *M. fortuitum-chelonae*
> *M. fortuitum-chelonei*
> *M. gastri*
> *M. gordonae*
> *M. habana*
> *M. haemophilum*
> *M. intracellularis*
> *M. kansasii*
> *M. leprae*
> *M. lepraemurium*
> *M. luciflavum*
> *M. marinum*
> *M. microti*
> *M. tuberculosis*
> *M. paratuberculosis*
> *M. phlei*
> *M. scrofulaceum*
> *M. simiae*
> *M. smegmatis*
> *M. szulgai*
> *M. terrea-nonchromogenicum-triviale*
> *M. tuberculosis*
> *M. tuberculosis* var. *avium*
> *M. tuberculosis* var. *bovis*
> *M. tuberculosis* var. *hominis*
> *M. ulcerans*
> *M. xenopi*

Myconostoc
> *M. gregarium*

Mycoplana
> *M. bullata*
> *M. dimorpha*

Mycoplasma
> *M. faucium*
> *M. fermentans*
> *M. hominis*
> *M. orale*
> *M. orale* type 1
> *M. pharyngis*
> *M. pneumoniae*
> *M. salivarium*

mycoplasma (mycoplasmas, mycoplasmata)
> T-strain m.

mycoplasmal
mycosis (mycoses)
> m. fungoides
> m. fungoides d'emblée

myelocyte
myeloperoxidase (MPO)
"my-nute" Phonetic for minute [small].
myoadenylate deaminase
myofibrilla (myofibrillae)
myofibrillar
myoglobulin
Myrtophyllum
> *M. hepatis*

"mytotic" Phonetic for mitotic.
myxovirus
Naegleria
nanogram(s) (ng)
NCA—nonspecific cross-reacting antigen
NCF—neutrophil chemotactic factor
Ne—norepinephrine
Necator
> *N. americanus*

necropsy
necroscopy
necrose, necrosed
necrosis (necroses)
> caseous n.
> cheesy n.
> colliquative n.
> gangrenous n.
> liquefaction n.

necrosis (necroses) (continued)
    liquefactive n.
    moist n.
    progressive emphysematous
      n.
    septic n.
necrotic
necrotomy
NED—no evidence of disease
Negri bodies
Neisseria
    N. catarrhalis
    N. caviae
    N. flavescens
    N. gonorrhoeae
    N. intracellularis
    N. lactamica
    N. lactamicus
    N. meningitides
    N. meningitidis
    N. mucosa
    N. ovis
    N. perflava
    N. pharyngis
    N. sicca
    N. subtiara
    N. tiara
Neisser-Wechsberg phenomenon
neoformation
neoformative
neomembrane
neomort
neoplasia
    gestational trophoblastic n.
    intraepithelial n.
    multiple endocrine n. (MEN)
neoplasm
    adrenal n.
    benign n.
    histoid n.
    malignant n.
    metastatic n.
    stromal cell n.
    trophoblastic n.
    vascular n.
neoplastic
"neu–" Phonetic for words begin-
    ning pneu–.

Neumann
    cells
    sheath
neuroblast
    sympathetic n.
neurocyte
neurocytology
neurodendrite
neurodendron
neurofiber
neurofibril
neurofilament
neurohistology
neurokeratin
neuron
neuropodion
neuropodium (neuropodia)
neutrophil
    band n.
    juvenile n.
    mature n.
    polymorphonuclear n.
    segmented n.
"new–" Phonetic for words begin-
    ning pneu–.
ng—nanogram(s)
Nickerson medium smear
β-nicotyrine [beta-]
"ni-dar-ee-an" Phonetic for cnidarian.
Niemann-Pick
    cells
    lipid
Nissl bodies
nitrite
nitrogen (N)
    blood urea n. (BUN)
    nonprotein n. (NPN)
    urea n.
nitrogen-fixing
nitrogenous
NK—natural killer
NK cells
NNM—Nicolle-Novy-MacNeal
    (medium)
Nocardia
    N. asteroides
    N. brasiliensis
    N. caviae

Nocardia (continued)
    N. intracellularis
    N. madurae
    N. minutissima
    N. asteroides
    N. otitidis-caviarum
    N. pelletieri
    N. tenuis
Nonne
    test
nonprotein nitrogen (NPN)
nonspecific
"noo–" Phonetic for words beginning pneu–.
norepinephrine
normoblast
    acidophilic n.
    basophilic n.
    intermediate n.
    orthochromatophilic n.
    polychromatophilic n.
Norris corpuscles
nosomycosis
noticeable
noxa (noxae)
NP—nasopharyngeal
NPDL—nodular, poorly differentiated lymphocytes
NR—nonreactive
NSQ—not sufficient quantity
"nu–" Phonetic for words beginning pneu–.
nuclear
    n. aggregate
    n. inclusion body
    n. pore alteration
    n. vacuolization
nucleated
nuclei (genitive and plural of nucleus)
nucleic
nucleiform
nucleoid
nucleolar
nucleoli (plural of nucleolus)
nucleoliform
nucleolin
nucleolinus
nucleolus (nucleoli)

nucleoprotein
nucleotide polymerase
oasis (oases)
Ochromyia
    O. anthropophaga
Octomitus
    O. hominis
Octomyces
    O. etiennei
Oestrus
    O. hominis
    O. ovis
OGTT—oral glucose tolerance test
oleaginous
oligodendrocyte
oligodendroglia
oligonucleotide
    o. probe
Onchocerca
    O. volvulus
O&P—ova and parasites
Opalski cell
opaque
    o. microscope
Opisthorchis
    O. felineus
    O. noverca
    O. viverrini
organism
    Arizona o.
    Rickett o.
    Vincent o.
organon (organa)
organum (organa)
Ornithodoros
    O. coriaceus
ortho
    o.-aminoazotoluene
osmicate
osmification
osmiophilic
osmiophobic
osmium (Os)
    o. tetroxide
osmolality
    calculated serum o.
    urine o.
osmolar

osmolarity
osmole (Osm)
osmolute
osmophilic
osmoreceptor
osmosis
Ostertag
    streptococcus of O.
Otomyces
    O. hageni
    O. purpureus
oxalate
oxyhemoglobin (HbO$_2$ [HBO2])
Oxyuris
    O. incognita
    O. vermicularis
P.—Pasteurella
    Plasmodium
    Proteus
pachymeninx (pachymeninges)
PaCO$_2$ [PaCO2]—arterial carbon dioxide partial pressure
PACO$_2$ [PACO2]—alveolar carbon dioxide partial pressure
PAF—platelet-activating factor
Pagano-Levin medium smear
Paget
    cell
PAH, PAHA—*p*-aminohippuric acid [p-, para-]
PAM—pulmonary alveolar macrophage(s)
panel
    urine drug p. (UDP)
p24 antigen test
PaO$_2$ [PaO2]—arterial partial pressure of oxygen (arterial pO$_2$)
PAO$_2$ [PAO2]—alveolar partial pressure of oxygen (alveolar pO$_2$)
Pap—Papanicolaou
PAP—prostatic acid phosphatase
Papanicolaou (Pap)
    smear
    stain
    test
paper
    blue litmus p.
    Congo red p.

paper (continued)
    filter p.
    indicator p.
    litmus p.
    red litmus p.
    test p.
papillomavirus
    human p. (HPV)
papovavirus
    lymphotropic p. (LPV)
Pappenheim
    hemoblast
    reagent
    stain
para
    p.-aminohippuric acid (PAH, PAHA) synthetase
    p.-dimethylaminoazobenzene
    p.-fluorophenylalanine
    p. hydroxyphenylpyruvic acid (PHPPA)
Paracoccidioides
    P. brasiliensis
Paracolobactrum
    P. aerogenoides
    P. arizonae
    P. coliforme
    P. intermedium
Paragonimus
    P. westermani
Paragordius
    P. cinctus
    P. tricuspidatus
    P. varius
Paramecium
    P. coli
Parasaccharomyces
    P. ashfordi
parasitic
parasitology
parathormone (PTH)
particulate
PAS—periodic acid−Schiff
PAS (periodic acid−Schiff) reaction
PAS (periodic acid−Schiff) test
Pasteurella
    P. haemolytica
    P. multocida

Pasteurella (continued)
    P. pestis
    P. pneumotropica
    P. pseudotuberculosis
    P. septica
    P. tularensis
    P. ureae
path—pathology
pathoanatomy
pathogenesis
pathogenetic
pathogenic
pathognomonic
pathognomy
pathologic, pathological
Pb—barometric pressure
PBG—porphobilinogen
PBL—peripheral blood lymphocytes
PBT_4—protein-bound thyroxine
PC—phosphocreatine
    platelet count
pCO_2 [pCO2]—carbon dioxide
    pressure
PCR—polymerase chain reaction
PDGF—platelet-derived growth
    factor
PDH—phosphate dehydrogenase
pearl
    epidermic p.'s
    epithelial p.'s
Pectobacterium
    P. carotovorum
Pediculus
    P. humanus
    P. humanus capitis
    P. humanus corporis
    P. humanus humanus
    P. humanus vestimentorum
    P. inguinalis
    P. pubis
    P. vestimenti
pediculus (pediculi) [anatomy]
PEF—peak expiratory flow
PEFR—peak expiratory flow rate
Pelger nuclear anomaly
penicillin-fast
Penicillium
    P. barbae

Penicillium (continued)
    P. bouffardi
    P. minimum
    P. montoyai
    P. notatum
    P. patulum
    P. spinulosum
Pentastoma
    P. constrictum
    P. denticulatum
    P. taenioides
Pentatrichomonas
    P. ardin delteili
peptidase
    leucine amino p.
Peptococcus
    P. anaerobius
    P. asaccharolyticus
    P. constellatus
    P. magnus
    P. prevotii
Peptostreptococcus
    P. anaerobius
    P. intermedius
    P. lanceolatus
    P. micros
    P. productus
Petri
    dish
    test
Petriellidium
    P. boydii
PFGE—pulsed field gradient gel
    electrophoresis
PFR—peak flow rate
PFT—pulmonary function test
pg—picogram(s)
PG—prostaglandin
PGD_2 [PGD2]—prostaglandin D_2
PGE_1 [PGE1]—prostaglandin E_1
PGE_2 [PGE2]—prostaglandin E_2
$PGF_{2\alpha}$ [PGF2-alpha]—prostaglan-
    din $F_{2\alpha}$ [F2-alpha]
PGG_2 [PGG2]—prostaglandin G_2
PGH—pituitary growth hormone
PGH_2 [PGH2]—prostaglandin H_2
PGI_2 [PGI2]—prostaglandin I_2
    [prostacyclin]

pH—hydrogen ion concentration
phagocyte
    mononuclear p.
phagocytosis
phagocytotic
phase
    p. microscope
phase-contrast
    p.-c. microscope
    p.-c. microscopy
phenomenon (phenomena)
    Anderson p.
    Bordet-Gengou p.
    cold agglutination p.
    Denys-Leclef p.
    d'Herelle p.
    erythrocyte adherence p.
    Gengou p.
    halisteresis p.
    Hamburger p.
    Hektoen p.
    Huebener-Thomsen-Frieden-
      reich p.
    iceberg p.
    immune-adherence p.
    Lewis p.
    Liacopoulos p.
    Liesegang p.
    Mills-Reincke p.
    Neisser-Wechsberg p.
    Pfeiffer p.
    prozone p.
    reclotting p.
    red cell adherence p.
    satellite p.
    Soret p.
    Theobald Smith p.
    Twort-d'Herelle p.
phenotype
    Bombay p.
pheochromocyte
Phialophora
    P. jeanselmi
    P. verrucosa
Philadelphia chromosome
phlebectomy
phlebotomist
phlebotomize

Phlebotomus
    P. argentipes
    P. chinensis
    P. intermedius
    P. macedonicum
    P. noguchi
    P. papatasi
    P. sergentii
    P. verrucarum
    P. vexator
phlebotomy
phosphatase
    acid p.
    alkaline p.
    serum p.
phosphate
phosphatidic acid
phosphatidylcholine-sterol *O*-acyl-
    transferase
phosphatidylethanolamine (PE)
phosphatidylinositol
phosphatidylserine (PS)
phosphorus (P) [noun]
phthalein
    alpha-naphthol p.
    orthocresol p.
Phthirus
    P. pubis
phymatorhusin
Physalia
physalides (plural of physalis)
physaliform
physaliphorous
physalis (physalides)
physallization
Physaloptera
    P. caucasica
    P. mordens
physiolysis
phytanic acid
phytanic acid α-hydroxylase [alpha-]
PI—phosphatidylinositol
Pick [eponym]
    bodies
    bundle
    cell
picogram(s) (pg)
picornavirus

Piedraia
 P. hortae
PIF—peak inspiratory flow
 prolactin-inhibiting factor
PIFR—peak inspiratory flow rate
pigment
 bile p.
 lipid p.
"pikno–" Phonetic for words beginning pykno–.
piliate
piliform
pipette
"piro–" Phonetic for words beginning pyro–.
Pityrosporon
 P. orbiculare
 P. ovale
 P. versicolor
PKU—phenylketonuria
PL—phospholipid
plaque
 Redlich-Fisher miliary p.'s
 senile p.'s
 talc p.'s
plaque-forming cell assay
plasma
 antihemophilic human p.
plasmodium
 exoerythrocytic p.
Plasmodium
 P. falciparum
 P. malariae
 P. ovale
 P. pleurodyniae
 P. vivax
 P. vivax minuta
plate
 cough p.
 Petri p.
pls—prostaglandin-like substance
PM—after death (L. post mortem)
 polymorph (white blood cell)
 postmortem
PMB—polymorphonuclear basophil
 (leukocyte)
PME—polymorphonuclear
 eosinophil (leukocyte)

PMN—polymorphonuclear neutrophil (leukocyte)
pneumatization
pneumobacillus
 Friedländer p.
pneumococcus (pneumococci)
Pneumocystis
 P. carinii
Pneumovirus
pO_2 [pO2]—partial pressure of oxygen
POA—pancreatic oncofetal antigen
"poik" Slang for poikilocyte.
polarization
polarizing microscope
 rectified p.m.
policeman [glass stirring rod and
 transfer tool]
policeman's tip
poly—polymorphonuclear leukocyte
polyemia
 p. aquosa
 p. hyperalbuminosa
 p. polycythaemica
 p. serosa
polymorphonuclear
 p. basophil
 p. eosinophil
 p. leukocyte
 p. neutrophil
polynuclear
polypiform
polyploid
polyploidy
polyribosome
polysaccharide
polysomaty
Ponfick shadow
Porocephalus
 P. armillatus
 P. clavatus
 P. constrictus
 P. denticulatus
Porter-Silber chromogens test
Portuguese man-o'-war
post
 p. mortem

"posted" Slang for autopsy (post mortem examination) performed.
postprandial
potassium (K)
    p. acetate
    p. acid tartrate
    p. alum
    p. *p*-aminobenzoate [p-, para-]
    p. aspartate and magnesium aspartate
    p. bicarbonate
    p. bichromate
    p. bitartrate
    p. bromide
    p. carbonate
    p. chlorate
    p. chloride
    p. citrate
    p. cyanide
    p. dichromate
    p. dihydrogen phosphate
    p. ferricyanide
    p. glucaldrate
    p. gluconate
    p. glycerophosphate
    p. guaiacolsulfonate
    p. hydroxide
    p. iodate
    p. iodide
    p. mercuric iodide
    p. metaphosphate
    p. nitrate
    p. oxalate
    p. penicillin G
    p. perchlorate
    p. permanganate
    p. phenoxymethyl penicillin
    p. phosphate
    p. phosphate, dibasic
    p. phosphate, monobasic
    radioactive p.
    p. sodium tartrate
    p. sorbate
    p. sulfate
    p. tartrate
    p. thiocyanate

PPD—purified protein derivative (of tuberculin)
PPD-S—purified protein derivative–standard
ppm—parts per million
PRA—plasma renin activity
precipitate
    alum p.
PRF—prolactin-releasing factor
PRH—prolactin-releasing hormone
principal [primary, main]
principle [rule]
PRIST—paper radioimmunosorbent test
pro—prothrombin
proerythrocyte
profibrinolysin
profile
    liver p.
projection
    p. x-ray microscope
prolactin
proliferate
prolymphocyte
promegaloblast
Propionibacterium
    P. acnes
prostaglandin (PG)
    p. D_2 [D2] (PGD_2)
    p. E_1 [E1] (PGE_1)
    p. E_2 [E2] (PGE_2)
    p. endoperoxide synthase
    p. $F_{2\alpha}$ [F2-alpha] ($PGF_{2\alpha}$)
    p. $F_{2\alpha}$ tromethamine [F2-alpha]
    p. G_2 [G2] (PGG_2)
    p. H_2 [H2] (PGH_2)
    p. I_2 [I2] (PGI_2) [prostacyclin]
    p. synthase
prostatic
    benign p. hyperplasia (BPH)
    benign p. hypertrophy (BPH)
proteidin
    pyocyanase p.
protein
    C-reactive p.
protein-glutamine γ-glutamyltransferase [gamma-]

proteinuria
    Bence Jones p.
Proteus
    P. inconstans
    P. mirabilis
    P. morganii
    P. Ox-2
    P. Ox-K
    P. rettgeri
    P. vulgaris
prothrombin
proton
    p. spectroscopy
Providencia
    P. alcalifaciens
    P. stuartii
P/S—polyunsaturated-saturated
    fatty acid [ratio]
Pseudamphistomum
    P. truncatum
Pseudomonas
    P. acidovorans
    P. aeruginosa
    P. alcaligenes
    P. cepacia
    P. diminuta
    P. eisenbergii
    P. fluorescens
    P. fragi
    P. mallei
    P. nonliquefaciens
    P. paucimobilis
    P. pseudoalcaligenes
    P. pseudomallei
    P. syncyanea
    P. vesicularis
    P. viscosa
PT—prothrombin time
PTH—parathyroid hormone
PTHS—parathyroid hormone secre-
    tion [rate]
PTT—partial thromboplastin time
PUFA—polyunsaturated fatty acid(s)
pulpy
punctation
puncture
    transethmoidal p.
pyknocyte

pyknometer
pyknometry
pyknomorphous
pyknotic
pyocyanase
pyrogen
pyroglobulin
PZ—pancreozymin
PZ-CCK—pancreozymin-cholecys-
    tokinin
q.n.s.—quantity not sufficient (L.
    quantum non satis)
quick test
"rabd–" Phonetic for words begin-
    ning rhabd–.
radicle [noun: branch of nerve or
    vessel]
radiography
    mass r.
    mass miniature r. (MMR)
radioimmunoassay (RIA)
radiolabeled
radionuclide
radioreceptor
Ramon
    flocculation test
rarefaction
    bone r.
RAST—radioallergosorbent test
rate
ratio
    albumin-globulin (A/G) r.
    ALT/AST r.
    dextrose-nitrogen (D/N) r.
    glucose-nitrogen (G/N) r.
    ketogenic-antiketogenic
        (K/A) r.
    lecithin-sphingomyelin (L/S)
        r.
    myeloid-erythroid (M/E) r.
    peak-to-total r.
    polymorphonuclear-lympho-
        cyte r.
    stimulation r. (SR)
RBC—red blood cell(s)
    red blood [cell] count
RBCV—red blood cell volume
RCV—red cell volume

RDW—red blood cell distribution
    width index
reaction
    false-negative r.
    false-positive r.
    foreign body r.
    Forssman antigen-antibody r.
    glycine-arginine r.
    Gruber r.
    Gruber-Widal r.
    Sanarelli-Shwartzman r.
    sedimentation r.
    Selivanoff (Seliwanow) r.
    Shwartzman r., generalized
    Shwartzman r., localized
    sigma r.
    Wassermann r.
    Weil-Felix r.
    Widal r.
reagent
    Sickledex r.
receptor
    adrenergic r.
    α-adrenergic r.'s [alpha-]
    β-adrenergic r.'s [beta-]
    alpha r.'s
    B-cell antigen r.'s
    beta r.'s
    complement r.'s [CR1,
        C3b/C4b r., CD35; CR2,
        C3d/C3bi r., C3dg, CD21;
        CR3, C3bi r., CD11b/18;
        CR4, C3bi r., CD11c/18;
        C3aR (C3a r.); C5aR
        (C5a r.); C1qR (C1q r.)]
    cholinergic r.'s
    T-cell antigen r.'s
record
    dental identification r.
Redlich-Fisher miliary plaques
reducing substance
Reed cells, Dorothy Reed cells
Reed-Sternberg cells
reflecting microscope
region
    constant (C) r.
    hinge r.
    homology r.'s

region (continued)
    hypervariable r.'s
    variable (V) r.
residuum (residua)
    gastric r.
"retic" Slang for reticulocyte (count).
reticulohistiocytary
reticulohistiocytoma
reticulosis
    pagetoid r.
Retortamonas
    R. intestinalis
Rettgerella
    R. rettgeri
RFLA—rheumatoid factor–like
    activity
RFS—renal function study
RH—releasing hormone
Rh—Rhesus
Rh
        antibody
        blood group
        factor
        immunization
        incompatibility
        isoantigen
Rhabditis
    R. hominis
rhabdovirus
Rheinberg
        microscope
rhesus (Rh)
    r. factor
Rhizoglyphus
    R. parasiticus
Rhizomucor
rhizopod
Rhizopus
    R. oryzae
    R. rhizopodoformis
Rh neg—Rhesus factor–negative
Rhodin fixative
Rhodotorula'
    R. rubra
Rh pos—Rhesus factor–positive
RIA—radioimmunoassay
Rickettsia
    R. akamushi

Rickettsia (continued)
  R. *akari*
  R. *australis*
  R. *burnetii*
  R. *canada*
  R. *conorii*
  R. *diaporica*
  R. *mooseri*
  R. *muricola*
  R. *nipponica*
  R. *orientalis*
  R. *pediculi*
  R. *prowazekii*
  R. *quintana*
  R. *rickettsii*
  R. *siberica*
  R. *sibiricus*
  R. *tsutsugamushi*
  R. *typhi*
  R. *wolhynica*
rickettsia (rickettsiae)
Rieder
  cell
  lymphocyte
rigidity
  postmortem r.
rigor
  instantaneous r. mortis
  r. mortis
RIHSA—radioactive iodinated
  human serum albumin
Ringer
  injection
  injection, lactated
  irrigation
  lactate
  mixture
  solution
  solution, lactated
"rinokladeum" Phonetic for *Rhin-
  ocladium.*
RIP—radioimmunoprecipitation
RIPA—radioimmunoprecipitation
  assay
RIST—radioimmunosorbent test
"rizo–" Phonetic for words beginning rhizo–.
RLC—residual lung capacity

RNA—ribonucleic acid
RNP—ribonucleoprotein
rocking microtome
roentgenography
  mass r.
Röhl marginal corpuscles
Roida
      tube
roll
  r. tube
Rotavirus (antigen groups A–F)
RP—reactive protein
Rp—pulmonary resistance
RPCF, RPCFT—Reiter protein
  complement fixation test
RPR—rapid plasma reagin (test)
RPR-CT—rapid plasma reagin circle
  card test
RRA—radioreceptor assay
RS—respiratory syncytial
RSV—respiratory syncytial virus
Runeberg
  formula
RUR—resin-uptake ratio
Russell
    bodies
    corpuscles
    double-sugar agar
Ruysch
    glomeruli
RV—residual volume
RVRA—renal vein renin activity
    renal vein renin assay
RVRC—renal vein renin concentra-
    tion
Rye classification of Hodgkin disease
SA—serum albumin
Saccharomyces
saccharomyces
Saccharomyces
  S. *albicans*
  S. *anginae*
  S. *apiculatus*
saccharomyces
  Busse s.
Saccharomyces
  S. *cantliei*
  S. *capillitii*

Saccharomyces (continued)
    S. carlsbergensis
    S. cerevisiae
    S. coprogenus
    S. epidermica
    S. galacticolus
    S. glutinis
    S. hominis
    S. lemonnieri
    S. mellis
    S. mycoderma
    S. neoformans
    S. pastorianus
Sala cells
Salmonella
    S. choleraesuis
    S. choleraesuis var. *kuzendorf*
    S. choleraesuis var. *typhisuis*
    S. derby
    S. durazzo
    S. enteritidis
    S. enteritidis serotype
      hirschfeldii
    S. enteritidis serotype
      paratyphi A
    S. enteritidis serotype
      schottmuelleri
    S. enteritidis serotype
      typhimurium
    S. hirschfeldii
    S. indiana
    S. minnesota
    S. montevideo
    S. muenchen
    S. newington
    S. oranienburg
    S. paratyphi
    S. paratyphi A
    S. paratyphi B
    S. paratyphi C
    S. schottmuelleri
    S. sendai
    S. serogroup D
    S. suipestifer
    S. typhi
    S. typhimurium
    S. typhisuis
    S. typhosa

Salmonella (continued)
    S. virginia
Salvia
    S. horminium
    S. sclarea
sarcoma (sarcomas, sarcomata)
    See in *Oncology and Hematology* section.
sarcomatoid
Sarcophaga
    S. carnaria
    S. dux
    S. fuscicauda
    S. haemorrhoidalis
    S. nificornis
    S. rubicornis
sarcoplasmic
Sarcoptes
    S. scabiei
SCA— single-chain antigen-binding
SCA proteins
scan
    bilirubin s.
    fluorescence s.
scanning
    s. microscope, s. electron
      microscope
    s. transmission electron
      microscopy
SCAT—sickle cell anemia test
Schaumann
    bodies
Schick
    test
Schilling
    blood count
    test
schistocyte
Schistosoma
    S. haematobium
    S. intercalatum
    S. japonicum
    S. mansoni
schistosome
schistosomiasis
Schizoblastosporion
schizogony
schlieren microscope

Schmidt
    test
Schmitz bacillus
Schmorl
    body
Schutz
    micrococcus
schwannoma
scirrhoid
scirrhous [adj.]
SCK—serum creatine kinase
"scopes" See under full name.
    microscope
    microspectroscope
    photomicroscope
    spectroscope
    supermicroscope
    ultramicroscope
Scopulariopsis
    S. americana
    S. aureus
    S. blochi
    S. brevicaulis
    S. cinereus
    S. koningi
    S. minimus
SCPK—serum creatine phosphoki-
    nase [now: serum creatine
    kinase (SCK)]
screen
    urine drug s. (UDS)
sectio (sectiones)
    s. cadavaris
section
    celloidin s.
    paraffin s.
    Pitres s.'s
sed rate—sedimentation rate
sediment
    s. tube
    urinary s.
sedimentation
    s. tube
sedimentation rate
    erythrocyte s.r.
    Rourke-Ernstein s.r.
    Westergren s.r.
    Wintrobe s.r.

sedimentation rate (continued)
    Zeta s.r.
segmented neutrophils (segs, seg-
    menteds)
segs—segmented neutrophils
SEM—scanning electron microscopy
"seng-ker" Phonetic for Zenker.
sensitization
    active s.
sequestrant
sequestration
    biochemical s.
sera (plural of serum)
serology
    diagnostic s.
serotonin
serotype
    heterologous s.
serous
Serratia
    S. indica
    S. kiliensis
    S. liquefaciens
    S. marcescens
    S. piscatorum
    S. plymuthica
    S. proteamaculans
    S. rubidaea
Sertoli
    cell
    column
    tumor
serum (serums, sera)
    s. acid phosphatase
    s. albumin
    s. alkaline phosphatase
    s. alpha-fetoprotein (AFP)
    blood s. [See also *blood
      serum.*]
    blood grouping s.'s
    pregnancy s.
    quality control s.
    s. urea nitrogen (SUN)
seta (setae)
setaceous
Sézary
    cell

SG—serum globulin
   specific gravity
SGOT—serum glutamic-oxaloacetic
   transaminase [now: AST]
SGPT—serum glutamic-pyruvic
   transaminase [now: ALT]
shadow
     Ponfick s.
shadow-casting
SHBD—serum hydroxybutyrate
   dehydrogenase
sheath
     Neumann s., s. of Neumann
Shigella
     S. alkalescens
     S. ambigua
     S. arabinotarda (type A,
       type B)
     S. boydii
     S. ceylonensis
     S. dispar
     S. dysenteriae
     S. etousae
     S. flexneri
     S. madampensis
     S. newcastle
     S. paradysenteriae
     S. parashigae
     S. schmitzii
     S. shigae
     S. sonnei
     S. wakefield
"shwah-no-mah" Phonetic for
   schwannoma.
SI—International System of Units
   (Fr. Système International d'U-
   nités)
sickle cell
signature
     tumor s.
simple
     s. microscope
sin–. See also words beginning
   cin–, syn–.
single-chain antigen-binding proteins (SCA proteins)
β-sitosterolemia [beta-]

SLD, SLDH—serum lactate dehydrogenase
sliding microtome
SMA—sequential multiple analyzer
   [SMA 6/60, SMA 12/60, SMA
   20/60]
SMAC ["smack"]—sequential multiple analyzer plus computer
   [SMAC 7, SMAC 12, SMAC
   20]
smear
     bronchoscopic s.
     fungi s.
     Papanicolaou (Pap) s.
     TB s.
     Tzanck s.
sodium (Na)
     s. acetarsol
     s. acetate
     s. acetazolamide
     s. acid citrate
     s. acid phosphate
     s. alginate
     s. alizarinsulfonate
     s. *p*-aminohippurate [p-,
       para-]
     s. *p*-aminosalicylate [p-,
       para-]
     s. amobarbital
     s. ampicillin
     s. *n*-amylpenicillinate
     s. antimonyltartrate
     s. antimonylthioglycolate
     s. arsenate
     s. ascorbate
     s. aurothiomalate
     s. aurothiosuccinate
     s. aurothiosulfate
     s. azide
     s. benzoate
     s. benzosulfimide
     s. bicarbonate
     s. biphosphate
     s. bisulfite
     s. borate
     s. bromide

sodium (Na) (continued)
s. butabarbital
s. calcium edetate, s. calci-
umedetate
s. caprylate
s. carbonate
s. caseinate
s. cellulose phosphate
s. chloride (Cl [NaCl])
s. citrate
s. colistimethate
s. cyclamate
s. dextrothyroxine
s. diphenylhydantoin
s. dithionate
s. dodecyl sulfate
exchangeable s.
s. fluoride
s. fluosilicate
s. folate
s. fusidate
s. glutamate
s. glycocholate
s. gold thiosulfate
s. hydrate
s. hydroxide
s. hypochlorite
s. hyposulfite
s. iodide
s. isoamylethyl barbiturate
s. lactate
s. lauryl sulfate
s. levothyroxine
s. metabisulfite
s. methicillin
s. monofluorophosphate
monohydrated s. carbonate
s. nitrate
s. nitroferricyanide
s. nitroprusside
s. oxacillin
s. oxybate
s. para-aminosalicylate
s. penicillin G
s. pentobarbital
s. perborate
s. phenobarbital
s. phenylethylbarbiturate

sodium (Na) (continued)
s. phenytoin
s. phosphate
s. phosphate, dibasic
s. phosphate, dried
s. phosphate, effervescent
s. phosphate, exsiccated
s. phosphate, monobasic
s. phytate
s. polyethylene sulfonate
s. polyphosphate
s. polystyrene sulfonate
potassium s. tartrate
s. propionate
s. pyroborate
s. pyrophosphate
s. pyrosulfite
s. salicylate
s. secobarbital
s. silicofluoride
s. stearate
s. stibocaptate
s. succinate
s. sulfacetamide
s. sulfadiazine
s. sulfate
s. sulfite
s. sulfite, anhydrous
s. sulfite, exsiccated
s. sulfoxone
s. tetraborate
s. tetradecyl sulfate
s. thiamylal
s. thiopental
s. thiosulfate
s. tolbutamide
s. trimetaphosphate
s. warfarin
Solanum carolinense
solation
solid
gas-s. chromatography (GSC)
solution
See also *fluid, liquid,* and
liquor.
formaldehyde s.
Ringer s., lactated Ringer s.

"soot-soo-ga-moo-shee" Phonetic
   for tsutsugamushi. See under
   Rickettsia and *disease*.
sorbic acid
sorbitol
Soret
   band
   effect
   phenomenon
sorter
SPBI—serum protein-bound iodine
SPCA—serum prothrombin conversion accelerator
SPE—serum protein electrophoresis
specific gravity
spectra (plural of spectrum)
spectroscope
   direct vision s.
spectroscopy
   infrared s.
   microabsorption s.
   proton s.
spectrum (spectra)
   absorption s.
   action s.
   chemical s.
   fluorescence s.
   gaseous s.
SPEP—serum protein electrophoresis
SPF—split products of fibrin
sp gr—specific gravity
spherocyte
spherocytosis
sphingomyelin
sphingosine
spirillum (spirilla)
Spirillum
   S. minus
Spirochaeta
   S. daxensis
   S. eurystrepta
   S. marina
   S. pallida
   S. plicatilis
   S. stenostrepta
   S. vincenti
spongiocyte

Sporothrix
   S. schenckii
Sporotrichum
   S. schenckii
sporozoa
sporozoite
spot
   Christopher s.
   chromatin s.
   cold s.
   embryonic s.
   eye s.
   germinal s.
   hot s.
   milk s.
   milky s.
   soldier's s.
   Tardieu s.
   tendinous s.
sputum
   s. tube
squamatization
squamous cell
SR—sedimentation rate
SRH—somatotropin-releasing hormone
SRT—sedimentation rate test
SSA—sulfosalicylic acid (test)
stab [German word for band, immature neutrophil]
Stadie-Riggs
   microtome
"staf-il-o-kok-is" Phonetic for
   Staphylococcus.
stain
   acid-Schiff s.
   alcian blue s.
   ATPase s.
   Bowie s.
   carbolfuchsin s.
   chlorazol black E s.
   Congo red s.
   cresyl violet s.
   eosin s.
   Giemsa s.
   Gomori s.
   Gomori methenamine silver
      nitrate s.

stain (continued)
    Gram s.
    Gram-Weigert s.
    hematoxylin and eosin
      (H&E) s.
    Jenner-Giemsa s.
    Leishman s.
    Masson s.
    Mayer hemalum s.
    May-Grünwald-Giemsa s.
    methenamine silver s.
    mucicarmine s.
    Papanicolaou s.
    Pappenheim s.
    periodic acid−Schiff (PAS) s.
    polychrome methylene blue s.
    quinacrine s.
    Romanovsky (Romanowsky)
      s.
    Truant s.
    van Gieson s.
    von Kossa s.
    Wade-Fite-Faraco s.
    Weigert s.
    Wright s.
    Ziehl-Neelsen s.
standardization
staph—staphylococcus
staphylococcus (staphylococci)
Staphylococcus
    S. albus
    S. aureus
    S. citreus
    S. epidermidis
    S. faecalis
    S. pyogenes
    S. pyogenes aureus
    S. pyogenes var. *albus*
    S. saprophyticus
    S. simulans
    S. viridans
staphylolysin
    α s., alpha s.
    β s., beta s.
    δ s., delta s.
    ε s., epsilon s.
    γ s., gamma s.

stercobilin
stercobilinogen
stereocilium (stereocilia)
stereoscopic
    s. microscope
sterilize
Sternberg
    giant cells
Sternberg-Reed cells
stippling
    basophilic s.
Stokvis
    test
stool
    s. culture
    s. guaiac
Strasburger cell plate
strata (plural of stratum)
stratiform
stratum (strata)
strep—streptococcal
    streptococci
Streptobacillus
    S. moniliformis
streptococcal groups A, B, G
Streptococcus
    S. agalactiae
    S. anginosus
    S. bovis
    S. cremoris
    S. durans
    S. equi
    S. equisimilis
    S. faecalis
    S. faecium
    S. lacticus
    S. lactis
    S. liquefaciens
    S. mitis
    S. mutans
    S. pneumoniae
    S. pyogenes
    S. salivarius
    S. uberis
    S. viridans
    S. zooepidemicus
    S. zymogenes

streptococcus (streptococci)
    alpha s.
    anhemolytic s.
    Bargen s.
    beta s.
    Fehleisen s.
    gamma s.
    hemolytic s.
    nonhemolytic s.
    s. of Ostertag
streptolysin
    s. O
Streptomyces
    S. madurae
    S. pelletieri
    S. somaliensis
Streptothrix
stria (striae)
stroboscopic
    s. microscope
Strong bacillus
Strongyloides
    S. stercoralis
STS—serologic test for syphilis
STT—serial thrombin time
study
    cytogenetic s.
    cytological s.
    enzyme s.
    erythrokinetic s.
    fat absorption s.
SUA—serum uric acid
substance
    anterior pituitary-like s.
    white s. of Schwann
    zymoplastic s.
subtle
Sudan
    S. I
    S. II
    S. III
    S. IV
    S. black
    S. yellow G
"sudo–" Phonetic for words begin-
    ning pseudo–.
SUDS—sudden unexplained death
    syndrome

SUN—serum urea nitrogen
suppression
survival
    red blood cell s.
"sut-el" Phonetic for subtle.
syn–. See also words beginning
    cin–, sin–.
syncytial
    s. alteration
    s. trophoblast
syndrome
    See in medical specialty sec-
      tions.
synovial
    s. stromal cells
Syphacia
    S. obvelata
syphilis
    serologic test for s. (STS)
Système International d'Unités (SI)
T_3 [T3]—triiodothyronine [test]
T_4 [T4]—thyroxine [test]
tache ["tahsh"]
    t. blanche ["blahnsh"]
taenia (taeniae) [anatomy: flat band]
taenia (taeniae) [tapeworm]
Taenia
    T. africana
    T. bremneri
    T. confusa
    T. cucurbitina
    T. hydatigena
    T. mediocanellata
    T. multiceps
    T. philippina
    T. saginata
    T. solium
taeniacides [a class of drugs]
taenial
taeniasis
taeniform
TAT—thromboplastin activation test
TB—tuberculin
TBG—thyroxine-binding globulin
TBII—thyrotropin-binding inhibito-
    ry immunoglobulin
TBP—thyroxine-binding protein
TBT—tolbutamide test

TC—total cholesterol
T cell [noun]
T-cell [adj.]
    T-c. antibody labeling
    T-c. antigen
    T-c. lymphoma
    T-c. marker(s)
    T-c. proliferation
TCGF—T-cell growth factor
TcR—T-cell receptor
TDA—TSH-displacing antibody
TDE—tetrachlorodiphenylethane
    (pesticide)
TDI—toluene-diisocyanate
TeBG—testosterone-estradiol–bind-
    ing globulin
technique
    See also *method.*
    direct fluorescent antibody t.
    double antibody t.
    double-layer fluorescent
       antibody t.
    enzyme-multiplied immuno-
       assay t. (EMIT)
    Ficoll-Hypaque t.
    fluorescent antibody t.
    Southern blot t.
    Western blot t.
    zinc sulfate centrifugal flota-
       tion t.
TEM—transmission electron
    microscopy
teratoblastoma
teratologic, teratological
teratoma (teratomas, teratomata)
    adult t.
    anaplastic malignant t.
    benign cystic t.
    cystic t.
    differentiated t.
    immature t.
    malignant t.
    mature t.
    sacrococcygeal t.
    solid t.
    tropoblastic malignant t.
    undifferentiated malignant t.
teratomatous

teratospermia
test
    Abrams t.
    acetic acid t.
    acetic acid and potassium
       ferrocyanide t.
    acetoacetic acid t.
    acetone t.
    acidified serum t.
    acidity reduction t.
    acid-lability t.
    acidosis t.
    acid phosphatase t.
    ACTH t.
    Adamkiewicz t.
    Adler t.
    adolase t.
    adrenaline t.
    adrenocortical inhibition t.
    agglutination t.
    A/G ratio t.
    albumin t.
    aldosterone t.
    alizarin t.
    alkali t.
    alkali denaturation t.
    alkaline phosphatase t.
    alkali tolerance t.
    alkaloid t.
    alpha amino nitrogen t.
    alpha-fetoprotein (AFP) t.
    amylase t.
    antibody screening t.
    antiglobulin t. (AGT)
    anti-Rho-D titer t.
    antistreptolysin O (ASO) t.
    antithrombin t.
    Apt t.
    arginine t.
    arginine stimulation t.
    arginine tolerance t. (ATT)
    Argo corn starch t.
    arylsulfatase t.
    Aschheim-Zondek (AZ) t.
    ascorbate cyanide t.
    ascorbic acid t.
    ASO (antistreptolysin O) t.
    automated reagin t. (ART)

test (continued)

BEI (butanol extractable iodine) t.
Bence Jones protein t.
Benedict t.
bentonite flocculation t.
beta-hCG t.
BG (Bordet-Gengou) t.
bile acid t.
bile acid tolerance t.
bile pigment t.
bile solubility t.
bilirubin t., direct
bilirubin t., indirect
bilirubin tolerance t.
biuret t.
bleeding time t.
blood urea nitrogen (BUN) t.
Bloor t.
blot t.
Bloxam t.
Boas t.
Bonanno t.
Bordet-Gengou (BG) t.
breath analysis t.
bromosulfalein t.
bromsulfophthalein (BSP) t.
butanol extractable iodine (BIE) t.
calcium t.
Calmette t.
CAMP t.
capillary fragility t.
carbohydrate tolerance t.
carbon dioxide combining power t.
carbon monoxide t.
cardiolipin t.
Casoni intradermal t.
Castellani t.
catecholamine t.
CEA (carcinoembryonic antigen) t.
cephalin-cholesterol flocculation t.
cephalin flocculation t.
cetylpyridium chloride t.
Chediak t.

test (continued)

cholesterol t.
cholesterol-lecithin flocculation t.
cholinesterase t.
chromogenic cephalosporin t.
coagulation t.
cold agglutinin t.
colloidal gold t.
complement fixation (CF) t.
conglutinating complement absorption t. (CCAT)
Congo red t.
Coombs t., direct
Coombs t., indirect
coproporphyrin t.
cortisone-glucose tolerance t.
C-reactive protein t.
creatine t.
creatinine t.
creatinine clearance t.
cyanide-nitroprusside t.
cysteine t.
D-dimer t.
deoxyribonuclease (DNase) t.
dexamethasone suppression t.
dextrose t.
DFA (direct fluorescent antibody) t.
Diagnex blue t.
Dick t.
differential t. for infectious mononucleosis
dinitrophenylhydrazine t.
diphtheria t.
direct antiglobulin t.
direct Coombs t.
direct fluorescent antibody (DFA) t.
direct immunofluorescence t.
dithionite t.
DNase (deoxyribonuclease) t.
Donath-Landsteiner t.
Duke t.
Duke bleeding time t.
D-xylose absorption t.
D-xylose tolerance t.
edrophonium chloride t.

test (continued)

Ehrlich t.

electrophoresis t.

ELISA (enzyme-linked immunosorbent assay) t.

Ellsworth-Howard t.

Epstein-Barr nuclear antigen t. (EBNA)

erythrocyte adherence t.

erythrocyte fragility t.

erythrocyte protoporphyrin (EP) t.

estrogen receptor assay (ERA) t.

estrogen stimulation t.

estrogen suppression t.

FANA (fluorescent antinuclear antibody) t.

fecal fat t.

Fehling t.

ferric chloride t.

Feulgen t.

fibrinogen t.

FIGLU excretion t.

Fishberg concentration t.

Fisher exact t.

fixation t.

flocculation t.

fluorescent antibody t.

fluorescent treponemal antibody (FTA) t.

fluorescent treponemal antibody absorption (FTA-ABS) t.

formol-gel t.

fragility t.

free urinary cortisol t.

Frei t.

Friedman t.

frog t.

FTA (fluorescent treponemal antibody) t.

FTA-ABS (fluorescent treponemal antibody absorption) t.

galactose tolerance t.

β-galactosidase t. [beta-]

Gerhardt t.

test (continued)

globulin t.

glucagon t.

glucagon response t.

glucagon stimulation t.

glucose t.

glucose suppression t.

glucose tolerance t. (GTT)

glycogen storage t.

glycosylated hemoglobin t.

gonadotropin-releasing hormone stimulation t.

Gravindex t.

guaiac t.

Guthrie t.

Ham t.

Hanger t.

Harrison t.

hatching t.

hemadsorption t.

hemadsorption inhibition t.

hemagglutination t.

hemagglutination inhibition (HI, HAI) t.

heme t.

Hemoccult t.

hemosiderin t.

hepatic function t.

heterophil antibody t.

Hicks-Pitney thromboplastin generation t.

Hinton t.

hippuric acid t.

Histalog t.

histamine t.

histamine flare t.

histamine stimulation t.

histidine loading t.

HIVAGEN t.

Hogben t.

homogentisic acid t.

Howard t.

17-hydroxycorticosteroid t.

5-hydroxyindoleacetic acid t.

icterus index t.

immunofluorescence t.

indican t.

indigo-carmine t.

test (continued)

    indirect antiglobulin t.
    indirect Coombs t.
    indirect hemagglutination t.
    indirect immunofluorescence
        t.
    indocyanine green t.
    indole t.
    insulin clearance t.
    insulin-glucose tolerance t.
    insulin tolerance t.
    interference t.
    inulin clearance t.
    in vitro t.
    iodine t.
    iodine I 131 uptake t., radio-
        active iodine uptake t.
    iron-binding capacity t.
    isoiodeikon t.
    isopropanol precipitation t.
    Ivy bleeding time t.
    Jones-Cantarow t.
    Kahn t.
    Katayama t.
    17-ketogenic steroid t.
    ketone body t.
    17-ketosteroid t.
    kidney function t.
    Kolmer t.
    Kunkel t.
    Kveim t.
    lactate dehydrogenase t.
    lactic acid t.
    lactose tolerance t.
    Ladendorff t.
    Lancefield precipitation t.
    Lang t. (for taurine)
    Lange t. (for acetone in urine)
    Lange colloidal gold t.
    LAP (leucine aminopepti-
        dase) t.
    latex fixation t.
    latex particle agglutination t.
    latex slide agglutination t.
    LE (lupus erythematosus) t.
    LE (lupus erythematosus)
        cell t.

test (continued)

    leucine aminopeptidase
        (LAP) t.
    leucine tolerance t.
    leukocyte adherence inhibi-
        tion t.
    Levinson t.
    levulose tolerance t.
    limulus lysate t.
    lipase t.
    lipid t.
    liver function t. (LFT)
    lupus erythematosus (LE)
        cell t.
    lymphocyte transfer t.
    magnesium t.
    malaria film t.
    male frog t., male toad t.
    mallein t.
    Malmejde t.
    mast cell degranulation t.
    mastic t.
    melanin t.
    methylene blue t.
    Metopirone t.
    microhemagglutination t. for
        Treponema pallidum
        (MHA-TP)
    microimmunofluorescence t.
    microprecipitation t.
    Middlebrook-Dubos hemag-
        glutination t.
    MIF (migration inhibitory
        factor) t.
    monocyte function t.
    Monospot t.
    Mono-Vac t.
    Mosenthal t.
    Motulsky dye reduction t.
    mucoprotein t.
    Murphy-Pattee t.
    NBT (nitroblue tetrazolium) t.
    niacin t.
    nicotine t.
    Ninhydrin t.
    nitrate utilization t.
    nitric acid t.
    nitrites t.

test (continued)

nitroblue tetrazolium (NBT) t.
nitroprusside t.
nonprotein nitrogen t.
Obermayer t.
Obermüller t.
occult blood t.
one-stage prothrombin time t.
osazone t.
osmotic fragility t.
pancreatic function t.
pancreozymin-secretin t.
P and P (prothrombin and proconvertin) t.
Pandy t.
Papanicolaou (Pap) t.
partial thromboplastin time (PTT) t.
PAS (periodic acid–Schiff) t.
paternity t.
Paul-Bunnell t.
Paul-Bunnell-Barrett t.
periodic acid–Schiff (PAS) t.
Petri t.
pH t.
phenolphthalein t.
phenolsulfonphthalein t.
phenylketonuria t.
phosphatase t.
phospholipid t.
phosphoric acid t.
Piazza t.
pineapple t.
pine wood t.
plasma ACTH t.
plasma cortisol t.
plasma hemoglobin t.
platelet aggregation t.
Porges-Meier t.
Porges-Salomon t.
porphobilinogen t.
porphyrin t.
potassium t.
precipitation t.
precipitin t.
pregnancy t.
prolactin t.
protein t.

test (continued)

protein-bound iodine t.
prothrombin t. (PT)
prothrombin-proconvertin (P and P) t.
provocative t.
pulmonary function t. (PFT)
purine bodies t.
qualitative fecal fat t.
quantitation t.
Quick t. (for liver function)
Quick tourniquet t. (for prothrombin time)
radioactive fibrinogen uptake t.
radioactive iodine (RAI) t.
radioimmunosorbent t. (RIST)
radioisotope renal excretion t.
RA latex fixation t.
rapid plasma reagin (RPR) t.'s
rapid serum amylase t.
reactone red t.
renal function t. (RFT)
renin stimulation t.
renin suppression t.
resorcinol t.
rheumatoid factor (RF) t.
Rose t.
rose bengal t.
Rose-Waaler t.
Rothera t.
Rotozyme t.
Rotter t.
Rous t.
Rowntree and Geraghty t.
RPR (rapid plasma reagin) t.
Sabin-Feldman dye t.
salicylic acid t.
Schick t.
Schilling t.
Schultze t.
screen t.
secretin t.
sedimentation t.
serologic t.
serologic t. for syphilis (STS)
serology t.

test (continued)

serum alkaline phosphatase t.
serum bilirubin t.
serum calcium t.
serum creatine kinase (CK) t.
serum creatinine t.
serum enzyme t.
serum globulin t.
serum phosphorus t.
Sia t.
sickle cell t.
sickling t.
silver nitroprusside t.
Sims-Huhner t.
SISI (short increment sensitivity index) t.
slide agglutination t.
slide flocculation t.
short increment sensitivity index (SISI) t.
SMA profile t. (SMA-12, SMA-21, etc.)
smear t.
sodium t.
soy bean t. (for urease)
specific gravity t.
spectroscopic t.
split renal function t.
starch hydrolysis t.
stool guaiac t.
streptolysin O t.
streptozyme t.
Sulkowitch t.
susceptibility t.
sweat t.
syphilis t.
T_3 [T3] suppression t.
Takata-Ara t.
Tardieu t.
tetrazolium t.
Thayer-Martin t.
thiamine t.
Thorn t.
thromboplastin generation t. (TGT)
Thudichum t.
thymol turbidity t.
thyroid antibody t.

test (continued)

thyroid function t. (TFT)
thyroid suppression t.
thyrotropin-releasing hormone stimulation t.
thyroxine-binding index t.
toad t.
tolbutamide tolerance t.
TPHA (*Treponema pallidum* hemagglutination) t.
TPI (*Treponema pallidum* immobilization) t.
treponemal antibody t. (TAT)
treponemal hemagglutination (TPHA) t.
Treponema pallidum complement fixation t.'s
Treponema pallidum hemagglutination (TPHA) t.
Treponema pallidum immobilization (TPI) t.
T_3 [T3] resin uptake t.
T_4 [T4] RIA t.
triiodothyronine (T_3 [T3]) uptake t.
Trousseau t.
trypsin t.
t. tube
tubular reabsorption of phosphate t.
two-stage prothrombin t.
tyrosine t.
Tzanck t.
Uffelmann t.
unheated serum reagin (USR) t.
urea t.
urea clearance t.
urea concentration t.
urea nitrogen t.
urease t.
Urecholine supersensitivity t.
uric acid t.
urine acetone t.
urobilinogen t.
van den Bergh t.
vanillylmandelic acid (VMA) t.

test (continued)
    Van Slyke t.
    VDRL (Venereal Disease
        Research Laboratories) t.
        [abbreviation not expand-
        ed]
    VMA (vanillylmandelic
        acid) t.
    Voges-Proskauer t.
    Volhard t.
    Wassermann t.
    Watson-Schwartz t.
    Westergren sedimentation
        rate t.
    Western blot t.
    Western blot electrotransfer t.
    Widal serum t.
    wire loop t.
    Xenopus t., *Xenopus laevis* t.
    xylose concentration t.
    zinc flocculation t.
    zinc turbidity t.
testosterone
tetraploidy
TG—thyroglobulin
        triglyceride
"thaleen" Phonetic for phthalein.
Thayer-Martin culture medium
THC—tetrahydrocannabinol
theliolymphocyte
thick-layer autoradiography
thin-layer chromatography (TLC)
        instant t.l.c. (ITLC)
thioglycolate (THIO) broth
"thir-us" Phonetic for *Phthirus.*
Thomsen
        antibody
Thomsen-Friedenreich
        antigen
thread
        mucous t.'s
thrombi (plural of thrombus)
thrombinogen
thromboagglutinin
thrombocytapheresis
thrombocytopoietic
thromboplastinogen

thrombosis
    See in *Cardiology* section.
thrombostasis
thrombosthenin
thrombotest
thrombus (thrombi)
    See also in *Cardiology* sec-
        tion.
    postmortem t.
Thudichum
    test
thymidine
thyroid-stimulating hormone (TSH)
TIBC—total iron-binding capacity
tidal volume (TV)
time (T)
        activated coagulation t., acti-
            vated clotting t. (ACT)
        activated partial thrombo-
            plastin t. (APTT, aPTT)
        bleeding t.
        bleeding t., secondary
        clot retraction t.
        clotting t.
        coagulation t.
        doubling t.
        euglobulin clot lysis t.
        filter bleeding t.
        generation t.
        Ivy bleeding t.
        one-stage prothrombin t.
        partial thromboplastin t.
            (PTT)
        prothrombin t. (PT)
        recalcification t.
        reptilase t.
        Russell viper venom t.
        sedimentation t.
        serum prothrombin t.
        Stypven t.
        template bleeding t.
        thrombin t. (TT), thrombin
            clotting t.
        turn-around time (TAT)
titer
        agglutination t.
        antihyaluronidase t.
        anti-Rho-D t.

titer (continued)
    CF antibody t.
    toxoplasmosis, other agents,
      rubella, cytomegalovirus,
      herpes simplex (TORCH)
      t.
titration
TLC—thin-layer chromatography
    total lung capacity
TMAb—thyroid microsomal anti-
    body
TMIF—tumor-cell migration–inhi-
    bition factor
TNF—tumor necrosis factor
TNTC—too numerous to count
togavirus
toluidine
    t. blue O
TORCH—toxoplasmosis, other
    agents, rubella, cytomegalovi-
    rus, herpes simplex [syndrome]
TORCH
    titer
Torula
    T. capsulatus
    T. histolytica
Torulopsis
    T. glabrata
Touton giant cells
Toxocara
    T. canis
    T. cati
    T. mystax
Toxoplasma
    T. gondii
    T. pyrogenes
TP—total protein
TPA—*Treponema pallidum* aggluti-
    nation
TPC—thromboplastic plasma com-
    ponent
TPCF—*Treponema pallidum* com-
    plement fixation
TPHA— *Treponema pallidum*
    hemagglutination assay
TPI—*Treponema pallidum* immobi-
    lization
TPI cardiolipin test

transferase
transferrin
transition
transmission electron microscopy
    (TEM)
Trematoda
    T. clonorchis
    T. dicrocoelium
    T. echinostoma
    T. fasciola
    T. fasciolopsis
    T. gastrodiscoides
    T. heterophyes
    T. metagonimus
    T. opisthorchis
    T. paragonimus
    T. schistosoma
trematode
Treponema
    T. calligyrum
    T. carateum
    T. genitalis
    T. macrodentium
    T. microdentium
    T. mucosum
    T. pallidum
    T. pertenue
    T. pintae
TRF—thyrotropin-releasing factor
TRH—thyrotropin-releasing hormone
Trichinella
    T. spiralis
Trichomonas
    T. buccalis
    T. hominis
    T. intestinalis
    T. pulmonalis
    T. tenax
    T. pulmonalis
    T. urethritis
    T. vaginalis
Trichophyton
    T. concentricum
    T. epilans
    T. faviforme
    T. ferrugineum
    T. mentagrophytes
    T. rosaceum

Trichophyton (continued)
    T. rubrum
    T. sabouraudi
    T. schoenleini
    T. schoenleinii
    T. sulfureum
    T. tonsurans
    T. verrucosum
    T. violaceum
Trichoptera
Trichosporon
    T. beigelii
    T. cutaneum
    T. pedrosianum
Trichostrongylus
    T. axei
    T. brevis
    T. colubriformis
    T. instabilis
    T. orientalis
    T. vitrinus
Trichothecium
    T. roseum
Trichuris
    T. trichiura
triglycerides
trinocular microscope
Triodontophorus
    T. diminutus
Trombicula
    T. autumnalis
    T. irritans
    T. tsalsahuatl
    T. vandersandi
trophospongium (trophospongia)
T_3 RU (resin uptake)
Trypanosoma
    T. brucei
    T. cruzi
    T. escomeli
    T. gambiense
    T. rangeli
    T. rhodesiense
tryptase
TSA—tumor-specific antigen
T_4SA [T4SA]—thyroxine-specific
    activity
"tseng-ker" Phonetic for Zenker.

TSH—thyroid-stimulating hormone
TSH-RF—thyroid-stimulating hormone–releasing factor
TSP—total serum protein
TSPAP—total serum prostatic acid
    phosphatase
TSR—thyroid-to-serum ratio
T-strain mycoplasma
TT—thrombin time
    total thyroxine
TTH—thyrotropic hormone
TTT—tolbutamide tolerance test
tube
    capillary t.
    t. cell
    Craigies t.
    discharge t.
    Durham t.
    electron multiplier t.
    fermentation t.
    Mett (Mette) test t.
    photomultiplier t. (PMT)
    Roida t.
    roll t.
    sediment t.
    sedimentation t.
    sputum t.
    test t.
    vacuum t.
    Veillon t.
    Wintrobe t.
tuberculin
    Koch t.
    Old t. (OT)
    purified protein derivative
      (PPD) t.
    Seibert t.
tuberculoid
tuberculosis (TB)
tubocurarine
tubulovesicle
tubulovesicular
tularemia
tumefaction
Tunga
    T. penetrans
turbidimetric
turbidimetry

Türk
    cell
    irritaion leukocyte
TV—tidal volume
12/60 (short for SMA 12/60 or
    chemistry 12/60)
two-dimensional
    t.-d. chromatography
two-emulsion autoradiography
Twort-d'Herelle phenomenon
type
    blood t.'s
typhoid
typing
    ABO t.
    ABO-Rh t.
Tyroglyphus
    T. siro
Tzanck
    cell
    smear
    test
UA—uric acid
    urinalysis
UBBC—unsaturated vitamin B_{12}-
    binding capacity
UC—urea clearance
UCG—urinary chorionic gonado-
    tropin
UDCA—ursodeoxycholic acid
UDP—urine drug panel
UDS—urine drug screen
UIBC—unsaturated iron-binding
    capacity
ULN—upper limit of normal
ultramicroscope
ultrasonic
    u. microscope
ultraviolet
    u. microscope
UN—urea nitrogen
uncia (unciae)
unctuous
unit
    See also in *General Medical
      Terms.*
    Allen-Doisy u.
    amboceptor u.

unit (continued)
    antigen u.
    Bethesda u.
    Bodansky u.
    CH_{50} [CH50] u.
    colony-forming u. (CFU)
    colony-forming u.–culture
      (CFU-C)
    colony-forming u.–erythroid
      (CFU-E)
    colony-forming u.–granulo-
      cyte-macrophage (CFU-
      GM)
    colony-forming u.–spleen
      (CFU-S)
    complement u.
    enzyme u.
    flotation u.
    Gutman u.
    hemolytic u.
    hemorrhagin u.
    international u. (IU)
    international u. of enzyme
      activity
    Karmen u.
    King u., King-Armstrong u.
    minimal hemolytic u.
    mouse u.
    pepsin u.
    plaque-forming u.
    rat u.
    Russell u.
    Shinowara-Jones-Reinhard u.
    SI (Système International) u.
    Somogyi u.
    sudanophobic u.
    Svedberg u.
    Svedberg flotation u.
    u. of thyrotrophic activity
    Todd u.
    toxic u., toxin u.
    turbidity-reducing u. (TRU)
    Wohlgemuth u.
Unna
    cell
U/P—urine-plasma [ratio]
UPG—uroporphyrinogen

uptake
    RAI (radioactive iodine) u.
    resin u.
urea nitrogen (UN)
Ureaplasma
    U. urealyticum
urine
    u. drug panel (UDP)
    u. drug screen (UDS)
urine urea nitrogen (UUN)
USR—unheated serum reagin (test)
UTBG—unbound thyroxine–binding globulin
UUN—urine urea nitrogen
vacuole
    autophagic v.
    contractile v.
    plasmocrine v.
    rhagiocrine v.
vacuum
    v. tube
van den Bergh
    test
vaporization
vaporize
Vaquez disease
Vaquez-Osler disease
vasalium
Vater-Pacini corpuscles
VC—vital capacity
VEE—vagina ectocervix and endocervix
VEE smear
Veillon
    tube
Veillonella
    V. alcalescens
    V. discoides
    V. orbiculus
    V. parvula
    V. reniformis
    V. vulvovaginitidis
venipuncture
vermicular
vermiculous
vermiform
vermifugal

Verneuil
    canals
Verticillium
    V. graphii
vial
Vibrio
vibrio (vibrios, vibriones)
Vibrio
    V. alginolyticus
    V. bulbulus
vibrio (vibrios, vibriones)
    Celebes v.
Vibrio
    V. cholerae
    V. cholerae-asiaticae
vibrio (vibrios, vibriones)
    cholera v.
Vibrio
    V. coli
    V. comma
    V. danubicus
vibrio (vibrios, vibriones)
    El Tor v.
Vibrio
    V. faecalis
    V. fetus
    V. finkleri
    V. ghinda
    V. jejuni
    V. massauah
    V. metchnikovii
    V. niger
vibrio (vibrios, vibriones)
    nonagglutinating (NAG) v's
    paracholera v's
Vibrio
    V. parahaemolyticus
    V. phosphorescens
    V. proteus
    V. septicus
    V. tyrogenus
vibrion
    v. septique
Vicia
    V. graminea
Vignal cells
villoglandular

viral
   v. load
virus
   adeno-associated v. (AAV)
   animal v.'s
   v. animatum
   arbor v.'s (arbovirus)
   attenuated v.
   Australian X disease v.
   bacterial v.
   Brunhilde v.
   Bunyamwera v.
   Bwamba fever v.
   C v.
   CA v.
   Cache valley v.
   California v.
   California encephalitis v.
   California myxoma v.
   Chikungunya v.
   Coe v.
   Colorado tick fever (CTF) v.
   coryza v.
   Coxsackie v. [now: coxsack-
     ievirus]
   croup-associated v.
   CTF (Colorado tick fever) v.
   cytomegalic inclusion dis-
     ease v.
   dengue v.
   DNA v.'s
   eastern equine encephalo-
     myelitis v.
   EB (Epstein-Barr) v.
   Ebola v.
   ECHO 28 v.
   EEE (eastern equine enceph-
     alomyelitis) v.
   EMC (encephalomyocardi-
     tis) v.
   encephalomyocarditis
     (EMC) v.
   enteric cytopathogenic
     bovine orphan (ECBO) v.
     [now: ecbovirus]
   enteric cytopathogenic dog
     orphan (ECDO) v. [now:
     ecdovirus]

virus (continued)
   enteric cytopathogenic
     human orphan (ECHO) v.
     [now: echovirus]
   enteric cytopathogenic mon-
     key orphan (ECMO) v.
     [now: ecmovirus]
   enteric cytopathogenic
     swine orphan (ECSO) v.
     [now: ecsovirus]
   enteric orphan v's
   entomopox v.
   epidemic keratoconjunctivi-
     tis v.
   Epstein-Barr v., EB v. (EBV)
   equine encephalomyelitis v.
   filterable v.
   v. fixé, fixed v.
   Guaroa v.
   hemadsorption v. (type 1,
     type 2)
   hepatitis A v. (HAV)
   hepatitis B v. (HBV)
   hepatitis C v. (HCV)
   hepatitis delta v.
   hepatitis E v.
   hepatitis G v. (HGV)
   hepatitis GB v. (HGBV,
     HGBV-A, HGBV-B,
     HGBV-C)
   herpangina v.
   herpes v. [pref: herpesvirus]
   herpes simplex v. (HSV)
   human immunodeficiency v.
     (HIV)
   human papilloma v. (papil-
     lomavirus)
   human T-cell leukemia/lym-
     phoma v. (HTLV) [now:
     HIV]
   human T-cell lymphotrophic
     v., (HTLV) [now: HIV]
   Ilheus v.
   inclusion conjunctivitis v.
   influenza v.
   Japanese B encephalitis v.
   JH (Johns Hopkins) v.
   Junin v.

virus (continued)
   Kumba v.
   Kyasanur Forest disease v.
   Lansing v.
   Lassa v.
   latent v.
   LCM (lymphocytic chori-
      omeninigitis) v.
   Leon v.
   lepori pox v.
   louping ill v.
   Lunyo v.
   lymphadenopathy-associated
      v. (LAV)
   lymphocytic choriomeningi-
      tis v. (LCM)
   lymphogranuloma venereum
      v.
   masked v.
   Mayaro v.
   measles v.
   Mengo v.
   Murray Valley encephalitis v.
   neurotrophic v.
   v. neutralization test
   newborn pneumonitis v.
   Newcastle disease v.
   non-A, non B-hepatitis v.
   O'nyong-nyong v.
   ornithosis v.
   Oropouche v.
   orphan v's
   papilloma v.
   pappataci fever v.
   parainfluenza v.
   parapox v.
   parinfluenza v.
   pharyngoconjunctival fever v.
   pneumonitis v.
   poliomyelitis v.
   polyoma v.
   Powassan v.
   pox v. (poxvirus)
   psittacosis v.
   rabies v.
   respiratory syncytial v. (RSV)
   Rift Valley fever v.
   RNA v.'s

virus (continued)
   RS (respiratory syncytial) v.
   rubella v.
   Russian spring-summer
      encephalitis v.
   salivary gland v.
   Semliki Forest v.
   Sendai v.
   Simbu v.
   simian v. (SV)
   Sindbis v.
   St. Louis encephalitis v.
   street v.
   Teschen v.
   Theiler v.
   tick-borne v.'s
   trachoma v.
   2060 v.
   Uganda S v.
   unorganized v.
   Uruma v.
   vaccinia v.
   vacuolating v.
   varicella-zoster v.
   variola v.
   VEE (Venezuelan equine
      encephalomyelitis) v.
   WEE (western equine
      encephalomyelitis) v.
   Wesselsbron v.
   western equine encephalo-
      myelitis v.
   West Nile v.
viscidity
viscose [noun or adj.]
viscosimeter
   Stormer v.
viscosimetry
viscosity
   absolute v.
viscous [adj.]
VLDL, VLDLP—very low-density
   lipoprotein
VMA—vanillylmandelic acid
Voges-Proskauer
   broth
volatile
volatilization

volatilize
volatilizer
Volhard
    test
volume
    inspiratory reserve v. (IRV)
von Bezold. See *Bezold.*
von Gierke. See *Gierke.*
von Jaksch. See *Jaksch.*
von Leyden. See *Leyden.*
von Mikulicz. See *Mikulicz.*
von Monakow. See *Monakow.*
von Willebrand (Willebrand)
    factor
von Zenker. See *Zenker.*
VP—vasopressin
    venipuncture
VPC—volume of packed cells
VT—tidal volume
Walthard cell
Warthin-Finkeldey cell
washing
    bronchial w.'s
WBC—white blood cell
    white blood [cell] count
WBC/hpf—white blood cell(s) per
    high-power field
WCC—white cell count
WD—well-differentiated
Weeks bacillus
Welch bacillus
Westergren method
Western
    blot electrotransfer test
West Nile
    virus
wet mount
Whipple
    test
Whitmore
    bacillus
    disease
    fever

Whitmore (continued)
    melioidosis
Widal
    reaction
    serum test
    syndrome
    test
Willebrand. See *von Willebrand.*
Wintrobe
    tube
WNL—within normal limits
Wuchereria
    W. bancrofti
    W. malayi
xanthochromia
xanthochromic
Xanthomonas
    X. maltophilia
xanthurenic acid
Xenopsylla
    X. cheopis
Xenopus
    X. laevis
x-ray
    x-r. microscope
    projection x-r. microscope
Yersinia
    Y. enterocolitica
    Y. pestis
    Y. pseudotuberculosis
"zank" Phonetic for Tzanck.
Zeiss counting cell
Zenker
    fixative
    fluid
    solution
zenkerize
zone
    z. of antemortem wound
zoning
zoonotic
ZSR—zeta sedimentation rate

Reference Values for Hematology

Test	Conventional Units	SI Units
Acid hemolysis (Ham test)	No hemolysis	No hemolysis
Alkaline phosphatase, leukocyte	Total score 14–100	Total score 14–100
Cell counts		
Erythrocytes		
Males	4.6–6.2 million/mm³	$4.6–6.2 \times 10^{12}$/L
Females	4.2–5.4 million/mm³	$4.2–5.4 \times 10^{12}$/L
Children (varies with age)	4.5–5.1 million/mm³	$4.5–5.1 \times 10^{12}$/L
Leukocytes, total	4500–11,000/mm³	$4.5–11.0 \times 10^{9}$/L
Leukocytes, differential counts	(percentages)	(absolute counts)
Myelocytes	0%	0/L
Band neutrophils	3–5%	$150–400 \times 10^{6}$/L
Segmented neutrophils	54–62%	$3000–5800 \times 10^{9}$/L
Lymphocytes	25–33%	$1500–3000 \times 10^{9}$/L
Monocytes	3–7%	$300–500 \times 10^{6}$/L
Eosinophils	1–3%	$50–250 \times 10^{6}$/L
Basophils	0–1%	$15–50 \times 10^{6}$/L
Platelets	150,000–400,300/mm³	$150–400 \times 10^{9}$/L
Reticulocytes	25,000–75,000/mm³	$25–75 \times 10^{9}$/L
	(0.5–1.5% of erythrocytes)	
Coagulation tests		
Bleeding time (template)	2.75–8.0 min	2.75–8.0 min
Coagulation time (glass tube)	5–15 min	5–15 min
D-dimer	<0.5 µg/mL	<0.5 mg/L
Factor VIII and other coagulation factors	50–150% of normal	0.5–1.5 of normal
Fibrin split products (Thrombo-Wellco test)	<10 µg/mL	<10 mg/L
Fibrinogen	200–400 mg/dL	2.0–4.0 g/L
Partial thromboplastin time, activated (aPTT)	20–35 s	20–35 s
Prothrombin time (PT)	12.0–14.0 s	12.0–14.0 s

285

Reference Values for Hematology (continued)

Test	Conventional Units	SI Units
Coombs test		
Direct	Negative	Negative
Indirect	Negative	Negative
Corpuscular values of erythrocytes		
Mean corpuscular hemoglobin (MCH)	26–34 pg/cell	26–34 pg/cell
Mean corpuscular volume (MCV)	80–96 μm^3	80–96 fL
Mean corpuscular hemoglobin concentration (MCHC)	32–36 g/dL	320–360 g/L
Haptoglobin	20–165 mg/dL	0.20–1.65 g/L
Hematocrit		
Males	40–54 mL/dL	0.40–0.54
Females	37–47 mL/dL	0.37–0.47
Newborns	49–54 mL/dL	0.49–0.54
Children (varies with age)	35–49 mL/dL	0.35–0.49
Hemoglobin		
Males	13.0–18.0 g/dL	8.1–11.2 mmol/L
Females	12.0–16.0 g/dL	7.4–9.9 mmol/L
Newborns	16.5–19.5 g/dL	10.2–12.1 mmol/L
Children (varies with age)	11.2–16.5 g/dL	7.0–10.2 mmol/L
Hemoglobin, fetal	<1.0% of total	<0.01 of total
Hemoglobin A_{1c}	3–5% of total	0.03–0.05 of total
Hemoglobin A_2	1.5–3.0% of total	0.015–0.03 of total
Hemoglobin, plasma	0.0–5.0 mg/dL	0.0–3.2 $\mu mol/L$
Methemoglobin	30–130 mg/dL	19–80 $\mu mol/L$
Sedimentation rate (ESR)		
Wintrobe: Males	0–5 mm/h	0–5 mm/h
Females	0–15 mm/h	0–15 mm/h
Westergren: Males	0–15 mm/h	0–15 mm/h
Females	0–20 mm/h	0–20 mm/h

Reference Values* for Blood, Serum, and Plasma

Analyte	Conventional Units	SI Units
Acetoacetate plus acetone		
Qualitative	Negative	Negative
Quantitative	0.3–2.0 mg/dL	30–200 µmol/L
Acid phosphatase, serum (thymolphthalein monophosphate substrate)	0.1–0.6 U/L	0.1–0.6 U/L
ACTH (see Corticotropin)		
Alanine aminotransferase (ALT) serum (SGPT)	1–45 U/L	1–45 U/L
Albumin, serum	3.3–5.2 g/dL	33–52 g/L
Aldolase, serum	0.0–7.0 U/L	0.0–7.0 U/L
Aldosterone, plasma		
Standing	5–30 ng/dL	140–830 pmol/L
Recumbent	3–10 ng/dL	80–275 pmol/L
Alkaline phosphatase (ALP), serum		
Adult	35–150 U/L	35–150 U/L
Adolescent	100–500 U/L	100–500 U/L
Child	100–350 U/L	100–350 U/L
Ammonia nitrogen, plasma	10–50 µmol/L	10–50 µmol/L
Amylase, serum	25–125 U/L	25–125 U/L
Anion gap, serum, calculated	8–16 mEq/L	8–16 mmol/L
Ascorbic acid, blood	0.4–1.5 mg/dL	23–85 µmol/L
Aspartate aminotransferase (AST) serum (SGOT)	1–36 U/L	1–36 U/L
Base excess, arterial blood, calculated	0 ± 2 mEq/L	0 ± 2 mmol/L
Bicarbonate		
Venous plasma	23–29 mEq/L	23–29 mmol/L
Arterial blood	21–27 mEq/L	21–27 mmol/L
Bile acids, serum	0.3–3.0 mg/dL	0.8–7.6 µmol/L
Bilirubin, serum		
Conjugated	0.1–0.4 mg/dL	1.7–6.8 µmol/L
Total	0.3–1.1 mg/dL	5.1–19.0 µmol/L

287

Reference Values* for Blood, Serum, and Plasma (continued)

Analyte	Conventional Units	SI Units
Calcium, serum	8.4–10.6 mg/dL	2.10–2.65 mmol/L
Calcium, ionized, serum	4.25–5.25 mg/dL	1.05–1.30 mmol/L
Carbon dioxide, total, serum or plasma	24–31 mEq/L	24–31 mmol/L
Carbon dioxide tension (Pco_2), blood	35–45 mm Hg	35–45 mm Hg
β-carotene, serum	60–260 μg/dL	1.1–8.6 μmol/L
Ceruloplasmin, serum	23–44 mg/dL	230–440 mg/L
Chloride, serum or plasma	96–106 mEq/L	96–106 mmol/L
Cholesterol, serum or ethylenediaminetetraacetic acid (EDTA) plasma		
Desirable range	<200 mg/dL	<5.20 mmol/L
Low-density lipoprotein (LDL) cholesterol	60–180 mg/dL	1.55–4.65 mmol/L
High-density lipoprotein (HDL) cholesterol	30–80 mg/dL	0.80–2.05 mmol/L
Copper	70–140 μg/dL	11–22 μmol/L
Corticotropin (ACTH), plasma, 8 AM	10–80 pg/mL	2–18 pmol/L
Cortisol, plasma		
8 AM	6–23 μg/dL	170–630 nmol/L
4 PM	3–15 μg/dL	80–410 nmol/L
10 PM	<50% of 8 AM value	<50% of 8 AM value
Creatine, serum		
Males	0.2–0.5 mg/dL	15–40 μmol/L
Females	0.3–0.9 mg/dL	25–70 μmol/L
Creatine kinase (CK), serum		
Males	55–170 U/L	55–170 U/L
Females	30–135 U/L	30–135 U/L
Creatine kinase MB isoenzyme, serum	<5% of total CK activity	<5% of total CK activity
	<5.0 ng/mL by immunoassay	<5.0 ng/mL by immunoassay
Creatinine, serum	0.6–1.2 mg/dL	50–110 μmol/L
Estradiol-17β, adult		
Males	10–65 pg/mL	35–240 pmol/L

Reference Values* for Blood, Serum, and Plasma (continued)

Analyte	Conventional Units	SI Units
Estradiol-17β, adult (continued)		
Females		
Follicular	30–100 pg/mL	110–370 pmol/L
Ovulatory	200–400 pg/mL	730–1470 pmol/L
Luteal	50–140 pg/rL	180–510 pmol/L
Ferritin, serum	20–200 ng/mL	20–200 μg/L
Fibrinogen, plasma	200–400 mgdL	2.0–4.0 g/L
Folate, serum	3–18 ng/mL	6.8–41 nmol/L
Erythrocytes	145–540 ng/mL	330–1220 nmol/L
Follicle-stimulating hormone (FSH), plasma		
Males	4–25 mU/mL	4–25 U/L
Females, premenopausal	4–30 mU/mL	4–30 U/L
Females, postmenopausal	40–250 mU/mL	40–250 U/L
Gamma-glutamyltransferase (GGT), serum	5–40 U/L	5–40 U/L
Gastrin, fasting, serum	0–100 pg/mL	0–100 mg/L
Glucose, fasting, plasma or serum	70–115 mg/dL	3.9–6.4 nmol/L
Growth hormone (hGH), plasma, adult, fasting	0–6 ng/mL	0–6 μg/L
Haptoglobin, serum	20–165 mg/dL	0.20–1.65 gm/L
Immunoglobulins, serum		
(see the *Reference Values for Immune Function* table)		
Iron, serum	75–175 μg/dL	13–31 μmol/L
Iron binding capacity, serum		
Total	250–410 μg/dL	45–73 μmol/L
Saturation	20–55%	0.20–0.55
Lactate		
Venous whole blood	5.0–20.0 mg/dL	0.6–2.2 mmol/L
Arterial whole blood	5.0–15.0 mg/dL	0.6–1.7 mmol/L
Lactate dehydrogenase (LD), serum	110–220 U/L	110–220 U/L

289

Reference Values* for Blood, Serum, and Plasma (continued)

Analyte	Conventional Units	SI Units
Lipase, serum	10–140 U/L	10–140 U/L
Lutropin (LH), serum		
Males	1–9 U/L	1–9 U/L
Females		
Follicular phase	2–10 U/L	2–10 U/L
Midcycle peak	15–65 U/L	15–65 U/L
Luteal phase	1–12 U/L	1–12 U/L
Postmenopausal	12–65 U/L	12–65 U/L
Magnesium, serum	1.3–2.1 mg/dL	0.65–1.05 mmol/L
Osmolality	275–295 mOsm/kg water	275–295 mOsm/kg water
Oxygen, blood, arterial, room air		
Partial pressure (Pao_2)	80–100 mm Hg	80–100 mm Hg
Saturation (Sao_2)	95–98%	95–98%
pH, arterial blood	7.35–7.45	7.35–7.45
Phosphate, inorganic, serum		
Adult	3.0–4.5 mg/dL	1.0–1.5 mmol/L
Child	4.0–7.0 mg/dL	1.3–2.3 mmol/L
Potassium		
Serum	3.5–5.0 mEq/L	3.5–5.0 mmol/L
Plasma	3.5–4.5 mEq/L	3.5–4.5 mmol/L
Progesterone, serum, adult		
Males	0.0–0.4 ng/mL	0.0–1.3 nmol/L
Females		
Follicular phase	0.1–1.5 ng/mL	0.3–4.8 nmol/L
Luteal phase	2.5–28.0 ng/mL	8.0–89.0 nmol/L
Prolactin, serum		
Males	1.0–15.0 ng/mL	1.0–15.0 µg/L
Females	1.0–20.0 ng/mL	1.0–20.0 µg/L

290

Reference Values* for Blood, Serum, and Plasma (continued)

Analyte	Conventional Units	SI Units
Protein, serum, electrophoresis		
Total	6.0–8.0 g/dL	60–80 g/L
Albumin	3.5–5.5 g/dL	35–55 g/L
Globulins		
Alpha$_1$	0.2–0.4 g/dL	2.0–4.0 g/L
Alpha$_2$	0.5–0.9 g/dL	5.0–9.0 g/L
Beta	0.6–1.1 g/dL	6.0–11.0 g/L
Gamma	0.7–1.7 g/dL	7.0–17.0 g/L
Pyruvate, blood	0.3–0.9 mg/dL	0.03–0.10 mmol/L
Rheumatoid factor	0.0–30.0 IU/mL	0.0–30.0 kIU/L
Sodium, serum or plasma	135–145 mEq/L	135–145 mmol/L
Testosterone, plasma		
Males, adult	300–1200 ng/dL	10.4–41.6 nmol/L
Females, adult	20–75 ng/dL	0.7–2.6 nmol/L
Pregnant females	40–200 ng/dL	1.4–6.9 nmol/L
Thyroglobulin	3–42 ng/mL	3–42 µg/L
Thyrotropin (hTSH), serum	0.4–4.8 µIU/mL	0.4–4.8 mIU/L
Thyrotropin-releasing hormone (TRH)	5–60 pg/mL	5–60 ng/L
Thyroxine (FT$_4$), free, serum	0.9–2.1 ng/dL	12–27 pmol/L
Thyroxine (T$_4$), serum	4.5–12.0 µg/dL	58–154 nmol/L
Thyroxine-binding globulin (TBG)	15.0–34.0 µg/mL	15.0–34.0 mg/L
Transferrin	250–430 mg/dL	2.5–4.3 g/L
Triglycerides, serum, 12-h fast	40–150 mg/dL	0.4–1.5 g/L
Triiodothyronine (T$_3$), serum	70–190 ng/dL	1.1–2.9 nmol/L
Triiodothyronine uptake, resin (T$_3$RU)	25–38%	0.25–0.38
Urate		
Males	2.5–8.0 mg/dL	150–480 µmol/L
Females	2.2–7.0 mg/dL	130–420 µmol/L

291

Reference Values* for Blood, Serum, and Plasma (continued)

Analyte	Conventional Units	SI Units
Urea, serum or plasma	24–49 mg/dL	4.0–8.2 nmol/L
Urea nitrogen, serum or plasma	11–23 mg/dL	8.0–16.4 nmol/L
Viscosity, serum	1.4–1.8 × water	1.4–1.8 × water
Vitamin A, serum	20–80 µg/dL	0.70–2.80 µmol/L
Vitamin B_{12}, serum	180–900 pg/mL	133–664 pmol/L

*Reference values may vary, depending on the method and sample source used.

Reference Values for Lymphocyte Subsets in Heparinized Whole Blood

Antigen(s) Expressed	Cell Type	Percentage	Absolute Cell Count
CD3	Total T cells	56–77%	860–1880
CD19	Total B cells	7–17%	140–370
CD3 and CD4	Helper-induced cells	32–54%	550–1190
CD3 and CD8	Suppressor-cytotoxic cells	24–37%	430–1060
CD3 and DR	Activated T cells	5–14%	70–310
CD2	E rosette T cells	73–87%	1040–2160
CD16 and CD56	Natural killer (NK) cells	8–22%	130–500
Helper/suppressor ratio: 0.8–1.8			

292

Reference Values* for Urine

Analyte	Conventional Units	SI Units
Acetone and acetoacetate, qualitative	Negative	Negative
Albumin		
Qualitative	Negative	Negative
Quantitative	10–100 mg/24 h	0.15–1.5 μmol/d
Aldosterone	3–20 μg/24 h	8.3–55 nmol/d
δ-Aminolevulinic acid (δ-ALA)	1.3–7.0 mg/24 h	10–53 μmol/d
Amylase	<17 U/h	<17 U/h
Amylase/creatinine clearance ratio	0.01–0.04	0.01–0.04
Bilirubin, qualitative	Negative	Negative
Calcium (regular diet)	<250 mg/24 h	<6.3 nmol/d
Catecholamines		
Epinephrine	<10 μg/24 h	<55 nmol/d
Norepinephrine	<100 μg/24 h	<590 nmol/d
Total free catecholamines	4–126 μg/24 h	24–745 nmol/d
Total metanephrines	0.1–1.6 mg/24 h	0.5–8.1 μmol/d
Chloride (varies with intake)	110–250 mEq/24 h	110–250 mmol/d
Copper	0–50 μg/24 h	0.0–0.80 μmol/d
Cortisol, free	10–100 μg/24 h	27.6–276 nmol/d
Creatine		
Males	0–40 mg/24 h	0.0–0.30 mmol/d
Females	0–80 mg/24 h	0.0–0.60 mmol/d
Creatinine	15–25 mg/kg/24 h	0.13–0.22 mmol/kg/d
Creatinine clearance (endogenous)		
Males	110–150 mL/min/1.73 m^2	110–150 mL/min/1.73 m^2
Females	105–132 mL/min/1.73 m^2	105–132 mL/min/1.73 m^2
Cystine or cysteine	Negative	Negative
Dehydroepiandrosterone (DHEA)		
Males	0.2–2.0 mg/24 h	0.7–6.9 μmol/d
Females	0.2–1.8 mg/24 h	0.7–6.2 μmol/d

Reference Values* for Urine (continued)

Analyte	Conventional Units	SI Units
Estrogens, total		
Males	4–25 µg/24 h	14–90 nmol/d
Females	5–100 µg/24 h	18–360 nmol/d
Glucose (as reducing substance)	<250 mg/24 h	<250 mg/d
Hemoglobin and myoglobin, qualitative	Negative	Negative
Homogentisic acid, qualitative	Negative	Negative
17-Ketogenic steroids		
Males	5–23 mg/24 h	17–80 µmol/d
Females	3–15 mg/24 h	10–52 µmol/d
17-Hydroxycorticosteroids		
Males	3–9 mg/24 h	8.3–25 µmol/d
Females	2–8 mg/24 h	5.5–22 µmol/d
5-Hydroxyindoleacetic acid		
Qualitative	Negative	Negative
Quantitative	2–6 mg/24 h	10–31 µmol/d
17-Ketosteroids		
Males	8–22 mg/24 h	28–76 µmol/d
Females	6–15 mg/24 h	21–52 µmol/d
Magnesium	6–10 mEq/24 h	3–5 mmol/d
Metanephrines	0.05–1.2 ng/mg creatinine	0.03–0.70 mmol/mmol creatinine
Osmolality	38–1400 mOsm/kg water	38–1400 mOsm/kg water
pH	4.6–8.0	4.6–8.0
Phenylpyruvic acid, qualitative	Negative	Negative
Phosphate	0.4–1.3 g/24 h	13–42 mmol/d
Porphobilinogen		
Qualitative	Negative	Negative
Quantitative	<2 mg/24 h	<9 µmol/d

Reference Values* for Urine (continued)

Analyte	Conventional Units	SI Units
Porphyrins		
Coproporphyrin	50–250 μg/24 h	77–380 nmol/d
Uroporphyrin	10–30 μg/24 h	12–36 nmol/d
Potassium	25–125 mEq/24 h	25–125 mmol/d
Pregnanediol		
Males	0.0–1.9 mg/24 h	0.0–6.0 μmol/d
Females		
Proliferative phase	0.0–2.6 mg/24 h	0.0–8.0 μmol/d
Luteal phase	2.6–10.6 mg/24 h	8–33 μmol/d
Postmenopausal	0.2–1.0 mg/24 h	0.6–3.1 μmol/d
Pregnanetriol	0.0–2.5 mg/24 h	0.0–7.4 μmol/d
Protein, total		
Qualitative	Negative	Negative
Quantitative	10–150 mg/24 h	10–150 mg/d
Protein/creatinine ratio	<0.2	<0.2
Sodium (regular diet)	60–260 mEq/24 h	60–260 mmol/d
Specific gravity		
Random specimen	1.003–1.030	1.003–1.030
24-hour collection	1.015–1.025	1.015–1.025
Urate (regular diet)	250–750 mg/24 h	1.5–4.4 mmol/d
Urobilinogen	0.5–4.0 mg/24 h	0.6–6.8 μmol/d
Vanillylmandelic acid (VMA)	1.0–8.0 mg/24 h	5–40 μmol/d

*Values may vary depending on the method used.

Reference Values for Serum Levels of Therapeutic Drugs

Analyte	Therapeutic Range	Toxic Concentrations	Brand Name(s)
Analgesics			
Acetaminophen	10–20 µg/mL	>250 µg/mL	Tylenol, Datril
Salicylates (including aspirin)	100–250 µg/mL	>300 µg/mL	Anacin, Bufferin
Antibiotics			
Amikacin	25–30 µg/mL	Peak >35 µg/mL	Amikin
		Trough >10 µg/mL	
Gentamicin	5–10 µg/mL	Peak >10 µg/mL	Garamycin
		Trough >2 µg/mL	
Tobramycin	5–10 µg/mL	Peak >10 µg/mL	Nebcin
		Trough >2 µg/mL	
Vancomycin	5–35 µg/mL	Peak >40 µg/mL	Vancocin
		Trough >10 µg/mL	
Anticonvulsants			
Carbamazepine	5–12 µg/mL	>15 µg/mL	Tegretol
Ethosuximide	40–100 µg/mL	>150 µg/mL	Zarontin
Phenobarbital	15–40 µg/mL	40–100 ng/mL (varies widely)	Luminal
Phenytoin	10–20 µg/mL	>20 µg/mL	Dilantin
Primidone	5–12 µg/mL	>15 µg/mL	Mysoline
Valproic acid	50–100 µg/mL	>100 µg/mL	Depakene
Antineoplastics and Immunosuppressives			
Cyclosporine	50–400 ng/mL	>400 ng/mL	Sandimmune
Methotrexate, high dose, 48-h	Variable	>1 µmol/L 48 h after dose	
Tacrolimus, whole blood	3–10 µg/L	>15 µg/L	Prograf
Bronchodilators and Respiratory Stimulants			
Caffeine	3–15 ng/mL	>30 ng/mL	NoDoz
Theophylline (aminophylline)	10–20 µg/mL	>20 µg/mL	Elixophyllin, Quibron

Reference Values for Serum Levels of Therapeutic Drugs (continued)

Analyte	Therapeutic Range	Toxic Concentrations	Brand Name(s)
Cardiovascular Drugs			
Amiodarone	1.0–2.0 µg/mL	>2.0 µg/mL	Cordarone
(obtain specimen more than 8 h after last dose)			
Digitoxin	15–25 ng/mL	>35 ng/mL	Crystodigin
(obtain specimen 12–24 h after last dose)			
Digoxin	0.8–2.0 ng/mL	>2.4 ng/mL	Lanoxin
(obtain specimen more than 6 h after last dose)			
Disopyramide	2–5 µg/mL	>7 µg/mL	Norpace
Flecainide	0.2–1.0 ng/mL	>1 ng/mL	Tambocor
Lidocaine	1.5–5.0 µg/mL	>6 µg/mL	Xylocaine
Mexiletine	0.7–2.0 ng/mL	>2 ng/mL	Mexitil
Procainamide	4–10 µg/mL	>12 µg/mL	Pronestyl
Procainamide plus N-acetyl-p-aminophenol (NAPA)	8–30 µg/mL	>30 µg/mL	
Propranolol	50–100 ng/mL	Variable	Inderal
Quinidine	2–5 µg/mL	>6 µg/mL	Cardioquin, Quinaglute
Tocainide	4–10 ng/mL	>10 ng/mL	Tonocard
Psychopharmacologic Drugs			
Amitriptyline	120–150 ng/mL	>500 ng/mL	Elavil, Triavil
Bupropion	25–100 ng/mL	Not applicable	Wellbutrin
Desipramine	150–300 ng/mL	>500 ng/mL	Norpramin
Imipramine	125–250 ng/mL	>400 ng/mL	Tofranil
Lithium	0.6–1.5 mEq/L	>1.5 mEq/L	Lithobid
(obtain specimen 12 h after last dose)			
Nortriptyline	50–150 ng/mL	>500 ng/mL	Aventyl, Pamelor

Reference Values for Toxic Substances

Analyte	Conventional Units	SI Units
Arsenic, urine	<130 µg/24 h	<1.7 µmol/d
Bromides, serum, inorganic	<100 mg/dL	<10 mmol/L
Toxic symptoms	140–1000 mg/dL	14–100 mmol/L
Carboxyhemoglobin, blood:	Saturation	
Urban environment	<5%	<0.05
Smokers	<12%	<0.12
Symptoms		
Headache	>15%	>0.15
Nausea and vomiting	>25%	>0.25
Potentially lethal	>50%	>0.50
Ethanol, blood	<0.05 mg/dL	<1.0 mmol/L
	<0.005%	
	>100 mg/dL	>22 mmol/L
Intoxication	>0.1%	
Marked intoxication	300–400 mg/dL	65–87 mmol/L
	0.3–0.4%	
Alcoholic stupor	400–500 mg/dL	87–109 mmol/L
	0.4–0.5%	
Coma	>500 mg/dL	>109 mmol/L
	>0.5%	
Lead, blood		
Adults	<25 µg/dL	<1.2 µmol/L
Children	<15 µg/dL	<0.7 µmol/L
Lead, urine	<80 µg/24 h	<0.4 µmol/d
Mercury, urine	<30 µg/24 h	<150 nmol/d

Reference Values for Cerebrospinal Fluid (CSF)

Test	Conventional Units	SI Units
Cells	<5/mm³, all mononuclear	<5 × 10⁶/L, all mononuclear
Protein electrophoresis	Albumin predominant	Albumin predominant
Glucose	50–75 mg/dL (20 mg/dL less than in serum)	2.8–4.2 mmol/L (1.1 mmol less than in serum)
IgG		
Children under 14	<8% of total protein	<0.08 of total protein
Adults	<14% of total protein	<0.14 of total protein
IgG index $\left(\dfrac{\text{CSF/serum IgG ratio}}{\text{CSF/serum albumin ratio}} \right)$	0.3–0.6	0.3–0.6
Oligoclonal banding on electrophoresis	Absent	Absent
Pressure, opening	70–180 mm H₂O	70–180 mm H₂O
Protein, total	15–45 mg/dL	150–450 mg/L

Reference Values for Semen

Test	Conventional Units	SI Units
Volume	2–5 mL	2–5 mL
Liquefaction	Complete in 15 min	Complete in 15 min
pH	7.2–8.0	7.2–8.0
Leukocytes	Occasional or absent	Occasional or absent
Spermatozoa		
Count	60–150 × 10⁶/mL	60–150 × 10⁶/mL
Motility	>80% motile	>0.80 motile
Morphology	80–90% normal forms	>0.80–0.90 normal forms
Fructose	>150 mg/dL	>8.33 mmol/L

Reference Values for Gastrointestinal Function

Test	Conventional Units
Bentiromide test	6-h urinary arylamine excretion >57% excludes pancreatic insufficiency
β-Carotene, serum	60–260 ng/dL
Fecal fat estimation	
Qualitative	No fat globules seen by high-power microscope
Quantitative	<6 g/24 h (>95% coefficient of fat absorption)
Gastric acid output	
Basal	
Males	0.0–10.5 mmol/h
Females	0.0–5.6 mmol/h
Maximum (after histamine or pentagastrin)	
Males	9.0–48.0 mmol/h
Females	6.0–31.0 mmol/h
Ratio: basal maximum	
Males	0.0–0.31
Females	0.0–0.29
Secretin test, pancreatic fluid	
Volume	>1.8 mL/kg/h
Bicarbonate	>80 mEq/L
D-xylose absorption test, urine	>20% of ingested dose excreted in 5 h

Reference Values for Immune Function

Test	Conventional Units	SI Units
Complement, Serum		
C3	85–175 mg/dL	0.85–1.75 gm/L
C4	15–45 mg/dL	150–450 mg/L
Total hemolytic (CH$_{50}$)	150–250 U/mL	150–250 U/mL
Immunoglobulins, Serum, Adult		
IgG	640–1350 mg/dL	6.4–13.5 g/L
IgA	70–310 mg/dL	0.70–3.1 g/L
IgM	90–350 mg/dL	0.90–3.5 g/L
IgD	0.0–6.0 mg/dL	0.0–60 mg/L
IgE	0.0–430 ng/dL	0.0–430 µg/L

Source:

All tables are from William Z. Borer, Reference Values for the Interpretation of Laboratory Tests. *In* Robert E. Rakel (ed.): Conn's Current Therapy 2000. Philadelphia, W.B. Saunders Company, 2000.

Sloane's
Medical
Word
Book

Part Two

Specialties

Cardiology

a—[as a subscript] symbol for arterial blood
A—[as a subscript] symbol for alveolar gas
A_2 [A2]—aortic second sound
AA—ascending aorta
A-a, $(A-a)O_2$, $P(A-a)O_2$—alveolar-arterial [oxygen gradient]
AAA—abdominal aortic aneurysm
AAI—arm-ankle index
AAS—aortic arch syndrome
AB—apex beat
A/B—apnea-bradycardia
A&B—apnea and bradycardia
ABC—airway-breathing-circulation [protocol]
    apnea, bradycardia, cyanosis
abdominal
    a. aortography
abdominocardiac reflex
abdominothoracic
    a. arch
ABE—acute bacterial endocarditis
Abée
    support
aberrancy
aberrant
    a. conduction
ABF—aortobifemoral [bypass]
ABG, ABGs—arterial blood gas(es)
ABI—ankle-brachial index
ablation
abluminal
abouchement
ABP—arterial blood pressure
Abrams
    heart reflex
abscess
    atheromatous a.
    embolic a.
    lung a.

abscess (continued)
    mediastinal a.
    metastatic a.
    myocardial a.
    pulmonary a.
    subpectoral a.
    subscapular a.
    thymic a.
ACA—anterior cerebral artery
ACBG—aortocoronary bypass graft
ACBGS—aortocoronary bypass graft surgery
ACBS—aortocoronary bypass surgery
ACC—American College of Cardiology
    anodal closure contraction
accelerated idioventricular rhythm
accentuation
    presystolic a.
access
    arteriovenous a.
    hemodialysis vascular a.
    vascular a.
    venovenous a.
accident
    cardiovascular a.
    cerebrovascular a. (CVA)
accretio
    a. cordis
    a. pericardii
ACD—absolute cardiac dullness
    anterior chest discomfort
ACE—angiotensin-converting enzyme
ACEIs—ACE inhibitors [a class of drugs]
ACG—angiocardiogram
    angiocardiography
    apexcardiogram

acid
    folic a.
acidosis
    lactic a.
acidotic
ACLS—advanced cardiac life support
acromicria
acrotic
acrotism
ACS—American College of Surgeons
    anodal closing sound
activated partial thromboplastin
    time (APTT, aPTT)
activator
    plasminogen a.
    single-chain urokinase-type
        plasminogen (scu-PA) a.
        (prourokinase)
    tissue plasminogen a. (t-PA,
        tPA, TPA)
    urinary plasminogen a., u-
        plasminogen a. (urokinase)
activity
    a.'s of daily living (ADL,
        ADLs)
    plasma renin a.
actodigin
ACVD—acute cardiovascular disease
    arteriosclerotic cardiovascular disease
    autoimmune collagen vascular disease
acyl coenzyme A
ADA—anterior descending artery
Adamkiewicz
    artery
Adams
    disease
Adams-Stokes
    disease
    syncope
    syndrome
ADC—anodal duration contraction
Addison
    disease
    planes
    point

addisonian
    a. syndrome
addisonism
ADG—atrial diastolic gallop
ADH—antidiuretic hormone
adiemorrhysis
adipositas
    a. cordis
ADL, ADLs—activities of daily living
adrenal
    a. adenoma
    a. cortex
    a. gland
    a. hyperplasia
    a. medulla
adrenaline
adrenergic
    a. agonists [a class of drugs]
    a. antagonist
    a. nervous system
    a. stimulant
adventitious
    a. sounds
Ae-H interval
aeremia
aerobic capacity
aeroembolism
AF—atrial fibrillation
Af—atrial flutter
AFBG—aortofemoral bypass graft
A-flutter [slang for atrial flutter]
AFP—atrial filling pressure
afterdepolarization
    delayed a. (DAD)
    early a. (EAD)
    late a.
afterload
    a. matching
    a. mismatching
    a.-reducing agent
    a. reduction
    ventricular a.
agent
    adrenergic blocking a.
agger
    a. valvae venae
β_2 agonist

agonist
> beta-2 a.
> cholinergic a.'s [a class of drugs]
> vascular serotonin 5-HT$_1$ [5-HT1] receptor a.'s [a class of drugs]

agonistic

AHA—American Heart Association

"ah-boosh-maw" Phonetic for abouchement.

AHD—arteriosclerotic heart disease
> atherosclerotic heart disease

air-cuff plethysmography

akinesis

Albini nodules

aldosteronoma

aldosteronopenia

aldosteronuria

Aldrich-Mees lines

alkalotic

alkaluria

Allen
> maneuver
> test

allotransplantation

alpha
> a.-galactosidase A

ALS—advanced life support

alternans
> auditory a.
> auscultatory a.
> a. of the heart
> mechanical a.

alternation

alveolar
> a. capillary membrane
> a. hypoventilation
> a. proteinosis

AMI—acute myocardial infarction

A-mode ultrasonography

amplitude
> a. image

ampulla (ampullae)
> a. of thoracic duct

analyzer
> pulse-height a.

anastomosis (anastomoses)
> See also *operation* and *procedure.*
> aorticopulmonary a.
> Baffe a.
> intermesenteric arterial a.
> portacaval a.
> splenorenal a.

Anel
> method
> operation

aneurysm
> abdominal a.
> abdominal aortic a. (AAA)
> aortic a.
> aortic arch a.
> aortic sinusal a.
> arteriovenous a.
> axial a.
> Bérard a.
> cardiac a.
> cylindroid a.
> cystogenic a.
> dissecting a.
> ectatic a.
> embolic a.
> embolomycotic a.
> endogenous a.
> erosive a.
> exogenous a.
> fusiform a.
> intrathoracic a.
> luetic a.
> mycotic a.
> Park a.
> peripheral a.
> phantom a.
> popliteal a.
> posterior inferior communicating artery (PICA) a.
> Pott a.
> Richet a.
> Rodrigues a.
> saccular a.
> silent a.
> a. of sinus of Valsalva
> subclinoid a.
> syphilitic a.

aneurysm (continued)
    thoracic a.
    thoracoabdominal aortic a.
    traumatic a.
    ventricular a.
aneurysmal
aneurysmatic
aneurysmectomy
aneurysmoplasty
aneurysmorrhaphy
aneurysmotomy
angina
    a. cordis
    a. decubitus
    a. dyspeptica
    a. equivalent
    exertional a.
    hypercyanotic a.
    hysterical a.
    intestinal a.
    a. inversa
    monocytic a.
    a. nervosa
    a. pectoris
    a. pectoris vasomotoria
    Plaut a.
    preinfarction a.
    Prinzmetal a.
    a. sine dolore
    unstable a.
    variant a. pectoris
    vasomotor a.
anginal
angioendothelioma
angioendotheliomatosis
    a. proliferans
    systemic proliferating a.
angiogranuloma
angiography
    aortic arch a.
    coronary a. (CA)
    digital subtraction a. (DSA)
    emission a.
    magnetic resonance a. (MRA)
    peripheral a.
    pulmonary a.
    radionuclide a.
    subtraction a.

angiokeratoma
    a. corporis diffusum
    a. corporis diffusum universale
    diffuse a.
angioneurectomy
angioplasty
    balloon a.
    coronary a.
    laser a.
    patch a.
    percutaneous transluminal a. (PTA)
    percutaneous transluminal coronary a. (PTCA)
    percutaneous transluminal renal a. (PTRA)
angioscopy
    fiberoptic a.
angiospasm
angiostomy
angiotelectasis
angiotensin
    a. II
    a. III
    a. amide
    a.-converting enzyme (ACE)
    a.-converting enzyme inhibitors (ACEIs) [a class of drugs]
    a. II receptor antagonists (AIIRAs) [a class of drugs]
angiotomy
angiotribe
angle
    costosternal a.
    QRST a.
angor
    a. nocturnus
    a. pectoris
Anichkov (Anitschkow)
    cell
    myocyte
annular
annuloplasty
    DeVega a.
    Kay a.
annulotomy

annulus (annuli) [compare: anulus]
anomalous
anomaly
    cor triatriatum a.
    Ebstein a.
    Shone a.
    Taussig-Bing a.
    Uhl a.
anorexia
    a. nervosa
anorexigenic
anoxia
    myocardial a.
    stagnant a.
anoxiate
antagonist
    adrenergic a.
    alpha-adrenergic a.
    beta-adrenergic a.
    calcium a.
anteroposterior
antiadrenergics [a class of drugs]
antibody (antibodies)
    See also in *Laboratory,*
    Pathology, and Chemistry
    Terms.
    B-cell a.
anticoagulant
    circulating a.
anticoagulants [a class of drugs]
antidiuretic
    a. hormone
antidiuretics [a class of drugs]
antigen (Ag)
    See also in *Laboratory,*
    Pathology, and Chemistry
    Terms.
    transplantation a.
antihyperlipidemic agents [a class
    of drugs]
antilipemics [a class of drugs]
antimuscarinics [a class of drugs]
antispasmodics [a class of drugs]
anulus (anuli) [compare: annulus]
"anurizm" Phonetic for aneurysm.
aorta (aortae)
    abdominal a.
    a. abdominalis

aorta (aortae) (continued)
    a. ascendens
    ascending a.
    bicuspal a.
    buckled a.
    a. chlorotica
    a. descendens
    descending a.
    descending thoracic a.
    dextropositioned a.
    double a.
    dynamic a.
    kinked a.
    overriding a.
    palpable a.
    pericardial a.
    primitive a.
    retroesophageal a.
    root of a.
    a. sacrococcygea
    straddling a.
    a. thoracalis
    thoracic a.
    throbbing a.
    ventral a.
aortic
    a. aneurysm
    a. arch
    a. arch angiography
    a. arteritis
    a. cross-clamp
    a. dissection
    a. embolism
    a. impedance
    a. insufficiency
    a. knob
    a. regurgitation
    a. septal defect
    a. sinus
    a. stenosis
    a. thrombosis
    a. valve
    a. valvulitis
    a. valvuloplasty
aortismus
    a. abdominalis
aortitis
    Döhle-Heller a.

aortitis (continued)
    luetic a.
    nummular a.
    rheumatic a.
    a. syphilitica
    a. syphilitica obliterans
    ulcerative a.
aortogram
    flush a.
    transbrachial arch a.
    translumbar a.
aortography
    abdominal a.
    catheter a.
    intravenous a.
    lumbar a.
    retrograde a.
    selective visceral a.
    thoracic a.
    translumbar a.
    venous a.
    visceral a.
aortotomy
    a. incision
AP—action potential
    angina pectoris
    aortic pressure
    apical pulse
APB—atrial premature beat
APC—atrial premature contraction
APD—action potential duration
    atrial premature depolariza-
      tion
apex (apices, apexes)
    a. cordis
apical
    a. impulse
apices (plural of apex)
apolipoprotein
    a. A-I
    a. B
    a. C-II
    a. D
    a. E (Apo-E)
apoplexy
apparatus
    suspensory a. of pleura

appearance
    angry a.
    beavertail a. of balloon profile
    bullneck a.
    coarse a.
    cobra-head a.
    cushingoid a.
    fine-speckled a.
    fish-flesh a.
    Florence flask a.
    frondlike a.
    ground-glass a.
    heterogeneous a.
    homogeneous a.
    lobulated saccular a.
    plucked-chicken a.
    reticulogranular a.
    shocklike a., shocky a.
    string-of-beads a.
    toxic a.
    trilayer a.
    whorled a.
appendage
    atrial a.
appendix (appendices)
    auricular a.
approach
    transthoracic a.
APTT, aPTT—activated partial
    thromboplastin time
Arantius
    body (bodies)
    nodules
arcade
    anomalous mitral a.
arch
    anastomotic a.
    aortic a.
    persistent right aortic a.
arctation
arcus
    a. aortae
    a. aorticus
ARD—acute respiratory disease
    acute respiratory distress
area (areae, areas)
    Bamberger a.
    cardiogenic a.

area (areae, areas) (continued)
    mitral valve a.
    portal a.
    pulmonary valve a.
    tricuspid valve a.
arrest
    cardiac a.
    circulatory a.
    sinus a.
    sudden cardiac a.
arrhythmia
    inotropic a.
    nodal a.
    phasic a.
    respiratory a.
    sinus a.
    vagus a.
    ventricular a.
arteria (arteriae)
    a. anastomotica
    a. lusoria
arterial
    a. blood flow
    a. calcification
    a. coupling
    a. line (A-line)
    a. pressure
    a. pulse
    a. thrombosis
arterialization
    a. of portal vein
arteriogram
    coronary a.
    femoral a.
    pruned-tree a.
    subclavian a.
    wedge a.
arteriography
    axillary a.
    brachiocephalic a.
    catheter a.
    cine coronary a.
    completion a.
    coronary a.
    digital subtraction a. (DSA)
    femoral a.
    mesenteric a.
    operative a.

arteriography (continued)
    peripheral a.
    pulmonary a.
    selective a.
arteriopathy
    hypertensive a.
arteriosclerosis
    cerebral a.
    coronary a.
    decrescent a.
    diffuse a.
    hyaline a.
    hypertensive a.
    infantile a.
    intimal a.
    Mönckeberg a.
    nodose a.
    nodular a.
    a. obliterans
    peripheral a.
    presenile a.
    senile a.
arteriosus
    patent ductus a.
    truncus a.
arteriotomy
    a. incision
arteriovenous
    a. fistula
    a. oxygen difference
    a. shunt
arteritis (arteritides)
    brachiocephalic a.
    coronary a.
    a. deformans
    a. hyperplastica
    necrosing a.
    necrotizing a.
    a. nodosa
    a. obliterans
    Takayasu a.
    a. umbilicalis
    a. verrucosa
artery
    brachial a.
    brachiocephalic a.
    carotid a.
    celiac a.

artery (continued)
    circumflex a.
    coronary a.
    epicardial coronary a.
    esophageal a.
    femoral a.
    iliac a.
    innominate a.
    intercostal a.
    interventricular a.
    marginal a.
    peripheral a.
    peroneal a.
    preventricular a.
    pulmonary a.
    renal a.
    subclavian a.
    tibial a.
arthritis (arthritides)
    Jaccoud a.
    rheumatoid a.
artifact
AS—aortic stenosis
    arteriosclerosis
ascending
    a. aorta
    a. venography
Aschner
    phenomenon
    reflex
    sign
    test
Aschoff
    bodies
    cell
    node
    nodule
assay
    D-dimer a.
asthenia
    neurocirculatory a.
asthma
    cardiac a.
    Elsner a.
    Heberden a.
    Rostan a.
asynchronism

atherosclerosis
    coronary a.
atherothrombosis
atm—atmosphere(s)
atresia
    aortic a.
    tricuspid a.
atria (plural of atrium)
atrial
    balloon a. septectomy
    balloon a. septostomy
    a. contraction
    a. enlargement
    a. fibrillation
    a. flutter
    a. infarction
    a. kick
    a. myocardial cell
    a. natriuretic peptide
    a. pacing
    percutaneous transluminal a.
        valvuloplasty (PTAV)
    a. premature contraction
        (APC)
    a. rhythm
    a. septal defect (ASD)
    a. septostomy
    a. septum
    a. standstill
    a. tachycardia
atrio-His
    pathway
    tract
atrioventricular
    a. block (AVB)
    a. bundle
    a. canal defect
    a. conduction
    a. dissociation
    a. flow rambling murmurs
    a. junction
    a. junctional escape beat
    a. junctional rhythm
    a. nodal reentrant tachycardia
    a. nodal reentry
    a. node artery
    a. septal defect
    a. valve

atrioventricularis communis
atrium (atria)
    common a.
    a. cordis
    a. dextrum
    a. of heart
    a. pulmonale
    pulmonary a.
    single a.
    a. sinistrum
atrophy
    cardiac a.
attack
    drop a.
    heart a.
augmentation
auscultatory
Austin Flint
    cavernous respiration
    murmur
    phenomenon
AV—aortic valve
AV, A-V (arteriovenous)
    AV anastomosis
    AV fistula
AV, A-V (atrioventricular)
    AV bundle
    AV conduction delay
    AV dissociation
    AV heart block
    AV refractory period
AVN—atrioventricular node
AVR—aortic valve replacement
AWI—anterior wall infarction
axillary
    a. arteriography
Ayerza
    disease
    syndrome
azygos
    a. vein
Babcock
    operation
Babinski
    syndrome
Babinski-Vaquez
    syndrome

Bachmann
    bundle
bacillus (bacilli)
    See in *Laboratory, Pathology, and Chemistry Terms.*
Bacillus
    See in *Laboratory, Pathology, and Chemistry Terms.*
backbleeding
backflow
bacterial
    b. endocarditis
    b. myocarditis
    b. pericarditis
bacterium (bacteria)
    See specific bacteria in *Laboratory, Pathology, and Chemistry Terms.*
Baffe anastomosis
baffle
    pericardial b.
    Senning-type of intra-atrial b.
Bainbridge
    reflex
Balke
    protocol
balloon
    b. angioplasty
    b. atrial septectomy
    b. atrial septostomy
    catheter b. valvuloplasty (CBV)
    b. tuboplasty
    b. valvuloplasty
ballooning
    b. mitral cusp
ballooning mitral cusp syndrome
Bamberger
    area
    bulbar pulse
    disease
    sign
Bamberger-Marie
    disease
    syndrome
band
    MB b.

bandage
See in *General Surgical Terms.*
Barley-Gibbon rib contractor
Barlow
syndrome
Bársony-Polgár syndrome
Basedow
disease
bathycardia
Baumgarten
murmur
Bayliss theory
Bazett formula
Bazin
disease
ulcer
B cell [noun]
B-cell [adj.]
B-c. antibody
Beale ganglion cell
beat
atrial b.
automatic b.
capture b.
combination b.
coupled b.'s
dependent b.
echo b.
ectopic b.
idioventricular b.
interference b.
mixed b.'s
nodal b.
paired b.'s
premature auricular b.
retrograde b.
summation b.
ventricular fusion b.
ventricular premature b.
Beau
disease
lines
syndrome
Beck
See also *Boeck, Bock.*
operation (I, II)
triad

bed
collateral vascular b.
vascular b.
Behier-Hardy
sign
symptom
benefited
benzothiazepines [a class of drugs]
Bérard
aneurysm
ligament
Bernheim
syndrome
beta
b. adrenoceptor
b.-2 agonist
b. blockers [a class of drugs]
b.-galactosidase
b. ray
b. thromboglobulin
Bezold (von Bezold)
ganglion
reflex
Bianchi
nodule
Bichat
membrane
tunic, tunica
bicuspidal
bicuspidate
bicuspidization
Bidder
ganglia
organ
Bier
spots
syndrome
bifascicular
bifurcation
b. of bundle of His
bigeminy
atrial b.
atrioventricular nodal b.
escape-capture b.
nodal b.
reciprocal b.
ventricular b.

binaural
> b. stethoscope

bioimplant

biopsy
> needle b.

BiPAP—bilateral positive airway pressure

bipolar
> augmented b. limb leads
> b. electrocardiogram (ECG, EKG)
> b. lead
> b. limb lead
> b. pacemaker

Björk-Shiley
> heart valve

blackout

Blalock
> operation

Blalock-Hanlon
> operation

Blalock-Taussig
> operation
> shunt

blast
> b. effect

bloater
> blue b. [emphysema]

block
> See also *heart block.*
> anodal b.
> antegrade b.
> anterograde b.
> atrioventricular b.
> brachial b.
> entrance b.
> exit b.
> fascicular b.
> first-degree atrioventricular (AV) b.
> heart b.
> interventricular b.
> intra-atrial b.
> intraventricular b.
> partial b.

blockage

blocker
> alpha-adrenergic b.

blocker (continued)
> alpha-adrenoceptor b.
> beta b.'s (β-blockers) [a class of drugs]
> calcium channel b.
> renin-angiotensin b.
> slow-channel b.'s [a class of drugs]

blood
> deoxygenated b.

blood flow study
> pulmonary b.f.s.

blood volume expanders [a class of drugs]

blow
> diastolic b.

BLS—basic life support

blue
> b. bloater [emphysema]

blush
> angiographic b.

Bock
> See also *Beck, Boeck.*
> ganglion
> nerve

body (bodies)
> Aschoff b.
> b. of rib
> b. of sternum

Boeck
> See also *Beck, Bock.*
> disease
> sarcoid, sarcoidosis

Boettcher. See *Böttcher.*

Bogros space

"boo-e-yo(z)" Phonetic for Bouillaud.

"boo-ve-ray" Phonetic for Bouveret.

border
> See also *limbus* and *margin.*
> inferior b. of heart
> left b. of cardiac dullness

borderline

Botallo
> duct
> foramen
> ligament

Bouillaud
> disease

Bouillaud (continued)
    sign
    syndrome
    tinkle
Bouveret
    disease
    syndrome
    tachycardia
bovine
    b. heterograft
Bowditch
    effect
    law
    phenomenon
Bozzolo
    sign
BP—blood pressure
bpm—beats per minute
brachial
brachiocephalic
    b. arteriography
Bracht-Wachter lesion
bradycardia
    Branham b.
    cardiomuscular b.
    clinostatic b.
    essential b.
    nodal b.
    physiologic b.
    postinfective b.
    sinoatrial b.
    sinus b.
    true b.
    vagal b.
bradyrhythmia
branch
    branches of bundle of His
    branches of suprascapular
      artery
    branches of vertebral artery
Branham
    bradycardia
    sign
Brauer
    operation
Braunwald
    sign

brawny
    b. edema
    b. induration
breach
breathing
    apneustic b.
    ataxic b.
    autonomous b.
    Biot b.
    bronchial b.
    Cheyne-Stokes b.
    continuous positive-pressure
      b. (CPPB)
    diaphragmatic b.
    frog b.
    glossopharyngeal b.
    intermittent positive-pres-
      sure b. (IPPB)
    Kussmaul b.
    labored b.
    mouth-to-mouth b.
    shallow b.
    suppressed b.
    vesicular b.
bridging
    myocardial b.
Bright
    murmur
Broadbent
    inverted sign
    sign
Brock
    infundibulectomy
Brockenbrough
    sign
bronchoplasty
bronchopulmonary
    b. lavage
"broo-ee" Phonetic for bruit.
Bruce
    stages I–VI
    treadmill protocol
bruit
    abdominal b.
    aneurysmal b.
    aortic b.
    carotid b.
    b. de canon ["duh kah-naw"]

bruit (continued)
    b. de choc ["duh shawk"]
    b. de clapotement ["duh
        klah-pot-maw"]
    b. de craquement ["duh
        krak-maw"]
    b. de cuir neuf ["duh kwer
        nuf"]
    b. de diable ["duh dee-ahbl"]
    b. de frolement ["duh frol-
        maw"]
    b. de lime ["duh leem"]
    b. de moulin ["duh moo-lah"]
    b. de parchemin ["duh
        parsh-maw"]
    b. de piaulement ["duh py-o-
        le-maw"]
    b. de rape ["duh rahp"]
    b. de rappel ["duh rah-pel"]
    b. de Roger ["duh roh-zha"]
    b. de scie ["duh se"]
    femoral b.
    Roger b.
    seagull b.
    systolic b.
    Verstraeten b.
Bryant
    ampulla
BTR—Bezold-type reflex
bubble
    b. ventriculography
Buckberg cardioplegia
Buerger
    disease
    exercises
    symptom
bulbospinal tract
bulbus
    b. aortae
    b. arteriosus
    b. caroticus
    b. cordis
    b. venae jugularis
bundle
    See also *tract*.
    atrioventricular (AV) b.
    Bachmann b.
    b. branch block

bundle (continued)
    b. branch reentry
    b. of His
    Keith b.
    Kent b.
    Kent-His b.
    sinoatrial b.
    b. of Stanley-Kent
    Thorel b.
Burns ligament
BVH—biventricular hypertrophy
bypass
    aortocoronary vein b.
    aortoiliac b.
    cardiopulmonary b.
    coronary artery b. (CAB)
    femoral-popliteal b.,
        femoropopliteal b.
    saphenous vein b.
CA—cardiac arrest
    cardiac arrhythmia
    carotid artery
    coronary angiography
    coronary arrest
    coronary artery
CAB—coronary artery bypass
CABG—coronary artery bypass graft
CACG—cineangiocardiogram
CAD—coronary artery disease
CAF—continuous atrial fibrillation
    coronary arteriovenous fistula
café coronary
caged-ball
    c.-b. prosthesis
    c.-b. valve
CAHD—coronary arteriosclerotic
    heart disease
    coronary atherosclerotic
        heart disease
calcification
    aortic c.
    coronary c.
    myocardial c.
    pericardial c.
    valvular c.
calcium (Ca)
    c. antagonists [a class of
        drugs]

calcium (Ca) (continued)
    c. channel blockers [a class
        of drugs]
    c. ion(s)
    c. paradox
    c. sign
    c. transient
Calori bursa
camera
        Anger c.
        gamma c.
Cammann
        stethoscope
CA (cardiac-apnea) monitor
canal
        pleuropericardial c.
        pleuroperitoneal c.
        van Horne c.
canalization [formation of canals,
    natural, pathologic, or surgical]
cannulate
cannulation, cannulization [intro-
    duction of a cannula]
capacity
        oxygen-diffusing c.
capillarectasia
capillaritis
capillaropathy
capillary (capillaries)
        Meigs c.
capneic
capsule
        perivascular fibrous c.
capture
        ventricular c.
carcinoid
    c. heart disease
    c. plaque
    c. syndrome
    c. tumor
    c. valve disease
carcinoma (carcinomas, carcinomata)
    See in *Oncology and Hema-
        tology* section.
Cardarelli
        sign
        symptom

cardiac
    c. catheterization
    c. output
    c. ventriculography
cardiac glycosides [a class of drugs]
cardiac risk factors (CRFs)
cardioangiography
    retrograde c.
cardiocirculatory
cardiodynamics
cardiodynia
cardiographic
cardiography
    M-mode c.
    radionuclide c.
    ultrasonic c.
cardiohepatic
cardiohepatomegaly
cardiokymographic
cardiokymography
cardiomegalia
    c. glycogenica circumscripta
cardiomegaly
    idiopathic c.
cardiomyopathy
    alcoholic c.
    Becker c.
    beer-drinker's c.
    cobalt c.
    dilated c.
    end-stage c.
    familial c.
    fatty c.
    hypertrophic c.
    hypertrophic obstructive c.
        (HOCM)
    idiopathic dilated c.
    infiltrative c.
    nephropathic c.
    nonobstructive hypertrophic
        c.
    obstructive hypertrophic c.
    restrictive c.
    thyrotoxic c.
    toxic c.
cardiopathy
    endocrine c.
cardioplasty

cardioplegic
    c. solution
cardioprotective agents [a class of drugs]
cardiorespiratory
    arrest
cardioselective
cardiotocograph
cardiotocography
cardiotonic
cardiotopometry
carditis
    rheumatic c.
    Sterges c.
carotid
    c. artery
    c. endarterectomy (CEA)
    c. pulse
    c. shudder
    c. sinus
Carpentier
    rings
    stent
CAST—Cardiac Arrhythmia Suppression Trial
catheter
    c. aortography
    c. arteriography
    c. balloon valvuloplasty (CBV)
catheterization
    cardiac c.
    hepatic vein c.
    Seldinger c.
catheterize
cava (plural of cavum)
CAVB—complete atrioventricular block
cavitis
cavity
    pericardial c.
cavum (cava)
    c. pectoris
    c. pericardii
    c. thoracis
CBBB—complete bundle branch block
CBF—coronary blood flow

CBV—catheter balloon valvuloplasty
    circulating blood volume
    corrected blood volume
CC—cardiac cycle
CCA—circumflex coronary artery
    common carotid artery
CCF—congestive cardiac failure
CD—cardiac disease
    cardiac dullness
CE—cardiac enlargement
CEA—carotid endarterectomy
cell
    See also in *Laboratory, Pathology, and Chemistry Terms.*
    B c.
    P c.
    T c.
Cell Saver Haemolite
Centurion blood pressure monitor
ceramidase deficiency
cerebrocardiac
CESD—cholesteryl ester storage disease
CF—cardiac failure
CFA—common femoral artery
challenge
    fluid c.
chamber
    cardiac c.'s
change
    E to A c.'s
    QRS c.
    QRST c.
    ST-segment c.
    T-wave c.
Charcot-Weiss-Baker
    syndrome
CHB—complete heart block
CHD—congenital heart disease
chest
    barrel c.
    flail c.
    funnel c.
Cheyne-Stokes
    respiration
CHF—congestive heart failure

Chiari
    disease
    network
    reticulum
    syndrome
cholesterol
    c. emboli syndrome
cholesterolemia
cholinergic
    c. agonists [a class of drugs]
chorda (chordae)
    c. tendineae cordis
chordal
chylomicron
chylopericarditis
chylopericardium
CI—cardiac index
    cardiac insufficiency
    coronary insufficiency
cicatrix (cicatrices)
CICU—coronary intensive care unit
CIHD—chronic ischemic heart disease
cin–. See also words beginning sin–, syn–.
cine
    c. coronary arteriography
cinedensigraphy
CIOH—chronic idiopathic orthostatic hypotension
circuitous
circulation
    extracorporeal c.
    systemic c.
circulatory
    c. arrest
    c. failure
circulus (circuli)
    c. arteriosus
circumflex
    c. artery
CK—creatine kinase
CL—chest and left arm (ECG lead)
clamp
    aortic cross-c.
classification
    DeBakey c. of aortic dissection (types I–III, IIIA, IIIB)

classification (continued)
    Keith-Wagener-Barker c. (groups 1–4)
    Killip c. (I–IV)
    New York Heart Association (NYHA) c. (classes I–IV, A–D)
claudication
    intermittent c.
    venous c.
click
    midsystolic c.
    mitral c.
closed
    transventricular c. valvotomy
clubbing
    c. of fingers
CMN—cystic medial necrosis
CMN-AA—cystic medial necrosis of the ascending aorta
CMO—cardiac minute output
CMV—continuous mechanical ventilation
CO—cardiac output
    coronary occlusion
coagulant effect
coagulants [a class of drugs]
coagulopathy
coarctation
    c. of the aorta
coarctotomy
coat
    white c. syndrome
COCl—cathodal-opening clonus
coenzyme
    c. A (CoA)
    c. Q 10 (CoQ 10)
coeur
    c. en sabot
coeur en sabot
collapse
    hemodynamic c.
collapsed lung
comes (comites)
commissurotomy
    mitral c.
    percutaneous mitral c. (PMC)

communis
    atrioventricularis c.
compensatory
competent
    c. vessel
competitive
    c. blood flow
completion arteriography
complex
    Eisenmenger c.
    Lutembacher c.
    QRS c.
    QRST c.
    QS c.
    ventricular c. (Q, R, S, T
      waves)
concomitant
    c. condition
    c. disease
    c. medical problem
    c. metabolic acidosis
    c. procedure
concretio
    c. cordis
conduction
    aberrant c.
    atrioventricular c.
    c. velocity
    decremental c.
    intraventricular c.
    ventricular c.
congestion
    circulatory c.
congestive
    c. heart failure (CHF)
consensus
contraction
    anodal closure c.
    anodal opening c.
    atrial premature c. (APC)
    automatic ventricular c.
    isometric c.
    isotonic c.
    nodal premature c.
    premature ventricular c.
      (PVC)
    supraventricular premature c.

contrast
    c. ventriculography
conus
    c. arteriosus
CoQ 10 (coenzyme Q 10)
cor
    c. adiposum
    c. arteriosum
    c. biloculare
    c. bovinum
    c. dextrum
    c. hirsutum
    c. juvenum
    c. mobile
    c. pendulum
    c. pseudotriloculare biatria-
      tum
    c. pulmonale
    c. sinistrum
    c. taurinum
    c. tomentosum
    c. triloculare biatriatum
    c. triloculare biventriculare
    c. venosum
    c. villosum
coronary
    c. angiography (CA)
    c. angioplasty
    c. arterial reserve
    c. arteriography
    c. artery ectasia
    c. artery occlusion
    c. atherosclerosis
    c. bifurcation
    c. bypass surgery
    café c.
    cine c. arteriography
    c. insufficiency
    c. ostial stenosis
    percutaneous transluminal c.
      angioplasty (PTCA)
    c. sinus
    c. steal
    c. stenosis
    c. thrombolysis
    c. thrombosis
    c. vascular resistance
coronary artery bypass graft (CABG)

coronary artery disease (CAD)
coronary heart disease (CHD)
corporeal
Corrigan
    disease
    pulse
    respiration
    sign
Corvisart
    disease
    facies
costovertebral
cough
    aneurysmal c.
coumarins [a class of drugs]
counterpulsation
    intra-aortic balloon c.
course
    arterial c., c. of artery
    venous c., c. of vein
coursing
CP—chest pain
    cor pulmonale
CPAP—continuous positive airway
    pressure
CPB—cardiopulmonary bypass
CPBS—cardiopulmonary bypass
    surgery
CPC—chronic passive congestion
CPE—cardiogenic pulmonary edema
CPI—coronary prognostic index
CPK—creatine phosphokinase
    [now: creatine kinase (CK)]
CPK-MB
CPPB—continuous positive-pres-
    sure breathing
CPR—cardiopulmonary resuscitation
CR—chest and right arm (ECG lead)
CRBBB—complete right bundle
    branch block
crescendo-decrescendo murmur
CRF—cardiac risk factor(s)
CRI—cardiac risk index
crisis (crises)
    hypertensive c.
crista (cristae)
    c. supraventricularis
    c. terminalis atrii dextri

cristal
cristate
criterion (criteria)
    Jones criteria
Crocq
    disease
cross-sectional echocardiography
crura (plural of crus)
crural
crus (crura)
    c. fasciculi atrioventricularis
        sinistrum
    c. fasciculi atrioventricularis
        dextrum
crux (cruces)
    c. of heart
CS—coronary sinus
CSIU—cardiac surgery intermedi-
    ate unit
CSR—Cheyne-Stokes respiration
CT—cardiothoracic
    contraction time
CTR—cardiothoracic ratio
CTZ—chlorothiazide
culprit
    c. lesion
    c. vessel
current
    K c.
curve
    Traube c.'s
Cushing
    effect
    phenomenon
    reaction
    response
cuspidate
cuspis (cuspides)
cutidure
cutiduris
CV—cardiovascular
CVD—cardiovascular disease
CVIU—cardiovascular intermediate
    unit
CVP—central venous pressure
CVR—cardiovascular-respiratory
    [system]
CVRD—cardiovascular renal disease

CVS—cardiovascular surgery
cardiovascular system
cyanosis
shunt c.
tardive c.
cyanotic
cyst
pericardial c.
DaCosta
syndrome
Dacron
graft
DAD—delayed after-depolarization
DAH—disordered action of the heart
data (plural of datum)
datum (data)
DBP—diastolic blood pressure
DC—direct current
DE—duration of ejection
Dean Ornish reversal diet
dearth
d. of evidence
d. of findings
d. of symptoms
DeBakey
graft
debilitation
decortication
arterial d.
defect
aorticopulmonary d.
aortic septal d.
atrial septal d.
atrioseptal d.
endocardial cushion d.
ostium primum d.
ostium secundum d.
septal d.
ventricular septal d.
defibrillated
defibrillation
deficit
deflection
atrial d.
His bundle d.
QRS d.
QS d.

degeneration
Mönckeberg d.
Quain d.
DeLee-Hillis
obstetric stethoscope
deleterious
d. effects
delirium (deliria)
postcardiotomy d.
Delorme
operation
delta
d. wave
de Musset
sign
de Mussy
point
sign
dependent
d. edema
depressants [a class of drugs]
cardiac d.
depression
ST d., ST-segment d.
systolic d.
unipolar d.
Desault
ligation
descending
d. venography
devastation
senile cortical d.
DeVega
annuloplasty
deviation
right axis d.
ST-T d.
device
Adams-DeWeese d.
dextrocardia
mirror-image d.
dg—decigram
DG—diastolic gallop
diabetes
type I d.
type 2 d.
diastasis
d. cordis

diastolic
    d. filling
    d. function
    d. motion
    d. overload
    d. pressure-time index
    d. pressure-volume relation
    d. reserve
    d. stiffness
diet
    Dean Ornish reversal d.
    Karell d.
    Kempner d.
    Pritikin d.
"diff" Slang for differential.
differential
    d. stethoscope
"dig" Slang for digitalis, digoxin.
digital
    d. subtraction angiography
        (DSA)
    d. subtraction arteriography
        (DSA)
digitalis
    d. effect
digitalis glycosides [a class of
    drugs]
dihydropyridines [a class of drugs]
"dij" Phonetic for "dig"; slang for
    digitalis, digoxin.
dimer
    D-d.
Dinamap
diphenylalkylamines [a class of
    drugs]
dire
    d. consequences
    d. straits
dis–. See also words beginning dys–.
discordance
    atrioventricular d.
    ventriculoarterial d.
discordant
discrete
    d. focal stenosis
    d. narrowing
    d. plaque

disease
    See also *syndrome.*
    Adams d.
    Adams-Stokes d.
    Addison d.
    Beau d.
    Bouveret d.
    Buerger d.
    congenital heart d.
    congestive heart d. (CHD)
    coronary artery d. (CAD)
    coronary heart d. (CHD)
    Corrigan d.
    Corvisart d.
    Crocq d.
    Duroziez d.
    Eisenmenger d.
    eosinophilic endomyocardial
        d.
    Favre d.
    Gaisböck d.
    Hamman d.
    Heller-Döhle d.
    Hodgson d.
    hypertensive heart d.
    hypertensive vascular d.
    ischemic heart d. (IHD)
    Krishaber d.
    Lenègre d.
    Lev d.
    Libman-Sacks d.
    Lutembacher d.
    Lyme d.
    Marie-Bamberger d.
    Pick d.
    pulmonary embolic d.
    pulmonary heart d.
    pulseless d.
    Raynaud d.
    rheumatic heart d.
    Roger d.
    Rougnon-Heberden d.
    Rummo d.
    small-vessel d.
    thyrotoxic heart d.
    valvular d., valvular heart d.
    von Willebrand d.
    Wenckebach d.

dissecting
 d. aortic aneurysm
 d. hematoma
dissociation
 atrioventricular (AV) d.
 electromechanical d.
 Mobitz-type atrioventricular
  d.
diuresis (diureses)
diuretic
 d. effect
diuretics [a class of drugs]
 cardiac d.
 loop d.
 osmotic d.
 potassium-sparing d.
DM—diastolic murmur
Docke murmur
DOE—dyspnea on exertion
Döhle
 disease
Doppler
 echocardiography
 effect
 interrogation
 phenomenon
 principle
 study
 ultrasonography
 ultrasound
dose
 loading d.
downstream
DP—diastolic pressure
drainage
 anomalous pulmonary
  venous d.
dressing
 See in *General Surgical
  Terms.*
Dressler
 beat
 disease
DSA—digital subtraction angiography
 digital subtraction arteriography

Duchenne
 muscular dystrophy
 sign
Duchenne-type muscular dystrophy
duct
 d. of Botallo
ductus (ductus)
 d. arteriosus
dupp. See *lubb-dupp.*
Duromedics
 valve
Duroziez
 disease
 murmur
 sign
DVT—deep vein thrombosis
 deep venous thrombosis
dynamic
 d. venous plethysmography
dys–. See also words beginning dis–.
dyskinetic
dyslipidosis
dyspnea
 cardiac d.
 exertional d.
 nocturnal d.
 orthostatic d.
 paroxysmal d.
 paroxysmal nocturnal d.
  (PND)
dysrhythmia
 sinus d.
dystrophy
 Duchenne d.
 Duchenne muscular d.
 Duchenne-type muscular d.
 myotonic d.
EB—escape beat
Ebstein
 angle
 anomaly
 disease
 malformation
EC—ejection click
ECBV—effective circulating blood
  volume
ECC—edema, clubbing, cyanosis
 extracorporeal circulation

ECG—electrocardiogram
electrocardiography
echo
e. delay time
ventricular e.
echocardiography
cross-sectional e.
Doppler e.
M-mode e.
real-time e.
two-dimensional e. (TDE)
echogenic
echogenicity
echogram
echographia
echoing
echolucent
echophony
echo time (TE)
ectopia
e. cordis
e. cordis abdominalis
e. cordis pectoral
edema
alveolar e.
brawny e.
cardiac e.
interstitial e.
nonpitting e.
pedal e.
pulmonary e.
subpleural e.
EDP—end-diastolic pressure
EDTA—ethylenediaminetetra-acetic
acid
ethylenediaminetetra-acetate
EDV—end-diastolic volume
Edwards
patch
EF—ejection fraction
EFE—endocardial fibroelastosis
effect [noun: result, outcome]
See also *phenomenon*.
Anrep e.
blast e.
Bohr e.
Bowditch e.
Cushing e.

effect [noun: result, outcome] (continued)
cyclosporine e.
deleterious e.'s
digitalis e.
diuretic e.
Doppler e.
Fahraeus-Lindqvist e.
Haldane e.
jet e.
Venturi e.
effect [verb: to produce, to bring
about]
to e. a cure
efficacious
efficacy
effusion
pericardial e.
EH—essential hypertension
Ehlers-Danlos
disease
syndrome
Einthoven
law
triangle
Eisenmenger
complex
disease
syndrome
tetralogy
ejection
e. fraction
e. phase indices
e. shell image
e. sound
EKG [pref: ECG]—electrocardiogram
electrocardiography
"eko–" Phonetic for words beginning echo–.
elasticity
electrical impedance plethysmography
electrocardiogram (ECG)
See also *electrocardiography* and *electrogram*.
bipolar e.
esophageal e.

electrocardiogram (ECG) (continued)
    intracardiac e.
    scalar e.
    twelve-lead e., 12-lead e.
    unipolar e.
electrocardiography (ECG)
    See also *electrocardiogram*
      and *electrogram.*
    fetal e.
    intrabronchial e.
    intracavitary e.
    precordial e.
    twelve-lead e., 12-lead e.
electrode
    See also *lead.*
    esophageal pill e.
electrodiagnosis
electrodiagnostic
electrodiagnostics
electrodialysis
electrodialyzer
electroendosmosis
electrogram
    See also *electrocardiogram.*
    atrial e.
    coronary sinus (CS) e.
    esophageal e.
    high right atrial (HRA) e.
    His bundle e. (HBE)
    intra-atrial e.
    intracardiac e.
    right ventricular e.
    right ventricular apical e.
    sinus node e.
electrography
electrokymogram (EKY)
electrokymograph
electrolyte
    e. imbalance
electrolytic
electromechanical
    e. coupling
    e. dissociation
    e. interval
electronic
    e. stethoscope
electrophysiologic

electrophysiology
    cardiac e.
electroversion
electrovert
elevation
    ST e., ST-segment e.
EM—ejection murmur
embolectomy
emboliform
embolism
    See also *embolus.*
    air e.
    bacterial e.
    coronary e.
    hematogenous e.
    paradoxical e.
    plasmodium e.
    pulmonary e.
    venous e.
embolization
    partial vein e. (PVE)
embolotherapy
embolus (emboli)
    See also *embolism.*
    cholesterol e.
    pantaloon e.
    platelet e.
    pulmonary e.
    shower of emboli
EMD—electromechanical dissociation
EMF—endomyocardial fibrosis
emission
    e. angiography
    single photon e. computed
      tomography (SPECT)
emphysema
    mediastinal e.
empyema
    e. of pericardium
    pulsating e.
endaortitis
    bacterial e.
endarterectomize
endarterectomy
    carotid e. (CEA)
    eversion e.
    transaortic e.

endarterial
endarteritis
    e. deformans
    Heubner specific e.
    e. obliterans
    e. proliferans
endarterium
endarteropathy
endartery
end-diastolic
endoaneurysmorrhaphy
endocardial
    e. cushion defect
    e. fibroelastosis
    e. fibrosis
    e. resection
    e. sclerosis
endocarditis
    acute bacterial e.
    bacterial e.
    e. benigna
    e. chordalis
    constrictive e.
    fungal e.
    gonococcal e.
    infective e.
    e. lenta
    Libman-Sacks e.
    Löffler e.
    malignant e.
    marantic e.
    mural e.
    mycotic e.
    nonbacterial thrombotic e.
    noninfective e.
    parietal e.
    e. parietalis fibroplastica
    plastic e.
    polypous e.
    prosthetic valve e.
    pulmonic e.
    pustulous e.
    rheumatic e.
    rickettsial e.
    septic e.
    subacute bacterial e.
    syphilitic e.
    tuberculous e.

endocarditis (continued)
    ulcerative e.
    valvular e.
    vegetative e.
    verrucous e.
    viridans e.
endomyocardial
    e. biopsy
    e. fibrosis
endophlebitis
    e. hepatica obliterans
    proliferative e.
endoscopic
    e. ultrasonography
endothelia (plural of endothelium)
endothelialization
endothelioid
endothelium (endothelia)
    vascular e.
end-systolic
    e.-s. counts
    e.-s. pressure-volume relation
    e.-s. stress-dimension relation
    e.-s. volume
eosinophilic
    e. endomyocardial disease
epicardial
epinephrine
epipleural
episode
    syncopal e.
episternal
episternum
epitheliitis
EPS—electrophysiology study
equation
    Nernst e.
    Starling e.
Erb
    point
Erben
    phenomenon
    reflex
    sign
Erdheim
    cystic medial necrosis
    disease
ergometer

ERP—effective refractory period
erratic
ESM—ejection-systolic murmur
esophageal
    e. stethoscope
esophagism
ESP—end-systolic pressure
ESV—end-systolic volume
eurhythmia
eversion
    e. endarterectomy
EVG—endovascular graft
Ewart
    sign
excavatum
    pectus e.
excitation
    anomalous e.
    atrioventricular e.
extrasystole
    auricular e.
    auriculoventricular e.
    infranodal e.
    interpolated e.
    nodal e.
    retrograde e.
    ventricular e.
FA—femoral artery
facies (facies)
    acromegalic f.
    Corvisart f.
    mitral f., mitrotricuspid f.
factor
    cardiac risk f.'s (CRFs)
    Hageman f.
    tissue plasminogen f.
failure
    high-output heart f.
    low-output heart f.
Fallot
    disease
    pentalogy of F.
    syndrome
    tetrad
    tetralogy of F.
    triad
    trilogy of F.

Fanconi-Albertini-Zellweger syn-
    drome
fascia (fasciae)
    popliteal f.
fasciculation
fasciculus (fasciculi)
Favre disease
female pseudo-Turner syndrome
femoral
    f. arteriography
    f. artery
femorocele
fenestrate
fenestration
    aortopulmonary f.
"fenomenon" Phonetic for phenom-
    enon.
"feo–" Phonetic for words begin-
    ning pheo–.
fetal
    f. electrocardiography
fever
    rheumatic f.
"fib" Slang for fibrillation.
fiber
    Purkinje f.
fiberoptic
    f. angioscopy
fibrillation
    atrial f.
    auricular f.
    ventricular f.
fibroelastosis
    endocardial f.
fibroma
    myxoid f.
    periapical f.
fibromatogenic
fibromatoid
fibromatosis
fibromatous
fibromectomy
fibromyxoma
fibrosis
    arteriocapillary f.
Fick
    formula
    method

Fick (continued)
    principle
Fiedler
    disease
    myocarditis
fishmouth
    f. mitral stenosis
fissure
    Henle f.
fistula (fistulas, fistulae)
    aortocaval f.
    aortoduodenal f.
    aortoenteric f.
    arteriovenous (AV) f.
    congenital coronary f.
    coronary artery f.
    Eck f.
    pulmonary arteriovenous f.
fistulectomy
fistulization
fistulotomy
Flack
    node
"flebektomee" Phonetic for phle-
    bectomy.
"flebitis" Phonetic for phlebitis.
"flebo–" Phonetic for words begin-
    ning phlebo–.
"fleg–" Phonetic for words begin-
    ning phleg–.
florid
flow
    effective pulmonary blood f.
    f. tract
flowmeter
    pulsed Doppler f.
fluctuation
fluid
    extravascular f.
flutter
    atrial f.
    auricular f.
    impure f.
    pure f.
    ventricular f.
flutter-fibrillation
focus (foci)

fold
    pleuroperitoneal f.
Fontan
    operation
foramen (foramina)
    Galen f.
    interatrial f. secundum
    f. of Lannelongue
    f. ovale cordis
    patent f. ovale
    f. venae cavae
    Vieussens f.
foraminal
force
    f.-frequency relation
    f.-length relation
    Starling f.
    f.-velocity relation
forceps
    Love-Gruenwald f.
formula
    See also *law* and *method.*
    Bazett f.
    Fick f.
    Gorlin f.
    Hamilton-Stewart f.
fossa (fossae)
    Mohrenheim f.
    f. ovalis cordis
    supraclavicular f.
    suprasternal f.
four-vessel angiography
F&R—force and rhythm (of pulse)
fragmentation
    f. of myocardium
Frank
    lead system
Fränkel (Fraenkel)
    treatment
Frank-Starling
    mechanism
fremitus
    pericardial f.
"freng-kuhl" Phonetic for Fränkel.
Frenkel
    See *Fränkel.*
fretum (freta)
    f. halleri

Friedreich
    sign
FRP—functional refractory period
fulguration
functional
    f. image
    f. imaging
fungus (fungi)
    See specific fungi in *Laboratory, Pathology, and Chemistry Terms.*
furrow
    atrioventricular f.
fusion
    f. beats
FVL—femoral vein ligation
Gaisböck
    disease
    syndrome
galactophlebitis
α-galactosidase A [alpha-]
β-galactosidase [beta-]
Galen
    foramen
    nerve
    veins
    ventricles
gallop
    atrial g.
    protodiastolic g.
    S_3 g. [S3]
    summation g.
    systolic g.
    ventricular g.
gamma
    g. camera
    g. ray
ganglial
ganglion (ganglia, ganglions)
    cardiac g.
    g. cardiaca
    Wrisberg g.
gas
    g. mediastinography
gastroesophageal
    g. reflux
gated
    g. system

GCA—giant cell arteritis
GE—General Electric
generator
    asynchronous pulse g.
    atrial synchronous pulse g.
    demand pulse g.
    fixed-rate pulse g.
    standby pulse g.
    ventricular-inhibited pulse g.
    ventricular-triggered pulse g.
George Lewis technique
Gibbon and Landis test
Gibson
    murmur
    vestibule
gland
    adrenal g.
Glenn
    operation
    procedure
    shunt
glomus (glomera)
    glomera aortica
    g. carotideum
glossopharyngeal
glutaraldehyde
    g.-tanned porcine heart valve
glycosaminoglycans [a class of drugs]
glycosides, cardiac [a class of drugs]
Goldblatt
    hypertension
    kidney
    phenomenon
gooseneck deformity
Gordon
    syndrome
Gorlin
    formula
Gorlin-Chaudhry-Moss
    syndrome
Gowers
    attack
    syndrome
gradient
    ventricular g.
graft
    autogenous vein g.

graft (continued)
  coronary artery bypass g.
    (CABG)
  cross-leg g.
  Dacron g.
  DeBakey g.
  femoropopliteal bypass g.
  Gore-Tex g.
  saphenous vein bypass g.
  Weavenit patch g.
Graham Steell
  murmur
great vessels
groove
  deltopectoral g.
Grüntzig (Gruentzig)
  catheter
  technique
Guéneau de Mussy point
HAE—hereditary angioneurotic
  edema
H-Ae interval
Hageman coagulation factor
Haller (von Haller)
  channel
  duct
  insula
Hamman
  disease
  murmur
  sign
  syndrome
Hampton
  hump
Hancock
  II porcine bioprosthesis
Harken
  rib spreader
Harrington
  operation
HASHD—hypertensive arteriosclerotic heart disease
HB—heart block
HCTZ—hydrochlorothiazide
HDL—high-density lipoprotein
headache
  nitroglycerin h.

heart
  armored h.
  athletic h.
  beriberi h.
  h. block
  bovine h.
  chaotic h.
  encased h.
  extracorporeal h
  h. failure
  fibroid h.
  flask-shaped h.
  frosted h.
  hyperthyroid h.
  hypoplastic h.
  intracorporeal h.
  irritable h.
  luxus h.
  h. murmur
  myxedema h.
  paracorporeal h.
  Quain fatty h.
  tabby cat h.
  Traube h.
  triatrial h.
  triocular h.
  h. valve
  vertical h.
  wandering h.
  wooden-shoe h.
heart block
  arborization h.b.
  atrioventricular h.b.
  2:1 AV (atrioventricular) h.b.
  bifascicular h.b.
  bundle-branch h.b.
  complete h.b.
  congenital h.b.
  divisional h.b.
  entrance h.b.
  exit h.b.
  fascicular h.b.
  first-degree h.b.
  incomplete h.b.
  interventricular h.b.
  intraventricular h.b.
  Mobitz h.b.
  partial h.b.

heart block (continued)
    peri-infarction h.b.
    sinoauricular h.b.
    subjunctional h.b.
    Wenckebach h.b.
heart failure
    backward h.f.
    congestive h.f.
    forward h.f.
    high-output h.f.
    left ventricular h.f.
    right ventricular h.f.
Heberden
    angina
Heller-Döhle
    disease
hematology
hemoptysis
    cardiac h.
hemorrhage
hemorrhagic
hemosiderosis
Henle
    fissure
    membrane
heparin
    low-molecular-weight h.'s [a
       class of drugs]
hepatic
    h. vein catheterization
hepatomegaly
Hess
    capillary test
heterograft
    porcine h.
HF—heart failure
hiatus
    aortic h.
high-density lipoprotein (HDL)
Hill
    sign
"hipo–" Phonetic for words begin-
    ning hypo–.
His [eponym]
    band
    bundle of H.
    bursa
    canal

His [eponym] (continued)
    disease
    duct
    spindle
    tubercle
    zones
His-Purkinje
    conduction
    system
    tissue
histocompatibility
HLDH—heat-stable lactate dehy-
    drogenase
HMG-CoA (3-hydroxy-3-methylglu-
    taryl–coenzyme A) reductase
    inhibitors [a class of drugs]
HMSAS—hypertrophic muscular
    subaortic stenosis
HOCM—hypertrophic obstructive
    cardiomyopathy
Hodgson disease
homeometric
HR—heart rate
HSA—human serum albumin
HT, htn—hypertension
Huchard
    disease
    sign
    symptom
Hufnagel
    operation
hump
    Hampton h.
Hunter
    canal
Hutinel disease
HVSD—hydrogen-detected ventric-
    ular septal defect
3-hydroxy-3-methylglutaryl–coen-
    zyme A (HMG-CoA) reductase
    inhibitors [a class of drugs]
hyperazotemia
hyperbetalipoproteinemia
    familial h.
hyperbradykininemia
hyperbradykininism
hypercholesterolemia
    essential h.

hypercholesterolemia (continued)
    familial h.
    polygenic h.
hypercholesterolemic
hyperchromaffinism
hyperdicrotic
hyperdicrotism
hyperdiuresis
hyperdynamia
hyperdynamic
hyperechoic
hyperelectrolytemia
hyperemia
    Bier passive h.
    constriction h.
hyperemic
hyperepinephrinemia
hypererythrocythemia
hyperferremia
hyperferremic
hyperfibrinogenemia
hyperglyceridemia
hyperglyceridemic
hyperheparinemia
hyperkalemia
hyperkinemic
hyperkinesia
hyperkinesis
hyperkinetic
hyperlipemia
    carbohydrate-induced h.
    combined fat- and carbohy-
      drate-induced h.
    endogenous h.
    essential familial h.
    familial fat-induced h.
    mixed h.
hyperlipidemia
hyperlipidemic
hyperlipoproteinemia
    acquired h.
    familial h. (types I–V, IIa, IIb)
hypermagnesemia
hypernatremia
hypernatremic
hyperosmolality
hyperosmolarity
hyperpermeability

hyperplasia
    intimal h.
hyperplasmia
hyperplastic
hyperpotassemia
hyperprebetalipoproteinemia
    familial h.
hyperreninemia
hyperreninemic
hyperresponsive
hyperresponsiveness
hypersaline
hypersensitivity
    carotid sinus h.
hypersphyxia
hypertension
    arterial h.
    essential h.
    portal h.
    pulmonary h.
    renovascular h.
    secondary h.
    vascular h.
hypertensive
    h. crisis
    h. heart disease
    h. pulmonary vascular disease
    h. renal disease
    h. vascular disease
hypertensor
hyperthrombinemia
hyperthyroidism
hypertonia
    h. polycythaemica
hypertonic
hypertonicity
hypertriglyceridemia
hypertrophic
hypertrophy
    ventricular h.
hypervascular
hyperventilation
hypervolemia
hypervolemic
hypoaldosteronemia
hypoaldosteronism
    hyporeninemic h.
    isolated h.

hypoaldosteronuria
hypocapnia
hypocapnic
hypocholesterolemia
hypocholesterolemic
hypodynamia
 h. cordis
hypodynamic
hypoechoic
hypoelectrolytemia
hypokalemia
hypokalemic
hypokinemia
hypokinesia
hypokinesis
hypokinetic
hypomagnesemia
hypoperfusion
hypopiesia
hypopietic
hypoplasia
 h. of aortic tract complexes
hypopotassemia
hypoprothrombinemia
hyporeninemia
hyporeninemic
hypostasis
hypostatic
hypotension
 arterial h.
 chronic idiopathic orthostat
  ic h.
 chronic orthostatic h.
 controlled h.
 familial orthostatic h.
 idiopathic orthostatic h.
 induced h.
 orthostatic h.
 postural h.
 vascular h.
 ventricular h.
hypotensive
hypothermia
hypothermic
hypotonia
hypotonic
hypovenosity
hypovolemia

hypovolemic
IA—intra-aortic
 intra-arterial
IABP—intra-aortic balloon pump
IADH—inappropriate antidiuretic
 hormone
IAS—interatrial septum
IASD—interatrial septal defect
IC—intermittent claudication
 isovolumic contraction
ICD—ischemic coronary disease
ICM—intercostal margin
ICT—isovolumic contraction time
ictal
ictus
 i. cordis
ID—internal diameter
idiopathic
IDL—intermediate-density lipopro-
 tein
IDVC—indwelling venous catheter
IHR—intrinsic heart rate
IHSS—idiopathic hypertrophic
 subaortic stenosis
IJP—internal jugular [vein] pressure
IJV—internal jugular vein
"iktus" Phonetic for ictus.
ILD—ischemic leg disease
 ischemic limb disease
IMA—internal mammary artery
image
 pulse echo i.
imaging
 See in *Radiology, Nuclear*
  Medicine, and Other
  Imaging section.
imbalance
 electrolyte i.
IMH—idiopathic myocardial hypertrophy
immunosuppressants [a class of
 drugs]
immunotherapy
impedance
 electrical i. plethysmography
 i. plethysmography
 i. venography
implantation

impressio (impressiones)
    i. cardiaca pulmonis
impression
impulse
    apex i.
    apical i.
    i. conduction
    ectopic i.
    episternal i.
    left parasternal i.
    point of maximal i. (PMI)
    right parasternal i.
incipient
    i. heart attack
incision
    aortotomy i.
    arteriotomy i.
    thoracotomy i.
incisura (incisurae)
    See also *notch.*
    i. apicis cordis
    i. cardiaca ventriculi
incisural
incisure
    See *incisura* and *notch.*
incompetence
incubus
index (indexes, indices)
    ankle-brachial i. (ABI)
    arm-ankle i. (AAI)
inductive plethysmography
infarct
infarctectomy
infarction
    anteroinferior myocardial i.
    anterolateral myocardial i.
    anteroseptal myocardial i.
    apical myocardial i.
    atrial i.
    cardiac i.
    diaphragmatic i.
    high-lateral myocardial i.
    inferolateral myocardial i
    lateral myocardial i.
    myocardial i. (MI)
    posterior myocardial i.
    posterolateral myocardial i.
    pulmonary i.

infarction (continued)
    right ventricular i.
    Roesler-Dressler i.
    septal myocardial i.
    silent myocardial i.
    subendocardial i.
    through-and-through myo-
        cardial i.
    transmural myocardial i.
inferior vena cava (IVC)
infundibula (plural of infundibulum)
infundibulectomy
    Brock i.
infundibuliform
infundibulum (infundibula)
    cardiac i.
    i. of heart
inhibitor
    HMG-CoA (3-hydroxy-3-
        methylglutaryl–coenzyme
        A) reductase i.'s [a class
        of drugs]
    phosphodiesterase III (PDE
        III) i.'s [a class of drugs]
inoperable
inotropes [a class of drugs]
INPV—intermittent negative-pres-
    sure assisted ventilation
inspiratory
    i. murmur
insufficiency
    aortic i.
    cardiac i.
    coronary i.
    mitral i.
    myocardial i.
    myovascular i.
    pseudoaortic i.
    tricuspid i.
    valvular i.
    venous i.
insult
    myocardial i.
interrogation
    Doppler i.
interval
    A-H i.
    atriocarotid i.

interval (continued)
    atrioventricular (AV) i.
    cardioarterial i.
    coupling i.
    escape i.
    H-Ae i.
    H-V i.
    P-A i.
    P-P i.
    PQ i.
    P-R i.
    Q-M i.
    QRST i.
    Q-T i.
    Q-U i.
    S_2–OS [S2–OS] i. [second sound to opening snap]
intervalvular
interventricular
intoxication
    digitalis i.
intrabronchial
    i. electrocardiography
intracardiac
    i. phonocardiography
intracavitary
    i. electrocardiography
intravascular
    i. coagulation
intravenous
    i. aortography
intraventricular
inversion
    T-wave i.
I&O—intake and output
iodoventriculography
Ionescu-Shiley
    valve
IPG—impedance plethysmography
IPPB—intermittent positive-pressure breathing
IPPV—intermittent positive-pressure ventilation
irregularity
    luminal i.
    i. of pulse
irritability
    ventricular i.

ischemia
    i. cordis intermittens
    myocardial i.
    subendocardial i.
ISD, ISDN—isosorbide dinitrate
isoelectric
    i. point
isotope
    i. ventriculography
ITP—idiopathic thrombocytopenic purpura
IV—interventricular
    intravascular
    intravenous
    intraventricular
IVC—inferior vena cava
IVCD—intraventricular conduction defect
IVCP—inferior vena cava pressure
IVCV—inferior venacavography
Ivemark syndrome
IVP—intraventricular pressure
IVS—interventricular septum
IVSD—interventricular septal defect
IWMI—inferior wall myocardial infarction
J—joule
Jaboulay
    method
Janeway
    lesion
    sphygmomanometer
    spots
Jaquet apparatus
Javid
    shunt
Jefferson
    syndrome
Jobst
    stockings
joint
    See in *Orthopedics and Sports Medicine* section.
judicious
Judkins technique
jugular
    j. pulse sphygmography
    j. venous distention (JVD)

jugular (continued)
    j. venous pressure (JVP)
    j. venous pulse (JVP)
junctional
    j. escape rhythm
juncture
    saphenofemoral j.
juxtaductal
    j. coarctation
JV—jugular vein
    jugular venous
JVP—jugular venous pressure
    jugular venous pulse
K—potassium
Karell
    diet
    treatment
Kartagener
    disease
    syndrome
    triad
Katz-Wachtel
    phenomenon
Kawasaki
    disease
    syndrome
Kay
    annuloplasty
KCl—potassium chloride
Kearns-Sayer
    syndrome
Keith
    bundle
    node
Keith-Wagener-Barker classification
    (groups 1–4)
Kerley
    A lines
    B lines
"ker on sa-bo" Phonetic for coeur
    en sabot.
Kimmelstiel-Wilson
    disease
    syndrome
kinetocardiogram (KCG)
kinetocardiography
kissing-balloon technique

Koch
    node
    triangle
Koerber-Salus-Elschnig syndrome
"ko-mees" Phonetic for comes.
Korotkoff
    method
    sounds
    test
Krishaber disease
Kronecker
    puncture
Krönig
    steps
"krus" Phonetic for crus.
Kussmaul
    disease
    pulse
    sign
    symptom
KWB—Keith, Wagener, Barker
    [classification, groups 1–4]
LA—left atrial
    left atrium
Labbé
    syndrome
labile
    l. blood pressure
labored breathing
laborious
lactate
    l. dehydrogenase (LDH)
lactic
    l. acid
    l. acidosis
lacticacidemia
LAD—left anterior descending
    [coronary artery]
LADA—left anterior descending
    artery
LAE—left atrial enlargement
LAH—left atrial hypertrophy
Larrey
    cleft
    ligation
laser
    l. angioplasty

law

    See also *principle* and *rule.*
    all-or-none l.
    Einthoven l.
    Laplace l.
    Ohm l.
    Starling l.

LBB—left bundle branch
LBBB—left bundle branch block
LBCD—left border of cardiac dullness
LCA—left circumflex coronary artery
    left carotid artery
LCF, LCx—left circumflex [coronary artery]
LCM—left costal margin
LD—living donor
LDA—left descending artery
LDH—lactate dehydrogenase
LDL—low-density lipoprotein
lead ["leed"]

    See also *electrode.*
    l. I (II, III)
    Accufix l.
    active fixation l.
    anterior precordial l.
    anterolateral l.
    anteroseptal l.
    atrial l.
    augmented bipolar limb l.'s
    augmented limb l.'s (aVF, aVL, aVR)
    aVL l.
    aVF l.
    aVR l.
    bipolar (standard) l.
    bipolar limb l.
    bipolar precordial l.
    CL (chest and left arm) l.
    CB (chest and back) l.
    CF (chest and left leg) l.
    chest l.
    CR (chest and right arm) l.
    deep limb l.
    direct l.
    ECG (electrocardiogram) l.
    electroencephalographic l.
    esophageal l.

lead ["leed"] (continued)

    Frank XYZ orthogonal l.
    indirect l.
    inferior l.
    inferior precordial l.
    inferolateral l.
    intracardiac l.
    lateral l.
    lateral precordial l.
    left precordial l.
    limb l.'s
    orthogonal Frank XYZ l.
    pacemaker l., pacing l.
    precordial l.'s (V_1–V_6)
    reversed arm l.
    right precordial l. (V_{3r}, V_{4r}, etc.)
    right-sided chest l.
    semidirect l.
    standard (bipolar) l.'s (I, II, III)
    sternal l.
    unipolar l.
    unipolar limb l.
    unipolar precordial l.
    V l.'s (V_1–V_6)
    ventricular l.
    Wilson l.'s
    XYZ Frank ECG l.

Leff

    stethoscope

lemniscus (lemnisci)
Lenègre

    disease
    syndrome

Leriche

    disease
    operation
    syndrome

lesion

    Baehr-Löhlein l.
    bird's nest l.
    Blumenthal l.
    Bracht-Wächter l.
    Janeway l.
    jet l.
    Löhlein-Baehr l.

Lev disease

Levine
 sign
LFA—left femoral artery
Libman-Sacks
 disease
 endocarditis
 syndrome
ligamentum (ligamenta)
ligation
 Desault l.
 proximal l.
ligature
 Woodbridge l.
Lillehei-Kaster
 valve
limb
 l. venography
limbal
limbic
limbus (limbi)
 See also *border* and *margin*.
 l. foraminis ovalis
 l. fossae ovalis
 l. fossae ovalis Vieussenii
 l. of Vieussens
limen (limina)
line
 anterior axillary l.
 Conradi l.
 Dobie l.
 Kerley A l.'s
 Kerley B l.'s
 Krause l.
 median axillary l.
 midaxillary l.
 midclavicular l.
 posterior axillary l.
 Z l.
linea (lineae)
lingula (lingulae)
 l. of left lung
lingular
lingulectomy
lipoprotein
 familial high-density l.
  (HDL) deficiency
 high-density l. (HDL)
 intermediate-density l. (IDL)

lipoprotein (continued)
 low-density l. (LDL)
 very low-density l. (VLDL)
Litten
 diaphragm phenomenon
 sign
Livierato
 reflex
 test
LLL—left lower lobe
loading dose
lobectomy
 sleeve l.
lobulated
lobulation
lobulus (lobuli)
 lobuli thymi
Löffler
 disease
 endocarditis
loop
 l. diuretics [a class of drugs]
 P l.
 QRS l.
 ventricular l.
low-density lipoprotein (LDL)
low-molecular-weight heparins [a
 class of drugs]
LPA—left pulmonary artery
LPV—left pulmonary vein
LSB—left sternal border
LSM—late systolic murmur
LSV—left subclavian vein
lubb-dupp
lumbar
 l. aortography
lumen (lumina)
 residual l.
luminal
lung
 l. transplantation
 shock l.
lunula (lunulae)
 lunulae of aortic valve
 lunulae of cusps of aortic
  valve
 lunulae of cusps of pulmonary valve

lunula (lunulae) (continued)
    lunulae of pulmonary valves
    lunulae of semilunar valves
        of aorta
    lunulae of valves of pulmo-
        nary trunk
    lunulae valvularum semilu-
        narium valvae aortae
    lunulae valvularum semilu-
        narium valvae trunci pul-
        monalis
Lutembacher
    complex
    disease
    syndrome
LV—left ventricle
LVAD—left ventricular assist device
LVDP—left ventricular diastolic
    pressure
LVE—left ventricular enlargement
LVEDP—left ventricular end-dias-
    tolic pressure
LVEF—left ventricular ejection
    fraction
LVET—left ventricular ejection time
LVF—left ventricular failure
LVH—left ventricular hypertrophy
LVP—left ventricular pressure
LVS—left ventricular strain
LVSP—left ventricular systolic
    pressure
LVSV—left ventricular stroke vol-
    ume
LVSW—left ventricular stroke work
Lyme
    disease
Lyon-Horgan
    operation
μ—micro- [prefix; alphabetized as
    m]
M_1—mitral first sound
M_2—mitral second sound
MA—mean arterial [blood pressure]
MABP—mean arterial blood pressure
machine
    heart-lung m.
macrocardius
macula (maculae)

magnetic
    m. moment
    m. relaxation time
    m. resonance angiography
        (MRA)
    m. resonance imaging (MRI)
    m. resonance signal
maladie
    m. de Roger ["duh ro-jay"]
malformation
    Ebstein m.
    Ebstein-like m. of mitral
        valve
    Taussig-Bing m.
    vascular m.
mammary artery
    left internal m.a. (LIMA)
    right internal m.a. (RIMA)
maneuver
    See also *method* and *tech-
        nique.*
    Mueller m.
    Valsalva m.
MAP—mean aortic pressure
    mean arterial pressure
Marfan
    sign
    syndrome
margin
    See also *border* and *limbus.*
    acute m. of heart
    left m. of heart
    obtuse m. of heart
    right m. of heart
margo (margines)
Marie-Bamberger disease
Martin
    bandage
Martorell
    syndrome
    ulcer
mask
    partial rebreathing m.
massage
    cardiac m.
    carotid sinus m.
    heart m.

Matas
    operation
"Maddox" Phonetic for Mattox.
Mattox
    maneuver
Maugeri
    syndrome
MAVIS—mobile artery and vein
    imaging system
MB bands
MBF—myocardial blood flow
MBP—mean blood pressure
MC—myocarditis
MCL—midclavicular line
MCT—mean circulation time
MD—myocardial damage
Meadox vascular graft
mechanism
    Frank-Starling m.
    reentrant m.
    Starling m.
median
    m. sternotomy
mediastina (plural of mediastinum)
mediastinal
    m. crunch
mediastinitis
mediastinography
    gas m.
    opaque m.
mediastinoscopic
mediastinoscopy
mediastinotomy
mediastinum (mediastina)
    anterior m.
    m. anterius
    inferior m.
    m. inferius
    m. medium
    middle m.
    posterior m.
    m. posterius
    superior m.
    m. superius
Meigs
    capillaries
membranate

membrane
    Henle m.
    Henle elastic m.
    Henle fenestrated m.
    Krause m.
    PTFE (polytetrafluoroethyl-
      ene) m.
mEq—milliequivalent(s)
MER—mean ejection rate
mercury (Hg)
    millimeters of m. (mm Hg)
Merendino technique
mesenteric
    m. arteriography
mesoaortitis
    m. syphilitica
metastasis (metastases)
    retrograde m.
method
    See also *maneuver* and *tech-
      nique.*
    Fick m.
    Korotkoff m.
    Orsi-Grocco m.
    Scarpa m.
MHR—maximal heart rate
MI—mitral incompetence
    mitral insufficiency
    myocardial infarction
microanastomosis
microaneurysm
microangiopathic
microangiopathy
microcalcification
microcalcificectomy
microcirculation
microcirculatory
microemboli (plural of microembo-
    lus)
microembolization
microembolus (microemboli)
    showers of microemboli
microinfarct
microlesion
microperfusion
microphone
    cardiac catheter-m.
microplethysmography

microthrombi (plural of
    microthrombus)
microthrombosis
microthrombus (microthrombi)
microvasculature
migration
    retrograde m.
MILIS—Multicenter Investigation
    for the Limitation of Infarct Size
mill-house murmur
milliequivalent(s) (mEq)
millijoule(s) (mJ)
millimeter(s) (mm)
    m.'s of mercury (mm Hg)
    m.'s of water (mm H_2O)
minute [small]
"mio–" Phonetic for words begin-
    ning myo–.
mitral
    m. annulus
    m. commissurotomy
    m. incompetence
    m. insufficiency
    m. opening snap
    percutaneous m. commis-
      surotomy (PMC)
    percutaneous transluminal
      m. valvuloplasty (PTMV)
    m. prolapse
    m. regurgitation
    m. stenosis
    m. valve
    m. valve prolapse
    m. valve prosthesis
    m. valvotomy
    m. valvulitis
    m. valvuloplasty
mitrale
    P m.
mJ—millijoule(s)
MLAP—mean left atrial pressure
mm Hg—millimeters of mercury
mm H_2O [mm H2O]—millimeters
    of water
M-mode
    M-m. cardiography
    M-m. echocardiogram
    M-m. echocardiography

M-mode (continued)
    M-m. scanning
MMR—myocardial metabolic rate
Mobitz
    AV heart block (I, II)
mode
    M-m.
modification
    Mason-Likar limb lead m.
Mönckeberg
    arteriosclerosis
    calcification
    degeneration
    mesarteritis
    sclerosis
    syndrome
Mondor
    disease
    syndrome
monitor
    Holter m.
monocrotic
monocrotism
monophasic
Moore
    operation
Morgagni
    disease
    foramen
    nodule
Morgagni-Adams-Stokes syndrome
Moschcowitz
    sign
    test
Moynahan
    syndrome (I, II)
MP—mean pressure
MPA—main pulmonary artery
MPAP—mean pulmonary arterial
    pressure
MR—mitral reflux
    mitral regurgitation
MRA—magnetic resonance angiog-
    raphy
MRAP—mean right atrial pressure
MRFIT—Multiple-Risk Factor
    Intervention Trial

MRVP—mean right ventricular
    pressure
μs—microsecond(s)
ms, msec—millisecond(s)
MS—mitral stenosis
MSER—mean systolic ejection rate
mucro (mucrones)
    m. sterni
Mueller
    See also *Müller.*
    maneuver
MUGA—multiple gated acquisition
    [scan]
Müller
    See also *Mueller.*
    sign
multi-infarct
mural
murmur
    amphoric m.
    aneurysmal m.
    aortic m.
    apex m.
    apical diastolic m.
    arterial m.
    attrition m.
    Austin Flint m.
    basal diastolic m.
    bellows m.
    blowing m.
    Bright m.
    cardiac m.
    cardiopulmonary m.
    cardiorespiratory m.
    Carey Coombs m.
    continuous m.
    cooing m.
    crescendo m.
    Cruveilhier-Baumgarten m.
    decrescendo m.
    deglutition m.
    diamond-shaped m.
    diastolic m.
    Duroziez m.
    dynamic m.
    ejection m.
    endocardial m.
    Eustace Smith m.

murmur (continued)
    exocardial m.
    expiratory m.
    Fisher m.
    Flint m.
    Fraentzel m.
    friction m.
    functional m.
    Gibson m.
    grades 1–6
    Graham Steell m.
    Hamman m.
    harsh m.
    hemic m.
    holosystolic m.
    hour-glass m.
    humming-top m.
    inorganic m.
    inspiratory m.
    lapping m.
    machinery m.
    Makins m.
    mitral m.
    musical m.
    nun m.
    obstructive m.
    organic m.
    pansystolic m.
    Parrot m.
    pericardial m.
    pleuropericardial m.
    prediastolic m.
    presystolic m.
    pulmonic m.
    reduplication m.
    regurgitant m.
    respiratory m.
    Roger m.
    seagull m.
    seesaw m.
    Steell m.
    stenosal m.
    Still m.
    subclavicular m.
    systolic m.
    to-and-fro m.
    Traube m.
    tricuspid m.

murmur (continued)
 venous m.
 vesicular m.
 water-wheel m.
muscle
 See also in *Orthopedics and
  Sports Medicine* section.
 cardiac m.
 diaphragmatic m.
 infrahyoid m.'s
 intercostal m.'s (external,
  internal)
 intercostal m.'s, innermost
 interspinal m.'s of thorax
 intertransverse m.'s, anterior
 intertransverse m.'s of thorax
 longissimus m. of thorax
 Oehl m.
 organic m.
 papillary m. of left ventricle
  (anterior, posterior)
 papillary m. of right ventricle (anterior, posterior)
 papillary m.'s of right ventricle, septal
 pectinate m.'s
musculus (musculi)
 See in *Orthopedics and
  Sports Medicine* section.
Mustard [eponym]
 vascular operation
MV—mitral valve
MVP—mitral valve prolapse
mycoplasmal
"my-nute" Phonetic for minute
  [small].
myocardial
 m. bridging
 m. concussion
 m. contractility
 m. depolarization
 m. disease
 m. edema
 m. failure
 m. fiber shortening
 m. function
 m. hibernation
 m. hypertrophy

myocardial (continued)
 m. imaging
 m. infarction
 m. ischemia
 m. metabolism
 m. necrosis
 m. oxygen consumption
 m. perfusion imaging
 m. perfusion scintigraphy
 m. perfusion study
 m. rupture
 m. stiffness
 m. stunning
 m. tension
 m. tissue
myocardiopathy
 alcoholic m.
 chagasic m.
 idiopathic m.
myocarditic
myocarditis
 acute bacterial m.
 acute isolated m.
 chronic m.
 diphtheritic m.
 fibrous m.
 Fiedler m.
 fragmentation m.
 giant cell m.
 idiopathic m.
 indurative m.
 infectious m.
 interstitial m.
 parenchymatous m.
 protozoal m.
 rheumatic m.
 rickettsial m.
 m. scarlatinosa
 toxic m.
 tuberculoid m.
 tuberculous m.
 viral m.
myocardosis
 Riesman m.
myocytolysis
 coagulative m.
myoendocarditis

myofibrosis
    m. cordis
myomalacia
    m. cordis
myopathia
    m. cordis
myopericarditis
myxoma (myxomas, myxomata)
    atrial m.
    m. of heart
    vascular m.
NBTE—nonbacterial thrombotic
    endocarditis
NCA—neurocirculatory asthenia
necrosis (necroses)
    arteriolar n.
    avascular n.
    coagulation n.
    coagulative n.
    contraction band n.
    coumarin n.
    cystic medial n.
    embolic n.
    Erdheim cystic medial n.
    fibrinoid n.
    ischemic n.
    medial n.
    subendocardial n.
    transmural n.
necrotic
necrotizing
    n. vasculitis
neointima
neovascular
neovascularization
Nernst
    equation
nerve
    parasympathetic n.
    sympathetic n.
    vagus n.
net
    See *network, plexus,* and *rete.*
    Chiari n.
network
    See *net, plexus,* and *rete.*
    Chiari n.
    Purkinje n.

neuritic
neuritis
    ischemic n.
neurocardiac
neurovascular
nidus (nidi)
nitrates [a class of drugs]
nodal
node
    Aschoff n.
    n. of Aschoff and Tawara
    atrioventricular (AV) n.
    Flack n.
    His-Tawara n.
    Osler n.
    SA (sinoatrial) n.
    sinoatrial n., sinuatrial n.,
        sinus n.
nodi (plural of nodus)
noduli (plural of nodulus)
nodulous [adj.]
nodulus (noduli)
nodus (nodi)
    n. atrioventricularis
    n. sinuatrialis
nonfunctioning
    n. heart valve
nonocclusive
Noonan syndrome
normostatic
notch
    See also *incisura.*
    anacrotic n.
    aortic n.
    dicrotic n.
    Sibson n.
NPB—nodal premature beat
NSR—normal sinus rhythm
nuclear
    n. angiography
    n. scintigraphy
"nur–" Phonetic for words begin-
    ning neur–.
NYHA (New York Heart Associa-
    tion) classification (I–IV)
O_2 [O2]—oxygen
obstruction
    vena cava o.

occlusion
> coronary o.
> mesenteric artery o.
> o. of renal artery
> thrombotic o.
> venous o. plethysmography

Oehler symptom

Öhnell
> X wave of O.

oleandrism

OM—obtuse marginal (coronary artery)

opaque
> o. mediastinography

operable

operation
> See also in *General Surgical Terms.*
> Anel o.
> Babcock o.
> Beck o. (I, II)
> Blalock o.
> Blalock-Hanlon o.
> Blalock-Taussig o.
> Brauer o.
> Delorme o.
> Fontan o.
> Harrington o.
> Hufnagel o.
> Jacobaeus o.
> Leriche o.
> Lyon-Horgan o.
> Matas o.
> Moore o.
> Mustard vascular o.
> Potts o.
> Potts-Smith-Gibson o.
> Rastelli o.
> Senning o.
> Vineberg o.
> Waterston o.

operative
> o. arteriography

OPG/CPA—oculoplethysmography/carotid phonoangiography

orthopnea
> three-pillow o.
> two-pillow o.

orthostatic
> o. hypotension

OS—opening snap

OSA—obstructive sleep apnea

Osborne
> wave

oscillation

oscillogram

oscillograph

Osler
> nodes
> sign

osmotherapy

osmotic diuretics [a class of drugs]

ostia (plural of ostium)

ostial [pertaining to opening, aperture, orifice]

ostium (ostia)
> o. aortae
> o. aorticum
> o. arteriosum cordis
> o. atrioventriculare dextrum
> o. atrioventriculare sinistrum
> o. cardiacum
> coronary o.
> persistent o. primum
> o. primum
> o. primum defect
> o. secundum
> o. secundum defect
> o. sinus coronarii
> sinusoidal o.
> o. trunci pulmonalis
> o. venae cavae inferioris
> o. venae cavae superioris
> o. venarum pulmonalium
> o. venosum cordis

overload
> aortic o.
> circulatory o.

oximeter
> finger o.
> intracardiac o.
> pulse o.

oximetry
> finger o.
> pulse o.

oxygen (O)
    molecular o. (O_2) [O2])
P—pulse
P_1—pulmonic first sound
P_2—pulmonic second sound
PA—pulmonary artery
PAC—pericarditis, arthropathy,
    camptodactyly (syndrome)
    premature atrial contraction
pacemaker
    Amtech-Killeen p.
    Arco p.
    artificial p.
    asynchronous p.
    Atricor p.
    bifocal demand p.
    Biotronik p.
    bipolar p.
    Chardak-Greatbatch p.
    Coratomic p.
    Cordis p.
    Cordis Atricor p.
    Cordis-Ectocor p.
    Cordis fixed-rate p.
    Cordis Ventricor p.
    CPI Maxilith p.
    CPI Minilith p.
    demand p.
    Ectocor p.
    Electrodyne p.
    endocardial bipolar p.
    epicardial p.
    General Electric p.
    implantable p.
    lithium p.
    Nathan p.
    nuclear p.
    Omni-Atricor p.
    Omni-Ectocor p.
    Omni-Stanicor p.
    radio frequency p. [also:
      radiofrequency]
    Stanicor p.
    Starr-Edwards p.
    Telectronic p.
    transvenous p.
    unipolar p.
    Ventricor p.

pacemaker (continued)
    wandering p.
    Zoll p.
    Zyrel p.
    Zytron p.
PAF—pulmonary arteriovenous fis-
    tula
PAFIB—paroxysmal atrial fibrillation
Paget-von Schroetter syndrome
PAH—pulmonary artery hypertension
PAL—posterior axillary line
palpitation
panangiitis
    diffuse necrotizing p.
PAOD—peripheral arterial occlu-
    sive disease
      peripheral arteriosclerotic
        occlusive disease
PAP—positive airway pressure
      pulmonary artery pressure
PAPVC—partial anomalous pulmo-
    nary venous connection
PAPVR—partial anomalous pulmo-
    nary venous return
PAR—pulmonary arteriolar resistance
paracentesis
    p. cordis
    p. pericardii
paradoxic, paradoxical
paraganglion (paraganglia)
    adrenergic p.
    aortic p.
    cardiac p.
    cholinergic p.
parasite
    See specific parasites in
      Laboratory, Pathology,
      and Chemistry Terms.
paroxysmal
    p. nocturnal dyspnea (PND)
pars (partes)
PAS—pulmonary artery stenosis
PASG—pneumatic antishock garment
PAT—paroxysmal atrial tachycardia
patch
    p. angioplasty
    Edwards p.
    MacCallum p.

patch (continued)
>Teflon p.

patent
>p. ductus arteriosus (PDA)
>p. foramen ovale

pathogen
>See specific pathogens in
>*Laboratory, Pathology,
>and Chemistry Terms.*

pathologic, pathological

pathway
>reentrant p.

PAWP—pulmonary artery wedge
pressure

PC—pulmonic closure

PCW—pulmonary capillary wedge
(pressure)

PD—patent ductus

PDA—patent ductus arteriosus
>posterior descending artery

PDE III (phosphodiesterase III)
inhibitors [a class of drugs]

pectus
>p. carinatum
>p. excavatum

PEEP—positive end-expiratory
pressure

pentalogy
>p. of Fallot

percutaneous
>p. mitral commissurotomy
>(PMC)
>p. transluminal angioplasty
>(PTA)
>p. transluminal atrial valvu-
>loplasty (PTAV)
>p. transluminal coronary
>angioplasty (PTCA)
>p. transluminal mitral valvu-
>loplasty (PTMV)
>p. transluminal renal angio-
>plasty (PTRA)

Perez
>sign

perforans (perforantes)

perfusion
>p. scintigraphy

periarteritis
>p. nodosa

pericardial
>p. calcification
>p. cyst
>p. effusion
>p. fluid
>p. friction
>p. knock
>p. peel
>p. window

pericarditis
>acute fibrinous p.
>adhesive p.
>amebic p.
>bacterial p.
>p. calculosa
>p. callosa
>carcinomatous p.
>constrictive p.
>p. with effusion
>p. epistenocardiaca
>p. externa et interna
>fibrous p.
>hemorrhagic p.
>idiopathic p.
>localized p.
>mediastinal p.
>neoplastic p.
>p. obliterans
>obliterating p.
>purulent p.
>rheumatic p.
>serofibrinous p.
>p. sicca
>suppurative p.
>tuberculous p.
>uremic p.
>p. villosa
>viral p.

pericardium
>adherent p.
>bread-and-butter p.
>calcified p.
>p. fibrosum
>fibrous p.
>parietal p.
>p. serosum

pericardium (continued)
 serous p.
 shaggy p.
 visceral p.
period
 Wenckebach p.
peripheral
 p. angiography
 p. arteriography
 p. vasodilators [a class of drugs]
 p. venography
peroneal
 p. artery
 p. nerve
 p. vein
Perthes
 test
petechia (petechiae)
PG—prostaglandin
PGE_1 [PGE1]—prostaglandin E_1
PGE_2 [PGE2]—prostaglandin E_2
PGH_2 [PGH2]—prostaglandin H_2
PGI_2 [PGI2]—prostaglandin I_2
 [prostacyclin]
PH—pulmonary hypertension
phenomenon (phenomena)
 See also *effect, reflex, sign,* and *test.*
 Aschner p.
 Ashman p.
 Austin Flint p.
 Cushing p.
 Doppler p.
 Erben p.
 first-set p.
 Gärtner p.
 Goldblatt p.
 Hering p.
 Katz-Wachtel p.
 Litten diaphragm p.
 no-reflow p.
 Raynaud p.
 R on T p.
 Schellong-Strisower p.
 second-set p.
 treadmill p.
 Wenckebach p.

pheochromocytoma
phlebectomy
phlebitis
phlebofibrosis
phlebogenous
phlebolith
phlebolithiasis
phleboplasty
phleborheography
phlebosclerosis
phlebothrombosis
phlegmasia
 p. alba dolens
 p. alba dolens puerperarum
 cellulitic p.
 p. cerulea dolens
 thrombotic p.
phonoangiography
 oculoplethysmography/carotid p. (OPG/CPA)
phonocardiography
 intracardiac p.
phosphodiesterase III (PDE III)
 inhibitors [a class of drugs]
physiologic, physiological
physiopathology
PICA—posterior inferior communicating artery
PICA aneurysm
Pick [eponym]
 disease
 syndrome
plaque
 atheromatous p.
 gelatinoid p.
plasma expanders [a class of drugs]
plasma protein fractions [a class of drugs]
plethysmograph
 body p.
 digital p.
 finger p.
plethysmography
 air-cuff p.
 dynamic venous p.
 electrical impedance p.
 impedance p. (IPG)
 inductive p.

plethysmography (continued)
    strain-gauge p.
    thermistor p.
    venous occlusion p.
pleura (pleurae)
    diaphragmatic p.
    p. diaphragmatica
    mediastinal p.
    p. mediastinalis
    parietal p.
    p. parietalis
    pericardiac p.
    p. pericardiaca
    pericardial p.
    visceral p.
    p. visceralis
plexus (plexus, plexuses)
    See also *net, network,* and
      rete.
    brachial p.
    cardiac p.
    p. cardiacus profundus
    p. cardiacus superficialis
    p. caroticus communis
    p. caroticus externus
    p. caroticus internus
    p. coronarius cordis
    perimuscular p.
    perimysial p.
    vascular p.
    p. venosus caroticus internus
    venous p.
plication
    caval p.
PM—pacemaker
    presystolic murmur
PMC—percutaneous mitral com-
    missurotomy
PMI—point of maximal impulse
    point of maximal intensity
P mitrale
PN—percussion note
PND—paroxysmal nocturnal dyspnea
pneumatocardia
pneumohemia
pneumohemopericardium
pneumohydropericardium
pneumohydrothorax

pneumomediastinum
pneumopericardium
pO$_2$ [pO2]—partial pressure of oxy-
    gen
point
    Erb p.
    isoelectric p.
    J p.
polyarteritis
    p. nodosa
polycythemia
    See in *Oncology and Hema-*
      tology section.
"poo-drahzh" Phonetic for poudrage.
porcine
    p. heterograft
    p. xenograft
position
    See in *General Surgical*
      Terms.
postcardiotomy
    p. syndrome
postmyocardial infarction
postpump syndrome
potassium-sparing diuretics [a class
    of drugs]
potential
    pacemaker p.
Pott
    aneurysm
    gangrene
Potts
    operation
Potts-Smith-Gibson
    operation
poudrage
PPB—positive-pressure breathing
PPH—primary pulmonary hyper-
    tension
P pulmonale syndrome
PPV—positive-pressure ventilation
PR—pulse rate
PRCs—packed red cells
precipitous
    p. drop [in blood pressure or
      laboratory indices]
    p. rise [in blood pressure or
      laboratory indices]

precordial
    p. electrocardiography
preejection
preponderance
    ventricular p.
principal [primary, main]
    p. aspect
    p. reason
    p. symptom
principle [rule]
    See also *law* and *rule.*
    Fick p.
probe
    scintillation p.
procedure
    See also *maneuver, method,*
        operation, and *technique.*
    Fontan p.
    Senning p.
process
prolapse
    mitral valve p.
prostaglandin (PG)
    See also in *Laboratory,*
        Pathology, and Chemistry
        Terms.
    p. E_1 [E1] (PGE_1)
    p. E_2 [E2] (PGE_2)
    p. H_2 [H2] (PGH_2)
    p. I_2 [I2] (PGI_2) [prostacyclin]
prosthesis (prostheses)
    See also *graft* and *valve.*
prothrombin
protocol
    Bruce treadmill p.
    Naughton treadmill p.
proton
    p. spectroscopy
pruned-tree
    p.-t. arteriogram
PS—pulmonary stenosis
pseudoanemia
    p. angiospastica
pseudocoarctation
    p. of the aorta
pseudo-Turner syndrome
PSG—peak systolic gradient
    presystolic gallop

PT—paroxysmal tachycardia
    physical therapist
    physical therapy
    pneumothorax
    prothrombin time
PTA—persistent truncus arteriosus
PTAV—percutaneous transluminal
    atrial valvuloplasty
PTCA—percutaneous transluminal
    coronary angioplasty
PTE—pulmonary thromboembolism
PTFE—polytetrafluoroethylene
    [See *Teflon* in *General Surgi-*
    cal Terms.]
PTMV—percutaneous transluminal
    mitral valvuloplasty
PTRA—percutaneous transluminal
    renal angioplasty
PTT—partial thromboplastin time
pulmoaortic
pulmonale
    P p.
    cor p.
pulmonary
    p. angiography
    p. arteriography
    p. artery wedge pressure
        (PAWP)
    p. edema
    p. ejection clicks
    p. hypertension
    p. infarction
    p. perfusion
    p. resection
    p. toilet
    transventricular p. valvotomy
    p. valvotomy
    p. veno-occlusive disease
pulmonectomy
pulmonic
    p. atresia
    p. stenosis
pulsatile
pulsation
    expansile p.
    suprasternal p.
pulse
    abdominal p.

pulse (continued)

    abrupt p.

    allorhythmic p.

    alternating p.

    anacrotic p.

    anadicrotic p.

    anatricrotic p.

    apical p.

    arachnoid p.

    atrial liver p.

    atrial venous p., atriovenous
        p.

    auriculovenous p.

    Bamberger bulbar p.

    biferious p., bisferious p.

    bigeminal p.

    cannon-ball p.

    capillary p.

    carotid p.

    catacrotic p.

    catadicrotic p.

    catatricrotic p.

    centripetal venous p.

    collapsing p.

    cordy p.

    Corrigan p.

    coupled p.

    decurtate p.

    p. deficit

    dicrotic p.

    digitalate p.

    dropped-beat p.

    elastic p.

    entoptic p.

    epigastric p.

    equal p.

    febrile p.

    filiform p.

    formicant p.

    frequent p.

    full p.

    funic p.

    gaseous p.

    gate p.

    guttural p.

    hard p.

    hepatic p.

    high-tension p.

pulse (continued)

    hyperdicrotic p.

    infrequent p.

    intermittent p.

    irregular p.

    jerky p.

    jugular p.

    jugular p. sphygmography

    Kussmaul p.

    Kussmaul Monneret p.

    labile p.

    low-tension p.

    Monneret p.

    monocrotic p.

    mouse tail p.

    nail p.

    paradoxical p.

    parvus et tardus p.

    pedal p.

    pistol-shot p.

    plateau p.

    polycrotic p.

    pulmonary p.

    quadrigeminal p.

    quick p.

    Quincke p.

    radial p.

    respiratory p.

    retrosternal p.

    Riegel p.

    running p.

    sharp p.

    short p.

    slow p.

    soft p.

    strong p.

    tense p.

    thready p.

    tremulous p.

    tricrotic p.

    trigeminal p.

    trip-hammer p.

    undulating p.

    unequal p.

    vagus p.

    venous p.

    ventricular venous p.

    vermicular p.

pulse (continued)
  vibrating p.
  water-hammer p.
  wiry p.
pulse-height analyzer
pulseless
  p. disease
pulsus (pulsus)
  p. abdominalis
  p. aequalis
  p. alternans
  p. biferiens
  p. bigeminus
  p. bisferiens
  p. celer
  p. contractus
  p. cordis
  p. debilis
  p. deficiens
  p. deletus
  p. differens
  p. duplex
  p. durus
  p. filiformis
  p. formicans
  p. fortis
  p. frequens
  p. heterochronicus
  p. intercurrens
  p. irregularis perpetuus
  p. magnus
  p. magnus et celer
  p. mollis
  p. monocrotus
  p. oppressus
  p. paradoxus
  p. parvus
  p. parvus et tardus
  p. plenus
  p. pseudo-intermittens
  p. rarus
  p. tardus
  p. trigeminus
  p. undulosus
  p. vacuus
  p. venosus
  p. vibrans

pump
  Emerson p.
puncture
  Kronecker p.
  pericardial p.
  sternal p.
Purkinje
  fibers
  network
purpura
  p. fulminans
purulent
puruloid
PVC—premature ventricular contraction
  pulmonary venous congestion
PVD—peripheral vascular disease
PVE—partial vein embolization
PVR—peripheral vascular resistance
  pulmonary vascular resistance
PVS—premature ventricular systole
PVT—paroxysmal ventricular tachycardia
PWI—posterior wall infarction
Px—pneumothorax
pyemia
  arterial p.
  portal p.
pylephlebitis
  adhesive p.
pyrogen
QRS
  alternans
  axis
  changes
  complex
  loop
  vector
  wave
Quain
  degeneration
  fatty heart
Quincke
  capillary pulsation
  pulse
  sign
RA—renal artery
  right atrial

RA— (continued)
    right atrium
RAD—right axis deviation
radiation
    r. pericarditis
radionuclide
    r. angiocardiography
    r. cardiography
    r. venography
    r. ventriculography
RAE—right atrial enlargement
RAH—right atrial hypertrophy
rale
    See in *Pulmonary Medicine*
        section.
ramose
ramus (rami)
RAP—right atrial pressure
RAS—renal artery stenosis
Rasmussen aneurysm
Rastelli
    operation
ratio
    cardiothoracic r.
    risk-benefit r.
    R/S r.
    ventilation-perfusion (V/Q) r.
ray
    β r.'s [beta]
    γ r.'s [gamma]
Raynaud
    disease
    phenomenon
RBB—right bundle branch
RBBB—right bundle branch block
RBP—resting blood pressure
RCA—radionuclide cerebral
  angiogram
    right coronary artery
real-time
    r.-t. echocardiography
receptor
    histamine H_1 r. [H1]
    histamine H_2 r. [H2]
    low-density lipoprotein
        (LDL) r.'s
reciprocal
red herring

reentrant
reentry
reflex
    See also in *Neurology and*
        Pain Management section.
    Abrams heart r.
    Bainbridge r.
    Bezold-Jarisch r.
    bregmocardiac r.
    carotid sinus r.
    diving r.
    Erben r.
    eyeball compression r., eye-
        ball-heart r.
    heart r.
    Livierato r.
    McDowall r.
    oculocardiac r.
    psychocardiac r.
    pulmonocoronary r.
    viscerocardiac r.
reflux
    abdominojugular r.
    hepatojugular (HJ) r.
refractory
    r. period
region
    antebrachial r., radial
    antebrachial r., ulnar
    antebrachial r., volar
    anterior antebrachial r.
    anterior brachial r.
    axillary r.
    lateral r. of neck
    precordial r.
    sternocleidomastoid r.
    subscapular r.
regurgitation
    aortic r.
    mitral r.
    pulmonic r.
    tricuspid r.
rehab—rehabilitation
reminiscent
renal
    percutaneous transluminal r.
        angioplasty (PTRA)

resection
> endocardial r.
> pulmonary r.
> septal r.

resistance
> capillary r.
> peripheral r.
> total peripheral r.
> vascular r.

resonance
> amphoric r.
> bell-metal r.
> cavernous r.
> cough r.
> cracked-pot r.
> shoulder-strap r.
> skodaic r.
> vesicular r.
> vocal r. (VR)
> whispering r.

respiration
> See also in the *Pulmonary Medicine* section.
> artificial r.
> Cheyne-Stokes r.
> Corrigan r.
> intermittent positive-pressure r. (IPPR)
> labored r.

respiratory
> r. arrest
> r. distress
> r. insufficiency

resuscitation
> cardiopulmonary r.

rete (retia)
> See also *net, network,* and *plexus.*
> r. arteriosum
> r. mirabile
> r. vasculosum
> r. venosum

retial

retrograde
> r. aortography
> r. cardioangiography

retrosternal

revascularization
> myocardial r.

RFA—right femoral artery

rheumatic
> r. fever
> r. heart disease

rhonchus (rhonchi)
> See in the *Pulmonary Medicine* section.

rhythm
> accelerated idioventricular r.
> agonal r.
> atrial r.
> atrioventricular r.
> cantering r.
> cardiac r.
> coronary sinus r.
> coupled r.
> ectopic r.
> escape r.
> gallop r.
> gallop r., systolic
> idioventricular r.
> junctional r.
> nodal r.
> pendulum r.
> quadruple r.
> reciprocal r.
> reciprocating r.
> reversed r.
> sinus r.
> sinusoidal r.
> train-wheel r.
> triple r.
> ventricular r.

rhythmic, rhythmical

rhythmicity

rib contractor
> Bailey r.c.
> Bailey-Gibbon r.c.
> Sellor r.c.

rib spreader
> Burford r.s.
> Harken r.s.
> Lemmon r.s.
> Lilienthal-Sauerbruch r.s.
> Rienhoff-Finochietto r.s.
> Tuffier r.s.

rib spreader (continued)
    Wilson r.s.
Richet
    aneurysm
Riesman
    myocardosis
rigor
    calcium r.
RIMA—right internal mammary
    anastomosis
    right internal mammary artery
ring
    atrial r.
    Carpentier r
    Effler r.
    vascular r.
"rithm" Phonetic for rhythm.
RLD—related living donor
RO, R/O—rule out
Roger
    bruit
    disease
    murmur
Rogers sphygmomanometer
ROMI—rule out myocardial infarc-
    tion
"romied" Slang for myocardial
    infarction ruled out.
"rongk–" Phonetic for words begin-
    ning rhonch–.
rotation
    clockwise r. of heart
    counterclockwise r. of heart
Roth
    spots
Rougnon-Heberden disease
RP—refractory period
    resting pressure
    rest pain
RPA—right pulmonary artery
RPV—right pulmonary vein
RSB—right sternal border
RSR—regular sinus rhythm
RSV—right subclavian vein
rub
    friction r.
    pericardial r.
    pleural r.

rub (continued)
    pleuritic r.
    pleuropericardial r.
rule
    See also *law* and *principle*.
    r. of bigeminy
    Liebermeister r.
    Rolleston r.
rumble
    diastolic r.
Rummo disease
runoff
RV—right ventricle
RVE—right ventricular enlargement
RVEDP—right ventricular end-
    diastolic pressure
RVH—right ventricular hypertrophy
RVR—renal vascular resistance
RVRA—renal vein renin activity
    renal vein renin assay
RVRC—renal vein renin concentra-
    tion
S_1–S_4 [S1–S4]—heart sounds (first
    through fourth)
SA—sinoatrial
    Stokes-Adams
SA attack
saddle
    s. emboli
salvo
SAM—systolic anterior motion
SAP—systemic arterial pressure
saphenofemoral
saphenous
sarcoidosis
    s. cordis
sarcoma (sarcomas, sarcomata)
    See in *Oncology and Hema-*
    tology section.
SAS—supravalvular aortic stenosis
Saunders
    disease
SBE—subacute bacterial endocarditis
SBP—systolic blood pressure
SC—subclavian (vein)
scale
    Borg s.

scan
    See also in *Radiology,
    Nuclear Medicine, and
    Other Imaging* section.
    B s.
    capillary blockade perfusion
      s.
    cardiac s.
    MUGA (multiple gated
      acquisition) s.
    perfusion s.
    thallium myocardial s.
    ventilation s.
    ventilation-perfusion (V/Q) s.
scanning
    ventilation-perfusion (V/Q) s.
Scarpa
    method
    triangle
schistosomiasis
scimitar
    s. shadow
    s. sign
    s. syndrome
scintigraphy
    myocardial perfusion s.
    nuclear s.
    perfusion s.
    thallium perfusion s.
    ventilation s.
scintillation
    s. camera
    s. scan
sclerogenous
sclerosis
    arterial s.
    s. circumscripta pericardii
    endocardial s.
    subendocardial s.
    valvular s.
    vascular s.
    venous s.
sclerostenosis
"scopes" See under full name.
    sphygmoscope
    stethoscope
scurvy

SD—septal defect
    sudden death
S/D—systolic-to-diastolic [ratio]
SDS—sudden death syndrome
seagull bruit
sedatives [a class of drugs]
    cardiac s.
    vascular s.
sedentary
segment
    PQ s.
    PR s.
    ST s.
    TP s.
    TP-Q s.
segmenta (plural of segmentum)
segmental
segmentum (segmenta)
Seldinger
    catheterization
selective
    s. arteriography
    s. venography
Sellor
    rib contractor
semilunar
Senning
    operation
    procedure
SEP—systolic ejection period
septa (plural of septum)
septal
    s. defect
    s. resection
septectomy
    balloon atrial s.
septi (genitive of septum)
septic
    s. embolization
    s. shock
septostomy
    atrial s.
    balloon atrial s.
septotomy
septum (septa)
    aorticopulmonary s.
    atrioventricular s. of heart
    bulbar s.

septum (septa) (continued)
    interatrial s. of heart
    interventricular s. of heart
    mediastinal s.
    s. primum
    s. secundum
    spurious s.
    s. of ventricles of heart, ven-
       tricular s.
sequela (sequelae)
SER—systolic ejection rate
serum (serums, sera)
    pericardial s.
SET—systolic ejection time
sheath
    femoral s.
Sheehan-Dodge technique
shock
    cardiac s.
    cardiogenic s.
    electric s.
    postoperative s.
Shone
    anomaly
    complex
    syndrome
shower
    s. of echoes
    s. of emboli
shunt
    aortopulmonary s.
    arteriovenous (AV) s.
    cardiovascular s.
    cavamesenteric s.
    dialysis s.
    Glenn s.
    intracardiac s.
    left-to-right s.
    portacaval s.
    portarenal s.
    postcaval s.
    right-to-left s.
    side-to-side s.
    Waterston s.
Sibson
    notch
    vestibule

sign
    See also *phenomenon, reflex,*
      and *test.*
    Auenbrugger s.
    Bamberger s.
    Béhier-Hardy s.
    Bouillaud s.
    Bozzolo s.
    Branham s.
    Braunwald s.
    Broadbent s.
    Broadbent inverted s.
    Brockenbrough s.
    Carvallo s.
    Cegka s.
    Corrigan s.
    Delbet s.
    de Musset s.
    Dorendorf s.
    Drummond s.
    Duchenne s.
    Duckworth s.
    Duroziez s.
    E s.
    Erben s.
    Ewart s.
    figure three s.
    Friedreich s.
    Glasgow s.
    Gunn s.
    Gunn crossing s.
    Hall s.
    Hamman s.
    Heim-Kreysig s.
    Hill s.
    Homans s.
    Hope s.
    jugular s.
    Kreysig s.
    Kussmaul s.
    Levine s.
    Litten s.
    Mahler s.
    McGinn-White s.
    Moschcowitz s.
    Müller s.
    Musset s.
    Nicoladoni s.

sign (continued)
    Oliver s.
    Osler s.
    Perez s.
    Pins s.
    Porter s.
    Potain s.
    Quénu-Muret s.
    Quincke s.
    reversed three s.
    Rivero-Carvello s.
    Robertson s.
    Rotch s.
    Sansom s.
    scimitar s.
    square root s.
    Sterles s.
    three s.
    Traube s.
    vein s.
    vital s.'s
    Wenckebach s.
    Williamson s.
silence
    electrical s.
silhouette
    cardiac s.
    cardiovascular s.
"sil-oo-et" Phonetic for silhouette.
sin–. See also words beginning
    cin–, syn–.
sinus (sinus, sinuses)
    s. aortae (Valsalvae)
    aortic s.
    s. arrest
    s. arrhythmia
    s. bradycardia
    carotid s.
    coronary s.
    s. of internal jugular vein,
        inferior
    s. of internal jugular vein,
        superior
    s. of Morgagni
    s. nodal reentry
    s. node
    oblique s. of pericardium
    s. pause

sinus (sinus, sinuses) (continued)
    pericardial s.
    Petit s.
    s.'s of pulmonary trunk
    s. rhythm
    s. tachycardia
    transverse s. of pericardium
    s. of Valsalva
    s. of venae cavae
    s. venosus defect
    venous s.
sinusoid
    myocardial s.'s
sinusoidal
sinusoidalization
situs (situs)
    s. inversus
    s. inversus thoracis
    s. inversus viscerum
    s. perversus
    s. transversus
SK—streptokinase
"sklero–" Phonetic for words begin-
    ning sclero–.
skodaic
    s. resonance
SKSD—streptokinase-streptodornase
sleeve
    s. lobectomy
slope
    E to F s.
slow-channel blockers [a class of
    drugs]
SM—systolic murmur
SMA—superior mesenteric artery
small-vessel disease
Smith
    sign
SN—suprasternal notch
snap
SOB—shortness of breath
sodium (Na)
    s. channel
    s. nitrite
"soo-fl," "soo-flay" Phonetic for
    souffle.
souffle
    cardiac s.

souffle (continued)
    fetal s.
    funic s., funicular s.
    umbilical s.
sound
    aortic second s. (A_2 [A2])
    atrial s.
    auscultatory s.'s
    bellows s.
    cardiac s.'s
    diastolic s.
    eddy s.'s
    ejection s.'s
    first heart s. (S_1 [S1])
    flapping s.
    fourth heart s. (S_4 [S4])
    friction s.
    gallop s. (S_3, S_4)
    heart s's (first through
      fourth, S_1–S_4 [S1 S4])
    Korotkoff s.
    metallic s.
    percussion s.
    pericardial friction s.
    physiologic s.'s
    pistol-shot s.
    pulmonic second s. (P_2 [P2])
    second s., aortic (A_2 [A2])
    second heart s. (S_2 [S2])
    second s., pulmonic (P_2 [P2])
    S_3 gallop s. [S3]
    S_4 gallop s. [S4]
    tick-tack s.'s
    vesicular breath s.'s
    water-wheel s.
    xiphisternal crunching s.
space
    Poiseuille s.
    retrocardiac s.
    third s.
    Virchow-Robin s.'s
spasm
    arterial s.
    coronary artery s.
    vascular s.
spatial
    s. vectorcardiography

spectroscopy
    proton s.
Spens syndrome
sphygmobologram
sphygmography
    jugular pulse s.
sphygmomanometer
    Erlanger s.
    Faught s.
    Janeway s.
    Riva-Rocci s.
    Rogers s.
    Staunton s.
    Tycos s.
sphygmoscope
    Bishop s.
spirometry
    Tri-Flow incentive s.
splenosis
    pericardial s.
splitting
    s. of heart sounds
spot
    milk s.
    Roth s.'s
    soldier's s.
SR—sinus rhythm
    systemic resistance
SS—subaortic stenosis
SSS—sick sinus syndrome
standstill
    atrial s.
    auricular s.
    cardiac s.
    respiratory s.
    sinus s.
    ventricular s.
Starling
    equation
    forces
    law
    mechanism
Starr-Edwards
    pacemaker
    valve
stasis
    venous s.
statins [a class of drugs]

status
    s. lymphaticus
    s. post [event]
    s. thymicolymphaticus
    s. thymicus
Staunton
    sphygmomanometer
steal
    subclavian s.
    s. syndrome
Steinert
    disease
    myotonic dystrophy
    syndrome
stenosed
stenosing
stenosis (stenoses)
    aortic s. (AS)
    aortic valve s.
    arterial s.
    buttonhole mitral s.
    calcified aortic s.
    carotid s.
    cicatricial s.
    congenital aortic s.
    coronary s.
    coronary ostial s.
    critical s.
    Dittrich s.
    fishmouth mitral s.
    granulation s.
    idiopathic hypertrophic
      subaortic s. (IHSS)
    mitral s.
    muscular subaortic s.
    muscular subvalvular s.
    myocardial infundibular s.
    preventricular s.
    pulmonary s.
    pulmonary artery s.
    pulmonary valve s.
    pulmonic s.
    renal artery s.
    subaortic s.
    subvalvular aortic s.
    supravalvular s.
    tricuspid s.
    valvular s.

stenosis (stenoses) (continued)
    valvular pulmonic s.
stent
    Carpentier s.
step
    Krönig s.'s
sternotomy
    median s.
sternum
    s. bifidum
    cleft s.
stethoscope
    binaural s.
    Cammann s.
    DeLee-Hillis obstetric s.
    differential s.
    electronic s.
    esophageal s.
    Leff s.
Still
    murmur
stimulation
    vagus s.
STK—streptokinase
stocking
    Jobst s.
    thromboembolic s.
Stokes
    collar
    syndrome
Stokes-Adams
    attack
    disease
    syndrome
strain-gauge plethysmography
streak
    fatty s.
stress
    s. film
    s. test
stria (striae)
striation
    tabby cat s.
    tigroid s.
stricturotomy
stroke
    back s.
ST segment [noun]

ST-segment [adj.]
    ST-s. alterans
    ST-s. changes
    ST-s. elevation
study
    opacification s.
subaortic
subclavian
    s. artery
subclavicular
sublingual
subtle
subtraction
    s. angiography
    s. venography
Sudeck
    critical point
"sudo–" Phonetic for words beginning pseudo–.
SUDS—sudden unexplained death syndrome
sulci (plural of sulcus)
sulciform
sulcus (sulci)
    aortic s.
    atrioventricular s.
    coronary s. of heart
    interatrial s.
    interventricular s. of heart
    longitudinal s. of heart
    pulmonary s. of thorax
    subclavian s., s. of subclavian artery
    s. of subclavian vein
    terminal s. of right atrium
    transverse s. of heart
    s. of vena cava
sump
    Baylor s.
superior
    s. vena cava (SVC)
support
    Abée s.
surgery
    See also *maneuver, method, operation, procedure,* and *technique.*
    cardiac s.

surgery (continued)
    cardiovascular s.
    open heart s.
    peripheral vascular s.
    thoracic s.
surgical procedure
    See *operation, procedure,* and *technique.*
survey
    Jenkins activity s.
"sut-el" Phonetic for subtle.
suture [material]
    See in *General Surgical Terms.*
suture [technique]
    See in *General Surgical Terms.*
SV—sinus venosus
    stroke volume
    subclavian vein
SVAS—supravalvular aortic stenosis
SVC—superior vena cava
SVR—systemic vascular resistance
SVT—supraventricular tachycardia
SW—stroke work
sympathetic
    s. ganglia
    s. nervous system
sympatholytics [a class of drugs]
symptom
    See also in *General Medical Terms.*
    Buerger s.
    constitutional s.
    equivocal s.
    Oehler s.
    premonitory s.
    prodromal s.
syn–. See also words beginning cin–, sin–.
synchondrosis (synchondroses)
    sternal s., s. sternalis
syncope
    Adams-Stokes s.
    s. anginosa
    cardiac s.
    carotid s.
    deglutition s.

syncope (continued)
    orthostatic s.
    postural s.
    vasovagal s.
syndrome
    See also *disease.*
    Adams-Stokes s.
    adrenogenital s.
    allergic vasculitis s.
    anginal s.
    aortic arch s.
    Ask-Upmark s.
    Ayerza s.
    Babinski s.
    Babinski-Vaquez s.
    ballooning mitral cusp s.
    Barlow s.
    Beau s.
    Bernheim s.
    Bouillaud s.
    Bouveret s.
    brachial s.
    bradycardia-tachycardia s.
    cardiofacial s.
    cervical rib s.
    cervicobrachial s.
    Charcot s.
    cholesterol emboli s.
    click s.
    click-murmur s.
    coronary failure s.
    coronary intermediate s.
    Dressler s.
    effort s.
    Eisenmenger s.
    floppy valve s.
    Gaisböck s.
    Gordon s.
    Gorlin-Chaudhry-Moss s.
    Gowers s.
    Holt-Oram s.
    leopard s., LEOPARD s.
    Leriche s.
    Libman-Sacks s.
    long QT s.
    Lown-Ganong-Levine s.
    Lutembacher s.
    Marfan s.

syndrome (continued)
    mitral valve prolapse s.
    myocardial postinfarction s.
    Noonan s.
    Paget-von Schroetter s.
    Pick s.
    postcardiac injury s.
    postcardiotomy s.
    postcardiotomy psychosis s.
    postinfarction s.
    postmyocardial infarction s.
    postpericardiotomy s.
    postpump s. (PPS)
    P pulmonale s.
    pseudo-Turner s.
    QT s.
    scimitar s.
    sick sinus s. (SSS)
    steal s.
    stiff heart s.
    straight back s.
    subclavian steal s.
    sudden unexplained death s.
    Takayasu s.
    Taussig-Bing s.
    thoracic outlet s.
    Touraine I s.
    Wolff-Parkinson-White s.
        (WPW)
    s. X
    XO s.
    XXXX s.
    XXXY s.
synechia (synechiae)
    s. pericardii
syphilis
    cardiovascular s.
system
    cardiovascular s.
    conducting s. of heart, con-
        duction s. of heart
    His-Purkinje s.
    vascular s.
systemic
    s. lupus erythematosus (SLE)
systole
    aborted s.
    arterial s.

systole (continued)
- atrial s.
- auricular s.
- extra s.
- frustrate s.
- hemic s.
- ventricular s.

systolic
- s. apical impulse
- s. click-murmur syndrome
- s. current
- s. function
- s. motion
- s. murmur
- s. pressure-time index
- s. reserve
- s. time interval

tachycardia
- alternating bidirectional t.
- antidromic t.
- atrial t.
- atrioventricular t.
- auricular t.
- nodal t.
- nonparoxysmal t.
- orthostatic t.
- paroxysmal ventricular t.
- reciprocating t.
- sinus t.
- supraventricular t.
- ventricular t.

tachysystole
- atrial t.
- auricular t.

Takayasu
- arteritis
- pulseless disease
- syndrome

TAMI—Thrombolysis and Angioplasty in Myocardial Infarction
[trial]

tamponade
- balloon t.
- cardiac t.
- chronic t.
- heart t.
- pericardial t.
- Rose t.

TAO—thromboangiitis obliterans

TAPVD—total anomalous pulmonary venous drainage

TAR—thrombocytopenia–absent
radius [syndrome]

Taussig-Bing
- disease
- malformation
- syndrome

Tawara node

TD—transverse diameter

TDF—thoracic duct fistula

technique
- See also *maneuver* and *method.*
- See also in *General Surgical Terms.*
- Creech t.
- George Lewis t.
- Gruentzig t.
- Judkins t.
- pulse echo t.
- Seldinger t.
- Sheehan-Dodge t.

TED, T.E.D. (thromboembolic disease) [T.E.D. is trademark form]
- hose
- stockings

TEE—transesophageal echocardiogram

Teflon
- patch

telangiectasis (telangiectases)

telangiitis

telangion

tendon
- Todaro t.

"tennis" Phonetic for Toennis.

test
- See also in *Laboratory, Pathology, and Chemistry Terms.*
- Allen t.
- antistreptozyme t.
- atrial pacing t.
- Balke-Ware t.
- carotid sinus t.
- collateral circulation t.

test (continued)
    D-dimer t.
    Dehio t.
    effort tolerance t.
    ergonovine t.
    exercise t.'s
    Gibbon and Landis t.
    graded exercise t. (GXT)
    Korotkoff t.
    lipid t.
    Livierato t.
    Master two-step exercise t.
    partial thromboplastin time
      (PTT) t.
    performance t.
    platelet aggregation t.
    prothrombin t. (PT)
    Quick tourniquet t. (for pro-
      thrombin time)
    radioactive fibrinogen
      uptake t.
    regitine t.
    serum enzyme t.
    stress t.
    thallium stress t.
    thromboplastin generation t.
      (TGT)
    tolerance t.
    tourniquet t.
    treadmill exercise t. (TET)
    treadmill stress t. (TST)
    Trendelenburg t.
    ultrasound t.
    Valsalva t.
"tet" Slang for tetralogy of Fallot.
tetralogy
    t. of Fallot
Teutleben ligament
TF—tactile fremitus
    tetralogy of Fallot
TGA—transposition of the great
    arteries
TGV—transposition of the great
    vessels
thallium (Tl)
    t. myocardial scan
    t. perfusion scintigraphy
    t. stress testing

theca (thecae)
    t. cordis
thecal
theorem
    Bayes t.
    Bernouilli t.
theory
    Bayliss t.
therapy
    anticoagulant t.
    antiplatelet t.
    collapse t.
    immunosuppressive t.
    intravenous t.
    thrombolytic t.
thermistor
    t. plethysmography
thermodilution
    t. technique
thiazides [a class of drugs]
third-spacing
thoracectomy
thoracentesis
thoracic
    t. aortography
    t. outlet syndrome
thoracostomy
    tube t.
thoracotomy
    t. incision
three-pillow orthopnea
threshold
thrill
    aneurysmal t.
    aortic t.
    diastolic t.
    presystolic t.
    systolic t.
thrombectomy
thrombi (plural of thrombus)
thromboangiitis
    t. obliterans
thromboaortopathy
    occlusive t.
thromboarteritis
    t. purulenta
thromboclastic
thrombocyst

thrombocytic
thrombocytopenia
    t. with absence of radius
thrombocytosis
thromboembolectomy
thromboendarterectomy
thrombogenic
thromboid
thrombokinase
thrombolysin
thrombolytics [a class of drugs]
thrombophlebitis
    iliofemoral t.
    t. migrans
    t. purulenta
    t. saltans
thrombose, thrombosed
thrombosis
    See also in *Cardiology* section.
    See also *thrombus.*
    agonal t.
    arterial t.
    atrophic t.
    ball-valve t.
    cardiac t.
    catheter-induced t.
    coronary t.
    creeping t.
    deep venous t. (DVT)
    dilatation t.
    intracardiac t.
    intraventricular t.
    marantic t., marasmic t.
    mural t.
    plate t., platelet t.
    propagating t.
    traumatic t.
    venous t.
thrombus (thrombi)
    See also *thrombosis.*
    agglutinative t.
    agonal t., agony t.
    annular t.
    antemortem t.
    ball t.
    ball-valve t.
    blood plate t., blood platelet t.

thrombus (thrombi) (continued)
    calcified t.
    canalized t.
    coral t.
    coronary t.
    currant jelly t.
    fibrin t.
    hyaline t.
    infective t.
    laminated t.
    lateral t.
    marantic t., marasmic t.
    mixed t.
    mural t.
    obstructive t.
    occluding t., occlusive t.
    organized t.
    pale t.
    parasitic t.
    parietal t.
    phagocytic t.
    pigmentary t.
    plate t., platelet t.
    primary t.
    propagated t.
    red t.
    saddle t.
    septic t.
    stratified t.
    traumatic t.
    valvular t.
    white t.
thymectomize
thymectomy
thyrotoxic heart disease
TI—tricuspid incompetence
    tricuspid insufficiency
Tietze
    disease
    syndrome
time (T)
    A-H conduction t.
    arm-lung t.
    circulation t.
    clot retraction t.
    echo t. (TE)
    ejection t.
    H-R conduction t.

time (T) (continued)
    H-V conduction t.
    intra-atrial conduction t.
    isovolumic relaxation t.
      (IVRT)
    left ventricular ejection t.
      (LVET)
    mean circulating t.
    occlusion t. (OT)
    P-A conduction t.
    P-H conduction t.
    rise t.
    sinoatrial conduction t.
      (SACT)
    sinoatrial recovery t. (SART)
    systolic ejection t. (SET)
    treadmill walking t.
    ventricular activation t.
TIMI—Thrombolysis in Myocardial
    Infarction [TIMI II trial]
tinkle
    Bouillaud t.
tissue
    His-Purkinje t.
    t. plasminogen activator (t-
      PA, tPA, TPA)
TLA—translumbar aortogram
TMI—threatened myocardial
    infarction
    transmural infarction
Todaro tendon
toilet
    pulmonary t.
tomography
    single photon emission com-
      puted t. (SPECT)
torsades de pointes
tortuous
    t. aorta
    t. veins
Touraine
    syndrome (I)
t-PA, tPA, TPA—tissue plasmino-
    gen activator
TPR—total pulmonary resistance
TPVR—total pulmonary vascular
    resistance
TR—tricuspid regurgitation

trabecula (trabeculae)
    trabeculae carneae cordis
    trabeculae cordis
trabecularism
trabeculate
trabeculation
tract
    See also *bundle.*
    atriohisian t.
tractus (tractus)
transaortic
    t. endarterectomy
translumbar aortography
transluminal
    percutaneous t. angioplasty
      (PTA)
    percutaneous t. atrial valvu-
      loplasty (PTAV)
    percutaneous t. coronary
      angioplasty (PTCA)
    percutaneous t. mitral valvu-
      loplasty (PTMV)
    percutaneous t. renal angio-
      plasty (PTRA)
transplantation
    heart t.
    lung t.
transposition
    t. of great vessels
transventricular
    t. closed valvotomy
    t. pulmonary valvotomy
Traube
    curves
    gallop rhythm
    heart
    heart murmur
    murmur
    sign
Traube-Hering waves
trauma (traumas, traumata)
traumatopnea
treadmill
    t. exercise test (TET)
    t. stress test (TST)
treatment
    Fränkel t.
    Karell t.

treatment (continued)
    Oertel t.
triad
    Beck t.
triangle
    Burger t.
    cardiohepatic t.
    Einthoven t.
    Scarpa t.
tricuspid
    t. atresia
    t. opening snap
    t. regurgitation
    t. stenosis
    t. valve
trifurcation
triglycerides
trigonal
trigonum (trigona)
    trigona fibrosa cordis
    t. fibrosum dextrum cordis
    t. fibrosum sinistrum cordis
trilogy
    t. of Fallot
troponin
    t. C
    t. I
    t. T
truncal
truncate
truncus (trunci)
    t. arteriosus
    t. brachiocephalicus
    t. fasciculi atrioventricularis
trunk
    brachiocephalic t.
TS—thoracic surgery
    tricuspid stenosis
TU—thiouracil
tubercle
    Lower t.
tubercula (plural of tuberculum)
tuberculoid
tuberculum (tubercula)
    t. intervenosum, t. intervenosum (Loweri)
    t. Loweri
tuberositas (tuberositates)

tuboplasty
    balloon t.
tumentia
tunic
    Bichat t.
tunica (tunicae)
    t. adventitia
    t. elastica interna
    t. intima vasorum
    t. media vasorum
    t. vasculosa
tunicate
turgor
    t. vitalis
Turner
    familial syndrome
    male syndrome
    phenotype with normal karyotype
    syndrome
    syndrome in females with normal X chromosome
T wave [noun]
T-wave [adj.]
    T-w. changes
    T-w. inversion
twelve-lead (12-lead) electrocardiography
two-dimensional
    t.-d. echocardiography (TDE)
two-pillow orthopnea
"u–" Phonetic for words beginning eu–.
Uhl anomaly
UK—urokinase
ultrasonic
    u. cardiography
ultrasonography
    A-mode u.
    Doppler u.
unit
    See also in *General Medical Terms* and *Laboratory, Pathology, and Chemistry Terms.*
    cardiac care u. (CCU)
    cardiology intensive care u. (CICU)

unit (continued)
>   coronary care u. (CCU)
>   coronary intensive care u.
>   (CICU)
>   critical care u. (CCU)
>   digitalis u.
>   intensive care u. (ICU)
>   intensive coronary care u.
>   (ICCU)
>   medical intensive care u.
>   (MICU)
>   peripheral resistance u. (PRU)
>   pulmonary intensive care u.
>   (PICU)
>   surgical intensive care u.
>   (SICU)

VA—ventriculoatrial
vagal
vagina (vaginae)
>   v. vasorum
vaginate
Valsalva
>   maneuver
>   sinus
valva (valvae)
>   v. aortae, v. aortica
>   v. atrioventricularis dextra
>   v. atrioventricularis sinistra
>   v. mitralis
>   v. pulmonaria
>   v. sinus venosi
>   v. tricuspidalis
>   v. trunci pulmonalis
valval, valvar
valvate
valve
>   v. of aorta, aortic v.
>   atrioventricular v.
>   bicuspid v.
>   bicuspid aortic v.
>   bicuspid pulmonary v.
>   cardiac v.'s
>   caval v.
>   coronary v.
>   v. of coronary sinus
>   eustachian v.
>   flail mitral v.
>   heart v.'s

valve (continued)
>   mitral v.
>   monocuspid aortic v.
>   parachute mitral v.
>   pulmonary v.
>   pulmonary trunk v., v. of
>   pulmonary trunk
>   quadricuspid aortic v.
>   quadricuspid pulmonary v.
>   semilunar v.
>   thebesian v.
>   tricuspid v.
>   v.'s of veins
valvectomy
valvotomy
>   mitral v.
>   pulmonary v.
>   transventricular closed v.
>   transventricular pulmonary v.
valvula (valvulae)
>   v. bicuspidalis
>   v. biscuspidalis (mitralis)
>   v. foraminis ovalis
>   v. mitralis
>   valvulae semilunares aortae
>   v. semilunaris
>   v. semilunaris anterior arte-
>   riae pulmonalis
>   v. semilunaris anterior trunci
>   pulmonalis
>   v. semilunaris dextra aortae
>   v. semilunaris dextra arteriae
>   pulmonalis
>   v. semilunaris dextra trunci
>   pulmonalis
>   v. semilunaris posterior aortae
>   v. semilunaris sinistra aortae
>   v. semilunaris sinistra arteri-
>   ae pulmonalis
>   v. semilunaris sinistra trunci
>   pulmonalis
>   v. sinus coronarii, v. sinus
>   coronarii (Thebesii)
>   v. tricuspidalis
>   v. venae cavae inferioris, v.
>   venae cavae inferioris
>   (Eustachii)
>   v. venosa

valvula (valvulae) (continued)
    v. vestibuli
valvular
    v. aortic stenosis
    v. stenosis
valvule
valvulectomy
valvulitis
    rheumatic v.
valvuloplasty
    aortic v.
    balloon v.
    catheter balloon v. (CBV)
    mitral v.
    percutaneous transluminal
        atrial v. (PTAV)
    percutaneous transluminal
        mitral v. (PTMV)
van Horne (van Hoorn, van Hoorne)
   canal
variant
    v. angina
variation
varicose
    v. vein
varicosity
varix (varices)
    anastomotic v.
    aneurysmal v., aneurysmoid v.
    arterial v.
    cirsoid v.
    gelatinous v.
vas (vasa)
    v. aberrans
vascular
    v. impedance
    v. resistance
    v. ring
    v. stenosis
vascularize
vasculitic
vasculopathy
vasculum (vascula)
    v. aberrans
vasiform
vasoconstriction
vasoconstrictive
vasoconstrictors [a class of drugs]

vasodilatation
vasodilators [a class of drugs]
vasoinhibitory
vasoligation
vasomotion
vasomotoricity
vasoneuropathy
vasoparalysis
vasoparesis
vasopressors [a class of drugs]
vasoreflex
vasorelaxation
vasosection
vasospasm
    refractory ergonovine-
        induced v.
vasospasmolytic
vasospastic
vasostimulant
vasotonia
vasotonic
vasovagal
VC—vena cava
VE—volumic ejection
vector
      P v.
      T v.
vectorcardiography (VCG)
    spatial v.
vegetation
      bacterial v.
      verrucous v.
vein
      azygos v.
      cephalic v.
      hepatic v. catheterization
      portal v.
      pulmonary v.
      saphenous v.
      varicose v.
vena cava (venae cavae)
      inferior v.c. (IVC)
      superior v.c. (SVC)
venacavogram
venacavography
      inferior v. (IVCV)
venacavotomy
venae cavae (plural of vena cava)

venectomy
venipuncture
venography
    ascending v.
    descending v.
    impedance v.
    limb v.
    peripheral v.
    radionuclide v.
    selective v.
    subtraction v.
venous
    v. aortography
    dynamic v. plethysmography
    v. hum
    v. occlusion plethysmography
    v. pressure
    v. pulse
    v. resistance
    v. return curve
    v. smooth muscle
    v. thromboembolism
    v. thrombosis
venovenostomy
"vent" Slang for ventricular.
ventilation
    arterial v.
    v.-perfusion (V/Q) ratio
    v. scintigraphy
    v. threshold
ventricle
    aortic v. of heart
    double-inlet v.
    double-outlet right v.
    v.'s of the heart
    left v. of heart
    right v. of heart
ventricular
    v. arrhythmia
    v. assist device
    v. contour
    v. dilatation
    v. ectopy
    v. end-diastolic volume
    v. end-systolic pressure
    v. fibrillation
    v. filling
    v. flutter

ventricular (continued)
    v. function
    v. fusion
    v. gradient
    v. hypertrophy
    v. interdependence
    v. mapping
    v. pacing
    v. performance
    v. premature beat
    v. premature contractions
    v. pressure-volume loop
    v. reentry
    v. relaxation
    v. rhythm
    v. septal defect
    v. septum
    v. systole
    v. tachyarrhythmia
    v. tachycardia
    v. wall motion
    v. wall shortening
ventriculi (plural of ventriculus)
ventriculoarterial
    v. coupling
ventriculography
    bubble v.
    cardiac v.
    contrast v.
    isotope v.
    radionuclide v.
ventriculomegaly
ventriculoplasty
ventriculovenostomy
ventriculus (ventriculi)
    v. cordis
    v. dexter cordis
    v. sinister cordis
Venturi
    effect
Verneuil
    canals
vertex (vertices)
    v. cordis
vertigo
    cardiovascular v.
vessel
    great v.'s

vestibule
    Gibson v.
    Sibson v.
VF—left leg (electrode)
    ventricular fibrillation
    ventricular fluid
VFP—ventricular fluid pressure
VG—ventricular gallop
VH—ventricular hypertrophy
VHD—valvular heart disease
vibration
    chest wall v.
videodensitometry
Vieussens
    foramen
villus (villi)
    pericardial v.
Vineberg
    operation
virus
    See specific viruses in *Laboratory, Pathology, and Chemistry Terms.*
visceral
    v. aortography
    selective v. aortography
visceropleural
vitium
    v. cordis
VLDL, VLDLP—very low-density lipoprotein
V leads: V_1–V_6 [V1–V6]
VMA—vanillylmandelic acid
von Bezold. See *Bezold.*
von Haller. See *Haller.*
von Willebrand (Willebrand)
    disease
    syndrome
vortex (vortices)
    v. cordis, v. of heart
VP—venipuncture
VPB—ventricular premature beat
VPC—ventricular premature complex
    ventricular premature contraction
VR—valve replacement
    vascular resistance

VS—ventricular septum
    vital signs
VSD—ventricular septal defect
VSS—vital signs stable
VSW—ventricular stroke work
VT—ventricular tachycardia
wandering
    w. pacemaker lead
Warren
    shunt
Waterston
    operation
    shunt
Watson-Alagille syndrome
wave
    A w.
    arterial w.
    C w.
    cannon w.
    catacrotic w., catadicrotic w.
    contraction w.
    cove-plane T w.
    dicrotic w.
    F w.
    fibrillary w.'s
    fibrillation w.'s
    Osborne w.
    oscillation w.
    overflow w.
    P w.
    papillary w.
    percussion w.
    peridicrotic w.
    predicrotic w.
    pre-excitation w.
    Q w.
    QRS w.
    R w.
    recoil w.
    respiratory w.
    S w.
    T w.
    tidal w.
    transverse w.
    Traube-Hering w.'s
    tricrotic w.
    U w.
    vasomotor w.

wave (continued)
 ventricular w.
 X w. of Öhnell
waveform
Weavenit
 patch graft
wedge
 w. resection
 w. pressure
Wenckebach
 cycle
 disease
 heart block
 period
 phenomenon
 sign
Willebrand. See *von Willebrand.*

Willebrand-Jürgens
 syndrome
Williams
 syndrome
Wolff-Parkinson-White syndrome
WPW—Wolff-Parkinson-White
 (syndrome)
Wrisberg
 ganglion
xenon (Xe)
 x. Xe 127
 x. Xe 133
"yoo–" Phonetic for words beginning eu–.
"zifoid" Phonetic for xiphoid.
Z lines
zone
 tendinous z.'s of heart

Dentistry
Includes Dental and Maxillofacial Surgery

AAA—amalgam
AADP—American Academy of
  Denture Prosthetics
AADR—American Academy of
  Dental Radiology
AADS—American Association of
  Dental Schools
AAE—American Association of
  Endodontists
AAID—American Academy of
  Implant Dentistry
AAO—American Association of
  Orthodontists
AAP—acute apical periodontitis
  American Academy of
    Pedodontics
  American Academy of Peri-
    odontology
AB—axiobuccal
ABC—axiobuccocervical
aberrant
  a. cementosis
  a. cementum
ABG—axiobuccogingival
ABL—axiobuccolingual
ablation
ablution
abocclusion
abrade
abrasio
  a. dentinum
abrasion
  acid a.
  bobby pin a.
  cervical a.
  dental a., denture a.
  dentifrice a.

abrasion (continued)
  gingival a.
  marginal a.
  occupational a.
  tooth a.
abrasive
  aluminum oxide a.
  diatomaceous silicon diox-
    ide a.
  a. disk
  FF a., FFF a. [degree of
    fineness]
  flint a.
  garnet a.
  iron oxide a.
  a. point
  polishing a.
  quartz a.
  silicon carbide a.
  silicon dioxide a.
  a. strip
  zirconium silicate a.
abscess
  alveolar a.
  apical a.
  Bezold (von Bezold) a.
  bicameral a.
  buccal space a.
  chronic a.
  cold a.
  dental a.
  dentoalveolar a.
  dry a.
  gingival a.
  interradicular a.
  lateral a.
  lateral root a.

377

abscess (continued)
    palatal a.
    parietal a.
    periapical a.
    pericemental a.
    pericoronal a.
    peridental a.
    periodontal a.
    periodontal infrabony a.
    phoenix a.
    pulp a., pulpal a.
    radicular a.
    recrudescent a.
    root a.
    sublingual space a.
    submandibular space a.
    submasseteric space a.
    submental space a.
    subperiosteal a.
    lateral alveolar a.
    tooth a.
    vestibular a.
abutment
    anterior a.
    auxiliary a.
    bombed a.
    bridge a.
    a. groove
    implant a.
    isolated a.
    multirooted a.
    a. post
    screw-type a.
    splinted a.
AC—axiocervical
aclusion
AD—axiodistal
ADA—American Dental Association
ADAA—American Dental Assis-
    tants Association
adamantine
adamantoblast
adamantoblastoma
adamas
    a. dentis
ADC—axiodistocervical
adenoameloblastoma
ADG—axiodistogingival

ADHA—American Dental Hygien-
    ists Association
adhesion
    sublabial a.
adhesive
    cyanoacrylate a.
    dental a., denture a.
ADI—axiodistoincisal
adjustment
    occlusal a.
admaxillary
ADO—axiodisto-occlusal
advancement
    maxillary a.
Aeby
    muscle
    plane
aerodontalgia
aerodontics
AG—axiogingival
agnathia
agnathous
agnathus
AI—axioincisal
Airbrasive
AL—axiolingual
ala (alae)
    a. nasi
Albrecht
    bone
    suture
alignment
    anatomical a.
    optimal a.
allotriodontia
alveolabial
alveolalgia
alveolar
    a. arch
    a. ridge
alveolate
alveolectomy
    transseptal a.
alveoli (genitive and plural of alve-
    olus)
alveolingual
alveolitis
    a. sicca dolorosa

alveoloclasia
alveolocondylean
alveolodental
alveololabial
alveololabialis
alveololingual
alveolomerotomy
alveolonasal
alveolopalatal
alveoloplasty
    interradicular a.
    intraseptal a.
alveolotomy
alveolus (alveoli)
    dental a.
    alveoli dentales mandibulae
    alveoli dentales maxillae
    alveoli dentis
alveolysis
amalgam
    copper a.
    dental a.
    retrograde a.
    silver a.
amalgamate
amalgamation
amalgamator
amelification
ameloblastoma
    acanthomatous a.
    basal cell a.
    cystic a.
    extraosseous a.
    follicular a.
    granular cell a.
    malignant a.
    multicystic a.
    peripheral a.
    plexiform a.
    plexiform unicystic a.
    solid a.
    unicystic a.
amelodentinal
amelogenesis
    a. imperfecta
amelogenic
anchorage

anesthesia
    See in *General Surgical Terms.*
angina
    Ludwig a.
anginal
"angkilo–" Phonetic for words beginning ankylo–.
angle
    antegonial a.
    Bennett a.
    Frankfort-mandibular plane a.
Angle [eponym]
    classification
ankylosed
ankylosis (ankyloses)
    dental a.
ankylotic
ankylotomy
anodontia
    partial a.
anomalad
anomaly
    Pierre Robin a.
antegonial
    a. angle
    a. notch
anterior
    a. palatine suture
antra (plural of antrum)
antrectomy
antrostomy
    intranasal a.
    radical maxillary a.
antrotomy
    sublabial a.
antrum (antra)
    a. of Highmore
ANUG—acute necrotizing ulcerative gingivitis
AP—axiopulpal
apertognathia
    Le Fort a. repair (I)
apex (apices, apexes)
    a. cuspidis
    a. cuspidis dentis
    flaring a.
    a. linguae, a. lingualis

apex (apices, apexes) (continued)
    a. radicis dentis
    radiographic a.
    root a.
apical
apices (plural of apex)
apicoectomy
apicolocator
apicostome
apicostomy
apophysis (apophyses)
apoxemena
apoxesis
appearance
    cotton-wool a.
    cystlike a.
    eggshell a.
    honeycomb a.
    lamina dura-like a.
    pigtail a.
    punched-out a.
    soap-bubble a.
    sun-ray a., sunray a.
    worm-eaten a.
appliance
    See also *prosthesis.*
apposition
approach
    transnasal a.
    transseptal a.
aqueduct
    fallopian a.
arch
    maxillary a.
    palatine a.
    zygomatic a.
arcus
    a. dentalis
    a. zygomaticus
atresia
atrophy
    gingival a.
attachment
    Gottlieb epithelial a.
attrition
AUG—acute ulcerative gingivitis
avulsion
    tooth a.

Babbitt metal
BAC—buccoaxiocervical
bacillus (bacilli)
    See in *Laboratory, Pathology, and Chemistry Terms.*
Bacillus
    See in *Laboratory, Pathology, and Chemistry Terms.*
bacterium (bacteria)
    See specific bacteria in *Laboratory, Pathology, and Chemistry Terms.*
band
    anchor b.
    elastic b. fication [of fracture]
    incisal b.
    orthodontic b.
    preformed b.
    premolar b.
    b. and spur retainer
bar
    fixation arch b.
barodontalgia
basifacial
basihyoid
BC—buccocervical
BD—buccodistal
beak
    b. of sphenoid bone
Begg
    light-wire differential force technique
    paralleling
    torque
Bell
    nerve
bell-crowned
Bennett
    angle
    movement
Bertin
    bone
    ossicles
BG—buccogingival
Bichat
    fat pad
    protuberance
bicuspidal

bicuspoid
bidental
bidentate
bimaxillary
biscuit
    hard b.
    medium b.
    soft b.
biscuiting
bisque
    hard b.
    low b.
    soft b.
bite
    balanced b.
    check b. [also: checkbite,
      check-bite]
    close b.
    convenience b.
    cross b. [also: crossbite,
      cross-bite]
    deep b.
    edge-to-edge b.
    end-to-end b.
    locked b.
    open b.
    raised b.
    rest b.
    scissors b.
    stork b.
    underhung b.
    wax b.
    X-b.
biteplane, bite-plane, bite plane
biteplate, bite-plate, bite plate
biterim, bite-rim, bite rim
bitewing, bite-wing, bite wing
BL—buccolingual
Black
    classification
black B, Sudan
bleaching
    coronal
"blef–" Phonetic for words begin-
    ning bleph–.
BLM (buccal-lingual-masticatory)
    dyskinesia

block
    infraorbital b.
blockout
BM—buccomesial
BO—bucco-occlusal
Bochdalek
    ganglion
    muscle
body (bodies)
    Bichat fatty b. of cheek
    b. of mandible
    b. of maxilla
    b. of sphenoid
    b. of tongue
Bondy
    mastoidectomy
Bonwill
    crown
    triangle
Boo-Chai craniofacial cleft
border
    See also *labium, limbus,* and
      margin.
    mucocutaneous b.
    vermilion b.
bow
    cupid's b.
    labial b.
bowl
    mastoid b.
Br—bridge
breath
    bad b.
bridge
    cantilever b.
    dentin b.
    removable b.
    stationary b.
bridou
Brophy
    operation
bruxism
buccal
    b. mucosa
    b. smear
    b. tube
buccally
buccoclination

buccolingually
bulb
    dental b.
burn-out
CA—cervicoaxial
cacodontia
calcification
Caldwell-Luc
    operation
canal
    alveolodental c.'s
    root c.
    zygomatico-orbital c.
canaliculus (canaliculi)
    canaliculi dentales
    incisor c.
canine
capsule
    cricoarytenoid articular c.
    dental c.
Carabelli
    cusp
    sign
    tubercle
carcinoma (carcinomas, carcinomata)
    See in *Oncology and Hematology* section.
caries
    arrested c.
    rampant c.
    senile dental c.
cariogenesis
cariogenic
cariogenicity
cariology
cariosity
cariostatic
carious
cartilage
    gingival c.
cavitary
    c. lesion
cavitas (cavitates)
    c. dentis
cavum (cava)
    c. dentis
C&B—crown and bridge

cell
    See in *Laboratory, Pathology, and Chemistry Terms.*
cellulitis
cementation
cementoperiostitis
cementosis
cementum
centric
    c. occlusion
    power c.
    c. relation
    true c.
ceramic
    dental c.'s
cervicoaxial
CFA—craniofacial abnormality
checkbite, check-bite, check bite
cheilosis
cheilotomy
cin–. See also words beginning sin–, syn–.
cingulectomy
cingulotomy
cingulum (cingula)
classification
    See also *index.*
    Angle c. of malocclusion
    Black c.
    Cummer c.
    Kennedy c.
    Skinner c.
    Tessier c. for clefts
cleft
    c. palate
coagulate
collum (colla)
    c. dentis
combined approach
    c.a. mastoidectomy
Commando
    operation
comminution
concentric
    c. pantomography
condensation
condylar

condyle
    c. of mandible
connector
conservative
    c. mastoidectomy
corona (coronae)
    c. dentis
coronal
coronoid
coronoidectomy
cortical
    c. mastoidectomy
corticalosteototomy
cotton-wool
    c.-w. appearance
CP&C—cast post and core
crepitation
crepitus
crest
crevice
    gingival c.
crevicular
cribra (plural of cribrum)
cribral
cribrate
cribration
cribriform
cribrum (cribra)
crista (cristae)
    c. buccinatoria
cristal
cristate
Crombie ulcer
crossbite, cross-bite, cross bite
crown
    Carmichael c.
    Davis c.
    dowel c.
crural
crusta (crustae)
    c. petrosa dentis
    c. radicis
crypt
    bony c.
    dental c.
    enamel c.
crypta (cryptae)

curettage
    subgingival c.
curettement
    root c.
cuspid
cuspidate
cuspis (cuspides)
    c. coronae
    c. dentales, c. dentis
cuticula (cuticulae)
    c. dentis
cuticular
cyst
    radicular c.
cytology
D—deciduous
DA—dental assistant
"da-breed-maw" Phonetic for
    débridement.
dam
    rubber d.
David
    disease
DB—distobuccal
DBO—distobucco-occlusal
DBP—distobuccopulpal
DC—distocervical
DDS, D.D.S.—Doctor of Dental
    Surgery
débridement
debris
dec—deciduous
deciduous
DEF, def—decayed, extracted, filled
DEF, def
    D. index
    D. rate
deglutition
Denonvilliers
    operation
dens (dentes)
    dentes acustici
    d. angulares
    dentes canini
    dentes decidui
    d. epistrophei
    dentes incisivi
    d. in dente

dens (dentes) (continued)
 d. invaginatus
 dentes molares
 dentes permanentes
 dentes premolares
 d. sapientiae
 d. serotinus
dentes (plural of dens)
dentia
 d. praecox
 d. tarda
denticle
 interstitial d.
dentin
 adventitious d.
 circumpulpar d.
 cover d.
 hereditary opalescent d.
 interglobular d.
 intermediate d.
 irregular d.
 mantle d.
 opalescent d.
 primary d.
 reparative d.
 sclerotic d.
 secondary d.
 sensitive d.
 tertiary d.
 transparent d.
dentinalgia
dentinogenesis
 d. imperfecta
dentition
 deciduous d.
 precocious d.
 predeciduous d.
 transitional d.
denture
 spoon d.
DG—distogingival
diastema (diastemata)
 anterior d.
dimension
 contact vertical d.
 occlusal vertical d.
 postural vertical d.
 rest vertical d.

dimension (continued)
 vertical d.
dis–. See also words beginning dys–.
discrepancy
disease
 See also *syndrome*.
 David d.
 Fauchard d.
 periodontal d.
 Riggs d.
 Spira d.
 Takahara d.
disharmony
 maxillomandibular d.
displacement
dissection
 blunt d.
 sharp d.
distal
DL—distolingual
DLA—distolabial
DLAI—distolabioincisal
DLI—distolinguoincisal
DLO—distolinguo-occlusal
DLP—distolinguopulpal
DMD, D.M.D.—Doctor of Dental
 Medicine
DMF (decayed, missing, filled) index
DO—disto-occlusal
DP—distopulpal
DPL—distopulpolingual
drilling
drip
 succinylcholine d.
duct
 parotid d.
 submandibular d.
 submaxillary d.
 Wharton d.
dys–. See also words beginning dis–.
dyskinesia
 BLM (buccal-lingual-masticatory) d.
EBF—elastic band fixation [of frac-
 ture]
EBF fixation of fracture
eburnation

eccentric
    e. pantomography
edentulism
edentulous
"ekselsimosis" Phonetic for exelcymosis.
"eksognatheon" Phonetic for exognathion.
"eksolever" Phonetic for exolever.
electrocautery
end
    e. tube
enucleation
enula
epiglottis
epignathous [adj.]
epignathus [noun]
epimandibular
epithelium (epithelia)
    dental e.
    oral e.
epulis (epulides)
    congenital e.
    e. fibromatosa, fibromatous e.
    e. fissurata
    giant cell e., e. gigantocellularis
    e. granulomatosa
    e. of newborn
equilibration
    occlusal e.
Erich
    operation
erythrodontia
evulsed
excavation
    dental e.
excementosis
excursion
    protrusive e.
    retrusive e.
exodontology
exolever
exostosis (exostoses)
    dental e.
extirpation
extrude
extrudoclusion

extrusion
exudation
FACD—Fellow of the American College of Dentists
"fatno–" Phonetic for words beginning phatno–.
Fauchard disease
faveolate
Fergusson
    incision
    operation
fetor
    f. exore
    f. oris
fibroma
    ameloblastic f.
    cementifying f.
    cemento-ossifying f.
    desmoplastic f.
    myxoid f.
fibromatosis
    f. gingivae
fibromyxoma
fibrosarcoma
    odontogenic f.
filtrum [part of larynx]
    See also *philtrum.*
    Merkel f. ventriculi
fistula (fistulas, fistulae)
    dental f.
    gingival f.
fistulous
fixation
    arch bar f.
    elastic band f. (EBF) of fracture
    intermaxillary f.
flange
    buccal f.
    labial f.
    lingual f.
flap
    f. operation
Fleischmann hygroma
FME—full-mouth extraction
FMS—full-mouth series
follicular

foramen (foramina)
    apical f. of root of tooth,
        apical f. of tooth
    f. apicis dentis
    greater palatine f.
    lesser palatine foramina
    mandibular f.
    mental f.
    foramina palatina minora
    f. radicis dentis
    Scarpa foramina
foraminal
form
    arch f.
    retention f.
    spherical f. of occlusion
    tooth f.
formula
    dental f.
fossa (fossae)
    glossoepiglottic f.
    Merkel f.
    occlusal f.
Fournier
    teeth
Franceschetti-Jadassohn syndrome
frena (plural of frenum)
frenal
frenulum (frenula)
frenum (frena)
    buccal f.
    lingual f.
    f. of tongue
Frey
    syndrome
Frey-Baillarger syndrome
frontoethmoidal
    f. suture
frontomalar
    f. suture
frontomaxillary
    f. suture
frontonasal
    f. suture
furca (furcae)
furcal
furcation
    denuded f.

furcation (continued)
    invaded f.
    f. invasion
    f. involvement
fusospirillary
fusospirillosis
G—gingival
GA—gingivoaxial
gauge
    bite g. [also: bitegage, bite-
        gage]
GBA—gingivobuccoaxial
gemination
Gilbert-Behçet syndrome
Gillies
    flap
    operation
gingiva (gingivae)
    alveolar g.
    areolar g.
    attached g.
    buccal g.
    cemental g.
    cemented g.
    cleft g.
    free g.
    interdental g.
    interproximal g.
    labial g.
    lingual g.
    marginal g.
    papillary g.
    septal g.
    unattached g.
gingivalgia
gingivally
gingival periodontal index (GPI)
gingivectomy
    Ochsenbein g.
gingivitis
    eruptive g.
    fusospirochetal g.
    herpetic g.
    marginal g.
    necrotizing ulcerative g.
gingivoaxial
gingivoglossitis
gingivosis

gingivostomatitis
    herpetic g.
GLA—gingivolinguoaxial
gland
    lingual g.
    Nuhn g.'s
    palatine g.
    parotid g.
    salivary g.
    sublingual g.
    submandibular salivary g.
    submaxillary g.
    Suzanne g.
glossectomy
glossoplasty
glossorrhaphy
glossotomy
gnathodynia
gnathoplasty
gnathoschisis
gomphiasis
Gorlin-Chaudhry-Moss
    syndrome
Goslee tooth
Gottlieb
    cuticle
    epithelial attachment
GP—gutta-percha
GPI—gingival periodontal index
granuloma
GT—gingiva, treatment of
gubernacula (plural of gubernaculum)
gubernacular
gubernaculum (gubernacula)
    g. dentis
Guérin
    fold
    fracture
    glands
    sinus
    valve
Günther
    syndrome
gutta-percha
Hajek
    operation
headgear
    Kloehn h.

Heath
    operation
hemimandibulectomy
hemimaxillectomy
hemisection
hemisectomy
herpes
    h. labialis
herpetic
Hertwig sheath
Highmore
    antrum
"hipo–" Phonetic for words begin-
    ning hypo–.
Hirschfeld
    canals
    disease
    method
horizontal
    h. tube
Horner
    teeth
Howship
    lacuna
Hutchinson
    syndrome
    teeth
    triad
hydrotherapy
hygienist
    dental h.
hygroma
    Fleischmann h.
hypercementosis
hyperdontia
hyperplasia
    cementum h.
    chronic perforating pulp h.
    denture h.
    Dilantin h.
    gingival h.
hyperplastic
hypertaurodontism
hypnodontics
hypocalcification
hypocone
hypoconid
hypoconule

hypoconulid
hypodontia
hypoglossal
hypoplasia
    craniofacial h.
    hereditary brown h. of enamel
    nasomaxillary h.
    h. of tooth
I—incisor, permanent
imbrication
immobilization
IMPA—incisal mandibular plane
   angle
impaction
impression
incision
    Risdon extraoral i.
incisive
    i. suture
inclination
index (indexes, indices)
    See also *classification.*
    decayed, extracted, filled
      (def) caries i.
    DMF (decayed, missing, or
      filled) i.
    gingival periodontal i. (GPI)
    palatal i.
    palatal height i.
    palatine i.
    palatomaxillary i.
    periodontal i.
    PMA (papilla, gingival mar-
      gin, and attached gingiva) i.
Indian
    operation
infection
    apical i.
    Vincent i.
Ingrassia
    apophysis
    process
    wings
injection
    nasopalatine i.
interfurca (interfurcae)
intermaxillary
    i. suture

internasal
    i. suture
interosseous
interpalatine
    i. suture
interradicular alveoloplasty
intranasal
    i. antrostomy
intrapulpal
intraseptal alveoloplasty
IP—incisioproximal
Italian
    operation
Jacob
    disease
Jacobson
    cartilage
Johanson-Blizzard syndrome
joint
    temporomandibular j. (TMJ)
Joseph
    operation
juga (plural of jugum)
jugale
jugate
jugomaxillary
jugum (juga)
Kazanjian
    operation
Kennedy
    classification
keratosis (keratoses)
    k. labialis
Killian
    operation
Killian-Freer
    operation
Körte-Ballance
    operation
LA—linguoaxial
labia (plural of labium)
labial
labially
labium (labia)
    See also *border, limbus,* and
      margin.
    l. mandibulare
    l. maxillare

labium (labia) (continued)
  labia oris
labrale
lacrimoconchal
  l. suture
lacrimoethmoidal
  l. suture
lacrimomaxillary
  l. suture
lacrimoturbinal
  l. suture
lacuna (lacunae)
  absorption l.
  Howship l.
  resorption l.
lacunar
lacunula (lacunulae)
lacunule
LAG—labiogingival
LAI—labioincisal
lamella (lamellae)
  enamel lamellae
lamellar
lamelliform
lamina (laminae)
  buccal l.
  buccogingival l.
  dental l.
  dentogingival l.
  labial l.
  labiodental l.
  labiogingival l.
  palatine l. of maxilla
laminar
larynx
layer
LD—linguodistal
LDDS—local dentist
ledging
Le Fort
  apertognathia repair (I)
lesion
  impaction l.
leukoedema
leukokeratosis
leukoplakia
  l. buccalis
  l. lingualis

leukoplakia (continued)
  oral l.
  ·   speckled l.
LG—linguogingival
LI—linguoincisal
limbus (limbi)
  See also *border, labium,* and
    margin.
  alveolar l. of mandible
  l. alveolaris mandibulae
  alveolar l. of maxilla
  l. alveolaris maxillae
line
  blue l.
  Burton l.
  calcification l.'s
  cervical l.
  Clapton l.
  contour l.'s
  copper l.
  Corrigan l.
  gingival l.
  gum l.
  lead l.
  mucogingival l.
  l. of occlusion
  l.'s of Owen
  Pickerill imbrication l.'s
  Retzius l.'s
  Salter incremental l's
lingual
linguale
lingually
lingula (lingulae)
  l. of lower jaw
  l. of mandible
  l. mandibulae
lingular
linguoplate
  palatal l.
LM—linguomesial
LO—linguo-occlusal
LP—linguopulpal
Luc
  operation
Ludwig
  angina
m—molar, deciduous

M—mesial
    molar, permanent
macrodont
macrodontia
macrodontic
macrogenia
macrogingivae
macrotooth (macroteeth)
macula (maculae)
macule
Malassez
    epithelial rests
malomaxillary
    m. suture
mamelon
mammillary
    m. suture
mandibula (mandibulae)
mandibular
    m. resection
mandibulectomy
margin
    See also *border, labium,* and
      limbus.
    alveolar m. of mandible
    alveolar m. of maxilla
    dentate m.
    free gingival m.
    free gum m.
    gingival m.
    gum m.
    incisal m.
    infraorbital m. of maxilla
    infraorbital m. of orbit
    lacrimal m. of maxilla
    lateral margin of orbit
    malar m.
    medial m. of orbit
    orbital m.
margo (margines)
mass
    Stent m.
massage
    gingival m.
mastication
    muscles of m.
masticatory

mastoid
    m. obliteration operation
    m. operation
    m. suture
mastoidectomy
    Bondy m.
    combined approach m.
    conservative m.
    cortical m.
    modified radical m.
    radical m.
    Schwartze m.
    simple m.
matrix (matrices)
    amalgam m.
maxilla (maxillae, maxillas)
maxillary
    radical m. antrostomy
    m. resection
maxillodental
maxillolabial
maxillomandibular
maxillotomy
MB—mesiobuccal
MBO—mesiobucco-occlusal
MBP—mesiobuccopulpal
median
    m. palatine suture
medicine
    oral m.
melanotrichia
    m. linguae
membrane
    dentinoenamel m.
    Nasmyth m.
    peridental m.
mentalis
mercury (Hg)
Merkel
    fossa
mesiad [adv.]
mesial [adj.]
mesially
mesiobuccal (MB)
mesiobucco-occlusal (MBO)
mesiobuccopulpal (MBP)
mesiocervical
mesioclination

mesioclusion
mesiodens (mesiodentes)
mesiodistal
mesiogingival (MG)
mesioincisodistal (MID)
mesiolabial (MLA)
mesiolabioincisal (MLAI)
mesiolingual (ML)
mesiolinguoincisal (MLI)
mesiolinguo-occlusal (MLO)
mesiolinguopulpal (MLP)
mesio-occlusal (MO)
mesio-occlusodistal (MOD)
mesiopalatal
mesiopulpal (MP)
mesiopulpolabial (MPLA)
mesiopulpolingual (MPL)
mesioversion
metaplasia
    m. of pulp
metodontiasis
MG—mesiogingival
microdont
microdontia
microdontic
micrognathia
micrognathism
micromandible
micromaxilla
microstomia
microsurgery
MID—mesioincisodistal
middle
    m. palatine suture
migration
    tooth m., pathologic
    tooth m., physiologic
milling-in
ML—mesiolingual
MLA—mesiolabial
MLAI—mesiolabioincisal
MLI—mesiolinguoincisal
MLO—mesiolinguo-occlusal
MLP—mesiolinguopulpal
MO—mesio-occlusal
MOD—mesio-occlusodistal
modified
    m. radical mastoidectomy

molar
Moon
    molars
    teeth
mouthwash
MP—mesiopulpal
MPL—mesiopulpolingual
MPLA—mesiopulpolabial
mucocele
mucogingival
mucosa
    buccal m.
    retromolar m.
    retrotuberosity m.
mucosal
mucosanguineous
mucoserous
Mueller
    See also *Müller.*
    operation
Mules
    operation
Müller
    See also *Mueller.*
    muscle
multicuspid
multirooted
Mummery
    pink tooth
mummification
muscle
    See also in *Orthopedics and*
        Sports Medicine section.
    buccinator m.
    canine m.
    depressor m. of angle of
        mouth
    depressor m. of lower lip
    depressor m. of septum of
        nose
    digastric m.
    facial and masticatory m.'s
    glossopalatine m.
    glossopharyngeal m.
    incisive m.'s of lip (inferior,
        lower, superior, upper)
    levator m. of palatine velum
    levator m. of upper lip

muscle (continued)
>levator m. of upper lip and ala of nose
>levator m. of velum palatinum
>masseter m.
>m.'s of mastication
>masticatory m.
>mylohyoid m.
>orbicular m. of mouth
>palatine m.'s
>pharyngopalatine m.
>platysma m.
>pterygoid m. (external, internal, lateral, medial)
>quadrate m. of lower lip
>quadrate m. of upper lip
>risorius m.
>Santorini m.
>sternocleidomastoid m.
>styloglossus m.
>temporal m.
>tensor m. of velum palatinum

musculus (musculi)
>See in *Orthopedics and Sports Medicine* section.

Mustardé
>flap
>otoplasty

nasal
>n. suture

Nasmyth membrane

nasofrontal
>n. suture

"natho–" Phonetic for words beginning gnatho–.

navel
>enamel n.

neck
>surgical n. of tooth

necrosis (necroses)
>exanthematous n.
>gangrenous pulp n.
>mandibular n.
>phosphorus n.

necrotic

necrotizing
>n. gingivitis
>n. sialometaplasia

nerve
>alveolar n.'s
>buccal n.
>buccinator n.
>dental n., inferior
>glossopalatine n.
>glossopharyngeal n.
>hypoglossal n.
>lingual n.
>mandibular n.
>masseteric n.
>maxillary n.
>mental n.
>palatine n.
>sublingual n.
>submaxillary n.'s

Neumann
>sheath

notch
>antegonial n.
>mandibular n.
>palatine n.

Nuhn glands

OC—occlusocervical

occlusion
>o., classes I–III
>abnormal o.
>acentric o.
>acquired eccentric o.
>afunctional o.
>anatomical o.
>anterior o.
>balanced o.
>buccal o.
>centric o.
>distal o.
>dynamic o.
>eccentric o.
>edge-to-edge o.
>equilibrated o.
>functional o.
>gliding o.
>habitual o.
>hyperfunctional o.
>ideal o.
>labial o.
>lateral o.
>lingual o.

occlusion (continued)
    locked o.
    mechanically balanced o.
    mesial o.
    neutral o.
    normal o.
    pathogenic o.
    physiologically balanced o.
    posterior o.
    postnormal o.
    prenormal o.
    protrusive o.
    retrusive o.
    skeletal o.
    spherical form of o.
    terminal o.
    traumatic o.
    traumatogenic o.
    working o.
Ochsenbein
    gingivectomy
ODD—oculodentodigital
ODD dysplasia
odontagra
odontalgia
    phantom o.
odontatrophia
odontectomy
odontiasis
odontocele
odontoceramic
odontocia
odontoclasis
odontogenesis
    o. imperfecta
odontoglyph
odontohyperesthesia
odontoloxia
odontonecrosis
odontoneuralgia
odontoplerosis
odontoptosis
odontorrhagia
odontosteophyte
odontotomy
odontotrypy
OFD—oral-facial-digital
    orofaciodigital

OFD dysplasia
OFD syndrome (I, II)
Ogston-Luc
    operation
"oolo–" Phonetic for words beginning ulo–.
operation
    See also in *General Surgical Terms.*
    Brophy o.
    Caldwell-Luc o.
    Commando o.
    Denonvilliers o.
    Erich o.
    Fergusson o.
    flap o.
    Gillies o.
    Hajek o.
    Heath o.
    Indian o.
    Italian o.
    Joseph o.
    Kazanjian o.
    Killian o.
    Killian-Freer o.
    Körte-Ballance o.
    Luc o.
    mastoid o.
    mastoid obliteration o.
    Mueller o.
    Mules o.
    Ogston-Luc o.
    osteoplastic frontal sinus o.
    palatal pushback o.
    Partsch o.
    radical antrum o.
    Regnoli o.
    Rose o.
    Rose-Thompson o.
    Skoog o.
    Tennison o.
    Tennison-Randall o.
    Tessier o.
opercula (plural of operculum)
opercular
operculate
operculectomy
operculitis

operculum (opercula)
    cartilaginous o.
    dental o.
oromandibular
oropharynx
orthopedics
    dental o.
    dentofacial o.
    functional jaw o.
os (ossa) [bone]
    See in *Orthopedics and*
       Sports Medicine section.
OS—oral surgery
ostectomy
osteocementum
osteodentin
osteodentinoma
osteoma
    o. dentale
    maxillary o.
osteomatoid
osteomatosis
osteo-odontoma
osteoperiostitis
    alveolodental o.
osteoplastic
    o. frontal sinus operation
osteotomy
otoplasty
    Mustardé o.
oulectomy
OVD—occlusal vertical dimension
overbite
    deep o.
    horizontal o.
    vertical o.
overdenture
overjut
overriding
Owen
    contour lines
    view
P—premolar
PA—pulpoaxial
pack
    oropharyngeal p.
palata (plural of palatum)

palatal
    p. height index
    p. index
palate
    cleft p.
    submucous cleft p.
palati (genitive of palatum)
palatine
    anterior p. suture
    p. bone
    p. index
    median p. suture
    middle p. suture
    posterior p. suture
    transverse p. suture
palatoethmoidal
    p. suture
palatomaxillary
    p. index
    p. suture
palatum (palata)
    p. durum
    p. durum osseum
    p. fissum
    p. molle
    p. ogivale
    p. osseum
pan-oral radiography
panoramic
    p. radiography
    p. tomography
Panorex
pantomography
    concentric p.
    eccentric p.
papilla (papillae)
    dental p., dentinal p., p. dentis
    gingival p., p. gingivalis
    p. incisiva, incisive p.
    interdental p.
    p. interdentalis
    interproximal p.
    retromolar p.
papillate
papillation
papilliferous
papilliform
Papillon-Lefèvre syndrome

parodontal
parodontid
parotid
partial
    p. pulpectomy
Partsch
    operation
pathogen
    See specific pathogens in
    Laboratory, Pathology,
    and Chemistry Terms.
pattern
    rugal p.
PBA—pulpobuccoaxial
PD—pulpodistal
PDI—periodontal disease index
pearl
    enamel p.
perforation
    root p.
pericementitis
    apical p.
pericementoclasia
perikyma (perikymata)
periodontics
periodontist
periodontitis
periodontium (periodontia)
    p. insertionis
    p. protectionis
    p. protectoris
periodontoclasia
periodontology
periodontosis
periosteum
    p. alveolare
pharyngeal
pharynx
phatnoma
phatnorrhagia
philtrum [vertical groove above
    upper lip; compare: filtrum]
PI—periodontal index
pigmentation
    gingival p.
pillar
    p.'s of soft palate

"pio–" Phonetic for words begin-
    ning pyo–.
PL—pulpolingual
PLA—pulpolabial
    pulpolinguoaxial
plane
    axial p. of tooth
    axiolabiolingual p.
    axiomesiodistal p.
    bite p. [also: biteplane,
      bite-plane]
    buccolingual p.
    cusp p.
    labiolingual p.
    mesiodistal p.
    occlusal p., p. of occlusion
    tooth p.
plaque
    dental p.
plate
    bite p. [also: biteplate, bite-
      plate]
    cortical p.
    dental p.
    lingual p.
    palatal p.
    spring p.
platysma
pliers
    crown-crimping p.
PM—pulpomesial
PMA—papillary, marginal, attached
   [prevalence of gingivitis]
poikilodentosis
polishing
polydontia
polysinusectomy
porcelain
    dental p.
porcelaneous
posterior
    p. palatine suture
pouch
    Rathke p.
PP—permanent partial
PR—prosthion
premaxillary
    p. suture

prisma (prismata)
>prismata adamantina

procedure
>See *maneuver, method, operation,* and *technique.*

process
>mastoid p.
>maxillary p.

profile
>prognathic p.
>retrognathic p.

prominence
>See *apophysis, process, protuberance* and *swelling.*

prophylactodontics

prophylaxis

prosthesis (prostheses)
>See also *appliance.*

prosthion (PR)

prosthodontics

prosthodontist

protrusion

protuberance

pulp
>coronal p.
>mummified p.
>necrotic p.
>radicular p.

pulpa (pulpae)
>p. coronale
>p. dentis
>p. radicularis

pulpal

pulpalgia

pulpectomy
>partial p.

pulpiform

pulpitis (pulpitides)
>anachoretic p.
>closed p.
>hyperplastic p.
>open p.

pulpless

pulpoaxial

pulpobuccoaxial

pulpodistal

pulpolabial

pulpolingual

pulpolinguoaxial

pulpomesial

pulpotomy

pulpy

pultaceous

purchase
>p. point

pushback
>palatal p.

putrescence

pyorrhea
>p. alveolaris
>paradental p.
>Schmutz p.

radectomy

radical [adj.]
>r. antrum operation
>r. mastoidectomy
>r. maxillary antrostomy
>modified r. mastoidectomy

radices (plural of radix)

radiciform

radicis (genitive of radix)

radicular

radiectomy

radiograph
>bite-wing r.
>extraoral r.
>intraoral r.
>panoramic r.
>periapical r.

radiography
>pan-oral r.
>panoramic r.

radiology
>dental r., oral r.

radiolucency

radisectomy

radix (radices)
>r. dentis

"ra-fee" Phonetic for raphe.

ramus (rami)

raphe (raphae)
>buccal r.
>r. palati
>palatine r.
>pterygomandibular r.
>r. pterygomandibularis

raphes (genitive of raphe)
Rathke
    pouch
ratio
    clinical crown-clinical root r.
record
    dental identification r.
region
    buccal r.
    infraorbital r.
    mental r.
    oral r.
    retromaxillary r.
    submandibular r.
    submaxillary r.
    submental r.
Regnoli
    operation
replantation
    intentional r.
reposition
resection
    mandibular r.
    maxillary r.
    submucosal r.
    submucous r. and rhinoplasty (SMRR)
restbite
restoration
    crown r.
retraction
    gingival r.
Retzius
    lines
    parallel striae
    stripes
rhagades [grammatically plural; no singular form]
rhinoplasty
    submucous resection and r. (SMRR)
rhizodontropy
rhizodontrypy
rhizoid
ridge
Rieger
    dysgenesis
Riggs disease

Risdon
    extraoral incision
"rizo–" Phonetic for words beginning rhizo–.
RMT—retromolar trigone
roentgentherapy
    intraoral r.
root
    r. curettement
    r. resection
root canal
root-splitting forceps
Rose [eponym]
    operation
    position
Rose-Thompson
    operation
    repair
rubber
    r. band [also: rubber-band]
ruga (rugae)
    rugae palatinae, palatine rugae
rugal pattern
rugate
Rutherfurd syndrome
sacculated
sacculi (genitive and plural of sacculus)
sacculiform
sacculus (sacculi)
    s. dentis
Salter
    incremental lines
saprodontia
sarcoma (sarcomas, sarcomata)
    See in *Oncology and Hematology* section.
scaling
    deep s.
    root s.
    subgingival s.
    ultrasonic s.
scan
    See in *Radiology, Nuclear Medicine, and Other Imaging* section.

Scarpa
    foramina
Schmutz pyorrhea
Schreger
    striae
Schwartze
    mastoidectomy
scissors-bite
sclerosis
    dentinal s.
"scopes" See under full name.
    microgonioscope
    odontoscope
    periodontoscope
section
    root s.
segmenta (plural of segmentum)
segmental
segmentum (segmenta)
semicrista (semicristae)
    s. incisiva
septa (plural of septum)
septal
    s. resection
septi (genitive of septum)
septum (septa)
    s. alveoli
    bucconasal s.
    deviated nasal s.
    dorsal median s.
    enamel s.
    gingival s.
    gum s.
    interalveolar s.
    interdental s.
    interradicular s.,
    s. linguae, lingual s.
    s. of tongue
sequestra (plural of sequestrum)
sequestral
sequestration
sequestrectomy
sequestrotomy
sequestrum (sequestra)
sheath
    dentinal s.
    Neumann s., s. of Neumann

shelf
    buccal s.
    dental s.
    palatal s.
    palatine s.
shoulder
    linguogingival s.
sign
    Burton s.
    Carabelli s.
    floating-tooth s.
    Hutchinson s.
    Roux s.
simple
    s. mastoidectomy
sin–. See also words beginning
    cin–, syn–.
"singul–" Phonetic for words
    beginning cingul–.
sinus (sinus, sinuses)
    dental s.
    oral s.
Skoog
    operation
SMR—submucous resection
SMRR—submucous resection and
    rhinoplasty
socket
    dry s.
sordes (sordes)
sore
    canker s.
    cold s. [pref: coldsore]
    denture s.
space
    apical s.
    s.'s in dentin
    interdental s.
    subgingival s.
    submaxillary s.
sphenomalar
    s. suture
sphenomaxillary
    s. suture
spheno-orbital
    s. suture
sphenovomerine
    s. suture

sphenozygomatic
    s. suture
sphincter
    s. oris
spicular
spiculated
spicule
spiculum
Spira disease
splint
    acrylic s.
    canine-to-canine lingual s.
spoon
    s. denture
spot
stability
    denture s.
stabilizer
    endodontic s.
stenocompressor
Stent [eponym]
    compound
    mass
Stim-U-Dents
stomatitis (stomatitides)
    acute necrotizing s.
    allergic s.
    angular s.
    aphthobullous s.
    s. aphthosa
    aphthous s.
    s. arsenicalis
    bismuth s.
    catarrhal s.
    contact s.
    denture s.
    epidemic s.
    epizootic s.
    erythematopultaceous s.
    s. exanthematica
    fusospirochetal s.
    gangrenous s.
    gonococcal s.
    gonorrheal s.
    herpetic s.
    infectious s.
    s. intertropica
    lead s.

stomatitis (stomatitides) (continued)
    s. medicamentosa
    membranous s.
    mercurial s.
    mycotic s.
    necrotizing ulcerative s.
    s. nicotina
    nonspecific s.
    s. prosthetica
    recurrent aphthous s.
    s. scarlatina
    s. scorbutica
    syphilitic s.
    traumatic s.
    tropical s.
    ulcerative s.
    uremic s.
    s. venenata
    vesicular s.
    Vincent s.
    vulcanite s.
stomatorrhagia
    s. gingivarum
strata (plural of stratum)
stratiform
stratum (strata)
    s. adamantinum
    s. eboris
stria (striae)
    Retzius parallel striae
    Schreger s.
striatal
subgingival
    s. curettage
sublabial
    s. antrotomy
submucosal
    s. resection
submucous
    s. cleft palate
    s. resection (SMR)
    s. resection and rhinoplasty
      (SMRR)
substance
    adamantine s. of tooth
    bony s. of tooth
substantia (substantiae)
    s. adamantina dentis

substantia (substantiae) (continued)
    s. eburnea dentis
sulci (plural of sulcus)
sulciform
sulculus (sulculi)
sulcus (sulci)
    alveolabial s.
    alveolingual s.
    alveolobuccal s.
    buccal s.
    gingival s.
    gingivobuccal s.
    gingivolingual s.
    greater palatine s. of maxilla
    greater palatine s. of palatine bone
    infraorbital s. of maxilla
    labiodental s.
    lingual s.
    mandibular s.
    median s. of tongue, s. medianus linguae
    mentolabial s.
    palatine sulci of maxilla
    sphenovomerian s.
    vomeral s.
supernumerary
suppuration
    alveodental s.
surgery
    dental s.
    dentofacial s.
    maxillofacial s.
    oral s.
    oral and maxillofacial s.
surgical procedure
suture [material]
    See in *General Surgical Terms.*
suture [technique]
    See in *General Surgical Terms.*
Suzanne gland
swelling
symphysis (symphyses)
syn–. See also words beginning cin–, sin–.

syndesmosis (syndesmoses)
    dentoalveolar s., s. dentoalveolaris
syndrome
    See also *disease.*
    Gorlin-Chaudhry-Moss s.
    Günther s.
    PHC s.
    Rutherfurd s.
    temporomandibular dysfunction s.
    temporomandibular joint (TMJ) s.
Takahara disease
tattoo
    amalgam t.
TE—tooth extracted
technique
    Begg light-wire differential force t.
teeth (plural of tooth)
temporomalar
    t. suture
temporozygomatic
    t. suture
Tennison
    operation
Tennison-Randall
    operation
Tessier
    operation
test
    See in *Laboratory, Pathology, and Chemistry Terms.*
therapy
    myofunctional t.
    pulp canal t.
    root canal t.
tic
    t. douloureux ["doo-loo-roo"]
tipping
TMJ—temporomandibular joint
TMJ syndrome
tomography
    panoramic t.
tongue
    adherent t.
    bifid t.

tongue (continued)
    cleft t.
    double t.
    split t.
    stippled t.
tooth (teeth)
    abutment t.
    accessional t.
    accessory t.
    acrylic resin t.
    anatomical t.
    anchor t.
    ankylosed t.
    anterior teeth
    artificial t.
    baby teeth
    back t.
    barred t.
    bicuspid t.
    brown opalescent t., heredi-
      tary
    buccal t.
    buck t.
    canine t.
    cheek t.
    cheoplastic t.
    Chiaie t.
    conical t.
    connate t.
    corner t.
    cross-bite t., crossbite t.
    cross-pin t.
    cuspid t., cuspidate t.
    cuspless t.
    cutting t.
    dead t.
    deciduous t.
    devital t., devitalized t.
    diatoric t.
    drifting t.
    embedded t.
    extruded t.
    eye t.
    fluoridated t.
    Fournier t.
    fused t.
    geminate t., geminated t.
    ghost t.

tooth (teeth) (continued)
    Goslee t.
    green t.
    hag t.
    hair t.
    hereditary brown opalescent t.
    Horner t.
    Hutchinson teeth
    hutchinsonian t.
    impacted t.
    incisor t.
    labial t.
    malacotic t.
    malposed t.
    mandibular t.
    maxillary t.
    metal insert t.
    migrating t.
    milk t.
    molar t.
    Moon t.
    morsal t.
    mottled t.
    mulberry t.
    multicuspid t.
    natal t.
    neonatal t.
    nonanatomic t.
    nonvital t.
    normally posed t.
    notched t.
    oral t.
    peg t., pegged t.
    peg-shaped t.
    pegtop t.
    permanent t.
    perpetually growing t., per-
      sistently growing t.
    pink t. of Mummery
    pinless t.
    plastic t.
    posterior t.
    predeciduous t.
    premature t.
    premilk t.
    premolar t.
    primary t.
    protruding t.

tooth (teeth) (continued)
    pulpless t.
    rake t.
    rootless t.
    rotated t.
    sclerotic t.
    screwdriver t.
    second t.
    shell t.
    snaggle t.
    spaced t.
    stomach t.
    straight-pin t.
    submerged t.
    succedaneous t.
    successional t.
    superior t.
    supernumerary t.
    supplemental t.
    syphilitic t.
    temporary t.
    tube t.
    Turner t.
    unerupted t.
    vital t.
    wandering t.
    wisdom t.
    zero-degree t.
toothache
tooth-borne
toothbrushing
toothed
toothpick
tophus (tophi)
    dental t.
tori (plural of torus)
torus (tori)
    buccal t.
    t. mandibulae
    t. mandibularis
    palatine t.
    t. palatinus
    supraorbital t.
traction
    elastic t.
    intermaxillary t.
    intraoral elastic t.
    maxillomandibular t.

transplantation
    tooth t.
transseptal
    t. alveolectomy
transverse
    t. palatine suture
    t. suture of Krause
trauma (traumas, traumata)
    occlusal t.
    periodontal t.
    potential t.
    primary occlusal t.
    secondary occlusal t.
traumatism
    occlusal t.
    periodontal t.
treatment
    preventive t., prophylactic t.
    root canal t.
trephination
    dental t.
TT—tooth, treatment of
tube
    buccal t.
    end t.
    horizontal t.
tubercula (plural of tuberculum)
tuberculoid
tuberculum (tubercula)
    t. coronae
    t. dentale, t. dentis
    t. geniale
    t. labii superioris
    t. mentale mandibulae
tuberositas (tuberositates)
    t. masseterica
    t. pterygoidea mandibulae
Turner
    tooth
    tooth hypoplasia
tympanomastoid
    t. suture
ulcer
    Crombie u.
Ullrich-Feichtiger
    syndrome
ulocace
"ulokahse" Phonetic for ulocace.

ulotomy
unit
> See also in *General Medical
> Terms* and *Laboratory,
> Pathology, and Chemistry
> Terms.*
>
> dental u.

UPP, UPPP—uvulopalatopharyngoplasty
uvula (uvulae)
uvular
uvularis
uvulectomy
velum (vela)
> Baker v.
> v. palati
> palatine v.
> v. palatinum

vermilion
> v. border

vestibular
vestibuloplasty
view
> panoramic v.

Vincent
> infection
> stomatitis

vinculum (vincula)
virus
> See specific viruses in *Labo-
> ratory, Pathology, and
> Chemistry Terms.*

vulcanite
wedge
> dental w.

Wharton
> duct

WHO—World Health Organization
xanthodontus
xanthoma (xanthomas, xanthomata)
> verruciform x.

X-bite
"yulo–" Phonetic for words beginning ulo–.
zone
> contact area z.
> coronal z.
> dentofacial z.
> neutral z.
> occlusal z.

zygomaticofrontal
> z. suture

zygomaticomaxillary
> z. suture

Dermatology

AAD—American Academy of Dermatology
ABC—aspiration biopsy cytology
Abernethy
    sarcoma
abradant
abrade
abscess
    follicular a.
    fungal a.
    Munro a.
    Monro a.
    Paget a., Paget a. syndrome
    Pautrier a.
    phlegmonous a.
    pulp a., pulpal a.
    subcutaneous a.
    subepidermal a.
    subungual a.
    sudoriparous a.
abtropfung
acanthamebiasis
acantholysis
    a. bullosa
acantholytic
acanthoma
    a. adenoides cysticum
    basal cell a.
    clear cell a.
    Degos a.
    a. inguinale
    pilar sheath a.
    a. tropicum
    a. verrucosa seborrheica
acanthosis
    malignant a. nigricans
    a. nigricans
    a. papulosa nigra
    a. seborrheica
    a. verrucosa
acari (plural of acarus)

acarian
acaricide
acarid
acarine
acarodermatitis
    a. urticarioides
acaroid
acarotoxic
ACD—allergic contact dermatitis
acetamidine
achromasia
achromia
    congenital a.
    consecutive a.
    a. parasitica
achromic
    a. nevus
acid
    trichloroacetic a.
aciduric
acne
    adolescent a.
    a. albida
    apocrine a.
    a. artificialis
    a. atrophica
    a. bacillus
    bromide a.
    a. cachecticorum
    a. cheloidalis
    chlorine a.
    a. ciliaris
    colloid a.
    comedo a.
    common a.
    a. conglobata, conglobate a.
    contact a.
    a. cosmetica
    cystic a., a. cystica
    a. decalvans
    a. detergicans

acne (continued)
   a. disseminata
   a. dorsalis
   epidemic a.
   a. erythematosa
   a. estivalis
   excoriated a.
   a. excoriée des filles, a.
      excoriée des jeunes filles
   a. frontalis
   a. fulminans
   a. generalis
   halogen a.
   a. hypertrophica
   a. indurata
   infantile a.
   a. inversa
   iodide a.
   a. keloid
   a. keloidalis, a. keloidalis
      nuchae
   a. keratosa
   lupoid a.
   a. mechanica, mechanical a.
   a. medicamentosa
   menstrual a.
   a. mentagra
   a. miliaris, miliary a.
   a. necrotica, a. necrotica
      miliaris
   a. necroticans et exulcerans
      serpiginosa nasi
   neonatal a., a. neonatorum
   nodulocystic a.
   occupational a.
   oil a.
   papular a., a. papulosa
   petroleum a.
   picker's a.
   pomade a.
   premenstrual a.
   a. punctata
   pustular a., a. pustulosa
   a. rosacea
   a. scorbutica
   a. scrofulosorum
   a. seborrheica
   a. simplex

acne (continued)
   steroid a.
   summer a.
   a. syphilitica
   systemic a.
   tar a.
   a. tarsi
   a. telangiectodes
   tropical a., a. tropicalis
   a. urticata
   a. varioliformis
   a. venenata
   a. vulgaris
acnegen
acnitis
acritochromacy
acrocyanosis
acrodermatitis
   a. chronica atrophicans
   a. continua
   a. enteropathica
   Hallopeau a.
   a. hiemalis
   papular a.
   a. papulosa infantum
   a. perstans
   pustular a.
   a. vesiculosa tropica
acrodermatosis (acrodermatoses)
acrodynia
acrohyperhidrosis
acrokeratoelastoidosis
acrokeratosis
   paraneoplastic a.
   a. verruciformis
acromelalgia
acromicria
acropachyderma
   a. with pachyperiostitis
acroparesthesia
   Nothnagel-type a.
   Schultze-type a.
acropigmentatio reticularis
acropurpura
acrospiroma
   eccrine a.
actinic
   a. elastosis

actinic (continued)
    a. keratosis
    a. porokeratosis
    a. reticuloid
    a. telangiectasis
actinicity
actiniform
actinism
actinobacillosis
actinolyte
actinometer
actinometry
actinomycelial
actinomycoma
actinomycotin
actinoneuritis
actinoquinol sodium
actinotherapeutics
actinotherapy
acuminatum (acuminata, acuminatae)
    condyloma acuminatum,
        condylomata acuminata
    verruca acuminata, verrucae
        acuminatae
acuminate
Adamantiades-Behçet syndrome
Addison
    disease
    keloid
    morphea
    pigmentation
Addison-Gull
    disease
addisonian
    a. syndrome
addisonism
adenocarcinoma
    sebaceous a.
adenoepithelioma
adenolipoma
adenolipomatosis
adenoma
    a. sebaceum
adenomatosis
    a. oris
adipofibroma
adipogenic
adipogenous

adiponecrosis
adiposalgia
adipositis
adjuvant
    Freund a.
    mycobacterial a.
adventitial
    a. dermis
afibrinogenemia
"af-tha" Phonetic for aphtha.
agminated
    a. follicles
"ahn mahs" Phonetic for en masse.
air
    liquid a.
albedo
    a. unguium
albinism
    a. I, a. II
    acquired a.
    Amish a.
    autosomal dominant oculo-
        cutaneous a.
    autosomal recessive ocular
        a. (AROA)
    brown a.
    complete imperfect a.
    complete perfect a.
    cutaneous a.
    Forsius-Eriksson–type ocu-
        lar a.
    localized a.
    Nettleship-Falls–type ocular
        a.
    ocular a. (OA)
    oculocutaneous a. (OCA)
    partial a.
    piebald a.
    red a.
    rufous a.
    tyrosinase-negative (ty-neg)
        oculocutaneous a.
    tyrosinase-positive (ty-pos)
        oculocutaneous a.
    xanthous a.
    X-linked ocular a. (Nettle-
        ship) (XOAN)
    yellow mutant (ym) a.

albinismus
    a. circumscriptus
    a. conscriptus
    a. totalis
    a. universalis
albinoidism
albinotic
Albright
    syndrome
Aldrich-Mees lines
Alibert
    disease
    keloid
    mentagra
allergic
    a. contact dermatitis (ACD)
    a. granuloma
    a. purpura
    a. urticaria
allergy
    atopic a.
    bacterial a.
    contact a.
    drug a.
    hereditary a.
    immediate a.
    physical a.
allylamines [a class of drugs]
aloe
aloetic
alopecia
    a. acquisita
    androgenetic a.
    a. areata
    a. capitis totalis
    cicatricial a.
    a. cicatrisata
    a. circumscripta
    congenital a.
    a. congenitalis
    congenital sutural a.
    congenital triangular a.
    a. disseminata
    drug a.
    favic a., favid a.
    female pattern a.
    follicular a.
    a. follicularis

alopecia (continued)
    a. hereditaria
    hereditary a.
    a. leprotica
    a. liminaris
    male pattern a.
    marginal a.
    a. marginalis
    mechanical a.
    a. medicamentosa
    a. mucinosa
    ophiasic a. areata
    a. orbicularis
    physiologic a.
    pityriasic a.
    postpartum a.
    a. prematura
    a. presenilis
    pressure a.
    roentgen a.
    a. seborrheica
    senile a.
    a. senilis
    a. symptomatica
    a. syphilitica
    a. totalis
    a. toxica
    traction a.
    a. traumatica
    a. triangularis congenitalis
    a. universalis
    x-ray a.
alpha
    a. nerve fibers
amatol
amelanosis
ameloblastoma
    melanotic a.
    pigmented a.
p-aminobenzoate (PAB) [p-, para-]
p-aminobenzoic acid (PABA) [p-,
    para-]
amyloidosis
    cutaneous a.
    a. cutis
ancylostomiasis
    cutaneous a.
    a. cutis

Andrews
disease
anesthesia
See in *General Surgical Terms.*
anetoderma
Jadassohn-Pellizari a.
Schweninger-Buzzi a.
angioendothelioma
angioendotheliomatosis
a. proliferans
systemic proliferating a.
angiofibroma
a. contagiosum tropicum
angiogranuloma
angiokeratoma
a. circumscriptum
a. corporis diffusum
a. corporis diffusum universale
diffuse a.
a. of Fordyce
a. of Mibelli
scrotal a., a. of scrotum
solitary a.
vulvar a., a. of vulva
angioleiomyoma
angiolupoid
angioma
cherry a.
hereditary hemorrhagic a.
infectious a.
a. pigmentosum
plane a.
plexiform a.
sclerosing a.
senile a.
a. serpiginosum
spider a.
stellate a.
strawberry a.
tuberous a.
angiomatoid
angiomatosis
Sturge-Weber a.
angioneurotic
a. edema
anhidrotics [a class of drugs]

anogenital
anomaly
Jordan a.
morning glory a.
anonychia
anthrarobin
antibromics [a class of drugs]
antigen (Ag)
Mitsuda a.
antihistamines [a class of drugs]
antihydrotics [a class of drugs]
antiseptics [a class of drugs]
antiserum
aphtha (aphthae)
Bednar a.
Mikulicz aphthae
aplasia
a. cutis congenita
apocrine
a. chromhidrosis
a. cystadenoma
a. gland(s)
a. metaplasia
appearance
cluster-of-grapes a.
cushingoid a.
enamel paint spot a.
finger-in-glove a.
ground-glass a.
hair-on-end a., hair-standing-on-end a.
slapped-cheek a., slapped-face a.
stuck-on a.
areata
alopecia a.
areatus
areola (areolae)
Chaussier a.
primary a.
vaccinal a.
areolate
Arndt-Gottron
disease
syndrome
arrector (arrectores)
a. pili, arrectores pilorum

arthritis (arthritides)
 psoriatic a.
arthropathia
 a. psoriatica
Asboe-Hansen
 disease
aspiration
asteatosis
 a. cutis
asthma
astringents [a class of drugs]
atheroma
 a. cutis
atheromatosis ·
 a. cutis
atopic
atopy
atrophic
 a. striae
atrophie ["ah-tro-fee"]
 a. blanche ["blahnsh"]
 a. noire ["nwahr"]
atrophoderma
 follicular a.
 macular a.
 neuritic a.
 a. striatum et maculatum
 a. vermicularis
 vermiculate a. of cheeks
atrophodermia
atrophy
 cutaneous a.
 striate a. of skin
Audouin microsporon
aula.
autoantibody
avulsion
"awla" Phonetic for aula.
azoles [a class of drugs]
BA—betamethasone acetate
bacillus (bacilli)
 See in *Laboratory, Pathology, and Chemistry Terms.*
Bacillus
 See in *Laboratory, Pathology, and Chemistry Terms.*
bacterid
 pustular b.

bacterium (bacteria)
 See specific bacteria in *Laboratory, Pathology, and Chemistry Terms.*
Baelz
 disease
Bäfverstedt syndrome
balanitis
 b. xerotica obliterans
baldness
 male pattern b.
Ballingall
 disease
band
 See *layer, line, streak,* and *stria.*
bandage
 See in *General Surgical Terms.*
barba (barbae)
 eczema barbae
 folliculitis barbae
 pseudofolliculitis barbae
 sycosis barbae
 tinea barbae
 trichophytosis barbae
Barber [eponym]
 psoriasis
barbula hirci
Barcoo
 disease
 rot
Bardet-Biedl
 syndrome
Bart syndrome
base
 b. of nail
Basedow
 disease
Basis soap
Bateman
 disease
 purpura
 syndrome
bath
 Aveeno b.
 infrared b.

Bazin
    disease
    ulcer
Beau
    lines
Beck
    See *Boeck.*
Becker
    nevus
bed
    nail b.
bedbug
Behçet
    disease
    syndrome
Beigel
    disease
benzoyl
    b. peroxide
benzylamines [a class of drugs]
Besnier
    prurigo
Besnier-Boeck
    disease
bilharzioma
Biobrane
    adhesive
    glove
    synthetic skin substitute
biopsy
    biochemical b.
    excisional b.
    punch b.
    shave b.
    total b.
    wedge b.
birthmark
    port wine stain b.
    strawberry b.
blackhead
Blancophor, blankophore
blastomycosis
    cutaneous b.
    systemic b.
bleeding
    punctate b.
blister
    blood b.

blister (continued)
    burn b.
    fever b.
    water b.
Bloch-Siemens-Sulzberger
    syndrome
blotch
    palpebral b.
blotchy
body (bodies)
    Bollinger b.'s
    Civatte b.
    colloid b.
    Lipschütz b.
    b. of sweat gland
Boeck
    disease
    itch
    sarcoid, sarcoidosis
    scabies
Boerhaave
    sweat glands
boil
    Madura b.
    salt water b., sea water b.
Bollinger
    bodies
    granules
Bourneville
    disease
    syndrome
Bourneville-Brissaud
    disease
Bourneville-Pringle
    syndrome
Bowen
    disease
    precancerous dermatosis
bowenoid
bracelet
Breslow
    classification
    thickness
Bretonneau
    angina
    disease
bridou

Brocq
    disease
    erythrose péribuccale pig-
        mentaire
    lupoid sycosis
    pseudopelade
Brooke
    disease
    tumor
bubo
    Frei b.
    gonorrheal b.
    indolent b.
    nonvenereal b.
    pestilential b.
    strumous b.
    venereal b.
bubon
    b. d'emblée
Buerger
    disease
bulla (bullae)
bullate
bullation
bullous
    b. congenital ichthyosiform
        erythroderma
    b. dermatosis
    b. erythema multiforme
    b. impetigo
    b. pemphigoid
bull's eye lesion
bumps
    goose b.
bunion
Burow
    solution
Buschke
    disease
    scleredema
butterfly
    b. rash
Bx—biopsy
café au lait spot
calcinosis
    c. circumscripta
    c. cutis

calor
    c. mordax
    c. mordicans
Canada-Cronkhite syndrome
cancer
    See also *carcinoma.*
    See also in *Oncology and
        Hematology* section.
    epidermal c.
candidiasis
    cutaneous c.
capillarectasia
capillaritis
capillaropathy
capillus (capilli)
carbunculoid
carcinoma (carcinomas, carcinomata)
    See also in *Oncology and
        Hematology* section.
    basal cell c.
    fungating c.
    hair-matrix c.
    c. in situ
    intraepidermal c.
    melanotic c.
    squamous cell c.
carotenoderma
Carrión
    disease
Casal
    collar
    necklace
caseous
    c. necrosis
Casoni
    intradermal test
    reaction
Castellani
    paint
caustic
caustics [a class of drugs]
cauterants [a class of drugs]
cavernous
    c. hemangioma
    c. lymphangioma
Cazenave
    disease
    lupus

Cazenave (continued)
    vitiligo
cell
    See also in *Laboratory,
        Pathology, and Chemistry
        Terms.*
    basal c.
    horny c.
    keratinized c.
    Lipschütz c.
    malpighian c.
    Merkel c.
    Schwann c.
    squamous c.
    Touton giant c.
    Tzanck c.
cellulitis
    clostridial c.
    eosinophilic c.
    gangrenous c.
    streptococcal c.
Celsus
    kerion
    papules
    vitiligo
ceramidase deficiency
chalazodermia
chancre
    erosive c.
    fungating c.
    indurated c.
    Ricord c.
    Rollet c.
    sporotrichotic c.
    sulcus c.
    tularemic c.
chancroid
chancroidal
chancrous
Chaoul
    tube
Charlouis
    disease
cheilitis
    actinic c.
    c. actinica
    allergic c.
    apostematous c.

cheilitis (continued)
    commissural c.
    exfoliativa c.
    glandularis apostematosa c.
    c. granulomatosa impetigi-
        nous c.
    Miescher granulomatous c.
    migrating c.
    mycotic c.
    c. venenata
chemabrasion
chemosurgery
    Mohs c.
chest
    fissured c.
chickenpox
chilblain
    necrotized c.
chloasma
    c. hepaticum
    c. periorale virginium
    c. phthisicorum
    c. traumaticum
chloroma
chlorosis
cholesterosis
    c. cutis
chondrodermatitis
    c. nodularis chronica helicis
chondroid
    c. syringoma
Christian-Weber
    disease
chromate
chromatophore
chromatosis
chromhidrosis
chromomycosis
Ciarrocchi
    disease
cicatrices (plural of cicatrix)
cicatricial
    c. alopecia
cicatrix (cicatrices)
    hypertrophic c.
    vicious c.
cin–. See also words beginning
    sin–, syn–.

circinate
Civatte
    bodies
    poikiloderma
Clark
    classification of malignant
      melanoma (levels I–V)
    levels (I–V)
classification
    Breslow c.
    Clark c. of malignant mela-
      noma (levels I–V)
    Lund-Browder c.
clavus (clavi)
    c. syphiliticus
Cloudman melanoma
Clouston syndrome
CMM—cutaneous malignant mela-
    noma
coarse
    c. texture
coldsore
collagenous
    c. plaques
collar
    Biett c.
    c. of pearls
    c. of Venus
comedo (comedones)
    See also *acne.*
    closed c.
    open c.
    solar c.
comedocarcinoma
comedogenic
complex
    EAHF (eczema, asthma, hay
      fever) c.
complexion
condyloma (condylomata)
    flat c.
    giant c.
    c. latum, condylomata lata
    pointed c.
    c. subcutaneum
condylomatoid
condylomatosis
condylomatous

contracture
    Dupuytren c.
contusion
cornu (cornua)
    c. cutaneum
cornual
cornuate
corona (coronae)
    c. seborrheica
    c. veneris
coronal
corps ["kor"]
    c. ronds
cortex (cortices)
    c. of hair shaft
corticis (genitive of cortex)
counterirritants [a class of drugs]
cracked heels
CREST—calcinosis cutis, Raynaud
    phenomenon, esophageal dys-
    function/hypermotility, sclero-
    dactyly, telangiectasia
    [syndrome]
crinis (crines)
Cronkhite-Canada syndrome
cryosurgery
cryptococcosis
    cutaneous c.
crystal violet
CTH—ceramide trihexoside
cunicular
curettement
cutaneous
    c. anthrax
    c. larva migrans
    c. leishmaniasis
    c. mucormycosis
    c. nevi
    c. vasculitis
cuticle
cuticular
cutis
    c. anserina
    c. elastica
    c. hyperelastica
    c. laxa
    c. marmorata

cutis (continued)
    c. marmorata telangiectatica
      congenita
    c. pendula
    c. pensilis
    c. rhomboidalis nuchae
    c. testacea
    c. unctuosa
    c. vera
    c. verticis gyrata
cyst
    dermoid c.
    epidermal c.
    epithelial c.
    hydatid c.
    mucous c.
    myxoid c.
    pheomycotic c.
    pilonidal c.
    popliteal c.
    sebaceous c.
    thyroglossal c.
    trichilemmal c.
cystoid
"da-breed-maw" Phonetic for
    débridement.
dactylitis
    d. strumosa
    d. syphilitica
    d. tuberculosa
Danbolt-Closs syndrome
Danielssen
    disease
Danielssen-Boeck
    disease
    sarcoidosis
Danlos
    disease
    syndrome
Darier
    disease
    sign
Darier-White
    disease
débridement
    enzymatic d.
    surgical d.

deficiency
    riboflavin d.
defluxio
    d. capillorum
    d. ciliorum
Degos
    disease
    syndrome
deodorants
dermabraded
dermabrader
    Iverson d.
    sandpaper d.
dermabrasion
dermamyiasis
    d. linearis migrans oestrosa
dermatitis (dermatitides)
    actinic d.
    d. aestivalis
    allergic d.
    allergic contact d.
    d. ambustionis
    ammonia d.
    ancylostome d.
    arsphenamine d.
    d. artefacta
    ashy d.
    atopic d.
    d. atrophicans
    autosensitization d.
    avian mite d.
    bather's d.
    berlock d., berloque d.
    bhiwanol d.
    blastomycetic d.
    d. blastomycotica
    brown-tail moth d.
    brucella d.
    d. bullosa
    d. bullosa striata pratensis
    d. calorica
    carcinomatous d.
    caterpillar d.
    cement d.
    cercarial d.
    chemical d.
    chigger d.
    chromate d.

dermatitis (dermatitides) (continued)
  chronic bullous d.
  d. combustionis
  d. congelationis
  contact d.
  d. contusiformis
  copra mite d.
  cosmetic d.
  d. cruris pustulosa et atroph-
    icans
  cumulative insult d.
  dhobie mark d.
  diaper d.
  dried fruit d.
  d. dysmenorrhoeica
  eczematous d.
  d. epidemica
  d. erythematosa
  d. escharotica
  d. excoriativa infantum
  d. exfoliativa epidemica
  d. exfoliativa neonatorum
  exfoliative d.
  exudative discoid and
    lichenoid d.
  factitial d.
  d. gangrenosa
  d. gangrenosa infantum
  d. hemostatica
  d. herpetiformis
  d. hiemalis
  d. hypostatica
  industrial d.
  d. infectiosa eczematoides
  infectious eczematous d.
  insect d.
  interdigital d.
  io-moth d.
  irritant d.
  Jacquet d.
  Leiner d.
  livedoid d.
  marine d.
  meadow d., meadow-grass d.
  d. medicamentosa
  moth d.
  d. multiformis
  mycotic d.

dermatitis (dermatitides) (continued)
  napkin d.
  nasal solar d.
  nickel d.
  d. nodosa
  d. nodularis necrotica
  nummular eczematous d.
  occupational d.
  onion mite d.
  d. papillaris capillitii
  papular d.
  d. pediculoides ventricosus
  Pelodera d.
  perfume d.
  periocular d.
  perioral d.
  photoallergic contact d.
  photocontact d.
  phototoxic d.
  phytophototoxic d.
  pigmented purpuric
    lichenoid d.
  poison ivy d.
  poison oak d.
  poison sumac d.
  precancerous d.
  primary irritant d.
  d. psoriasiformis nodularis
  purpuric pigmented
    lichenoid d.
  radiation d.
  rat mite d.
  d. repens
  rhabditic d.
  rhus d.
  roentgen-ray d.
  schistosome d.
  seborrheic d.
  d. seborrheica
  d. simplex
  d. skiagraphica
  d. solaris
  stasis d.
  d. striata pratensis bullosa
  swimmer's d.
  d. traumatica
  trefoil d.
  uncinarial d.

dermatitis (dermatitides) (continued)
    d. vegetans
    d. venenata
    d. verrucosa
    verrucose d., verrucous d.
    vesicular d.
    weeping d.
    x-ray d.
dermatodysplasia
    d. verruciformis
dermatofibroma
    d. protuberans
dermatofibrosarcoma
    d. protuberans
dermatofibrosis
    d. lenticularis disseminata
dermatolysis
    d. palpebrarum
dermatomycosis
    blastomycetic d.
    d. furfuracea
    d. microsporina
    d. trichophytina
dermatophytosis
    d. furfuracea
dermatoplasty
    Thompson d.
dermatosis (dermatoses)
    acarine d.
    acute febrile neutrophilic d.
    angioneurotic d.
    ashy d. of Ramirez
    Auspitz d.
    Bowen precancerous d.
    d. cenicienta
    cholinogenic d.
    chronic bullous d. of child-
        hood
    chronic hemosideric d.
    contact d.
    juvenile plantar d.
    lichenoid d.
    meadow grass d.
    menstrual d.
    neutrophilic d.
    occupational d.
    palmoplantar d.
    d. papulosa nigra

dermatosis (dermatoses) (continued)
    precancerous d.
    progressive pigmentary d.
    purpuric d.
    radiation d.
    rhythmical d.
    Schamberg d.
    seborrheic d.
    stasis d.
    subcorneal pustular d.
    Unna d.
    vulvar d.
dermatozoon (dermatozoa)
dermatozoonosis
dermoid
desiccate
desiccation
    electric d.
desiccative
desmoplastic
    d. trichoepithelioma
desquamation
    furfuraceous d.
    membranous d.
    siliquose d.
Devergie
    disease
DHA—dihydroxyacetone
DHAP—dihydroxyacetone phosphate
Dick
    reaction
    test
digital
    d. fibromatosis
digitate
    d. warts
dis–. See also words beginning dys–.
discoid
    d. lupus erythematosus
discrete
    d. lesion
    d. nodule
disease
    See also *syndrome*.
    Addison d.
    Addison-Gull d.
    Alibert d.
    Andrews d.

disease (continued)
    Arndt-Gottron d.
    Asboe-Hansen d.
    Ballingall d.
    Bazin d.
    Beigel d.
    Besnier-Boeck d.
    Besnier-Boeck-Schaumann d.
    Boeck d.
    Bourneville d.
    Bourneville-Brissaud d.
    Bowen d.
    Brooke d.
    Buerger d.
    Carrión d.
    Cazenave d.
    Charlouis d.
    Christian-Weber d.
    Ciarrocchi d.
    Danielssen d.
    Darier d.
    Darier-White d.
    Degos d.
    Devergie d.
    Duhring d.
    Dukes d.
    extramammary Paget d.
    Favre d.
    Filatov-Dukes d.
    Fordyce d.
    Fox d.
    Fox-Fordyce d.
    Frei d.
    Gaucher d.
    Gibert d.
    Gilchrist d.
    Habermann d.
    Hailey-Hailey d.
    Hallopeau d.
    Hand-Schüller-Christian d.
    Hansen d.
    Hartnup d.
    Hebra d.
    Hodgkin d.
    Hünermann d.
    Hutchinson d.
    Hyde d.
    Jadassohn d.

disease (continued)
    Johnson-Stevens d.
    Kalischer d.
    Kaposi d.
    Kawasaki d.
    Köbner d.
    Kyrle d.
    Landouzy d.
    Lane d.
    Leiner d.
    Leloir d.
    Letterer-Siwe d.
    Lewandowsky-Lutz d.
    Lipschütz d.
    Lobo d.
    Lortat-Jacobs d.
    Lutz-Miescher d.
    Lutz-Splendore-Almeida d.
    Majocchi d.
    Meleda d.
    Mibelli d.
    Milton d.
    Mitchell d.
    Mucha d.
    Mucha-Habermann d.
    Neumann d.
    Nicolas-Favre d.
    Niemann-Pick d.
    Osler d.
    Osler-Vaquez d.
    Paget d.
    pink d.
    Puente d.
    Quincke d.
    Quinquaud d.
    Rayer d.
    Raynaud d.
    Recklinghausen d.
    Reclus d.
    Reiter d.
    Ritter d.
    Robinson d.
    Robles d.
    Schamberg d.
    Senear-Usher d.
    Sjögren d.
    Sticker d.
    Sutton d.

disease (continued)
    Symmers d.
    Taenzer d.
    Underwood d.
    Urbach-Oppenheim d.
    vagabond's d.
    Weber d.
    Weber-Christian d.
    White d.
    Winkler d.
    Witkop-Von Sallman d.
    Woringer-Kolopp d.
    Zahorsky d.
dissecting
    d. cellulitis
disseminated
    d. granuloma annulare
    d. lupus erythematosus (DLE)
    d. porokeratosis
    d. rosacea
    d. xanthoma
dot
    See *macula, macule,* and *spot.*
down [lanugo]
dressing
    See in *General Surgical*
      Terms.
DSAP— disseminated superficial
    actinic porokeratosis
Dubreuilh precancerous melanosis
Ducrey
    test
Duhring
    disease
    pruritus
Dukes
    disease
Dupuytren
    contracture
dynamometer
    Collins d.
dys–. See also words beginning dis–.
dyshidrosis
    trichophytic d.
dyskeratosis
    d. congenita
    d. follicularis
dyskeratotic

dystrophic
    d. epidermolysis bullosa
    d. palmoplantar hyperker-
      atosis
dystrophy
    median canaliform d. of the
      nail
    twenty-nail d.
EACD—extrinsic allergic contact
    dermatitis
EAHF—eczema, asthma, hay fever
EB—epidermolysis bullosa
ecchymoma
ecchymosis (ecchymoses)
    multiple e.'s
    old e.
    Roederer e.
    scattered e.'s
echovirus (serotypes 1–7, 9, 11–18,
    20–27, 29–34)
ECM—erythema chronicum migrans
ecthyma
    e. contagiosum
    e. gangrenosum
    e. syphiliticum
ectodermal
    e. dysplasia
ectodermosis
    e. erosiva pluriorificialis
ectozoon (ectozoa)
eczema
    allergic e.
    e. articulorum
    atopic e.
    e. barbae
    e. capitis
    e. craquelé
    e. crustosum
    e. diabeticorum
    dyshidrotic e.
    e. epilans
    e. epizootica
    e. erythematosum
    flexural e.
    follicular e.
    e. herpeticum
    e. hypertrophicum
    infantile e.

eczema (continued)
    e. intertrigo
    lichenoid e.
    linear e.
    e. madidans
    e. marginatum
    e. neuriticum
    e. nummulare
    e. papulosum
    e. parasiticum
    pustular e.
    e. pustulosum
    e. rubrum
    e. scrofuloderma
    e. seborrheicum
    e. siccum
    e. solare
    e. squamosum
    stasis e.
    e. tyloticum
    e. vaccinatum
    e. verrucosum
    e. vesiculosum
    weeping e.
eczematogenic
edema
    angioneurotic e.
    cyclic e.
    epidermal e.
    hereditary angioneurotic e.
      (HANE)
    Milton e.
    nonpitting e.
    pedal e.
    periorbital e.
"efelis" Phonetic for ephelis.
effect [noun: result, outcome]
    Deelman e.
    isomorphic e.
    Köbner (Koebner) e.
effluvium
    anagen e.
    telogen e.
"efidrosis" Phonetic for ephidrosis.
"egzema" Phonetic for eczema.
Ehlers-Danlos
    disease
    syndrome

"eksan–" Phonetic for words beginning exan–.
"eksema" Phonetic for eczema.
elastosis
    actinic e.
    e. senilis
electrocautery
electromagnetic
    e. radiation
electron
    e. beam therapy
    e. microscopy
elephantiasis
    e. arabicum
    e. asturiensis
    e. filariensis
    e. graecorum
    e. leishmaniana
    lymphangiectatic e.
    e. neuromatosa
    e. nostras
    e. telangiectodes
emollients [a class of drugs]
emphysema
    subcutaneous e.
emulsion
    Pusey e.
EN—erythema nodosum
endothelioma
    e. capitis
    e. cutis
Engman
    dermatitis
    disease
ENL—erythema nodosum leprosum
en masse
entirety
entomophthoromycosis
eosinophilic
    e. cellulitis
    e. fasciitis
    e. granuloma
    e. spongiosis
ephelis
ephidrosis
    e. cruenta
epicuticle
epidermatoplasty

epidermidalization
epidermodysplasia
    e. verruciformis
epidermoid
epidermolysis
    e. acquisita
    e. bullosa
    e. bullosa dystrophica, poly-
       dysplastic
    e. bullosa, junctional
    e. bullosa simplex
    toxic bullous e.
epidermolytic
    e. hyperkeratosis
epidermophytosis
    e. cruris
    e. interdigitale
epidermotropic
    e. reticulosis
epilate
epistasis
epistatic
epithelia (plural of epithelium)
epithelialize, epithelialized
epitheliitis
epithelioma
    e. adenoides cysticum
    basal cell e.
    e. capitis
    Malherbe calcifying e.
    e. molluscum
epithelium (epithelia)
    tegumentary e.
eponychium
"erisipelas" Phonetic for erysipelas.
"erithema" Phonetic for erythema.
"erithro–" Phonetic for words
    beginning erythro–.
erosio
    e. interdigitalis blasto-
       mycetica
erosion
eruption
    bullous e.
    creeping e.
    crustaceous e.
    erythematous e.
    Kaposi varicelliform e.

eruption (continued)
    maculopapular e.
    papulosquamous e.
    petechial e.
    pustular e.
    serum e.
    squamous e.
    tubercular e.
    vesicular e.
    vesiculopustular e.
erysipelas
    ambulant e.
    coast e.
    gangrenous e.
    e. grave internum
    idiopathic e.
    migrant e.
    e. perstans
    phlegmonous e.
    e. pustulosum
    e. verrucosum
    e. vesiculosum
    zoonotic e.
erythema
    e. ab igne
    acrodynic e.
    acute infectious e.
    e. annulare
    e. annulare centrifugum
    e. annulare rheumaticum
    e. a pudore
    e. arthriticum
    e. bullosum
    e. caloricum
    e. chromicum figuratum
       melanodermicum
    e. chronicum migrans
    circinate syphilitic e.
    e. circinatum
    e. contusiformis
    e. dyschromicum perstans
    e. elevatum diutinum
    e. endemicum
    e. exudativum
    e. figuratum
    e. fugax
    e. gyratum repens
    e. induratum

erythema (continued)
    e. infectiosum
    e. intertrigo
    e. iris
    Jacquet e.
    e. marginatum
    e. marginatum rheumaticum
    migratory e.
    Milian e.
    e. multiforme
    e. multiforme bullosum
    e. multiforme exudativum
    e. necrolytica migrans
    e. neonatorum
    e. neonatorum toxicum
    e. nodosum
    e. nodosum leprosum
    e. nodosum migrans
    e. nodosum syphiliticum
    e. nuchae
    nummular e.
    palmar e.
    e. palmare hereditarium
    papuloerosive e.
    e. papulosum
    e. paratrimma
    pellagroid e.
    e. pernio
    e. perstans
    e. pudicitiae
    e. punctatum
    rheumatic e.
    e. scarlatiniforme
    e. simplex
    e. solare
    e. streptogenes
    e. subitum
    e. toxicum
    e. toxicum neonatorum
    e. traumaticum
    e. urticans
    e. venenatum
erythematosus
    discoid lupus e.
    systemic lupus e. (SLE)
erythemogenic
erythrasma
    Baerensprung e.

erythrism
erythristic
erythrocyanosis
    e. crurum puellaris
    e. frigida
    e. frigida crurum puellarum
    e. supramalleolaris
erythroderma
    atopic e.
    congenital ichthyosiform e.
    e. desquamativum
    exfoliative e.
    e. ichthyosiforme congenitum
    lymphomatous e.
    e. psoriaticum
    Sézary e.
    e. squamosum
erythrokeratodermia
    progressive symmetrical ver-
      rucous e.
    e. variabilis
erythromelalgia
erythroplakia
erythroplasia
    e. of Queyrat
erythroprosopalgia
erythrose
    e. péribuccale pigmentaire
      of Brocq
erythrosis
    e. of Bechterew
eschar
    burn e.
escharotic
"eskar" Phonetic for eschar.
exanthem
    vesicular e.
exanthema (exanthemata)
    Boston e.
    e. subitum
excoriation
    necrotic e.
"exema" Phonetic for eczema.
extractor
    Amico e.
    comedo e.
    Schamberg e.
    Unna e.

extractor (continued)
    Walton e.
extramammary Paget disease
exulceratio
    e. simplex
Fabry
    disease
    syndrome
facies (facies)
    f. hepatica
    myxedematous f.
"fajedenah" Phonetic for phagedena.
fasciitis
    exudative f.
    necrotizing f.
    nodular f.
    proliferative f.
    pseudosarcomatous f.
favid
Favre disease
Favre-Racouchot syndrome
favus
    f. circinatus
    f. herpeticus
    f. herpetiformis
    f. pilaris
Fegeler syndrome
felon
    bone f.
    deep f.
    subcutaneous f.
    subcuticular f.
    subperiosteal f.
    thecal f.
female pseudo-Turner syndrome
"fenomenon" Phonetic for phenom-
    enon.
Ferguson-Smith–type epithelioma
fester
fiber
    A-alpha nerve f.
    Herxheimer f.'s
fibrinoid
    f. necrosis
fibroblast
fibroma
    f. cutis
    f. lipomatodes

fibroma (continued)
    f. molle
    f. pendulum
    perifollicular f.
    periungual f.
    senile f.
    telangiectatic f.
    f. xanthoma
fibromatogenic
fibromatoid
fibromatosis
    f. colli
fibromatous
fibromectomy
fibrosis
fibrous
    f. histiocytoma
    f. papule fibroxanthoma
Fiessinger-Leroy-Reiter
    syndrome
Fiessinger-Rendu
    syndrome
figure
    flame f.
"fi-ko-mi-co-sis" Phonetic for phy-
    comycosis.
Filatov-Dukes disease
filiform
    f. tumor
    f. wart
fissure
flame
    f. figure
flammeus nevus
flesh
    goosebump f.
"flikt–" Phonetic for words begin-
    ning phlyct–.
florid
"foit" Phonetic for Voigt and Voit.
follicle
    pilosebaceous f.
    sebaceous f.
    tertiary f.
folliclis
follicular
    f. eczema
    f. lichen planus

follicular (continued)
  f. mucinosis
  f. psoriasis
folliculitis
  f. abscedens et suffodiens
  agminate f.
  f. barbae
  f. cheloidalis
  f. cruris atrophicans
  f. decalvans
  f. decalvans cryptococcia
  f. decalvans et lichen spinu-
    losus
  f. gonorrhoeica
  industrial f.
  f. keloidalis
  f. nares perforans
  oil f.
  f. ulerythematosa reticulata
  f. varioliformis
foot (feet)
  athlete's f.
foot tetter
Forchheimer spots
Fordyce
  disease
  granule
  spots
foveolar
foveolate
Fox
  disease
  impetigo
Fox-Fordyce disease
fragilitas
  f. crinium
  f. unguium
Franceschetti-Jadassohn syndrome
freckle
  melanotic f. of Hutchison
Frei
  bubo
fulguration
fungi (plural of fungus)
fungicidal
fungicide
fungiform
fungistasis

fungistat
fungistatic
fungus (fungi)
  See also specific fungi in
    *Laboratory, Pathology,
    and Chemistry Terms.*
  beefsteak f.
  cutaneous f.
  umbilical f.
furunculosis
furunculus (furunculi)
  f. vulgaris
fusus (fusi)
  cortical fusi
  fracture fusi
"fy-ko-my-co-sis" Phonetic for phycomycosis.
galactophlysis
galvanic
  g. epilator
gangrene
  cutaneous g.
  disseminated cutaneous g.
  Fournier g.
  gaseous g.
  Raynaud g.
  wet g.
Gaucher
  disease
Gerhardt
  disease
  phenomenon
  reaction
  test for acetoacetic acid
giant cell
  g.c. arteritis
  g.c. epulis
  g.c. granuloma
Gibert
  disease
  pityriasis
Gilchrist
  disease
  mycosis
gland
  apocrine g.
  sebaceous g.
  sweat g.

glomus (glomera)
    g. body
    g. cell
    cutaneous g.
    digital g.
    neuromyoarterial g.
    g. tumor
glossitis
    g. areata exfoliativa
    g. dissecans
    Hunter g.
    g. migrans
    g. parasitica
    parenchymatous g.
    rhomboid g.
    g. rhomboidea mediana
Goltz
    syndrome
Goltz-Gorlin
    syndrome
gonitis
    fungous g.
Gorlin
    syndrome
Gorlin-Goltz
    syndrome
Gottron
    papules
    sign
    syndrome
Gougerot
    triad
Gougerot-Blum
    disease
    syndrome
Gougerot-Carteaud
    syndrome
Gowers
    panatrophy
Graham Little
    syndrome
granulate
granule
    Bollinger g.'s
granuloma
    g. annulare
    g. endemicum
    g. fissuratum

granuloma (continued)
    g. fungoides
    g. gangraenescens
    Hodgkin g.
    g. inguinale
    lipoid g.
    lycopodium g.
    Majocchi g.
    g. malignum
    Miescher actinic g.
    g. multiforme
    g. pyogenicum
    g. sarcomatodes
    g. telangiectaticum
    g. trichophyticum
    g. venereum
granulomatosis
    Miescher-Leder g.
granulomatous
    g. reaction
    g. rosacea
    g. vasculitis
Greither
    syndrome
Grönblad-Strandberg
    syndrome
Günther
    syndrome
guttate
    g. psoriasis
GV—gentian violet
gyrose
Haber
    syndrome
Habermann
    disease
HAE—hereditary angioneurotic
    edema
Haemophilus
Hailey-Hailey
    disease
hairy
    h. nevus
    h. tongue
Hallopeau
    acrodermatitis
    disease

Hallopeau-Siemens
    syndrome
Hamilton
    bandage
    pseudophlegmon
    test
Hand-Schüller-Christian
    disease
    syndrome
hangnail
Hanot
    disease
    syndrome
Hansen
    disease
Harada
    disease
    syndrome
Hartnup
    disease
    syndrome
Hebra
    disease
    ointment
    pityriasis
    prurigo
heliotherapy
helminthiasis
    h. elastica
helotomy
hemangioma
    capillary h.
    cavemous h.
    h. congenitale
    h. hypertrophicum cutis
    sclerosing h.
    h. simplex
    strawberry h.
    h.-thrombocytopenia syndrome
    verrucous h.
hemophilus
hemorrhage
hemorrhagic
hemostatics [a class of drugs]
Henoch
    disease
    purpura

Henoch-Schönlein
    purpura
    syndrome
herald
    patch
    plaque
Herlitz
    disease
    syndrome
Hermansky-Pudlak syndrome
herpes
    h. catarrhalis
    h. digitalis
    h. facialis
    h. farinosus
    h. febrilis
    h. generalisatus
    h. genitalis
    h. gestationis
    h. gladiatorum
    h. labialis
    h. menstrualis
    h. mentalis
    nasal h.
    h. odeus
    h. phlyctaenodes
    h. praepuffalis
    h. progenitalis
    h. recurrens
    h. simplex recurrens
    h. tonsurans
    h. tonsurans maculosus
    h. vegetans
    wrestler h.
    h. zoster oticus
    h. zoster varicellosus
herpesvirus
    herpes whitlow h.
Herxheimer
    fibers
    reaction
    spirals
heterotrichosis
    h. superciliorum
hexamethyl violet
hidradenitis
    h. axillaris
    h. suppurativa

hidradenitis (continued)
    suppurative h.
hidradenoma
    h. papilliferum
hidrorrhea
"hipo–" Phonetic for words beginning hypo–.
histiocyte
hives
Hodgkin
    disease
    granuloma
Hofmann violet
homme
    h. rouge
homologous
HOOD—hereditary osteo-onycho-dysplasia
hookworm
Howel-Evans
    syndrome
Hünermann
    disease
Hunt
    syndrome
hunterian
    h. chancre
Hutchinson
    disease
    freckle
    lentigo
    syndrome
    triad
Hyde
    disease
hydroa
    h. aestivale
    h. febrile
    h. gestationis
    h. gravidarum
    h. puerorum
    h. vacciniforme
    h. vesiculosum
hygroma
    h. colli
    cystic h.
    h. cysticum
hyperacanthosis

hypercarotenemia
hyperhidrosis
    axillary h.
    gustatory h.
    h. lateralis
    unilateral h.
hyperhidrotic
hyperimmunoglobulinemia
    h. E
hyperkcratinization
hyperkeratosis
    h. congenitalis palmaris et plantaris
    epidermolytic h.
    h. excentrica
    h. figurata centrifuga atrophica
    h. follicularis in cutem penetrans
    h. follicularis vegetans
    h. linguae
    palmoplantar h.
    h. penetrans
    h. subungualis
    h. universalis congenita
hyperliposis
hypermelanotic
hyperonychia
hyperpigmentation
hyperplasia
    angiolymphoid h. with eosinophilia
    basal cell h.
    congenital sebaceous gland h.
    cutaneous lymphoid h.
    sebaceous h.
    verrucous h.
hyperplastic
hypersensitivity
    atopic h.
hypersteatosis
hypertrichosis
    h. lanuginosa
    h. universalis
hypha (hyphae)
hyphal
hypoderm
hypodermolithiasis

hypohidrosis
hypomelanism
hypomelanosis
    hereditary h.
    idiopathic guttate h.
    h. of Ito
hyponychial
hyponychom
hyponychium
hypopigmentation
hypopigmenter
hypoplasia
    h. cutis congenita
hypotrichiasis
hypotrichosis
ichthyismus
    i. exanthematicus
ichthyoid
ichthyosiform
    i. erythroderma
ichthyosis
    i. congenita
    i. cornea
    follicular i.
    i. follicularis
    i. hystrix
    lamellar i.
    linear i.
    i. linguae
    nacreous i.
    i. palmaris
    i. palmaris et plantaris
    i. plantaris
    i. sauroderma
    i. scutulata
    i. sebacea cornea
    senile i.
    i. serpentina
    i. simplex
    i. spinosa
    i. thysanotrichica
    i. vulgaris
icterus
id [secondary skin eruption]
    reaction
I&D—incision and drainage
idiopathic
    i. thrombocytopenic purpura

"ikthe–" Phonetic for words beginning ichthy–.
impetigo
    Bockhart i.
    i. bullosa
    bullous i.
    i. contagiosa
    i. eczematodes
    follicular i.
    Fox i.
    furfuraceous i.
    i. herpetiformis
    i. neonatorum
    i. simplex
    i. staphylogenes
    i. syphilitica
    i. variolosa
incontinentia
    i. pigmenti
    i. pigmenti achromians
indurated
    i. cellulitis
    i. lymphangitis
infection
    fungal i.
infiltration
    adipose i.
    cellular i.
    inflammatory i.
    lymphocytic i.
inoculation
integument
integumentum
    i. commune
interface
    dermoepidermal i.
intertrigo
    i. labialis
    i. saccharomycetica
intimitis
    proliferative i.
itch
    Boeck i.
    dhobie i.
    grain i.
    Moeller i.
    seven-year i.
    swimmer's i.

Jacob
  ulcer
Jacquet
  dermatitis
  erythema
Jadassohn
  anetoderma
  disease
  sebaceous nevus
  testerma
Jadassohn-Lewandowsky
  law
  syndrome
Jadassohn-Pellizari
  anetoderma
Jadelot
  furrows
  lines
Janeway
  lesion
  spots
jaundice
Johnson-Stevens
  disease
junction
  dermoepidermal i.
junctional
  j. epidermolysis bullosa
  j. nevus
juvenile
  j. hyaline fibromatosis
  j. lentigo melanoma
  j. xanthogranuloma
Kalischer
  disease
Kaposi
  disease
  sarcoma
  varicelliform eruption
  xeroderma
Kawasaki
  disease
  syndrome
Keller
  ultraviolet test
keloid
  Addison k.

keratitis
  amebic k.
  interstitial k.
keratoderma
  k. blennorrhagica
  k. climactericum
  k. palmare et plantare
  plantar k.
  punctate k.
  symmetric k.
keratolysis
  k. exfoliativa
  k. neonatorum
  pitted k.
  k. plantare sulcatum
keratolytics [a class of drugs]
keratoma
  k. diffusum
  k. hereditaria mutilans
  k. malignum congenitale
  k. palmare et plantare
  k. plantare sulcatum
  k. senile
keratomycosis
  k. linguae
keratosis (keratoses)
  actinic k.
  arsenical k.
  aural k.
  k. blennorrhagica
  k. diffusa fetalis
  k. follicularis
  k. follicularis contagiosa
  gonorrheal k.
  inverted follicular k.
  lichenoid k.
  lichen planus-like k.
  nevoid k.
  k. nigricans
  k. obliterans
  k. palmaris et plantaris
  k. pilaris
  k. pilaris atrophicans
  k. pilaris atrophicans faciei
  k. pilaris rubra
  k. punctata
  k. rubra figurata
  seborrheic k.

keratosis (keratoses) (continued)
    k. seborrheica
    senile k.
    k. senilis
    solar k.
    stucco k.
    k. suprafollicularis
    tar k.
    k. universalis congenita
    k. vegetans
kerion
    k. celsi
    Celsus k.
Kienböck-Adamson
    points
Klauder
    syndrome
Köbner (Koebner)
    disease
    effect
    phenomenon
koilonychia
Koplik
    spots
kraurosis
    k. penis
    k. vulvae
Kveim
    test
Kyrle
    disease
lacerate, lacerated
lacuna (lacunae)
lacunula (lacunulae)
lacunule
lame foliacée ["lahm fol-yah-say"]
lamella (lamellae)
    cornoid l.
lamellar
    l. exfoliation
    l. granules
    l. ichthyosis
lamelliform
lamina (laminae)
laminar
lamination
lamp
    black light fluorescent l.

lamp (continued)
    black ray l.
    carbon arc l.
    cold quartz l.
    fluorescent sun l.
    hot quartz l.
    quartz l.
    quartz-iodine l.
    xenon arc l.
Landouzy
    disease
    purpura
Lane
    disease
Langhans
    cells
    layer
larva (larvae)
    cutaneous l. migrans
    l. migrans
larval
Lassar
    betanaphthol paste
    plain zinc paste
Lauth violet
law
    Jadassohn-Lewandowsky l.
layer
    See also *line, streak,* and
      stria.
    Langhans l.
    malpighian l.
Leiner
    dermatitis
    disease
leiomyoma (leiomyomas, leiomy-
    omata)
    l. cutis
    multiple cutaneous l.'s
leishmaniasis
    cutaneous l.
    mucocutaneous l.
    l. recidivans
leishmanoid
    dermal l.
    post–kala-azar dermal l.
Leloir disease
lentiginosis

lentiginous
lentigo (lentigines)
 l. maligna
 nevoid lentigines
 senile lentigines
 l. senilis
 l. simplex
 solar lentigines
lepra
 l. alba
 l. alphoides
 l. alphos
 l. anaesthetica
 l. arabum
 l. conjunctivae
 l. graecorum
 l. maculosa
 l. mutilans
 l. nervorum
 l. nervosa
 l. tuberculoides
 Willan l.
leprosy
 Asturian l.
 borderline l.
 borderline lepromatous l.
 borderline tuberculous l.
 cutaneous l.
 diffuse l. of Lucio
 dimorphous l.
 histoid l.
 indeterminate l.
 intermediate l.
 lazarine l.
 lepromatous l.
 Lombardy l.
 Lucio l.
 macular l.
 maculoanesthetic l.
 neural l.
 nodular l.
 polar lepromatous l.
 pure neural l.
 reactional l.
 spotted l.
 subclinical l.
 subpolar lepromatous l.
 trophoneurotic l.

leprosy (continued)
 tuberculoid l.
 uncharacteristic l.
 virchowian l.
 water-buffalo l.
leprotic
lesion
 blueberry muffin l.
 Cole herpetiform l.
 disseminated l.
 herpetiform l. of Cole
 initial syphilitic l.
 Janeway l.
 sessile l.
 shagreen l.
Letterer-Siwe
 disease
leukemia
 l. cutis
leukoderma
 l. acquisitum centrifugum
 l. colli
 genital l.
 occupational h.
 postinflammatory l.
 syphilitic l.
leukonychia
leukopathia
 acquired l.
 congenital l.
 l. punctata reticularis symmetrica
 l. unguium
leukopathy
 symmetric progressive l.
leukotrichia
Lewandowsky
 nevus elasticus
Lewandowsky-Lutz
 disease
lice (plural of louse)
lichen
 l. albus
 l. amyloidosus
 l. annularis
 l. aureus
 l. chronicus simplex
 l. corneus hypertrophicus

lichen (continued)
    l. fibromucinoidosus
    l. frambesianus
    l. leprosus
    l. myxedematosus
    l. nitidus
    l. obtusus corneus
    l. pilaris
    l. planopilaris
    l. planus
    l. planus actinicus
    l. planus, acute bullous
    l. planus annularis
    l. planus atrophicus
    l. planus, bullous
    l. planus erythematosus
    l. planus et acuminatus
        atrophicans
    l. planus follicularis
    l. planus, hypertrophic
    l. planus hypertrophicus
    l. planus subtropicum
    l. planus tropicum
    l. planus verrucosus
    l. planus, vesiculobullous
    l. ruber acuminatus
    l. ruber moniliformis
    l. ruber planus
    l. sclerosus
    l. sclerosus et atrophicus
    l. scrofulosorum
    l. scrofulosus
    l. simplex chronicus
    l. spinulosus
    l. striatus
    l. tropicus
    l. urticatus
lichenificatio
    l. gigantea
lichenoid
    l. amyloidosis
    l. dermatosis
    l. phase
light
    actinic l.
    infrared l.
    ultraviolet l.
    Wood l.

line
    See also *layer, streak,* and
        stria.
    Beau l.
    Futcher l.
    Morgan l.
    Pastia l.'s
    Voigt l.'s
linea (lineae)
    lineae albicantes
lipedema
lipoatrophy
lipoblast
lipogranulomatosis
lipoidosis
Lipschütz
    bodies
    cell
    disease
    erythema
    ulcer
livedo
    l. annularis
    l. racemosa
    l. reticularis
    l. reticularis idiopathica
    l. reticularis symptomatica
    l. telangiectatica
Lobo
    disease
Lortat-Jacobs
    disease
louse (lice)
    body l.
    clothes l.
    crab l.
    head l.
    pubic l.
    sucking l.
lues
    l. nervosa
    l. tarda
    l. venerea
"luko–" Phonetic for words begin-
    ning leuko–.
Lund-Browder
    burn scale

lunula (lunulae)
    l. of nail
    l. unguis
lupus
    Cazenave l.
    chilblain l.
    discoid l.
    disseminated follicular l.
    disseminated l. erythematosus
    l. erythematodes
    l. erythematosus (LE)
    l. erythematosus, chilblain
    l. erythematosus, cutaneous
    l. erythematosus, discoid
      (DLE)
    l. erythematosus discoides
    l. erythematosus disseminatus
    l. erythematosus, hypertrophic
    l. erythematosus hyper-
      trophicus
    l. erythematosus profundus
    l. erythematosus tumidus
    l. fibrosus
    l. hypertrophicus
    l. livido
    l. miliaris disseminatus faciei
    l. pernio
    photosensitive l. erythemato-
      sus
    l. profundus
    l. serpiginosus
    systemic l. erythematosus
      (SLE)
    transient neonatal systemic
      l. erythematosus
    l. tuberculosus
    l. tumidus
    l. verrucosus
    l. vorax
    l. vulgaris
Lutz-Miescher
    disease
Lutz-Splendore-Almeida
    disease
Lyell
    disease
    syndrome

lymphangioma
    l. cavernosum
    l. circumscriptum
    l. cysticum
    l. tuberosum multiplex
    l. xanthelasmoideum
lymphangitic
    l. sporotrichosis
lymphangitis
    l. carcinomatosa
lymphedema
    l. praecox
    l. tarda
lymphocytoma
    l. cutis
lymphogranuloma
    l. benignum
    l. inguinale
    l. venereum
lymphogranulomatosis
    l. cutis
    l. inguinalis
    l. maligna
lymphoma
    cutaneous T-cell l.
    l. cutis
    T-cell l., cutaneous
lymphomatoid
    l. granulomatosis
    l. papulosis
    l. vasculitis
lymphomatous
lymphosarcomatosis
maceration
macula (maculae)
    See also *macule* and *spot.*
    maculae atrophicae
    cerebral m.
    maculae ceruleae
    m. solaris
macular
maculate
maculation
macule
    See also *macula* and *spot.*
    ash-leaf m.
    lance-ovate m.
maculopapular

maculovesicular
Majocchi
    disease
    granuloma
    purpura
mal
    m. de Meleda
    m. morado
    m. perforant du pied
Malherbe
    calcifying epithelioma
malpighian
    m. cells
    m. layer
mamanpian
mammiform
mammilla (mammillae)
mammillated
mammillation
mammilliform
mammose
Manson
    pyosis
marbleization
margin
    hidden m. of nail
    m. of nail, free
    m. of nail, hidden
    m. of nail, lateral
margo (margines)
mastocytoma
    solitary m.
mastocytosis
    malignant m.
matricectomy
matrix (matrices)
    hair m.
    nail m.
    m. unguis
Mauriac
    syndrome
medulla (medullae)
    m. of hair shaft
medullated
medullation
medusae
    caput m.
megalonychia

Meirowsky phenomenon
melanoderma
    m. cachecticorum
    parasitic m.
    senile m.
melanodermatitis
melanoleukoderma
    m. colli
melanoma
    acral lentiginous m.
    amelanotic m.
    benign juvenile m.
    juvenile m.
    lentigo maligna m.
    malignant m.
    nodular m.
    spindle cell m.
    subungual m.
    superficial spreading m.
melanosis
    addisonian m.
    m. cachecticorum
    m. circumscripta precan-
      cerosa
    m. lenticularis progressiva
    periorbital m.
    pustular m.
    Riehl m.
melanotic [pertaining to melanin]
melanotrichia
melasma
    m. universale
Meleda
    disease
Melkersson
    syndrome
Melkersson-Rosenthal
    syndrome
membrane
    basement m.
meningococcemia
mentagra
    Alibert m.
Merkel
    cell
    cell carcinoma
methyl
    m. violet

MF—mycosis fungoides
Mibelli
    angiokeratoma
    disease
    porokeratosis
    syndrome
microabscess
    Pautrier m.
microadenoma
microlesion
micronychia
microsporosis
    m. capitis
Miescher
    actinic granuloma
    granulomatous cheilitis
migratory
    m. erythema
Mikulicz (von Mikulicz)
    aphthae
Milian
    erythema
    sign
    syndrome
miliaria
    m. alba
    apocrine m.
    m. crystallina
    m. papulosa
    m. profunda
    m. propria
    pustular m.
    m. pustulosa
    m. rubra
    m. vesiculosa
milium (milia)
    colloid m.
    multiple eruptive milia
    m. neonatorum
millijoule(s) (mJ)
Milton
    disease
    edema
    urticaria
"mio–" Phonetic for words beginning myo–.
Mitchell
    disease

Mitsuda
    antigen
    reaction
    test
mixed connective tissue disease
mJ—millijoule(s)
Moeller
    itch
Mohs
    chemosurgery
    procedure
    surgery
    technique
molluscum
    cholesterinic m.
    m. contagiosum
    m. epitheliale
    m. fibrosum
    m. giganteum
    m. lipomatodes
    m. pendulum
    m. sebaceum
    m. simplex
    m. varioliformis
    m. verrucosum
mongolian
    m. macule
    m. spot
Monro
    abscess
morphea
    acroteric m.
    m. alba
    m. atrophica
    m. flammea
    m. guttata
    herpetiform m.
    m. linearis
    m. nigra
morpio, morpion (morpiones)
Mortimer
    disease
    malady
mottled
Mucha
    disease
Mucha-Habermann
    disease

Mucha-Habermann (continued)
    syndrome
mucinosis
    follicular m.
    papular m.
Muckle-Wells
    syndrome
mulberry
    m. lesion
    m. pattern
Munro
    abscess
    microabscess
muscle
    See also in *Orthopedics and*
      Sports Medicine section.
    cutaneous m.
    dermal m.
mycetoma
    actinomycotic m.
    eumycotic m.
mycosis (mycoses)
    cutaneous m.
    m. cutis chronica
    m. favosa
    m. framboesioides
    m. fungoides
    m. fungoides d'emblée
    m. interdigitalis
myeloperoxidase (MPO) deficiency
myocutaneous
myxoma (myxomas, myxomata)
    lipomatous m.
nail
    double-edge n.
    eggshell n.
    hang n. [pref: hangnail]
    ingrown n.
    parrot beak n.
    pitted n.'s
    reedy n.
    spoon n.
    turtle-back n.
nail bed
nail nipper
    Amico n.n.
necklace
    Casal n.

necrobiosis
    n. lipoidica
    n. lipoidica diabeticorum
necrobiotic
    n. xanthogranuloma
necrolysis
    toxic epidermal n.
necrosis (necroses)
    cold-induced n.
    pressure n.
    n. progrediens
    radiation n.
    radium n.
necrotic
Nelson
    syndrome
neodymium (Nd)
    n.:yttrium-aluminum-garnet
      (Nd:YAG) laser
nerve
Netherton
    syndrome
Neumann
    disease
neuritic
neuritis
neurocutaneous
neurodermatitis
    circumscribed n.
    n. disseminata
    disseminated n.
    exudative n.
    localized n.
    nummular n.
neuroepidermal
neurofibromatosis
neurolipomatosis
    n. dolorosa
neuroma
    n. cutis
    false n.
    nevoid n.
    n. telangiectodes
neuromatosis
neuromatous
neuronevus
nevoid
    n. lentigo

nevoid (continued)
    n. telangiectasia
nevus (nevi)
    achromic n.
    n. acneiformis unilateris
    amelanotic n.
    n. anemicus
    n. angiectodes
    n. angiomatodes
    angiomatous n.
    n. arachnoideus
    n. araneosus
    n. araneus
    n. avasculosus
    balloon cell n.
    basal cell n.
    bathing trunk n.
    Becker n.
    blue n.
    blue rubber bleb n.
    capillary n.
    n. cavernosus
    cellular n.
    cellular blue n.
    n. cerebelliformis
    chromatophore n. of Naegeli
    comedo n.
    n. comedonicus
    compound n.
    connective tissue n.
    n. depigmentosus
    dermal n.
    dermoepidermal n.
    dysplastic n.
    n. elasticus
    n. elasticus of Lewandowsky
    epidermal n.
    epithelial nevi
    n. epitheliomatocylindro-
        matosus
    erectile n.
    fatty n.
    n. fibrosus
    n. flammeus
    n. follicularis
    n. fragarius
    n. fuscoceruleus acromiodel-
        toideus

nevus (nevi) (continued)
    n. fuscoceruleus ophthalmo-
        maxillaris
    giant congenital pigmented n.
    giant hairy n.
    giant pigmented n.
    hair follicle n.
    hairy n.
    halo n.
    hard n.
    hepatic n.
    honeycomb n.
    intradermal n.
    n. of Ito, Ito n.
    Jadassohn n.
    Jadassohn-Tièche n.
    junction n., junctional n.
    linear n.
    n. lipomatodes superficialis
    n. lipomatosus
    n. lipomatosus cutaneus
        superficialis
    lymphatic n.
    n. lymphaticus
    n. maculosis
    malignant blue n.
    marginal n.
    n. maternus
    melanocytic n.
    mixed n.
    n. mollusciformis
    n. molluscum
    n. morus
    multiplex n.
    n. nervosus
    neural n., neuroid n.
    nevocellular n.
    nevocytic n.
    nevus cell n.
    nodular connective tissue n.
    nonpigmented n.
    nuchal n.
    oral epithelial n.
    n. of Ota, Ota n.
    n. papillaris
    n. papillomatosus
    pigmented hairy epidermal n.
    pigmented n., n. pigmentosus

nevus (nevi) (continued)
    n. pilosus
    plane n.
    polyploid n.
    port-wine n.
    n. profundus
    raspberry n.
    n. sanguineus
    sebaceous n., n. sebaceus
    sebaceous n. of Jadassohn
    segmental n.
    n. simplex
    soft n.
    spider n.
    n. spilus
    n. spilus tardus
    spindle and epithelioid cell n.
    spindle cell n.
    Spitz n.
    n. spongiosus albus mucosae
    stellar n.
    straight hair n.
    strawberry n.
    subcutaneous n.
    Sutton n.
    n. syringocystadenosus
       papilliferus
    n. tardus
    n. unilateralis comedonicus
    n. unius lateralis
    n. unius lateris
    Unna n.
    vascular n., n. vascularis, n.
       vasculosus
    n. vascularis fungosus
    n. venosus
    venous n.
    n. verrucosus
    verrucous n.
    n. vinosus
    vulvar n.
    white sponge n.
    zoniform n.
Nicolas-Favre
    disease
nocardiosis
nodi (plural of nodus)
nodular

nodularity
nodulated
nodulation
noduli (plural of nodulus)
nodulous [adj.]
nodulus (noduli)
nodus (nodi)
NSHD—nodular sclerosing Hodg-
    kin disease
"nur–" Phonetic for words begin-
    ning neur–.
ochronosis
    exogenous o.
    ocular o.
oculocutaneous
    o. albinism
ointment
    Hebra o.
    Jarisch o.
    Whitfield o.
onchocerciasis
"onik–" Phonetic for words begin-
    ning onych–.
"on moss" Phonetic for en masse.
onychauxis
onychectomy
onychia
    o. lateralis
    o. maligna
    monilial o.
    o. parasitica
    o. periungualis
    o. sicca
    syphilitic o.
onychodystrophy
onychogryphosis
onycholysis
onychomycosis
    dermatophytic o.
onychorrhexis
onychosis
onychotomy
operation
    See in *General Surgical*
       Terms.
ophiasis
Osler
    disease

Osler (continued)
    nodes
    sign
    syndrome II
    triad
Osler-Vaquez
    disease
Osler-Weber-Rendu
    disease
    syndrome
osseous
    o. syphilis
    o. yaws
osteodermia
osteohypertrophic nevus flammeus
osteoma
    o. cutis
osteomatoid
osteomatosis
osteotelangiectasia
overgrowth
    fungal o.
PAB—*p*-aminobenzoate [p-, para-]
PABA—*p*-aminobenzoic acid [p-, para-]
PAC—papular acrodermatitis of childhood
pachyderma
    p. lymphangiectatica
pachydermoperiostosis
    p. plicata
PAFD—percutaneous abscess and fluid drainage
Paget
    abscess, abscess syndrome
    disease
paint
    Castellani p.
pallor
palmar
panatrophy
    Gowers p.
panniculalgia
panniculitis
    nodular nonsuppurative p.
panniculus (panniculi)
    p. adiposus

papilla (papillae)
    p. corii
    dermal p., p. dermatis, p. dermis
    hair p.
    nerve p.
    p. pili
    skin p.
    tactile papillae
papillary
papillate
papillation
papilliferous
papilliform
papilloma
    cutaneous p.
    p. diffusum
    intracanalicular p.
    p. lineare
    p. venereum
    warty p.
papillomatosis
    malignant p. of Degos
Papillon-Lefèvre syndrome
pappose
papular
    p. acrodermatitis
    p. urticaria
papulation
papule
    Celsus p.
    Gottron p.'s
    prurigo p.
    split p.
papulosis
    bowenoid p.
    lymphomatoid p.
para
    p.-aminobenzoate (PAB)
    p.-aminobenzoic acid (PABA)
parakeratosis [compare: porokeratosis]
    p. ostracea
    p. papulosa
    p. psoriasiformis
    p. scutularis
    p. variegata

parapsoriasis
    p. acuta
    acute p.
    atrophic p.
    p. atrophicans
    chronic p.
    p. en plaques
    p. guttata, guttate p.
    large-plaque p.
    p. lichenoides
    p. lichenoides chronica
    p. maculata
    poikilodermic p., poikiloder-
       matous p.
    retiform p.
    small-plaque p.
    p. variegata
    p. varigata
    p. varioliformis
    p. varioliformis acuta
    p. varioliformis chronica
parasite
    See specific parasites in
       Laboratory, Pathology,
       and Chemistry Terms.
parasitic
paronychia
    p. tendinosa
parrot
    p. beak nail
Pasini-Pierini
    syndrome
paste
    Lassar p.
    Veiel p.
patch
    herald p.
    shagreen p.
pathogen
    See specific pathogens in
       Laboratory, Pathology,
       and Chemistry Terms.
Pautrier
    abscess
PCT—porphyria cutanea tarda
peau
    p. de chagrin (Fr. shagreen
       skin)

peau (continued)
    p. d'orange (Fr. orange peel
       skin)
pedicular
pediculicides
pediculosis
    p. capillitii
    p. capitis
    p. corporis
    p. inguinalis
    p. palpebrarum
    p. pubis
    p. vestimenti
    p. vestimentorum
pediculous
pedicure
peduncular
pedunculated
peel
    chemical p.
    facial p.
peeling
PEG—polyethylene glycol
pellagra
pemphigoid
    bullous p.
pemphigus
    p. acutus
    p. erythematosus
    p. foliaceus
    p. gangrenosus
    p. hemorrhagicus
    p. malignus
    p. neonatorum
    p. syphiliticus
    p. vegetans
    p. vulgaris
periadenitis
    p. mucosa necrotica recurrens
periadnexal
    p. dermis
periarteritis
    p. gummosa
    p. nodosa
perifolliculitis
    p. capitis abscedens et suffo-
       diens
    superficial pustular p.

periorificial
    p. lentiginosis
petechia (petechiae)
PG—pyoderma gangrenosum
phagedena
    sloughing p.
    tropical p.
phakoma
phenomenon (phenomena)
    Arthus p., p. of Arthus
    Chase-Sulzberger p.
    Köbner (Koebner) p.
    Lucio p.
    Meirowsky p.
    Raynaud p.
    Sulzberger-Chase p.
phlyctena (phlyctenae)
phlyctenar
phlyctenoid
phthiriasis
    p. capitis
    p. corporis
    p. inguinalis
    pubic p.
phycomycosis
    subcutaneous p.
phyma (phymata)
piedra
    black p.
    white p.
pigment
    age p.
    melanotic p.
pigmentation
    addisonian dermal p.
pigmented
"pikno–" Phonetic for words beginning pykno–.
pilial
piliform
pilonidal
pilus (pili)
    pili annulati
    p. annulatus
    pili canaliculi
    p. cuniculatus
    pili incarnati
    pili incarnati recurvi

pilus (pili) (continued)
    p. incarnatus
    pili multigemini
    pili torti, p. tortus
    pili trianguli et canaliculi
pink disease
pityriasis
    p. alba
    p. amiantacea
    p. capitis
    p. circinata
    p. circinata et marginata
    p. furfuracea
    Gibert p.
    Hebra p.
    p. lichenoides
    p. lichenoides et varioliformis acuta
    p. linguae
    p. maculata
    p. pilaris
    p. rosea
    p. rotunda
    p. rubra
    p. rubra pilaris
    p. sicca
    p. simplex
    p. steatoides
    p. versicolor
planar
    p. xanthoma
plantar
    p. dermatosis, juvenile
    p. fibromatosis
    p. hyperkeratosis
    p. inoculum
    p. nevi
    p. wart
plaque
    herald p.
    Hutchinson p.'s
    shagreen p.
plate
    nail p.
PML—polymorphous light eruption
pock
pockmark

"po-do-rahnj" Phonetic for peau
    d'orange.
"po-duh-shah-grah" Phonetic for
    peau de chagrin.
poikiloderma
    p. atrophicans vasculare
    Civatte p.
    p. congenitale
point
    Kienböck-Adamson p.'s
poison
    contact p.
    corrosive p.
    p. ivy
    p. oak
    p. sumac
poliosis
    p. eccentrica
pollinosis
polyarteritis
    p. nodosa
polyenes [a class of drugs]
polyp
    lipomatous p.
polypoid
pomphoid
pompholyx
pomphus
pori (genitive and plural of porus)
porokeratosis [compare: parakerato-
    sis]
    disseminated superficial
      actinic p.
    p. of Mibelli
    p. palmaris et plantaris dis-
      seminata
poroma
porphyria
    p. cutanea tarda hereditaria
    p. variegata
portwine marks
porus (pori)
    p. sudoriferus
Posada mycosis
pressure ring
    Walsh p.r.
procedure
    Mohs p.

protoporphyria
    erythropoietic p.
PRP—pityriasis rubra pilaris
prurigo
    p. agria
    Besnier p., p. of Besnier
    p. chronica multiformis
    p. estivalis
    p. ferox
    p. gestationis
    p. of Hebra
    Hutchinson summer p.
    melanotic p.
    p. mitis
    nodular p.
    p. nodularis
    polymorphic p.
    p. simplex
    summer p. of Hutchinson
    p. universalis
    p. vulgaris
    winter p.
pruritus
    p. ani
    Duhring p.
    p. gravidarum
    p. hiemalis
    p. scroti
    senile p., p. senilis
    uremic p.
    p. vulvae
pseudofolliculitis
    p. barbae
pseudo-Turner syndrome
pseudoxanthoma
    p. elasticum
psoralens [a class of drugs]
psoriasis
    annular p.
    p. annularis
    p. annulata
    p. arthopica
    arthritic p.
    p. arthropathica
    Barber p.
    p. buccalis
    p. circinata
    circinate p.

psoriasis (continued)
    p. diffusa
    discoid p.
    p. discoidea
    p. discoides
    erythrodermic p.
    exfoliative p.
    p. figurata
    figurate p.
    flexural p.
    follicular p.
    p. follicularis
    generalized pustular p.
    p. guttata
    guttate p.
    p. gyrata
    gyrate p.
    inverse p.
    p. inveterata
    p. linguae
    localized pustular p.
    nummular p.
    p. nummularis
    p. ostracea
    ostraceous p.
    palmar p.
    p. palmaris et plantaris
    p. of palms and soles
    p. punctata
    pustular p.
    rupioid p.
    p. rupioides
    seborrheic p.
    p. universalis
    volar p.
    p. vulgaris
    Zumbusch p.
psorophthalmia
pterygium (pterygia)
    p. unguis
pubic
    p. lice
    p. phthiriasis
    p. trichomycosis
Puente disease
pulicicide
pultaceous
punctate

pura (plural of pus)
puris (genitive of pus)
purpura
    actinic p.
    allergic p.
    p. angioneurotica
    p. annularis telangiectodes
    autoimmune thrombocytopenic p.
    p. bullosa
    p. cachectica
    drug p.
    essential p.
    factitious p.
    p. iodica
    Landouzy p.
    p. maculosa
    Majocchi p.
    mechanical p.
    p. nervosa
    orthostatic p.
    p. pigmentosa chronica
    psychogenic p.
    p. pulicosa
    p. rheumatica
    senile p., p. senilis
    p. simplex
    steroid p.
    symptomatic p., p. symptomatica
    p. urticans
    p. variolosa
purulent
puruloid
pus (pura)
"pussy" Slang for pustular, puslike.
pustula (pustulae)
    p. maligna
pustular
pustule
pustulosis
    p. palmaris
    p. vacciniformis acuta
PUVA—psoralens and ultraviolet A
pyknotic
pyoderma
    p. chancriforme faciei
    p. faciale

pyoderma (continued)
    p. gangrenosum
    streptococcal p.
    p. ulcerosum tropicalum
    p. vegetans
    p. verrucosum
pyosis
    Corlett p., p. of Corlett
pyrethrins
Quincke
    angioedema
    disease
    edema
    I syndrome
Quinquaud
    disease
radiation
    r. dermatitis
    electromagnetic r.
    r. erythema
    r. spectrum
    ultraviolet r.
radices (plural of radix)
radiciform
radicis (genitive of radix)
radionuclide
radix (radices)
    r. pili
    r. unguis
ranula
Rayer disease
Raynaud
    disease
    gangrene
    phenomenon
    syndrome
reaction
    Bloch r.
    cutaneous r.
    dopa r.
    foreign body r.
    Goetsch skin r.
    Herxheimer r.
    id r.
    Jones-Mote r.
    Mitsuda r.
    wheal and erythema r.,
        wheal and flare r.

receptor
    contact r.
    cutaneous r.
    pain r.
    pressure r.
    sensory r.
    tactile r.
    touch r.
Recklinghausen (von Reckling-
    hausen)
    disease
    disease, central, type II
Reclus disease
reflex
    erector spinae r.
    pilomotor r.
Reiter
    disease
    syndrome
Rendu-Osler-Weber
    disease
    syndrome
rete (retia)
    dermal r.
    malpighian r.
retial
reticular
    r. dermis
    r. erythematous mucinosis
reticulosis
    epidermotropic r.
    lipomelanotic r.
    medullary r.
    pagetoid r.
reticulum (reticula)
retiform
    r. parapsoriasis
retinoids [a class of drugs]
retraction
rhacoma
rhagades [grammatically plural; no
    singular form]
rhagadiform
rhus dermatitis
Richner-Hanhart
    syndrome
Riley-Smith
    syndrome

ringworm
  r. of axillae
  r. of the beard
  black-dot r.
  r. of the body
  crusted r.
  r. of the face
  r. of the feet
  gray-patch r.
  r. of the groin
  r. of the hand
  honeycomb r.
  hypertrophic r.
  r. of the nails
  r. of the scalp
Ritter
  disease
"rizo–" Phonetic for words begin-
    ning rhizo–.
Robinson
  disease
Robles disease
Rollet
  chancre
rosacea
  granulomatous r.
Rosenbach
  erysipeloid
roseola
  r. infantum
rosette
  EAC r.
Rothmann-Makai
  syndrome
Rothmund
  syndrome
Rothmund-Thomson
  syndrome
rubeosis
ruber
ruberous
rubescent
rubor
ruborous
rubrous
Rud
  syndrome

rudiment
  hair r.
rufous
rupia
  r. escharotica
rupial
rupioid
sarcoid
  Boeck s., s. of Boeck
  Darier-Roussy s.
  Spiegler-Fendt s.
sarcoma (sarcomas, sarcomata)
  See also in *Oncology and
      Hematology* section.
  Abernethy s.
  adipose s.
  Kaposi s.
  melanotic s.
  multiple idiopathic hemor-
      rhagic s.
  pseudo-Kaposi s.
sarcomatosis
  s. cutis
sarcomatous
scabicides [a class of drugs]
scabies
  Boeck s.
  Norwegian s.
scale
  Lund-Browder burn s.
scaling
  s. nodule
  s. plaque
scan
  See in *Radiology, Nuclear
      Medicine, and Other
      Imaging* section.
scapus (scapi)
  s. pili
scarification
scarify
Schäfer
  syndrome
Schamberg
  dermatosis
  disease
  progressive pigmented pur-
      puric dermatosis

schistosomiasis
Schmidt
   syndrome
Schönlein
   disease
   purpura
Schönlein-Henoch
   disease
   purpura
   syndrome
Schultz
   angina
   disease
   syndrome
Schultze
   acroparesthesia
Schultze-type acroparesthesia
schwannoma
scleredema
   s. adultorum
   Buschke s.
   s. neonatorum
sclerema
   s. neonatorum
scleroadipose
sclerodactylia
   s. annularis ainhumoides
sclerodermatomyositis
sclerodermatous
sclerodermitis
sclerose
sclerosed
sclerosis
   miliary s.
sclerostenosis
sclerous
scrofuloderma
   s. gummosa
   papular s.
   pustular s.
   tuberculous s.
   ulcerative s.
   verrucous s.
scurvy
seborrhea
   s. adiposa
   s. capitis
   s. congestiva

seborrhea (continued)
   s. corporis
   eczematoid s.
   s. faciei
   s. furfuracea
   s. generalis
   nasolabial s.
   s. nigricans
   s. oleosa
   s. sicca
seborrheal
seborrheic
   s. dermatitis
   s. keratosis
Senear-Usher
   disease
   syndrome
senile
   s. keratosis
   s. lentigines
   s. purpura
sensitization
   active s.
separation
   eschar s.
serpiginous
serum (serums, sera)
   blister s.
Sézary
   erythroderma
   reticulosis
   syndrome
shaft
   hair s.
shagreen
"shangker" Phonetic for chancre.
"shangkroid" Phonetic for chancroid.
shingles
"shogren" Phonetic for Sjögren.
"shwah-no-mah" Phonetic for
   schwannoma.
sign
   See also *phenomenon, reflex,*
     and *test.*
   Auspitz s.
   Crowe s.
   Darier s.
   Dennie s.

sign (continued)
    Elliot s.
    Gottron s.
    Leser-Trélat s.
    Milian s.
    Nikolsky s.
    Osler s.
    Pastia s.
    Raynaud s.
    Silex s.
    Thomson s.
Silex
    sign
silicone
    s. granuloma
sin–. See also words beginning
    cin–, syn–.
sinus (sinus, sinuses)
    barber's hair s.
    s. unguis
Sjögren
    disease
    syndrome
skin
    alligator s.
    bronzed s.
    citrine s.
    collodion s.
    crocodile s.
    elastic s.
    farmers' s.
    fish s.
    freeze-dried s.
    glabrous s.
    glossy s.
    India rubber s.
    lax s., loose s.
    lyophilized s.
    marble s.
    nail s.
    parchment s.
    piebald s.
    pig s.
    porcupine s.
    sailors' s.
    shagreen s.
"sklero–" Phonetic for words begin-
    ning sclero–.

SLE—systemic lupus erythematosus
slough
sloughing
"sluff" Phonetic for slough.
"sluffing" Phonetic for sloughing.
smear
    Tzanck s.
soap
    Basis s.
SOAP—Subjective, Objective,
    Assessment, Plan [format for
    medical reports]
sola (plural of solum)
solar
solum (sola)
    s. unguis
"sor–" Phonetic for words begin-
    ning psor–.
sore
    bed s.
    canker s.
    chrome s.
    Cochin s.
    cold s. [pref: coldsore]
    Delhi s.
    desert s.
    Gallipoli s.
    hard s.
    mixed s.
    Naga s.
    oriental s.
    pressure s.
    primary s.
    soft s.
    umballa s.
    veldt s.
    venereal s.
Spanlang-Tappeiner
    syndrome
spiral
    Herxheimer s.'s
splinter
    s. hemorrhage
sponge
    white s. nevus
spoon
    s. nail

spot
>See also *macula* and *macule.*
>ash leaf s.
>blue s.
>café au lait s.
>cayenne pepper s.
>cold s.
>De Morgan s.
>Forchheimer s.
>Fordyce s.
>hot s.
>Koplik s.'s
>liver s.
>mongolian s.
>mulberry s.
>orange s.
>pain s.
>pink s.
>rose s.
>sacral s.
>shin s.
>temperature s.
>typhoid s.
>warm s.

squamate
squamous cell
SSSS—staphylococcal scalded skin
>syndrome
stain
>alcian blue s.
>Brown-Brenn s.
>Giemsa s.
>Hotchkiss-McManus s.
>Masson trichrome s.

staining
staphylococcal scalded skin syndrome (SSSS)
steatocystoma
>s. multiplex
Stevens-Johnson
>disease
>syndrome
Sticker disease
stomatitis (stomatitides)
>s. medicamentosa
strata (plural of stratum)
stratification

stratum (strata)
>s. corneum epidermidis
>s. corneum unguis
>s. malpighii
streak
>See also *layer, line,* and *stria.*
stria (striae)
>See also *layer, line,* and
>*streak.*
>striae albicantes
>striae atrophicae
>striae distensae
>Wickham s.
striatal
Sturge
>disease
>syndrome
Sturge-Weber
>disease
>encephalotrigeminal
>angiomatosis
>syndrome
styptics
subcutaneous
subcuticular
"sudo–" Phonetic for words beginning pseudo–.
sulciform
sulcus (sulci)
>sulci cutis
>s. of matrix of nail
>sulci of skin
Sulzberger-Garbe syndrome
sumac
>swamp s.
suppurative
surgery
>laser s.
>Mohs s.
Sutton
>disease
>nevus (nevi)
Sutton-Rendu-Osler-Weber
>syndrome
suture [material]
>See in *General Surgical Terms.*

suture [technique]
    See in *General Surgical
       Terms.*
swimmer's
    s. dermatitis
    s. itch
sycosiform
    s. tinea barbae
sycosis
    bacillogenic s.
    s. barbae
    coccogenic s.
    s. contagiosa
    s. framboesia
    s. framboesiaeformis
    hyphomycotic s.
    lupoid s.
    nonparasitic s.
    s. nuchae necrotisans
    parasitic s.
    s. staphylogenes
    s. vulgaris
Symmers
    disease
symptom
    See also in *General Medical
       Terms.*
    Sklowsky s.
syn–. See also words beginning
    cin–, sin–.
syndrome
    See also *disease.*
    Abt-Letterer-Siwe s.
    Albright s.
    Albright-McCune-Sternberg
      s.
    Alibert-Bazin s.
    ataxia-telangiectasia s.
    Bäfverstedt s.
    Bazex s.
    Bloch-Siemens-Sulzberger s.
    Bourneville s.
    Bourneville-Pringle s.
    Buschke-Ollendorff s.
    Danlos s.
    Degos s.
    Degos-Delort-Tricot s.
    Ehlers-Danlos s.

syndrome (continued)
    Felty s.
    Fiessinger-Leroy-Reiter s.
    Fiessinger-Rendu s.
    Gianotti-Crosti s.
    Goltz s.
    Goltz-Gorlin s.
    Gorlin-Goltz s.
    Gougerot s.
    Gougerot-Blum s.
    Gougerot-Carteaud s.
    Graham Little s.
    Greither s.
    Grönblad-Strandberg s.
    Günther s.
    Haber s.
    Hallopeau-Siemens s.
    Hartnup s.
    Henoch-Schönlein s.
    Howel-Evans s.
    intestinal polyposis–cutane-
      ous pigmentation s.
    Jadassohn-Lewandowsky s.
    Kasabach-Merritt s.
    keratitis-ichthyosis-deafness
      (KID) s.
    KID s.
    Klauder s.
    Klippel-Trénaunay s.
    Klippel-Trénaunay-Weber s.
    leopard s., LEOPARD s.
    Libman-Sacks s.
    Lyell s.
    Mauriac s.
    Melkersson s.
    Melkersson-Rosenthal s.
    Milian s.
    Muckle-Wells s.
    multiple lentigines s.
    Nelson s.
    Netherton s.
    pseudo-Turner s.
    Riley-Smith s.
    Rothmann-Makai s.
    Rothmund s.
    Rothmund-Thomson s.
    Rud s.
    Schäfer s.

syndrome (continued)
    Sézary s.
    Sjögren s.
    Sjögren-Larsson s.
    Stevens-Johnson s.
    Stryker-Halbeisen s.
    Sutton-Rendu-Osler-Weber s.
    Sweet s.
    Touraine III s.
    Touraine-Solente-Golé s.
    Unna-Thost s.
    Waterhouse-Friderichsen s.
    Weber-Christian s.
    Weber-Cockayne s.
    Werner s.
syphilitic
syringocystadenoma
    s. papilliferum
system
    integumentary s.
systemic
    s. lupus erythematosus (SLE)
tabes
    t. dorsalis
tabetic
tache ["tahsh"]
    t. bleuâtres ["bloo-ahtr"]
    t. noire ["nwahr"]
    t.'s noire sclérotiques
        ["sklay-ro-teek"]
Taenzer
    disease
"tahsh" Phonetic for tache.
tattoo
taut
    t. skin
T cell [noun]
T-cell [adj.]
technique
    See also in *General Surgical
        Terms.*
    Mohs t.
tela (telae)
    t. subcutanea
    t. submucosa
telangiectasia
    spider t.
    unilateral nevoid t.

telangiectasis (telangiectases)
    spider t.
    stellate t.
telar
test
    See also in *Laboratory,
        Pathology, and Chemistry
        Terms.*
    basophil degranulation t.
    coccidioidin skin t.
    Draize t.
    Frei t.
    Ito-Reenstierna t.
    Jadassohn-Bloch t.
    Keller ultraviolet t.
    Kolmer t.
    Kveim t.
    lepromin t.
    Mitsuda t.
    Tzanck t.
tetter
    brawny t.
    honeycomb t.
textus (textus)
thelerethism
thelium (thelia)
therapy
    See also *treatment.*
    grenz ray t.
    light t.
    photodynamic t.
    PUVA (psoralens and ultra-
        violet A light) t.
"theri–" Phonetic for words begin-
    ning phthiri–.
Thibierge-Weissenbach syndrome
Thompson
    dermatoplasty
Thomson
    disease
    poikiloderma congenitale
    scattering
    sign
tinea
    t. amiantacea
    t. axillaris
    t. barbae
    t. capitis

tinea (continued)
    t. ciliorum
    t. circinata
    t. corporis
    t. cruris
    t. decalvans
    t. favosa
    t. furfuracea
    t. glabrosa
    t. imbricata
    t. inguinalis
    t. kerion
    t. manuum
    t. nigra
    t. nodosa
    t. pedis
    t. profunda
    t. sycosis
    t. tarsi
    t. tonsurans
    t. unguium
    t. versicolor
tissue
    scar t.
toenail
"tool grah" Phonetic for tulle gras.
tophus (tophi)
    t. syphiliticus
torulus (toruli)
    toruli tactiles
"tosh" Phonetic for tache.
Touraine
    syndrome (III)
trauma (traumas, traumata)
treatment
    See also *therapy.*
    Castellani t.
    Gennerich t.
    Goeckerman t.
    light t.
    oatmeal t.
triad
    Gougerot t.
    Hutchinson t.
trichoepithelioma
    t. papillosum multiplex
trichomycosis
    t. axillaris

trichomycosis (continued)
    t. chromatica
    t. favosa
    t. nigra
    t. nodosa
    t. palmellina
    t. pustulosa
    t. rubra
trichophytosis
    t. barbae
    t. capitis
    t. corporis
    t. cruris
    t. unguium
trichorrhexis
    t. invaginata
    t. nodosa
trichrome
    t. vitiligo
tuber (tubers, tubera)
tubercle
tubercula (plural of tuberculum)
tuberculate, tuberculated
tuberculation
tuberculid
    micronodular t.
    papular t.
    papulonecrotic t.
    rosacea-like t.
tuberculitis
tuberculization
tuberculoderma
tuberculoid
tuberculosis (TB)
    t. colliquativa
    t. colliquativa cutis
    cutaneous t.
    t. cutis
    t. cutis indurativa
    t. cutis lichenoides
    t. cutis miliaris disseminata
    t. cutis orificialis
    t. cutis verrucosa
    t. fungosa cutis
    t. lichenoides
    t. miliaris cutis
    t. miliaris disseminata
    miliary t.

tuberculosis (TB) (continued)
    orificial t.
    papulonecrotic t.
    t. papulonecrotica
    t. of skin
    t. verrucosa cutis
    warty t.
tuberculum (tubercula)
tuberosis
tuberositas (tuberositates)
tubiferous
tularemia
tumentia
tumescent
tumor
    Abrikosov (Abrikossoff) t.
    benign t.
Turner
    familial syndrome
    male syndrome
    phenotype with normal
      karyotype
    syndrome
    syndrome in females with
      normal X chromosome
Turner-Keiser
    syndrome
tylosis
    t. ciliaris
    t. palmaris et plantaris
Tzanck
    cell
    smear
    test
ulcer
    chancroid u.
    decubitus u.
    Lipschütz u.
    Meleney chronic undermin-
      ing u.
ulcera (plural of ulcus)
ulcerate
ulcerating
ulceration
    ischemic u.
ulcerative
ulcus (ulcera)
    u. ambulans

ulcus (ulcera) (continued)
    u. ambustiforme
    u. durum
    u. interdigitale
    u. molle cutis
    u. scorbuticum
    u. syphiliticum
    u. vulvae acutum
ulerythema
    u. acneiforma
    u. centrifugum
    u. ophryogenes
    u. sycosiforme
Ullrich-Turner
    syndrome
ultraviolet
    u. A (UVA)
Underwood disease
unguent
unguenta (plural of unguentum)
unguenti (genitive of unguentum)
unguentum (unguenta)
unguis (ungues)
    u. incarnatus
unit
    See also in *General Medical*
      Terms and *Laboratory,*
      Pathology, and Chemistry
      Terms.
    pilosebaceous u.
    skin test u.
Unna
    boot
    cell
    dermatosis
    disease
    nevus
    syndrome
Unna-Thost
    syndrome
Urbach-Oppenheim disease
urethritis
    gonorrheal u.
urticaria
    acute u.
    aquagenic u.
    u. bullosa
    bullous u.

urticaria (continued)
    cholinergic u.
    chronic u.
    cold u.
    contact u.
    endemic u.
    u. endemica
    u. epidemica
    u. factitia
    factitious u.
    giant u.
    u. gigantea
    heat u.
    hemorrhagic u.
    u. hemorrhagica
    heredofamilial u.
    light u.
    u. medicamentosa
    Milton u.
    u. multiformis endemica
    papular u.
    u. papulosa
    u. perstans
    u. photogenica
    u. pigmentosa
    pressure u.
    solar u.
    u. solaris
    u. subcutanea
    subcutaneous u.
UV—ultraviolet
UVA—ultraviolet A
UVB—ultraviolet B
UVL—ultraviolet light
vaccine
vaccinia
    v. gangrenosa
vagabond's disease
vallecula (valleculae)
    v. unguis
vallecular
vallum (valla)
    v. unguis
varicella
    v. gangrenosa
    pustular v.
    v. pustulosa

varicelliform
    Kaposi v. eruption
variola
    v. crystallina
    v. inserta
    v. miliaris
    v. minor
    v. mitigata
    v. pemphigosa
    v. siliquosa
    v. vera
    v. verrucosa
vascular
    v. endothelium
    v. hamartoma
    v. hemophilia
    v. nevus
    v. spider
    v. tumor
vasculitic
vasculitis
    granulomatous v.
    livedoid v.
    lymphomatoid v.
    necrotizing v.
    nodular v.
    septic v.
    urticarial v.
vasoconstriction
vellus
    v. hair
    v. olivae
Venus
    collar of V.
Verneuil
    neuroma
verruca (verrucae)
    v. acuminata, verrucae
        acuminatae
    v. digitata
    v. filiformis
    v. glabra
    v. mollusciformis
    v. necrogenica
    v. peruana
    v. peruviana
    v. plana
    v. plana juvenilis

verruca (verrucae) (continued)
    v. plantaris
    v. seborrheica
    v. senilis
    v. simplex
    v. tuberculosa
    v. vulgaris
verrucosis
    lymphostatic v.
verruga
    v. peruana
vesicants
vesicatory
vesicobullous
vesicular
    v. bullous pemphigoid
    v. dermatophytid
    v. ringworm
    v. stomatitis
vesiculated
vesiculiform
vesiculobullous
vesiculopapular
vesiculopustular
vibesate
vibex (vibices)
vibratory
    v. angioedema
Vinson syndrome
virus
    See also in *Laboratory,*
      Pathology, and Chemistry
      Terms.
    enteric cytopathogenic
      human orphan (ECHO) v.
      [now: echovirus]
    measles v.
visceral
    v. syphilis
vitiligines (plural of vitiligo)
vitiliginous
vitiligo (vitiligines)
    v. capitis
    Cazenave v.
    Celsus v.
    circumscribed v.
    perinevic v.

Vogt-Koyanagi
    syndrome
Vogt-Koyanagi-Harada
    syndrome
Vohwinkel syndrome
Voigt
    boundary lines
von Recklinghausen. See *Reckling-*
    hausen.
von Zumbusch. See *Zumbusch.*
vortex (vortices)
    vortices pilorum
Walsh
    pressure ring
wart
    anatomical w.
    filiform w.
    mosaic w.
    mucocutaneous w.
    necrogenic w.
    periungual w.
    pitch w.
    plantar w.
    seborrheic w.
    seed w.
    telangiectatic w.
    tuberculous w.
    venereal w.
warty
    w. dyskeratoma
    w. tuberculosis
Weber-Christian
    disease
    panniculitis
    syndrome
Wells
    syndrome
Werner
    syndrome
White [eponym]
    disease
whitlow
Whitmore
    disease
    fever
    melioidosis
Wilks
    disease

Wilson
    disease
    lichen
Winkler disease
Witkop-Von Sallman disease
Wood [eponym]
    lamp
    light
Woringer-Kolopp disease
xanthism
xanthochromia
xanthochromic
xanthoerythrodermia
    x. perstans
xanthogranulomatosis
xanthogranulomatous
xanthoma (xanthomas, xanthomata)
    diabetic x., x. diabeticorum
    disseminated x., x. dissemi-
       natum
    eruptive x., x. eruptivum
    generalized plane x.
    juvenile x.
    x. multiplex
    x. palpebrarum
    planar x., plane x., x. planum
    x. striatum palmare
    tendinous x., x. tendinosum
    tuberoeruptive x.
    x. tuberosum, x. tuberosum
       multiplex, tuberous x.
    verruciform x.
xanthosis
    x. cutis
    x. diabeticorum

xanthous
xeroderma
    follicular x.
    Kaposi x., x. of Kaposi
    x. pigmentosum
xerosis
    x. cutis
X-linked
    X.-l. cutis laxa
    X.-l. hypogammaglobuline-
       mia
    X.-l. ichthyosis
    X.-l. recessive inheritance
Zahorsky disease
"zank" Phonetic for Tzanck.
Zinsser-Cole-Engman syndrome
Zinsser-Engman-Cole syndrome
zona (zonae)
    z. dermatica
    z. epithelioserosa
    z. facialis
zonal
zonary
zone
    Head z.'s
    z.'s of hyperalgesia
    z. of hyperemia
    hyperesthetic z.
    keratogenous z.
    papillary z.
    vascular z.
zonesthesia
Zumbusch (von Zumbusch)
    psoriasis

Gastroenterology

AAC—antibiotic-associated colitis
AAD—antibiotic-associated diarrhea
AAPMC—antibiotic-associated
    pseudomembranous colitis
Aaron
        sign
AAS—acute abdominal series
Abbe
        intestinal anastomosis
        small-bowel operation
abdomen
abdominal
        a. abscess
        a. aortic aneurysm
        a. crisis
        a. decompression
        a. inguinal ring
abdominalgia
        periodic a.
abdominocardiac reflex
abdominocentesis
abdominocystic
abdominoperineal
        a. resection (APR)
abdominovesical
        a. pouch
abenteric
abscess
        amebic a.
        anorectal a.
        appendiceal a.
        bile duct a.
        biliary a.
        cholangitic a.
        crypt a.
        diaphragmatic a.
        diverticular a.
        Douglas a.
        entamebic a.
        epiploic a.
        fecal a.

abscess (continued)
        filarial a.
        helminthic a.
        hepatic a.
        intersphincteric a.
        intra-abdominal a.
        ischiorectal a.
        liver a.
        midabdominal a.
        pancreatic a.
        parapancreatic a.
        pelvirectal a.
        perianal a.
        pericholecystic a.
        perirectal a.
        peritoneal a.
        pilonidal a.
        postcecal a.
        preperitoneal a.
        protozoal a.
        psoas a.
        retrocecal a.
        retroesophageal a.
        retroperitoneal a.
        splenic a.
        stercoraceous a., stercoral a.
        subaponeurotic a.
        subhepatic a.
        subperitoneal a.
        subphrenic a.
        suprahepatic a.
        tympanitic a.
absorption
abuse
        laxative a.
acanthocytosis
acanthosis
        malignant a. nigricans
        a. nigricans
ACBE—air contrast barium enema
ACD—adult celiac disease

ACG—American College of Gastroenterology
achalasia
    cricopharyngeal a.
    pelvirectal a.
    sphincteral a.
achlorhydria
    a. apepsia
achlorhydric
acholuria
acholuric
achylia
    a. gastrica haemorrhagica
    a. pancreatica
achymia
acid
    amino a.
    hydrochloric a.
    saturated fatty a. (SFA)
    unsaturated fatty a.
acidic
acidophilus [*Lactobacillus acidophilus*]
acidophilus milk
acini (plural of acinus)
acinic
aciniform
acinitis
acinose [adj.]
acinotubular
acinous [adj.]
acinus (acini)
    liver a.
    pancreatic a.
acoprosis
acoprous
acrodermatitis
    a. enteropathica
acromphalus
ACS—American College of Surgeons
action
activated charcoal
Adamantiades-Behçet syndrome
Addison
    planes
    point

adenasthenia
    a. gastrica
adenitis
    mesenteric a.
adenocarcinoma
    gastric a.
adenohypersthenia
    a. gastrica
adenoma
    papillary a.
    tubulovillous a.
    villous a.
adenomatous
    a. polyposis
adipohepatic
adipolytic
adipopectic
adipopexis
adynamic
    a. ileus
aeroperitonia
aerosialophagy
aerosis
AGA—American Gastroenterological Association
aganglionic
agastria
agastric
AGE—acute gastroenteritis
β_2 agonist
agonist
    beta-2 a.
    cholinergic a.'s [a class of drugs]
air
    a. cushion
    a. insufflation
    a. swallowing
air-fluid level
"akahlazeea" Phonetic for achalasia.
Åkerlund
    deformity
"a-ky-lee-a" Phonetic for achylia.
albuminocholia
alimentation
alkalinity
allergy
    food a.

allergy (continued)
    gastrointestinal a.
Allingham
    colotomy
    fissure
    operation
    rectum excision
    ulcer
alpha
    a.-dextrinase
Alport
    syndrome
alvus
amasesis
amblygeustia
amebiasis
    intestinal a.
ampulla (ampullae)
    a. of gallbladder
    a. hepatopancreatica
    a. of Vater
Amussat
    operation
    valve
anal
    a. canal
    a. manometry
    a. sphincter
analysis
    gastric a.
anastomosis (anastomoses)
    See also *operation* and *pro-cedure.*
    Billroth a., Billroth I a., Billroth II a.
    Braun a.
    enteric a.
    esophagojejunal a.
    peristaltic a.
    rectosigmoid a.
    Roux-en-Y a.
Andersen
    disease
    syndrome
    triad
Andresen
    diet

anesthesia
    See in *General Surgical Terms.*
angina
    abdominal a.
    a. abdominalis
    a. dyspeptica
    intestinal a.
anginal
angiocholitis
    a. proliferans
angiography
    biliary a.
angioma
angiomatoid
angiomatosis
angle
    duodenojejunal a.
    ileocolic a.
annular
anococcygeal
anocutaneous
    a. fistula
anoderm
anogenital
anomalotrophy
anomaly
anopelvic
anoperineal
anoplasty
anorectal
anorectitis
anorectoplasty
    Laird-McMahon a.
anorexia
    a. nervosa
anorexigenic
anoscopy
antacids [a class of drugs]
antagonist
    histamine H_2 a.'s [a class of drugs]
antecolic
    a. gastrectomy
anticholinergics [a class of drugs]
antiemetics [a class of drugs]
antimesenteric
antinauseants [a class of drugs]

antiperistalsis
antiperistaltics [a class of drugs]
antispasmodics [a class of drugs]
antra (plural of antrum)
antral
    a. resection
antroduodenectomy
antrum (antra)
    duodenal a.
anus
    imperforate a.
APC—adenomatous polyposis coli
apepsia
    achlorhydria a.
aponeurosis (aponeuroses)
    perineal a.
    superficial perineal a.
apparatus
    Golgi a.
appearance
    cobblestone a.
    cobblestone-like a.
    ground-glass a.
    picket fence a.
appendalgia
appendectomy
appendical
appendiceal
appendicealgia
appendicectasis
appendicism
appendicitis
    acute a.
    a. by contiguity
    chronic a.
    fulminating a.
    gangrenous a.
    a. granulosa
    helminthic a.
    a. larvata
    myxoglobulosis a.
    necropurulent a.
    nonobstructive a.
    a. obliterans
    perforating a.
    perforative a.
    stercoral a.
    subperitoneal a.

appendicitis (continued)
    suppurative a.
    syncongestive a.
    verminous a.
appendiclausis
appendicocecostomy
appendicocele
appendicoenterostomy
appendicolith
appendicolithiasis
appendicolysis
appendicopathia
appendicopathy
appendicosis
appendicostomy
appendix (appendices)
    vermiform a.
appendolithiasis
appetite
    perverted a.
APR—abdominoperineal resection
arch
    arterial a.'s of colon
    arterial a.'s of ileum
    arterial a.'s of jejunum
    Treitz a.
area (areae, areas)
    areae gastricae
arteria (arteriae)
    a. lusoria
arterialization
    a. of portal vein
arteriography
    celiac a.
arthritis (arthritides)
    chylous a.
    colitic a.
    dysenteric a.
    enteropathic reactive a.
    villous a.
ASGE—American Society for Gas-
    trointestinal Endoscopy
aspiration
atony
    chronic intestinal a.
ATPase—adenosine triphosphatase
ATPase (adenosine triphosphatase)
    inhibitors [a class of drugs]

atresia
> biliary a.
> esophageal a.
> ileal a.
> pyloric a.

atrophy
> gastric mucosal a.

Aub-Dubois
> standards
> table

Auerbach
> ganglion (ganglia)
> node
> plexus

autocholecystectomy
autosplenectomy
avenolith
bacillus (bacilli)
> See in *Laboratory, Pathology, and Chemistry Terms.*

Bacillus
> See in *Laboratory, Pathology, and Chemistry Terms.*

bacterium (bacteria)
> See specific bacteria in *Laboratory, Pathology, and Chemistry Terms.*

Balfour
> gastroenterostomy

Ballance sign
balloon
> b. manometry
> b. tamponade

ballotable
ballottement
> abdominal b.

band
> See also *layer* and *line.*
> cholecystoduodenal b.
> Ladd b.
> Lane b.

bandage
> See in *General Surgical Terms.*

Banti
> disease
> splenic anemia
> syndrome

Bard
> syndrome

bariatrics
barium (Ba)
Barrett
> esophagus
> syndrome
> ulcer

Bársony-Polgár syndrome
Bauhin
> gland
> valve

Baumgarten
> cirrhosis
> syndrome

BE—barium enema
Beck
> gastrostomy

Beck-Jianu
> gastrostomy

bed
> stomach b.

Behçet
> disease
> syndrome

bellyache
Belsey
> Mark II fundoplication
> Mark IV operation
> Mark V operation
> repair

benzimidazoles, substituted [a class of drugs]
Bernard
> canal
> duct

Bernstein
> test

Best
> operation

beta
> b.-2 agonist
> b.-sitosterolemia

bezoar
Bi—bismuth
bicarbonate
> b. of soda, sodium b.

Biesiadecki fossa

bile acid sequestrants [a class of drugs]
biliary
    b. angiography
    b. hypoplasia
Billroth
    anastomosis (I, II)
    cord
    gastrectomy
    gastroduodenoscopy
    gastroenterostomy (I, II, III)
    gastrojejunostomy
    hypertrophy
    operation (I, II)
    strands
    venae cavernosae
binge
bingeing and purging
biopsy
    transrectal b.
Blatin
    sign
    syndrome
blindgut
bloat
block
    portal b.
blockage
blocker
    H_2 b.'s [a class of drugs]
    starch b.
blood
    occult b.
Bloodgood
    operation
Blumberg
    sign
BM—bowel movement
Boas
    algesimeter
    point
    sign
    test meal
Bochdalek
    foramen
    gap
    hernia

body (bodies)
    Mallory b.
    malpighian b.'s of spleen
    b. of pancreas
    Savage perineal b.
    b. of stomach
Boeck
    See *Beck.*
Boerhaave
    syndrome
Bogros space
"boo-shahr(z)" Phonetic for Bouchard.
"boo-ton" Phonetic for bouton.
"boo-ve-ray" Phonetic for Bouveret.
"boo-yaw," "boo-yawn" Phonetic for bouillon.
Borrmann gastric cancer typing system (types I–IV)
Bouchard
    disease
bouillon
bouton
    b. en chemise
Bouveret
    syndrome
Bouveret-Duguet ulcer
bowel
    gangrenous b.
    greedy b.
    b. movement (BM)
    b. obstruction
    b. sounds
Bowen
    disease
Boyden
    sphincter
    test
    test meal
bradyphagia
bradytrophia
bradytrophic
brash
    water b.
BRAT—bananas, rice cereal, applesauce, toast [diet]
Braun
    anastomosis

Braune
    muscle
    valve
Braun and Jaboulay
    gastroenterostomy
breach
breath
    liver b.
bridle
Brinton
    disease
Broesike fossa
bronchoesophageal
    b. fistula
bronchopancreatic
    b. fistula
"broo-ee" Phonetic for bruit.
"bru-ee" Phonetic for bruit.
bruit
    See in *Cardiology* and *Pulmonary Medicine* sections.
Brunner
    gland hamartoma
    glands
"brwe" Phonetic for bruit.
BS—bowel sounds
BSN—bowel sounds normal
bubble
    Garren-Edwards gastric b.
Budd-Chiari
    disease
    syndrome
bulb
    duodenal b.
bulimia
    b. nervosa
bulk-producing laxatives [a class of drugs]
Burnett
    syndrome
burping
Byler
    disease
bypass
    percutaneous biliary b.
CAG—chronic atrophic gastritis
Cal, Kcal—kilocalorie
calculous [adj.]

Calot
    operation
Campylobacter fetus enteritis
Canada-Cronkhite syndrome
canal
canaliculus (canaliculi)
    bile canaliculi, biliary canaliculi
    c. bilifer
    pseudobile c.
cancer
    See also *carcinoma.*
    See also in *Oncology and Hematology* section.
    colorectal c.
Cannon
    point
    ring
cap
    phrygian c.
capillariasis
    intestinal c.
CAPS—caffeine, alcohol, pepper, spicy foods
CAPS-free diet
capsule
    enteric c.
    Glisson c.
caput (capita)
    c. medusae
carcinoma (carcinomas, carcinomata)
    See also in *Oncology and Hematology* section.
    adenoid cystic c.
    bile duct c.
    biliary c.
    colorectal c.
    esophageal c.
    hepatocellular c.
    hilar c.
    liver cell c.
    oat cell c.
    pancreatic c.
    peritoneal c.
carcinomatosis
    c. peritonei
cardia
    c. of stomach

cardioesophageal
cardiohepatic
cardiohepatomegaly
Carnot
    function
    test
Caroli
    disease
catheter
    needle c. jejunostomy
CBD—common bile duct
CCC—chronic calculous cholecystitis
CCP—chronic calcifying pancreatitis
CD—common duct
    cystic duct
CDE—common duct exploration
cecectomy
cecocolic
cecocolon
cecocolopexy
cecocolostomy
cecocystoplasty
cecofixation
cecoileostomy
cecopexy
cecoplication
cecoptosis
cecorrhaphy
cecosigmoidostomy
cecotomy
CEG—chronic erosive gastritis
celiac
    c. arteriography
    c. disease
    c. sprue
celiocentesis
celioenterotomy
celiogastrotomy
celioparacentesis
celiorrhaphy
celiotomy
    c. incision
    vaginal c.
    ventral c.
cell
    See also in *Laboratory,
    Pathology, and Chemistry
    Terms.*

cell (continued)
    acinar c.
    goblet c.
    Paneth c.
celotomy
centrilobular
Chagas
    disease
Chagas-Cruz
    disease
chalasia
charcoal
    activated c.
Chiari
    disease
    syndrome
Chilaiditi
    sign
    syndrome
cholangiectasis
cholangioadenoma
cholangiocarcinoma
cholangiocholecysto-choledochecto-
    my
cholangioenterostomy
cholangiogram
    endoscopic retrograde c.
    intraoperative c.
    intravenous c.
    operative c.
    percutaneous transhepatic c.
    retrograde c.
    transhepatic c.
    T-tube c.
cholangiography
    cystic duct c.
    delayed operative c.
    direct percutaneous transhe-
        patic c.
    endoscopic c.
    endoscopic retrograde c.
        (ERC)
    fine-needle transhepatic c.
        (FNTC)
    intraoperative c.
    intravenous c. (IVC)
    operative c.
    percutaneous hepatobiliary c.

cholangiography (continued)
    percutaneous transhepatic c.
      (PTC)
    postoperative c.
    transabdominal c.
    transhepatic c. (TC)
    T-tube c.
cholangiohepatitis
cholangiohepatoma
cholangiojejunostomy
    intrahepatic c.
cholangioma
cholangiopancreatography
    endoscopic retrograde c.
      (ERCP)
cholangiostomy
cholangiotomy
cholangitis
    catarrhal c.
    c. lenta
cholecystalgia
cholecystatony
cholecystectasia
cholecystectomy
cholecystic
cholecystitis
    acute c.
    acute acalculous c.
    chronic c.
    c. cystica
    c. emphysematosa
    emphysematous c.
    follicular c.
    gaseous c.
    c. glandularis proliferans
cholecystocele
cholecystocolonic
cholecystocolostomy
cholecystocolotomy
cholecystoduodenostomy
cholecystoenterostomy
cholecystoenterotomy
cholecystogastric
cholecystogastrostomy
cholecystogogic
cholecystogram
cholecystography
    intravenous c.

cholecystography (continued)
    oral c.
    post–fatty meal c.
cholecystoileostomy
cholecystointestinal
cholecystojejunostomy
cholecystokinetic
cholecystolithiasis
cholecystolithotomy
cholecystolithotripsy
cholecystopathy
cholecystopexy
cholecystoptosis
cholecystopyelostomy
cholecystorrhaphy
cholecystosis
    hyperplastic c.
cholecystostomy
cholecystotomy
choledochal
    c. sphincterotomy
choledochitis
choledochocele
choledochocystostomy
choledochodochorrhaphy
choledochoduodenostomy
choledochogram
choledochography
choledocholith
choledocholithiasis
choledocholithotomy
choledocholithotripsy
choledochorrhaphy
choledochoscopy
choledochosphincterotomy
choledochostomy
choledochotomy
choledochus
cholelith
cholelithiasis
cholelithic
cholelithotomy
cholelithotripsy
cholelithotrity
cholemesis
cholemia
cholemic

cholepathia
  c. spastica
choleperitoneum
cholera
  bilious c.
  c. morbus
  c. nostras
cholescintigraphy
  radionuclide c.
cholestasis
  familial intraheptic c.
cholinergic
  c. agonists [a class of drugs]
chromoscopy
  gastric c.
chylangioma
chylaqueous
chyle
chylectasia
chyloperitoneum
chylorrhea
chyluria
CIBD—chronic inflammatory
  bowel disease
cicatricial
cin–. See also words beginning
  sin–, syn–.
circular
  Livaditis c. myotomy
cirrhosis
  biliary c.
  calculus c.
  cardiac c.
  Glisson c.
  Maixner c.
cirrhotic
CIS—carcinoma in situ
cistern
Clark
  sign
classification
  Astler-Coller modification
    of Dukes c.
  Borrmann c.
  Dukes c. (A, B, B_2, C_1, C_2)
    [B2, C1, C2]
  McNeer c.

cloaca (cloacae)
  congenital c.
  persistent c.
cloacal
CLOtest
coffee-grounds
  c-g. vomit, c.-g. vomitus
colectomy
colic
  biliary c.
  bilious c.
  crapulent c.
  gallstone c.
  gastric c.
  hepatic c.
  intestinal c.
  mucous c.
  pancreatic c.
  pseudomembranous c.
  saburral c.
  stercoral c.
  vermicular c.
  verminous c.
colicky pain
colitis (colitides)
  adaptive c.
  amebic c.
  balantidial c.
  collagenous c.
  c. cystica profunda
  c. cystica superficialis
  diversion c.
  fulminating c.
  granulomatous c.
  c. gravis
  infectious c.
  mucous c.
  myxomembranous c.
  c. polyposa
  pseudomembranous c.
  segmental c.
  transmural c.
  tuberculous c.
  ulcerative c.
  uremic c.
collum (colla)
  c. vesicae biliaris
colocecostomy

colocentesis
colocholecystostomy
coloclysis
colocolostomy
colocutaneous
colofixation
coloileal
colon
    c. ascendens
    ascending c.
    c. descendens
    descending c.
    distal c.
    irritable c.
    lead-pipe c.
    pelvic c. of Waldeyer
    proximal c.
    redundant c.
    c. resection (CR)
    sigmoid c.
    c. sigmoideum
    spastic c.
    thrifty c.
    transverse c.
    c. transversum
    unstable c.
colonalgia
colonization
    jejunal c.
    stool c.
colonopathy
colonorrhagia
colonorrhea
colonoscopy
    fiberoptic c.
colopexy
coloplication
coloproctectomy
coloproctostomy
coloptosis
colorectostomy
colorrhaphy
colosigmoidostomy
colostomy
    end c.
    end-to-side ileotransverse c.
    ileotransverse c.
    Wangensteen c.

colotomy
    Allingham c.
colovesical
    c. fistula
columna (columnae)
    columnae anales
    columnae rectales
competent
    c. bowel
complex
    Golgi c.
computed
    c. tomography (CT)
computerized
    c. axial tomography (CAT)
constipation
    gastrojejunal c.
Cooper
    hernia
    ligament hernioplasty
Courvoisier
    gallbladder
    gastroenterostomy
    law
    sign
CR—colon resection
cremasteric
crepitus
CREST—calcinosis cutis, Raynaud
    phenomenon, esophageal dys-
    function/hypermotility, sclero-
    dactyly, telangiectasia
    [syndrome]
Crigler-Najjar
    disease
    syndrome
Crohn
    disease
Cronkhite-Canada syndrome
CRS—colorectal surgery
Cruveilhier
    sign
Cruz-Chagas
    disease
crypt
    anal c.
    c.'s of Lieberkühn
    Luschka c.'s

crypt (continued)
    c. of Morgagni
    mucous c.'s of duodenum
    multilocular c.
crypta (cryptae)
cryptectomy
cryptitis
cryptoglandular
cryptolith
cryptosporidiosis
    biliary c.
Curschmann
    disease
curvature
    greater c.
    lesser c.
Cushing
    ulcer
Cushing-Rokitansky ulcer
cyst
    choledochal c.
    omental c.
cystectomy
cystic
    c. duct cholangiography
cystocolostomy
cystoduodenostomy
cystogastrostomy
cystojejunostomy
    Roux-en-Y c.
cystorectocele
decompression
    intestinal d.
Degos
    disease
    syndrome
dehydrogenase
    lactic d.
delayed
    d. operative cholangiography
Demerol [anesthetic agent]
demucosatio
    d. intestini
dentate
DePage-Janeway
    gastrostomy
DES—diffuse esophageal spasm

descending
    d. colon
Desjardins
    point
α-dextrinase [alpha-]
diabetic
    d. autonomic neuropathy
    d. gastroparesis
    d. ketoacidosis
diastase
    pancreatic d.
diet
    Andresen d.
    Atkins d.
    CAPS-free d.
    Ebstein d.
    Giordano-Giovannetti d.
    gluten-free d.
    high-protein d.
    Jarotsky d.
    low-carbohydrate d.
    Meulengracht d.
    paleolithic d.
    reducing d.
    Sippy d.
dieting
    yo-yo d.
Dieulafoy
    disease
    erosion
    theory
    triad
digestive
    d. tube
    d. tract
dilatation
    esophageal d.
Diogenes syndrome
direct
    d. percutaneous transhepatic
        cholangiography
dis–. See also words beginning dys–.
discrete
    d. lesion
    d. masses
    d. narrowing
    d. nodule
    d. organ enlargement

disease
  See also *syndrome.*
  Bowen d.
  Brinton d.
  Byler d.
  Caroli d.
  celiac d.
  Chagas d.
  Chagas-Cruz d.
  Crohn d.
  Cruveilhier d.
  Cruz-Chagas d.
  Degos d.
  extramammary Paget d.
  Gee d.
  Gee-Herter d.
  Gee-Thaysen d.
  Glénard d.
  graft-versus-host d. (GVHD)
  Gross d.
  Hanot d.
  hepatobiliary tract d.
  Herter-Heubner d.
  Heubner-Herter d.
  Hirschsprung d.
  Hodgkin d.
  inflammatory bowel d. (IBD)
  irritable bowel d. (IBD)
  Kohlmeier-Degos d.
  Mackenzie d.
  Ménétrier d.
  Mya d.
  Ohara d.
  Paget d.
  Patella d.
  Payr d.
  peptic ulcer d. (PUD)
  Reichmann d.
  Rossbach d.
  Tangier d.
  Thaysen d.
  Wassilieff d.
  Whipple d.
  Wolman d.
"disfajea" Phonetic for dysphagia.
DISIDA—diisopropyliminodiacetic
  acid

disorder
  appetite d.
  motility d.
distomiasis
  intestinal d.
diversion
  d. colitis
diverticula (plural of diverticulum)
diverticulae [incorrect spelling/pro-
    nunciation of diverticula]
diverticular
diverticulectomy
  vesical d.
diverticuli [incorrect spelling/pro-
    nunciation of diverticula]
diverticulitis
diverticulogram
diverticulosis
  jejunal d.
diverticulum (diverticula)
  epiphrenic d.
  hepatic d.
  hypopharyngeal d.
  jejunal d.
  Meckel d.
  midesophageal d.
  pharyngoesophageal d.
  Rokitansky d.
  supradiaphragmatic d.
  Zenker d.
double-contrast
  d.-c. barium enema
  d.-c. roentgenography
double pyloroplasty
doughy
  d. abdomen
  d. consistency
DPC—delayed primary closure
drainage
  duodenal d.
  percutaneous transhepatic
    biliary d. (PTBD)
dressing
  See in *General Surgical
    Terms.*
drip
  intragastric d.

duct
    biliary d.
    common bile d.
    extrahepatic bile d.
    hepatic d.
    Wirsung d.
ductography
    peroral retrograde pancreati-
        cobiliary d.
ductus (ductus)
    d. choledochus
Duhamel operation
Dukes
    classification (A, B, B_2, C_1,
      C_2 [B2, C1, C2])
dumping
    d. syndrome
duodenal
    d. atresia
    d. diverticula
    d. drainage
    d. ileus
    d. obstruction
    d. tube
    d. ulcer
duodenectomy
duodenitis
duodenocholangeitis
duodenocholecystostomy
duodenocholedochotomy
duodenocolic
duodenocystostomy
duodenoduodenostomy
duodenoenterostomy
duodenogram
duodenography
    hypotonic d.
duodenohepatic
duodenoileostomy
duodenojejunostomy
duodenolysis
duodenorrhaphy
duodenoscopy
duodenostomy
duodenotomy
duodenum
D&V—diarrhea and vomiting
dys–. See also words beginning dis–.

dysentery
    amebic d.
    bacillary d.
    balantidial d.
    bilharzial d.
    catarrhal d.
    ciliary d.
    ciliate d.
    flagellate d.
    Flexner d.
    fulminant d.
    giardiasis d.
    helminthic d.
    malarial d.
    protozoal d.
    scorbutic d.
    Shiga d.
    Sonne d.
    spirillar d.
    sporadic d.
    viral d.
dysgeusia
dyskinesia
    biliary d.
dyskinetic
dysphagia [difficulty swallowing]
    d. lusoria
    oropharyngeal d.
    sideropenic d.
dysphagic
dyspragia
    angiosclerotica
    d. intermittens
    intestinalis
ECHO—enteric cytopathogenic
    human orphan [now: echovirus]
Eckhout
    vertical gastroplasty
E. coli—Escherichia coli
edema
    alimentary e.
edematous
EEC—enteropathogenic *Escherich-
    ia coli*
EFA, EFAs—essential fatty acid(s)
effect [noun: result, outcome]
    See *phenomenon, reflex,* and
      sign.

efferent
EG—esophagogastrectomy
Ehlers-Danlos
    disease
    syndrome
EIEC—enteroinvasive *Escherichia coli*
electrocholecystectomy
electrocholecystocausis
electrogastrograph
emission
    positron e. tomography (PET)
cmollient laxatives [a class of drugs]
end
    e. colostomy
    e. ileostomy
    e.-to-side ileotransverse
        colostomy
endocholedochal
endometriosis
    e. of colon
endomorph
endomorphic
endomorphy
endoscopic
    e. cholangiography
    percutaneous e. gastrostomy
        (PEG)
    e. retrograde cholangiogra-
        phy (ERC)
    e. retrograde cholangiopan-
        creatography (ERCP)
    e. ultrasonography
endoscopy
endothelia (plural of endothelium)
endothelioma
endothelium (endothelia)
endotracheal (ET)
    e. intubation
enema
    air contrast barium e.
    barium e.
    cleansing e.
    high e.
    Hypaque e.
"en-sed" Phonetic for NSAID (non-
    steroidal anti-inflammatory
    drug).

enterectasis
enterectomy
enterically
enteritis
    bacterial e.
    choleriform e.
    cicatrizing e.
    e. cystica chronica
    e. gravis
    e. necroticans
    e. nodularis
    e. polyposa
    Escherichia coli e.
    granulomatous e.
    leishmanial e.
    myxomembranous e.
    pellicular e.
    phlegmonous e.
    protozoan e.
    pseudomembranous e.
    radiation e.
    regional e.
    segmental e.
    streptococcus e.
    ulcerative e.
enteroanastomosis
enterocele
enterocentesis
enterocholecystostomy
enterocholecystotomy
enterocleisis [closure, occlusion]
enteroclysis [injection, introduction]
enterocolectomy
enterocolitis
    hemorrhagic e.
    necrotizing e.
    pseudomembranous e.
    regional e.
enterocolostomy
enteroenterostomy
    Parker-Kerr e.
enterogastritis
enterolith
enterolithiasis
enteromycosis
    e. bacteriacea
enteronitis
    polytropous e.

enteropathy
> gluten e.
> protein-losing e.

enteropexy
enteroplasty
enteroptosis
enterorrhaphy
enterostomy
> gun-barrel e.
> Witzel e.

enterotomy
> e. incision

enterovesical
> e. fistula

enterozoon (enterozoa)
eosinophilic
> e. gastroenteropathy
> e. granuloma

EPEC—enteropathogenic *Escherichia coli*
epigastric
epigastrium
epiploenterocele
epiploon
epiplopexy
epiploplasty
epiplorrhaphy
epithelia (plural of epithelium)
epitheliitis
epithelium (epithelia)
> surface e.
> visceral e.

ERC—endoscopic retrograde cholangiography
ERCP—endoscopic retrograde cholangiopancreatography
erosion
> Dieulafoy e.

eructation
> nervous e.

"esofa–" Phonetic for words beginning esopha–.
esophageal
> e. atresia
> e. sphincter
> e. stethoscope
> e. varices

esophagectomy

esophagism
esophagitis
> acute corrosive e.
> e. dissecans superficialis
> herpetic e.
> infectious e.
> monilia e.
> peptic e.
> reflux e.
> thrush e.

esophagocele
esophagocologastrostomy
esophagoduodenostomy
esophagoenterostomy
esophagofundopexy
esophagogastrectomy (EG)
esophagogastroanastomosis
esophagogastroplasty
esophagogastroscopy
esophagogastrostomy
esophagojejunostomy
esophagolaryngectomy
esophagomalacia
esophagometer
esophagomycosis
esophagomyotomy
> Heller e.

esophagopharynx
esophagoplasty
esophagoplication
esophagoptosis
esophagosalivation
esophagospasm
esophagostenosis
esophagostoma
esophagostomy
esophagotomy
esophagraphy
esophagus
> Barrett e.

ET—endotracheal
état
> é. mammelonné

ETEC—enterotoxic *Escherichia coli*
euchlorhydria
eucholia
euchylia
eupepsia

eupeptic
euperistalsis
excavatio (excavationes)
    e. rectouterina
    e. rectovesicalis
excavation
    ischiorectal e.
    rectoischiadic e.
    rectouterine e.
    rectovesical e.
excrement
exenteritis
external
    e. proctotomy
extramammary Paget disease
extremitas (extremitates)
extremity
    anterior e. of spleen
    posterior e. of spleen
Faber
    anemia
    syndrome
facies (facies)
    f. hepatica
FAP—familial adenomatous polyposis
fascia (fasciae)
    f. lata, fasciae latae
    rectovaginal f.
    rectovesical f.
    Scarpa f.
fecal
    f. continence
    f. fluid
    f. impaction
    f. incontinence
    f. leukocytes
fecalith
    appendiceal f.
feces [grammatically plural; no singular form]
fecopurulent
feeding
    tube f.
Felty syndrome
"fenomenon" Phonetic for phenomenon.

fiberoptic
    f. colonoscopy
fiberscopic
fibroblast
fibrogastroscopy
fibrosis
    hepatic f.
filling defect
fine-needle
    f-n. transhepatic cholangiography
Finney
    operation
    pyloroplasty
fissura (fissurae)
    f. in ano
fissural
fissure
    anal f.
    f. in ano
fistula (fistulas, fistulae)
    anal f.
    f. in ano
    aortoduodenal f.
    aortoenteric f.
    bronchobiliary f.
    bronchocsophageal f.
    cholecystoduodenal f.
    chylous f.
    congenital urethrorectal f.
    Eck f.
    enterocolic f.
    enteroenteric f.
    enterovaginal f.
    enterovesical f.
    esophagobronchial f.
    esophagotracheal f.
    gastrocolic f.
    gastrojejunal f.
    gastrojejunocolic f.
    jejunocolic f.
    mucus f.
    perirectal f.
    rectolabial f.
    rectovaginal f.
    tracheoesophageal f.
    vesicocolonic f.
    vesicointestinal f.

fistula (fistulas, fistulae) (continued)
    vesicorectal f.
    vulvorectal f.
fistulectomy
fistuloenterostomy
fistulogram
fistulography
fistulotomy
"fitobezor" Phonetic for phytobezoar.
Fitz
    law
    syndrome
flat plate
    f.p. of abdomen
flatulence
flatus
"flegmon" Phonetic for phlegmon.
Flexner
    dysentery
flexura (flexurae)
flexure
    splenic f.
flora
    intestinal f.
fluctuation
fluid
fluke
    intestinal f.
flux
    bilious f.
    celiac f.
FNTC—fine-needle transhepatic cholangiography
focus (foci)
    dysplastic f.
fold
    pleuroperitoneal f.
follicle
    Lieberkühn f.
folliculus (folliculi)
food poisoning
foramen (foramina)
    f. of Bochdalek
    f. of Bochdalek hernia
    Duverney f.
    Morgagni f., morgagnian f.
    f. of Morgagni hernia
    pleuroperitoneal f.

foramen (foramina) (continued)
    f. of Winslow
foraminal
foreign body (FB)
    retained f.b. (RFB)
formation
    Gothic arch f.
Forssell sinus
fossa (fossae)
    duodenal f.
    epigastric f.
    Gruber-Landzert f.
    Hartmann f.
    ischiorectal f.
    Landzert f.
    pararectal f.
    retrocolic f.
    subsigmoid f.
    Treitz f.
    f. vesicae biliaris
Fothergill
    sign
foveola (foveolae)
    f. gastricae
foveolar
foveolate
FPC—familial polyposis coli
FPP—familial paroxysmal poly-
    serositis
Frank
    operation
Fredet-Ramstedt
    operation
    pyloromyotomy
"fren–" Phonetic for words begin-
    ning phren–.
frena (plural of frenum)
frenal
frenulum (frenula)
    See also *frenum.*
    f. of duodenal papilla
    f. of ileocolic valve
    f. of Morgagni
frenum (frena)
    See also *frenulum.*
    f. of Morgagni
    f. of valve of colon

Frey
    gastric pits
    hairs
Friderichsen-Waterhouse syndrome
FUDR, FUdR—5-fluorouracil deoxyribonucleoside [now: floxuridine]
functional
    f. anastomosis
fungus (fungi)
    See specific fungi in *Laboratory, Pathology, and Chemistry Terms.*
funicular
funiculate
funiculus (funiculi)
    hepatic f. of Rauber
gag reflex
gallstone
gallstone-solubilizing agents [a class of drugs]
GALT—gastrointestinal-associated lymphoid tissue
    gut-associated lymphoid tissue
gamma
    g.-aminobutyric acid (GABA)
    g. heavy chain disease
    g. interferon
Gamna
    nodules
Gandy-Gamna nodules
ganglial
ganglion (ganglia, ganglions)
    Troisier g.
gastralgia
    appendicular g.
gastrectomy
    antecolic g.
    Billroth g.
    physiologic g.
    Roux-en-Y g.
    von Haberer-Aguirre g.
gastric
    g. acid
    g. actinomycosis
    g. adenocarcinoma
    g. anoxia

gastric (continued)
    g. atrophy
    g. balloon implantation
    g. bubble
    g. by-pass surgery
    g. carcinoma
    g. chromoscopy
    g. dilation
    g. duplication
    g. dysfunction
    g. dysrhythmia
    g. emptying
    g. freezing
    g. hyperemia
    g. hypersecretion
    g. ileus
    g. inhibitory polypeptides
    g. lavage
    g. mucosal barrier
    g. neurectomy
    g. outlet obstruction
    g. parietography
    g. pseudolymphoma
    g. resection (GR)
    g. retention
    g. rupture
    g. stasis
    g. teratoma
    g. ulcer
    g. varices
    g. volvulus
gastric acid inhibitors [a class of drugs]
gastritis
    antral g.
    atrophic g.
    catarrhal g.
    cirrhotic g.
    emphysematous g.
    eosinophilic g.
    erosive g.
    exfoliative g.
    follicular g.
    giant hypertrophic g.
    g. granulomatosa fibroplastica
    granulomatous g.
    hyperpeptic g.
    hypertrophic g

gastritis (continued)
    idiopathic g.
    interstitial g.
    mycotic g.
    nonerosive g.
    phlegmonous g.
    polypous g.
    pseudomembranous g.
    purulent g.
    superficial g.
    suppurating g.
    suppurative g.
    syphilitic g.
    tuberculous g.
    uremic g.
gastrocele
gastrocolic
gastrocolitis
gastrocolostomy
gastrocolotomy
gastrodiaphanoscopy
gastrodiaphany
gastroduodenal
gastroduodenectomy
gastroduodenoenterostomy
gastroduodenoscopy
    Billroth g.
gastroduodenostomy
gastroenteritis
    eosinophilic g.
gastroenteroanastomosis
gastroenterocolostomy
gastroenterologic
gastroenteroplasty
gastroenterostomy (GE)
    Balfour g.
    Billroth g., Billroth I (II, III)
      g.
    Braun and Jaboulay g.
    Courvoisier g.
    Heineke-Mikulicz g.
    Hofmeister g.
    Polya g.
    Roux g.
    Roux-en-Y g.
    Schoemaker g.
    von Haberer-Finney g.
    Wölfler g.

gastroenterotomy
gastroepiploic
gastroesophageal
    g. reflux
gastroesophagostomy
gastrogalvanization
gastrogastrostomy
gastrogavage
gastrohepatic
gastroileitis
gastroileostomy
gastrointestinal (GI)
    g.-associated lymphoid tissue
    g. fistula
    g. fungal balls
    g. immunodeficiency syn-
      drome
    g. peptide hormone
    g. reflux
    g. smooth muscle
gastrojejunocolic
gastrojejunostomy
    Billroth g.
    Roux-en-Y g.
gastrolysis
gastromegaly
gastromyotomy
gastropexy
gastroplasty
    Eckhout vertical g.
    Mason g.
gastroplication
gastroptosis
gastropylorectomy
gastropyloric
gastrorrhaphy
gastrorrhea
    g. continua chronica
gastrorrhexis
gastroscopy
gastrosia
    g. fungosa
gastrosplenic
gastrostomy
    Beck g.
    Beck-Jianu g.
    DePage-Janeway g.
    Janeway g.

gastrostomy (continued)
Kader g.
Martin g.
Marwedel g.
percutaneous endoscopic g.
(PEG)
plug g.
Spivack g.
Ssabanejew-Frank g.
Stamm g.
Witzel g.
gastrosuccorrhea
digestive g.
g. mucosa
gastrotomy
gastroxynsis
g. fungosa
GB—gallbladder
GBS—gallbladder series
GE—gastroenterology
gastroenterostomy
Gee disease
Gee-Herter disease
Gee-Herter-Heubner
disease
Gee-Thaysen disease
GER—gastroesophageal reflux
GERD—gastroesophageal reflux
disease
GET—gastric emptying time
GET ½—gastric emptying half-time
GFD—gluten-free diet
GI—gastrointestinal
giardiasis
intestinal g.
Gibbon
hernia
GIP—gastrointestinal polyposis
GIS—gastrointestinal system
GIT—gastrointestinal tract
gland
Brunner g.
Galeati g.
Lieberkühn g.
malpighian g.'s
Theile g.
glandula (glandulae)
glandular

glandule
glandulous [adj.]
Glénard disease
Glisson
capsule
cirrhosis
disease
glissonitis
globus (globi)
esophageal g.
g. hystericus
gluten
g. enteropathy
g.-free diet
g. sensitivity
Goldstein
disease
hematemesis
Golgi
apparatus
complex
gonococcal
g. proctitis
gonorrhea
rectal g.
Gowers
attack
syndrome
Goyrand hernia
GR—gastric resection
graft-versus-host disease (GVHD)
granule
zymogen g.
granulomatosis
lipophagic intestinal g.
Gross disease
GRP—gastrin-releasing peptide
Gruber-Landzert fossa
GSE—gluten-sensitive enteropathy
guarding
gun-barrel enterostomy
gustatory
gutter
paracolic g.
H₂ blockers [a class of drugs]
Hampton
line

hanging
    h. panniculus
Hanot
    cirrhosis
    disease
    syndrome
Hanot-Chauffard syndrome
Hartmann
    operation
haustra coli
haustration
haustrum (haustra)
    cecal h.
    haustra coli, haustra of colon
Hawes-Pallister-Landor syndrome
Hayem
    icterus
    jaundice
healing
    h. by first intention
    h. by granulation
    h. by second intention
    h. per primam intentionem
        (L. by first intention)
    h. per secundam intentionem
        [L. by second intention]
heaves
    dry h.
Heineke-Mikulicz
    gastroenterostomy
    operation
    pyloroplasty
Heister
    diverticulum
    fold
    valve
Heller
    disease
    esophagomyotomy
    myotomy
    operation
    plexus
Helvetius ligaments
hematemesis
    Goldstein h.
    h. puellaris
heme
hemicolectomy

hemigastrectomy
    h. and vagotomy (H&V)
hemihepatectomy
hemipylorectomy
hemoptysis
hemorrhage
    petechial h.
hemorrhagic
hemorrhoidal
hemorrhoidectomy
hepatectomy
hepatic
    h. flexure
hepaticocholedochostomy
hepaticodochotomy
hepaticoduodenostomy
hepaticoenterostomy
hepaticogastrostomy
hepaticojejunostomy
hepaticoliasis
hepaticolithotomy
hepaticolithotripsy
hepaticopulmonary
    h. fistula
hepaticostomy
hepaticotomy
hepatitis (hepatitides)
    h. A
    alcoholic h.
    anicteric h.
    h. B
    h. B virus
    non-A h.
    non-B h.
    serum h.
    viral h.
hepatobiliary
    percutaneous h. cholangiog-
        raphy
    h. tract disease
hepatocarcinogenesis
hepatocarcinogenic
hepatocarcinoma
hepatocele
hepatocholangeitis
hepatocholangiocarcinoma
hepatocholangioduodenostomy
hepatocholangioenterostomy

hepatocholangiogastrostomy
hepatocholangiojejunostomy
hepatocholangiostomy
hepatocholangitis
hepatocholangiocystoduodenostomy
hepatocirrhosis
hepatocystis
hepatoduodenostomy
hepatoenterostomy
hepatogastric
hepatomegaly
hepatorrhaphy
hepatosplenomegaly
hepatostomy
hepatotomy
hepatotoxic
hepatotoxicity
hernia
    diaphragmatic h.
    hiatal h., hiatus h.
    Morgagni h.
    spigelian h.
    Treitz h.
hernial
hernioid
hernioplasty
    Cooper ligament h.
herniorrhaphy
herpes
    anorectal h.
Herter
    disease
    infantilism
Herter-Heubner disease
Hesselbach
    hernia
    ligament
    triangle
Heubner-Herter
    disease
Hey
    hernia
    ligament
hiatal, hiatus
    h. hernia
hiatus
    esophageal h.

HIDA—hepatoiminodiacetic acid
    [scan]
Hill
    posterior gastropexy
"hipo–" Phonetic for words begin-
    ning hypo–.
Hirschsprung disease
histamine H_2 antagonists [a class of
    drugs]
histocompatibility
Hodgkin
    disease
Hofmeister
    gastroenterostomy
    operation
Holthouse hernia
Horsley
    anastomosis
    gastropexy
    pyloroplasty
    suture
Horton-Devine
    operation
Houston
    valve
HPS—hypertrophic pyloric stenosis
HRF—histamine-releasing factor
Hueter
    maneuver
Hunter
    line
H&V—hemigastrectomy and vagot-
    omy
hydrocele
    inguinal h.
hydrocholeretics [a class of drugs]
hydroperitoneum
hydrops
    h. abdominis
Hypaque [contrast medium]
    enema
    swallow
hyperabsorption
hyperacid
hyperacidity
hyperadiposis
hyperalimentation
    total parenteral h.

hyperalimentosis
hyperalkalinity
hypercatharsis
hypercathartic
hypercholia
hyperchylia
hyperdistention
hyperechoic
hyperemesis
        h. hiemis
hyperemetic
hyperesthesia
        gustatory h.
hyperesthetic
hypergastrinemia
hyperhepatia
hyperingestion
hyperkoria
hypermotility
hypernutrition
hyperorexia
hyperosmotic laxatives [a class of
        drugs]
hyperpancreorrhea
hyperpepsia
hyperpepsinemia
hyperpepsinia
hyperpepsinuria
hyperperistalsis
hyperphagia
hyperphagic
hyperpipecolatemia
hyperplasia
        focal adenomyomatous h. of
            gallbladder
        focal nodular h. (FNH) of
            liver
        polypoid h.
hyperplastic
        h. polyp
hyperposia
hyperproteinemia
hyperproteosis
hypersecretion
        gastric h.
hypersplenism
hypertrophy
        Billroth h.

hypesthesia
hypoactive
        h. bowel sounds
hypoactivity
hypoalimentation
hypochlorhydria
hypocholuria
hypochondria (plural of hypochon-
        drium)
hypochondriac
hypochondriacal
hypochondrium (hypochondria)
hypochylia
hypodiaphragmatic
hypoesthesia
        gustatory h.
hypofunction
hypoganglionosis
hypogastric
hypogastroschisis
hypohepatia
hypolactasia
hypometabolic
hypometabolism
hypomotility
hypomyxia
hypopancreatism
hypopancreorrhea
hypopepsia
hypopepsinia
hypoperistaltic
hypophosphatasia
hypophrenic
hypophrenium
hypoplasia
hypoposia
hyposplenism
hyposteatolysis
hyposteatosis
hypothesis (hypotheses)
        Keller h.
hypothrepsia
hypotonic
        h. duodenography
Hyrtl
        sphincter
IC—irritable colon

ichthyismus
    i. exanthematicus
icterus
idiopathic
ileac [pertaining to ileus or ileum
    (bowel)]
ileal [pertaining to ileum (bowel)]
    i. conduit diversion
ileectomy
ileitis
        distal i.
        prestomal i.
        regional i.
        terminal i.
ileocecostomy
ileocecum
ileocolic
ileocolitis
    i. ulcerosa chronica
ileocolostomy
ileocolotomy
ileoileostomy
ileojejunitis
        granulomatous i.
        nongranulomatous i.
ileoproctostomy
ileorectal
ileorectostomy
ileorrhaphy
ileosigmoid
ileosigmoidostomy
ileostomy
        end i.
        Kock i.
ileotomy
ileotransverse
    i. colostomy
    end-to-side i. colostomy
ileum [bowel]
        terminal i.
ileus
        adynamic i.
        gallstone i.
        gastric i.
        meconium i.
        paralytic i.
        spastic i.
iliohypogastric

ilioinguinal
immunoglobulin (Ig)
    secretory i. A
impaction
    fecal i.
impressio (impressiones)
    i. esophagealis hepatis
impression
incarceration
incision
    celiotomy i.
    enterotomy i.
    LaRoque herniorrhaphy i.
    smile i., smiling i.
incontinence
    fecal i.
    sphincteric i.
incontinent
incontinentia
    i. alvi
indigestion
inertia
    colonic i.
infantile
    i. celiac disease
infarction
    intestinal i.
inguinoabdominal
inguinocrural
inhibitor
    ATPase (adenosine triphos-
        phatase) i.'s [a class of
        drugs]
    gastric acid i.'s [a class of
        drugs]
    proton pump i.'s [a class of
        drugs]
inoperable
insufficiency
    pancreatic i.
    pyloric i.
insula (insulae)
    insulae of Peyer
internal
    i. proctotomy
    i. sphincterotomy
intestinal
    i. atresia

intestinal (continued)
    i. lymphangiectasia
    i. metaplasia
    i. obstruction
    i. peptides
    i. perfusion
intraductal
intrahepatic
    i. cholangiojejunostomy
intraoperative
    i. cholangiography
intravenous
    i. cholangiography (IVC)
    i. cholecystography
intussusception
intussusceptum
intussuscipiens
IO—intestinal obstruction
IP—intraperitoneal
irritable bowel disease (IBD)
ischemia
    mesenteric i.
    midgut i.
ischioanal
ischiorectal
island
    i.'s of Langerhans
islet
    Langerhans i.
IV—intravenous
IVC—intravenous cholangiogram
Jaboulay
    pyloroplasty
Jackson
    membrane
    veil
Janeway
    gastrostomy
jaundice
    cholestatic j.
    nonobstructive j.
    obstructive j.
Jaworski
    bodies
    corpuscles
    test
jejunal
jejunectomy

jejunitis
jejunocecostomy
jejunocolostomy
jejunogastric
jejunoileitis
jejunoileostomy
jejunoileum
jejunojejunostomy
jejunoplasty
jejunorrhaphy
jejunostomy
    needle catheter j.
jejunotomy
jejunum
Jonnesco
    fold
    fossa
    operation
Joseph
    See *Sister Joseph.*
Judd
    pyloroplasty
junction
    esophagogastric j.
juvenile
    j. polyposis
Kader
    gastrostomy
    operation
"kalazea," "ka-la-zhuh" Phonetic
    for chalasia.
Karroo syndrome
Kasai
    operation
Katayama
    disease
    syndrome
Kcal, Cal—kilocalorie
Keller
    hypothesis
kilocalorie (kcal, Cal)
KLS—kidneys, liver, spleen
Kock
    ileostomy
    pouch
    reservoir
Kohlmeier-Degos
    disease

"kol–" Phonetic for words beginning chol–.
"kolee–" Phonetic for words beginning chole–, choli–, coli–.
König
    syndrome
Kraske
    operation
Kunkel syndrome
"kyl–" Phonetic for words beginning chyl–.
lactase
    adult l. deficiency
    l. deficiency
    intestinal l. deficiency
lacteal
    central l.
lactovegetarian
lactovegetarianism
lactulose
lacuna (lacunae)
    l. of muscles
lacunar
Laird-McMahon
    anorectoplasty
lamina (laminae)
    proper l. of mesentery
    l. propria
    vascular l. of stomach
laminar
lamp
    Wood l.
Landzert fossa
Lane
    band
laparocholecystotomy
laparocolectomy
laparocolostomy
laparocolotomy
laparoenterostomy
laparoscopy
laparosplenectomy
laparosplenotomy
laparotomy
LaRoque
    herniorrhaphy incision
    technique

Larrey-Weil
    disease
larva (larvae)
    l. currens
    visceral l. migrans
larval
lavage
    gastric l.
law
    Fitz l.
laxatives [a class of drugs]
    bulk-producing l.
    emollient l.
    hyperosmotic l.
    stimulant l.
    stool-softening l.
    surfactant l.
layer
    See also *band* and *line*.
    submucous l. of colon
leiomyoma (leiomyomas, leiomyomata)
    bizarre l.
    epithelioid l.
    parasitic l.
    Zenker l.
lesion
    annular l.
    bull's eye l.
    Councilman l.
    doughnut l.
    napkin-ring l.
    precancerous l.
    ring-like l.
    sessile l.
    target l.
    trophic l.
levator (levatores)
    l. ani
Lieberkühn
    ampulla
    crypts
    follicles
    glands
lien
    l. accessorius
    l. mobilis
lienal

lienculus, lienunculus
lienectomy
lienitis
lienocele
lienomalacia
lienomedullary
lienomyelogenous
lienomyelomalacia
lienopancreatic
lienopathy
lienorenal
lienunculus, lieenulus
ligament
      falciform l.
      fallopian l.
      gastrohepatic l.
      Treitz l.
limb
line
      See also *band* and *layer*.
      anococcygeal l., white
      anocutaneous l.
      anorectal l.
      Conradi l.
      dentate l.
      l. of Douglas
      Hampton l.
      Hilton white l.
      Hunter l.
      Poupart l.
      semicircular l. of Douglas
      l. of Toldt, white l. of Toldt
linea (lineae)
      l. alba
      l. nigra
linear
      l. proctotomy
linguatuliasis
linitis
      l. plastica
lipodystrophia
      l. intestinalis
lipodystrophy
      intestinal l.
lipophagia
      l. granulomatosis
lipophagic
lipophagy

liquefy
liquid
liquor (liquors, liquores)
      l. entericus
      l. gastricus
      l. pancreaticus
Littré-Richter hernia
Livaditis
      circular myotomy
liver
      biliary cirrhotic l.
      l. dysfunction
      l. scan
LLQ—left lower quadrant
lobe
      caudate l. of liver
      l. of liver, left
      l. of liver, right
      quadrate l. of liver
      Riedel l.
      l.'s of liver
lobectomy
lobi (plural of lobus)
lobulation
      portal l.
lobule
      l. of pancreas
      portal l.
lobuli (plural of lobulus)
lobulization
lobulose
lobulus (lobuli)
lobus (lobi)
loop
      afferent l.
      efferent l.
      intestinal l.
      jejunal l.
      Roux-en-Y l.
      terminal ileal l.
Lotheissen-McVay technique
lumbocolostomy
lumbocolotomy
lumen (lumina)
LUQ—left upper quadrant
Luschka
      cystic gland

lymphogranuloma
   l. venereum
lymphonodulus (lymphonoduli)
   lymphonoduli splenici
Macewen
   operation
Mackenzie
   disease
macrocolon
MAI—*Mycobacterium avium-intracellulare*
Mallory-Weiss
   syndrome
   tear
malpighian
   m. bodies
mammillated
mammillation
mammilliform
mammose
maneuver
   See also *method.*
   Hoguet m.
   Hueter m.
Mann-Williamson ulcer
Manson
   disease
   schistosomiasis
margin
   crenate m. of spleen
   cristate m. of spleen
   inferior m. of liver
   obtuse m. of spleen
   m. of pancreas, superior
margo (margines)
Martin
   gastrostomy
Marwedel
   gastrostomy
Mary Joseph
   See *Sister Joseph.*
Mason
   gastroplasty
Mattox
"Maddox" Phonetic for Mattox.
Mattox
   maneuver
mature, matured

Maydl
   operation
McKenzie
   See *Mackenzie.*
MCT—medium-chain triglyceride
   [oil]
McVay
   operation
MDR—minimum daily requirement
meal
   barium m.
Meckel
   diverticulum
   scan
meckelectomy
meconium
   m. ileus
   m. peritonitis
medusae
   caput m.
megacolon
   acquired m.
   acquired functional m.
   acute m.
   aganglionic m.
   congenital m.
   m. congenitum
   idiopathic m.
   toxic m.
megaloesophagus
megalogastria
melanin
melanosis
   m. coli
melena
   m. neonatorum
   m. spuria
   m. vera
melenemesis
melenic [pertaining to melena,
   blood in the stool]
membranate
membrane
   croupous m.
   Debove m.
   false m.
   Jackson m.
Ménétrier disease

mesenterectomy
mesenteric
    m. adenitis
    m. fibromatosis
mesenteriolum
mesenteriopexy
mesenteriorrhaphy
mesenteriplication
mesenteritis
mesenterium
mesentorrhaphy
mesoappendicitis
mesoappendix
mesocecum
mesocoloplication
mesogastric
mesogastrium
        dorsal m.
        ventral m.
mesorectum
mesosigmoid
mesosigmoidopexy
metastasis (metastases)
method
        See also *maneuver.*
        Jenckel cholecystoduo-
            denostomy m.
        McArthur m.
        Morison m.
        Nimeh m.
        Sippy m.
microfilariasis
microgastria
microvillus (microvilli)
midepigastric
"mik" Slang for Mikulicz.
Mikulicz (von Mikulicz)
        operation
"mio–" Phonetic for words begin-
    ning myo–.
molimen (molimina)
MOM—milk of magnesia
Moore
        syndrome
morcellement
        m. operation
Morgagni
        columns

Morgagni (continued)
        crypts
        frenulum
        hernia
        retinaculum
        sinus
        valves
Morison
        pouch
"mor-sel-maw" Phonetic for mor-
    cellement.
Moschcowitz
        operation
Mosse syndrome
motility
        colon m.
        m. disorder
        esophageal m.
        gastrointestinal (GI) m.
        ineffective esophageal m.
            (IEM)
        reduced m.
MTT—mean transit time
mucilaginous
mucocutaneous
        m. fistula
        m. hemorrhoid
mucoenteritis
mucoid
mucosa
        antral m.
        colonic m.
        duodenal m.
        esophageal m.
        gastric m.
        gastroduodenal m.
        jejunal m.
mucosal
mucosanguineous
mucoserous
mucositis
mucous [adj.]
        m. fistula
        m. membrane
mucus [noun]
multilocular
        m. crypt

Munro
    point
Murphy
    sign treatment
muscle
    See also in *Orthopedics and Sports Medicine* section.
    Braune m.
    diaphragmatic m.
    external oblique m.
    Gavard m.
    iliopsoas m.
    interfoveolar m.
    interspinal m.'s of loins
    levator ani m.
    oblique m. of abdomen (external, internal)
    obturator m. (external, internal)
    Ochsner m.
    Oddi m.
    organic m.
    m.'s of pelvic diaphragm
    perineal m.'s, m.'s of perineum
    pleuroesophageal m.
    psoas m. (greater, smaller)
    pubicoperitoneal m.
    pubococcygeal m.
    puborectal m.
    pyloric sphincter m.
    pyramidal m.
    rectus m.
    sphincter m. of anus (external, internal)
    sphincter m. of bile duct
    sphincter m. of hepatopancreatic ampulla
    sphincter m. of pancreatic duct
    sphincter m. of pylorus
    suspensory m. of duodenum
    transverse m. of abdomen
    transverse perineal m. (deep, superficial)
    transverse m. of perineum (deep, superficial)
    m. of Treitz

muscle (continued)
    visceral m.
muscularis
    m. mucosa
    m. propria
musculus (musculi)
    See also *muscle.*
    See also in *Orthopedics and Sports Medicine* section.
    musculi abdominis
    m. levator ani
    m. pubococcygeus
    m. puborectalis
    m. rectococcygeus
    m. rectus abdominis
    m. sphincter ani
    m. transversus abdominis
Mya disease
myasthenia
    m. gastrica
mycoplasmal
mycosis (mycoses)
    m. intestinalis
myoneurosis
    colic m.
    intestinal m.
myotomy
    Heller m.
    Livaditis circular m.
myxoneurosis
    intestinal m.
myxorrhea
    m. intestinalis
nasogastric
    n. intubation
    n. suction
nasojejunal
nausea
nauseant
nauseate
nauseated
nauseous
navel
    blue n.
NEC—necrotizing enterocolitis
necrosis (necroses)
    Balser fatty n.
    bridging n.

necrosis (necroses) (continued)
    caseous n.
    central n.
    cheesy n.
    colliquative n.
    enzymatic fat n.
    fat n.
    focal n.
    gangrenous n.
    gummatous n.
    icteric n.
    infectious pancreatic n.
    liquefaction n.
    liquefactive n.
    massive hepatic n.
    moist n.
    peripheral n.
    piecemeal n.
    progressive emphysematous
      n.
    septic n.
    subacute hepatic n.
    submassive hepatic n.
necrotic
necrotizing
    n. enterocolitis (NEC)
needle
    n. catheter jejunostomy
Nembutal [anesthetic agent]
neomembrane
neorectum
neostigmine
    n. methylsulfate
neostomy
nerve
    anal n.'s, inferior
    hypogastric n.
    hypogastric n. of Latarjet
    iliohypogastric n.
    n. of Latarjet
    n.'s to levator ani muscle
    phrenic n.
    splanchnic n.'s
    vagus n.
nesidiectomy
"neu–" Phonetic for words begin-
    ning pneu–.

neurectomy
    gastric n.
"new–" Phonetic for words begin-
    ning pneu–.
NG—nasogastric
Nissen
    fundoplication
    operation
node
    shotty n.
    Sister Mary Joseph n.
    Troisier n.
    Virchow n.
nodular
nodularity
nodulated
nodulation
nodule
    Gamna n.'s
    Gandy-Gamna n.'s
    Sister Mary Joseph n.
nonfunctioning
    n. gallbladder
nonocclusive
    n. intestinal infarction
nonperforating
    n. ulcer
nonsteroidal anti-inflammatory drugs
    (NSAIDs) [a class of drugs]
nonvisualization
"noo–" Phonetic for words begin-
    ning pneu–.
notch
    angular n. of stomach
    n. of gallbladder
    gastric n.
NSAIA—nonsteroidal anti-inflam-
    matory agent
NSAID, NSAIDs—nonsteroidal
    anti-inflammatory drug(s) [a
    class of drugs]
"nu–" Phonetic for words beginning
    pneu–.
NUD—non-ulcer dyspepsia
nux
    n. vomica
N&V—nausea and vomiting
NVD—nausea, vomiting, diarrhea

obesity
  alimentary o.
  exogenous o.
  morbid o.
obstruction
  biliary tract o.
  intestinal o.
  small-bowel o.
occlusion
  enteromesenteric o.
  hepatic vein o.
OCG—oral cholecystogram
Ochsner
  ring
  treatment
Oddi sphincter
Ohara
  disease
oleandrism
Olympus model GTF-A gastrocamera
omenta (plural of omentum)
omental
omentitis
omentovolvulus
omentum (omenta)
omphalocele
O&P—ova and parasites
operation
  See also in *General Surgical
    Terms.*
  Abbe small-bowel o.
  Allingham o.
  Amussat o.
  Belsey Mark IV o., Belsey
    Mark V o.
  Best o.
  Billroth I o., Billroth II o.
  Bloodgood o.
  Calot o.
  Duhamel o.
  Finney o.
  Frank o.
  Fredet-Ramstedt o.
  Hartmann o.
  Heineke-Mikulicz o.
  Heller o.
  Hofmeister o.
  Horton-Devine o.

operation (continued)
  Jonnesco o.
  Kader o.
  Kasai o.
  Kraske o.
  Macewen o.
  Maydl o.
  McVay o.
  Mikulicz o.
  Moschcowitz o.
  Nissen o.
  Polya o.
  Ramstedt o.
  Soave o.
  Ssabanejew-Frank o.
  string o.
  Swenson o.
  Wangensteen o.
operative
  o. cholangiography
  delayed o. cholangiography
oral
  o. cholecystography
organomegaly
oscillation
Osler
  syndrome II
ostia (plural of ostium)
ostial [pertaining to opening, aperture, orifice]
ostium (ostia)
  o. appendicis vermiformis
  o. ileocecale
  o. pyloricum
  o. valvae ilealis
ostomy. See specific procedure.
  colostomy
  gastrostomy
  ileostomy
  jejunostomy
  neostomy
  proctostomy
  sigmoidostomy
ostreotoxism
overgrowth
  candidal o.
  yeast o.

Paget
    disease
pancolectomy
pancreas (pancreata)
    aberrant p.
    p. accessorium
    accessory p.
    annular p.
    divided p.
    p. divisum
    lesser p.
    unciform p.
    Willis p.
    Winslow p.
pancreatectomy
pancreatic
pancreaticobiliary
    peroral retrograde p. ductography
pancreatis (genitive of pancreas)
pancreatitis
    acute p.
    acute hemorrhagic p.
    calcereous p.
    centrilobar p.
    chronic p.
    chronic relapsing p.
    edematous p.
    interstitial p.
    mumps p.
    perilobar p.
    purulent p.
pancreatogenous
pancreatography
    endoscopic retrograde p.
pancreatomegaly
pancreatotomy
panendoscopy
panniculalgia
panniculus (panniculi)
    hanging p.
panproctocolectomy
papilla (papillae)
    anal p.
    bile p.
    duodenal p.
    duodenal p., major
    duodenal p., minor

papilla (papillae) (continued)
    p. duodeni major
    p. duodeni minor
    ileal p.
    p. ilealis
    p. ileocaecalis, ileocecal p.
    major duodenal p.
    minor duodenal p.
    p. of Santorini
    p. of Vater
papillary
papillate
papillation
papilliferous
papilliform
papilloma
    villous p.
papillosphincterotomy
papule
    moist p., mucous p.
paralysis (paralyses)
    esophageal p.
paraproctitis
parasite
    See specific parasites in *Laboratory, Pathology, and Chemistry Terms.*
parasitic
paries (parietes)
parietitis
parietography
    gastric p.
parietosplanchnic
parietovisceral
Parker-Kerr
    enteroenterostomy
pars (partes)
Patella disease
Paterson
    syndrome
Paterson-Brown-Kelly
    syndrome
Paterson-Kelly
    syndrome
pathogen
    See specific pathogens in *Laboratory, Pathology, and Chemistry Terms.*

pattern
    rugal p.
Patterson
    See *Paterson.*
Payr
    disease
    method
    syndrome
PBC—primary biliary cirrhosis
PCS—portacaval shunt
PCT—portacaval transposition
PE—pharyngoesophageal
pecten (pectines)
    p. of anal canal, p. analis
pectenitis
pectenotomy
pectinate
PEG—percutaneous endoscopic
    gastrostomy
pelvirectal
penicilli (plural of penicillus)
penicilliary
penicillus (penicilli)
    penicilli arteriae lienalis
    penicilli arteriae splenicae
peptic
percutaneous
    direct p. transhepatic
      cholangiography
    p. endoscopic gastrostomy
      (PEG)
    p. hepatobiliary cholangiog-
      raphy
    p. transhepatic biliary
      drainage (PTBD)
    p. transhepatic cholangiog-
      raphy (PTC)
    p. transhepatic portography
perforation
    pyloroduodenal p.
periappendicitis
    p. decidualis
pericholecystitis
    gaseous p.
peridiverticular
peridiverticulitis
periesophageal
periesophagitis

perigastric
perineum
    anterior p.
    posterior p.
    watering-can p.
perirectal
peristalsis
    mass p.
    retrograde p.
    reversed p.
peristaltic
peritoneal
    p. cavity, greater
    p. cavity, lesser
    p. lavage
peritoneum
    visceral p.
peritonitis
    bacterial p.
    chylous p.
    coccidioidal p.
    fungal p.
    granulomatous p.
    parasitic p.
    sclerosing p.
    tuberculous p.
perityphlitis
    p. actinomycotica
periumbilical
peroral
    p. retrograde pancreaticobil-
      iary ductography
per primam intentionem (L. by first
    intention)
per secundam intentionem (L. by
    second intention)
Pertik diverticulum
PET—positron emission tomogra-
    phy [scan]
PG—prostaglandin
PGE_2 [PGE2]—prostaglandin E_2
pharyngoesophageal
phenomenon (phenomena)
    See also *reflex* and *sign.*
    Anderson p.
    Kanagawa p.
phlegmon
phlegmonous

phren
phrenalgia
phrenectomy
phrenemphraxis
phrenicectomized
phrenicectomy
phreniclasia
phreniclasis
phrenic nerve
phrenicoexeresis
phreniconeurectomy
phrenicotomy
phrenicotripsy
phrenocolic
phrenocolopexy
phrenodynia
phrenogastric
phrenoglottic
phrenohepatic
phrenoplegia
phrenoptosis
phrenospasm
phrenosplenic
physalopteriasis
physiologic, physiological
    p. gastrectomy
phytobezoar
piecemeal
pigment
    bile p.
pile
    prostatic p.
    sentinel p.
    thrombosed p.
PIPIDA—para-isopropyliminodi-
    acetic acid technetium 99m
    hepatobiliary
PIPIDA
    hepatobiliary scan
    scan
plate
    anal p.
pleurocholecystitis
pleurovisceral
plexus (plexus, plexuses)
    enteric p.
    myenteric p.

plica (plicae)
    p. duodenalis
    p. epigastrica
    p. ileocecalis
    p. umbilicalis
plug
    p. gastrostomy
Plummer
    treatment
Plummer-Vinson
    syndrome
PMC—pseudomembranous colitis
pneumatosis
    p. cystoides intestinalis
    p. cystoides intestinorum
    intestinal p.
    p. intestinalis
pneumoenteritis
pneumography
    retroperitoneal p.
pneumoperitonitis
pneumoradiography
    retroperitoneal p.
PNI—Prognostic Nutritional Index
Polya
    gastroenterostomy
    operation
polyp
    adenomatous p.
    colonic p.
    hyperplastic p.
    inflammatory p.
    intestinal p.
    mucosal p.
polypectomy
polypi (plural of polypus)
polypiform
polypoid
polyposis
    p. coli
    p. gastrica
    p. intestinalis
    p. ventriculi
polypus (polypi)
    p. cysticus
    p. hydatidosus
pons (pontes)
    p. hepatis

ponticulus (ponticuli)
    p. hepatis
porcelain
    p. gallbladder
pori (genitive and plural of porus)
porta (portae)
    p. hepatis
    p. lienis
    p. omenti, p. of omentum
    p. of spleen
portacaval
portal
    p. portography
    p. venography
portography
    percutaneous transhepatic p.
    portal p.
    splenic p.
    umbilical p.
portosystemic shunt
porus (pori)
    p. galeni
position
    See in *General Surgical Terms.*
positron
    p. emission tomography (PET)
post–fatty meal cholecystography
postoperative
    p. cholangiography
postprandial
pouch
    Hartmann p.
    Heidenhain p.
    Koch p.
    Morison p.
    pararectal p.
    Physick p.'s
    Zenker p.
procedure
    See also *maneuver, method, operation,* and *technique.*
    Puestow-Gillesby p.
proctalgia
    p. fugax
proctectasia
proctectomy

proctocolectomy
proctocolitis
proctocystocele
proctocystoplasty
proctocystotomy
proctologic
proctology
proctoperineoplasty
proctopexy
proctoplasty
proctoptosis
proctorrhaphy
proctoscopy
proctosigmoidectomy
proctosigmoiditis
proctosigmoidoscopy
proctostenosis
proctostomy
proctotomy
    external p.
    internal p.
    linear p.
proctovalvotomy
properitoneal
prostaglandin (PG)
    See also in *Laboratory, Pathology, and Chemistry Terms.*
    p. E_2 [E2] (PGE_2)
proton pump inhibitors [a class of drugs]
pruritus
    p. ani
PS—pyloric stenosis
PSC—primary sclerosing cholangitis
pseudoleukemia
    p. gastrointestinalis
pseudomyxoma
    p. peritonei
psoas
    p. abscess
    p. fascia
    p. muscle
    p. sign
psorenteritis
psychogenic
PTC—percutaneous transhepatic cholangiography

PUD—peptic ulcer disease
pull-through
    ileoanal p.-t. anastomosis
    p.-t. operation
pulpa (pulpae)
    p. lienis
    p. splenica
puncture
    epigastric p.
    Marfan epigastric p.
purge
purging
    bingeing and p.
purpura
    p. abdominalis
    Henoch p.
    Henoch-Schönlein p.
    Schönlein p.
    Schönlein-Henoch p.
P&V—pyloroplasty and vagotomy
pyloric
    p. string sign
pyloristenosis
pyloroduodenitis
pylorogastrectomy
pyloromyotomy
    Fredet-Ramstedt p.
pyloroplasty
    double p.
    Finney p.
    Heineke-Mikulicz p.
    Horsley p.
    Jaboulay p.
    Judd p.
    Ramstedt p.
    vagotomy and p. (V&P)
    p. and vagotomy (P&V)
pyloroptosis
pyloroscopy
pylorospasm
    congenital p.
    reflex p.
pylorostomy
pylorotomy
pylorus
pyoderma
    p. gangrenosum
rabbit stools

radiation
    r. colitis
    r. enteropathy
    r. gastritis
    r. hepatitis
radioallergosorbent
radionuclide
    r. cholescintigraphy
"ra-fee" Phonetic for raphe.
Ramstedt
    operation
    pyloroplasty
ramus (rami)
Ranson criteria [for severity of
    acute pancreatitis]
raphe (raphae)
    abdominal r.
    anogenital r.
    median r. of perineum
raphes (genitive of raphe)
RE—regional enteritis
receptaculum (receptacula)
    r. chyli
    r. Pecqueti
receptor
    gustatory r.
    histamine H_1 r. [H1]
    histamine H_2 r. [H2]
    taste r.
recess
recessus (recessus)
rectal
    r. valvotomy
rectocele
rectocystotomy
rectosigmoid
rectotomy
rectum
reflex
    See also *phenomenon* and
       sign.
    See also in *Neurology and*
       Pain Management section.
    anal r.
    anal wink r.
    deglutition r.
    epigastric r.
    gag r.

reflex (continued)
  gastrocolic r.
  gastroileac r.
  gastroileal r.
  ileogastric r.
  myenteric r.
  perianal r.
  rectal r.
  renointestinal r.
  somatointestinal r.
  swallowing r.
  vesicointestinal r.
  wink r.
reflux
  esophageal r.
  r. esophagitis
  gastroesophageal r. (GER)
region
  abdominal r.
  hypochondriac r.
  hypogastric r.
  inguinal r.
  lateral abdominal r.
  perineal r.
  suprainguinal r.
  umbilical r.
  urogenital r.
Reichmann
  disease
  syndrome
resection
  abdominoperineal r. (APR)
  antral r.
  colon r. (CR)
  gastric r. (GR)
  massive bowel r. syndrome
residuum (residua)
  gastric r.
resonance
  hydatid r.
  tympanic r.
  tympanitic r.
  vesiculotympanic r.
  wooden r.
retching
rete (retia)
retial
retrocecal

retrograde
  endoscopic r. pancreatography
  peroral r. pancreaticobiliary ductography
retroperitoneal
  r. pneumography
  r. pneumoradiography
RFB—retained foreign body
rhagades [grammatically plural; no singular form]
RI—regional ileitis
Riedel
  lobe
RIH—right inguinal hernia
ring
  Cannon r.
  lower esophageal contraction r.
  Ochsner r.
  Schatzki r.
RLQ—right lower quadrant
roentgenography
  double-contrast r.
Roger
  reflex
Rokitansky
  disease
  diverticulum
  hernia
Rokitansky-Aschoff sinus
Rossbach
  disease
rotavirus
  r. gastroenteritis
Rotor syndrome
Roux
  gastroenterostomy
Roux-en-Y
  anastomosis
  cystojejunostomy
  gastrectomy
  gastroenterostomy
  gastrojejunostomy
  operation
rudiment
  hepatic r.

ruga (rugae)
    rugae gastricae
    rugae of stomach
rugal pattern
rugate
rugose, rugous
rule
    Goodsall r.
rumble
RUQ—right upper quadrant
Rusconi anus
Ruysch
    disease
    veins
sacculated
sacculation
    cecal s.'s
    colic s.'s
    s.'s of colon
sacculi (genitive and plural of sac-
    culus)
sacculiform
sacculus (sacculi)
    sacculi of Beale
"Sah-bah-ne-yev" Phonetic for Ssa-
    banejew.
saline
    s. laxatives
saliva
salivary
sarcoma (sarcomas, sarcomata)
    See also in *Oncology and
        Hematology* section.
    Kupffer cell s.
sarcomatous
sarcomphalocele
Saunders
    disease
SBFT—small bowel follow-through
    [x-ray]
scan
    See also in *Radiology,
        Nuclear Medicine, and
        Other Imaging* section.
    hepatobiliary s.
    HIDA (hepatoiminodiacetic
        acid) s.
    liver s.

scan (continued)
    liver-spleen s.
    Meckel s.
    PIPIDA hepatobiliary s.
    spleen s.
Scarpa
    fascia
schistosomiasis
Schmidt
    diet
Schoemaker
    gastroenterostomy
Schultz
    angina
    disease
    syndrome
sclerosing
    s. cholangitis
    s. peritonitis
sclerosis
    gastric s.
    systemic duodenal s.
sclerotherapy
"scopes" See under full name.
    stethoscope
scybala (plural of scybalum)
scybalous
scybalum (scybala)
section
    abdominal s.
    perineal s.
sedatives [a class of drugs]
    gastric s.
    intestinal s.
segmenta (plural of segmentum)
segmental
segmentum (segmenta)
"seng-ker" Phonetic for Zenker.
sentinel pile
sepsis
    s. intestinalis
septum (septa)
    cloacal s.
    rectovesical s.
    tracheoesophageal s.
    urorectal s.
shelf
    Blumer s.

shelf (continued)
    mesocolic s.
    rectal s.
Shouldice herniorrhaphy
shunt
    Linton s.
    portosystemic s.
    transjugular intrahepatic
       portosystemic s. (TIPS)
Shwachman-Diamond syndrome
sialorrhea
    s. pancreatica
"sibah–" Phonetic for words begin-
    ning scyba–.
sigmoidectomy
sigmoiditis
sigmoidoproctostomy
sigmoidorectostomy
sigmoidoscopy
sigmoidostomy
sigmoidotomy
sigmoidovesical
sign
    See also *phenomenon* and
      reflex.
    Aaron s.
    auscultatory s.'s
    Blatin s.
    Blumberg s.
    Boas s.
    bowler hat s.
    Boyce s.
    Carman s.
    Carman-Kirklin s.
    Carman-Kirklin meniscus s.
    Carnett s.
    Chilaiditi s.
    coiled spring s.
    Cole s.
    colon cutoff s.
    Courvoisier s.
    crescent s.
    Dew s.
    double-bubble s.
    E s.
    echo s.
    Federici s.
    Haudek s.

sign (continued)
    Hennings s.
    Horn s.
    Kantor string s.
    Kehr s.
    Klemm s.
    Lennhoff s.
    Leser-Trélat s.
    McBurney s.
    Meltzer s.
    meniscus s.
    Mercedes-Benz s.
    Mexican hat s.
    moulage s.
    Murphy s.
    niche s.
    obturator s.
    psoas s.
    pyloric string s.
    Rosenbach s.
    Rovighi s.
    Rovsing s.
    Stierlin s.
    Strauss s.
    string s.
    string-of-beads s.
    Sumner s.
    Trimadeau s.
    Zugsmith s.
"sike–" Phonetic for words begin-
    ning psych .
sin–. See also words beginning
    cin–, syn–.
singultation
singultous [adj.]
singultus [noun]
    s. gastricus nervosus
sinus (sinus, sinuses)
    anal s.
    s. anales
    draining s.
    Forssell s.
    s. lienis
    pilonidal s.
    pleuroperitoneal s.
    rectal s.
    Rokitansky-Aschoff s.
    s. of spleen, splenic s.

Sister Joseph, Sister Mary Joseph
    node
    nodule
β-sitosterolemia [beta-]
situs (situs)
    s. inversus
    s. inversus abdominalis
    s. inversus viscerum
    s. perversus
    s. transversus
"skibah–" Phonetic for words
    beginning scyba–.
"sklero–" Phonetic for words begin-
    ning sclero–.
slurry
smile, smiling
    s. incision
Soave
    operation
    procedure
solution
"soo-fl," "soo-flay" Phonetic for
    souffle.
"sor–" Phonetic for words begin-
    ning psor–.
sordes (sordes)
    s. gastricae
souffle
    splenic s.
sound
    succussion s.'s
space
    Traube semilunar s.
spasm
    diffuse esophageal s.
    esophageal s.
spastic
    s. colon
sphincter
    anal s.
    s. ani
    s. of bile duct
    cardiac s.
    cardioesophageal s.
    s. of common bile duct
    duodenal s.
    esophagogastric s.
    external s. of anus

sphincter (continued)
    gastroesophageal s.
    Glisson s.
    Hyrtl s.
    ileal s.
    internal s. of anus
    Oddi s.
    pharyngoesophageal s.
    prepyloric s.
    pyloric s.
    rectal s.
sphincterectomy
sphincteric
sphincterismus
sphincteritis
sphincteroplasty
sphincteroscopy
sphincterotomy
    choledochal s.
    internal s.
Spivack
    gastrostomy
splenic
    s. flexure
    s. portography
    s. venography
splenocele
splenocleisis
splenolaparotomy
splenopexy
splenoportal venography
splenorrhagia
spot
    epigastric s.
sprue
    tropical s.
SS—soapsuds [enema]
Ssabanejew-Frank
    gastrostomy
    operation
SSE—soapsuds enema
Stamm
    gastrostomy
stasis
    ileal s.
    venous s.
status
    s. gastricus

status (continued)
    nutrition s.
steatorrhea
steatosis
Steinert
    disease
    myotonic dystrophy
    syndrome
stenosis (stenoses)
    adult pyloric s.
    anorectal s.
    antral s.
    congenital hypertrophic
      pyloric s.
    cystic duct s.
    esophageal s.
    hypertrophic pyloric s.
    papillary s.
    pyloric s.
stercolith
stercoraceous
stercoral
stercoroma
stercorous
stercus (stercora)
stethoscope
    esophageal s.
stimulant laxatives [a class of drugs]
Stokvis
    disease
    test
Stokvis-Talma syndrome
stomach
    cup-and-spill s.
    leather bottle s.
stool
    acholic s.
    bilious s.
    caddy s.
    s. culture
    currant jelly s.
    fatty s.
    s. guaiac
    lienteric s.
    mucous s.
    pea soup s.
    pipe-stem s.
    rabbit s.'s

stool (continued)
    ribbon s.'s
    rice-water s.'s
    sago-grain s.
    silver s.
    spinach s.
stool-softening laxatives [a class of
    drugs]
Strachan
    disease
    syndrome
Strachan-Scott syndrome
strand
    Billroth s.'s
strata (plural of stratum)
stratiform
stratum (strata)
    submucous s. of colon
    submucous s. of rectum
    submucous s. of small intes-
      tine
    submucous s. of stomach
streak
    See *line.*
stria (striae)
    See *line.*
string
    s. operation
string sign
submucous
    s. layer of colon
    s. ulcer
substituted benzimidazoles [a class
    of drugs]
succagogue
succi (plural of succus)
succorrhea
succus (succi)
    s. entericus
    s. gastricus
    s. pancreaticus
succussion
    s. splash
Sudeck
    critical point
"sudo–" Phonetic for words begin-
    ning pseudo–.
sulci (plural of sulcus)

sulciform
sulcus (sulci)
   s. of umbilical vein
suppository
   glycerin s.
surfactant laxatives [a class of drugs]
suture [material]
   See in *General Surgical*
    Terms.
suture [technique]
   See also in *General Surgical*
    Terms.
   Horsley s.
swallow
   barium s.
   Hypaque s.
Swenson
   operation
Symington body
symptom
   See also in *General Medical*
    Terms.
   crossbar s. of Fränkel
syn–. See also words beginning
   cin–, sin–.
syndrome
   See also *disease.*
   afferent loop s.
   bacterial overgrowth s.
   Banti s.
   Barrett s.
   Bazex s.
   Behçet s.
   blind loop s.
   Boerhaave s.
   bowel bypass s.
   Budd-Chiari s.
   Chinese restaurant s. (CRS)
   Courvoisier-Terrier s.
   Dubin-Johnson s.
   dumping s.
   Ehlers-Danlos s.
   functional bowel s.
   Gardner s.
   gastrocardiac s.
   gastrojejunal loop obstruc-
    tion s.
   Gee-Herter-Heubner s.

syndrome (continued)
   Glénard s.
   glioma-polyposis s.
   Hanot-Rössle s.
   intestinal polyposis–cutane-
    ous pigmentation s.
   irritable bowel s. (IBS)
   König s.
   Maffucci s.
   malabsorption s.
   Mallory-Weiss s.
   massive bowel resection s.
   Meigs s.
   Ogilvie s.
   Oldfield s.
   Osler s.
   pancreaticohepatic s.
   Paterson s.
   Paterson-Brown-Kelly s.
   Paterson-Kelly s.
   Peutz-Jeghers s.
   Plummer-Vinson s.
   postcholecystectomy s.
   short-bowel s.
   short-gut s.
   sump s.
   Turcot s.
   wasting s.
   Wermer s.
   Zellweger s.
   Zollinger-Ellison s. (ZES)
synechtenterotomy
syphilis
   anorectal s.
system
   portal s.
tabes
   t. mesaraica
   t. mesenterica
tabetic
taenia (taeniae) [anatomy: flat band]
   taeniae coli
   t. omentalis
   taeniae pylori
   taeniae of Valsalva
taeniacides [a class of drugs]
taenial
taeniasis

taeniform
tampon
    Corner t.
tamponade
    esophageal t.
    esophageal balloon t.
    esophagogastric t.
Tangier disease
TC—transhepatic cholangiography
TE—tracheoesophageal
tear
    Mallory-Weiss t.
technique
    See *maneuver* and *method.*
    See also in *General Surgical*
      Terms.
TEF—tracheoesophageal fistula
tela (telae)
    t. subserosa intestini tenuis
telangiectasia
    hemorrhagic t.
telangiectasis (telangiectases)
telar
tenia (teniae)
    See also *taenia [flat band].*
    t. coli
    t. mesocolica
    t. omentalis
tenial
teniamyotomy
test
    See also in *Laboratory,*
      Pathology, and Chemistry
      Terms.
    acid clearance t.
    acid reflux t.
    alkaline phosphatase t.
    Althausen t.
    bentiromide t.
    Bernstein t.
    bile acid tolerance t.
    Carnot t.
    Congo red t.
    Diagnex blue t.
    D-xylose absorption t.
    D-xylose tolerance t.
    fecal fat t.
    gallbladder function t.

test (continued)
    gastric function t.
    gastrointestinal blood loss t.
    glucose absorption t.
    Gmelin t.
    heme t.
    Hemoccult t.
    histamine t.
    hydrogen breath t.
    lactose tolerance t.
    liver function t. (LFT)
    Lundh t.
    motility t.
    Moynihan t.
    pineapple t.
    qualitative fecal fat t.
    Quick t. (for liver function)
    radioallergosorbent t. (RAST)
    Sahli t.
    Salomon t.
    Schilling t.
    secretin t.
    secretin-pancreozymin t.
    serum bilirubin t.
    stool guaiac t.
    string t.
    Szabo t.
    Töpfer t.
    Trousseau t.
    Udránszky t.
    vitamin A absorption t.
    xylose tolerance t.
test meal
    Boas t.m.
    Boyden t.m.
    Dock t.m.
    Ehrmann alcohol t.m.
    Ewald t.m.
    Fischer t.m.
    Leube t.m.
    motor t.m.
    Riegel t.m.
    Salzer t.m.
Thaysen disease
thelium (thelia)
therapy
    See also *treatment.*
    alimentary t.

therapy (continued)
>> diet t.
threshold
>> swallowing t.
thrombi (plural of thrombus)
thrombose, thrombosed
thrombosis
>> See also in *Cardiology* section.
>> See also *thrombus*.
>> mesenteric t.
thrombus (thrombi)
>> See also *thrombosis*.
>> bile t.
thymus
time (T)
>> colonic transit t.
>> gastric emptying t.
>> occlusion t. (OT)
>> transit t.
TIPS—transjugular intrahepatic portosystemic shunt
TNM—tumor, nodes, metastases [tumor staging system]
Toldt
>> line, white line
tomography
>> computed t. (CT)
>> computerized axial t. (CAT)
>> positron emission t. (PET)
>> ultrasonic t.
"too-mur" Phonetic for tumeur.
torsion
tortuous
>> t. bowel
TPN—total parenteral nutrition
TPPN—total peripheral parenteral nutrition
trabecula (trabeculae)
>> trabeculae lienis
>> trabeculae of spleen, trabeculae splenicae
trabecularism
trabeculate
trabeculation
tract
>> alimentary t.
>> biliary t.

tract (continued)
>> digestive t.
>> gastrointestinal (GI) t.
>> intestinal t.
transabdominal
>> t. cholangiography
transhepatic
>> t. cholangiography (TC)
>> direct percutaneous t. cholangiography
>> fine-needle t. cholangiography (FNTC)
>> percutaneous t. biliary drainage (PTBD)
>> percutaneous t. cholangiography (PTC)
>> percutaneous t. portography
trauma (traumas, traumata)
treatment
>> See also *therapy*.
>> Murphy t.
>> Ochsner t.
Treitz
>> arch
>> fossa
>> hernia
>> ligament
>> muscle
trichobezoar
truncal
truncate
truncus (trunci)
>> t. celiacus
>> trunci intestinales
"tseng-ker" Phonetic for Zenker.
TT—transit time
T tube, T-tube
>> T-t. cholangiography
tube
>> digestive t.
>> duodenal t.
>> t. feeding
tuberculoid
tuberculosis (TB)
>> esophageal t.
>> ileocecal t.
>> intestinal t.
>> t. of intestines

tuberculous
t. peritonitis
tuberosity
omental t. of liver
tubi (plural of tubus)
tubulus (tubuli)
tubus (tubi)
t. digestorius
Tuerck. See *Türck*.
tumeur
t. pileuse
tumor
cystic t.
desmoid t.
islet cell t.
tunic
fibrous t. of liver
mucous t.
muscular t.
pharyngeal t., pharyngobasi-
lar t.
tunica (tunicae)
t. adventitia
t. fibrosa
t. mucosa
t. muscularis
t. serosa
tunicate
Türck
zone
tympanites
false t.
tympany
t. of the stomach
typhlectomy
typhlostomy
typhlotomy
"u–" Phonetic for words beginning
eu–.
UDCA—ursodeoxycholic acid
UGI—upper gastrointestinal
UGI
endoscopy
study
tract
ulcer
Cushing u.
duodenal u.

ulcer (continued)
esophageal u.
gastric u.
jejunal u.
peptic u.
postbulbar u.
stercoral u.
stomal u.
stress u.
submucous u.
ulcera (plural of ulcus)
ulcerate
ulcerating
ulceration
tracheal u.
ulcerative
ulcerogenic
ulcus (ulcera)
u. penetrans
u. ventriculi
ultrasonic
u. tomography
ultrasonography
endoscopic u.
umbilical
u. portography
unit
See also in *General Medical
Terms* and *Laboratory,
Pathology, and Chemistry
Terms*.
pepsin u.
unrest
peristaltic u.
vagal
vaginal
v. celiotomy
vagotomy
hemigastrectomy and v.
(H&V)
pyloroplasty and v. (P&V)
vagus
valva (valvae)
v. ilealis
v. ileocaecalis
valve
anal v.'s
v. of colon

valve (continued)
  ileocecal v., ileocolic v.
  v. of Macalister
  Morgagni v.'s
  pyloric v.
  semilunar v.'s of Morgagni
  semilunar v.'s of colon
  semilunar v.'s of rectum
  sigmoid v.'s of colon
  spiral v. of cystic duct
  spiral v. of Heister
valvotomy
  rectal v.
valvula (valvulae)
  valvulae anales
  v. processus vermiformis
  v. spiralis (Heisteri)
valvule
valvulectomy
van den Bergh
  disease
  test
variation
varix (varices)
  esophageal v.
vasospasmolytic
vasospastic
vasovagal
venography
  portal v.
  splenic v.
  splenoportal v.
venter (ventres)
ventral
  v. celiotomy
ventralis
ventrocystorrhaphy
vermiform
Verner-Morrison syndrome
vertical
  Eckhout v. gastroplasty
vesica (vesicae)
  v. biliaris
  v. fellea
vesical [adj.: pertaining to the bladder]
  v. compliance
  v. diverticulectomy

vesical [adj.: pertaining to the bladder] (continued)
  v. exstrophy
  v. external sphincter dyssynergia (VSD)
  v. fibrosis
  v. fistula
  v. neck
vesicointestinal
vesicula (vesiculae)
  v. bilis, v. fellea
vessel
  hypogastric v.
vestige
vestigial
villi (plural of villus)
villiferous
villose, villous [adj.]
  v. adenoma
  v. arthritis
  v. papilloma
villosity
villus (villi)
  colonic villi
  intestinal villi, villi intestinales
  jejunal villi
  villi of small intestine
vinculum (vincula)
  See *frenulum* and *frenum*.
Vinson syndrome
VIP—vasoactive intestinal polypeptide
virus
  See specific viruses in *Laboratory, Pathology, and Chemistry Terms*.
visceral
  v. larva migrans
  v. leishmaniasis
  v. schistosomiasis
visceralgia
visceromegaly
visceroparietal
visceroperitoneal
visceroptosis
volvulus
  v. of colon

volvulus (continued)
   gastric v.
   v. neonatorum
vomit
   bilious v.
   black v.
   coffee-grounds v.
vomiting
   cyclic v.
   dry v.
   explosive v.
   fecal v.
   hysterical v.
   periodic v.
   pernicious v.
   projectile v.
   recurrent v.
   stercoraceous v.
vomito
   v. negro
vomitus
   coffee-grounds v.
   v. cruentus
   v. matutinus
von Haberer-Aguirre
   gastrectomy
von Haberer-Finney
   gastroenterostomy
von Rokitansky. See *Rokitansky*.
V&P—vagotomy and pyloroplasty
Waldeyer colon
Wangensteen
   colostomy
   operation
wart
   venereal w.
Wassilieff disease
wave
   peristaltic w.
web
   esophageal w.
wedge
   w. resection
Weil
   disease
   syndrome

Wermer
   syndrome
Whipple
   disease
   syndrome
   triad
white
   w. line of Toldt
Wilson
   muscle
Winslow
   pancreas
Wirsung duct
Witzel
   enterostomy
   gastrostomy
Wölfler
   gastroenterostomy
Wolman disease
Yersinia
   Y. enteritis
"yoo–" Phonetic for words beginning eu–.
yo-yo dieting
Zenker
   diverticulum
   leiomyoma
   pouch
Zieve syndrome
Zollinger-Ellison (ZE)
   syndrome
   tumor
zone
   epigastric z.
   hemorrhoidal z.
   hypogastric z.
   papillary z.
   rugae z.
   transformation z.
   Türck z.
zymogen
   z. granules
   lab z.
zymosis
   z. gastrica

Infectious Diseases and Immunology
Includes Allergy

AAI—American Association of
  Immunologists
AAV—adeno-associated virus
Ab—antibody
abscess
    bilharziasis a.
    brain a.
    caseous a.
    cheesy a.
    Dubois a.
    entamebic a.
    eosinophilic a.
    filarial a.
    fungal a.
    gangrenous a.
    gas a.
    helminthic a.
    metastatic tuberculous a.
    miliary a.
    nocardial a.
    Pautrier a.
    phlegmonous a.
    pneumococcic a.
    Pott a.
    protozoal a.
    pyemic a.
    pyogenic a.
    scrofulous a.
    septicemic a.
    spirillar a.
    sterile a.
    streptococcal a.
    strumous a.
    syphilitic a.
    thymic a.
    tropical a.
    tuberculous a.

abscess (continued)
    verminous a.
absorption
acanthamebiasis
acantholytic
acarian
ACD—allergic contact dermatitis
acervuline
acetin
Achilles
    bursitis
achromic
acne
    contact a.
    occupational a.
    a. venenata
acrodermatitis
actinic
actinomycosis
    cervicofacial a.
    pulmonary a.
actinomycotin
actinophytosis
action
    cumulative a.
activation
    lymphocyte a.
activator
    polyclonal a.
activity
ACVD—autoimmune collagen vas-
    cular disease
Addison
    disease
Addison-Gull
    disease

507

ADE—acute disseminated
    encephalitis
ADEM—acute disseminated
    encephalomyelitis
adenitis
    acute epidemic infectious a.
    acute infectious a.
    Bartholin a.
    cervical a.
    phlegmonous a.
    syphilitic inguinal a.
    tuberculous a.
    vestibular a.
adenosine
    a. deaminase
    a. diphosphate (ADP)
    a. kinase
    a. monophosphate (AMP)
    a. triphosphate (ATP)
adenoviral
adiaspiromycosis
adjuvant
    Freund a.
    immunologic a.
    pertussis a.
adrenal cortical steroids, adrenocor-
    tical steroids [a class of drugs]
adrenaline
ADS—antibody-deficient syndrome
AdV—adenovirus
AEA—allergic extrinsic alveolitis
aeroallergen
aeroplankton
affinity
    functional a.
    a. labeling
African meningitis
Ag—antigen
AGA—acute gonococcal arthritis
agammaglobulinemia
    Bruton a.
agent
    virus-inactivating a.
Agent Orange
agglutination
    passive a.
agglutinative

agglutinin
    cold a.
    febrile a.
agglutinogenic
agglutinophilic
aggregated human IgG (AHuG)
aggregation
    familial a.
AID—acute infectious disease
AIDS—acquired immunodeficiency
    syndrome
airborne
airway
    a. reactivity
alastrim
alastrimic
alimentation
alkylamines [a class of drugs]
allelic
    a. exclusion
allergenic extracts [a class of drugs]
allergic
    a. bronchopulmonary
      aspergillosis
    a. contact dermatitis (ACD)
    a. granuloma
    a. granulomatosis
    a. orchitis
    a. purpura
    a. rhinitis
    a. salute
    a. shiner
    a. urticaria
allergist
allergization
allergize
allergoid
allergologic, allergological
allergologist
allergology
allergosis
allergy
    atopic a.
    bacterial a.
    bronchial a.
    cold a.
    contact a.
    delayed a.

allergy (continued)
    drug a.
    food a.
    gastrointestinal a.
    hereditary a.
    humoral a.
    immediate a.
    intrinsic a.
    latent a.
    nasal a.
    physical a.
    pollen a.
    polyvalent a.
    seasonal a.
    spontaneous a.
alloimmune
alloimmunization
allosensitization
allotoxin
allotype
    Am a.
    Gm a.
    Km a.
    latent a.
    nominal a.
    simple a.
    a. suppression
allotypic
    a. determinant
allylamines [a class of drugs]
Almeida
    disease
alpha
    a.-difluoromethylornithine
    a.-fetoprotein (AFP)
    a.-helix
    a.-hemolytic streptococci
    a.-interferon
    a.-methyldopa
    a.-streptococci
    a.-$_1$-thymosin
alpha chain disease
alpha heavy chain disease
alveolitis
    allergic a.
amebicides [a class of drugs]
p-aminobenzoate (PAB) [p-, para-]

p-aminobenzoic acid (PABA) [p-, para-]
aminoglycosides [a class of drugs]
21-aminosteroids [a class of drugs]
"amp" Slang for ampicillin.
"amp and gent" Slang for ampicillin and gentamicin.
"anafil–" Phonetic for words beginning anaphyl–.
analogue [anatomical, chemical]
anamnesis
anamnestic
    a. response
anaphylactic
anaphylactogen
anaphylactogenesis
anaphylactogenic
anaphylatoxin
    a. inactivator
anaphylaxis
    heterocytotropic a.
    homocytotropic a.
anemia
    autoimmune hemolytic a.
    fish tapeworm a.
    hemolytic a.
    Leishman a.
    pernicious a.
anergy
    cutaneous a.
    negative a.
    positive a.
angiitis
    necrotizing a.
angiogram
    fluorescein a.
angioleiomyoma
angiolupoid
angioma
    infectious a.
angiomatoid
angiomatosis
"angkilo–" Phonetic for words beginning ankylo–.
ankylosing
    a. hyperostosis
    a. spondylitis
anorexigenic

antagonist
  histamine H₁ a.'s [a class of
    drugs]
anthelmintics [a class of drugs]
anthracic
anthraconecrosis
anthracyclines [a class of drugs]
anthroponosis
antibiotics [a class of drugs]
  aminoglycoside a.
  bactericidal a.
  bacteriostatic a.
  broad-spectrum a.
  carbapenem a.
  cephalosporin a.
  fluoroquinolone a.
  glycopeptide a.
  β-lactam a. [beta-]
  lincosamide a.
  macrolide a.
  oral a.
  polyene a.
  sulfonamide a.
  tetracycline a.
  topical a.
antibody (antibodies)
  See also in *Laboratory,
    Pathology, and Chemistry
    Terms.*
  anti-basement membrane a.
  anticytoplasmic a.
  antimitochondrial a.
  antinuclear a. (ANA)
  antipeptide a.
  antireceptor a.
  anti-T-cell a.
  auto–anti-idiotypic a.
  autoimmune a.
  autologous a.
  blocking a.
  combining-site a.
  complement-fixing a.
  cross-reacting a.
  cytophilic a.
  a. deficiency syndrome
  a.-dependent cell–mediated
    cytotoxicity
  Donath-Landsteiner a.

antibody (antibodies) (continued)
  enhancing a.
  a. excess
  heteroclitic a.
  heterogenetic a.
  heterophile a.
  homocytotropic a.
  humoral a.
  hybrid a.
  hybridoma a.
  isophil a.
  maternal a.
  monoclonal a.
  neutralizing a.
  nonprecipitation a.
  skin-sensitizing a.
  Thomsen a.
  TSH-displacing a.
  warm-reactive a.
anticoagulant
  circulating a.
antigen (Ag)
  See also in *Laboratory,
    Pathology, and Chemistry
    Terms.*
  allogeneic a.
  alum-precipitated a.
  a.-antibody complex
  autologous a.
  bacterial a.
  a.-binding capacity
  carcinoembryonic a. (CEA)
  Chido-Rodgers a.
  cross-reacting a.
  cryptococcal a.
  differentiation a.
  Duffy a.
  endogenous a.
  a. excess
  exogenous a.
  Forssman a.
  H a.
  hepatitis a., hepatitis-associ-
    ated a. (HAA) [now: hep-
    atitis B surface antigen]
  hepatitis B core a. (HBcAg)
  hepatitis B e a. (HBeAg)

antigen (Ag) (continued)
hepatitis B surface a.
(HBsAg)
heterogeneic a.
heterophile a.
histocompatibility a.
homologous a.
human leukocyte a. (HLA)
human thymus lymphocyte a.
Ia a.
idiotypic a.
isophile a.
leukocyte common a.
Ly a.
lymphocyte function–associated a. 1 (LFA-1)
lymphocyte function–associated a. 2 (LFA-2)
lymphocyte function–associated a. 3 (LFA-3)
Mitsuda a.
O a.
oncofetal a.
organ-specific a.
Oz a.
plasma cell a.
a. presentation
a.-presenting cell
proliferating cell nuclear a.
QA a.
skin-specific histocompatibility a.
surface a.
synthetic a.
T-cell a.
thymus-dependent a.
thymus-independent a.
transplantation a.
tumor-associated a.
tumor-specific a.
viral capsid a.
antigenic
a. antibody lattice formation
a. binding receptor
a. competition
a. determinant
a. drift
a. modulation

antigenic (continued)
a. shift
a. variation
antihistamines [a class of drugs]
antinauseants [a class of drugs]
antiperiodics [a class of drugs]
antiphlogistics [a class of drugs]
antipyretics [a class of drugs]
antisense drugs [a class of drugs]
antiserum
monospecific a.
monovalent a.
multivalent a.
polyvalent a.
Reenstierna a.
antitoxins [a class of drugs]
antituberculous agents [a class of
drugs]
antivirals [a class of drugs]
aphtha (aphthae)
Bednar a.
Behçet a.
cachectic a.
a. febriles
a. tropicae
aphthosis
Touraine a.
apocrine
apolipoprotein
a. E (Apo-E)
appearance
toxic a.
APPG—aqueous procaine penicillin
G
arachnodactyly
contractural a.
arcade
vascular a.
ARD—arthritis and rheumatic disease
arteritis (arteritides)
giant cell a.
Takayasu a.
arthritis (arthritides)
atypical mycobacterial a.
bacterial a.
candidal a.
crystal a.

arthritis (arthritides) (continued)
    degenerative a.
    dysenteric a.
    enteropathic a.
    erosive a.
    fungal a.
    gonococcal a.
    gouty a.
    gram-negative bacilli a.
    hemochromatotic a.
    hemorrhagic a.
    infectious a.
    inflammatory a.
    Lyme a.
    meningococcal a.
    monoarticular a.
    a. mutilans
    mycobacterial a.
    neuropathic a.
    nongonococcal bacterial a.
    noninflammatory a.
    ochronotic a.
    palindromic a.
    postinfectious a.
    psoriatic a.
    purulent a.
    pyogenic a.
    reactive a.
    rheumatoid a.
    rubella a.
    sarcoid a.
    senescent a.
    septic a.
    traumatic a.
    tuberculous a.
    vital a.
arthropathy
    Charcot a.
    gonococcal a.
Asboe-Hansen
    disease
Aschoff
    cell
    nodule
Ascoli
    reaction
    test
    treatment

aspergillosis
    allergic bronchopulmonary a.
aspergillustoxicosis
assay
    enzyme-linked immunosorbent a. (ELISA)
    hemolytic plaque a.
    immunofluorescence a. (IFA)
    immunoradiometric a. (IRMA)
    Jerne plaque a.
    plaque-forming cell a.
    polyethylene glycol precipitation a.
    radioimmunoprecipitation a. (RIPA)
    Raji cell a.
    staphylococcal protein A binding a.
Assmann
    tuberculous infiltrate
asteatosis
asthma
    allergic a.
    Millar a. [stridorous laryngismus]
ataxia
    Leyden a.
    a.-telangiectasia
atheroma
atheromatosis
atopic
atopy
atrium (atria)
    a. of infection
atrophy
    syphilitic spinal muscular a.
aula.
Australia antigen (Au)
autoantibody
    antiplatelet a.
    Donath-Landsteiner cold a.
    incomplete a.
    warm a.
autoimmune disease (AID)
autosplenectomy
"awla" Phonetic for aula.
azoles [a class of drugs]

AZT—azidothymidine [now: zidovudine]
Babinski
    syndrome
Babinski-Vaquez
    syndrome
bacille Calmette-Guérin (BCG) vaccine
bacillus (bacilli)
    See in *Laboratory, Pathology, and Chemistry Terms.*
Bacillus
    See in *Laboratory, Pathology, and Chemistry Terms.*
bacteremia
    puerperal b.
bacteremic
bacteria (plural of bacterium)
bactericidal
bacteriolysis
    immune b.
bacteriolytic
bacteriophage
    lambda b.
bacteriophagia
bacteriophagic
bacteritic
bacterium (bacteria)
    See also specific bacteria in *Laboratory, Pathology, and Chemistry Terms.*
    resistant b.
balanitis
    b. xerotica obliterans
Baló
    concentric encephalitis
    concentric sclerosis
    concentric syndrome
    disease
    syndrome
Bancroft filariasis
Bannister
    disease
Barcoo
    disease
    rot
Bayle
    disease

B cell [noun]
B-cell [adj.]
    B-c. antigen receptors
    B-c. lymphoma
BCG (bacille Calmette-Guérin) vaccine
Bearn-Kunkel-Slater syndrome
Behçet
    disease
    syndrome
Behring (von Behring)
    B. law
    B. serum
Bekhterev-Strümpell spondylitis
Bence Jones
    body
    protein
benzylamines [a class of drugs]
Besnier
    prurigo
beta
    b.-interferon
    b.-lactams [a class of drugs]
    b.-2-microglobulin
    b.-pleated sheet
BHAPs—bisheteroarylpiperazines [a class of drugs]
Biernacki sign
bilharzial
bilharziosis, bilharziasis
binding
    b. constant
    b. protein
biocidal
biohazard
biotoxin
bisheteroarylpiperazines (BHAPs) [a class of drugs]
bivalency
    monogamous b.
blast
    b. transformation
blastomycosis
    cutaneous b.
    systemic b.
Blatin
    sign
    syndrome

blocker
    H_1 b.'s [a class of drugs]
blood groups
    ABO
    Duffy
    Kell-Cellano
    Kidd
    Lutheran
    MNSs
    Rh
blotch
    palpebral b.
blotting
    Northern b.
    Southern b.
    Western b.
Bodechtel-Guttmann
    disease
body (bodies)
    anti-immune b.
    Bollinger b.'s
    Cowdry intranuclear inclu-
      sion b. (type A, type B)
    cytomegalic inclusion b.
    cytoplasmic inclusion b.
    fuchsin b.
    Gamna-Favre b.
    glass b.
    hematoxylin b.
    inclusion b.
    Leishman-Donovan b.
    Lipschütz b.
    Prowazek-Greeff b.
    psittacosis inclusion b.
    reticulate b.
    Russell b.
    trachoma b.'s
Bollinger
    bodies
    granules
"boo-ton" Phonetic for bouton.
Borsieri
    line
    sign
Bostock
    disease
botulism
    food-borne b.

bouton
    b. de Bagdad
    b. de Biskra
    b. d'Orient
    b. en chemise
brain
    b. abscess
Breda
    disease
breeding
    random b.
Brehmer
    method
    treatment
Bretonneau
    angina
    disease
Brill
    disease
Brion-Kayser
    disease
broad-spectrum antibiotics [a class
    of drugs]
bronchoalveolar
    b. lavage
bronchomoniliasis
"broo-ee" Phonetic for bruit.
Bruce
    septicemia
bruit
    See in *Cardiology* and *Pul-
    monary Medicine* sections.
bubo
    Frei b.
    gonorrheal b.
    indolent b.
    nonvenereal b.
    pestilential b.
    strumous b.
    venereal b.
bubonic
Buerger
bunyavirus
bursitis
    anserine b.
    iliopectineal b.
    ischiogluteal b.
    prepatellar b.

bursitis (continued)
    septic b.
    traumatic b.
    trochanteric b.
butterfly
    b. rash
button
    Biskra b.
cachexia
CAH—chronic active hepatitis
CAHC—chronic active hepatitis
    with cirrhosis
Cairns
    syndrome
calcinosis
California encephalitis (CE)
Calmette
    vaccine
calor
Campylobacter fetus enteritis
cancer
    See in *Oncology and Hematology* section.
candidiasis
    bronchial c.
    cutaneous c.
    pulmonary c.
capacity
    antigen-binding c.
capillariasis
    intestinal c.
Caplan
    nodules
    syndrome
capsaicin
Capsicum, capsicum
capsule
    articular c.
capsulitis
    adhesive c.
carbacephems [a class of drugs]
carcinoembryonic antigen (CEA)
carcinoma (carcinomas, carcinomata)
    See in *Oncology and Hematology* section.
cardiomegaly
cardiomyopathy

carrier
    active c.
    chronic c.
    contact c.
    convalescent c.
    healthy c.
    intermittent c.
Carter
    mycetoma
cartilage
    articular c.
cascade
Casoni
    intradermal test
    reaction
CAST—color allergy screening test
Castellani
    bronchitis
    disease
CDC—Centers for Disease Control
    and Prevention
celiac
    c. disease
    c. sprue
cell
    See also in *Laboratory, Pathology, and Chemistry Terms.*
    accessory c.
    adherent c
    antigen-presenting c.
    Aschoff c.
    B c.
    blast c.
    bone marrow c.
    cytotoxic c.
    dendritic epidermal c.
    enterochromaffin c.
    epithelioid c.
    follicular dendritic c.
    helper c.
    helper T c.'s
    hematopoietic stem c.
    homozygous typing c.
    hybrid c.
    hyperchromatic c.
    immunologically competent c.

cell (continued)
  inclusion c.
  inducer c.
  intracytoplasmic inclusion c.
  K c.
  killer c.
  Kupffer c.
  Langerhans c.
  Langhans c.
  LE c.
  lymphoreticular c.
  M c.
  mast c.
  maturation B c.
  c.-mediated immunity
  mediator c.
  mononuclear c.
  myeloid c.
  NK (natural killer) c.
  nonadherent c.
  null c.
  phagocytic c.
  plaque-forming c.'s
  plasma c.
  pre-B c.
  prickle c.
  Reed-Sternberg giant c.
  sinusoidal endothelial c.
  spindle-shaped c.
  stem c.
  suppressor c.
  T c.
  target c.
  T-cytotoxic c.
  thymic epithelial c.
  thymus nurse c.
  T-suppressor c.
  veiled c.
  white c.'s, white blood c.'s
    (WBCs)
cell-mediated immunity (CMI)
cellular
  c. immune deficiency
  c. immunity
cellulitis
  eosinophilic c.
  gaseous c.
  streptococcal c.

Centers for Disease Control and
    Prevention (CDC)
cephalosporins [a class of drugs]
cephamycins [a class of drugs]
CFA—complete Freund adjuvant
CFIDS—chronic fatigue immune
    deficiency syndrome
CFS—chronic fatigue syndrome
Chagas
      disease
Chagas-Cruz
      disease
chancre
chancroid
chancroidal
chancrous
Charlin syndrome
Charlouis
      disease
Chauffard
      syndrome
Chauffard-Still
      syndrome
chemosuppression
chemotherapy
      combination c.
chickenpox
chilblain
Child
      hepatic risk classification
        (A–C)
CHL—chloramphenicol
Chlamydia sepsis
chloroma
chlorosis
cholangitis
      sclerosing c.
cholera
      Asiatic c.
      bilious c.
      European c.
      c. fulminans
      c. infantum
      c. morbus
      c. nostras
chondritis
      auricular c.

chorea
    Sydenham c.
choreal
chromate
chromatophore
chromatosis
chromhidrosis
chromomycosis
chromosome
    c. walking
chyluria
CID—combined immunodeficiency
    disease
    cytomegalic inclusion disease
CIDS—cellular immune deficiency
    syndrome
cin–. See also words beginning
    sin–, syn–.
cirrhosis
    Laënnec c.
CJD—Creutzfeldt-Jakob disease
classification
    Gell and Coombs c. (types
       I–IV)
    International Labor Organi-
       zation (ILO) C. of Pneu-
       moconioses
    Lukes-Collins c. of non-
       Hodgkin lymphoma
CM—capreomycin
    chloroquine-mepacrine
CMI—cell-mediated immunity
    cellular-mediated immune
       [response]
    cytomegalic inclusion
CML—cell-mediated lympholysis
CMV—cytomegalovirus
coccidioidomycosis
    primary extrapulmonary c.
cognate
    c. interaction
    c. recognition
colitis (colitides)
    amebic c.
    balantidial c.
    ulcerative c.
collagen
    c. disease

collagen (continued)
    intimal c.
    c. vascular disease
colonization
colony count
colony-stimulating factors [a class
    of drugs]
Colorado tick fever
column
    Morgagni c.
combined immunodeficiency disease
communicable disease
complement
    c. deficiency
    c. deviation
    c. level
    c.-mediated anaphylaxis
    c. receptors [CR1, CR2, CR3,
       CR4, C1qR, C3aR, C5aR]
    c. sequence
    c. test
complex
    EAHF (eczema, asthma, hay
       fever) c.
    Golgi c.
ConA—concanavalin A
concentrate
    lyophilized c.
concomitant
    c. condition
condyloma (condylomata)
    flat c.
    giant c.
    c. latum, condylomata lata
    pointed c.
condylomatosis
conformational
    c. determinant
connective tissue disease
contracture
    Dupuytren c.
Corbus
    disease
corpuscle
    Hassall c.
corticosteroids [a class of drugs]
COX-2 (cyclooxygenase-2) inhibi-
    tors [a class of drugs]

coxsackievirus (group A, group B)
CP—chloroquine and primaquine
CPPD—calcium pyrophosphate
    dihydrate (crystals)
CQ—chloroquine-quinine
CR1, C3b/C4b r., CD35; CR2,
    C3d/C3bi r. C3dg, CD21;
    CR3, C3bi r., CD11b/18; CR4,
    C3bi r., CD11c/18; C3aR (C3a
    r.); C5aR (C5a r.); C1qR (C1q
    r.) [various complement recep-
    tor designations]
craniotabes
Creutzfeldt-Jakob
    disease
    syndrome
criterion (criteria)
    Jones criteria
Crohn
    disease
CRP—C-reactive protein
Cruz
    trypanosomiasis
Cruz-Chagas
    disease
cryptococcal
    c. meningitis
    c. meningoencephalitis
cryptococcosis
    cutaneous c.
    pulmonary c.
cryptoplasmic
cryptopyic
cryptosporidiosis
    biliary c.
cryptostromosis
cryptotoxic
crystal
    Charcot-Leyden c.
cuffing
culprit
    c. organism
Curtis–Fitz-Hugh syndrome
cutaneous
    c. anthrax
    c. larva migrans
    c. leishmaniasis

cutis
    c. elastica
    c. hyperelastica
    c. laxa
CVD—collagen vascular disease
cyclo—cyclophosphamide
cyclooxygenase-2 (COX-2) inhibi-
    tors [a class of drugs]
cysticercosis
cytochalasin
    c. B
cytomegalovirus (CMV)
cytometry
    flow c.
cytoprotective agents [a class of
    drugs]
cytotoxic
    c. T lymphocyte
    c. T lymphocyte precursor
dactylitis
    d. strumosa
    d. syphilitica
    d. tuberculosa
Danielssen-Boeck
    disease
    sarcoidosis
Danysz
    effect
    phenomenon
Dawson encephalitis
DDC, ddC—dideoxycytidine
deficiency
    acquired C1 inhibitor d.
    adenosine deaminase d.
    C7 d.
    cytochrome b d.
    factor D (H, I) d.
    IgA d.
    IgM d.
    immunoglobulin d.
    kappa chain d.
    leukocyte adhesion d.
    riboflavin d.
    tyrosine aminotransferase d.
    X-linked hypogammaglobu-
        linemia with growth hor-
        mone d.

defluxio
    d. capillorum
    d. ciliorum
deformity
    swan neck d.
delta
    d. antigen
    d. hepatitis
Dennie-Marfan syndrome
dense-deposit disease
dentinogenesis
    d. imperfecta
de Quervain
    disease
    syndrome
    tenosynovitis
dermabrader
    Iverson d.
    sandpaper d.
dermamyiasis
    d. linearis migrans oestrosa
dermatitis (dermatitides)
    allergic d.
    allergic contact d.
    atopic d.
    contact d.
    cosmetic d.
    dhobie mark d.
    industrial d.
    meadow d., meadow-grass d.
    nickel d.
    occupational d.
    perfume d.
    photoallergic contact d.
    photocontact d.
dermatosis (dermatoses)
    occupational d.
desensitization
    anaphylactic d.
desmoplastic
    d. trichoepithelioma
determinant
    antigenic d.
    conformational d.
    hidden d.
    immunogenic d. I
    isoallotypic d.
    isotypic d.

determinant (continued)
    Kern isotypic d.
    Km allotypic d.
    Mcg isotypic d.
    Oz isotypic d.
    sequential d.
Devergie
    disease
DFU—dideoxyfluorouridine
DH—delayed hypersensitivity
DHT—dihydrotestosterone
diabetes
    juvenile-onset d.
    d. mellitus
"diff" Slang for differential.
differential
differentiation
    thymus cell d.
digitate
    d. warts
dilatation
    sinusoidal d.
dis–. See also words beginning dys–.
discrete
    d. disease
disease
    See also *syndrome.*
    Addison d.
    Almeida d.
    alpha chain d.
    autoimmune d. (AID)
    Bannister d.
    Behçet d.
    Bodechtel-Guttmann d.
    Breda d.
    Brill d.
    Brion-Kayser d.
    celiac d.
    Chagas d.
    Chagas-Cruz d.
    Charlouis d.
    collagen d.
    collagen vascular d.
    connective tissue d.
    Corbus d.
    Crohn d.
    Cruz-Chagas d.
    dense-deposit d.

disease (continued)
 Dukes d.
 Durand-Nicholas-Favre d.
 endocrine d.
 Favre d.
 Filatov-Dukes d.
 Forestier d.
 Francis d.
 gamma heavy chain d.
 Gaucher d.
 graft-versus-host d. (GVHD)
 Graves d.
 Gumboro d.
 Hansen d.
 heavy chain d.
 HIB (*Haemophilus influenzae* type b) d.
 His-Werner d.
 Hodgkin d.
 Hurst d.
 immunodeficiency d.
 inflammatory bowel d. (IBD)
 Isambert d.
 Jakob-Creutzfeldt d.
 Jüngling d.
 Kashin-Beck d.
 Kawasaki d.
 Kellgren d.
 Lancereau-Mathieu d.
 Larrey-Weil d.
 Legg-Calvé-Perthes d.
 Leiner d.
 Leyden d.
 Lipschütz d.
 Lobo d.
 Lutz-Splendore-Almeida d.
 Lyme d.
 lysosomal storage d.
 mixed connective tissue d.
 mu heavy chain d.
 Newcastle d.
 Nicolas-Favre d.
 Ohara d.
 Osgood-Schlatter d.
 Parkinson d.
 Poncet d.
 Posada-Wernicke d.
 Ramsay Hunt d.

disease (continued)
 Reclus d.
 Ritter d.
 Rust d.
 San Joaquin Valley d.
 Schottmüller d.
 sickle cell d.
 Stanton d.
 Still d.
 Sylvest d.
 Takahara d.
 tsutsugamushi d.
 von Willebrand d.
 Wassilieff d.
 wasting d.
 Whipple d.
 Whytt d.
 Wilson d.
disequilibrium
 linkage d.
disorder
 immunoproliferative d.
dissecting
 d. cellulitis
disseminated
 d. candidiasis
 d. cytomegalovirus
dissociation
 d. constant
distribution
 Sips d.
DLE—disseminated lupus erythematosus
Döhle
 disease
 inclusion bodies
Donath-Landsteiner
 syndrome
dose
 loading d.
DPVNS—diffuse pigmented villonodular synovitis
DT—diphtheria [vaccine] and tetanus toxoids [vaccine]
dT—diphtheria [booster] and tetanus toxoids [vaccine]
DTH—delayed-type hypersensitivity

Dubois
  abscesses
  disease
  sign
Ducrey
  test
duct
  thoracic d.
Duffy
  antigen
  blood group
Dukes
  disease
Duncan
  disease
  syndrome
Durand-Nicholas-Favre
  disease
Dutton
  disease
  relapsing fever
dynamometer
  Collins d.
dys–. See also words beginning dis–.
dysentery
  amebic d.
  bacillary d.
  balantidial d.
  bilharzial d.
  catarrhal d.
  ciliary d.
  ciliate d.
  flagellate d.
  Flexner d.
  fulminant d.
  giardiasis d.
  helminthic d.
  malarial d.
  protozoal d.
  scorbutic d.
  Shiga d.
  Sonne d.
  spirillar d.
  sporadic d.
  viral d.
dysfunction
  myocardial d.
  sensorineural d.

dysgenesis
  reticular d.
dyshidrosis
  trichophytic d.
dyskeratosis
  d. congenita
  d. follicularis
dystrophic
  d. epidermolysis bullosa
  d. palmoplantar hyperker-
    atosis
EAA—extrinsic allergic alveolitis
EACD—extrinsic allergic contact
  dermatitis
EAHF—eczema, asthma, hay fever
EB—Epstein-Barr [virus]
EBNA—Epstein-Barr nuclear antigen [test]
EBV—Epstein-Barr virus
ECHO—enteric cytopathogenic
  human orphan [now: echovirus]
echovirus (serotypes 1–7, 9, 11–18,
  20–27, 29–34)
Economo. See von Economo.
ecthyma
  e. contagiosum
  e. gangrenosum
  e. syphiliticum
ectodermal
  e. dysplasia
ectodermosis
edema
  angioneurotic e.
  hereditary angioneurotic e.
    (HANE)
edematous
EEE—eastern equine encephalomyelitis
effect [noun: result, outcome]
  See also phenomenon, reac-
    tion, and sign.
  contrast e.
  cumulative e.
  Danysz e.
  Lyon e.
effluvium
  anagen e.
  telogen e.

effusion
    pleural e.
elastosis
electromagnetic
electron
    e. microscopy
elephantiasis
    e. leishmaniana
    lymphangiectatic e.
    e. neuromatosa
    e. nostras
    e. telangiectodes
EMB—ethambutol
embolism
    bacterial e.
    plasmodium e.
emulsion
encephalitic
encephalitis (encephalitides)
    California e.
    eastern equine e.
    herpes simplex e.
    Japanese B e.
    Murray Valley e.
    Russian spring-summer e.
    St. Louis e.
    tick-borne e.
    viral e.
    western equine e.
    West Nile e.
encephalomyelitis
    disseminated e.
    eastern equine e. (EEE)
    Kelly e.
    Venezuelan equine e. (VEE)
    western equine e. (WEE)
endocarditis
    acute bacterial e.
    bacterial e.
    gonococcal e.
    infective e.
    Libman-Sacks e.
    mycotic e.
    septic e.
    subacute bacterial e.
    syphilitic e.
    tuberculous e.
endothelialization

endothelioid
"en-sed" Phonetic for NSAID (non-steroidal anti-inflammatory drug).
enteritis
    regional e.
enteropathy
    gluten-sensitive e.
entomophthoromycosis
environment
environmental
    e. allergies
eosinophil
eosinophilic
    e. cellulitis
    e. exudates
    e. fasciitis
    e. spongiosis
epidermodysplasia
    e. verruciformis
epidermolysis
    e. acquisita
    e. bullosa
    e. bullosa dystrophica, poly-dysplastic
    e. bullosa, junctional
    e. bullosa simplex
    toxic bullous e.
epidermolytic
    e. hyperkeratosis
epidermophytosis
    e. cruris
    e. interdigitale
epidermotropic
    e. reticulosis
epinephrine
epithelioma
    e. capitis
Epstein
    disease
    syndrome
equilibrium
    e. constant
    e. dialysis
erosio
    e. interdigitalis blasto-mycetica
erosion

eruption
  bullous e.
  creeping e.
  crustaceous e.
  erythematous e.
  Kaposi varicelliform e.
  maculopapular e.
  papulosquamous e.
  petechial e.
  pustular e.
  serum e.
  squamous e.
  tubercular e.
  vesicular e.
  vesiculopustular e.
erythematosus
  discoid lupus e.
  disseminated lupus e. (DLE)
  systemic lupus e. (SLE)
erythroblastosis
  e. fetalis
erythroderma
  atopic e.
  congenital ichthyosiform e.
  e. desquamativum
  exfoliative e.
  e. ichthyosiforme congenitum
  lymphomatous e.
  e. psoriaticum
  Sézary e.
  e. squamosum
esophagitis
  Candida e.
  herpetic e.
  infectious e.
  monilia e.
  thrush e.
esophagomycosis
ethanolamines [a class of drugs]
excoriation
  necrotic e.
exogenous
exophytic
extractor
  Amico e.
  comedo e.
  Schamberg e.
  Unna e.

extractor (continued)
  Walton e.
extrapulmonary
  e. tuberculosis
exuberant
  e. infection
exulceratio
  e. simplex
facies (facies)
  f. hepatica
  tabetic f.
  typhoid f.
factor
  albumin-autoagglutinating f.
  allogeneic effect f.
  angiogenesis f.
  colony-stimulating f. (CSF)
  decay-accelerating f.
  D, H, I deficiency f.
  eosinophil chemotactic f.
  epithelial thymic-activating f.
  Hageman f.
  hepatocyte-stimulating f.
  IgG rheumatoid f.
  IgM rheumatoid f.
  leukocyte inhibitory f.
  lymphocyte-activating f.
  macrophage-activating f.
  migration inhibitory f.
  nephritic f.
  neutrophil chemotactic f.
  osteoclast-activating f.
  rhesus (Rh) f.
  T-cell growth f.
  thymus-replacing f.
  tumor necrosis f.
"fago–" Phonetic for words beginning phago–.
fasciitis
  exudative f.
  necrotizing f.
  nodular f.
  proliferative f.
  pseudosarcomatous f.
fastigium
favid
Favre disease
FCA—Freund complete adjuvant

Felty syndrome
"fenomenon" Phonetic for phenomenon.
"fenotype" Phonetic for phenotype.
fester
α-fetoprotein (AFP) [alpha-]
fever
    cat-scratch f.
    Colorado tick f.
    hay f.
    hemorrhagic f.
    Malta f.
    Mediterranean f.
    mosquito-borne f.
    Oroya f.
    paratyphoid f.
    Q f.
    quinine f.
    quintana f.
    rat-bite f.
    relapsing f.
    rheumatic f.
    Rift Valley f.
    Rocky Mountain spotted f.
    saddleback f.
    San Joaquin f.
    scarlet f.
    South African tick f.
    South American hemorrhagic f.
    Southeast Asian f.
    spotted f.
    streptobacillary f.
    tick f.
    typhoid f.
    typhus f.
    undulant f.
    valley f.
    West Nile f.
    yellow f.
FIA—Freund incomplete adjuvant
fibrinoid
    f. necrosis
fibroblast
fibroma
    histiocytic f.
fibromatosis
    f. colli

fibrosis
Fiessinger-Leroy
    syndrome
"Fifer" Phonetic for Pfeiffer.
figure
    flame f.
"fi-ko-mi-co-sis" Phonetic for phycomycosis.
filarial
filariasis
    bancroftian f.
    brugian f.
    lymphatic f.
    occult f.
    periodic f.
    timorian f.
filaricidal
Filatov-Dukes
    disease
fissure
Fitz-Hugh
    syndrome
Fitz-Hugh–Curtis
    syndrome
flame
    f. figure
"flegmon" Phonetic for phlegmon.
Flexner
    dysentery
    serum
"flikt–" Phonetic for words beginning phlyct–.
florid
    f. infection
fluorescein
    f. isothiocyanate
fluorescence
    f.-activated cell sorter
    f. enhancement
    f. quenching
fluoroquinolones [a class of drugs]
focus (foci)
food poisoning
foot (feet)
    Hong Kong f.
    tropical immersion f.
Forchheimer spots
Forestier disease

Fournier
> disease
> gangrene
> syphiloma

fragilitas
> f. crinium
> f. unguium

fragment
> Fab f.
> Fabc f.
> Facb f.
> Fb f.
> Fc f.
> Fv f.
> Klenow f.
> restriction f.
> Spengler f.

Francis disease

freckle
> melanotic f. of Hutchison

Frei
> antigen
> bubo
> disease
> test

Friderichsen-Waterhouse syndrome

Friedländer
> bacillus pneumonia
> disease
> pneumonia

fulguration

fulminant

fungi (plural of fungus)

fungicidal

fungicide

fungiform

fungistasis

fungistat

fungistatic

fungus (fungi)
> See also specific fungi in
> *Laboratory, Pathology,*
> *and Chemistry Terms.*
> opportunistic f.
> pathogenic f.
> subcutaneous f.
> systemic f.

FUO—fever of undetermined origin
> fever of unknown origin

furunculus (furunculi)
> f. vulgaris

fusion
> protoplast f.

"fy-ko-my-co-sis" Phonetic for phy-
> comycosis.

gallium (Ga)
> g. scanning

galvanic
> g. epilator

gametocytemia

gamma
> g. globulin
> g. heavy chain disease
> g. interferon

gammopathy
> monoclonal g.
> polyclonal g.

Gamna
> nodules

Gandy-Gamna nodules

Gasser
> syndrome

Gaucher
> disease

GC—gonococcus

GCA—giant cell arteritis

"gee-ya bah-ray" Phonetic for Guil-
> lain-Barré.

gene
> g. bank
> cell interaction (CI) g.'s
> g. code
> g. complex
> env g.
> gag g.
> H g., histocompatibility g.
> immune response (Ir) g.'s
> immune supressor (Is) g.'s
> immunoglobulin g.'s
> g. mapping
> marker g.
> pol g.
> tat g.

generation time

genetic
> g. code

geneticist

Ghon
> complex
> focus
> lesion
> tubercle

giant cell
> g.c. arteritis
> g.c. epulis
> g.c. granuloma

giardiasis
> intestinal g.

Gilchrist
> disease
> mycosis

gingivitis
> gonococcal g.

gland
> Philip g.'s

globulin
> antidiphtheritic g.
> antitoxic g.
> D antigen immune g.
> gamma g.
> human gamma g.
> immune serum g.

glomerulonephritis
> acute post-streptococcal g.

glossitis
> g. areata exfoliativa
> g. dissecans
> Hunter g.
> g. migrans
> g. parasitica
> parenchymatous g.
> rhomboid g.
> g. rhomboidea mediana

glucocorticoids [a class of drugs]

glycopeptides [a class of drugs]

gonitis
> fungous g.

gonorrhea
> oropharyngeal g.
> pharyngeal g.
> rectal g.

gout
> tophaceous g.

graft
> g. rejection

graft-versus-host disease (GVHD)

granule
> Birbeck g.
> Bollinger g.'s

granulomatosis
> allergic g.
> lymphomatoid g.

Graves
> disease

Griesinger
> disease

group
> Kell-Cellano blood g.
> Kidd blood g.
> Lutheran blood g.

Gubler-Robin typhus

Guillain-Barré
> polyneuritis
> syndrome

Gumboro disease

GVHD—graft-versus-host disease

GVHR—graft-versus-host reaction

H_1 blockers [a class of drugs]

Haemophilus

Haenel symptom

hairy
> h. nevus
> h. tongue

Hamman-Rich
> disease
> syndrome

Hansen
> disease

HAV—hepatitis A virus

Hawes-Pallister-Landor syndrome

Hayem
> corpuscles

hay fever

HB—hepatitis B

HBLV—human B lymphotropic virus

HBV—hepatitis B virus

HDCV—human diploid cell
> (rabies) vaccine

heavy chain disease

Hecht
    phenomenon
    pneumonia
Hektoen phenomenon
helminthiasis
    h. elastica
helper cell
hemagglutination
    passive h.
hemangioma
    capillary h.
    cavernous h.
    h. congenitale
    h. hypertrophicum cutis
    sclerosing h.
    h. simplex
    strawberry h.
    verrucous h.
hemocytoblast
hemoglobinuria
    paroxysmal cold h.
    paroxysmal nocturnal h.
hemolysin
hemolysis
    passive h.
hemophilus
    See in *Laboratory, Pathology, and Chemistry Terms.*
hemorrhage
hemorrhagic
HEPA—high-efficiency particulate air [filter]
hepatitis (hepatitides)
    h. A
    acute h.
    aggressive h.
    autoimmune h.
    h. B
    h. B antigen
    h. B virus
    h. C
    chronic h.
    h. D
    delta h.
    drug-induced h.
    h. E
    fulminant h.
    h. G

hepatitis (hepatitides) (continued)
    giant cell h.
    infectious h.
    non-A h.
    non-A, non-B h.
    non-B h.
    peliosis h.
    serum h.
    syphilitic h.
    viral h.
hepatomegaly
heredolues
heredoluetic
heredosyphilis
heredosyphilitic
herpes
    anorectal h.
    buccal h.
    h. catarrhalis
    h. corneae
    h. digitalis
    h. disseminatus
    h. facialis
    h. farinosus
    h. febrilis
    h. generalisatus
    genital h.
    h. genitalis
    h. gestationis
    h. gladiatorum
    h. zoster
    h. iridis
    h. labialis
    lingual h.
    h. meningoencephalitis
    menstrual h.
    h. menstrualis
    h. mentalis
    nasal h.
    h. neonatalis
    neuralgic h.
    ocular h.
    h. odeus
    h. ophthalmicus
    orofacial h. simplex
    h. oticus
    pharyngeal h.
    h. pharyngitis

herpes (continued)
  h. phlyctaenodes
  h. praepuffalis
  h. praeputialis
  h. progenitalis
  h. recurrens
  recurrent h.
  h. simplex recurrens
  h. tonsurans
  h. tonsurans maculosus
  h. varicella-zoster virus
  h. vegetans
  wrestler h.
  h. zoster oticus
  h. zoster varicellosus
herpesvirus
  h. B
  h. simian B
herpetic
  h. proctitis
  h. whitlow
herpetiformis
  dermatitis h.
Herxheimer
  fever
  fibers
  reaction
  spirals
heterotrichosis
  h. superciliorum
Heubner
  disease
hexamethyl violet
HIB—*Haemophilus influenzae* type b
HIB disease
HIB polysaccharide vaccine
hidradenitis
  h. axillaris
  h. suppurativa
  suppurative h.
hidradenoma
  h. papilliferum
Hildenbrand
  disease
  typhus
"hipo–" Phonetic for words beginning hypo–.

histamine
  h. challenge
histamine H_1 antagonists [a class of drugs]
histaminergic
histiocyte
histiocytic
  h. lymphoma
  h. panniculitis
  h. reticulosis
histiocytoma
  h. cuffs
  h. cutis
  eruptive h.
  fibrous h.
  juvenile h.
  lipoid h.
  malignant fibrous h.
histiocytosis
  atypical h.
  cephalic h.
  malignant h.
  h. X
histioid
histocompatibility
  h. complex
histocompatible
histoincompatibility
histoincompatible
histopathology
histoplasmosis
  disseminated h.
  ocular h.
His-Werner
  disease
Hitzig
  syndrome
HIV—human immunodeficiency virus
hives
HIV protease inhibitors [a class of drugs]
HL—histocompatibility locus
Hodgkin
  disease
  granuloma
  lymphoma
Hofmann violet

homme
    h. rouge
homologous
hookworm
hormone
    thymic h.
HPV—human papillomavirus
HRF—histamine-releasing factor
HS—herpes simplex
HSV—herpes simplex virus
HSV encephalopathy
HTLV—human T-cell lymphotrophic virus [now: HIV]
humoral
    h. immune response
    h. immunity
Hunt
    syndrome
hunterian
    h. chancre
Hurst disease
Hutchinson
    disease
    mask
    syndrome
    teeth
    triad
HV—herpesvirus
hybridization
    DNA h.
    in situ h.
hybridoma
    B lymphocyte h.
    T lymphocyte h.
hydroa
    h. aestivale
    h. febrile
    h. gestationis
    h. gravidarum
    h. puerorum
    h. vacciniforme
    h. vesiculosum
hyperemia
    conjunctival h.
hyperemic
hypereosinophilia
hyperergia

hypergammaglobulinemia
    M-component h.
    monoclonal h.
    polyclonal h.
hyperglobulinemia
hyperhistidinemia
hyperhistidinuria
hyperimmune
    h. globulin
hyperimmunity
hyperimmunoglobulinemia
    h. E
hyperkeratosis
    h. congenitalis palmaris et plantaris
    epidermolytic h.
    h. excentrica
    h. figurata centrifuga atrophica
    h. follicularis in cutem penetrans
    h. follicularis vegetans
hyperleukocytosis
hyperneocytosis
hyperorthocytosis
hyperplasia
    angiofollicular mediastinal lymph node h.
    benign mediastinal lymph node h.
    follicular h.
    giant follicular h.
    giant lymph node h.
    inflammatory h.
    lymphoid h.
    mesangial h.
    pseudoepitheliomatous h.
    Schwann h.
hyperplastic
hyperpyrexia
hyperpyrexial
hypersensitive
hypersensitivity
    h., types I–IV
    atopic h.
hypersensitization
hypersplenism
hypersusceptibility

hypertoxic
hypertoxicity
hypertriglyceridemia
hypoallergenic
hypocomplementemic
hypodermiasis
hypoergia
hypoergic
hypogammaglobulinemia
    acquired h.
    congenital h.
    lymphopenic h.
    physiologic h.
    primary h.
    secondary h.
    Swiss-type h.
    transient h.
hypolymphemia
hyporeactive
hyposensitive
hyposensitivity
hyposensitization
hyposensitize
hypothesis (hypotheses)
    unitarian h.
HZ—herpes zoster
HZV—herpes zoster virus
icterus
ID—immunodeficiency
    Infectious Disease [service]
    infectious disease(s)
idiopathic
    i. thrombocytopenic purpura
IDU—idoxuridine
IEM—immune electron microscopy
Ig—immunoglobulin [IgA, IgD,
    IgE, IgG, IgM]
IH—infectious hepatitis
"ikso–" Phonetic for words begin-
    ning ixo–.
IL—interleukin [IL-1, IL-2, IL-3]
IL-2R—interleukin-2 receptor
IM—infectious mononucleosis
imaging
    See in *Radiology, Nuclear
    Medicine, and Other
    Imaging* section.

immune
    i. deviation
    i. elimination
    i. hemolysis
    i. interferon
    i. neutropenia
    i. paralysis
    i. serum
    i. serum globulin
    i. suppression
    i. surveillance
immunity
    herd i.
    humoral i.
    passive i.
immunization
    passive i.
    prophylactic i.
immunoassay
    solid-phase i.
immunodeficiency
    acquired i. syndrome (AIDS)
    acquired primary i.
    cellular i.
    i. disease
    human i.
    primary i.
    thymus-dependent i.
    X-linked hyper-IgM i.
immunodiffusion
    radial i.
immunoelectrophoresis
    rocket i.
immunofluorescence
    direct i.
    indirect i.
    i. microscopy
immunoglobulin (Ig)
    i. A (IgA)
    i. alpha chain
    Bence Jones monoclonal i.
    i. class
    i. class switching
    i. delta chain
    i. domain
    i. epsilon chain
    i. fold
    i. G (IgG)

immunoglobulin (Ig) (continued)
    i. gamma chain
    i. gene rearrangement
    i. genes
    i. heavy chain
    i. kappa chain
    i. lambda chain
    i. light chain
    membrane i.
    monoclonal i.
    i. mu chain
    secretory i. A
    i. subclass
    i. superfamily
    thyroid-binding inhibitory i.
      (TBII)
    thyroid-stimulating i.
    thyrotropin-binding inhibito-
      ry i. (TBII)
    TSH-binding inhibitory i.
immunologic
    i. imbalance
    i. memory
    i. surveillance
immunosuppressants [a class of
    drugs]
immunosuppression
immunosuppressive
immunotherapy
impetigo
    i. bullosa
    bullous i.
    i. contagiosa
    i. eczematodes
    follicular i.
    Fox i.
    furfuraceous i.
    i. herpetiformis
    i. neonatorum
    i. simplex
    i. staphylogenes
    i. syphilitica
    i. variolosa
inclusion
    i. bodies
incubation
indolent

indurated
    i. cellulitis
    i. lymphangitis
infantile
    i. celiac disease
infection
    abortive i.
    airborne i.
    bacterial i.
    concurrent i.
    contact i.
    covert i.
    cryptosporidial i.
    cysticercosis i.
    direct i.
    dormant i.
    Epstein-Barr virus i.
    focal i.
    hepatitis B virus i.
    herpes simplex i.
    herpes zoster i.
    iatrogenic i.
    indirect i.
    intercurrent i.
    latent i.
    local i.
    metazoan i.
    nonspecific i.
    nosocomial i.
    opportunistic i.
    parasitic i.
    perinatal i.
    phycomycotic i.
    protozoan i.
    puerperal i.
    pyogenic i.
    retrograde i.
    secondary i.
    silent i.
    slow i.
    subclinical i.
    toxoplasmosis, other agents,
      rubella, cytomegalovirus,
      herpes simplex (TORCH)
      i.
    transcervical i.
    transforming i.
    transplacental i.

infection (continued)
    tunnel i.
    viral i.
    water-borne i.
infectious mononucleosis
infiltration
    adipose i.
    cellular i.
    inflammatory i.
    lymphocytic i.
    mesentery i.
    parenchymal i.
inflammatory
INH—isonicotine hydrazine inhibitor
    isonicotinic acid hydrazide
      (isoniazid)
inhibitor
    COX-2 (cyclooxygenase-2)
      i.'s [a class of drugs]
    HIV protease i.'s [a class of
      drugs]
    non-nucleoside reverse
      transcriptase i.'s (NNR-
      TIs) [a class of drugs]
    protease i.'s [a class of drugs]
    reverse transcriptase (RT)
      i.'s [a class of drugs]
inoculate
inoculation
in situ
    i.s. hybridization
integument
integumentum
    i. commune
interleukin
    i. 1 (IL-1)
    i. 2 (IL-2)
    i. 2R (IL-2R)
    i. 3 (IL-3)
intertrigo
    i. labialis
    i. saccharomycetica
intimitis
    proliferative i.
intracranial
intrinsic
    i. affinity
    i. association constant

invariant
    i. chain
    I i.
IP—incubation period
IS—immune serum
Isambert disease
ISG—immune serum globulin
ISH—icteric serum hepatitis
isoelectric
    i. focusing
    i. point
isolation
itch
    Boeck i.
    dhobie i.
    grain i.
    seven-year i.
ITP—idiopathic thrombocytopenic
    purpura
IV—intravenous
ixodiasis
ixodic
JA—juvenile arthritis
Jakob
    disease
Jakob-Creutzfeldt
    disease
    syndrome
Japanese B encephalitis
jaundice
Jeanselme nodules
Joest bodies
joint
    See in *Orthopedics and
      Sports Medicine* section.
JRA—juvenile rheumatoid arthritis
jugulation
jugulodigastric
junctional
    j. epidermolysis bullosa
    j. nevus
Jüngling disease
juvenile
    j.-onset diabetes
    j. rheumatoid arthritis
"kahk–," "kak–" Phonetic for words
    beginning cac–, cach–.

Kahler
    disease
Kaposi
    disease
    sarcoma
    varicelliform eruption
    xeroderma
Kashin-Beck disease
Katayama
    disease
    syndrome
Kawasaki
    disease
    syndrome
Kellgren disease
keloid
    Addison k.
"kemo–" Phonetic for words beginning chemo–.
keratitis
    amebic k.
    dendritic k.
    interstitial k.
keratoconjunctivitis
    k. sicca
keratoderma
    k. blennorrhagica
keratolysis
    k. exfoliativa
    k. neonatorum
keratoma
    k. diffusum
    k. hereditaria mutilans
    k. malignum congenitale
    k. palmare et plantare
    k. plantare sulcatum
    k. senile
keratomycosis
    k. linguae
keratosis (keratoses)
    k. blennorrhagica
    k. follicularis contagiosa
    gonorrheal k.
kerion
    k. celsi
    Celsus k.
KM—kanamycin

Koch
    bacillus
    lymph node
Koplik
    sign
    spots
kraurosis
    k. penis
    k. vulvae
KV—kanamycin and vancomycin
Kveim
    reaction
Kyasanur Forest
    disease
"kyl–" Phonetic for words beginning chyl–.
kyphosis
    Scheuermann juvenile k.
labrocyte
β-lactams [beta-] [a class of drugs]
lambda
    l. bacteriophage
Lancereau-Mathieu disease
Landouzy
    disease
Landry
    syndrome
Landry-Guillain-Barré
    syndrome
Langhans
    cells
    layer
Larrey-Weil
    disease
larva (larvae)
    l. currens
    cutaneous l. migrans
    l. migrans
    ocular l. migrans
    visceral l. migrans
larval
latent
    l. infection
latex
    l. allergy
Lauth violet
LAV—lymphadenopathy-associated virus

law
>Behring l.
>von Behring (Behring) l.

lazaroids [a class of drugs]
lazy leukocyte syndrome (LLS)
LED—lupus erythematosus disseminatus
Leede-Rumpel phenomenon
Legg-Calvé-Perthes
>disease

legionella (legionellae)
>l. pneumonia

Leiner
>disease

Leishman
>anemia

Leishman-Donovan
>bodies

leishmaniasis
>l. recidivans
>visceral l.

Leloir disease
lentivirus
Lépine-Froin syndrome
lepra
>l. alba
>l. alphoides
>l. alphos
>l. anaesthetica
>l. arabum
>l. conjunctivae
>l. graecorum
>l. maculosa
>l. mutilans
>l. nervorum
>l. nervosa
>l. tuberculoides
>Willan l.

leprostatics [a class of drugs]
leprosy
>Asturian l.
>borderline l.
>borderline lepromatous l.
>borderline tuberculous l.
>cutaneous l.
>diffuse l. of Lucio
>dimorphous l.
>histoid l.

leprosy (continued)
>indeterminate l.
>intermediate l.
>lazarine l.
>lepromatous l.
>Lombardy l.
>Lucio l.
>macular l.
>maculoanesthetic l.
>neural l.
>nodular l.
>polar lepromatous l.
>pure neural l.
>reactional l.
>spotted l.
>subclinical l.
>subpolar lepromatous l.
>trophoneurotic l.
>tuberculoid l.
>uncharacteristic l.
>virchowian l.
>water-buffalo l.

leprotic
Leredde
>syndrome

lesion
>cavitary pulmonary l.
>Cole herpetiform l.
>Councilman l.
>Ghon primary l.
>herpetiform l. of Cole
>initial syphilitic l.

leukemia
>See in *Oncology and Hematology* section.

leukocyte
>l. inhibitory factor
>passenger l.
>polymorphonuclear l. leukocytoclastic

leukocytic
leukocytosis
>mononuclear l.

leukoencephalopathy
>multifocal progressive l.
>progressive multifocal l.

leukoerythroblastosis

leukopenia
    basophil l.
    basophilic l.
    congenital l.
    eosinophilic l.
    lymphocytic l.
    malignant l.
    monocytic l.
    neutrophilic l.
    pernicious l.
leukoplakia
    hairy l.
Leyden
    ataxia
    disease
LGV—lymphogranuloma venereum
lice (plural of louse)
lichenificatio
lincosamides [a class of drugs]
line
    Aldrich-Mees l.'s
    Borsieri l.
    Mees l.'s
    Pastia l.'s
lipedema
lipoatrophy
lipoblast
lipogranulomatosis
lipoidosis
lipophagia
    l. granulomatosis
lipophagy
Lipschütz
    bodies
    cell
    disease
    ulcer
listerial
listerism
livedo
    l. annularis
    l. racemosa
    l. reticularis
    l. reticularis idiopathica
    l. reticularis symptomatica
    l. telangiectatica
LLS—lazy leukocyte syndrome
loading dose

Lobo
    disease
locus (loci)
    minor histocompatibility l.
    l. minoris resistentiae
    T l.
Löffler
    disease
    endocarditis
    eosinophilia
    pneumonia
    syndrome
louse (lice)
    body l.
    clothes l.
    crab l.
    head l.
    pubic l.
    sucking l.
LP—lumbar puncture
lues
    l. nervosa
    l. tarda
    l. venerea
Lukes-Collins classification
"luko–" Phonetic for words beginning leuko–.
lupus
    discoid l.
    l. erythematosus (LE)
    l. nephritis
    systemic l. erythematosus (SLE)
Lutz-Splendore-Almeida
    disease
Lyb antigens
Lyell
    disease
    syndrome
Lyme
    disease
lymph
    l. node
    l. nodule
lymphangioma
    l. cavernosum
    l. circumscriptum
    l. cysticum

lymphangioma (continued)
l. tuberosum multiplex
l. xanthelasmoideum
lymphangitic
l. sporotrichosis
lymphangitis
l. carcinomatosa
lymphatic
lymphedema
l. praecox
l. tarda
lymphocyte
l.-activating factor (LAF)
l. recirculation
suppressor T l.
l. transformation
lymphocytoma
l. cutis
lymphogranuloma
l. benignum
l. venereum
lymphogranulomatosis
l. cutis
l. inguinalis
l. maligna
lymphoma
adult T-cell leukemia l.
African l.
B-cell l.
Burkitt l.
Burkitt-like l.
cutaneous T-cell l.
diffuse l.
follicular l.
follicular center cell l.
giant follicle l.
giant follicular l.
granulomatous l.
histiocytic l.
Hodgkin l.
large cell l.
Lennert l.
lymphoblastic l.
lymphocytic l.
lymphocytic l., poorly differentiated
lymphocytic l., well-differentiated

lymphoma (continued)
malignant l.
Mediterranean l.
mixed lymphocytic-histiocytic l.
nodular l.
non-Hodgkin l.
null-type non-Hodgkin's l.
pleomorphic l.
sclerosing l.
signet-ring cell l.
small B-cell l.
stem cell l.
T-cell l.'s.
T-cell l., convoluted
T-cell l., cutaneous
T-cell l., small lymphocytic
U-cell (undefined) l.
undifferentiated l.
lymphomatous
lymphosarcoma
fascicular l.
sclerosing l.
lysis
reactive l.
lysosomal storage disease
Lyt antigens
MAC—*Mycobacterium avium* complex
macroglobulinemia
Waldenström m.
macrolides [a class of drugs]
macrophage
activated m.
alveolar m.
suppressor m.
macula (maculae)
macule
maculopapular
MAI—*Mycobacterium avium-intracellulare*
maladie
m. du sommeil ["due somay"]
malaise
mamanpian
Manson
disease

Manson (continued)
    hemoptysis
    pyosis
    schistosomiasis
Marburg
    disease
    hemorrhagic fever
mask
    Hutchinson m.
mast cell
mastocytosis
    diffuse m.
    diffuse cutaneous m.
    malignant m.
    systemic m.
McKrae
    herpesvirus
M-CSF—macrophage colony-stim-
    ulating factor
measles
    atypical m.
    bastard m.
    black m.
    confluent m.
    French m.
    German m.
    hemorrhagic m.
    three-day m.
medication
    prophylactic m.
medicine
    environmental m.
Medin
    disease
    poliomyelitis
medium (media, mediums)
    HAT m.
melanoma
melanotic [pertaining to melanin]
melasma
    m. universale
membrane
    basement m.
    croupous m.
    diphtheritic m.
    false m.
meningitic

meningitis (meningitides)
    acute aseptic m.
    acute septic m.
    African m.
    aseptic m.
    Bacteroides m.
    basal m.
    m. of the base, basilar m.
    benign lymphocytic m.
    benign recurrent endotheli-
        oleukocytic m.
    brucellar m.
    m. carcinomatosa
    cerebral m.
    cerebrospinal m.
    chemical m.
    chronic posterior basic m.
    m. circumscripta spinalis
    cryptococcal m.
    curable serous m.
    eosinophilic m.
    epidemic cerebrospinal m.
    external m.
    gonococcal m.
    granulomatous m.
    gummatous m.
    herpetic m.
    influenzal m.
    internal m.
    leptospiral m.
    localized tuberculous m.
    lymphocytic m.
    meningococcal m.
    meningococcic m.
    metastatic m.
    Mollaret m.
    mumps m.
    mycobacterial m.
    mycotic m.
    m. necrotoxica reactiva
    neonatal m.
    occlusive m.
    m. ossificans
    otitic m.
    otogenic m.
    parameningococcus m.
    plague m.
    plasmodial m.

meningitis (meningitides) (continued)
    pneumococcal m.
    posterior m.
    posterior basic m.
    post-traumatic m.
    purulent m.
    pyogenic m.
    Quincke m.
    rheumatic m.
    sarcoid m.
    septicemic m.
    m. serosa
    m. serosa circumscripta
    m. serosa circumscripta cystica
    serous m.
    serum m.
    simple m.
    spinal m.
    staphylococcal m.
    sterile m.
    streptococcal m.
    suppurative m.
    m. sympathica
    syphilitic m.
    torula m., torular m.
    trypanosomal m.
    tubercular m., tuberculous m.
    typhoid m.
    viral m.
    Wallgren aseptic m.
    yeast m.
metastasis (metastases)
    biochemical m.
    contact m.
    miliary m.
methyl
    m. violet
MHC—major histocompatibility complex
microabscess
    Pautrier m.
microfilariasis
microglobulin β_2
microsporosis
    m. capitis
"miel–" Phonetic for words beginning myel–.

Mikulicz (von Mikulicz)
    syndrome
Mikulicz-Radecki
    syndrome
Mikulicz-Sjögren
    syndrome
Mills-Reincke phenomenon
mitogen
    pokeweed m.
    T-cell m.
Mitsuda
    antigen
    reaction
    test
mixed connective tissue disease
MLNS—mucocutaneous lymph node syndrome
molecular
    m. mimicry
Mollaret meningitis
molluscum
    m. bodies
    m. contagiosum
monobactams [a class of drugs]
monoclonal
    m. antibody (MAb)
monocyte
monoinfection
mononucleosis
    infectious m.
monotherapy
morphea
    acroteric m.
    m. alba
    m. atrophica
    m. flammea
    m. guttata
    herpetiform m.
    m. linearis
    m. nigra
mosquito (mosquitoes)
MPA—methylprednisolone acetate
MRSA—methicillin-resistant *Staphylococcus aureus*
MTX—methotrexate
mucinosis
    follicular m.
    papular m.

mucocutaneous
    m. candidiasis
    m. herpes simplex
mu heavy chain disease
multisensitivity
mumps
    m. meningoencephalitis
murine
    m. T-cell phenotype
Murray Valley
    disease
    encephalitis
muscle
    See in *Orthopedics and*
      Sports Medicine section.
musculus (musculi)
    See in *Orthopedics and*
      Sports Medicine section.
mushroom worker's
    disease
    syndrome
mutation
    somatic m.
mycetoma
    actinomycotic m.
    eumycotic m.
mycobacteriosis
mycobacterium (mycobacteria)
mycoplasmal
    m. pneumonia
myelitis
    acute syphilitic m.
    amyotrophic syphilitic m.
    tuberculous m.
myeloperoxidase (MPO) deficiency
myelophthisis
myelosyphilis
myositis
    m. ossificans
myxoma (myxomas, myxomata)
    infectious m.
myxovirus
National Institute of Allergy and
    Infectious Diseases (NIAID)
NCA—nonspecific cross-reacting
    antigen
necrosis (necroses)
    bacillary n.

necrosis (necroses) (continued)
    septic n.
    syphilitic n.
necrotic
neomembrane
nephritis (nephritides)
    Heymann n.
    Masugi n.
nephropathia
    n. epidermica
nephropathy
    human immunodeficiency
      virus–associated n. [HIV-]
neuritic
neuritis
    diphtheric n.
    influenzal n.
    leprous n.
    malarial n.
    malarial multiple n.
    rheumatic n.
    syphilitic n.
    tabetic n.
neuroallergy
neuroamebiasis
neuroborreliosis
neuroimmunologic
neuroimmunology
neurolabyrinthitis
    viral n.
neurolues
neurosyphilis
    asymptomatic n.
    congenital n.
    ectodermogenic n.
    juvenile n.
    latent n.
    meningeal n.
    meningovascular n.
    mesodermogenic n.
    parenchymatous s.
    paretic n.
    tabetic n.
neurotabes
    n. diabetica
neurovaccine
nevoid
    n. lentigo

nevoid (continued)
    n. telangiectasia
Newcastle
    disease
Nezelof
    syndrome
NIAID—National Institute of Allergy and Infectious Diseases
NIAMD—National Institute of Arthritis and Metabolic Diseases
Nicolas-Favre
    disease
nidus (nidi)
NK—natural killer
NK cells
NNRTIs—non-nucleoside reverse transcriptase inhibitors [a class of drugs]
node
    mesenteric n.
    shotty n.
nodosa
    periarteritis n.
nodular
nodularity
nodulated
nodulation
nodule
    Gamna n.'s
    Gandy-Gamna n.'s
    glial n.
non-nucleoside reverse transcriptase inhibitors (NNRTIs) [a class of drugs]
nonspecific
nonsteroidal anti-inflammatory drugs (NSAIDs) [a class of drugs]
norlupinanes [a class of drugs]
noxa (noxae)
NSAID, NSAIDs—nonsteroidal anti-inflammatory drug(s) [a class of drugs]
nucleoside
    n. analogue
    n. phosphorylase
"nur–" Phonetic for words beginning neur–.

nvCJD—new variant Creutzfeldt-Jakob disease
occult
ochronosis
    exogenous o.
    ocular o.
"ofthal–" Phonetic for words beginning ophthal–.
Ohara
    disease
ointment
    Hebra o.
    Whitfield o.
oligosaccharide
    asparagine-linked o.
onchocerciasis
opisthorchosis
organism
    transgenic o.
Osgood-Schlatter
    disease
    syndrome
osseous
    o. syphilis
    o. yaws
osteitis
    o. deformans
osteoarthritis
    o. deformans
    o. deformans endemica
    endemic o.
    erosive o.
    hyperplastic o.
    hypertrophic o.
    interphalangeal o.
    primary generalized hypertrophic o.
osteoarthropathy
    tabetic o.
osteochondritis
    o. dissecans
osteomyelitis
    salmonella o.
    tuberculous spinal o.
    typhoid o.
    o. variolosa
osteonecrosis
osteophyte

osteoporosis
    juxta-articular o.
osteotabes
Ouchterlony
    method
overgrowth
    candidal o.
    fungal o.
    yeast o.
overload
Oz
    O. antigen
    O. isotypic determinant
PAB—*p*-aminobenzoate [p-, para-]
PABA—*p*-aminobenzoic acid [p-, para-]
pachyderma
    p. lymphangiectatica
pachydermoperiostosis
    p. plicata
Pahvant Valley
    fever
    plague
paint
    Castellani p.
pallor
panatrophy
panencephalitis
    Pette-Döring p.
    subacute sclerosing p.
p24 antigen test
papulosis
    bowenoid p.
    lymphomatoid p.
para
    p.-aminobenzoate (PAB)
    p.-aminobenzoic acid (PABA)
paralysis (paralyses)
    ascending tick p.
    Erb syphilitic spinal p.
    Kussmaul p., Kussmaul-
      Landry p.
    parotitic p.
    postdiphtheric p.
    Pott p.
    syphilitic spastic spinal p.
    tick p.

parasite
    See specific parasites in
      Laboratory, Pathology,
      and Chemistry Terms.
parasitic
parenchyma
    hepatic p.
paresis
Parinaud
    syndrome
paronychia
    p. tendinosa
Parrot [eponym]
    disease
    nodes
    pseudoparalysis
    sign
    syndrome (I, II)
    syphilitic osteochondritis
    ulcer
paste
    Lassar p.
    Veiel p.
patch
    Peyer p.'s
    p. test
pathogen
    See specific pathogens in
      Laboratory, Pathology,
      and Chemistry Terms.
pathognomonic
pathway
    lipoxygenase p.
PBZ—pyribenzamine
PCA—passive cutaneous anaphylaxis
PCP—*Pneumocystis carinii* pneumonia
Pecquet
    cistern
    duct
    reservoir
pedicular
pediculosis
    p. capillitii
    p. capitis
    p. corporis
    p. inguinalis
    p. palpebrarum

pediculosis (continued)
    p. pubis
    p. vestimenti
    p. vestimentorum
pediculous
pemphigoid
    bullous p.
pemphigus
    p. acutus
    p. erythematosus
    p. foliaceus
    p. gangrenosus
    p. hemorrhagicus
    p. malignus
    p. neonatorum
    p. syphiliticus
    p. vegetans
    p. vulgaris
pen—penicillin
penems [a class of drugs]
penicillins [a class of drugs]
peptide
    chemotactic p.
    signal p.
perennial
periadenitis
    p. mucosa necrotica recurrens
periadnexal
    p. dermis
periarteritis
    p. gummosa
    p. nodosa
perifolliculitis
    p. capitis abscedens et suffo-
        diens
    superficial pustular p.
perihepatitis
    gonococcal p.
periorificial
    p. lentiginosis
pesticemia
pestilential
Pfeiffer
    disease
PG—prostaglandin
PGD_2 [PGD2]—prostaglandin D_2
PGE_2 [PGE2]—prostaglandin E_2

PGL—persistent generalized lym-
    phadenopathy
phagocyte
phagocytosis
phagocytotic
pharyngitis
    gonococcal p.
    streptococcal p.
phenomenon (phenomena)
    See also *effect, reaction,* and
        sign.
    anaphylactoid p.
    Anderson p.
    Arthus p., p. of Arthus
    booster p.
    Chase-Sulzberger p.
    cheek p.
    Danysz p.
    Debré p.
    fall-and-rise p.
    first-set p.
    Hata p.
    Hecht p.
    Hektoen p.
    Leede-Rumpel p.
    Leichtenstern p.
    LE (lupus erythematosus)
        cell p.
    Liacopoulos p.
    Matuhasi-Ogata p.
    Mills-Reincke p.
    Pfeiffer p.
    Raynaud p.
    Rumpel-Leede p.
    Sanarelli p.
    satellite p.
    Schramm p.
    Schultz-Charlton p.
    second-set p.
    Shwartzman p.
    Sulzberger-Chase p.
    vacuum p.
phenotype
    Bombay p.
    dominant p.
    McLeod p.
    murine T-cell p.
Philip glands

phlegmon
phlyctenulosis
    allergic p.
    tuberculous p.
phycomycosis
physalopteriasis
pian
    p. bois
    hemorrhagic p.
Picchini syndrome
piggyback
piggybacking
pilonidal
pinworm
    human p.
piperidines [a class of drugs]
pityriasis
    p. alba
    p. amiantacea
    p. capitis
    p. circinata
    p. circinata et marginata
    p. furfuracea
    Hebra p.
    p. lichenoides
    p. lichenoides et vario-
      liformis acuta
    p. linguae
    p. maculata
    p. pilaris
    p. rosea
    p. rotunda
    p. rubra
    p. rubra pilaris
    p. sicca
    p. simplex
    p. steatoides
    p. versicolor
planar
    p. xanthoma
plantar
    p. fibromatosis
    p. hyperkeratosis
    p. inoculum
    p. nevi
plaque-forming cell assay
pleocytosis
    mononuclear p.

plot
    Sips p.
    Wu-Kabat p.
PMR—polymyalgia rheumatica
pneumococcal
    p. meningitis
pneumonia
    eosinophilic p.
    Friedländer p.
    giant cell p.
    Legionella pneumophila p.
    Pneumocystis carinii p. (PCP)
    staphylococcal p.
pneumonitis
    hypersensitivity p.
    lymphoid interstitial p.
Pneumovax
    P. 23
POA—pancreatic oncofetal antigen
pock
pockmark
poikiloderma
    Civatte p.
    p. congenitale
polio—poliomyelitis
poliosis
    p. eccentrica
poliovirus
pollen
pollination
pollinosis
pollution
polyarteritis
    p. nodosa
polyarthritis
polyarthropathy
polyarthrosis
polychondritis
    relapsing p.
polychondropathia
polychondropathy
polyclonal
    p. hypergammaglobulinemia
    p. hyperglobulinemia
polymyalgia
    p. rheumatica
polyploid
polysaccharide

polyserositis
    idiopathic p.
    periodic p.
    recurrent p.
    tuberculous p.
pomphoid
pompholyx
pomphus
Poncet
    disease
    rheumatism
poroma
Posada-Wernicke disease
postnatal
Pott
    abscess
    disease
PPD—purified protein derivative
    (of tuberculin)
PPD-S—purified protein deriva-
    tive–standard
precipitate
    immune p.
precipitin
    p. curve
    p. reaction
PRIST—paper radioimmunosorbent
    test
procedure
    Cleveland p.
proctitis
    p. obliterans
    pseudoinfectious p.
    traumatic p.
prodroma (plural of prodromon)
prodromal
prodromata [incorrect term for pro-
    droma, plural of prodromon]
prodrome
prodromic
prostaglandin (PG)
    See also in *Laboratory,*
        Pathology, and Chemistry
        Terms.
    p. D$_2$ [D2] (PGD$_2$)
    p. E$_2$ [E2] (PGE$_2$)
protease inhibitors [a class of drugs]

protein
    A, G, S p.
    Bence Jones p.
protoporphyria
    erythropoietic p.
pseudoxanthoma
    p. elasticum
PST—penicillin, streptomycin,
    tetracycline
PTH—post-transfusion hepatitis
PTM—post-transfusion mononucle-
    osis
pubic
    p. lice
Puente disease
pulmonary
    p. anthrax
    p. ascariasis
    p. aspergillosis
    p. blastomycosis
    p. candidiasis
    p. cryptococcosis
    p. eosinophilia
    p. histoplasmosis
    p. mucormycosis
    p. nodulosis
purpura
    anaphylactoid p.
    autoimmune thrombocytope-
        nic p.
    Henoch p.
    Henoch-Schönlein p.
    Schönlein p.
    Schönlein-Henoch p.
pus (pura)
    p. tube
pyoderma
    p. gangrenosum
pyomyositis
    tropical p.
pyosis
pyrogen
    endogenous p.
pyroglobulin
PZA—pyrazinamide
Q fever
Quervain. See *de Quervain.*
quiescent

Quincke
    meningitis
quinolizidines [a class of drugs]
RA—rheumatoid arthritis
rabies
radiation
    r. spectrum
radioallergosorbent
radioimmunoassay (RIA)
radioimmunoelectrophoresis
radioimmunosorbent
radionuclide
Ramsay Hunt
    disease
    syndrome
ranula
RAST—radioallergosorbent test
rate
    Westergren sedimentation r.
ratio
    helper-suppressor cell r.
    polymorphonuclear-lympho-
        cyte r.
Raynaud
    disease
reaction
    See also *effect, phenomenon,*
        and *sign.*
    acute phase r.
    allergic r.
    allograft r.
    anaphylactic r.
    anaphylactoid r.
    antigen-antibody r.
    antiglobulin r.
    Arthus r.
    Arthus-type r.
    delayed hypersensitivity r.
    delayed-type hypersensitivi-
        ty r.
    Forssman antigen-antibody r.
    graft-versus-host r. (GVHR)
    Herxheimer r.
    homograft r.
    hypersensitivity r.
    immediate hypersensitivity r.
    immune r.
    immunity r.

reaction (continued)
    Jarisch-Herxheimer r.
    Jones-Mote r.
    Kveim r.
    Mantoux r.
    Mitsuda r.
    Prausnitz-Küstner (P-K) r.
    quantitative precipitin r.
    Schultz-Charlton r.
    Schultz-Dale r.
    wheal and erythema r.,
        wheal and flare r.
receptor
    B-cell antigen r.'s
    complement r.'s [CR1,
        C3b/C4b r., CD35; CR2,
        C3d/C3bi r., C3dg, CD21;
        CR3, C3bi r., CD11b/18;
        CR4, C3bi r., CD11c/18;
        C3aR (C3a r.); C5aR
        (C5a r.); C1qR (C1q r.)]
    Fc r.'s
    histamine H_1 r. [H1]
    histamine H_2 r. [H2]
    homing r.
    IgE r.'s
    immune adherence r.
    polyimmunoglobulin r.
    T-cell antigen r.'s
    transferrin r.
Recklinghausen-Appelbaum
    disease
Reclus disease
red herring
region
    framework r.
renal
    r. toxicity
    r. transplant
    r. transplantation
reservoir
    r. of infection
resistance
    drug r.
    multidrug r., multiple drug. r.
response
    allergic r.
    anamnestic r.

reticula (plural of reticulum)
reticuloendothelial
    r. blockade
    r. system
reticuloendotheliosis
    leukemic r.
reticulohistiocytosis
    multicentric r.
reticulum (reticula)
    r. cell carcinoma
    endoplasmic r.
retiform
    r. parapsoriasis
retinitis
    cytomegalovirus r.
retroperitoneal
retrovirus
    lymphotropic r.
reverse transcriptase (RT) inhibitors
    [a class of drugs]
RFLA—rheumatoid factor–like
    activity
Rh—Rhesus
Rh
    antibody
    blood group
    factor
    immunization
    incompatibility
    isoantigen
rhacoma
rhesus (Rh)
    r. factor
rheumatic
    r. disease
    r. factor
rheumatism
    palindromic r.
    Poncet r.
rheumatoid
    r. arthritis
    r. factor
    r. nodule
    r. vasculitis
rhinitis
    allergic r.
Rh neg—Rhesus factor–negative

rhodamine
    r. isothiocyanate
Rh pos—Rhesus factor–positive
rhus dermatitis
RIA—radioimmunoassay
"rino–" Phonetic for words begin-
    ning rhino–.
RIP—radioimmunoprecipitation
RIPA—radioimmunoprecipitation
    assay
RIST—radioimmunosorbent test
Ritter
    disease
"rizo–" Phonetic for words begin-
    ning rhizo–.
RNP—ribonucleoprotein
Roger
    reaction
    symptom
Rosenbach
    erysipeloid
roseola
    r. infantum
rosette
    E, EA, EAC r.
rotavirus
    r. gastroenteritis
RPR—rapid plasma reagin (test)
RT (reverse transcriptase) inhibitors
    [a class of drugs]
rubella
rubelliform
rubeola
Rumpel-Leede
    phenomenon
    sign
    test
rupia
    r. escharotica
Russian
    spring-summer encephalitis
Rust [eponym]
    disease
    syndrome
RW—ragweed
saccharide
    O-linked s.

sacroiliitis
    pyogenic s.
saliva
salivary
Sanarelli phenomenon
San Joaquin fever
San Joaquin Valley disease
sarcoma (sarcomas, sarcomata)
    See also in *Oncology and
        Hematology* section.
    immunoblastic s. of B cells
    immunoblastic s. of T cells
    Kaposi s.
    multiple idiopathic hemor-
        rhagic s.
sarcomatosis
    s. cutis
sarcomatous
sarcosepsis
sarcosis
sarcosporidiosis
SBE—subacute bacterial endocarditis
SCA—single-chain antigen-binding
SCA proteins
scabies
    Boeck s.
scan
    See in *Radiology, Nuclear
        Medicine, and Other
        Imaging* section.
scarify
scheme
    Kauffmann-White s.
Schick
    reaction
    sign
    test
Schilder
    disease
    encephalitis
schistosomiasis
Schottmüller (Schottmueller)
    disease
    fever
Schramm phenomenon
SCIDS—severe combined immuno-
    deficiency syndrome
scleradenitis

scleredema
    s. neonatorum
sclerema
    s. neonatorum
sclerodactylia
    s. annularis ainhumoides
sclerosis
    multiple s. (MS)
    progressive systemic s. (PSS)
    systemic s.
scrofuloderma
    s. gummosa
    papular s.
    pustular s.
    tuberculous s.
    ulcerative s.
    verrucous s.
scurvy
secretor
secretory
    s. component deficiency
    s. compound
    s. IgA
sed rate—sedimentation rate
self-limited, self-limiting
semen
sepsis
    s. agranulocytica
septic
    s. arthritis
septicemia
    acute fulminating meningo-
        coccal s.
    perinatal s.
septicemic
septic shock
sequence
    consensus s.
    Shine-Dalgarno s.
    signal s.
sequestra (plural of sequestrum)
sequestral
sequestration
sequestrum (sequestra)
serositis (serositides)
    adhesive s.
    multiple serositides
serous

serpiginous
serum (serums, sera)
    active s.
    s. albumin
    s. amyloid A component
    s. amyloid P component
    antianthrax s.
    antibotulinus s.
    anticholera s.
    anticomplementary s.
    anticrotalus s.
    antidiphtheria s.
    antiglobulin s.
    antilymphocyte s. (ALS)
    antimeningococcus s.
    antipneumococcus s.
    antirabies s.
    antisnakebite s.
    antitetanic s. (ATS)
    antithymocyte s.
    antitoxic s.
    bacteriolytic s.
    Behring s.
    convalescence s., convalescent s., convalescents' s.
    despeciated s.
    foreign s.
    heterologous s.
    homologous s.
    hyperimmune s.
    immune s.
    inactivated s.
    lymphatolytic s.
    monospecific s.
    monovalent s.
    North American antisnakebite s.
    polyvalent s.
    pooled s.
    Sclavo s.
    s. sickness
    specific s.
    s. urate level
    s. uric acid
    von Behring (Behring) s.
Sézary
    syndrome
SH—sinus histiocytosis

"shangker" Phonetic for chancre.
"shangkroid" Phonetic for chancroid.
shock
    anaphylactic s.
    anaphylactoid s.
    bacteremic s.
    endotoxic s.
    endotoxin s.
    histamine s.
    septic s.
    toxic s.
Shwartzman-Sanarelli phenomenon
sickle cell
    s.c. disease
sickness
    acute serum s.
    chronic serum s.
    drug-induced serum s.
    serum s.
"sifilis" Phonetic for syphilis.
"sifilo–" Phonetic for words beginning syphilo–.
sigmoidoscopy
sign
    See also *effect, phenomenon,* and *reaction.*
    Anghelescu s.
    Biederman s.
    Blatin s.
    Borsieri s.
    Brudzinski s.
    Brunati s.
    cardinal s.'s (of inflammation)
    clavicular s.
    contralateral s.
    Demarquay s.
    Dew s.
    Dubois s.
    echo s.
    Elliot s.
    Filipovitch s.
    floating-tooth s.
    Goggia s.
    Hatchcock s.
    Higouménaki s.
    Hoyne s.
    Hutchinson s.
    Kerandel s.

sign (continued)
    Koplik s.
    Krisovski s.
    Lennhoff s.
    Marfan s.
    Mirchamp s.
    palmoplantar s.
    Parrot s.
    Pastia s.
    Remak s.
    Romaña s.
    Rovighi s.
    Rumpel-Leede s.
    Schick s.
    Silex s.
    Sisto s.
    Thomson s.
    Tresilian s.
    trolley-track s.
    Wimberger s.
    Winterbottom s.
    Yergason s.
Silex
    sign
sin–. See also words beginning
    cin–, syn–.
single-chain antigen-binding pro-
    teins (SCA proteins)
sinus (sinus, sinuses)
    lymph s.'s, lymphatic s.'s
    marginal s., s. marginalis
    medullary s.'s
sinusoidal
sinusoidalization
Sips
    distribution
    plot
"sklero–" Phonetic for words begin-
    ning sclero–.
skull
    hot-cross-bun s.
    natiform s.
SLE—systemic lupus erythematosus
SM—streptomycin
SOD—superoxide dismutase [now:
    orgotein]
South African tick fever
South African tick typhus

South American hemorrhagic fever
Southeast Asian mosquito-borne
    hemorrhagic fever
spectrum (spectra)
    antibiotic s.
    broad-s. antibiotic
spherocytosis
spirochete
    nontreponemal s's.
spirometry
    Tri-Flow incentive s.
spondylitis
    ankylosing s.
spondylosis
    s. deformans
sporotrichosis
sporotrichotic
sporozoite
sporozooid
spot
    Christopher s.
    Forchheimer s.
    Koplik s.'s
    rose s.
    typhoid s.
sputum
SSP, SSPE—subacute sclerosing
    panencephalitis
SSSS—staphylococcal scalded skin
    syndrome
ST—skin test
stadium (stadia)
    s. acmes
    s. augmenti
    s. caloris
    s. decrementi
    s. defervescentiae
    s. fluorescentiae
    s. frigoris
    s. incrementi
    s. invasionis
    s. sudoris
stain
    alcian blue s.
    fluorescent auramine-rho-
      damine s.
    Giemsa s.
    Gram-Weigert s.

stain (continued)
    hematoxylin and eosin
       (H&E) s.
    Hotchkiss-McManus s.
    immunoperoxidase s.
    Masson trichrome s.
    methenamine silver s.
    mucicarmine s.
    phloxine-tartrazine s.
    reticulin s.
    toluidine blue s.
    Ziehl-Neelsen s.
staining
    immunoperoxidase s.
Stanton disease
staph—staphylococcus
staphylococcal scalded skin syn-
    drome (SSSS)
staphylococcosis
status
    s. criticus
steatocystoma
    s. multiplex
steatosis
    macrovesicular s.
    microvesicular s.
stigma (stigmas, stigmata)
    syphilitic s.'s
stigmatic
stigmatism
stigmatization
Still
    disease
Still-Chauffard syndrome
St. Louis encephalitis
STM—streptomycin
stomatitis (stomatitides)
    gonococcal s.
    gonorrheal s.
    infectious s.
    mycotic s.
    syphilitic s.
    s. venenata
Strachan
    disease
    syndrome
Strachan-Scott syndrome

strep—streptococcal
    streptococci
streptococcal groups A, B, G
streptogramins [a class of drugs]
Strümpell-Leichtenstern
    disease
    encephalitis
    hemorrhagic encephalitis
STS—serologic test for syphilis
STU—skin test unit
subluxation
"sudo–" Phonetic for words begin-
    ning pseudo–.
sulfonamides [a class of drugs]
sumac
    swamp s.
suppression
suppurative
surveillance
    immune s., immunological s.
Swyer-James
    syndrome
Swyer-James-Macleod
    syndrome
sycosiform
sycosis
    bacillogenic s.
    coccogenic s.
    s. contagiosa
    s. framboesia
    s. framboesiaeformis
    hyphomycotic s.
    lupoid s.
    nonparasitic s.
    s. nuchae necrotisans
    parasitic s.
    s. staphylogenes
    s. vulgaris
Sylvest disease
symptom
    See also in *General Medical
       Terms.*
    cardinal s.
    Castellani-Low s.
    characteristic s.
    delayed s.
    pathognomonic s.
    precursor s.

symptom (continued)
 prodromal s.
 Roger s.
 signal s.
 Sklowsky s.
syn–. See also words beginning
 cin–, sin–.
syndrome
 See also *disease.*
 acquired immunodeficiency
  s. (AIDS)
 allergic vasculitis s.
 antibody deficiency s.
 Babinski s.
 Babinski-Vaquez s.
 bacterial overgrowth s.
 bare lymphocyte s.
 Bearn-Kunkel s.
 Bearn-Kunkel-Slater s.
 Bruns s.
 Caner-Decker s.
 Caplan s.
 Charcot s.
 Chauffard s.
 Chauffard-Still s.
 Chédiak-Higashi s.
 Churg-Strauss s.
 cold agglutinin s.
 CREST s.
 Creutzfeldt-Jakob s.
 CRST s.
 Curtis-Fitz-Hugh s.
 Cushing s.
 Cushing s. medicamentosus
 de Quervain s.
 DiGeorge s.
 Duncan s.
 Ehlers-Danlos s.
 eosinophilic s.
 Felty s.
 Fiessinger-Leroy s.
 Fitz-Hugh s.
 Fitz-Hugh–Curtis s.
 gay bowel s.
 Good s.
 Goodpasture s.
 Guillain-Barré s.
 hyper IgE s.

syndrome (continued)
 hyper IgM s.
 immunodeficiency s.
 Jakob-Creutzfeldt s.
 marfanoid hypermobility s.
 mastocytosis s.
 Mauriac s.
 Mikulicz-Radecki s.
 Mikulicz-Sjögren s.
 mucocutaneous lymph node
  s. (MLNS)
 Nezelof s.
 occipital horn s.
 overlap s.
 postcardiotomy s.
 post-transfusion s.
 primary fibromyalgia s.
 Ramsay Hunt s.
 Reiter s.
 runting s.
 scalded skin s., staphylococcal
 s. of sea-blue histiocytes
 Sézary s.
 Shwachman s.
 Shwachman-Diamond s.
 sicca s.
 Stewart-Treves s.
 Still-Chauffard s.
 tarsal tunnel s.
 Tietze s.
 TORCH (toxoplasmosis,
  other agents, rubella,
  cytomegalovirus, herpes
  simplex) s.
 total allergy s.
 toxoplasmosis, other agents,
  rubella, cytomegalovirus,
  herpes simplex (TORCH)
  s.
 transfusion s.
 ulnar tunnel s.
 wasting s.
 Weil s.
 Wiskott-Aldrich s.
 X-linked lymphoprolifera-
  tive s.

syphilis
    acquired s.
    anorectal s.
    cardiovascular s.
    cerebrospinal s.
    congenital s.
    s. of conjunctiva
    s. d'emblée
    early s.
    early latent s.
    endemic s.
    gummatous s.
    s. hereditaria tarda
    s. of iris
    late s.
    late benign s.
    late latent s.
    latent s.
    meningovascular s.
    noduloulcerative s.
    nonvenereal s.
    parenchymatous s.
    prenatal s.
    primary s.
    secondary s.
    serologic test for s. (STS)
    tertiary s.
syphilitic
syringocystadenoma
    s. papilliferum
systemic
    s. lupus erythematosus (SLE)
    s. sclerosis
    s. vasculitis
TA-AIDS—transfusion-associated
    AIDS
tabes
    t. dorsalis
    hereditary t.
    t. infantum
    t. mesaraica
    t. mesenterica
tabetic
tache ["tahsh"]
    t. blanche ["blahnsh"]
    t. noire ["nwahr"]
    t.'s noire sclérotiques
        ["sklay-ro-teek"]

taeniacides [a class of drugs]
taenial
taeniasis
"tahsh" Phonetic for tache.
Takahara disease
TAO—thromboangiitis obliterans
TB—tuberculosis
T cell [noun]
T-cell [adj.]
    T-c. antibody labeling
    T-c. antigen
    T-c. lymphoma
    T-c. marker(s)
    T-c. proliferation
TCGF—T-cell growth factor
TCMI—T-cell–mediated immunity
TcR—T-cell receptor
technetium (Tc)
    t. diphosphonate
    t. pertechnetate
technique
    Rebuck skin window t.
telangiectasia
    ataxia-t.
    hereditary hemorrhagic t.
    t. lymphatica
telangiectasis (telangiectases)
tendon
    Achilles t.
tenosynovitis
    de Quervain t.
    gonococcic t.
    gonorrheal t.
    infectious t.
    tuberculous t.
terminator
    DNA-chain t.
tertiary
    t. granule
    t. structure
test
    See also in *Laboratory,*
        Pathology, and Chemistry
        Terms.
    ACTH stimulation t.
    agglutination t.
    augmented histamine t.
    blot t.

test (continued)

    complement fixation (CF) t.
    Coombs t.
    Dick t.
    Draize t.
    electrotransfer t.
    ELISA (enzyme-linked
      immunosorbent assay) t.
    Envacor t.
    Epstein-Barr nuclear antigen
      t. (EBNA)
    fluorescent antinuclear anti-
      body (FANA) t.
    fluorescent treponemal anti-
      body absorption (FTA-
      ABS) t.
    Foshay t.
    Frei t.
    Ham t.
    Heaf t.
    HIVAGEN t.
    immunofluorescence t.
    intracutaneous t.
    intracutaneous tuberculin t.
    intradermal t.
    Mantoux t.
    Mantoux skin t.
    mast cell degranulation t.
    microimmunofluorescence t.
    Mitsuda t.
    Monospot t.
    Mono-Vac t.
    mucin clot t.
    mumps skin t.
    neutralization t.
    nitroblue tetrazolium dye t.
    paperadioimmunosorbent t.
    patch t.
    Paul-Bunnell t.
    PCA (passive cutaneous
      anaphylaxis) t.
    PPD (purified protein deriv-
      ative) t.
    provocative t.
    radioallergosorbent t. (RAST)
    radioimmunosorbent t.
      (RIST)

test (continued)

    rapid plasma reagin (RPR)
      circle card t.
    rheumatoid arthritis (RA) t.
    rheumatoid factor (RF) t.
    ring t.
    RPR (rapid plasma reagin) t.
    Sabin-Feldman dye t.
    scarification t.
    Schick t.
    scratch t.
    serologic t.
    serologic t. for syphilis (STS)
    skin t.
    skin-puncture t.
    streptozyme t.
    susceptibility t.
    syphilis t.
    tine t., tine tuberculin t.
      (Rosenthal)
    transcriptase reverse t.
    tuberculin t.
    tuberculin patch t.
    tuberculin t., Sterneedle
    tuberculin titer t.
    tuberculosis t.
    VDRL (Venereal Disease
      Research Laboratories) t.
      [abbreviation not expand-
      ed]
    virus neutralization t.
    Vollmer t.
    Wassermann t.
    Wassermann-fast t.
    Wassermann reaction t.
    Western blot t.
    Winn t.

testing

    histocompatibility t.

tetracyclines [a class of drugs]

tetter

    brawny t.
    honeycomb t.

thalassemia

    sickle cell t.

theory

    Fisher-Race t.
    germ-line t.

theory (continued)
    side-chain t.
    template t.
therapy
    fever t.
    heat t.
    heterovaccine t.
    immunization t.
    immunosuppressive t.
    maggot t.
    malarial t.
    protective t.
    vaccine t.
thienamycins [a class of drugs]
Thomsen
    antibody
thrombi (plural of thrombus)
thrombocytopenia
thrombosis
    See also *thrombus.*
    See also in *Cardiology* section.
    infective t.
thrombus (thrombi)
    See also *thrombosis.*
    infective t.
    parasitic t.
    phagocytic t.
    septic t.
thrush
thymic
    t. hypoplasia
    t. peptide
    t. transplantation
thymopathy
thymus
thymus-dependent
thymus-independent
thyroiditis
    Hashimoto t.
    lymphocytic t.
tick paralysis
time (T)
    generation t.
    lead t.
tinea
    t. amiantacea
    t. axillaris

tinea (continued)
    t. capitis
    t. ciliorum
    t. circinata
    t. corporis
    t. cruris
    t. decalvans
    t. favosa
    t. furfuracea
    t. glabrosa
    t. imbricata
    t. inguinalis
    t. kerion
    t. manuum
    t. nigra
    t. nodosa
    t. pedis
    t. profunda
    t. sycosis
    t. tarsi
    t. tonsurans
    t. unguium
    t. versicolor
tissue
    gut-associated lymphoid t. (GALT)
titer
    toxoplasmosis, other agents, rubella, cytomegalovirus, herpes simplex (TORCH) t.
titration
TMP—trimethoprim
tolerance
    immune t.
    immunologic t.
tongue
    baked t.
tophus (tophi)
    gouty tophi
    t. syphiliticus
TORCH—toxoplasmosis, other agents, rubella, cytomegalovirus, herpes simplex [syndrome]
TORCH
    infection
    titer
"tosh" Phonetic for tache.

Touraine
    aphthosis
Touton giant cells
toxic shock
toxin
    antitetanus t.
toxoids [a class of drugs]
toxoplasmosis
    ocular t.
trachoma (trachomata)
TRAIDS—transfusion-related AIDS
transfer
    passive t.
transfusion
    exchange t.
transplantation
    bone marrow t.
treatment
    empiric t.
    preventive t., prophylactic t.
treponematosis
treponemiasis
triad
    Hutchinson t.
trichinosis
trichoepithelioma
    t. papillosum multiplex
trichomycosis
    t. axillaris
    t. chromatica
    t. favosa
    t. nigra
    t. nodosa
    t. palmellina
    t. pustulosa
    t. rubra
trichophytosis
    t. corporis
    t. cruris
    t. unguium
trichorrhexis
    t. invaginata
    t. nodosa
trichrome
    t. vitiligo
"trikinosis" Phonetic for trichinosis.
TRNG—tetracycline-resistant *Neisseria gonorrhoeae*

trypanosomiasis
    Cruz t.
tryptase
tsutsugamushi
    disease
tube
    pus t.
tubercular
tuberculocidal
tuberculocide
tuberculoid
tuberculosis (TB)
    abdominal t.
    active t.
    acute miliary t.
    adrenal t.
    adult t.
    aerogenic t.
    anthracotic t.
    attenuated t.
    atypical t.
    avian t.
    basal t.
    t. of bone
    t. of bones and joints
    bronchogenic t.
    bronchopneumonic t.
    caseous t.
    cerebral t.
    cestodic t.
    childhood t.
    chronic fibroid t.
    chronic ulcerative t.
    t. colliquativa
    t. colliquativa cutis
    cutaneous t.
    t. cutis
    t. cutis indurativa
    t. cutis lichenoides
    t. cutis miliaris disseminata
    t. cutis orificialis
    t. cutis verrucosa
    cystic t. of bones
    disseminated t.
    endogenous t.
    endothelial t.
    esophageal t.
    extrapulmonary t.

tuberculosis (TB) (continued)
    extrathoracic t.
    exudative t.
    fibrocaseous t.
    fibrosing t.
    t. fungosa cutis
    gastrointestinal t.
    genital t.
    genitourinary t.
    glandular t.
    hematogenous t.
    hilus t.
    ileocecal t.
    t. indurativa
    inhalation t.
    intestinal t.
    t. of intestines
    intrathoracic t.
    t. of kidney and bladder
    laryngeal t.
    t. of larynx
    latent t.
    t. lichenoides
    t. of lungs
    t. luposa
    t. of lymph nodes
    lymphogenous t.
    lymphoid t.
    meningeal t.
    t. miliaris cutis
    t. miliaris disseminata
    miliary t.
    minimal t.
    moderately advanced t.
    open t.
    oral t.
    orificial t.
    t. orificialis
    papulonecrotic t.
    t. papulonecrotica
    postprimary t.
    primary t.
    primary inoculation t.
    productive t.
    pulmonary t.
    quiescent t.
    reinfection t.
    renal t.

tuberculosis (TB) (continued)
    t. of serous membranes
    skeletal t.
    t. of skin
    spinal t., t. of spine
    surgical t.
    tracheobronchial t.
    t. ulcerosa
    warty t.
tuberculostatic
tuberculotic
tuberosis
tularemia
tumor
    Burkitt t.
    Burkitt-like t.
    Buschke-Löwenstein t.
    t. immunity
    t.-specific antigen
tylosis
    t. ciliaris
    t. palmaris et plantaris
typhus
    African tick t.
    Australian tick t.
    benign t.
    canine t.
    chigger-borne t.
    classic t.
    collapsing t.
    t. degenerativus amstelo-
        damensis
    endemic t.
    epidemic t.
    epidemic louse-borne t.
    European t.
    exanthematic t. of São Paulo
    t. exanthematique, exanthe-
        matous t.
    flea-borne t.
    Gubler-Robin t.
    Indian tick t.
    Kenya tick t.
    latent t.
    louse-borne t.
    Manchurian t.
    Mexican t.
    mite-borne t.

typhus (continued)
>t. mitior
>Moscow t.
>murine t.
>North Asian tick t.
>North Queensland tick t.
>petechial t.
>Queensland tick t.
>rat t.
>recrudescent t.
>rural t.
>scrub t.
>shop t.
>Siberian tick t.
>São Paulo t.
>South African tick t.
>sporadic t.
>tick t., tickborne t.
>Toulon t.
>tropical t.
>urban t.

tyrosine
>t. aminotransferase deficiency

UCTS—undifferentiated connective tissue syndrome

ulcer
>corneal u.
>decubitus u.
>Meleney chronic undermining u.

ulcera (plural of ulcus)

ulcerative
>u. colitis

ulcus (ulcera)
>u. ambulans

ulerythema
>u. acneiforma
>u. centrifugum
>u. ophryogenes
>u. sycosiforme

unit
>See also in *General Medical Terms* and *Laboratory, Pathology, and Chemistry Terms.*
>international u. of immunological activity
>international u. of penicillin

unit (continued)
>Lf u.
>Noon pollen u.
>u. of penicillin
>tuberculin u. (TU)

Urbach-Oppenheim disease

urethritis
>gonorrheal u.

urticaria

uveitis

vaccinatum
>eczema v.

vaccine
>attenuated v.
>BCG (bacille Calmette-Guérin) v.
>*Haemphilus influenzae* b conjugate v. (HhCV)
>*Haemphilus influenzae* b polysaccharide v. (HhPV)
>pertussis v.
>polyvalent v.
>Sabin v.
>Salk v.
>smallpox v.
>typhoid v.
>vital v.

vaccines [a class of drugs]

vaccinia
>v. gangrenosa
>v. immune globulin

vacuolar
>v. myelopathy

vagabond's disease

varicella
>v. bullosa
>v. gangrenosa
>v. inoculata pustulosa
>v.-zoster immune globulin (VZIG)
>v.-zoster virus

variola
>v. crystallina
>v. inserta
>v. miliaris
>v. minor
>v. mitigata
>v. pemphigosa

variola (continued)
  v. siliquosa
  v. vera
  v. verrucosa
varix (varices)
  lymph v., v. lymphaticus
vasculitis
  granulomatous v.
  hypersensitivity v.
  livedoid v.
  lymphomatoid v.
  necrotizing v.
  nodular v.
  septic v.
  urticarial v.
vasodilators [a class of drugs]
VDS—venereal disease–syphilis
vector
  expression v.
VEE—Venezuelan equine encephalomyelitis
venereal
  v. disease (VD)
Venezuelan equine encephalitis
Venezuelan equine encephalomyelitis
Venus
  collar of V.
vermicides [a class of drugs]
vermicular
vermiculation
vermiculous
vermiform
vermifugal
vermifuges
Verneuil
  disease
verruga
  v. peruana
vertebral
  v. artery
  v. compression fracture
  v. osteomyelitis
vesicular
  v. bullous pemphigoid
  v. dermatophytid
  v. ringworm
  v. stomatitis

vesiculobullous
vesiculopapular
vesiculopustular
VH—viral hepatitis
vibratory
  v. angioedema
vibriocidal
viral
  v. load
Virchow-Hassall body
virosis (viroses)
virus
  See also in *Laboratory,*
    Pathology, and Chemistry
    Terms.
  attenuated v.
  California encephalitis v.
  California myxoma v.
  Colorado tick fever (CTF) v.
  Coxsackie v. [now: coxsack-
    ievirus]
  CTF (Colorado tick fever) v.
  DNA v.'s
  eastern equine encephalo-
    myelitis v.
  EB (Epstein-Barr) v.
  Ebola v.
  EEE (eastern equine enceph-
    alomyelitis) v.
  enteric cytopathogenic
    human orphan (ECHO) v.
    [now: echovirus]
  equine encephalomyelitis v.
  hepatitis A v. (HAV)
  hepatitis B v. (HBV)
  hepatitis C v. (HCV)
  hepatitis delta v.
  hepatitis E v.
  hepatitis G v. (HGV)
  hepatitis GB v. (HGBV,
    HGBV-A, HGBV-B,
    HGBV-C)
  herpes v. [pref: herpesvirus]
  herpes simplex v. (HSV)
  herpes zoster v.
  human T-cell lymphotrophic
    v., (HTLV) [now: HIV]

virus (continued)
    LCM (lymphocytic chori-
      omeninigitis) v.
    lymphadenopathy-associated
      v. (LAV)
    lymphocytic choriomeningi-
      tis v. (LCM)
    neurotrophic v.
    v. neutralization test
    non-A, non B-hepatitis v.
    Norwalk v.
    RNA v.'s
    St. Louis encephalitis v.
    tick-borne v.'s
visceral
    v. larva migrans
    v. leishmaniasis
    v. schistosomiasis
VMR—vasomotor rhinitis
VNS—villonodular synovitis
Vogt-Koyanagi
    syndrome
Vogt-Koyanagi-Harada
    syndrome
vomiting
    explosive v.
    projectile v.
von Behring. See *Behring.*
von Economo
    disease
    encephalitis
von Leyden. See *Leyden.*
"vookereriasis" Phonetic for
    wuchereriasis.
vox (voces)
    v. cholerica
VZ—varicella-zoster
VZIG—varicella-zoster immune
    globulin
VZV—varicella-zoster virus
Wallgren aseptic meningitis
wart
    anatomical w.
    filiform w.
    mosaic w.
    mucocutaneous w.
    necrogenic w.
    periungual w.

wart (continued)
    pitch w.
    plantar w.
    telangiectatic w.
    tuberculous w.
    venereal w.
warty
    w. dyskeratoma
    w. tuberculosis
Wassermann
    fast test
Wassilicff disease
wasting disease
Weber-Christian
    disease
    panniculitis
WEE—western equine encephalo-
    myelitis
Wegner
    disease
    sign
Weil
    syndrome
Weingarten syndrome
Wells
    syndrome
Werner-His disease
Western
    blot electrotransfer test
    blot test
    blotting
western equine encephalitis (WEE)
West Nile
    encephalitis
    fever
Whipple
    disease
whitlow
Whitmore
    disease
    fever
    melioidosis
WHO—World Health Organization
Whytt
    disease
Widal
    reaction
    serum test

Widal (continued)
    syndrome
    test
Wilks
    disease
window
    skin w.
Wissler-Fanconi
    syndrome
Woringer-Kolopp
    disease
World Health Organization (WHO)
WRE—whole ragweed extract
wuchereriasis

xeroderma
    follicular x.
    x. pigmentosum
yellow fever
zeta
    z. potential
    z. sedimentation rate
zoonosis (zoonoses)
zoonotic
zoster
    dermatomal z.
    disseminated z.
    herpes z.
    z. immune globulin
    varicella z.

Internal Medicine
Includes Endocrinology and Metabolism

A_{1c} [A1C]—hemoglobin A_{1c} [glyco-
    sylated hemoglobin]
AAI—acute adrenal insufficiency
abdominocardiac reflex
Abercrombie
    degeneration
    syndrome
abetalipoproteinemia
ABG, ABGs—arterial blood gas(es)
ABO
    blood groups
    compatibility
    incompatibility
Abrami
    disease
Abrikosov (Abrikossoff)
    tumor
abscess
    caseocavernous a.
    chronic a.
    Dubois a.
    eosinophilic a.
    gangrenous a.
    glandular a.
    lymphatic a.
absorption
    fat a.
    intestinal a.
    iron a.
abuse
    alcohol a.
    elder a.
    ethanol a.
    laxative a.
    tobacco a.
acanthocytosis

acanthosis
    malignant a. nigricans
    a. nigricans
acapnial
acapnic
acarbia
accident
    cardiovascular a.
    cerebrovascular a. (CVA)
acervuline
acetonemic
acetonuria
Achard-Thiers syndrome
Achilles
    bursitis
achlorhydric
achondroplasia
achondroplastic
achrestic
achromocytosis
acid
    alpha-lipoic a. (ALA)
acidism
acid-maltase deficiency
acidophilus milk
acidosis
    carbon dioxide a.
    compensated a.
    diabetic a.
    hypercapnic a.
    hyperchloremic a.
    lactic a.
    metabolic a.
    non-anion gap a.
    nonrespiratory a.
    renal tubular a. (types 1, 2, 4)
    respiratory a.

acidosis (continued)
    starvation a.
    uremic a.
acidotic
aciduria
    β-aminoisobutyric a.
    glutamic a.
    glycolic a.
    L-glyceric a.
    paradoxical a.
    xanthurenic a.
aciduric
acinus (acini)
    liver a.
    pancreatic a.
    thyroid acini
Acosta
    disease
acoustic
acroarthritis
acrocyanosis
acrodermatitis
    a. chronica atrophicans
    a. enterohepatica
acrodynia
acrohyperhidrosis
acrohypothermy
acrokeratosis
    paraneoplastic a.
acromegalic
acromegalogigantism
acromelalgia
acrometagenesis
acromicria
acropachyderma
    a. with pachyperiostitis
acroparesthesia
    Nothnagel-type a.
    Schultze-type a.
acrotic
acrotism
acrotrophodynia
acrotrophoneurosis
ACT—activated coagulation time
ACTH—adrenocorticotropic hor-
    mone
ACTH-RF—ACTH-releasing factor
ACTH stimulation test

actinotoxin
action
    See also *effect* and *phenom-
        enon.*
    cumulative a.
activated coagulation time (ACT)
activated partial thromboplastin
    time (APTT, aPTT)
activity
    a.'s of daily living (ADL,
        ADLs)
    nonsuppressible insulin-like a.
acute demyelinating disease
acute on chronic
    a.o.c. illness
    a.o.c. symptoms
ACVD—autoimmune collagen vas-
    cular disease
ADA—American Diabetes Associa-
    tion
Adamantiades-Behçet syndrome
adamantinoma
    pituitary a.
Adams-Stokes
    disease
    syndrome
Addison
    anemia
    crisis
    disease
Addison-Biermer anemia
addisonian
    a. anemia
    a. crisis
    a. syndrome
addisonism
adenectopia
adenia
    angibromic a.
    leukemic a.
adenic
adenine phosphoribosyl transferase
    (APRT) deficiency
adenitis
    phlegmonous a.
adenocarcinoma
adenocele
adenocellulitis

adenocystoma
    papillary a. lymphomatosum
adenodynia
adenofibroma
    pseudomucinous a.
    serous a.
adenofibrosis
adenogenous
adenohypophysial
adenolymphitis
adenolymphocele
adenolymphoma
adenoma
    acinar a.
    adamantinum a.
    adnexal a.
    adrenocortical a.
    apocrine a.
    bronchial a.
    chromophobe a.
    chromophobic a.
    clear cell a.
    colloid a.
    cortical a
    cystic a.
    duct a.
    fetal a.
    hepatocellular a.
    islet cell a.
    langerhansian a.
    liver cell a.
    macrofollicular a.
    mesonephric a.
    microfollicular a.
    mucoid cell a.
    multiple endocrine a.
    oncocytic a.
    pituitary a.
    pseudomucinous a.
    renal cortical a.
    a. sebaceum
    a. simplex
    a. substantiae corticalis
      suprarenalis
    toxic thyroid a.
    tubulovillous a.
    water-clear cell a.
    wolffian a.

adenomalacia
adenomatosis
    erosive a. of nipple
    fibrosing a.
    multiple endocrine a. (MEA)
    pancreatic-islet a.
    pluriglandular a.
    polyendocrine a.
    pulmonary a.
adenomegaly
adenomyomatous
adenomyosis
adenoncus
adenopathy
    cervical a.
adenosis
    florid a.
adenosquamous
adenous
adiposis
    a. dolorosa
    a. hepatica
    a. tuberosa simplex
    a. universalis
adiposuria
adipsia
adipsous
adjuvant
ADL, ADLs—activities of daily liv-
    ing
adrenal
    a. adenoma
    a. cortex
    a. crisis
    a. gland
    a. hyperplasia
    a. hypoplasia
    a. insufficiency
    Marchand a.
    a. medulla
    a. steroids
    a. virilism
adrenal cortical steroids, adrenocor-
    tical steroids [a class of drugs]
adrenalinemia
adrenalinogenesis
adrenoceptive
adrenocorticohyperplasia

adrenocorticotropic hormone (ACTH)
adrenogenic
adrenogenital
    a. syndrome
adrenoreceptor
adynamia
    a. episodica hereditaria
aeropathy
"a-feem-ee-a" Phonetic for aphemia.
afibrinogenemia
"af-tha" Phonetic for aphtha.
AGA—acute gonococcal arthritis
aganglionic
agerasia
ageusia
    central a.
    conduction a.
    peripheral a.
ageusic
AGG—agammaglobulinemia
agglutinin
    cold a.
    febrile a.
aggregation
    familial a.
AGH—amenorrhea-galactorrhea
   hypothyroidism
aglycosuric
agnea
agonist
    cholinergic a.'s [a class of
      drugs]
agonistic
agranulocytosis
agrypnotic
AGS—adrenogenital syndrome
ague
Ahumada-del Castillo syndrome
AIDS—acquired immunodeficiency
   syndrome
AILD—angioimmunoblastic lymphadenopathy with dysproteinemia
air
    a. bed
    a. curtain
    a. embolism
    a. hunger

airsickness
akathisia
"a-kon-dro-plaz-ee-a" Phonetic for
   achondroplasia.
ALA—alpha-lipoic acid
alactasia
Alajouanine
   disease
   syndrome
Albright
   syndrome
albuminocholia
albuminoptysis
albuminoreaction
albuminorrhea
albuminuretic
alcoholemia
aldosteronism
   idiopathic a.
   juvenile a.
   primary a.
   pseudoprimary a.
   secondary a.
aldosteronoma
aldosteronopenia
aldosteronuria
Aldrich-Mees
   lines
aleukemic
aleukia
   a. hemorrhagica
aleukocytic
alexic
alkalosis
   acapnial a.
   altitude a.
   carbon dioxide a.
   compensated a.
   congenital gastrointestinal a.
   hypokalemic a.
   metabolic a.
   respiratory a.
alkalotic
alkaluria
alkaptonuric
alkylate
alkylation

Allen
    paradoxical law
    treatment
allergic
allergy
    drug a.
allotriogeustia
allotriophagy
alpha
    a.-dextrinase
    a.-L-fucosidase
    a.-galactosidase A
    1,4-a.-glucan branching
      enzyme
    a.-keto acid dehydrogenase
    a.-mannosidase
    a.-methylacetoacetyl CoA
      thiolase
Alström
    disease
    syndrome
alymphia
Alzheimer disease
amanitine
amastia
amatol
amaurosis
    albuminuric a.
    diabetic a.
    a. fugax
    uremic a.
amazia
amebiasis
    hepatic a.
amine
    aromatic a.
aminoacidemia
aminoacidopathy
aminoaciduria
    imidazole a.
    overflow a.
    renal a.
    transport a.
γ-aminobutyric acid (GABA)
    [gamma-]
ϵ-aminocaproic acid [epsilon-]
β-aminoisobutyricaciduria [beta-]
δ-aminolevulinic acid (ALA) [delta-]

ammonemia
"amp" Slang for ampicillin.
"amp and gent" Slang for ampicillin
    and gentamicin.
amphetamines [a class of drugs]
amyloidosis
    Andrade-type a.
    cutaneous a.
    a. cutis
    Indiana-type a.
    Iowa-type a.
    kidney a.
    a. of larynx
    a. of multiple myeloma
    Portuguese-type a.
    renal a.
amylosuria
amyotrophy
    diabetic a.
anabolic
"anafil " Phonetic for words begin-
    ning anaphyl–.
anaphylactic
anaphylactogen
anaphylactogenesis
anaphylactogenic
anaphylatoxin
anaphylaxis
    heterocytotropic a.
    homocytotropic a.
anasarca
ancillary
    a. measures
    a. therapy
Anders
    disease
Andersen
    disease
    syndrome
    triad
Andrade
    indicator
    syndrome
androgenic
androgenization
androgenized
androgenous
androgens [a class of drugs]

anemia

    achlorhydric a.
    achrestic a.
    acquired sideroblastic a.
    ancylostome a.
    aplastic a.
    arctic a.
    asiderotic a.
    atrophic a.
    autoimmune hemolytic a.
    Baghdad spring a.
    Banti a.
    Biermer-Ehrlich a.
    breast a.
    a. of chronic disease
    Chvostek a.
    congenital a. of newborn
    congenital dyserythropoietic
        a.
    congenital nonspherocytic
        hemolytic a.
    constitutional aplastic a.
    Cooley a.
    Coombs-negative immune
        hemolytic a.
    crescent cell a.
    Czerny a.
    Diamond-Blackfan a.
    Dresbach a.
    Edelmann a.
    enzyme deficiency hemolyt-
        ic a.
    erythroblastic a. of childhood
    Faber a.
    familial erythroblastic a.
    Fanconi a.
    febrile pleiochromic a.
    fish tapeworm a.
    fragmentation hemolytic a.
    globe cell a.
    glucose-6-phosphate dehy-
        drogenase deficiency a.
    hemolytic a.
    Herrick a.
    hyperchromic a.
    hypochromic a.
    a. hypochromica sidero-
        chrestica hereditaria

anemia (continued)

    hypoplastic a.
    hypoplastic a., congenital
    icterohemolytic a.
    immunohemolytic a.
    Israels-Wilkinson a.
    Jaksch a.
    Larzel a.
    lead a.
    Lederer a.
    Leishman a.
    leukoerythroblastic a.
    lysolecithin hemolytic a.
    macrocytic a.
    malignant a.
    Mediterranean a.
    megaloblastic a.
    meniscocytic a.
    microcytic a.
    microdrepanocytic a.
    microelliptopoikilocytic a. of
        Rietti, Greppi, and Micheli
    myelophthisic a.
    myelosclerotic a.
    a. neonatorum
    normochromic a.
    normocytic a.
    ovalocytary a.
    pernicious a.
    pernicious a., juvenile
    physiologic a.
    a. pseudoleukemica infantum
    pyridoxine-responsive a.
    pyruvate-kinase deficiency a.
    radiation a.
    sex-linked hypochromatic a.
        of Rundles and Falls
    sickle cell a.
    sideremic a.
    sideroblastic a.
    sideropenic a.
    spherocytic a.
    target cell a.
    thrombopenic a.
    thrombotic microangiopathic
        hemolytic a.
    toxic a.
    traumatic a.

anemia (continued)
>triose-phosphate isomerase deficiency a.
>tunnel a.
>unstable hemoglobin hemolytic a.
>von Jaksch a.
>Wills a.
>x-ray a.

anergy

angiitis
>visceral a.

angina
>a. cordis
>a. diphtheritica
>monocytic a.
>a. nervosa
>a. pectoris
>Plaut a.
>pseudomembranous a.
>Schultz a.
>ulceromembranous a.
>vasomotor a.

anginal

angioendothelioma

angioendotheliomatosis
>a. proliferans
>systemic proliferating a.

angiogranuloma

angiography
>four-vessel a.

angioimmunoblastic
>a. lymphadenopathy with dysproteinemia (AILD)
>a. lymphadenopathy

angiolupoid

angioma
>tuberous a.

angiomatoid

angiomatosis
>hemorrhagic familial a.

angioneurotic

angiopasmodic disease

angioplasty

"angkilo–" Phonetic for words beginning ankylo–.

anhidrotics [a class of drugs]

ankylosing
>a. spondylitis

anomalotrophy

anomaly
>Chédiak-Higashi a.
>Chédiak-Steinbrinck-Higashi a.
>Chiari a.
>Ebstein a.
>Hegglin a.
>Huët-Pelger nuclear a.
>Jordan a.
>May-Hegglin a.
>Pelger-Huët a.
>Pelger-Huët nuclear a.
>Steinbrinck a.
>Undritz a.

anorectics [a class of drugs]

anorexia nervosa

anorexiants [a class of drugs]

anorexigenic

anorexigenics [a class of drugs]

antagonist
>metabolic a.

anthracic

anthraconecrosis

anthracotic

antibiotics [a class of drugs]
>aminoglycoside a.
>bactericidal a.
>bacteriostatic a.
>broad-spectrum a.
>carbapenem a.
>cephalosporin a.
>fluoroquinolone a.
>glycopeptide a.
>β-lactam a. [beta-]
>lincosamide a.
>macrolide a.
>oral a.
>polyene a.
>sulfonamide a.
>tetracycline a.
>topical a.

antibody (antibodies)
>See also in *Laboratory, Pathology, and Chemistry Terms.*

antibody (antibodies) (continued)
    antimitochondrial a.
    thyroglobulin a.
    thyroid microsomal a.'s
    TSH-displacing a.
anticholinergics [a class of drugs]
anticoagulant
    circulating a.
antidiuretic
    a. hormone
antidopaminergics [a class of drugs]
antidotes [a class of drugs]
antifolate
antigen (Ag)
    See also in *Laboratory,*
    Pathology, and Chemistry
    Terms.
    ABO a.
    carcinoembryonic a. (CEA)
    Kell a.
    Kidd a.
    transplantation a.
antihistamines [a class of drugs]
antihyperlipidemic agents [a class of drugs]
antilipemics [a class of drugs]
antimuscarinics [a class of drugs]
antinauseants [a class of drugs]
antipyretics [a class of drugs]
antitoxins [a class of drugs]
α_1-antitrypsin [alpha-1-]
APA—aldosterone-producing adenoma
Apert
    hirsutism
aphasia
    Broca a.
apnea
    deglutition a.
    sleep a.
apolipoprotein C-II (apo C-II) deficiency, familial
apparatus
    inhalation therapy a.
appearance
    cushingoid a.
    toxic a.

APTT, aPTT—activated partial thromboplastin time
arborization
    cervical mucus a.
area (areae, areas)
    body surface a. (BSA)
areolitis
Arg—arginine
armamentarium
Armstrong
    disease
Arnold
    nerve reflex cough syndrome
arrested
    a. growth and development
arteritis (arteritides)
    temporal a.
arthralgia
    acromegalic a.
    nonspecific a.
    periodic a.
    a. saturnina
arthritis (arthritides)
    crystal a.
    degenerative a.
    erosive a.
    gouty a.
    a. hiemalis
    hypertrophic a.
    Jaccoud a.
    juvenile a.
    Lyme a.
    Marie-Strümpell a.
    a. nodosa
    nondeforming a.
    psoriatic a.
    rheumatoid a.
    tuberculous a.
arthropathy
    diabetic a.
asbestos
Ascher
    syndrome
Aschoff
    cell
    nodule
ascites
    chylous a.

ascites (continued)
    dialysis a.
    gelatinous a.
    nephrogenic a.
ASIM—American Society of Internal Medicine
asphyxia
    autoerotic a.
    sexual a.
    symmetric a.
asphyxiation
aspiration
    a. pneumonia
assay
    estrogen receptor a. (ERA)
    glycosylated hemoglobin a.
    hemoglobin A_{1c} a. [A1C]
asthenia
    a. gravis hypophyseogenea
    muscle a.
asthma
    Heberden a.
atelectasis
atelectatic
atrial
    a. fibrillation
    a. flutter
atrophy
    cyanotic a.
    fat replacement a.
    inactivity a.
    multisystem a.
    tubular a.
attack
    apnea a.
    Stokes-Adams a.
Aufrecht
    disease
aura
autologous
    a. transfusion
autotransfusion
avitaminosis
    conditioned a.
    a. D
Ayerza
    disease
Baber syndrome

Babinski-Fröhlich syndrome
bacillus (bacilli)
    See in *Laboratory, Pathology, and Chemistry Terms.*
Bacillus
    See in *Laboratory, Pathology, and Chemistry Terms.*
bacterium (bacteria)
    See specific bacteria in *Laboratory, Pathology, and Chemistry Terms.*
Bair-Hugger Convective Warming Unit
Baló
    disease
Bamberger
    disease
Bancroft filariasis
Bannister
    disease
Banti
    disease
    splenic anemia
    syndrome
Bar [eponym]
    syndrome
baresthesia
baresthesiometer
bariatrics
Barré
    sign
barrel
    b. chest
Bartter-Schwartz syndrome
Basedow
    disease
    goiter
    pseudoparaplegia
    syndrome
    triad
basophilia
    pituitary b.
    punctate b.
basophilism
    Cushing b.
    pituitary b.
bath
    paraffin b.

B cell [noun]
B-cell [adj.]
    B-c. lymphoma
Bearn-Kunkel-Slater syndrome
Beauvais
    disease
Beck
    See *Boeck*.
Becker
    phenomenon
    sign
Begbie
    disease
Behçet
    disease
    syndrome
    triple symptom complex
Behr
    disease
Bekhterev-Strümpell spondylitis
Bell
    palsy
belly
    prune-b. syndrome
Bence Jones
    body
    myeloma
    protein
    proteinuria
bends
Benedict-Roth
    apparatus
benefited
Bennett
    disease
    leukemia
Berardinelli syndrome
Berger
    disease
    focal glomerulonephritis
Bernard-Soulier syndrome
Besnier-Boeck
    disease
beta
    b.-aminoisobutyricaciduria
    b.-galactosidase
    b.-methylcrotonylglycinuria
    b.-sitosterolemia

Biermer
    anemia
    disease
Biernacki sign
bilharzial
bilharziosis, bilharziasis
biliary
    b. atresia
    b. cirrhosis
biliuria
binge
bingeing and purging
Bing-Neel syndrome
BiPAP—bilateral positive airway
    pressure
birthmark
    port wine stain b.
bisalbuminemia
Blackfan-Diamond
    anemia
    syndrome
blanket
    hypothermic b.
blast
    b. chest
    b. effect
    lung b.
blister
    burn b.
    fever b.
bloater
    blue b. [emphysema]
block
    b. resection
blockade
blocker
    alpha-adrenergic b.
    alpha-adrenoceptor b.
    beta b.'s (β-blockers) [a
      class of drugs]
    calcium channel b.
    H_2 b.'s [a class of drugs]
    slow-channel b.'s [a class of
      drugs]
    starch b.
blue
    b. bloater [emphysema]
Blumberg sign

Blumenthal
    disease
BMG—benign monoclonal gam-
    mopathy
Bock
    ganglion
    nerve
Bodian-Schwachman syndrome
body (bodies)
    creola b.
    Gamna-Gandy b.
    ketone b.
    Mallory b.
Boeck
    See *Bock.*
    disease
    sarcoid, sarcoidosis
Boerhaave
    syndrome
Bohr
    effect
    equation
Bonnot gland
"boo-e-yo(z)" Phonetic for Bouillaud.
"boo-shahr(z)" Phonetic for
    Bouchard.
"boo-shahr-dah(z)" Phonetic for
    Bouchardat.
"boo-yaw," "boo-yawn" Phonetic
    for bouillon.
Boston sign
botulism
    food-borne b.
Bouchard
    disease
    nodes
    nodules
    sign
Bouchardat
    treatment
Bouillaud
    disease
    syndrome
bouillon
Bowen
    disease
Bradley
    disease

bradykinesia
bradykinetic
branched-chain α-keto acid dehy-
    drogenase [alpha-]
brancher deficiency
brawny
    b. edema
    b. induration
breath
    lead b.
    liver b.
breathing
    apneustic b.
    ataxic b.
    autonomous b.
    Biot b.
    bronchial b.
    Cheyne-Stokes b.
    continuous positive-pressure
      b. (CPPB)
    diaphragmatic b.
    frog b.
    glossopharyngeal b.
    intermittent positive-pres-
      sure b. (IPPB)
    Kussmaul b.
    labored b.
    shallow b.
    suppressed b.
    vesicular b.
Breda
    disease
Brehmer
    method
    treatment
Brennemann
    syndrome
Bretonneau
    angina
    disease
Brill
    disease
Brill-Symmer
    disease
Brill-Zinsser
    disease
Brinton
    disease

Brion-Kayser
disease
brittle diabetes
broad-spectrum antibiotics [a class
of drugs]
Broca
amnesia
bronchi (plural of bronchus)
bronchitis
bronchospasm
bronchus (bronchi)
See in *Pulmonary Medicine*
section.
"broo-ee" Phonetic for bruit.
Bruhl
disease
bruit
See also in *Cardiology* and
Pulmonary Medicine sec-
tions.
carotid b.
cranial b.
Bruton
agammaglobulinemia
disease
BS—blood sugar
Budd
cirrhosis
jaundice
Budd-Chiari
disease
syndrome
Buerger
disease
exercises
symptom
bulimia
b. nervosa
bullosis
b. diabeticorum
Bürger-Grütz syndrome
Burkitt
lymphoma
tumor
burn
brush b.
chemical b.
first-degree b.

burn (continued)
flash b.
fourth-degree b.
full-thickness b.
high-tension b.
immersion b.
partial-thickness b.
powder b.
radiation b.
second-degree b.
thermal b.
third-degree b.
Busse-Buschke
disease
butterfly
b. rash
Byler
disease
byssinosis
cachectic
cachexia
addisonian c.
amyotrophic c.
cardiac c.
Grawitz c.
hypothalamic pituitary c.
neurogenic c.
café au lait spot
café coronary
CAH—chronic active hepatitis
congenital adrenal hyperplasia
CAHC—chronic active hepatitis
with cirrhosis
caisson disease
Cal, Kcal—kilocalorie
calcemia
calcinosis
c. interstitialis
c. universalis
calcium (Ca)
c. carbonate
calor
c. febrilis
c. fervens
c. innatus
c. internus

cancer
See also *carcinoma*.
See also in *Oncology and Hematology* section.
acinous c.
adenoid c.
c. atrophicans
cellular c.
cerebriform c.
colorectal c.
dendritic c.
dermoid c.
endothelial c.
epidermal c.
epithelial c.
fungous c.
glandular c.
hematoid c.
c. in situ
Lobstein c.
medullary c.
melanotic c.
retrograde c.
scirrhous c.
solanoid c.
spider c.
tubular c.
villous duct c.
withering c.
Cannon
law
syndrome
theory
Caplan
nodules
syndrome
carbamoyl phosphate synthetase (CAPS) deficiency
carcinoembryonic antigen (CEA)
carcinoma (carcinomas, carcinomata)
See also in *Oncology and Hematology* section.
acinous c.
adenocystic c.
adenoid cystic c.
c. adenomatosum
adrenal c.
alveolar c.

carcinoma (carcinomas, carcinomata) (continued)
ampullary c.
anaplastic c.
basal cell c.
c. basocellulare
basosquamous cell c.
bronchioalveolar c.
bronchiolar c.
bronchogenic c.
cavitated c.
cerebriform c.
chorionic c.
colloid c.
comedo c.
corpus c.
cribriform c.
c. cutaneum
cylindrical c.
cylindrical cell c.
ductal c.
c. durum
embryonal c.
encephaloid c.
c. en cuirasse
epibulbar c.
epidermoid c.
epithelial c.
c. epitheliale adenoides
erectile c.
c. erysipeloides
exophytic c.
c. exulcere
c. fibrosum
gelatiniform c.
gelatinous c.
giant cell c.
c. gigantocellulare
glandular c.
granulosa cell c.
hair-matrix c.
hematoid c.
hepatocellular c.
Hürthle cell c.
hyaline c.
hypernephroid c.
infiltrating ductal cell c.
c. in situ

carcinoma (carcinomas, carcinomata)
(continued)
intraepidermal c.
intraepithelial c.
Kulchitzky cell c.
lenticular c.
c. lenticulare
lipomatous c.
lobular c.
c. mastitoides
medullary c.
c. melanodes
melanotic c.
metastatic c.
c. molle
mucinous c.
c. muciparum
c. mucocellulare
mucoepidermoid c.
c. mucosum
c. myxomatodes
nasopharyngeal c.
nevoid basal cell c.
c. nigrum
oat cell c.
c. ossificans
osteoid c.
papillary c.
periportal c.
preinvasive c.
prickle cell c.
pultaceous c.
radiogenic c.
renal cell c.
c. sarcomatodes
schneiderian c.
scirrhous c.
c. scroti
signet-ring cell c.
c. simplex
solanoid c.
spheroidal cell c.
spindle cell c.
c. spongiosum
squamous c.
squamous cell c.
string c.
c. telangiectaticum

carcinoma (carcinomas, carcinomata)
(continued)
c. telangiectodes
transitional cell c.
c. tuberosum
tuberous c.
verrucous c.
c. villosum
cardiac risk factors (CRFs)
cardiomegaly
"carfol–" Phonetic for words beginning with carphol–.
carpal
carphologia
carphology
Carrión
disease
CAS—chronic alcohol syndrome
Casal
collar
necklace
Cassidy
syndrome
Cassidy-Scholte
syndrome
Castellani
disease
cat-scratch disease
cauda (caudae)
c. equina
CAV—congenital adrenal virilism
croup-associated virus
cavitis
Cawthorne maneuver
CCC—chronic calculous cholecystitis
CCP—chronic calcifying pancreatitis
celiac
c. disease
cell
See also in *Laboratory, Pathology, and Chemistry Terms.*
bone marrow c.
daughter c.
germinal c.
Kupffer c.
Leydig c.
parent c.

cell (continued)
    somatic c.
    target c.
    transducer c.
    transitional c.
cellulitis
    gaseous c.
center
    poison control c.
central
    c. nervous system (CNS)
cephalopathy
ceramidase deficiency
cerebrovascular
    c. accident (CVA)
CESD—cholesteryl ester storage
    disease
CFIDS—chronic fatigue immune
    deficiency syndrome
CFP—cystic fibrosis of pancreas
CFS—chronic fatigue syndrome
CG—choking gas (phosgene)
CHA—congenital hypoplastic ane-
    mia
    chronic hemolytic anemia
Chagas
    disease
chagoma
chamber
    decompression c.
change
    Alzheimer neurofibrillary c.'s
Charcot
    cirrhosis
    fever
    triad
Charcot-Weiss-Baker
    syndrome
Chauffard
    syndrome
Chauffard-Still
    syndrome
Chédiak-Higashi
    disease
    syndrome
Chédiak-Steinbrinck-Higashi anom-
    aly
chelate

chelating agents [a class of drugs]
chelation
chemotherapy
    combination c.
Chiari
    disease
    syndrome
Chiari-Arnold syndrome
Child
    hepatic risk classification
        (A–C)
chlorosis
cholangiohepatitis
cholangitis
    catarrhal c.
    c. lenta
cholecystitis
    acute acalculous c.
cholemia
    familial c.
    Gilbert c.
cholemic
cholepathia
    c. spastica
cholera
    Asiatic c.
    bilious c.
    c. morbus
    c. nostras
cholestasis
    familial intraheptic c.
cholesterol
cholesterolemia
cholesterosis
cholesteryl ester storage disease
cholinergic
    c. agonists [a class of drugs]
chondromatosis
chondrosarcoma
chondrosarcomatosis
chondrosarcomatous
choreal
choriocarcinoma
chorioepithelioma
    c. malignum
choriomeningitis
    lymphocytic c.
    pseudolymphocytic c.

Christian
    disease
    syndrome
Christmas
    disease
    factor
chromomycosis
chromosome
    Philadelphia c.
Chvostek
    anemia
chylemia
CID—combined immunodeficiency
    disease
    cytomegalic inclusion disease
CIDS—continuous insulin delivery
    system
cin–. See also words beginning
    sin–, syn–.
cirrhogenous
cirrhosis
    alcoholic c.
    atrophic c.
    biliary c.
    Budd c.
    Charcot c.
    congenital hepatic c.
    Cruveilhier-Baumgarten c.
    cryptogenic c.
    Glisson c.
    Hanot c.
    Laënnec c.
    macronodular c.
    Maixner c.
    micronodular c.
    obstructive c.
    pericholangiolitic c.
    portal c.
    Todd c.
cirrhotic
Clark
    sign
Clarke-Hadfield
    syndrome
classification
    See also *index*.
    Child c. of hepatic risk

classification (continued)
    Fredrickson and Lees c.
      (phenotypes I–V)
    Karnofsky status c. [score
      0–100]
    Lund-Browder c.
    TNM (tumor, node, metasta-
      sis) c.
    van Heuven anatomical c. of
      diabetic retinopathy
claudication
    intermittent c.
    venous c.
climacterium
    c. praecox
clostridial
    c. myonecrosis
CoA—coenzyme A
coagulation
    diffuse intravascular c. (DIC)
coagulopathy
    disseminated intravascular c.
      (DIC)
coat
    white c. syndrome
code
    genetic c.
    molecular c.
coffee-grounds
    c-g. vomit, c.-g. vomitus
cogwheel
    c. sign
colic
    renal c.
    stercoral c.
    ureteral c.
    uterine c.
colicky pain
collagen
    c. disease
    c. vascular disease
Colorado tick fever
coma
    diabetic c.
    hyperosmolar nonketotic c.
    hypoglycemic c.
comatose

combined immunodeficiency disease
complex
    Ghon c.
    Parkinson dementia c.
Concato
    disease
concomitant
    c. disease
    c. medical problem
    c. metabolic acidosis
consensus
contracture
    Dupuytren c.
convulsion
    hypoglycemic c.
Cooley
    anemia
    disease
Cooper
    disease
copper storage disease
cor
    c. pulmonale
    c. triatriatum
Cori
    disease
coronary
    café c.
corticoreticular
corticosteroids [a class of drugs]
Corvisart
    disease
corynebacteria
coryza
costalgia
coumarins [a class of drugs]
Courvoisier
    law
    sign
Cowden
    disease
    syndrome
COX-2 (cyclooxygenase-2) inhibitors [a class of drugs]
coxsackievirus (group A, group B)
CPC—chronic passive congestion
crescendo-decrescendo murmur

CREST—calcinosis cutis, Raynaud phenomenon, esophageal dysfunction/hypermotility, sclerodactyly, telangiectasia [syndrome]
cretinism
CRF—cardiac risk factor(s)
Crigler-Najjar
    disease
    syndrome
crisis (crises)
    adrenal c.
    adrenocortical c.
    sickle cell c.
criterion (criteria)
    Ranson criteria for severity of acute pancreatitis
Crocq
    disease
Crohn
    disease
Crouzon
    disease
    syndrome
CRP—C-reactive protein
CRS—Chinese restaurant syndrome
Cruveilhier
    sign
Cruveilhier-Baumgarten
    cirrhosis
    syndrome
cryptogenic
cryptopodia
cryptopyic
cryptorchidism
cryptotoxic
CS—chondroitin sulfate
CSA—chondroitin sulfate A
CTH—ceramide trihexoside
Curschmann
    disease
curse
    Ondine's c.
Curtius syndrome
Cushing
    basophilism
    disease
    effect

Cushing (continued)
    phenomenon
    pituitary basophilism
    reaction
    response
    syndrome
    syndrome medicamentosus
cushingoid
cutaneous
    c. vasculitis
cutis
    c. verticis gyrata
CVA—cerebrovascular accident
cyanosis
cycle
    growth c.
    Krebs-Henseleit urea c.
cyclooxygenase-2 (COX-2) inhibi-
    tors [a class of drugs]
cystomyoma
cystomyxoadenoma
cystomyxoma
cystosarcoma
    c. phylloides
cytology
    exfoliative c.
cytomegalic inclusion disease (CID,
    CMID)
cytomegalovirus (CMV)
cytomycosis
Czerny anemia
DA—degenerative arthritis
dactylolysis
    d. spontanea
Dalrymple
    disease
    sign
DAN—diabetic autonomic neuropa-
    thy
Danbolt-Closs syndrome
dance
    St. Vitus d.
Darling
    disease
David
    disease
dawn effect, dawn phenomenon
Dawson inclusion

DDAVP—desmopressin acetate
    [trademarked name]
dearth
    d. of evidence
    d. of findings
    d. of symptoms
debilitated
    d. patient
    d. state
debilitating
    d. illness
debilitation
debilitative
    d. disease
Debove
    disease
degeneration
    amyloid d.
    Armanni-Ehrlich d.
    hepatolenticular d.
    hyaline d.
Degos
    disease
    syndrome
Dejerine-Sottas
    disease
delirium (deliria)
    acute d.
    collapse d.
    febrile d.
    d. grave
    low d.
    d. mussitans
    oneiric d.
    organic d.
    postcardiotomy d.
    senile d.
    d. sine delirio
    substance-induced d.
    substance intoxication d.
    substance withdrawal d.
    toxic d.
    traumatic d.
    d. tremens (DTs)
Delphian node
delta
    d.-aminolevulinic acid (ALA)

dementia
    myxedematous d.
de Mussy
    point
    sign
demyelinating disease
demyelination
deoxyribose
dependent
    d. edema
de Quervain
    thyroiditis
Dercum
    disease
dermatitis (dermatitides)
    livedoid d.
dermatosis (dermatoses)
    acute febrile neutrophilic d.
    neutrophilic d.
    radiation d.
Dermograft-TC
Desjardins
    point
determination
    sweat chloride d.
devastation
    senile cortical d.
DEXA—dual energy x-ray absorp-
    tiometry [scan]
α-dextrinase [alpha-]
dextrose
DF—desferrioxamine
DFO—deferoxamine
DHE—dihydroergotamine
DHT—dihydrotachysterol
diabetes
    adult-onset d.
    d. alternans
    brittle d.
    class A d.
    d. insipidus
    insulin-dependent d. (IDD)
    insulin-dependent d. melli-
      tus (IDDM)
    juvenile-onset d.
    Lancereaux d.
    latent d.

diabetes (continued)
    maturity-onset d. of the
      young (MODY)
    d. mellitus
    non–insulin-dependent d.
      (NIDD) [also: noninsulin-
      dependent]
    non–insulin-dependent d.
      mellitus (NIDDM) [also:
      noninsulin-dependent]
    obesity-associated d.
    overt d.
    pregnancy d., d. of pregnancy
    secondary d.
    type I d.
    type 2 d.
diabetic
    d. ketoacidosis
Diamond-Blackfan
    anemia
    syndrome
diaphragma
    d. sellae
DIC—diffuse intravascular coagula-
    tion
    disseminated intravascular
      coagulation
diet
    Ebstein d.
dieting
    yo-yo d.
"diff" Slang for differential.
differential
differentiation
    cellular d.
Di Guglielmo
    syndrome
DIMOAD—diabetes insipidus, dia-
    betes mellitus, optic atrophy,
    deafness [syndrome]
Diogenes
    syndrome
diplococcemia
dipsosis
dis–. See also words beginning dys–.
discrete
    d. thyromegaly

disease
    See also *syndrome.*
    Abrami d.
    Acosta d.
    acute demyelinating d.
    Adams-Stokes d.
    Addison d.
    Alzheimer d.
    Anders d.
    Andersen d.
    angiospasmodic d.
    Armstrong d.
    Aufrecht d.
    Australian X d.
    autoimmune d. (AID)
    Ayerza d.
    Balo d.
    Bannister d.
    Banti d.
    Basedow d.
    Beauvais d.
    Begbie d.
    Behçet d.
    Behr d.
    Bennett d.
    Berger d.
    Besnier-Boeck d.
    Besnier-Boeck-Schaumann d.
    Blumenthal d.
    Boeck d.
    Bowen d.
    Bradley d.
    Breda d.
    Brill d.
    Brill-Symmer d.
    Brill-Zinsser d.
    Brinton d.
    Brion-Kayser d.
    Bruhl d.
    Buerger d.
    Busse-Buschke d.
    Byler d.
    caisson d.
    Carrión d.
    Castellani d.
    cat-scratch d.
    celiac d.
    Chagas d.

disease (continued)
    cholesteryl ester storage d.
    Christmas d.
    collagen d.
    collagen vascular d.
    combined immunodeficiency
      d.
    Concato d.
    Cooper d.
    Crocq d.
    Crohn d.
    Curschmann d.
    cytomegalic inclusion d.
      (CID, CMID)
    Darling d.
    David d.
    Debove d.
    Degos d.
    Dejerine-Sottas d.
    demyelinating d.
    Dercum d.
    Dressler d.
    Durand d.
    Ebstein d.
    Economo (von Economo) d.
    end-stage renal d. (ESRD)
    euthyroid Graves d.
    Fabry d.
    Fenwick d.
    Filatov d.
    Flajani d.
    Forbes d.
    Friedländer d.
    Gaisböck d.
    Gamna d.
    Gamstorp d.
    Gandy-Nanta d.
    Gaucher d.
    Gilbert d.
    Gilchrist d.
    Glénard d.
    glycogen storage d.
    Graves d.
    Gull d.
    Hand-Schüller-Christian d.
    Hanot d.
    Hansen d.
    Hartnup d.

disease (continued)
    Hashimoto d.
    Heberden d.
    Heerfordt d.
    hemolytic d.
    heredoconstitutional d.
    Hers d.
    Hirschsprung d.
    Hodgkin d.
    Horton d.
    Huchard d.
    Huntington d.
    Hutinel d.
    Iceland d.
    I-cell d.
    Itsenko d.
    Jodbasedow d.
    Kahler d.
    Keshan d.
    Kirkland d.
    Klippel d.
    Krabbe d.
    Krishaber d.
    Kufs d.
    Kussmaul-Maier d.
    Kyrle d.
    Lancereau-Mathieu d.
    Landouzy d.
    Larrey-Weil d.
    legionnaires' d.
    Letterer-Siwe d.
    Lignac d.
    Lignac-Fanconi d.
    Luft d.
    Lyme d.
    Mackenzie d.
    maple syrup urine d. (MSUD)
    Marie d.
    Marsh d.
    mast cell d.
    Mathieu d.
    Meige d.
    Meleda d.
    Ménière d.
    Mikulicz d.
    Milton d.
    Möbius d.
    Monge d.

disease (continued)
    Morquio d.
    Münchmeyer d.
    Niemann d.
    Niemann-Pick d.
    Ohara d.
    Ollier d.
    Opitz d.
    Ormond d.
    Osler d.
    Osler-Vaquez d.
    parenchymatous d.
    Parkinson d.
    Parrot d.
    Parry d.
    Parsons d.
    Pavy d.
    Pfeiffer d.
    Pick d.
    pink d.
    Plummer d.
    Pompe d.
    Poncet d.
    Posada-Wernicke d.
    Pott d.
    Poulet d.
    pulseless d.
    Raynaud d.
    Reclus d.
    Reed-Hodgkin d.
    Refsum d.
    Reiter d.
    rheumatic heart d.
    Riedel d.
    Rokitansky d.
    Runeberg d.
    Rust d.
    Sandhoff d.
    San Joaquin Valley d.
    Schaumann d.
    Schottmüller d.
    Shaver d.
    Sheehan d.
    Simmonds d.
    Sjögren d.
    Smith-Strang d.
    St. Anthony's d.
    Sternberg d.

disease (continued)
    Still d.
    Strümpell-Marie d.
    Stuart-Bras d.
    Stuart-Prower factor defi-
      ciency d.
    Swift d.
    Symmers d.
    Takahara d.
    Tangier d.
    Tay-Sachs d.
    Thaysen d.
    Underwood d.
    Urbach-Wiethe d.
    Vaquez d.
    Vaquez-Osler d.
    von Economo d.
    von Gierke d.
    von Recklinghausen d.
    von Willebrand d.
    Weil d.
    Weir Mitchell
    Werlhof d.
    Werner d.
    Wernicke d.
    Whipple d.
    Widal-Abrami d.
    Wilkins d.
    Willis d.
    Wilson d.
    Winkler d.
    zymotic d.
disorder
    appetite d.
    eating d.
dissection
    block d.
distomiasis
    hemic d.
    hepatic d.
diuresis (diureses)
DKA—diabetic ketoacidosis
DLE—disseminated lupus erythe-
    matosus
doll's eye
    test
Donath-Landsteiner
    syndrome

dot
    Schüffner d.
doughy
    d. abdomen
    d. consistency
dowager's hump
DR—diabetic retinopathy
Dresbach
    anemia
    syndrome
Dressler
    disease
Dubois
    abscesses
    disease
Duchenne
    sign
duct
    müllerian d.
    Wirsung d.
    wolffian d.
Duncan
    disease
    syndrome
Dupuytren
    contracture
    fascia
    hydrocele
    suture
Durand
    disease
DVT—deep vein thrombosis
    deep venous thrombosis
dwarf
    achondroplastic d.
    hypopituitary d.
    Laron d.
    Paltauf d.
dwarfism
    pituitary d.
dys–. See also words beginning dis–.
dysautonomia
    Riley-Day d.
dysbetalipoproteinemia
dyschondroplasia
dyscrasia
    blood d.
    lymphatic d.

dyslipidosis
dysostosis
    d. multiplex
dysplasia
    olfactogenital d.
dysponderal
dyspragia
dystonia
dysuria
EB—Epstein-Barr [virus]
Ebstein
    anomaly
    diet
    disease
    malformation
EBV—Epstein-Barr virus
ecphyma
    e. globulus
ectodermal
    e. dysplasia
ectodermosis
    e. erosiva pluriorificialis
edema
    brawny e.
    Milroy e.
    Milton e.
    nonpitting e.
    pedal e.
    Pirogoff e.
    prehepatic e.
    Reinke e.
edematous
edentulous
EDTA—ethylenediaminetetra-acetate
    ethylenediaminetetra-acetic
        acid
effect [noun: result, outcome]
    See also *reaction* and *phe-
        nomenon.*
    additive e.
    blast e.
    Bohr e.
    cumulative e.
    Cushing e.
    cyclosporine e.
    cytopathic e.
    cytoprotective e.
    Haldane e.

effect [noun: result, outcome] (con-
    tinued)
    placebo e.
    pressure e.
    Somogyi e.
    Staub-Traugott e.
    Wolff-Chaikoff e.
effect [verb: to produce, to bring
    about]
    to e. a cure
effusion
EHC—essential hypercholesterolemia
EHL—endogenous hyperlipidemia
Ehlers-Danlos
    disease
    syndrome
Ekbom syndrome
"eksan–" Phonetic for words begin-
    ning exan–.
elastofibroma
    e. dorsi
electrolyte
    e. imbalance
electrolytic
ellipsoid
    e. of spleen
emphysema
    subcutaneous e.
encephalopathy
    hepatic e.
    Wernicke e.
endarteritis
endocarditis
    acute bacterial e.
    bacterial e.
    gonococcal e.
    infective e.
    subacute bacterial e.
endocrinotropic
endomorph
endomorphic
endomorphy
endothelialization
endothelioid
end-stage renal disease (ESRD)
enema
    sedative e.

"en-sed" Phonetic for NSAID (nonsteroidal anti-inflammatory
drug).
enteritis
 e. necroticans
eosinopenia
eosinophilia
 Löffler e.
eosinophilopoietin
epidermolysis
 e. bullosa
epididymis
epididymitis
epilepsy
 abdominal e.
 catamenial e.
 gelastic e.
epistaxis
 Gull renal e.
epsilon
 e.-aminocaproic acid
equation
 Bohr e.
ERA—estrogen receptor assay
Erdheim
 disease
 syndrome
eructation
erythematosus
 disseminated lupus e. (DLE)
erythremia
erythrocytosis
 leukemic e.
 e. megalosplenica
erythrogenesis
 e. imperfecta
erythroid
erythroneocytosis
erythropenia
erythropoietin
esophagitis
"estriasis" Phonetic for oestriasis.
eunuch
eunuchism
 pituitary e.
eunuchoidism
euthymic
euthyroidism

Evans
 syndrome
exanthem
 e. subitum
excavatum
 pectus e.
exhaustion
exogenous
 e. obesity
Faber
 anemia
 syndrome
Fabry
 disease
 syndrome
facies (facies)
 acromegalic f.
 cushingoid f.
 f. hepatica
 moon f.
 myxedematous f.
 Parkinson f., parkinsonian f.
facioscapulohumeral
 f. dystrophy
factor
 cardiac risk f.'s (CRFs)
 von Willebrand f.
Fanconi
 anemia
 disease
 pancytopenia
 syndrome
Farber
 disease
 syndrome
fasciitis
 diffuse f.
 eosinophilic f.
 necrotizing f.
fastigium
FBS—fasting blood sugar
Felty syndrome
"fenil–" Phonetic for words beginning phenyl–.
"fenomenon" Phonetic for phenomenon.
Fenwick
 disease

"feo–" Phonetic for words beginning pheo–.
fetor
    f. hepaticus
fever
    breakbone f.
    etiocholanolone f.
    Haverhill f.
    hay f.
    phlebotomus f.
    quartan f.
    quotidian f.
    rheumatic f.
fiber
    Purkinje f.
fibroadenoma
fibroadenosis
fibrocystic
fibrolymphoangioblastoma
fibromyalgia
fibromyoma
fibromyositis
fibromyxosarcoma
fibrosis
    cystic f. (CF)
fibrous
    f. dysplasia
    f. plaque
Fiessinger-Leroy-Reiter
    syndrome
"Fifer" Phonetic for Pfeiffer.
FIGLU—formiminoglutamic acid
Filatov
    disease
fire
    St. Anthony's f.
fissure
fistula (fistulas, fistulae)
Fitz
    law
    syndrome
Fitz-Hugh–Curtis
    syndrome
flagellosis
Flajani disease
flattening
    f. of diaphragm
"flebitis" Phonetic for phlebitis.

fleckmilz
flight
    f. into disease
florid
fluctuation
"foke-mahn" Phonetic for Volkmann.
folliculosis
Fölling
    disease
    phenylketonuria
food poisoning
    Bacillus cereus f.p.
    enterococcal f.p.
"fool" Phonetic for Pfuhl.
foot (feet)
    burning feet
Forbes
    disease
forme (formes)
    f. fruste, formes frustes
    f. tardive
formiminoglutamic acid (FIGLU)
formula
    Berkow f.
fortification
    f. spectrum
fracture
    cough f.
fragilitas
    f. sanguinis
Frey
    syndrome
Frey-Baillarger syndrome
Friedländer disease
α-L-fucosidase [alpha-]
fungus (fungi)
    See specific fungi in *Laboratory, Pathology, and Chemistry Terms.*
FUO—fever of undetermined origin
    fever of unknown origin
Gaffky
    scale
    table
Gaisböck
    disease
    syndrome

gait
    helicopod g.
galactophlebitis
α-galactosidase A [alpha-]
β-galactosidase [beta-]
galactotoxism
gamma
    g.-aminobutyric acid (GABA)
    g. chain disease
    g. globulin
    g.-glutamylcysteine syn-
       thetase (deficiency)
    g.-glutamyl transpeptidase
    g. interferon
    g. rays
    g. streptococci
Gamna
    disease
Gamstorp disease
Gandy-Gamna
    disease
    nodules
    spleen
Gandy-Nanta disease
ganglial
ganglion (ganglia, ganglions)
    Troisier g.
ganglionitis
    acute posterior g.
gangliosidosis (gangliosidoses)
    generalized g.
    GM_1 g. [GM1]
    GM_2 g. [GM2]
    GM_2 g. (types I–III)
    GM_2 g., variant AB
    GM_2 g., variant B
    GM_2 g., variant O
gangrene
    Raynaud g.
gastroma
Gaucher
    disease
    splenomegaly
gavage
    g. feeding
GCA—giant cell arteritis
genitalia [grammatically plural; no
    singular form]

genome
    mitochondrial g.
geographic, geographical
geographic tongue
GFD—gluten-free diet
GH—growth hormone
GHD—growth hormone deficiency
GH-RF—growth hormone–releas-
    ing factor
giant cell
Gierke (von Gierke)
    disease
gigantism
    hyperpituitary g.
    pituitary g.
Gilbert
    cholemia
    disease
    sign
    syndrome
Gilchrist
    disease
GITT—glucose-insulin tolerance test
Gjessing syndrome
gland
    adrenal g.
    endocrine g.
    exocrine g.
    master g.
    parathyroid g.
    pineal g.
    pituitary g.
    Sigmund g.'s
    suprahyoid accessory thy-
      roid g.
    suprarenal g.
    thymus g.
    thyroid g.
glandula (glandulae)
glandular
glandule
glandulous [adj.]
Glénard disease
glioblastoma
    g. multiforme
Glisson
    cirrhosis
    disease

globulinuria
glomerulocapillary
  g. sclerosis
glomerulosclerosis
  intercapillary g.
glossopharyngeal
1,4α-glucan branching enzyme
  [-alpha-]
glucan-1,4α-glucosidase [-alpha-]
α-1,4-glucosidase deficiency [alpha-]
γ-glutamylcysteine synthetase deficiency [gamma-]
γ-glutamyl transpeptidase [gamma-]
γ-glutamyl transpeptidase deficiency [gamma-]
glycogen storage disease
glycosaminoglycans [a class of
  drugs]
Gn-RH—gonadotropin-releasing
  hormone
goiter
  adenomatous g.
  cabbage g.
  colloid g.
  cystic g.
  endemic g.
  exophthalmic g.
  familial g.
  fibrous g.
  follicular g.
  intrathoracic g.
  myxedematous g.
  nodular g.
  papillomatous g.
  parenchymatous g.
  substernal g.
  thoracic g.
  toxic g.
gonadotropin
  pituitary g.
gonadotropin-releasing hormone
  (Gn-RH)
    g.-r.h. analogues [a class of
      drugs]
Goodpasture
  syndrome
Gordon
  syndrome

gout
  abarticular g.
  articular g.
  calcium g.
  chalky g.
  latent g.
  lead g.
  misplaced g.
  oxalic g.
  polyarticular g.
  renal g.
  retrocedent g.
  rheumatic g.
  saturnine g.
  tophaceous g.
Gradenigo
  syndrome
grading
Graefe (von Graefe)
  sign
granuloblastosis
granuloma
  amebic g.
  eosinophilic g.
  Hodgkin g.
  g. inguinale
  necrotic g.
  pyogenic g.
granulomatosis
  beryllium g.
  bronchocentric g.
  g. infantiseptica
  lymphomatoid g.
  g. siderotica
granulopoiesis
granulosa
Graves
  disease
  disease, ophthalmic
gray-out
Greenfield
  disease
  syndrome
Grey Turner
  sign
GRF—gonadotropin-releasing factor
  growth hormone–releasing
    factor

GRH—growth hormone–releasing hormone
Gross leukemia
growth
    g. cycle
    g. fraction
    g. hormone
GSE—gluten-sensitive enteropathy
GSH—growth-stimulating hormone
GT—glucose tolerance
GTH—gonadotropic hormone
GTT—glucose tolerance test
Gubler icterus
Guéneau de Mussy point
Gull
    disease
    renal epistaxis
Günther
    syndrome
GVHD—graft-versus-host disease
GVHR—graft-versus-host reaction
gynecomastia
Hadfield-Clarke syndrome
Haemophilus
Haff disease
hairy cell leukemia
hallucination
    See in *Psychiatry* section.
hamartoma
    chondromatous h.
    leiomyomatous h.
Hand [eponym]
    disease
    syndrome
Hand-Schüller-Christian
    disease
    syndrome
Hanot
    cirrhosis
    disease
    syndrome
Hanot-Chauffard syndrome
Hartnup
    disease
    syndrome
Hashimoto
    disease
    struma

Hashimoto (continued)
    thyroiditis
Haven syndrome
Hawes-Pallister-Landor syndrome
Hayem
    icterus
    jaundice
HB—hepatitis B
HBO—hyperbaric oxygen
HBV—hepatitis B virus
headache
    cluster h.
    exertional h.
    Horton h.
    jolt h.
    meningeal h.
    migraine h.
    muscle contraction h.
    neuralgic h.
    nitroglycerin h.
    paraplegic h.
    postconcussional h.
    pressor h.
    spinal fluid loss h.
    tension h.
    thunderclap h.
    traction h.
    traumatic h.
    vascular h.
heaves
    dry h.
Heberden
    angina
    asthma
    disease
    nodes
    nodosities
    rheumatism
Hedinger syndrome
Heerfordt
    disease
    syndrome
helicine
helicoid
helicopod
    h. gait
heliosis

heliotherapy
helminthiasis
    cutaneous h.
    h. elastica
    h. wuchereri
hemangioendothelioma
hemangiomatosis
    systemic h.
hematinics [a class of drugs]
hematocrit (Hct, hct)
hematology
hematoma
    epidural h.
hematopoietics [a class of drugs]
hemoglobinemia
hemolytic
    h. anemia
    h. disease
hemophilia
    h. A
    h. B
    h. C
    Leyden h. B
    h. neonatorum
    vascular h.
hemophilus
    See in *Laboratory, Patholo-
    gy, and Chemistry Terms.*
hemoptysis
hemorrhage
hemorrhagic
hemosiderosis
    transfusional h.
Henle loop
Henoch-Schönlein
    purpura
    syndrome
hepar
    h. adiposum
    h. lobatum
heparan-α-glucosaminide *N*-acetyl-
    transferase [-alpha-]
hepatalgia
hepatatrophia
hepatic
    h. encephalopathy
hepatism

hepatitis (hepatitides)
    h. A
    acute h.
    aggressive h.
    alcoholic h.
    anicteric h.
    autoimmune h.
    h. B
    h. B virus
    h. C
    chronic h.
    h. D
    drug-induced h.
    h. E
    fulminant h.
    h. G
    giant cell h.
    infectious h.
    non-A h.
    non-A, non-B h.
    non-B h.
    peliosis h.
    serum h.
    syphilitic h.
    viral h.
hepatization
hepatodynia
hepatodystrophy
hepatomegaly
hepatotoxic
hepatotoxicity
heredoconstitutional disease
heredopathia
    h. atactica polyneuritiformis
hermaphroditism
hernia
    hiatal h., hiatus h.
herpes
    h. catarrhalis
    h. generalisatus
    h. genitalis
    h. gestationis
    h. labialis
    h. meningoencephalitis
    h. neonatalis
    h. varicella-zoster virus
Herrick anemia
Hers disease

Herter
  disease
hGH—human growth hormone
hiatal, hiatus
  h. hernia
hiatus
hidradenitis
  h. axillaris
  h. suppurativa
  suppurative h.
high-density lipoprotein (HDL)
hilum (hila)
  h. hepatis
  h. lienale
  h. of lymph node
  h. lymphoglandulae
  h. nodi lymphatici
  h. nodi lymphoidei
  h. splenicum
hilus (hili). See *hilum.*
"hipo–" Phonetic for words beginning hypo–.
Hirschsprung disease
hirsutism
  Apert h.
  idiopathic h.
histiocytosis
  h. X
histocompatibility
HIV—human immunodeficiency
  virus
HMG-CoA (3-hydroxy-3-methylglu-
  taryl–coenzyme A) reductase
  inhibitors [a class of drugs]
Hodgkin
  disease
  granuloma
  lymphoma
hormone
Horton
  arteritis
  cephalalgia
  disease
  headache
  syndrome
hot
  h. caudate lobe
  h. thyroid nodule

Houssay-Biasotti syndrome
hPFSH—human pituitary follicles-
  timulating hormone
hPG—human pituitary gonadotropin
HPT—hyperparathyroidism
H-shaped vertebra
Huchard
  disease
  sign
  symptom
Huët-Pelger nuclear anomaly
Huntington
  chorea
  disease
Hürthle
  cell
  cell adenoma
  cell carcinoma
  cell tumor
Hutinel disease
hydrocarbon
  aromatic h.
hydrocytosis
hydrogen (H)
hydromyelia
hydronephrosis
3-hydroxy-3-methylglutaryl–coenzyme A (HMG-CoA) reductase
  inhibitors [a class of drugs]
p-hydroxyphenylpyruvic acid
  (PHPPA) [p-, para-]
hymenolepiasis
hyperadenosis
hyperadiposis
hyperadrenalism
hyperadrenocorticism
hyperalbuminemia
hyperalbuminosis
hyperaldosteronemia
hyperaldosteronuria
hyperalimentation
  total parenteral h.
hyperalimentosis
hyperalonemia
hyperalphalipoproteinemia
hyperaminoacidemia
hyperammonemia
hyperammonuria

hyperandrogenism
hyperazotemia
hyperazoturia
hyperbaric
    h. chamber
    h. oxygen
hyperbarism
hyperbetalipoproteinemia
    familial h.
hyperbilirubinemia
    congenital h.
    conjugated h.
    constitutional h.
    hereditary nonhemolytic h.
    h. I
    neonatal h.
    unconjugated h.
hyperbilirubinemic
hyperbradykininemia
hyperbradykininism
hypercalcemia
    familial hypocalciuric h.
    idiopathic h.
hypercalcitoninemia
hypercalciuria
    absorptive h.
    idiopathic h.
    renal h.
    resorptive h.
    secondary h.
hypercapnia
hypercapnic
hypercarotenemia
hypercatabolic
hypercatabolism
hyperchloremic
hyperchloruria
hypercholesterolemia
    essential h.
    familial h.
    polygenic h.
hypercholesterolemic
hyperchromatism
    macrocytic h.
hypercorticalism
hypercorticism
hypercreatinemia
hypercryalgesia

hypercryesthesia
hypercupremia
hypercupriuria
hyperdipsia
hypereccrisia
hypereccritic
hyperelectrolytemia
hyperemesis
    h. hiemis
hyperemetic
hyperemia
    Bier passive h.
    constriction h.
hyperemic
hyperepinephrinemia
hyperestrogenemia
hyperestrogenism
hyperestrogenosis
hyperexcretory
hyperferremia
hyperferremic
hyperfibrinogenemia
hyperfiltration
hyperfunction
hyperfunctioning
hypergammaglobulinemia
hyperglandular
hyperglobulinemia
hyperglucagonemia
hyperglycemia
hyperglycemic
hyperglyceridemia
hyperglyceridemic
hyperglycerolemia
    infantile-type h.
    juvenile-type h.
    microdeletion-type h.
hyperglycinemia
    ketotic h.
    nonketotic h.
hyperglycistia
hyperglycogenolysis
hyperglycorrhachia
hyperglycosuria
hypergonadism
hypergonadotropic
hyperguanidinemia
hyperhemoglobinemia

hyperhemolytic
hyperheparinemia
hyperhidrosis
    axillary h.
    gustatory h.
    h. lateralis
    unilateral h.
hyperhidrotic
hyperhistidinemia
hyperhistidinuria
hyperhormonism
hyperhydration
hyperhydroxyprolinemia
Hypericum
    H. perforatum
hyperimidodipeptiduria
hyperingestion
hyperinsulinar
hyperinsulinemia
hyperinsulinism
    alimentary h.
    functional h.
    iatrogenic h.
hyperiodemia
hyperisotonia
hyperisotonic
hyperisotonicity
hyperkalemia
hyperketosis
hyperkoria
hyperlactacidemia
hyperlecithinemia
hyperleukocytosis
hyperleydigism
hyperlipemia
    carbohydrate-induced h.
    combined fat- and carbohy-
      drate-induced h.
    endogenous h.
    essential familial h.
    familial fat-induced h.
    mixed h.
hyperlipidemia
hyperlipidemic
hyperlipoproteinemia
    acquired h.
    familial h. (types I–V, IIa, IIb)
hyperlithemia

hyperlithic
hyperlithuria
hyperlycinemia
hypermagnesemia
hypermedication
hypermetabolic
hypermetabolism
    extrathyroidal h.
hypermetaplasia
hypermineralization
hypernatremia
hypernatremic
hypernitremia
hypernutrition
hyperorexia
hyperornithemia
hyperosmolality
hyperosmolarity
hyperoxemia
hyperoxia
hyperoxic
hyperoxidation
hyperpancreorrhea
hyperparathyroidism
    nutritional secondary h.
    primary h.
    secondary h.
    tertiary h.
hyperpexia
hyperphagia
hyperphagic
hyperphenylalaninemia
    malignant h.
    maternal h.
    persistent h.
    transient h.
hyperphosphatasemia
    chronic congenital idiopath-
      ic h.
    h. tarda
hyperphosphatemia
hyperphosphaturia
hyperphosphoremia
hyperpinealism
hyperpipecolatemia
hyperpituitarism
    basophilic h.
    eosinophilic h.

hyperplasia
    adrenal cortical h., adreno-
      cortical h.
    angiofollicular mediastinal
      lymph node h.
    benign mediastinal lymph
      node h.
    C-cell h.
    congenital adrenal h. (CAH)
    congenital adrenocortical h.
    follicular h.
    giant follicular h.
    giant lymph node h.
    inflammatory h.
    islet cell h.
    Leydig cell h.
    nodular adrenal h.
    lipoid adrenal h.
    lymphoid h.
    nodular adrenocortical h.
    ovarian stromal h.
    pseudoepitheliomatous h.
    Schwann h.
    thymic medullary h.
hyperplasmia
hyperplastic
hyperpolypeptidemia
hyperposia
hyperpotassemia
hyperprebetalipoproteinemia
    familial h.
hyperprogesteronemia
hyperproinsulinemia
hyperprolactinemic
hyperprolactinism
hyperprolinemia
    h., type I, type II
    familial h.
hyperproteinemia
hyperproteosis
hyperpyremia
hyperpyretic
hyperpyrexia
    fulminant h.
    heat h.
    malignant h.
hyperpyrexial
hyperreninemia

hyperreninemic
hypersalemia
hypersaline
hyperserotonemia
hypersomatotropism
hypersomia
hypersomnia
    continuous h.
    paroxysmal h.
    periodic h.
hypersomnolence
hypersplenism
hypersthenuria
hypersuprarenalism
hypersusceptibility
hypertensive
hypertestosteronism
hyperthecosis
    testoid h.
hyperthermal
hyperthermia
hyperthrombinemia
hyperthymism
hyperthyroid
hyperthyroidism
    apathetic h.
    factitious h.
    iatrogenic h.
    iodine-induced h.
    masked h.
    primary h.
    secondary h.
hyperthyroxinemia
hypertoxic
hypertoxicity
hypertransfusion
hypertrichosis
    h. lanuginosa
hypertriglyceridemia
hypertrophy
    Marie h.
hypertyrosinemia
hyperuresis
hyperuricemia
hyperuricemic
hyperuricuria
hyperventilation
hypervitaminosis

hypervitaminotic
hypnotoxin
hypoadrenalism
hypoadrenocorticism
    pituitary h.
    secondary h.
hypoalbuminemia
hypoalbuminosis
hypoaldosteronemia
hypoaldosteronism
    hyporeninemic h.
    isolated h.
hypoaldosteronuria
hypoalphalipoproteinemia
hypoandrogenism
hypoazoturia
hypobarism
hypobaropathy
hypobilirubinemia
hypocalcipectic
hypocalcipexy
hypocalciuria
hypocapnia
hypocapnic
hypochloremia
hypochloremic
hypochloridation
hypochlorization
hypochloruria
hypocholesterolemia
hypocholesterolemic
hypocholuria
hypochromia
    idiopathic h.
hypocitremia
hypocitruria
hypocomplementemic
hypocorticalism
hypocorticism
hypoelectrolytemia
hypoepinephrinemia
hypoferremia
hypoferrism
hypofibrinogenemia
hypogammaglobulinemia
hypoglandular
hypoglucagonemia
hypoglycemia

hypoglycemic
hypoglycemosis
hypoglycin (A or B)
hypoglycogenolysis
hypogonadism
    pituitary h.
hypohepatia
hypohidrosis
hypohormonal
hypohydration
hypohydrochloria
hypoinsulinemia
hypoinsulinism
hypoiodidism
hypokalemia
hypokalemic
hypolactasia
hypoleydigism
hypolipemia
hypolipidemic
hypoliposis
hypolymphemia
hypomagnesemia
hypometabolic
hypometabolism
    euthyroid h.
hyponatremia
hyponatremic
hyponatruria
hypo-osmolality
hypopancreatism
hypopancreorrhea
hypoparathyroid
hypoparathyroidism
    familial h.
hypophosphaturia
hypophysioprivic
hypophysiotropic
hypopiesia
hypopietic
hypopituitarism
    postpartum hemorrhagic h.
hypoplasia
    granulocytic h.
hypoposia
hypopotassemia
hypopotassemic

hypoproteinemia
    prehepatic h.
hypoproteinemic
hypoproteinia
hypoproteinic
hypoproteinosis
hypoprothrombinemia
hyporeactive
hyporeninemia
hyporeninemic
hyposecretion
hyposmolarity
hyposomatotropism
hyposplenism
hypostasis
hypostatic
hyposuprarenalism
hypotension
    chronic idiopathic orthostat-
      ic h.
    chronic orthostatic h.
    idiopathic orthostatic h.
    orthostatic h.
    postural h.
    vascular h.
hypotensive
hypothalamic
hypothalamus
hypothermia
    endogenous h.
    induced h.
    moderate h.
    profound h.
    regional h.
hypothermic
hypothrepsia
hypothrombinemia
hypothyroid
hypothyroidism
    familial goitrous h.
    hypothalamic h.
    infantile h.
    postoperative h.
    primary h.
    tertiary h.
hypotonia
hypotonic
hypotryptophanic

hypovitaminosis
hypovolemia
hypovolemic
HZ—herpes zoster
HZV—herpes zoster virus
^{131}I—radioactive iodine [iodine I 131]
IADH—inappropriate antidiuretic
    hormone
iatrogenic
IC—intermittent claudication
ICD—ischemic coronary disease
Iceland disease
I-cell disease
ichthyosis
ictal
icteric
icterus
    bilirubin i.
    i. castrensis gravis
    i. castrensis levis
    i. catarrhalis
    choluric hemolytic i. with
      splenomegaly
    cythemolytic i.
    i. gravis
    Gubler i.
    Hayem i.
    i. hemolyticus
    i. infectiosus
    i. praecox
    i. simplex
    spirochetal i.
    i. typhoides
    urobilin i.
    i. viridans
ictus
IDD—insulin-dependent diabetes
IDDM—insulin-dependent diabetes
    mellitus
idiopathic
IDL—intermediate-density lipopro-
    tein
α-L-iduronidase deficiency [alpha-]
IEM—inborn error of metabolism
IGF-1—insulin-like growth factor-1
IGT—impaired glucose tolerance
IHO—idiopathic hypertrophic
    osteoarthropathy

"ikthe–" Phonetic for words beginning ichthy–.

"iktus" Phonetic for ictus.

illness
- acute on chronic i.
- debilitating i.
- refractory i.

IM—infectious mononucleosis
- internal medicine

Imerslund
- syndrome

Imerslund-Graesbeck
- syndrome

Imerslund-Najman-Graesbeck
- syndrome

immunodeficiency
- acquired i. syndrome (AIDS)

immunoglobulin (Ig)
- thyroid-binding inhibitory i. (TBII)
- thyroid-stimulating i.
- thyrotropin-binding inhibitory i. (TBII)
- TSH-binding inhibitory i.

immunosuppressants [a class of drugs]

immunosuppression

immunosuppressive

incarnatio
- i. unguis

inclusion
- Dawson i.

incubation

index (indexes, indices)
- See also *classification.*
- free thyroxin i. (FTI)

infantilism
- idiopathic i.
- proportionate i.
- thyroid i.

infarction
- anteroinferior myocardial i.
- anterolateral myocardial i.
- anteroseptal myocardial i.
- apical myocardial i.
- atrial i.
- cardiac i.
- diaphragmatic i.

infarction (continued)
- high-lateral myocardial i.
- inferolateral myocardial i
- lateral myocardial i.
- myocardial i. (MI)
- posterior myocardial i.
- posterolateral myocardial i.
- pulmonary i.
- right ventricular i.
- Roesler-Dressler i.
- septal myocardial i.
- silent myocardial i.
- subendocardial i.
- through-and-through myocardial i.
- transmural myocardial i.

infection
- invasive burn i.

influenza
- i. A
- i. B
- i. C
- i. virus (A–C) [also: influenzavirus]
- clinical i.

influenzal

INH—isonicotinic acid hydrazide (isoniazid)

inhibition
- contact i.

inhibitor
- COX-2 (cyclooxygenase-2) i.'s [a class of drugs]
- factor VIII i.
- HMG-CoA (3-hydroxy-3-methylglutaryl–coenzyme A) reductase i.'s [a class of drugs]

inoculate

inoculation

INPV—intermittent negative-pressure assisted ventilation

insenescence

insensible
- i. fluid output

insipidus
- diabetes i.

insolation
    asphyxial i.
    hyperpyrexial i.
insufficiency
    acute adrenocortical i.
    anterior pituitary i.
    chronic adrenocortical i.
    pancreatic i.
insult
    hemorrhagic i.
intermittent
    i. claudication
    i. porphyria
intoxication
    bongkrek i.
    digitalis i.
    manganese i.
    water i.
IPG—impedance plethysmography
iritis
    diabetic i.
    gouty i.
islet
    i. of Langerhans
isolation
    pulmonary i.
ITP—idiopathic thrombocytopenic
    purpura
Itsenko disease
IV—intravenous
IV cocktail
Ivemark syndrome
Jaccoud
    arthritis
    arthropathy
    fever
    sign
    syndrome
Jansky-Bielschowsky syndrome
jargonaphasia
jaundice
    constitutional j.
    hemolytic j.
    hemorrhagic j.
    nonobstructive j.
    obstructive j.
    transfusion j.

Jellinek
    sign
    symptom
Jobst
    stockings
Job syndrome
Jodbasedow disease
Joffroy
    sign
joint
    See in *Orthopedics and
        Sports Medicine* section.
judicious
jugulation
jugulodigastric
juvenile
    j.-onset diabetes
    j. rheumatoid arthritis
KA—ketoacidosis
"kahk–," "kak–" Phonetic for words
    beginning cac–, cach–.
Kahler
    disease
Kaposi
    disease
    sarcoma
    varicelliform eruption
    xeroderma
Karnofsky
    rating scale
    status
    tumor grading
KB—ketone body
Kcal, Cal—kilocalorie
"kemo–" Phonetic for words begin-
    ning chemo–.
Kendall
    method
    rank correlation coefficient
    tau
Keshan disease
α-keto acid dehydrogenase [alpha-]
ketoacidosis
    diabetic k.
ketone bodies
ketotic
kilocalorie (kcal, Cal)

Kimmelstiel-Wilson
    disease
    syndrome
kinetics
    cell population k.
Kirkland
    disease
Klemperer
    disease
Klippel disease
koilonychia
"kolee–" Phonetic for words beginning chole–, choli–, coli–.
König
    syndrome
"kor–" Phonetic for words beginning cor– and chor–.
Krabbe
    disease
    hypoplasia
    leukodystrophy
    syndrome
Krishaber
    disease
Kufs
    disease
Kunkel
    syndrome
Kussmaul
    breathing
    disease
    respiration
Kussmaul-Maier disease
"kvos-tek" Phonetic for Chvostek.
KW—Kimmelstiel-Wilson [syndrome]
kyphosis
Kyrle
    disease
Labbé
    syndrome
labored breathing
laborious
lactacidemia
lactase
    adult l. deficiency
    l. deficiency
    intestinal l. deficiency

lactation
lactic
    l. acid
    l. acidosis
lacticacidemia
lactosuria
lactulose
Laënnec
    cirrhosis
    disease
Lancereau-Mathieu
    disease
Landouzy
    disease
    dystrophy
    purpura
    type
Langerhans
    cells
    granules
    islands
    islets (islets of Langerhans)
laparotomy
Laron
    dwarf
    syndrome
Larrey-Weil
    disease
larvate
laryngotracheobronchitis
Larzel anemia
latent
    l. diabetes mellitus
lathyrism
lathyritic
lathyrogen
lathyrogenic
latrodectism
LATS—long-acting thyroid stimulator
Launois
    syndrome
Launois-Cléret
    syndrome
Laurence-Biedl
    syndrome
Laurence-Moon
    syndrome

Laurence-Moon-Biedl
    law
    syndrome
law
    Courvoisier l.
    Fitz l.
Lawrence-Seip syndrome
lazaroids [a class of drugs]
LD—living donor
LDH—lactate dehydrogenase
LED—lupus erythematosus dissem-
    inatus
Leede-Rumpel phenomenon
Legal
    disease
legionnaires'
    l. disease
    l. pneumonia
leiomyoma (leiomyomas, leiomy-
    omata)
Leishman
    anemia
Lépine-Froin syndrome
leptospirosis
    l. icterohemorrhagica
Leriche
    disease
    syndrome
lesion
    Armanni-Ebstein l.
    Blumenthal l.
    cold l.
    Councilman l.
    Ebstein l.
    hot l.
    indiscriminate l.
    irritative l.
    ring-wall l.
lethargic
Letterer-Siwe
    disease
leukemia
    acute lymphoblastic l. (ALL)
    acute nonlymphocytic l.
      (ANLL)
    acute promyelocytic l.
    adult T-cell l.
    aleukemic l.

leukemia (continued)
    aleukocythemic l.
    aplastic l.
    basophilic l.
    blast cell l.
    blastic l.
    Burkitt-type acute lym-
      phoblastic l.
    chronic granulocytic l.
    chronic lymphocytic l. (CLL)
    chronic myelocytic l. (CML)
    l. cutis
    embryonal l.
    eosinophilic l.
    granulocytic l.
    Gross l.
    hairy cell l.
    hemoblastic l.
    hemocystoblastic l.
    hemocytoblastic l.
    histiocytic l.
    leukopenic l.
    lymphatic l.
    lymphoblastic l.
    lymphocytic l.
    lymphogenous l.
    lymphoid l.
    lymphoidocytic l.
    lymphosarcoma cell l.
    mast cell l.
    megakaryocytic l.
    micromyeloblastic l.
    monocytic l.
    myeloblastic l.
    myelocytic l.
    myelogenous l.
    myeloid l.
    myeloid granulocytic l.
    myelomonocytic l.
    Naegeli l.
    nonlymphocytic l.
    plasma cell l.
    plasmacytic l.
    prolymphocytic l.
    promyelocytic l.
    reticuloendothelial cell l.
    Rieder cell l.
    Schilling l.

leukemia (continued)
    smoldering l.
    splenomedullary l.
    splenomyelogenous l.
    stem cell l.
    subleukemic l.
    undifferentiated cell l.
leukolymphosarcoma
Leyden
    hemophilia B
Leydig cell
LFT—liver function test
Libman-Sacks
    endocarditis
    syndrome
Liebermeister
    rule
Lignac
    disease
    syndrome
Lignac-Fanconi
    disease
    syndrome
line
    blue l.
    Burton l.
    Clapton l.
    copper l.
    Corrigan l.
    lead l.
linitis
    l. plastica
lipoatrophy
lipodystrophia
    l. progressiva
lipoprotein
    familial high-density l.
      (HDL) deficiency
    high-density l. (HDL)
    intermediate-density l. (IDL)
    l. lipase (LPL)
    low-density l. (LDL)
    Lp(a) l.
    l. metabolism
    very low-density l. (VLDL)
    l. X
lipoprotein lipase (LPL) deficiency,
    familial

lipotropics [a class of drugs]
livedo
    l. reticularis
liver
    amyloid l.
    brimstone l.
    cirrhotic l.
    l. dysfunction
    lardaceous l.
    l. scan
Lloyd syndrome
lobe
    l.'s of thyroid gland
lobectomy
    thyroid l.
lobulation
    portal l.
locus (loci)
    l. minoris resistentiae
Löffler
    eosinophilia
    syndrome
Lorain-Levi dwarf
low-density lipoprotein (LDL)
lues
    l. hepatis
Luft
    disease
    syndrome
lumbago
    ischemic l.
Lund-Browder burn scale
lupus
    discoid l.
    drug-induced l.
    l. erythematosus (LE)
    hydralazine l.
    l. nephritis
    l. pernio
    l. profundus
    systemic l. erythematosus
      (SLE)
luteinizing hormone (LH)
Lyme
    arthritis
    disease
lymphadenectasis
lymphadenhypertrophy

lymphadenia
    l. ossea
lymphadenitis
    caseous l.
    paratuberculous l.
lymphadenocyst
lymphadenopathy
    angioimmunoblastic l.
    angioimmunoblastic l. with
        dysproteinemia (AILD)
    dermatopathic l.
    giant follicular l.
    immunoblastic l.
    subcarinal l.
    tuberculous l.
lymphangiogram
lymphatic
lymphedema
    l. praecox
lymphoblastoma
    giant follicular l.
lymphoglandula (lymphoglandulae)
lymphogranuloma
    l. venereum
lymphoma
    See in *Oncology and Hema-
        tology* section.
lymphomatous
lymphonodus (lymphonodi)
lymphopathia
    l. venereum
lymphosarcoma
    fascicular l.
    Kundrat l.
    lymphocytic l.
    sclerosing l.
lymphosarcomatosis
MAC—*Mycobacterium avium* com-
    plex
Mackenzie
    disease
Macleod
    capsular rheumatism
    syndrome
macrodystrophia
    m. lipomatosa progressiva
macrogenitosomia
    m. praecox

macroglobulinemia
    Waldenström m.
macrosomatia
    m. adiposa congenita
maculation
    pernicious m.
maculopapular
Madelung
    disease
    lipoma
    neck
    syndrome
MAI—*Mycobacterium avium-intra-
    cellulare*
mal
    m. de mer [seasickness]
    m. rouge
maladie
    m. des jambes ["dah zhahb"]
    m. de plongeurs ["duh plaw-
        zhoor"]
malaise
malformation
Malta fever
maneuver
    See also *method.*
    Heimlich m.
Mann
    sign
α-mannosidase [alpha-]
Marañon
    syndrome (I, II, III)
Marburg
    disease
    hemorrhagic fever
marche à petits pas [small steps]
Marchiafava-Micheli
    disease
    syndrome
Marfan
    sign
    syndrome
Marie
    disease
    hypertrophy
    sign
    syndrome (I, II)

Marie-Strümpell
    disease
    spondylitis
·   syndrome
Maroteaux-Lamy
    disease
    syndrome (I, II)
"marsh ah peh-tee pah" Phonetic
    for marche à petits pas.
Marshall
    syndrome
Marsh disease
masculinization
masculinize
masculinizing
mask
    m. facies
    Parkinson m.
mast cell disease
Mathieu disease
maturity
    m.-onset diabetes of the
        young (MODY)
Mauriac
    syndrome
McArdle
    disease
    syndrome
McKenzie
    See *Mackenzie.*
MCT—medullary carcinoma of thy-
    roid
MEA—multiple endocrine adeno-
    matosis
measles
measurement
    skinfold m.'s
MEDAC—multiple endocrine defi-
    ciency–autoimmune candidiasis
mediastinitis
medical
    m. thyroidectomy
medicine
    geriatric m.
    hyperbaric m.
    internal m.
medullated
medullation

medusae
    caput m.
Meige disease
melanoma
    lentigo maligna m.
    malignant m.
    nodular m.
    superficial spreading m.
melanosis
    m. coli
melanotic [pertaining to melanin]
melasma
    m. addisonii
    m. suprarenale
Meleda
    disease
melenemesis
melenic [pertaining to melena,
    blood in the stool]
mellitus
    diabetes m.
membrane
    nuclear m.
MEN—multiple endocrine neoplasia
Ménière
    disease
    syndrome
meningococcemia
meningotyphoid
meniscocytosis
Menkes
    disease
    syndrome
menometrorrhagia
menopause
menorrhagia
menstrual
meralgia
    m. paresthetica
Merseburg triad
mesangiocapillary
mesenteric
    m. adenitis
mesenteritis
metagonimiasis
metamorphosis
    fatty m.
metaphase

metaplasia
  myeloid m.
  pseudopyloric m.
  squamous m.
metastasis (metastases)
methemoglobinemia
  acquired m.
  congenital m.
  hereditary m.
  toxic m.
methemoglobinemic
methemoglobinuria
method
  See also *maneuver.*
  Fick m.
α-methylacetoacetyl CoA thiolase [alpha-]
β-methylcrotonylglycinuria [beta-]
methylene blue
Mibelli
  disease
  syndrome
microadenopathy
microalbuminuria
micronodular
microsplenia
microsplenic
"middle-shmertz" Phonetic for mittelschmerz.
"miel–" Phonetic for words beginning myel–.
migraine
  abdominal m.
  acute confusional m.
  m. without aura
  m. with aura
  basilar m., basilar artery m.
  Bickerstaff m.
  classic m.
  common m.
  complicated m.
  epileptic m.
  familial hemiplegic m.
  fulgurating m.
  hemiplegic m.
  hormonal m.
  menstrual m.
  neurologic m.

migraine (continued)
  ocular m.
  ophthalmic m.
  ophthalmoplegic m.
  retinal m.
migraineur
migrainoid
migrainous
Mikulicz (von Mikulicz)
  disease
  syndrome
Mikulicz-Radecki
  syndrome
Mikulicz-Sjögren
  syndrome
millibar(s) (mb, mbar)
millimeter(s) (mm)
  m.'s of mercury (mm Hg)
  m.'s of water (mm H_2O)
Milton
  disease
  edema
Minamata
  disease
  syndrome
mineralocorticoids [a class of drugs]
"mio–" Phonetic for words beginning myo–.
mitral
  m. insufficiency
  m. regurgitation
  m. stenosis
  m. valve
mittelschmerz [pain with ovulation]
MLNS—mucocutaneous lymph node syndrome
MM—multiple myeloma
mm H_2O [mm H2O]—millimeters of water
Möbius
  disease
  sign
  syndrome (I, II)
MODY—maturity-onset diabetes of the young
Mondor
  disease
  syndrome

Monge
    disease
    syndrome
monitor
    apnea m.
mononucleosis
    infectious m.
monosymptomatic
monotherapy
moon face, moon facies
Moore
    syndrome
morbidity
Morel
    disease
    syndrome
Morel-Wildi syndrome
Morquio
    disease
    sign
    syndrome
Morquio-Brailsford syndrome
Morquio-Ullrich
    disease
    syndrome
Morris syndrome
mosaicism
    XO/XY m.
Moschcowitz
    disease
    sign
    test
Mosse syndrome
M period
MPS—mucopolysaccharidosis
Muckle-Wells
    syndrome
mucolipid
mucolipidosis
mucopolysaccharidosis
    (mucopolysaccharidoses) (MPS)
        m. I–XIII (MPS I–XIII)
        m. IH (MPS I H)
        m. IH/S (MPS I H/S)
        m. IS (MPS I S)
mucopolysacchariduria
mucositis
    m. necroticans agranulocytica

mucoviscidosis
müllerian
    m. duct
    m. mixed tumor
multinodular
multiple sclerosis (MS)
multisystem
    m. disease
Münchausen
    by proxy syndrome
    syndrome
Münchmeyer disease
murmur
    heart m.
muscarine
muscarinic
muscarinism
muscle
    See in *Orthopedics and*
        Sports Medicine section.
musculus (musculi)
    See in *Orthopedics and*
        Sports Medicine section.
mutagen
mutagenesis
mutagenic
mutation
    spontaneous genetic m.
mutism
myalgia
myasthenia
    m. gravis
    m. gravis pseudoparalytica
myasthenic
myatonia
    m. congenita
mycoplasmal
mycosis (mycoses)
    m. fungoides
    Gilchrist m.
    splenic m.
myelinolysis
    central pontine m.
myeloid
myeloidosis
myeloma
    See in *Oncology and Hema-*
        tology section.

myelomatosis
myelosarcoma
myelosarcomatosis
myelosclerosis
myelosis
    aleukemic m.
    aplastic m.
    chronic nonleukemic m.
    erythremic m.
    funicular m.
    nonleukemic m.
myelosuppression
myelosuppressive
myoadenylate (AMP) deaminase
    deficiency
myocardial
    m. contractions
    m. infarction
    m. ischemia
myocarditis
    acute bacterial m.
    acute isolated m.
    chronic m.
    diphtheritic m.
    fibrous m.
    idiopathic m.
    rheumatic m.
    tuberculoid m.
    tuberculous m.
myoedema
myofascial
myoglobinuria
myoglobulinuria
myokymia
myolysis
    m. cardiotoxica
myonecrosis
myopathy
    Cushing disease m.
myositis
    m. ossificans
myringitis
myxadenitis
myxocystoma
myxoma (myxomas, myxomata)
    cystic m.
    m. fibrosum
    m. sarcomatosum

Naegeli
    syndrome
nanism
    Paltauf n.
narcosis
    nitrogen n.
    prolonged n.
NCA—neurocirculatory asthenia
neck
    bull n.
    Madelung n.
    webbed n.
    wry n.
necrobiosis
    n. lipoidica
    n. lipoidica diabeticorum
necrobiotic
necrosis (necroses)
    bland n.
    cold-induced n.
    decubital n.
    focal n.
    mercurial n.
    phosphorus n.
    postpartum pituitary n.
    pressure n.
    quiet n.
    simple n.
    spontaneous n.
necrotic
"nefrosis" Phonetic for nephrosis.
Nelson
    syndrome
nephroptosis
nephropyelitis
nephrosclerosis
nephrosclerotic
nephrosis (nephroses)
nephrotic
nervous
    n. breakdown
nesidiectomy
"neu–" Phonetic for words begin-
    ning pneu–.
neuralgia
    postherpetic n.
neuralgic
neurasthenia

neurastheniac
neurasthenic
neuritic
neuritis
    dietetic n.
    influenzal n.
    rheumatic n.
neuroacanthocytosis
neuroblastoma
neuroendocrinology
neurogenic
    n. bladder
neurolabyrinthitis
neurolathyrism
neuroleptic
neuromyasthenia
neuromyopathic
neuromyositis
neuromyotonia
neuropathy
    diabetic n.
    myxedematous n.
    peripheral n.
neutropenia
    chronic benign n. of child-
        hood
    chronic hypoplastic n.
    congenital n.
    cyclic n.
    familial benign chronic n.
    hypersplenic n.
    idiopathic n.
    Kostmann n.
    malignant n.
    neonatal n., transitory
    periodic n.
    peripheral n.
    primary splenic n.
    transitory neonatal n.
nevus (nevi)
    See in *Dermatology* section.
"new–" Phonetic for words begin-
    ning pneu–.
NIAMD—National Institute of
    Arthritis and Metabolic Diseases
NIDD—non–insulin-dependent dia-
    betes

NIDDM—non–insulin-dependent
    diabetes mellitus
nidus (nidi)
Niemann
    disease
    splenomegaly
nod
    bishop's n.
node
    Bouchard n.
    Heberden n.
    lymph n.
    Osler n.
    Parrot n.
    Schmorl n.
nodular
nodularity
nodulated
nodulation
nodule
    cold n.
    Gamna n.'s
    Gandy-Gamna n.'s
    hot n.
noduli (plural of nodulus)
nodulous [adj.]
nodulus (noduli)
non-anion gap acidosis
nonlymphocytic
Nonne-Milroy-Meige syndrome
nonsteroidal anti-inflammatory drugs
    (NSAIDs) [a class of drugs]
"noo–" Phonetic for words begin-
    ning pneu–.
Noonan syndrome
norepinephrine
Norman-Wood syndrome
NPH—neutral protamine Hagedorn
    (insulin)
NSAIA—nonsteroidal anti-inflam-
    matory agent
NSAID, NSAIDs—nonsteroidal
    anti-inflammatory drug(s) [a
    class of drugs]
NSHD—nodular sclerosing Hodg-
    kin disease
NTG—nontoxic goiter

"nu–" Phonetic for words beginning pneu–.
nucleoprotein
"nur–" Phonetic for words beginning neur–.
NYHA (New York Heart Association) classification (I–IV)
O_2 [O2]—oxygen
OA—osteoarthritis
obesity
    adrenocortical o.
    adult-onset o.
    alimentary o.
    endogenous o.
    exogenous o.
    hyperinsulinar o.
    o. of hyperinsulinism
    hyperplastic-hypertrophic o.
    hypertrophic o.
    hypoplasmic o.
    hypothalamic o.
    hypothyroid o.
    lifelong o.
    morbid o.
    simple o.
obstructive
    o. sleep apnea (OSA)
"ofthal–" Phonetic for words beginning ophthal–.
OGTT—oral glucose tolerance test
Ohara
    disease
oleandrism
oligodipsia
oligophrenia
    phenylpyruvic o.
oligophrenic
oligoptyalism
omentitis
omphalophlebitis
omphalorrhagia
omphalorrhea
oophoritis
    o. parotidea
operation
    See in *General Surgical Terms.*
ophthalmic Graves disease

ophthalmoplegia
    diabetic o.
    hyperthyroid o.
    thyrotoxic o.
Opitz
    disease
    syndrome
Ormond
    disease
os (ossa) [bone]
    See in *Orthopedics and Sports Medicine* section.
OSAS—obstructive sleep apnea syndrome
Osler
    disease
    nodes
    sign
    syndrome II
    triad
Osler-Vaquez
    disease
Osler-Weber-Rendu
    disease
    syndrome
osteitis
    o. deformans
    o. fibrosa cystica
osteoarthritis
    o. deformans
    o. deformans endemica
    endemic o.
    erosive o.
    hyperplastic o.
    hypertrophic o.
    interphalangeal o.
    primary generalized hypertrophic o.
osteochondrodysplasia
osteochondrodystrophia
    o. deformans
osteochondrodystrophy
    o. familial
osteodystrophy
    Albright hereditary o.
    parathyroid o.
    renal o.

osteogenesis
    endochondral o.
    o. imperfecta (OI), types I–IV
    o. imperfecta congenita (OIC)
    o. imperfecta cystica
    o. imperfecta tarda (OIT)
    periosteal o.
osteomalacic
osteonecrosis
osteopenia
osteopetrosis
osteophagia
osteoporosis
osteoporotic
ostia (plural of ostium)
ostial [pertaining to opening, aperture, orifice]
ostium (ostia)
    o. primum
    o. secundum
ostreotoxism
otorrhea
overhydration
overload
    iron o.
overtransfusion
overweight
Owren
    deficiency
    disease
oxalate
oxalosis
oximeter
    finger o.
    pulse o.
oximetry
    finger o.
    pulse o.
oxygen (O)
    high-pressure o.
    hyperbaric o. (HBO)
    molecular o. (O_2) [O2])
oxygenation
    apneic o.
    hyperbaric o.
Paget-von Schroetter syndrome
pagophagia

"pake–" Phonetic for words beginning pachy–.
paleospinothalamic
    p. tract
pallor
palpation
palpitation
palsy
    Bell p.
Paltauf dwarf
PAN—periarteritis nodosa
pancreas (pancreata)
    aberrant p.
    p. accessorium
    accessory p.
    annular p.
    divided p.
    p. divisum
    lesser p.
    unciform p.
    Willis p.
    Winslow p.
pancreatic
pancreatis (genitive of pancreas)
pancytopenia
    congenital p.
    Fanconi p.
panneuritis
    p. epidemica
panniculalgia
para
    p.-hydroxyphenylpyruvic acid (PHPPA)
paradoxic, paradoxical
paraganglion (paraganglia)
    adrenergic p.
    aortic p.
    cardiac p.
    cholinergic p.
paralysis (paralyses)
    p. agitans
    alcoholic p.
    arsenical p.
    Bell p.
    diver's p.
    familial hyperkalemic periodic p.

paralysis (paralyses) (continued)
  familial hypokalemic periodic p.
  hyperkalemic periodic p.
  hypokalemic periodic p.
  lead p.
  narcosis p.
  normokalemic periodic p.
  p. notariorum
  occupational p.
  periodic p., thyrotoxic
  pressure p.
  serum p.
  tourniquet p.
  Vernet p.
parameningeal
paramyotonia
  p. congenita
paraplegia
parasite
  See specific parasites in
  *Laboratory, Pathology,
  and Chemistry Terms.*
paraspinal
parathormone (PTH)
parathyroid
parathyroidectomy (PTX)
parathyroidoma
parathyroprival
parathyroprivia
parenchymatous disease
paresis
paresthesia
Parkinson
  complex
  crisis
  disease
  facies
  mask
  rigidity
  sign
  syndrome
parkinsonian
parkinsonism
  drug-induced p.
  postencephalitic p.
  postencephalitis p.
  primary p.

parkinsonism (continued)
  secondary p.
  vascular p.
parotitis
  p. phlegmonosa
Parrot [eponym]
  disease
parrot
  p. tongue
Parry
  disease
pars (partes)
Parsons disease
Paterson
  syndrome
Paterson-Brown-Kelly
  syndrome
Paterson-Kelly
  syndrome
pathema (pathemas, pathemata)
pathogen
  See specific pathogens in
  *Laboratory, Pathology,
  and Chemistry Terms.*
pathologic, pathological
Patterson
  See *Paterson.*
Pavy
  disease
Payr
  disease
  sign
PBC—primary biliary cirrhosis
PD—Parkinson disease
PDR—proliferative diabetic retinopathy
Pecquet
  cistern
  duct
  reservoir
pectus
  p. excavatum
Pel-Ebstein
  disease
  fever
  pyrexia
  symptom
Pelger nuclear anomaly

pellagra
  p. sine pellagra
  typhoid p.
pemphigus
  p. erythematosus
  p. foliaceus
  p. neonatorum
  p. vegetans
  p. vulgaris
Pendred
  disease
  syndrome
penicilli (plural of penicillus)
penicilliary
penicillus (penicilli)
  penicilli arteriae lienalis
  penicilli arteriae splenicae
Pepper [eponym]
  neuroblastoma
  syndrome
  type
periarteritis
  p. nodosa
period
  G_2 p. [G2]
peripheral
  p. vasodilators [a class of
    drugs]
peritoneum
perityphlitis
Perthes
  test
pesticemia
pestilential
pestis
  p. ambulans
  p. bubonica
  p. siderans
Pfeiffer
  disease
Pfuhl
  sign
PG—prostaglandin
PGE_2 [PGE2]—prostaglandin E_2
PGH—pituitary growth hormone
PGL—persistent generalized lymphadenopathy

phenomenon (phenomena)
  See also *effect* and *reaction*.
  anaphylactoid p.
  Becker p.
  Danysz p.
  dawn p.
  fall-and-rise p.
  first-set p.
  halisteresis p.
  Hecht p.
  Hering p.
  Leede-Rumpel p.
  LE (lupus erythematosus)
    cell p.
  Lucio p.
  paradoxical diaphragm p.
  Raynaud p.
  Rumpel-Leede p.
  second-set p.
  Somogyi p.
  Staub-Traugott p.
phenylketonuria (PKU)
  p. II
  p. III
  atypical p.
  maternal p.
Philadelphia chromosome
phlebitis
phosphate
phosphatidosis
photon
photophobia
photoscan
phototherapy
PHP—primary hyperparathyroidism
      pseudohypoparathyroidism
phthisis
  diabetic p.
  p. pancreatica
physiologic, physiological
phytanic acid α-hydroxylase [alpha-]
piarhemia
Pick [eponym]
  adenoma
  atrophy
  cell
  disease
  syndrome

pickwickian syndrome
piggyback
piggybacking
pill-rolling
pineal
pink disease
pink puffer [emphysema]
pityriasis
    p. alba
    p. lichenoides et varioliformis
    p. rosea
    p. rubra pilaris
pleurocholecystitis
pleurohepatitis
plumbism
plumbotherapy
Plummer
    disease
    sign
Plummer-Vinson
    syndrome
PMR—polymyalgia rheumatica
pneumonia
    pneumococcal p.
    Pneumocystis carinii p. (PCP)
Pneumovax
    P. 23
PNI—Prognostic Nutritional Index
pO$_2$ [pO2]—partial pressure of oxygen
podagra
podagral
point
    trigger p.
poison
    puffer p.
    shellfish p.
poison control center (PCC)
poisoning
    beryllium p.
    mushroom p.
poliomyelitis
    bulbar p.
pollinosis
polyarteritis
    p. nodosa
polyarthritis
polyarthropathy

polyarthrosis
polychondritis
polychondropathia
polychondropathy
polycythemia
    p. hypertonica
    inappropriate p.
    myelopathic p.
    primary p.
    relative p.
    p. rubra
    p. rubra vera
    secondary p.
    splenomegalic p.
    spurious p.
    stress p.
    p. vera
polydipsia
polyendocrinopathy
polymyalgia
    p. rheumatica
polymyositis
    trichinous p.
polyneuritis
    acute febrile p.
    acute idiopathic p.
    acute infective p.
    acute postinfectious p.
    alcoholic p.
    anemic p.
    ascending p.
    p. cerebralis menieriformis
    cranial p.
    diabetic p.
    endemic p., p. endemica
    p. gallinarum
    Guillain-Barré p.
    infectious p.
    Jamaica ginger p.
    postinfectious p.
    p. potatorum
    progressive hypertrophic p.
    triorthocresyl phosphate p.
polyneuropathy
    erythredema p.
    uremic p.
polyopsia
polyostotic

polyphagia
polyposis
    p. coil syndrome
polyuria
Pompe disease
Poncet
    disease
    rheumatism
pork insulin
Posada-Wernicke disease
postmastectomy
Pott
    gangrene
    syndrome (I, II)
Poulet disease
PPBS—postprandial blood sugar
PPD—purified protein derivative
    (of tuberculin)
PPD-S—purified protein deriva-
    tive–standard
PPV—positive-pressure ventilation
precipitous
    p. drop [in blood pressure or
      laboratory indices]
    p. rise [in blood pressure or
      laboratory indices]
precocious
precocity
principal [primary, main]
    p. aspect
    p. reason
    p. symptom
principle [rule]
proctalgia
    p. fugax
proctitis
    epidemic gangrenous p.
profound
    p. anemia
prolactin
prostaglandin (PG)
    See also in *Laboratory,*
      Pathology, and Chemistry
      Terms.
    p. E_2 [E2] (PGE_2)
prostaglandins [a class of drugs]
protein
    Bence Jones p.

proteinemia
    Bence Jones p.
    broad-beta p.
    floating-beta p.
proteinosis
    lipoid p.
    tissue p.
proteinuria
    Bence Jones p.
    orthostatic p.
prothrombin
prune-belly syndrome
pruritus
    p. ani
pseudoacanthosis
    p. nigricans
pseudohemophilia
    p. hepatica
pseudo-Hurler
    disease
    polydystrophy
pseudoleukemia
    p. lymphatica
pseudoxanthoma
    p. elasticum
psilosis
psittacosis
psoas
    p. sign
psychogenic
PTH—parathyroid hormone
    post-transfusion hepatitis
PTHS—parathyroid hormone secre-
    tion [rate]
PTM—post-transfusion mononucle-
    osis
PTT—partial thromboplastin time
PTU—propylthiouracil
PTX—parathyroidectomy
puberty
    delayed p.
    precocious p.
PUD—peptic ulcer disease
puffer
    chubby p. syndrome
    pink p. [emphysema]
pulmonary
    p. toilet

pulseless
　　p. disease
pulsus (pulsus)
　　p. alternans
　　p. paradoxus
purge
purging
　　bingeing and p.
purpura
　　p. cachectica
　　cocktail p.
　　dependent nonthrombocy-
　　　　topenic p.
　　p. hemorrhagica
　　hypergammaglobulinemic p.
　　hyperglobulinemic p.
　　p. hyperglobulinemica
　　idiopathic p.
　　idiopathic thrombocytopenic
　　　　p. (ITP)
　　Landouzy p.
　　nonpalpable p.
　　nonthrombocytopenic p.
　　orthostatic p.
　　palpable p.
　　p. rheumatica
　　secondary thrombocytopenic
　　　　p.
　　senile p., p. senilis
　　p. simplex
　　steroid p.
　　symptomatic p., p. sympto-
　　　　matica
　　thrombocytopenic p. (TP)
　　p. thrombolytica
　　thrombopenic p.
　　thrombotic p.
　　thrombotic thrombocytope-
　　　　nic p.
　　thrombotic thrombohemolyt-
　　　　ic p.
　　p. variolosa
　　vascular p.
　　Waldenström hyperglobu-
　　　　linemic p.
pustule
pyemia
　　arterial p.

pyemia (continued)
　　cryptogenic p.
pyomyositis
　　tropical p.
pyrazolopyrimidines [a class of
　　drugs]
pyrexia (pyrexiae)
　　heat p.
　　Pel-Ebstein p.
pyrexial
pyrogen
pyuria
　　abacterial p.
PZI—protamine zinc insulin
Quincke
　　angioedema
　　disease
　　edema
　　puncture
　　I syndrome
RA—rheumatoid arthritis
radiation
　　r. hepatitis
　　ionizing r.
　　r. necrosis
　　nonionizing r.
　　occupational r.
　　photochemical r.
　　r. sickness
　　r. syndrome
radioallergosorbent
radionuclide
radioreceptor
rale
　　See in *Pulmonary Medicine*
　　　　section.
Ramond
　　point
　　sign
Ranson criteria [for severity of
　　acute pancreatitis]
ranula
　　pancreatic r.
ratio
　　ketogenic-antiketogenic
　　　　(K/A) r.
Raymond
　　See also *Ramond.*

Raymond (continued)
    apoplexy
Raynaud
    disease
    gangrene
    phenomenon
    syndrome
RDS—respiratory distress syndrome
reaction
    See also *effect* and *phenomenon.*
    Mantoux r.
    Weil-Felix r.
receptor
    adrenergic r.
    α-adrenergic r.'s [alpha-]
    β-adrenergic r.'s [beta-]
    alpha r.'s
    beta r.'s
    histamine H_1 r. [H1]
    histamine H_2 r. [H2]
    insulin r.'s
    low-density lipoprotein
        (LDL) r.'s
    progesterone r.
    volume r.'s
Recklinghausen (von Recklinghausen)
    disease
    disease, central, type II
    disease of bone
Recklinghausen-Appelbaum
Reclus disease
rectum
Reed-Hodgkin disease
reflex
    See also *phenomenon, sign,*
        and *test.*
    See also in *Neurology and
        Pain Management* section.
    Somogyi r.
refractory
    r. anemia
    r. illness
Refsum
    disease
    syndrome

regurgitation
    aortic r.
Reichmann
    disease
    syndrome
Reiter
    disease
    syndrome
renal
    r. transplant
    r. transplantation
Rendu-Osler-Weber
    disease
    syndrome
resection
    block r.
resistance
    insulin r.
resonance
    hydatid r.
    tympanic r.
    tympanitic r.
    vesiculotympanic r.
    wooden r.
respiration
    See also in the *Pulmonary
        Medicine* section.
    Cheyne-Stokes r.
    Kussmaul r.
response
    Arthus r.
resuscitation
retching
reticula (plural of reticulum)
reticuloendotheliosis
    leukemic r.
reticuloendothelium
reticulohistiocytoma
reticulum (reticula)
    endoplasmic r.
    sarcoplasmic r.
retinal
    r. detachment
retroperitoneal
rheumatic
    r. heart disease
rheumatism
    Heberden r.

rheumatism (continued)
    MacLeod capsular r.
    Poncet r.
rheumatoid
    r. arthritis
rhonchus (rhonchi)
    See in the *Pulmonary Medi-cine* section.
RIA—radioimmunoassay
Richards-Rundle syndrome
Richner-Hanhart syndrome
rickets
Riedel
    disease
    struma
    thyroiditis
Riley-Day
    dysautonomia
    syndrome
Rimbaud-Passouant-Vallat syndrome
ring
    Kayser-Fleischer r.
    Schatzki r.
robertsonian translocation
Roger
    reaction
    symptom
Rokitansky
    disease
    diverticulum
Romaña sign
Romberg sign
"rongk–" Phonetic for words begin-ning rhonch–.
Rosenbach
    sign
Rosenthal
    syndrome
roseoliform
    r. exanthem
roseolus
Roth
    spots
Rothmann-Makai
    syndrome
Rotor
    syndrome

RR-HPO—rapid recompression–high-pressure oxygen
RTA—renal tubular acidosis
rubelliform
rubra
Rud
    syndrome
Rumpel-Leede
    phenomenon
    sign
    test
Rundles-Falls
    anemia
    syndrome
Runeberg
    anemia
    disease
    type
rupia
rupial
rupioid
Rust [eponym]
    disease
    phenomenon
    sign
    syndrome
SAA—severe aplastic anemia
sacculated
sacculi (genitive and plural of sac-culus)
sacculiform
sacculus (sacculi)
    sacculi of Beale
saddleback fever
salicylates [a class of drugs]
salicylism
"samo–" Phonetic for beginning psammo–.
Sandhoff disease
Sanfilippo
    disease
    syndrome
sanies (sanies)
sarcoid
    Darier-Roussy s.
sarcoidosis
    beryllium s.

sarcoma (sarcomas, sarcomata)
    See also in *Oncology and Hematology* section.
    glandular s.
    idiopathic multiple pigmented hemorrhagic s.
    Kaposi s.
sarcomatoid
sarcomatous
sarcosinemia
Saunders
    disease
SBE—subacute bacterial endocarditis
SC—sickle cell
scale
    Karnofsky s.
    Lund-Browder burn s.
scalenus anticus syndrome
scan
    See also in *Radiology, Nuclear Medicine, and Other Imaging* section.
    thyroid s.
scarlatina
SCAT—sickle cell anemia test
Schaumann
    bodies
    disease
    sarcoid, sarcoidosis
    syndrome
Schirmer test
schistosomiasis
    cutaneous s.
    hepatic s.
Schmidt
    diet
    syndrome
Schmorl
    node
Schottmüller (Schottmueller)
    disease
    fever
Schüffner
    dots
Schüller
    disease
    syndrome

Schüller-Christian
    disease
    syndrome
Schultz
    angina
Schultze
    acroparesthesia
Schultze-type acroparesthesia
Schwachman syndrome
schwannoma
Schwartz-Bartter syndrome
SCIDS—severe combined immunodeficiency syndrome
scintillating scotoma
scleradenitis
scleritis
sclerodactylia
    s. annularis ainhumoides
sclerogenous
sclérose en plaques
sclerosis
    amyotrophic lateral s. (ALS)
    multiple s. (MS)
scoleciasis
scotodinia
scotoma (scotomata)
scrofula
scurvy
sed rate—sedimentation rate
"sefa–" Phonetic for words beginning cepha–.
Seip-Lawrence
    syndrome
Selye
    adaptation syndrome
    syndrome
seminome
Senear-Usher
    disease
    syndrome
senile
    s. cataract
    s. dementia
sensorium
    general s.
sensory
    s. deficit

sepsis
    s. lenta
    puerperal s.
septicophlebitis
septicopyemia
septic shock
serositis (serositides)
    adhesive s.
    multiple serositides
serous
serpiginous
serum (serums, sera)
    anticrotalus s.
    antirabies s.
    antitoxic s.
    s. sickness
"sfero–" Phonetic for words beginning sphero–.
Shaver disease
Sheehan
    disease
    syndrome
shelf
    Blumer s.
shingles
shock
    burn s.
    electric s.
    hemorrhagic s.
    hypoglycemic s.
    hypovolemic s.
    insulin s.
    irreversible s.
    postoperative s.
    septic s.
    traumatic s.
"shogren" Phonetic for Sjögren.
"shov-stek," "shvo-stek" Phonetic for Chvostek.
Shwachman-Diamond syndrome
"shwah-no-mah" Phonetic for schwannoma.
sialadenitis
sialidosis
sialoadenitis
sialoangiitis
sialometaplasia

sialorrhea
    s. pancreatica
sickle cell
    s.c. anemia
    s.c. disease
    s.c. trait
sickness
    high-altitude s.
    motion s.
Sidbury syndrome
sideroblastic
"sifilis" Phonetic for syphilis.
"sifilo–" Phonetic for words beginning syphilo–.
sigmoidoscopy
Sigmund glands
sign
    See also *phenomenon, reflex,* and *test.*
    Ballance s.
    Ballet s.
    Barré s.
    Becker s.
    Blumberg s.
    Boston s.
    Bozzolo s.
    Burton s.
    cardinal s.'s (of inflammation)
    Carnett s.
    Chilaiditi s.
    cogwheel s.
    commemorative s.
    Cope s.
    Corrigan s.
    Courvoisier s.
    Cowen s.
    Cullen s.
    Dalrymple s.
    d'Espine s.
    Dixon Mann s.
    Duchenne s.
    Duckworth s.
    Enroth s.
    Erb s.
    Federici s.
    Gilbert s.
    Goggia s.
    Gorlin s.

sign (continued)
    Graefe (von Graefe) s.
    Grey Turner s.
    Griffith s.
    Grocco s.
    Gubler s.
    Gunn s.
    Guyon s.
    Heberden s.'s
    Homans s.
    Horn s.
    Hoyne s.
    Jendrassik s.
    jugular s.
    Kehr s.
    Kernig s.
    Knies s.
    Kocher s.
    Lennhoff s.
    Livierato s.
    Lucas s.
    Mann s.
    Marie s.
    McBurney s.
    Means s.
    Möbius s.
    Myerson s.
    Nikolsky s.
    objective s.'s
    obturator s.
    Osler s.
    Parkinson s.
    Pemberton s.
    Pfuhl s.
    physical s.'s
    Plummer s.
    pseudo-Graefe s.
    psoas s.
    puddle s.
    Quant s.
    Riesman s.
    Robertson s.
    Rommelaere s.
    Rovsing s.
    Rumpel-Leede s.
    setting-sun s.
    Simon s.
    Snellen s.

sign (continued)
    soft s.'s
    spinal s.
    Stellwag s.
    Sternberg s.
    Strauss s.
    subjective s.'s
    Suker s.
    Sumner s.
    Troisier s.
    Turner s.
    Unschuld s.
    vital s.'s
    Wilder s.
"sike–" Phonetic for words beginning psych–.
silicatosis
siliconoma
silicosis
silicotuberculosis
"silosis" Phonetic for psilosis.
Simmonds
    disease
    syndrome
Simon
    disease
simultanagnosia
sin–. See also words beginning cin–, syn–.
sinus (sinus, sinuses)
    draining s.
    lymph s.'s, lymphatic s.'s
    marginal s., s. marginalis
    medullary s.'s
    traumatic s.
Sipple syndrome
"sitakosis" Phonetic for psittacosis.
β-sitosterolemia [beta-]
situs (situs)
    s. solitus
Sjögren
    disease
    syndrome
"skis–" Phonetic for words beginning schis–.
"sklero–" Phonetic for words beginning sclero–.
SLE—systemic lupus erythematosus

sleep apnea
  obstructive s.a. (OSA)
  s.a. syndrome
Smith-Strang disease
SOB—shortness of breath
SOD—superoxide dismutase [now: orgotein]
somatization
somatotropin
somnambulism
Somogyi
  effect
  phenomenon
  reflex
sonofluoroscopy
"soo-chee," "soo-shee" Phonetic for sushi.
"soo-fl," "soo-flay" Phonetic for souffle.
sore
  bed s.
  pressure s.
souffle
  splenic s.
sound
  Korotkoff s.
spasticity
spectrum (spectra)
  broad-s. antibiotic
  fortification s.
S period
spermatogenesis
spherocytosis
sphingolipidosis
  cerebral s.
  late-onset cerebral s.
spinocerebellar
spleen
  accessory s.
  Gandy-Gamna s.
  lardaceous s.
splenadenoma
splenalgia
splenatrophy
splenauxe
splenculus
splenectasis
splenelcosis

splenemia
splenemphraxis
spleneolus
splenepatitis
splenetic
splenic
  s. flexure syndrome
splenicterus
splenitis
  spodogenous s.
splenocolic
splenocyte
splenodynia
splenogenous
splenogram
splenogranulomatosis
  s. siderotica
splenography
splenohepatomegaly
splenokeratosis
splenolymphatic
splenolysin
splenolysis
splenoma
splenomalacia
splenomedullary
splenomcgaly
  Gaucher s.
  hemolytic s.
  hypercholesterolemic s.
  myclophthisic s.
  Niemann s.
  siderotic s.
  spodogenous s.
splenometry
splenomyelogenous
splenomyelomalacia
splenonephric
splenonephroptosis
splenoparectasis
splenophrenic
splenoptosis
splenorrhagia
splenotoxin
splenotyphoid
splenulus
splinter
  s. hemorrhage

spondylarthritis
spondylitis
    von Bechterew-Strümpell s.
sporotrichotic
spot
    café au lait s.
    epigastric s.
    Janeway s.
    Roth s.'s
    shin s.
    trigger s.
SSS—sick sinus syndrome
ST—survival time
stadium (stadia)
    s. acmes
    s. augmenti
    s. caloris
    s. decrementi
    s. defervescentiae
    s. fluorescentiae
    s. frigoris
    s. incrementi
    s. invasionis
    s. sudoris
stage
    Tanner s.
staging
    TNM (tumor, node, metasta-
      sis) s.
St. Anthony's
    disease
    fire
stasis syndrome
statins [a class of drugs]
status
    s. asthmaticus
    s. calcifames
    s. choleraicus
    s. degenerativus
    s. epilepticus
    s. lymphaticus
    nutrition s.
    s. parathyroprivus
    s. praesens
    s. thymicolymphaticus
    s. thymicus
steal
    s. syndrome

steatorrhea
Steinbrinck anomaly
Stein-Leventhal syndrome
Stellwag sign
stenosis (stenoses)
    pulmonic s.
Sternberg
    disease
    giant cells
sternutatio
    s. convulsiva
stigma (stigmas, stigmata)
    malpighian s.'s
stigmatic
stigmatism
stigmatization
Still
    disease
Stokes
    collar
Stokes-Adams
    attack
stomatitis (stomatitides)
    acute necrotizing s.
    allergic s.
    angular s.
    aphthobullous s.
    s. aphthosa
    aphthous s.
    s. arsenicalis
    bismuth s.
    catarrhal s.
    contact s.
    denture s.
    epidemic s.
    epizootic s.
    erythematopultaceous s.
    s. exanthematica
    fusospirochetal s.
    gangrenous s.
    gonococcal s.
    gonorrheal s.
    herpetic s.
    infectious s.
    s. intertropica
    lead s.
    s. medicamentosa
    membranous s.

stomatitis (stomatitides) (continued)
    mercurial s.
    mycotic s.
    necrotizing ulcerative s.
    s. nicotina
    nonspecific s.
    s. prosthetica
    recurrent aphthous s.
    s. scarlatina
    s. scorbutica
    syphilitic s.
    traumatic s.
    tropical s.
    ulcerative s.
    uremic s.
    s. venenata
    vesicular s.
    Vincent s.
    vulcanite s.
stomatocytosis
stool
    s. guaiac
strabismus
strata (plural of stratum)
stratiform
stratum (strata)
    s. corneum
streptococcal groups A, B, G
streptolysin
    s. O
streptozyme test
stria (striae)
striatal
stroke
    exertional heat s.
    heat s.
    sun s. [pref: sunstroke]
struma
    s. basedowificata
    Hashimoto s.
    s. lymphomatosa
    s. ovarii
    Riedel s.
Strümpell
    disease
Stuart-Bras
    disease
    syndrome

Stuart-Prower factor deficiency disease
stupor
    benign s.
    Cairns s.
    catatonic s.
stuporous
St. Vitus dance
subaortic
subarachnoid
subcu, subq—subcutaneous
subcutaneous
subdural
subphrenic
substrate
subtle
sucrosemia
"sudo–" Phonetic for words beginning pseudo–.
SUDS—sudden unexplained death syndrome
Suker
    sign
sulfhemoglobinemia
sulfonylureas [a class of drugs]
sunstroke
superoxide
sushi
sustentaculum (sustentacula)
    s. lienis
"sut-el" Phonetic for subtle.
Sutton-Rendu-Osler-Weber
    syndrome
Swift disease
Swyer
    syndrome
Symmers
    disease
sympathochromaffin
symptom
    See also in *General Medical Terms.*
    accessory s.
    acute on chronic s.'s
    assident s.
    cardinal s.
    concomitant s.
    consecutive s.

symptom (continued)
    constitutional s.
    direct s.
    equivocal s.
    factitious s.
    localizing s.'s
    negative s.
    objective s.
    presenting s.
    rational s.
    reflex s.
    static s.
    subjective s.
    sympathetic s.
    systemic s.
syn–. See also words beginning
    cin–, sin–.
synapsis
syncope
    carotid sinus s.
    cough s.
    defecation s.
    deglutition s.
    micturition s.
    tussive s.
    vasovagal s.
syndrome
    See also *disease.*
    Abderhalden-Fanconi s.
    Abercrombie s.
    Achard-Thiers s.
    acquired immunodeficiency
      s. (AIDS)
    Adams-Stokes s.
    addisonian s.
    adrenogenital s.
    Ahumada-del Castillo s.
    Albers-Schönberg s.
    Albright s.
    Albright-McCune-Sternberg
      s.
    alcohol withdrawal s.
    Aldrich s.
    Alzheimer s.
    androgenital s.
    anginal s.
    anorexia-cachexia s.
    aortic arch s.

syndrome (continued)
    Arakawa-Higashi s.
    argentaffinoma s.
    Arias s.
    Ascher s.
    Ayerza s.
    Baber s.
    Banff s.
    Bar s.
    Bard-Pick s.
    Barlow s.
    Bartter s.
    Bartter-Schwartz s.
    basal cell nevus s.
    Bassen-Kornzweig s.
    Bearn-Kunkel s.
    Bearn-Kunkel-Slater s.
    Behçet s.
    Bernard s.
    Bernard-Horner s.
    Bernard-Sergent s.
    Bloom s.
    Blum s.
    Boerhaave s.
    Bouillaud s.
    Brennemann s.
    Brunsting s.
    Budd-Chiari s.
    burning feet s.
    Caplan s.
    carcinoid s.
    Cassidy s.
    Cassidy-Scholte s.
    cervical rib s.
    cervicobrachial s.
    Charcot s.
    Chauffard s.
    Chauffard-Still s.
    Chédiak-Higashi s.
    Chiari-Frommel s.
    Chinese restaurant s. (CRS)
    chorioretinopathy and pitu-
      itary dysfunction (CPD) s.
    chubby puffer s.
    Clarke-Hadfield s.
    Conn s.
    CPD (chorioretinopathy and
      pituitary dysfunction) s.

syndrome (continued)
    Cruveilhier-Baumgarten s.
    Cushing s.
    Cushing s. medicamentosus
    defibrination s.
    Degos s.
    Di Guglielmo s.
    DIDMOAD s.
    Dresbach s.
    dysglandular s.
    ectopic ACTH s.
    Ehlers-Danlos s.
    endocrine polyglandular s.
    Evans s.
    Faber s.
    Fanconi s.
    Felty s.
    Fiessinger-Leroy-Reiter s.
    Fitz s.
    Fitz-Hugh–Curtis s.
    Forbes Albright s.
    Friedmann vasomotor s.
    Gaisböck s.
    galactorrhea-amenorrhea s.
    Gardner s.
    Glanzmann s.
    Goodpasture s.
    Gopalan s.
    Gordon s.
    Gradenigo s.
    Guillain-Barré s.
    Gunther s.
    gynecomastia-aspermato-
      genesis s.
    Hamman-Rich s.
    Harris s.
    Hartnup s.
    Hayem-Widal s.
    Heerfordt s.
    Heidenhain s.
    hemopleuropneumonic s.
    Hench-Rosenberg s.
    Henoch-Schönlein s.
    hepatorenal s.
    Hermansky-Pudlak s.
    Hines-Bannick s.
    Horton s.
    Hunter s.

syndrome (continued)
    Hurler s.
    hydralazine lupus s.
    hyperventilation s.
    hyperviscosity s.
    Imerslund s.
    Imerslund-Graesbeck s.
    Imerslund-Najman-Graes-
      beck s.
    s. of inappropriate antidi-
      uretic hormone (SIADH)
      secretion
    Job s.
    Kallmann s.
    Kartagener s.
    Kawasaki s.
    Kimmelstiel-Wilson s.
    Kleine-Levin s.
    Klinefelter s.
    Kocher s.
    König s.
    Laron s.
    Launois s.
    Launois-Cléret s.
    Laurence-Biedl s.
    Laurence-Moon s.
    Laurence-Moon-Biedl s.
    Läwen-Roth s.
    lazy leukocyte s. (LLS)
    leopard s., LEOPARD s.
    Leriche s.
    Lesch-Nyhan s.
    Lignac s.
    Lignac-Fanconi s.
    Löffler s.
    Löwe s.
    Luft s.
    lymphoproliferative s.
    Macleod s.
    malabsorption s.
    male Turner s.
    malignant hyperthermia s.
    Marchiafava-Micheli s.
    Marfan s.
    Marie s. (I, II)
    Maroteaux-Lamy s.
    MEN s.
    Ménière s.

syndrome (continued)
    Mikulicz s.
    Mikulicz-Radecki s.
    Mikulicz-Sjögren s.
    Minkowski-Chauffard s.
    Morquio s.
    Muckle-Wells s.
    multiple endocrine neoplasia
      (MEN) s.
    Münchausen s.
    Nelson s.
    neurocutaneous s.
    nevoid basaloma s.
    Noonan s.
    Osler s.
    Paget-von Schroetter s.
    pancreatic insufficiency s.
    pancreaticohepatic s.
    Parkinson s.
    parkinsonian s.
    Paterson s.
    Paterson-Brown-Kelly s.
    Paterson-Kelly s.
    pickwickian s.
    Plummer-Vinson s.
    polyglandular s.
    polyposis coli s.
    postcholecystectomy s.
    post-lumbar puncture s.
    postperfusion s.
    post-transfusion s.
    Prader-Willi s.
    primary fibromyalgia s.
    prune-belly s.
    Reifenstein s.
    Reiter s.
    Rénon-Delille s.
    restless legs s.
    Reye s.
    Rh-null s.
    Richter s.
    Riley-Day s.
    Romberg-Paessler s.
    Rosenbach s.
    Rothmann-Makai s.
    Rotor s.
    Rovsing s.
    rubella s.

syndrome (continued)
    Rud s.
    runting s.
    Sanfilippo s.
    scalenus s.
    scalenus anticus s.
    Schaumann s.
    Scheie s.
    Schmidt s.
    s. of sea-blue histiocytes
    Senear-Usher s.
    Sézary s.
    Sjögren s.
    sleep apnea s.
    stasis s.
    steal s.
    Stein-Leventhal s.
    Stevens-Johnson s.
    Strachan-Scott s.
    Sutton-Rendu-Osler-Weber s.
    Takayasu s.
    thoracic outlet s.
    Tietze s.
    toxic shock s.
    transfusion s.
    Troisier s.
    Troisier-Hanot-Chauffard s.
    Turner s.
    Turner s., male
    Vernet s.
    von Hippel-Lindau s.
    Wallenberg s.
    Waterhouse-Friderichsen s.
    Weil s.
    Weinstein s.
    Wermer s.
    Werner s.
    Willebrand s.
    Wiskott-Aldrich s.
    withdrawal s.
    Wolfram s.
synthesis
    DNA s.
    protein s.
system
    kallikrein-kinin s.
    TNM (tumor, node, metasta-
      sis) staging s.

systemic
>s. lupus erythematosus (SLE)

systolic

T_3 [T3]—triiodothyronine [test]

T_4 [T4]—thyroxine [test]

tabes
>diabetic t.
>
>t. dorsalis

tabetic

tachyarrhythmias

Takahara disease

Takayasu
>arteritis
>
>pulseless disease
>
>syndrome

tamponade

Tangier disease

TAO—thromboangiitis obliterans

tardive
>t. akathisia
>
>t. dyskinesia (TD)
>
>t. dystonia

Tay-Sachs disease

TB—tuberculosis

TBG—thyroxine-binding globulin

TBII—thyrotropin-binding inhibitory immunoglobulin

TBP—thyroxine-binding protein

TBSA—total body surface area

TDA—TSH-displacing antibody

technique
>See *maneuver* and *method.*

TED, T.E.D. (thromboembolic disease) [T.E.D. is trademark form]
>hose
>
>stockings

telalgia

telangiectasis (telangiectases)
>spider t.
>
>stellate t.

telangiitis

telangion

template

tendinitis

test
>See also in *Laboratory, Pathology, and Chemistry Terms.*

test (continued)
>alpha-fetoprotein (AFP) t.
>
>cellophane tape t.
>
>diabetes t.
>
>doll's eye t.
>
>estrogen receptor assay (ERA) t.
>
>glucose tolerance t. (GTT)
>
>glycosylated hemoglobin t.
>
>Hanger-Rose skin t.
>
>Hemoccult t.
>
>Hickey-Hare t.
>
>Hoesch t.
>
>indirect hemagglutination t.
>
>iodine I 131 uptake t., radioactive iodine uptake t.
>
>Kveim-Siltzbach t.
>
>latex agglutination t.
>
>liver function t. (LFT)
>
>pancreatic function t.
>
>pulmonary function t. (PFT)
>
>Quick t. (for liver function)
>
>radioactive iodine (RAI) t.
>
>radioallergosorbent t. (RAST)
>
>renal function t. (RFT)
>
>rheumatoid arthritis (RA) t.
>
>rheumatoid factor (RF) t.
>
>Sabin-Feldman dye t.
>
>Schirmer t.
>
>sickle cell t.
>
>Staub-Traugott t.
>
>streptozyme t.
>
>sugar t.
>
>T_3 [T3] suppression t.
>
>thyroid antibody t.
>
>thyroid function t. (TFT)
>
>thyroid suppression t.
>
>thyrotropin-releasing hormone stimulation t.
>
>T_3 [T3] resin uptake t.
>
>T_4 [T4] RIA t.
>
>triiodothyronine (T_3 [T3]) uptake t.
>
>Wassermann t.
>
>Werner t.
>
>Widal t.

tetanus

tetany
> hyperventilation t.
> parathyroid t.
> parathyroprival t.
> rheumatic t.
> thyroprival t.

tetralogy
> t. of Fallot

TG—toxic goiter

Thaysen disease

thelalgia

thelarche

therapy
> deleading t.
> diathermic t.
> diet t.
> endocrine t.
> endocrine ablative t.
> gene t.
> hormonal t., hormone t.
> hyperbaric oxygen t.
> hypoglycemic t.
> immunosuppressive t.
> intravenous t.
> maggot t.
> oral rehydration t. (ORT)
> replacement t.
> specific t.
> substitution t.
> substitutive t.
> supportive t.
> thyroid replacement t., thyroxine replacement t.

thermography

thiazolidinediones [a class of drugs]

Thibierge-Weissenbach syndrome

"thi-sis" Phonetic for phthisis.

thoracic
> t. outlet syndrome

thrombi (plural of thrombus)

thromboangiitis
> t. obliterans

thromboarteriosclerosis
> t. obliterans

thrombocyst

thrombocytasthenia

thrombocythemia

thrombocytic

thrombocytopathic

thrombocytopathy

thrombocytopenic purpura (TP)

thrombocytopoietic

thrombogenic

thromboid

thrombolytics [a class of drugs]

thrombopenia

thrombophlebitis
> iliofemoral t.
> iliofemoral t., postpartum
> t. saltans

thrombose, thrombosed

thrombosis
> See also *thrombus.*
> See also in *Cardiology* section.
> agonal t.
> atrophic t.
> cardiac t.
> creeping t.
> deep venous t. (DVT)
> marantic t., marasmic t.

thrombus (thrombi)
> See also *thrombosis.*
> marantic t., marasmic t.
> traumatic t.

thrush

thunderclap headache

thymine

thymolipoma

thymopathy

thymus

thyroid
> aberrant t.
> accessory t.
> t. crisis
> t. deficiency
> ectopic t.
> t. gland
> intrathoracic t.
> lingual t.
> t. lobectomy
> t. nodule
> retrosternal t., substernal t.
> t.-stimulating hormone
> t. storm

thyroidectomy
    medical t.
thyroidism
thyroiditis
    de Quervain's t.
    ligneous t.
thyroid-stimulating hormone (TSH)
thyrophyma
thyroprival
thyrotoxicosis
    t. factitia
tic
    t. douloureux ["doo-loo-roo"]
Tietze
    disease
    syndrome
time (T)
    lead t.
    median survival t.
    tincture of t.
tincture
    t. of time
tinnitus
    t. aurium
    clicking t.
    Leudet t.
    nervous t.
    nonvibratory t.
    objective t.
    vibratory t.
"ti-sis" Phonetic for phthisis.
TNM—tumor, nodes, metastases
    [tumor staging system]
Todd
    cirrhosis
tolerance
    drug t.
    glucose t.
    impaired glucose t. (IGT)
Tommaselli
    disease
    syndrome
tongue
    amyloid t.
    antibiotic t.
    choreic t.
    geographic t.
    parrot t.

tonsillitis
tophaceous
tophus (tophi)
    gouty tophi
topographic, topographical
torticollis
tourniquet
    t. paralysis
toxicosis
toxic shock
    t.s. syndrome (TSS)
TPN—total parenteral nutrition
TPPN—total peripheral parenteral
    nutrition
tracheitis
trachelagra
tracheobronchitis
trait
    sickle cell t.
    thalassemia t.
translocation
    robertsonian t.
transplantation
    allogeneic marrow t.
trauma (traumas, traumata)
treatment
    conservative t.
    empiric t.
    expectant t.
    hyperbaric oxygen t.
    Paul t.
    preventive t., prophylactic t.
    symptomatic t.
    Yeo t.
trematode
trematodiasis
tremor
    action t.
    arsenic t.
    coarse t.
    essential t.
    intention t.
    pill-rolling t.
    rest t.
    resting t.
treponemiasis
TRF—thyrotropin-releasing factor
TRH—thyrotropin-releasing hormone

triad
>   Falta t.
>   Hutchinson t.
>   Merseburg t.
>   Whipple t.

trichocephaliasis
trichorrhexis
>   t. nodosa

trichostrongylosis
trichuriasis
trigeminal
>   t. neuralgia

triglycerides
"trik–" Phonetic for trich–.
"triko–" Phonetic for words beginning tricho–.
trismus
"trofedema" Phonetic for trophedema.
Troisier
>   ganglion
>   node
>   sign
>   syndrome

Troisier-Hanot-Chauffard syndrome
trophedema
truncal
truncate
truncus (trunci)
>   t. arteriosus

T$_4$SA [T4SA]—thyroxine-specific activity
TSH—thyroid-stimulating hormone
TSH-RF—thyroid-stimulating hormone–releasing factor
TTH—thyrotropic hormone
TTP—thrombotic thrombocytopenic purpura
TU—thiouracil
tuber (tubers, tubera)
tubercle
>   Farre t.

tubercula (plural of tuberculum)
tubercular
tuberculate, tuberculated
tuberculation
tuberculitis
tuberculization

tuberculocidal
tuberculocide
tuberculoid
tuberculosis (TB)
>   active t.
>   adult t.
>   attenuated t.
>   atypical t.

tuberculostatic
tuberculotic
tuberculous
>   t. peritonitis

tuberculum (tubercula)
>   t. thyroideum inferius
>   t. thyroideum superius

tuberositas (tuberositates)
tuberosity
>   omental t. of liver
>   omental t. of pancreas

tubular
>   t. proteinuria

tularemia
tumor
>   Burkitt t.
>   fungating t.
>   Grawitz t.
>   Hürthle cell t.
>   islet cell t.
>   mixed-tissue t.
>   mucinous t.
>   müllerian mixed t.
>   nonresponsive t.
>   radiocurable t.
>   radioresistant t.
>   radiosensitive t.
>   responsive t.
>   serous t.
>   solid t.
>   Wilms t.

tympanites
>   false t.

type
>   Runeberg t.

typhoid
typhoidette
"ty-sis" Phonetic for phthisis.
"u–" Phonetic for words beginning eu–.

ulcer
>aphthous u.
>cutaneous u.
>decubitus u.
>duodenal u.
>Meleney chronic undermining u.
>Parrot u.
>peptic u.
>serpiginous u.

ulcera (plural of ulcus)
ulcerative
>u. colitis

ulcerogenic
ulcus (ulcera)
>u. penetrans

ultrasound
>Doppler u.

unconsciousness
Underwood disease
Undritz anomaly
undulant fever
unit
>See also in *General Medical Terms* and *Laboratory, Pathology, and Chemistry Terms.*
>burn u.
>intensive care u. (ICU)
>intensive coronary care u. (ICCU)
>international insulin u.
>medical intensive care u. (MICU)
>parathyroid u.
>pulmonary intensive care u. (PICU)

Unschuld sign
"unukizm" Phonetic for eunuchism.
uptake
>radioactive iodine u.

uracil
Urbach-Wiethe disease
ureterocele
urethra
uricosuria
urinary
urine

urobilinemia
urobilinogenemia
urobilinuria
urogram
urolithiasis
urticaria
UTBG—unbound thyroxine–binding globulin
"uthanazea" Phonetic for euthanasia.
"uthiroid" Phonetic for euthyroid.
utricle
uveitis
uveomeningitis
vaccination
>smallpox v.

vaccinia
>v. gangrenosa

vaginosis
vagotomy
vagovagal
vanadiumism
varicella
>v.-zoster virus

varix (varices)
>lymph v., v. lymphaticus

vasculum (vascula)
>v. aberrans

vasomotoricity
vasoneuropathy
vasovagal
venereal
Verner-Morrison syndrome
Vernet
>paralysis (paralyses)
>syndrome

Verneuil
verruca (verrucae)
>v. peruana
>v. vulgaris

verrucous
vertebra (vertebrae)
>H-shaped v.

vertebral
vertiginous
vertigo
>arteriosclerotic v.
>benign paroxysmal positional v.

vertigo (continued)
    benign paroxysmal postural v.
    cardiac v.
    cardiovascular v.
    disabling positional v.
    essential v.
    paroxysmal positional v.
    positional v., postural v.
    subjective v.
    vestibular v.
VH—viral hepatitis
vibex (vibices)
vibration
    chest wall v.
villose, villous [adj.]
    v. duct cancer
Vinson syndrome
vinyl chloride
viricidal
virilism
    adrenal v.
    prosopopilary v.
virion
virosis (viroses)
virus
    See also in *Laboratory,*
      Pathology, and Chemistry
      Terms.
    Coxsackie v. [now: coxsack-
      ievirus]
    hepatitis A v. (HAV)
    hepatitis B v. (HBV)
    hepatitis C v. (HCV)
    hepatitis E v.
    hepatitis G v. (HGV)
    hepatitis GB v. (HGBV,
      HGBV-A, HGBV-B,
      HGBV-C)
    herpes v. [pref: herpesvirus]
    herpes zoster v.
    influenza v.
    non-A, non B-hepatitis v.
    oncogenic v.
    RNA v.'s
vitium
    v. conformationis
    v. primae formationis
VMA—vanillylmandelic acid

voces (plural of vox)
vocis (genitive of vox)
voiding
Volkmann
    contracture
vomit
    bilious v.
    black v.
    coffee-grounds v.
vomiting
    cyclic v.
    dry v.
    explosive v.
    hysterical v.
    periodic v.
    pernicious v.
    projectile v.
    recurrent v.
vomitus
    coffee-grounds v.
    v. matutinus
von Gierke. See *Gierke.*
von Recklinghausen. See *Reckling-*
    hausen.
von Rokitansky. See *Rokitansky.*
von Willebrand (Willebrand)
    disease
    factor
    factor deficiency
    syndrome
"vos-tek" Phonetic for *Chvostek.*
vox (voces)
    v. cholerica
Waldenström
    macroglobulinemia
    syndrome
Wallenberg syndrome
Wartenberg
    disease
    neuralgia
Wassermann
wasting
    w. syndrome
WDLL—well-differentiated lym-
    phocytic lymphoma
Weber-Christian
    syndrome

Weil
    disease
    syndrome
Weinstein syndrome
Weir Mitchell
    disease
    treatment
Werlhof disease
Wermer
    syndrome
Werner
    disease
    syndrome
    test
Wernicke
    aphasia
    disease
    encephalopathy
    syndrome
Wernicke-Korsakoff
    psychosis
    syndrome
Westphal-Strümpell
    disease
    pseudosclerosis
wheezing
Whipple
    disease
    syndrome
    triad
whitlow
whooping cough
Widal-Abrami disease
Wilkins disease
Willebrand. See *von Willebrand.*
Willebrand-Jürgens
    syndrome
Willis
    disease
    pancreas
Wills anemia
Wilms tumor
Wilson
    disease
Winkler disease
Winslow pancreas
Wirsung duct
Witts anemia

wolffian
    w. duct
Wolfram
    syndrome
Wright
    syndrome
xanthinuria
xanthinuric
xanthogranulomatosis
xanthogranulomatous
xanthoma (xanthomas, xanthomata)
    diabetic x., x. diabeticorum
    eruptive x., x. eruptivum
    generalized plane x.
    planar x., plane x., x. planum
    x. striatum palmare
    tendinous x., x. tendinosum
    tuberoeruptive x.
    x. tuberosum, x. tuberosum
        multiplex, tuberous x.
xanthosis
    x. diabetica
    x. diabeticorum
xanthurenic
    x. aciduria
xanthurenic acid
xenogeneic
xerocytosis
xeroderma pigmentosum
xiphoiditis
yellow fever
Yeo treatment
"yoo–" Phonetic for words begin-
    ning eu–.
Young
    syndrome
yo-yo dieting
"zero–" Phonetic for words begin-
    ning xero–.
"zheel-bare" Phonetic for Gilbert
    [Nicolas Augustin Gilbert].
Zieve syndrome
"zifoid" Phonetic for xiphoid.
zincalism
Zollinger-Ellison (ZE)
    syndrome
    tumor

zona (zonae)
    z. fasciculata
    z. glomerulosa
    z. reticularis
zonal
zonary

zone
    Head z.'s
    z.'s of hyperalgesia
zoster sine herpete
zymolysis
zymotic disease

Neurology and Pain Management

AAMD—age-associated memory disorder
AAN—American Academy of Neurology
AAO3, AAOx3—awake, alert, and oriented times three [to time, place, and person]
abaptiston
abasia
    choreic a.
    paralytic a.
    paroxysmal trepidant a.
    spastic a.
    trembling a.
    a. trepidans
abasic
Abbe
    neurectomy
ABEP—auditory brain stem evoked potential
abetalipoproteinemia
abient
ability
    primary mental a.
    verbal a.
ABMT—autologous bone marrow transplantation
ABR—auditory brain stem response
ABS—acute brain syndrome
abscess
    brain a.
    cerebellar a.
    cerebral a.
    dural a.
    embolic a.
    epidural a.
    extradural a.
    frontal a.
    intracranial a.

abscess (continued)
    intradural a.
    intramedullary a.
    metastatic a.
    otic cerebral a.
    otogenic a.
    Pott a.
    subarachnoid a.
    subdural a.
    subgaleal a.
    temporal lobe a.
    thecal a.
absence
    atypical a. seizure
    complex a. seizure
    a. epilepsy
    myoclonic a.
    a. seizure
    subclinical a. seizure
absentia
    a. epileptica
absinthe
abterminal
abulia
    cyclic a.
abulic
acalculia
acanthesthesia
acanthocytosis
accessory
    a. nerve
accident
    cerebrovascular a. (CVA)
accommodation
    reflex a., a. reflex
ACD—anticonvulsant drug
ACDF—anterior cervical diskectomy and fusion

acetylcholinesterase (AChE) inhibitors [a class of drugs]
α-*N*-acetylgalactosaminidase [alpha-]
AChE (acetylcholinesterase) inhibitors [a class of drugs]
acheiria
Achilles
    jerk
    reflex
    tendon
achromatopsia
acousma
acousmatagnosis
acousmatamnesia
Acrel ganglion
acroagnosis
acroanesthesia
acrobrachycephaly
acrocephalosyndactyly
acrodynia
acrodysesthesia
acroesthesia
acrognosis
acrohypothermy
acromelalgia
acroneuropathy
acroneurosis
acroparalysis
acroparesthesia
    Nothnagel-type a.
    Schultze-type a.
acropathy
    amyotrophic a.
    ulcerative mutilating a.
acrotrophodynia
acrotrophoneurosis
act
    reflex a.
action
    a. potential
    reflex a.
activation
    epileptic a.
activity
    alpha wave a.
    asynchronous a.
    background a.
    beta wave a.

activity (continued)
    continuous muscle fiber a.
    delta wave a.
    discrete a.
    electrical a.
    end-plate a.
    epileptiform a.
    insertion a., insertional a.
    intermittent rhythmic delta a.
    involuntary a.
    polymorphic delta a.
    pseudomotor a.
    salaam a.
    spike and wave a.
    spontaneous a.
    synchronous a.
    theta wave a.
    triggered a.
    voluntary a.
aculalia
acupuncture
Adamantiades-Behçet syndrome
adamantinoma
    pituitary a.
addiction
ADE—acute disseminated
    encephalitis
ADEM—acute disseminated
    encephalomyelitis
adenocarcinoma
adenohypophysectomy
adenohypophysial
adenoma
    a. sebaceum
adhesio
    a. interthalamica
adhesion
    interthalamic a.
adiadochokinesia
adiadochokinesis
adiaphoria
Adie
    pupil
    syndrome
adiposis
    a. cerebralis
    a. dolorosa
    a. tuberosa simplex

adipositas
> a. cerebralis

adiposity
> cerebral a.

adneural

ADR—absence of deep reflexes

adrenaline

Adson
> maneuver
> procedure
> suction tube
> syndrome
> test

adventitial

adynamia
> a. episodica hereditaria

AER—auditory evoked response

aero-asthenia

aerocele
> epidural a.
> intracranial a.

"a-feem-ee-a" Phonetic for aphemia.

affect [noun: state of mind]
> apathetic a.
> bland a.
> blunted a.
> congruent a.
> constricted a.
> depressed a., depressive a.
> euphoric a.
> flat a.
> impaired a.
> inappropriate a.
> labile a.
> restricted a.

affective

affectivity

affectomotor

African meningitis

AFS—Alzheimer fugue state

aftercurrent

afterdischarge

afterimpression

aftermovement

afterpotential
> negative a.
> positive a.
> a. wave

aftersensation

agenesia
> a. corticalis

agenesis
> callosal a.

agent
> myoneural blocking a.
> neuromuscular blocking a.

ageusia
> central a.
> conduction a.
> peripheral a.

agnea

agnosia
> apraxic a.
> body-image a.
> developmental a.
> digital a.
> face a., facial a.
> finger a.
> a. for faces
> geometrical a.
> gustatory a.
> ideational a.
> localization a.
> nonsymbolic visual a.
> position a.
> spatial a.
> symbolic visual a.
> tactile a.
> time a.
> topographical a.
> visual a.
> visual-spatial a., visuospatial a.

agonist
> muscarinic a.'s [a class of drugs]
> narcotic a.'s [a class of drugs]
> narcotic a.-antagonists [a class of drugs]
> vascular serotonin 5-HT$_1$ [5-HT1] receptor a.'s [a class of drugs]

agrammatica

agrammatism

agrammatologia

agraphesthesia

agraphia
>   absolute a.
>   acoustic a.
>   a. amnemonica
>   a. atactica
>   cerebral a.
>   jargon a.
>   literal a.
>   mental a.
>   motor a.
>   optic a.
>   sensory a.
>   verbal a.

agraphic
agyria
agyric
"ah-mi-el–" Phonetic for words
>   beginning amyel–.
"ah-mi-o–" Phonetic for words
>   beginning amyo–.
"ah-ser-vu-lus" Phonetic for acervu-
>   lus.
Aicardi syndrome
aid
>   prosthetic speech a.
>   speech a.
air
>   a. encephalography
>   a. myelography
akatamathesia
akatanoesis
akathisia
akinesia
>   a. algera
>   cerebral a.
>   Nadbath a.
>   spinal a.
>   Van Lint a.
akinesis
akinesthesia
Akureyri
>   disease
ala (alae)
>   a. cerebelli
>   a. cinerea
Alajouanine
>   disease
>   syndrome

alalia
>   a. cophica
>   developmental a.
>   a. organica
>   a. physiologica
>   a. prolongata
alalic
Alexander
>   disease
alexia
>   aphasic a.
>   cortical a.
>   Dejerine a.
>   developmental a.
>   geometric a.
>   isolated a.
>   motor a.
>   musical a.
>   occipital a.
>   optical a.
>   parietal a.
>   pure a.
>   semantic a.
>   sensory a.
>   subcortical a.
>   symbolic a.
>   tactile a.
>   verbal a.
>   a. with agraphia
>   a. without aphasia
alexic
algesia
algesic
algesichronometer
algesimeter
algesimetry
algesiogenic
algesthesia
algesthesis
algiomotor
algiomuscular
algiovascular
allesthesia
>   visual a.
allochiral
allochiria
allodynia

allograft
 nerve a.
allokinesis
allokinetic
Alpers
 disease
 polioencephalopathy
alpha
 a.-*N*-acetylgalactosaminidase
 a.-galactosidase A
 a. nerve fibers
alveus (alvei)
 a. hippocampi, a. of hippocampus
Alzheimer
 dementia
 disease
 primary degenerative
  dementia
 sclerosis
 syndrome
amaurosis
amaurotic
 a. familial idiocy (AFI)
ambilevosity
ambilevous
ambisinister
ambisinistrous
amblyaphia
ambulation
ameloblastoma
 pituitary a.
amimia
 amnesic a.
 ataxic a.
γ-aminobutyrate [gamma-]
γ-aminobutyric acid (GABA)
 [gamma-]
Ammon
 horn
amnemonic
amnesia
 affective a.
 anterograde a.
 auditory a.
 Broca a.
 concussion a.
 elective a.

amnesia (continued)
 graphokinetic a.
 hysterical a.
 immunologic a.
 incomplete a.
 infantile a.
 Korsakoff a.
 lacunar a.
 localized a.
 mimokinetic a.
 olfactory a.
 patchy a.
 postconcussion a.
 posthypnotic a.
 psychogenic a.
 retroactive a.
 retrograde a.
 systematic a.
 tactile a.
 transient global a.
amnesiac
amnesic
amnestic
Amnioplastin
amphetamines [a class of drugs]
amusia
 amnesic a.
 instrumental a.
 motor a.
 receptive a.
 sensory a.
 tonal a.
amyelia
amyelotrophy
amygdala
 a. of cerebellum
amygdalohippocampectomy
amyloid
amyostasia
amyostatic
amyosthenia
amyosthenic
amyotonia
 a. congenita
 Oppenheim a.
amyotrophia
amyotrophic

amyotrophy
>Aran-Duchenne a.
>diabetic a.
>neuralgic a.
>neuritic a.
>primary progressive a.
>progressive nuclear a.
>syphilitic a.

analeptics [a class of drugs]

analgesia
>neurolept a. [pref: neurolept-analgesia]
>conduction a.
>congenital a.
>electrical a.
>hysterical a.
>obstetric a.
>perineural a.

analgesics [a class of drugs]

anarithmia

anarthria
>a. literalis

anastomosis (anastomoses)
>See also *operation* and *procedure.*
>faciohypoglossal a.
>hypoglossal-facial nerve a.
>meningeal arterial a.'s
>nerve a.
>ventriculocisternal a.

Anders
>disease

André Thomas sign

anencephalia

anencephalic

anencephalohemia

anencephalous

anencephaly

anesthecinesia, anesthekinesia

anesthesia
>See also in *General Surgical Terms.*
>angiospastic a.
>bulbar a.
>compression a.
>a. dolorosa
>facial a.
>gauntlet a.

anesthesia (continued)
>girdle a.
>glove a.
>glove and stocking a.
>gustatory a.
>hysterical a.
>nausea a.
>olfactory a.
>pressure a.
>tactile a.
>thalamic hyperesthetic a.
>traumatic a.
>visceral a.

anesthetic

anesthetic agents
>Amytal
>benzocaine
>Brevital
>Demerol
>Dilaudid
>Duranest
>lidocaine HCl
>Marcaine HCl
>morphine
>Nembutal
>Novocain
>Xylocaine with epinephrine

anesthetize

aneurysm
>arterial a.
>arteriovenous a.
>berry a.
>caroticocavernous a.
>Charcot-Bouchard a.
>cirsoid a.
>fusiform a.
>innominate a.
>intracavernous a.
>intracranial a.
>miliary a.
>mycotic a.
>racemose a.

angiography
>carotid a.
>cerebral a.
>peripheral a.
>spinal cord a.
>vertebral a.

angiokeratoma
    a. corporis diffusum
    a. corporis diffusum universale
    diffuse a.
angioma
    a. arteriale racemosum
    a. cavernosum
    cavernous a.
    cerebral a.
    encephalic a.
    spinal a.
    a. venosum racemosum
angiomatoid
angiomatosis
    cephalotrigeminal a.
    oculoencephalic a.
    Sturge-Weber a.
angiomyolipoma
angioneurectomy
"angkilo–" Phonetic for words beginning ankylo–.
angle
angophrasia
"angzietas" Phonetic for anxietas.
anisocoria
ankylosed
ankylosis (ankyloses)
    operative a.
ankylotic
anodynes [a class of drugs]
anomaly
    Aristotle a.
    craniovertebral a.'s
    Jordan a.
anomia
anorthography
anosmia
anosmic
anosognosia
anoxia
    diffuse cerebral a.
ansa (ansae)
    a. of Galen
    a. of Haller
    Henle a.
    a. of lenticular nucleus
    a. of Vieussens

ansa (ansae) (continued)
    a. of Wrisberg
ansate
ansotomy
anterior
    a. cervical diskectomy and fusion (ACDF)
    a. rhizotomy
    a. thalamotomy
anticoagulated
anticonvulsant
anticonvulsants [a class of drugs]
anticonvulsive
antiepileptic drugs (AEDs) [a class of drugs]
"anurizm" Phonetic for aneurysm.
Apert
    disease
    syndrome
aphasia
    ageusic a.
    amnemonic a.
    amnesic a.
    amnestic a.
    anosmic a.
    apractic a.
    association a.
    associative a.
    Broca a.
    color name a.
    crossed a.
    efferent motor a.
    finger a.
    gestural a.
    global a.
    kinetic motor a.
    monoglot a.
    musical a.
    paroxysmal a.
    puerperal a.
    pure motor a.
    visual a.
    Wernicke a.
aphonia
    hysterical a.
    a. paralytica
    a. paranoica
    spastic a.

apicectomy
apicotomy
aplasia
> a. axialis extracorticalis congenita

apnea
> chemoreceptor a.
> deglutition a.
> hypersomnia sleep a.
> induced a.
> initial a.
> late a.
> a. neonatorum
> obstructive sleep a.
> postanesthesia a.
> sleep a.
> traumatic a.

apophyseal
apophysis (apophyses)
> See also *process* and *protuberance.*
> cerebral a.
> a. cerebri
> genial a.

apoplexy
> Broadbent a.
> cerebellar a.
> cerebral a.
> fulminating a.
> ingravescent a.
> meningeal a.
> pituitary a.
> pontile a.
> Raymond a.
> thrombotic a.

apparatus
> spine a.

appearance
appendicular
> a. ataxia

appendix (appendices)
> a. cerebri

apperception
apperceptive
apprehension
> a. test

approach
> transcranial a.

apractic
apraxia
> agnosic a.
> akinetic a.
> a. algera
> amnestic a.
> congenital a.
> cortical a.
> developmental a.
> geometric a.
> ideational a.
> ideokinetic a.
> ideomotor a.
> innervation a.
> limb-kinetic a.
> motor a.
> oculomotor a.
> optic a.
> sensory a.
> tongue a.
> transcortical a.
> trunk a.
> visual a.

apraxic
aqueduct
> cerebral a.
> a. of midbrain
> a. of Sylvius
> a. of the vestibule

aqueductus
> a. cerebri
> a. vestibuli

arachnitis
arachnoid
arachnoidea
> a. encephali
> a. spinalis

arachnoideae
arachnoiditis
> basal a.
> a. of cerebral hemispheres
> cisternal a.
> opticochiasmatic a.
> optochiasmatic a.
> a. of posterior cerebral fossa
> spinal a.

Aran
> law

Aran-Duchenne
    amyotrophy
    disease
    muscular atrophy
Arantius
    ventricle
arbor
    a. medullaris vermis
    a. vitae cerebelli
arch
    neural a.
    parieto-occipital a.
archipallial
archipallium
area (areae, areas)
    associative a.
    auditory cortical a.
    auditory projection a.
    auditory psychic a.
    autonomic a.
    Broca a.
    Brodmann a.
    central speech a.
    cortical 4S a.
    cortical gustatory a.
    cortical oculomotor a.
    cortical speech a.
    cortical tactile a.
    cortico-oculocephalogyric a.
    entorhinal a.
    extrapyramidal motor a.
    first motor speech a.
    Flechsig a.
    a. of Forel, areae foreli
    frontal a.
    fronto-orbital a.
    gustatory receiving a.
    Hines strip a.
    Obersteiner-Redlich a.
    parastriate a.
    a. paraterminalis
    Patrick trigger a.'s
    postcentral a.
    a. postpterygoidea
    a. postrema
    prefrontal a.
    premotor a.
    a. pterygoidea

area (areae, areas) (continued)
    recipient a.
    silent a.
    somatosensory a.
    temporal a.
    vagus a.
    Wernicke a.
areflexia
Argyll Robertson
    See also *pseudo-Argyll*
      Robertson.
    pupil
    sign
arhinencephalia
Aristotle anomaly
Armstrong
    disease
Arnold-Chiari
    deformity
    syndrome
arteriogram
arteriography
    carotid a.
    cerebral a.
    spinal a.
    vertebral a.
arteriosclerosis
    cerebral a.
arteritis (arteritides)
    cranial a.
    temporal a.
artery
    basilar a.
    callosomarginal a.
    carotid a.
    cerebellar a.
    cerebral a.
    choroidal a.
    communicating a.
    a. of Heubner, Heubner a.
    lenticulostriate a.
    pericallosal a.
    thalamostriate a.
    vertebral a.
arthritis (arthritides)
    meningococcal a.
    neurogenic a.
    neuropathic a.

arthritis (arthritides) (continued)
    rheumatoid a.
AS—arteriosclerosis
asemasia
asemia
    a. graphica
    a. mimica
    a. verbalis
Asherson syndrome
assessment
    Dubowitz Neurological A.
astasia
    a.-abasia
    atonia-a.
astatic
astereocognosy
astereognosia
astereopsis
asthenia
    muscle a.
    neurotic a.
astrocytoma
    a. diffusum
astrocytomatosis cerebri
astroglia
astroid
asymbolia
    tactile a.
asynchronism
asynergia
asynergy
    appendicular a.
    axial a.
    axioappendicular a.
    progressive cerebellar a.
    progressive locomotor a.
    truncal a.
    verbal a.
atactic
atactiform
ataxia
    acute tabetic a.
    adult onset a.
    appendicular a.
    autonomic a.
    Briquet a.
    Broca a.
    Bruns frontal a.

ataxia (continued)
    bulbar a.
    central a.
    cerebellar a.
    cerebellofugal degeneration a.
    cerebral a.
    cervical a.
    dentate cerebellar a.
    diphtheric a.
    dynamic a.
    equilibratory a.
    Fergusson and Critchley a.
    Friedreich a.
    frontal a.
    hereditary cerebellar a.
    Holmes a.
    hysterical a.
    intermittent a.
    intrapsychic a.
    kinetic a.
    labyrinthic a.
    Leyden a.
    limb kinetic a.
    locomotor a.
    Marie a.
    motor a.
    nonequilibratory a.
    nutritional spinal a.
    optic a.
    periodic a.
    polyneuritic spinocerebellar a.
    postural a.
    professional a.
    progressive a.
    proprioceptive a.
    pseudotabetic a.
    psychomotor a.
    Saenger-Brown a.
    sensory a.
    spastic a.
    spinal a.
    spinocerebellar a.
    static a.
    a.-telangiectasia
    thermal a.
    vasomotor a.
    vestibular a.
ataxiagram

ataxiagraph
ataxiamnesic
ataxiaphasia
atelencephalia
atelomyelia
atheroma
    cerebral a.
athetoid
athetosis
    bilateral a.
    congenital a.
    posthemiplegic a.
    unilateral a.
atlas [C1 vertebra]
atonia
    a.-astasia
atonic
atonicity
atony
    muscle a.
atremia
atrophy
    alcoholic cerebral a.
    Aran-Duchenne muscular a.
    cerebellar a.
    Charcot-Marie-Tooth a.
    circumscribed a. of brain
    convolutional a.
    Cruveilhier a.
    degenerative a.
    Dejerine-Sottas a.
    denervated muscle a.
    Duchenne-Aran muscular a.
    Erb a.
    facioscapulohumeral a.
    familial spinal muscular a.
    fat replacement a.
    Fazio-Londe a.
    Hoffmann a.
    Hunt a.
    idiopathic muscular a.
    infantile a.
    Jadassohn muscular a.
    lamellar cerebellar a.
    Landouzy-Dejerine a.
    lobar a.
    multisystem a.
    myelopathic muscular a.

atrophy (continued)
    myotonic a.
    neural a.
    neuritic muscular a.
    neurogenic a.
    neuropathic a.
    neurotic a.
    neurotrophic a.
    olivopontocerebellar a.
    olivoubrocerebellar a.
    paraneoplastic cerebellar a.
    Parrot a. of the newborn
    peroneal a.
    Pick convolutional a.
    progressive diffuse cerebro-
      cortical a.
    progressive nuclear muscle a.
    pseudohypertrophic muscu-
      lar a.
    pseudomyopathic spinal
      muscular a.
    scapuloperoneal muscular a.
    spinoneural a.
    spinopontine a.
    syphilitic spinal muscular a.
    trophoneurotic a.
    von Leber a.
    Vulpian a.
    Werdnig-Hoffmann a.
    Zimmerlin a.
attack
    apnea a.
    cerebellar a.
    cyclical epileptic a.
    decerebrate a.
    drop a.'s
    epileptic a.
    epileptiform a.
    focal a.
    myoclonic a.
    posterior a.
    tonic cerebellar a.
    transient carotid ischemic a.
    uncinate a.
    vasovagal a.
Aubert
    phenomenon

audiometry
    brain stem evoked response
      (BSER) a.
auditory
    a. nerve
    a. nuclei
augmentation
aula
aura
autocerebrospinal
autokinesis
autokinetic
    a. visible light phenomenon
automatism
    epileptic a.
    postepileptic a.
    postictal a.
    vigil ambulatory a.
autonomic
autonomy
AVM—arteriovenous malformation
axis [C2 vertebra]
axon
axonopathy
Ayala
    equation
    index
    quotient
Ayer test
Ayer-Tobey test
Azorean
    disease
Baastrup
    disease
    syndrome
Babès
    nodes
    nodules
    tubercles
Babinski
    law
    phenomenon
    reflex
    sign
    syndrome
Babinski-Fröhlich syndrome
Babinski-Nageotte syndrome

Babinski-Vaquez
    syndrome
bacillus (bacilli)
    See in *Laboratory, Patholo-*
    gy, and Chemistry Terms.
Bacillus
    See in *Laboratory, Patholo-*
    gy, and Chemistry Terms.
bacterium (bacteria)
    See specific bacteria in *Lab-*
    oratory, Pathology, and
    Chemistry Terms.
Bailey
    conductor
Baillarger
    bands
    lines
    sign
    striae
    stripes
    syndrome
Bálint syndrome
Ballet
    disease
    sign
ballism
ballismus
Baló
    concentric encephalitis
    concentric sclerosis
    concentric syndrome
    disease
    syndrome
Bamberger
    disease
banana
    b. sign
band
    See *frenulum* and *vinculum.*
    See also *line* and *stria.*
bandage
    See in *General Surgical*
    Terms.
baragnosis
Bárány
    pointing test
    positional vertigo
    sign

Bárány (continued)
 syndrome
 test
barbaralalia
barbiturates [a class of drugs]
barbotage
Bard
 sign
Bardet-Biedl syndrome
Barker
 point
Barkman reflex
barognosis
Barré
 pyramidal sign
 sign
Barré-Guillain syndrome
Barré-Liéou syndrome
Bársony-Polgár syndrome
Bársony-Teschendorf syndrome
Bartholin
 anus
Bärtschi-Rochaix syndrome
barylalia
base
 b. of brain
 b. of skull
Basedow
 pseudoparaplegia
 syndrome
bases (plural of basis)
basial
basialis
basialveolar
basicranial
basilaris
 b. cranii
basinasial
basioccipital
basion
basirhinal
basis (bases)
 b. capituli
 b. pontis
basisphenoid
basitemporal
basivertebral

Bassen-Kornzweig
 disease
 syndrome
Bastian
 law
 syndrome
Bastian-Bruns
 law
 sign
bathyesthesia
bathyhyperesthesia
bathyhypesthesia
Batten-Mayou
 disease
Battle
 sign
Bayle
 disease
Beck
 syndrome
Becker
 dystrophy
Becker-type muscular dystrophy
Bekhterev (Bechterew)
 band
 deep reflex
 layer
 line
 nucleus
 nystagmus
 reaction
 reflex
 sign
 test
Bekhterev-Mendel reflex
Bell
 law
 nerve
 palsy
 phenomenon
 sign
Bell-Magendie law
Benedek reflex
Benedikt syndrome
benzodiazepines [a class of drugs]
Berger
 paresthesia
 rhythm

Berger (continued)
    wave
Bergeron
    chorea
    disease
Bergmann
    cells
    cords
    fibers
Bernard
    puncture
    syndrome
Bernard-Horner syndrome
Bernhardt
    disease
    paresthesia
Bernhardt-Roth syndrome
beta
    b.-galactosidase
Betz
    cell area
    cells
Bevan Lewis cells
Biber-Haab-Dimmer
    dystrophy
Bichat
    canal
    fissure
    foramen
Biedl
    disease
Biemond
    syndrome (type I, type II)
Biernacki sign
bifrontal
bilateral
    b. vagotomy
Billroth
    disease
Bing
    reflex
    sign
Bing-Neel syndrome
Binswanger
    dementia
    disease
    encephalitis
biodynamics

biopsy
    bone marrow b.
    nerve b.
    trephine b.
Biot
    breathing
    breathing sign
    respiration
    sign
bipolar
    b. cautery
birth
    b. palsy
    b. paralysis
Bischof
    corona
    crown
    myelotomy
    operation
    test
bitemporal
biventer
    b. cervicis
blackout
blepharospasm
blindness
    pure word b.
block
    cerebrospinal fluid b.
    meningeal b.
    spinal subarachnoid b.
    stellate b.
    sympathetic b.
    ventricular b.
    vertebral b.
blockade
blocker
    neuromuscular b.
Blocq
    disease
blood-brain barrier
blood flow study
    cerebral b.f.s.
blood patch
Blumenau
    nucleus
Blumenbach
    clivus

Blumenbach (continued)
    plane
    process
board
    alphabet b.
Boas
    algesimeter
Bodechtel-Guttmann
    disease
body (bodies)
    Hirano b.
    Lipschütz b.
    b. of Luys
    pineal b.
    psammoma b.
    Schmorl b.
    b. of sphenoid
    b. of Vicq d'Azyr
Boeck
    See *Beck*.
Bonhoeffer
    sign
    symptom
Bonnet
    sign
    syndrome
Bonnier syndrome
bony
    b. suture
"boo-ton" Phonetic for bouton.
border
    See also *limbus* and *margin*.
    lambdoid b.
Bordier-Fränkel sign
boss
    frontal b.
bossing
    b. of cranium
Bourneville
    disease
    syndrome
Bourneville-Brissaud
    disease
Bourneville-Pringle
    syndrome
bouton
    b. en passage ["ahn pah-sahj"]

bouton (continued)
    b. en passant ["ahn pah-sahn"]
brachial plexus
brachiofaciolingual
brachium (brachia)
    anterior conjunctival b.
    b. of colliculus
    b. of mesencephalon
    b. pontis
brachybasia
brachycephalic
brachycephaly
brachycranic
bradykinesia
bradykinetic
bradylalia
bradylexia
bradylogia
bradyphasia
bradyphrasia
bradyphrenia
bradypragia
bradyteleokinesis
Bragard sign
brain
    b. abscess
    base of b.
    b. cicatrix
    b. death
    b. disorder
    hernia of b.
    b. laceration
    organic b. syndrome
    b. pressure
    b. purpura
    b. sand
    b. scan
    b. scanning
    softening of the b.
    b. stem
    b. swelling
    b. syndrome
    b. wave
Brain [eponym]
    quadrupedal reflex
    reflex
brain-damaged

brain-dead
brain death
    b.-d. protocol electroen-
      cephalogram (EEG)
brain stem
    b.s. auditory evoked poten-
      tial (BAEP)
    b.s. crisis
    b.s. evoked response (BSER)
    b.s. evoked response
      (BSER) audiometry
    b.s. infarction
    b.s. ischemia
branch
    branches of vertebral artery
Bravais-jacksonian epilepsy
bredouillement
bregma
bregmatic
"breh-dwe-maw" Phonetic for bre-
    douillement.
Briquet
    ataxia
    syndrome
Brissaud
    reflex
Brissaud-Sicard syndrome
Bristowe syndrome
Broadbent
    apoplexy
    law
Broca
    amnesia
    aphasia
    area
    ataxia
    center
    convolution
    fissure
    gyrus
    motor speech area of the
      brain
    space
Brodmann areas
Brompton
    cocktail
"broo-ee" Phonetic for bruit.
Browning vein

Brown-Séquard
    lesion
    paralysis
    syndrome
    treatment
Brudzinski
    reflex
    sign
bruit
    See also in *Cardiology* and
      Pulmonary Medicine sec-
      tions.
    carotid b.
    cranial b.
    spinal b.
Bruns
    ataxia
    disease
    sign
    syndrome
Brushfield-Wyatt
    disease
    syndrome
bruxism
"brwe" Phonetic for bruit.
BS—Babinski sign
BSE—bilateral, symmetrical, and
    equal
BSER—brain stem evoked response
BSF—basal skull fracture
BT—brain tumor
bubble
    b. ventriculography
bulbonuclear
bulbopontine
bundle
    See also *fasciculus* and *tract.*
    Helweg b.
    lateral pontine b.
    Meynert b.
Burdach tract
Burns amaurosis
burst
    bilaterally synchronous b.
C1 through C7—cervical vertebrae
    1–7
CA—carotid artery
cacogeusia

café au lait spot
calcarine
calcification
    intracranial c.
California encephalitis (CE)
callosal
callosomarginal
calvaria (calvariae)
calvarium [incorrect term for calvaria]
CAM—computer-assisted myelography
campotomy
camptocormia
camptocormy
campus of Wernicke
canal
    caudal c.
    spinal c.
canaliculus (canaliculi)
    canaliculi caroticotympanici
    mastoid c., mastoid c. for
        Arnold nerve
    c. mastoideus
Canavan
    spongy degeneration
Canavan-van Bogaert-Bertrand
    disease
cancer
    See also *carcinoma.*
    See also in *Oncology and*
        Hematology section.
    dendritic c.
Cannon
    law
    theory
Cantelli sign
capacity
    mental c.
carcinoma (carcinomas, carcinomata)
    See in *Oncology and Hematology* section.
carcinomatosis
    meningeal c.
    c. of meninges
"carfol–" Phonetic for words beginning carphol–.

carotid
    c. angiography
    c. compression tonography
    c. endarterectomy (CEA)
    c. ischemia
carphologia
carphology
cataphoria
cataphoric
cataplectic
cataplexie
    c. du réveil
cataplexis
cataplexy
catapophysis
catatonia
catatonic
catechol-*O*-methyl transferase
    (COMT)
cat-eye, cat's eye
    c-e. reflex
cauda (caudae)
    c. cerebelli
    c. equina
caudatolenticular
caudectomy
cautery
    bipolar c.
    Birtcher c.
    Mils c.
cava (plural of cavum)
cavernous
    c. sinus thrombosis
cavity
    Meckel c.
cavum (cava)
    c. epidurale
    c. septi pellucidi
    c. subarachnoideale
    c. subdurale
    c. vergae
Cawthorne maneuver
CBS—chronic brain syndrome
CCA—common carotid artery
CCF—carotid cavernous fistula
CDR—clinical dementia rating
CE—cerebral edema
CEA—carotid endarterectomy

cell
> See also in *Laboratory, Pathology, and Chemistry Terms.*
> glitter c.
> Golgi c.
> Hortega c.
> microglial c.

cella
> c. lateralis ventriculi lateralis
> c. media ventriculi lateralis

center
> Broca c.

central
> c. nervous system (CNS)

central nervous system
> c.n.s. disease

centrencephalic
centriciput
centrilobular
centripetal
CEP—cortical evoked potential
cephalalgia
cephalhematocele
> Stromeyer c.

cephalhematoma
> c. deformans

cephalhydrocele
cephalocele
cephalocentesis
cephalogram
cephalogyric
cephalomegaly
cephalomeningitis
cephalomotor
cephalopathy
cephaloplegia
cephalorhachidian
cephalotomy
CERA—cortical evoked response audiometry
cerebellar
cerebellifugal
cerebellipetal
cerebellitis
cerebellofugal
cerebello-olivary
cerebellopontine

cerebellopontine
cerebellopontine angle tumor
cerebelloretinal
cerebellorubral
cerebellorubrospinal
cerebellospinal
cerebellum
cerebral
> c. angiography
> c. arteriography
> c. gammography
> c. pneumography
> c. sinusography
> c. ventriculography

cerebralgia
cerebrasthenia
cerebration
> unconscious c.

cerebriform
cerebrifugal
cerebripetal
cerebritis
> saturnine c.

cerebrocardiac
cerebrocentric
cerebrocerebellar
cerebrocuprein
cerebrogalactose
cerebrogalactoside
cerebrohyphoid
cerebroid
cerebrology
cerebroma
cerebromacular
cerebromalacia
cerebromedullary
> c. tube

cerebromeningeal
cerebromeningitis
cerebro-ocular
cerebropathia
> c. psychica toxemica

cerebropathy
cerebrophysiology
cerebropontile
cerebrorachidian
cerebrosclerosis
cerebroscopy

cerebrosidosis
cerebrosis
cerebrospinal
     c. fluid (CSF)
cerebrospinant
cerebrostomy
cerebrotendinous
cerebrotomy
cerebrotonia
cerebrovascular
     c. accident (CVA)
cerebrum
ceroid
ceroid lipofuscin
ceroid lipofuscinosis
     Finnish-type c.
     Hagberg-Santavuori variant
        of c.
     Jansky-Bielschowsky–type c.
     Kufs-type c.
cervical
     anterior c. diskectomy and
        fusion (ACDF)
     c. laminectomy
     c. plexus
     c. sympathectomy
cervicomedullary
Cestan
     sign
     syndrome
Cestan-Chenais
     syndrome
Cestan-Raymond
     syndrome
Cetacaine [anesthetic agent]
Chaddock
     reflex
     sign
change
     Alzheimer neurofibrillary c.'s
character
     epileptic c.
Charcot
     disease
     gait
     triad
Charcot-Bouchard aneurysm

Charcot-Marie
     atrophy
     type
Charcot-Marie-Tooth
     atrophy
     disease
     type
     syndrome
Charcot-Marie-Tooth-Hoffmann
     syndrome
chemical
     c. sympathectomy
chemonucleolysis
chemopallidectomy
chemopallidothalamectomy
chemopallidotomy
chemothalamectomy
chemothalamotomy
CHI—closed head injury
Chiari
Chiari-Arnold syndrome
Chiari-type malformation
chiasma (chiasmata)
     See *commissura.*
chiasmal
chiasmatic
cholesteatoma
     intracranial c.
cholinesterase inhibitors [a class of
     drugs]
chondroma
chordoma
chorea
     atonic c.
     automatic c.
     Bergeron c.
     button-maker's c.
     chronic c.
     c. cordis
     c. cruciata
     dancing c.
     diaphragmatic c.
     c. dimidiata
     Dubini c.
     electric c.
     epidemic c.
     c. festinans
     fibrillary c.

chorea (continued)
    c. gravidarum
    c. gravis
    habit c.
    hemilateral c.
    hemiplegic c.
    Henoch c.
    hereditary c.
    Huntington c.
    hyoscine c.
    hysterical c.
    imitative c.
    infective c.
    c. insaniens
    jumping c.
    juvenile c.
    laryngeal c.
    limp c.
    local c.
    c. major
    malleatory c.
    maniacal c.
    methodic c.
    mimetic c.
    c. minor
    c. mollis
    Morvan c.
    c. nocturna
    c. nutans
    one-sided c.
    paralytic c.
    polymorphous c.
    posthemiplegic c.
    prehemiplegic c.
    procursive c.
    rheumatic c.
    rhythmic c.
    rotary c.
    saltatory c.
    Schrötter c.
    c. scriptorum
    senile c.
    simple c.
    Sydenham c.
    tetanoid c.
    tic c.
choreal
choreic

choreiform
choreoathetoid
choreoathetosis
    paroxysmal familial c.
    paroxysmal kinesogenic c.
choreoid
choriomeningitis
    lymphocytic c.
    pseudolymphocytic c.
choroidectomy
Christensen-Krabbe
    disease
    poliodystrophy
Chvostek
    sign
    symptom
    test
CI—cerebral infarction
cicatrix (cicatrices)
    brain c.
    meningocerebral c.
cin–. See also words beginning
    sin–, syn–.
cinerea
cingula (plural of cingulum)
cingulate
cingulectomy
cingulotomy
cingulum (cingula)
CIPN—chronic idiopathic peripher-
    al neuropathy
circle
    c. of Willis
circulation
    vertebral-basilar c.
circulus (circuli)
    c. arteriosus cerebri
circumstantiality
cistern
    anterolateral cerebellar c.
    cerebellomedullary c.
    chiasmatic c.
    c. of corpus callosum
    c. of fossa of Sylvius
    Golgi c.'s
    c. of great cerebral vein
    c. of lateral fossa of cerebrum
    c. of Pecquet

cistern (continued)
    pontine c.
    subarachnoidal c.
    supracallosal c.
    c. of Sylvius
cisterna (cisternae)
    c. magna
    c. Sylvii
    c. valleculae lateralis cerebri
    c. venae magnae cerebri
cisternal
    c. arachnoiditis
    c. puncture
cisternography
    metrizamide c.
    oxygen c.
    radionuclide c.
cisternomyelography
CJD—Creutzfeldt-Jakob disease
Clarke
    column
    dorsal nucleus
    collateral bundle
classification
    See also *index*.
    Frankel c. (groups A–E)
    Goldstein c.
    Head c.
    Hunt and Hess neurological c.
    Kleist c.
    Luria c.
Claude
    hyperkinesis sign
    syndrome
Claude-Lhermitte syndrome
claustrum (claustra)
clava
claval
clavate
clinoid
clivus
    basilar c.
    Blumenbach c.
clonic
clonism
Clonopin [now: Klonopin]
clonus
    ankle c.

Cloward
    drill
    operation
CMT—Charcot-Marie-Tooth [atrophy, disease, syndrome]
CN—cranial nerve
CND—congenital neuromuscular disorder
CNS—central nervous system
CNV—conduction nerve velocity
coagulator
    Malis c.
Cockayne
    disease
    syndrome
Cogan
    disease
    syndrome
cognition
cognitive
cogwheel
    c. gait
    c. phenomenon
    c. rigidity
    c. sign
cogwheeling
Collet
    syndrome
Collet-Sicard
    syndrome
colliculi (plural of colliculus)
colliculitis
colliculus (colliculi)
    facial c.
    inferior c.
Colorado tick fever
column
    Gowers c.
coma
    epileptic c.
comatose
comes (comites)
commissura (commissurae)
    c. alba medullae spinalis
    c. anterior cerebri
    c. cerebelli
    c. grisea medullae spinalis
    c. habenularum

commissural
    c. myelotomy
commissure
    Meynert c.
commotio
    c. cerebri
    c. spinalis
compensatory
complex
    Parkinson dementia c.
computed
    cranial c. tomography (CCT)
    c. tomography (CT)
computerized
    c. axial tomography (CAT)
COMS—chronic organic mental
    syndrome
COMT—catechol-O-methyl trans-
    ferase
COMT inhibitors [a class of drugs]
concussion
    acceleration c.
    compression c.
conduction
    c. velocity
    nerve c.
confabulation
confluens
    c. sinuum
confusion
congestion
    cerebral c.
connector
    Rochester c.
constellation
    c. of symptoms
contraction
    Gowers c.
contrast
    positive c. encephalography
    c. ventriculography
contraversion
    ocular c.
contrecoup
contusion
    cerebral c.
conus
    c. medullaris

convexobasia
convolution
    Broca c.
    c. of cerebrum
    c.'s of Gratiolet
    Heschl c.
    occipitotemporal c.
    Zuckerkandl c.
convulsant
convulsibility
convulsion
    audiogenic c.
    choreic c.
    clonic c.
    coordinate c.
    epileptiform c.
    febrile c.
    hypoglycemic c.
    hysterical c., hysteroid c.
    infantile c.
    jackknife c.
    mimetic c.
    mimic c.
    myoclonic c.
    puerperal c.
    salaam c.
    static c.
    tetanic c.
    tonic-clonic c.
    toxic c.
    traumatic c.
    uremic c.
convulsive
Corning
    puncture
cornu (cornua)
    cornua of spinal cord
cornual
cornuate
cornucommissural
corona (coronae)
    c. radiata
coronal
    c. suture
corpora (plural of corpus)
corporis (genitive of corpus)
corpus (corpora)
    corpora amylacea

corpus (corpora) (continued)
    corpora arenacea
    c. callosum
    c. striatum
corpuscallostomy, corpus callostomy
cortex (cortices)
    agranular c.
    auditory c.
    cerebellar c., c. cerebellis
    c. cerebelli, c. of cerebellum
    cerebral c.
    c. cerebri, c. of cerebrum
    cingulate c.
    driftwood c.
    entorhinal c.
    frontal premotor c.
    interpyramidal c.
    limbic c.
    periamygdaloid c.
    precentral motor c.
    premotor c.
    sensorimotor c.
    somatosensory c.
    supplementary motor c.
corticectomy
cortices (plural of cortex)
corticis (genitive of cortex)
corticoafferent
corticoautonomic
corticobulbar
corticocerebral
corticodiencephalic
corticoefferent
corticomesencephalic
corticopeduncular
corticopontine
corticospinal
corticothalamic
costotransversectomy
costovertebral
Cotte
    operation
Cotugno
    disease
coxsackievirus (group A, group B)
CP—cerebral palsy
    closing pressure
CPI—congenital pain indifference

CPM—central pontine myelinolysis
CR—corneal reflex
cracked pot note
craniad [adv.]
cranial [adj.]
    c. computed tomography
      (CCT)
    c. sutures
cranialis
craniamphitomy
craniectomy
cranioacromial
cranioaural
craniocele
craniocerebral
craniomalacia
craniomeningocele
craniopharyngioma
cranioplasty
craniopuncture
craniorachischisis
    c. totalis
cranioschisis
craniosclerosis
cranioscopy
craniospinal
craniostenosis
craniostosis
craniosynostosis
craniotabes
craniotonoscopy
craniotopography
craniotympanic
craniovertebral
cranitis
cranium
cretinism
Creutzfeldt-Jakob
    disease
    syndrome
crisis (crises)
    brain stem c.
    Lundvall blood c.
crossed reflex
cross-leg Patrick maneuver
Crouzon
    disease
    syndrome

crura (plural of crus)
crural
crus (crura)
    c. I, c. II
    c. cerebelli ad pontem
    c. cerebri
Cruveilhier
    atrophy
    disease
    fossa
    joint
    paralysis
cryohypophysectomy
cryothalamectomy
cryothalamotomy
cryptococcoma
cryptogenic
    c. drop attacks
cryptomerorachischisis
CSC—blow-on-blow (Fr. coup sur coup)
CSF—cerebrospinal fluid
CSF rhinorrhea
CSH—chronic subdural hematoma
CSLR—crossed straight leg raising [test]
cubital
    c. tunnel syndrome
cue [signal, hint, suggestion]
    verbal c.'s
culmen (culmina)
    c. cerebelli, c. of cerebellum
    c. monticuli
culprit
    c. lesion
cuneate
cuneus
curettement
Cushing
    medulloblastoma
    tumor
CV—cerebrovascular
CVA—cerebrovascular accident
CVD—cerebrovascular disease
CVI—cerebrovascular insufficiency
CVOD—cerebrovascular occlusive disease
cyanosis

cybernetics
cyclothymia
cyclothymiac
cyclothymic
cyclothymosis
cyst
    colloid c.
cysticercosis
cytomegalic inclusion disease (CID, CMID)
DAN—diabetic autonomic neuropathy
Dana
    operation
dance
    St. Vitus d.
Dandy-Walker
    deformity
    syndrome
Darkschewitsch
    fibers
    nucleus
Dawson encephalitis
DDD—degenerative disk disease
dearth
    d. of evidence
    d. of findings
    d. of symptoms
debilitated
    d. patient
    d. state
debilitating
    d. illness
debilitative
    d. disease
Debré-Sémélaigne syndrome
decerebellation
decerebrate
    d. rigidity
decerebration
decision
    Durham d.
declive
    d. monticuli cerebelli
decompression
    cerebral d.
    subtemporal d.
    trigeminal d.

decompressive laminectomy
decortication
decursus
    d. fibrarum cerebralium
decussatio (decussationes)
    See *commissura.*
decussation
    Forel d.
    fountain d. of Meynert
deficit
    reversible ischemic neuro-
      logic d.
degeneration
    alcoholic cerebellar d.
    axonal d.
    cerebellar d.
    Holmes d.
    spongiform d.
    striatonigral d.
    wallerian d.
Degos
    disease
    syndrome
Deiters
    phalanges
Dejerine
    disease
    sign
    syndrome
Dejerine-Klumpke
    palsy
    paralysis
    syndrome
Dejerine-Landouzy
    dystrophy
Dejerine-Lichtheim phenomenon
Dejerine-Roussy syndrome
Dejerine-Sottas
    atrophy
    disease
    syndrome
Dejerine-Thomas atrophy
de la Camp sign
demented
dementia
    alcoholic d.
    Alzheimer d.
    arteriosclerotic d.

dementia (continued)
    Binswanger d.
    boxer's d.
    catatonic d.
    chronic d.
    epileptic d.
    hebephrenic d.
    hydrocephalic d.
    d. infantilis
    d. myoclonica
    myxedematous d.
    paralytic d.
    d. paralytica
    d. paranoides
    paretic d.
    d. praecocissima
    d. praecox
    d. praesenilis
    presenile d.
    progressive d.
    d. pugilistica
    semantic d.
    senile d.
    static d.
    subcortical d.
    terminal d.
    toxic d.
    vascular d.
Demerol [anesthetic agent]
de Morsier
    syndrome
de Morsier-Gauthier
    syndrome
demyelinate
demyelination
dendrite
Dennie-Marfan syndrome
dens (dentes)
    d. axis
dentate
    d. suture
depressants [a class of drugs]
depression
    involutional d.
    Leão spreading d.
    pacchionian d.
    postdormital d.
    unipolar d.

depressive
depressor
    Cushing d.
deranencephalia
Dercum
    disease
derencephalocele
derencephalus
derencephaly
De Sanctis-Cacchione
    syndrome
descending
    d. root tractotomy
deterioration
devastation
    senile cortical d.
Devic
    disease
    syndrome
DHE—dihydroergotamine
diachesis
diadochokinesia
diadochokinetic
"diakesis" Phonetic for diachesis.
diaphragma
    d. sellae
diastematocrania
diencephalic
diencephalic syndrome
diencephalohypophysial
diencephalon
digitatio (digitationes)
Dilaudid [anesthetic agent]
Dimitri
    disease
diplegia
    atonic-astatic d.
    flaccid d.
    Förster d.
    infantile d.
    spastic d.
diploë
dis–. See also words beginning dys–.
disc
    See *disk.*
discectomy [pref: diskectomy]
disci (genitive and plural of discus)
disciform ["disiform"]

discitis [pref: diskitis]
discopathy
discrete
    d. downward drifting [of
        raised limb against gravity]
    d. slowing [on EEG]
    d. weakness
discrimination
discus (disci)
disease
    See also *syndrome.*
    Akureyri d.
    Alpers d.
    Alzheimer d.
    Anders d.
    Aran-Duchenne d.
    Azorean d.
    Ballet d.
    Batten d.
    Batten-Mayou d.
    Biedl d.
    Binswanger d.
    Blocq d.
    Bodechtel-Guttmann d.
    Bourneville d.
    Bourneville-Brissaud d.
    Brushfield-Wyatt d.
    Canavan-van Bogaert-
      Bertrand d.
    central nervous system d.
    Charcot d.
    Charcot-Marie-Tooth d.
    Christiansen-Krabbe d.
    Cotugno d.
    Creutzfeldt-Jakob d.
    Crouzon d.
    Cushing d.
    cytomegalic inclusion d.
      (CID, CMID)
    Dercum d.
    Dimitri d.
    Down d.
    Dubini d.
    Dubois d.
    Duchenne d.
    Duchenne-Aran d.
    Economo (von Economo) d.
    Erb d.

disease (continued)
- Erb-Charcot d.
- Erb-Goldflam d.
- Erb-Landouzy d.
- Eulenburg d.
- Fahr d.
- Flatau-Schilder d.
- Friedreich d.
- Fürstner d.
- Gamstorp d.
- Gerlier d.
- Gilles de la Tourette d.
- Goldflam d.
- Goldflam-Erb d.
- Gowers d.
- Guinon d.
- Hartnup d.
- Heine-Medin d.
- Henneberg d.
- Hoffa-Kastert d.
- Hunt d.
- Huntington d.
- Hurst d.
- Janet d.
- Kalischer d.
- Klippel d.
- Koshevnikoff d.
- Krabbe d.
- Kufs d.
- Kugelberg-Welander d.
- Kümmell-Verneuil d.
- Leigh d.
- Leyden d.
- Little d.
- Machado-Joseph d.
- Marchiafava-Bignami d.
- Menkes d.
- Merzbacher-Pelizaeus d.
- Mills d.
- Mitchell d.
- Mouchet d.
- moyamoya d.
- neuropathic joint d.
- Niemann-Pick d.
- Parkinson d.
- Pelizaeus-Merzbacher d.
- Pick d.
- pink d.

disease (continued)
- Ramsay Hunt d.
- Rendu-Osler-Weber d.
- Romberg d.
- Roth (Rot) d.
- Roth-Bernhardt d.
- Sachs d.
- Schilder d.
- Schmorl d.
- Scholz d.
- Scholz-Greenfield d.
- Simmonds d.
- Sjögren d.
- small-vessel d.
- Sottas d.
- Spielmeyer-Vogt d.
- St. Anthony's d.
- Steinert d.
- Strümpell d.
- Sturge d.
- Sturge-Weber d.
- Sturge-Weber-Dimitri d.
- Tay-Sachs d.
- Thomsen d.
- Tourette d.
- Unverricht d.
- van Bogaert-Bertrand d.
- van Bogaert-Nyssen-Peiffer d.
- Vogt d.
- Vogt-Spielmeyer d.
- von Economo d.
- von Hippel-Lindau d.
- von Recklinghausen d.
- Weber d.
- Weir Mitchell
- Werdnig-Hoffmann d.
- Wernicke d.
- white matter d.
- Whytt d.
- Wilson d.
- Winkelman d.
- Ziehen-Oppenheim d.

"disfajea" Phonetic for dysphagia.
"disfazea" Phonetic for dysphasia.
"disfonia" Phonetic for dysphonia.
"disfrasia" Phonetic for dysphrasia.
"disiform" Phonetic for disciform.

disk

> *Note: Some specialists and references prefer* disc.

    herniated d.
    intervertebral d.
    protruded d.
    ruptured d.

diskectomy
    anterior cervical d. and
      fusion (ACDF)

diskiform

diskogram

disorder
    affective d.
    alcoholic brain d.'s
    anxiety d.
    arteriosclerotic brain d.
    autonomic d.
    brain d.
    epileptoid personality d.
    equilibratory d.
    extrapyramidal d.
    somatoform pain d.

distribution
    stocking-glove d.

dolichocephalic

dolichocephalism

doll's eye
    reflex
    sign
    test

doll's head
    maneuver
    phenomenon

dominance

dopaminergics [a class of drugs]

Dorello
    canal

dorsa (plural of dorsum)

dorsad [adv.]

dorsal [adj.]
    d. rhizotomy

dorsi (genitive of dorsum)

dorsomedial
    d. thalamotomy

dorsum (dorsa)
    d. sellae

Down [eponym]
    disease
    syndrome

downgoing

DP—dementia praecox

drawer sign

dressing
    See in *General Surgical Terms.*

DREZ (dorsal root entry zone) lesion

drop
    d. attacks
    d. spells

DSA—digital subtraction angiography

DTP—distal tingling on pressure

DTRs—deep tendon reflexes

Dubini
    chorea
    disease

Dubowitz
    evaluation
    examination
    Neurological Assessment
    score

Duchenne
    disease
    dystrophy
    muscular dystrophy
    paralysis
    syndrome

Duchenne-Aran
    disease
    muscular atrophy
    sign

Duchenne-Erb
    paralysis
    syndrome

Duchenne-Landouzy
    dystrophy

Duchenne-Landouzy–type dystrophy

Duchenne-type muscular dystrophy

ductus (ductus)
    d. perilymphatici

Duncan ventricle

dural
    d. incision

dura mater
    d.m. encephali
    d.m. of brain
    d.m. of spinal cord
    d.m. spinalis
duramatral
duraplasty
Duret
    hemorrhage
    lesion
duroarachnitis
dys–. See also words beginning dis–.
dysarthria
    ataxic d.
    d. literalis
    spastic d.
    d. syllabaris spasmodica
dysarthric
dysbasia
    d. angiosclerotica
    d. angiospastica
    d. intermittens angiosclerotica
    d. lordotica progressiva
    d. neurasthenica intermittens
dyscalculia
dyscephaly
dyschiria
dysdiadochokinesia
dysergia
dysgraphia
dyskinesia
    d. algera
dyskinetic
dyslalia
dyslexia
dysmetria
dysnomia
dysosmia
dysphagia [difficulty swallowing]
dysphagic
dysphasia [difficulty with speech]
dysphonia
dysphonic
dysphrasia
dysphylaxia
dyspraxia
dysprosody

dysrhythmia
    cortical d.
    paroxysmal cerebral d.
dyssymbolia
dyssynergia
    d. cerebellaris myoclonica
    d. cerebellaris progressiva
dystaxia
    d. agitans
    d. cerebralis infantilis
dystectia
dystonia
    cranial d.
    d. musculorum deformans
    segmental d.
    torsion d.
dystrophia
    d. myotonica
dystrophy
    autosomal-dominant distal d.
    Becker d.
    Becker-type muscular d.
    Duchenne d.
    Duchenne muscular d.
    Duchenne-type muscular d.
    Emery-Dreifuss d.
    Erb d.
    facioscapulohumeral d.
    Fröhlich adiposogenital d.
    juvenile progressive muscu-
        lar d.
    Landouzy-Dejerine d.
    Leyden-Möbius
    limb-girdle d.
    muscular d.
    myotonic d.
    oculocerebrorenal d.
    oculopharyngeal d., ocu-
        lopharyngeal muscular d.
    reflex sympathetic d.
    scapulohumeral d.
    scapuloperoneal d.
    thyroneural d.
    X-linked muscular d.
Eaton-Lambert syndrome
ecchordosis physaliphora
echoencephalogram

echoencephalograph
    midline e.
echoencephalography
echogenic
echogenicity
echogram
echographia
echokinesis
echolucent
echomatism
echomotism
echopathy
echopraxia
echopraxis
echovirus (serotypes 1–7, 9, 11–18,
    20–27, 29–34)
Economo. See *von Economo.*
ED—epileptiform discharge
edema
    cerebral e.
    Huguenin e.
    interstitial e.
EEE—eastern equine encephalomy-
    elitis
EEG—electroencephalogram
    electroencephalography
effect [noun: result, outcome]
    See also *phenomenon.*
    clasp-knife e.
    Mierzejewski e.
    Orbeli e.
efferent
Ekbom syndrome
"eko–" Phonetic for words begin-
    ning echo–.
electroacupuncture
electroanalgesia
electroanesthesia
electrocerebral inactivity
electrocorticogram
electrocorticography
electrode
    See also *lead.*
    dual e. lead [EEG]
    multi-e. lead [EEG]
electrodermal
electrodiagnosis
electrodiagnostic

electrodiagnostics
electroencephalogram (EEG)
    brain death protocol e.
    flat e.
    isoelectric e.
electroencephalography (EEG)
electroencephalograph
electrogram
electrography
electrogustometer
electrogustometry
electromyogram (EMG)
    integrated e. (IEMG)
    single-fiber e. (SFEMG)
    ureteral e.
electromyograph
electromyography (EMG)
    needle e.
electroneurography
electroneurolysis
electroneuromyography
electronystagmogram (ENG)
electronystagmography
electrophysiologic
electrospectrogram
electrospectrography
electrospinogram
electrospinography
electrostimulation
electrostriatogram
electrotherapist
electrotonic
electrotonus
electrovagogram
emboliform
embolism
    cerebral e.
embolus (emboli)
Emery-Dreifuss dystrophy
EMG—electromyogram
    electromyography
emission
    positron e. tomography (PET)
emprosthotonos
empyema
    subdural e.
encephalalgia
encephalatrophy

encephalemia
encephalic
encephalitic
encephalitis (encephalitides)
    acute demyelinating e.
    acute disseminated e.
    acute necrotizing e.
    American e.
    arbovirus e.
    Baló concentric e.
    boutonneuse e.
    bulbar e.
    Calabrian e.
    California e.
    cerebellar e.
    Condorelli e.
    demyelinating e.
    diffuse sclerosing e.
    eastern e.
    eastern equine e.
    eastern North American e.
    Economo e.
    hemorrhagic e.
    e. hemorrhagica superior
    herpes simplex e.
    inclusion body e.
    Japanese B e.
    e. lethargica
    limbic e.
    Mengo e.
    mumps e.
    Murray Valley e.
    e. neonatorum
    otic e.
    perivenous e.
    postexanthematous e.
    Russian spring-summer e.
    Schilder e.
    Sicilian e.
    e. siderans
    St. Louis e.
    Strümpell-Leichtenstern e.
    tick-borne e.
    torula e.
    typhoid e.
    varicella e.
    Venezuelan equine e.
    viral e.

encephalitis (encephalitides) (continued)
    von Economo e.
    western e.
    western equine e.
    West Nile e.
encephaloarteriography
encephalocele
encephalocoele
enccphalocystocele
encephalocystomeningocele
encephalogram
encephalography
    air e.
    fractional e.
    gamma e.
    positive contrast e.
encephalolith
encephaloma
encephalomalacia
    periventricular e.
encephalomeningitis
encephalomeningocele
encephalomeningopathy
encephalomyelitis
    eastern equine e. (EEE)
    Kelly e.
    parainfectious e.
    western equine e. (WEE)
encephalomyelocele
encephalomyeloneuropathy
encephalomyelopathy
encephalomyeloradiculitis
encephalomyeloradiculoneuritis
encephalomyeloradiculopathy
encephalon
encephalonarcosis
encephalopathy
    alcoholic e.
    anoxic e.
    Creutzfeldt-Jakob presenile e.
    demyelinating e.
    hepatic e.
    hypercalcemic e.
    hypoxic e.
    Leigh e.
    metabolic e.
    postanoxic e.

encephalopathy (continued)
    progressive multifocal e.
    spongiform e.
    toxic e.
    uremic e.
    Wernicke e.
encephalopuncture
encephalopyosis
encephaloradiculitis
encephalorrhagia
encephalosclerosis
encephaloscopy
encephalosepsis
encephalosis
encephalospinal
encephalothlipsis
encephalotomy
encephalotrigeminal
    e. angiomatosis
endarterectomy
    carotid e. (CEA)
endarteritis
    syphilitic cerebral e.
ENG—electronystagmogram
    electronystagmography
engram
en passage ["ahn pah-sahj"]
en passant ["ahn pah-sahn"]
"en-sed" Phonetic for NSAID (non-steroidal anti-inflammatory drug).
"ensef–" Phonetic for words beginning enceph–.
enuresis [urinary incontinence, bed-wetting]
    epileptic e.
EPC—epilepsia partialis continua
ependyma
ependymal
ependymitis
ependymoblast
ependymoblastoma
ependymocyte
ependymocytoma
ependymoma
ependymopathy
"epi" Slang for epinephrine.
epicritic

epidermoid
epidermoidoma
epidural
    e. abscess
    e. empyema
    e. hemorrhage
epilepsia
    e. gravior
    e. major
    e. minor
    e. mitior
    e. nutans
    e. partialis continua
    e. procursiva
    e. rotatoria
    e. tarda
epilepsy
    abdominal e.
    absence e.
    Bravais-jacksonian e.
    catamenial e.
    cortical e.
    corticoreticular e.
    cryptogenic e.
    diurnal e.
    focal e.
    grand mal e.
    hysterical e.
    idiopathic e.
    jacksonian e.
    juvenile myoclonic e.
    Lafora-type of e.
    larval e.
    latent e.
    limbic e.
    matutinal e.
    menstrual e.
    musicogenic e.
    myoclonus e.
    nocturnal e.
    petit mal e.
    photosensitive e.
    physiologic e.
    primary e.
    procursive e.
    psychic e.
    psychomotor e.
    reflex e.

epilepsy (continued)
    rolandic e.
    secondary e.
    seesaw e.
    sensory e.
    serial e.
    sylvian e.
    symptomatic e.
    tardy e.
    temporal lobe e.
    tonic e.
    traumatic e.
    uncinate e.
    Unverricht-Lundborg type of
      e.
epileptic
    e. equivalent
    e. seizure
epileptiform
epileptogenic
epileptogenous
epileptoid
epileptologist
epileptology
epileptosis
epinephrine
epineural
epineurial
epineurium
episode
    psycholeptic e.
    syncopal e.
episthotonos
epithalamic
epithalamus
epithelia (plural of epithelium)
epitheliitis
epithelioma
    e. myxomatodes psammosum
epithelium (epithelia)
    mesenchymal e.
    nerve e.
EPP—end-plate potential
"eppy" Slang for epinephrine.
EPS—extrapyramidal signs
    extrapyramidal symptoms
EPSP—excitatory postsynaptic
  potential

ER—evoked response
Erb
    atrophy
    disease
    dystrophy
    palsy
    progressive muscular dystro-
      phy
    pseudohypertrophic muscu-
      lar dystrophy
    sclerosis
    spastic paraplegia
    syndrome
Erb-Charcot disease
Erb-Duchenne paralysis
Erb-Goldflam disease
Erb-Landouzy disease
Erb-Oppenheim-Goldflam syndrome
Erdheim
    tumor
erratic
erythrochromia
erythromelalgia
    e. of the head
erythroprosopalgia
ESB—electrical stimulation to brain
état
    é. marbré
    é. lacunaire
    é. criblé
    é. dysmelinique
ethmoidolacrimal
    e. suture
ethmoidomaxillary
    e. suture
Eulenburg disease
eupraxia
eupraxic
evaluation
    Dubowitz e.
examination
    Dubowitz e.
excitability
    proprioceptive e.
excitomotor
exteroceptive
extracranial

extradural
    e. venography
extramedullary
extrapyramidal
eye
    doll's e.'s
fabere
facetectomy
facies (facies)
    Marshall Hall f.
    myasthenic f.
    myopathic f.
    paralytic f.
    Parkinson f., parkinsonian f.
    tabetic f.
Fahr
    disease
Fajersztajn
    sign
fallopian
    f. aqueduct
    f. artery
    f. hiatus
    f. neuritis
Fallopius
    aqueduct of F.
falx
    f. cerebelli
    f. cerebri
Fañana
    glia of F.
fascia (fasciae)
    dentate f.
fascicular
fasciculated
fasciculation
fasciculitis
fasciculus (fasciculi)
    See also *bundle* and *tract.*
    f. aberrans of Monakow
    f. cuneatus
    f. of Foville
    f. of Gowers
    f. gracilis
    f. lenticularis
    f. of Rolando
fastigium

Fazio-Londe
    atrophy
    disease
    syndrome
F&D—fixed and dilated
feeblemindedness
female pseudo-Turner syndrome
"fenil–" Phonetic for words beginning phenyl–.
"fenomenon" Phonetic for phenomenon.
"feo–" Phonetic for words beginning pheo–.
Fergusson and Critchley ataxia
festination
fiber
    Darkschewitsch f.
fibra (fibrae)
fibril
fibrilla (fibrillae)
fibrillar, fibrillary
fibrillated
fibroblastoma
    meningeal f.
fibroma
    f. cavernosum
fibromatogenic
fibromatoid
fibromatosis
fibromatous
fibromectomy
figure
    fortification f
"fi-ko-mi-co-sis" Phonetic for phycomycosis.
fila (plural of filum)
filament
filamentum (filamenta)
filum (fila)
    f. of spinal dura mater
    f. terminale
fire
    St. Anthony's f.
Fisher
    syndrome
fissura (fissurae)
    f. cerebri lateralis sylvii

fissure
> Broca f.
> calcarine f.
> dentate f.
> Monro f.
> Pansch f.
> Rolando f.
> f. of Sylvius

fistula (fistulas, fistulae)
> caroticocavernous f.
> cerebrospinal fluid f.

"fizeo–" Phonetic for words beginning physio–.

Flatau
> disease
> law
> syndrome

Flatau-Schilder
> disease

flavectomy

"flebitis" Phonetic for phlebitis.

Flechsig
> area
> bundle
> fasciculi
> tract

floccillation

flocculus

flow
> cerebral blood f.

fluctuation

fluid
> See also *liquor.*
> cerebrospinal f. (CSF)
> straw-colored f.
> xanthochromic f.

focus (foci)
> epileptogenic f.
> mirror f.
> secondary epileptogenic f.

"foit" Phonetic for Voigt and Voit.

Foix
> paramedian syndrome
> syndrome

Foix-Alajouanine
> disease
> syndrome

"foke-mahn" Phonetic for Volkmann.

"fokt" Phonetic for Vogt.

fold
> Veraguth f.

folium (folia)
> f. cacuminis
> folia cerebelli
> f. vermis

fontanelle
> See also *fonticulus.*
> anterior f.
> anterolateral f.
> Casser f., casserian f., Casserio f.
> frontal f.
> Gerdy f.
> occipital f.
> posterolateral f.
> quadrangular f.
> sagittal f.
> sphenoidal f.
> triangular f.

fonticulus (fonticuli)
> f. quadrangularis
> f. triangularis

foot (feet)
> dangle f.
> drop f. [also: footdrop]

footdrop

foramen (foramina)
> arachnoid f.
> f. caecum medullae oblongatae
> f. cecum ossis frontalis
> emissary f.
> f. ethmoidale anterius
> f. ethmoidale posterius
> f. ovale basis cranii
> f. ovale ossis sphenoidalis
> interventricular f.
> jugular f.
> f. of Key and Retzius
> Luschka f.
> Magendie f.
> f. magnum
> f. of Monro
> neural f.
> f. occipitale magnum
> f. ovale ossis sphenoidalis

foramen (foramina) (continued)
    oval f. of sphenoid bone
    f. of Pacchioni, pacchionian f.
    Retzius f.
    f. rotundum ossis sphenoidalis
    f. spinosum
    f. Vesalii, f. of Vesalius
    f. of Vicq d'Azyr
foraminal
foraminotomy
forceps
    Love-Gruenwald f.
forebrain
foreconscious
Forel decussation
formatio (formationes)
    f. alba
    f. grisea
    f. hippocampalis
    f. reticularis pontis
    f. vermicularis
formation
    hippocampal f.
    medullary reticular f.
fornix (fornices)
    f. cerebri
Förster-Penfield
    operation
fortification
    f. spectrum
fossa (fossae)
    cerebellar f.
    cerebral f.
    cranial f.
    f. cranii anterior
    f. cranii media
    f. cranii posterior
    Cruveilhier f.
    frontal f.
    hypophyseal f.
    lateral f. of brain
    f. of Pacchioni
    posterior f.
fossula (fossulae)
    f. of vestibular window
Fothergill
    disease
    neuralgia

Foville
    fasciculus (fasciculus of
      Foville)
    syndrome
    tract
fractional
    f. encephalography
fracture
    compound skull f.
    dentate f.
    hangman's f.
    temporal bone f.
    transcervical f.
fraise
    diamond f.
Francke
    striae
Franke
    tabes operation
Frankel
    See also *Frenkel.*
    classification (groups A–E)
Frazier-Spiller
    operation
frena (plural of frenum)
frenal
"freng-kuhl" Phonetic for Frankel
    and Frenkel.
Frenkel
    See also *Frankel.*
    exercises
    movements
    symptoms
    tracks
    treatment
frenulum (frenula)
    See also *vinculum.*
    f. of anterior medullary velum
    f. cerebelli
    f. of Giacomini
frenum (frena)
    See *frenulum* and *vinculum.*
Friderichsen-Waterhouse syndrome
Friedmann
    complex
    disease
    vasomotor syndrome

Friedreich
    ataxia
    disease
    foot
    tabes
Fröhlich (Froehlich)
    dystrophy
Froin
    syndrome
frons
    f. cranii
frontal
    f. lobotomy
    f. suture
frontolacrimal
    f. suture
fronto-occipital
    f-o. tract
frontoparietal
    f. suture
frontosphenoid
    f. suture
frontotemporal
frontozygomatic
    f. suture
fugue
    epileptic f.
    f. state
funicular
funiculate
funiculi (genitive and plural of
    funiculus)
funiculitis
funiculus (funiculi)
    f. cuneatus
    funiculi of spinal cord
    f. ventralis
furor
    f. epilepticus
Fürstner
    disease
fusion
    anterior cervical diskectomy
      and f. (ACDF)
"fwah" Phonetic for Foix.
"fy-ko-my-co-sis" Phonetic for phy-
    comycosis.
gag reflex

gait
    antalgic g.
    ataxic g.
    calcaneous g.
    cerebellar g.
    Charcot g.
    cogwheel g.
    double-step g.
    drag-to g.
    drunken g.
    duck g.
    equine g.
    festinating g.
    footdrop g.
    four-point g.
    glue-footed g.
    gluteal g.
    gluteus maximus g.
    gluteus medius g.
    heel-toe g.
    helicopod g.
    hemiplegic g.
    listing g.
    myopathic g.
    Oppenheim g.
    paraparetic g.
    Petren g.
    reeling g.
    scissors g.
    skater's g.
    spastic equinus g.
    staggering g.
    stamping g.
    star g.
    steppage g.
    swing-through g.
    swing-to g.
    tabetic g.
    tandem g.
    three-point g.
    Todd g.
    Trendelenburg g.
    two-point g.
    waddling g.
gait and station
α-galactosidase A [alpha-]
β-galactosidase [beta-]

galea
- g. aponeurotica
- tendinous g.

galeatus

galvanopalpation

gamma
- g.-aminobutyrate
- g.-aminobutyric acid (GABA)
- g. encephalography
- g.-glutamylcysteine synthetase (deficiency)

gammography
- cerebral g.

Gamstorp disease

ganglial

ganglion (ganglia, ganglions)
- basal ganglia
- ganglia of facial nerve
- gasserian g.
- Meckel g.
- trigeminal g.

ganglionectomy

ganglioneuroblastoma

ganglioneuroma
- dumbbell g.
- hourglass g.

gangliosympathectomy

Ganser
- commissure

Garcin syndrome

Gardner
- operation

Gastaut
- disease
- syndrome

gastric
- g. neurectomy

GBA—ganglionic-blocking agent

GCS—Glasgow Coma Scale

"geel duh lah too-ret" Phonetic for
Gilles de la Tourette.

"gee-naw" Phonetic for Guinon.

"gee-ya bah-ray" Phonetic for Guillain-Barré.

gegenhalten

Gélineau syndrome

generalization

genicula (plural of geniculum)

geniculate

geniculate body

geniculocalcarine

geniculocalcarine tract

geniculotemporal

geniculum (genicula)

genu
- g. corporis callosi
- g. nervi facialis

Gerhardt
- sign

Gerlier disease

Gerstmann syndrome

Gill
- operation

Gilles de la Tourette
- disease
- syndrome

glabella

glabellar [adj.]
- g. tap reflex
- g. tap sign

gland
- pineal g.
- pituitary g.

glaserian fissure

Glasgow
- Coma Scale (GCS)
- score
- sign

glia
- cytoplasmic g.
- g. of Fañana
- fibrillary g.

glial

glioblastoma
- giant cell g.
- magnocellular g.
- g. multiforme

gliocytoma

gliofibrilla

gliofibrillary

gliofibrosarcoma

gliogenous

glioma
- astrocytic g.
- ependymal g.
- extramedullary g.

glioma (continued)
    ganglionic g.
    heterotopic g.
    malignant peripheral g.
    g. multiforme
    pontine g.
    g. sarcomatosum
gliomatosis
gliomatous
gliomyoma
gliomyxoma
glioneuroma
gliophagia
gliopil
gliosa
gliosarcoma
gliosis
    basilar g.
    cerebellar g.
    diffuse g.
    hemispheric g.
    hypertrophic nodular g.
    isomorphic g.
    lobar g.
    perivascular g.
    progressive subcortical g.
    spinal g.
    unilateral g.
gliosome
globus (globi)
    g. pallidus
glomerulus (glomeruli)
γ-glutamylcysteine synthetase deficiency [gamma-]
glycorrhachia
Goldflam
    disease
Goldflam-Erb
    disease
Goldstein
    classification
    syndrome
Goldstein-Reichmann syndrome
Golgi cells
Goll tract
Gombault
    degeneration
    neuritis

Gordon
    reflex
    sign
    symptom
Gowers
    column
    contraction
    disease
    fasciculus
    phenomenon
    sign
    tract
Gradenigo
    syndrome
Gradenigo-Lannois
    syndrome
grand mal
    g.m. epilepsy
    g.m. seizure
graphesthesia
grasp reflex
Grashey aphasia
Grasset-Gaussel phenomenon
gray
    g. matter
gray-out
groove
    g. of Lucas
GSR—galvanic skin response
guard
    Sachs g.
Gubler
    hemiplegia
    paralysis
    sign
    tumor
Gubler-Millard paralysis
Guidi canal
Guillain-Barré
    polyneuritis
    reflex
    syndrome
Guinon
    disease
gumma (gummas, gummata)
gummate
gummatous
GVHD—graft-versus-host disease

GVHR—graft-versus-host reaction
gyrectomy
gyrencephalic
gyri (plural of gyrus)
gyrometer
gyrose
gyrospasm
gyrus (gyri)
    Broca g.
    cingulate g.
    cuneolingual g.
    deep transitional g.
    dentate g.
    external orbital g.
    fusiform g.
    hippocampal g.
    internal orbital g.
    marginal g.
    parahippocaudal g.
    parasplenial g.
    postrolandic g.
    precentral g.
    prerolandic g.
    retrosplenal g.
    g. of Retzius
    splenial g.
    straight g.
    subcalcarine g.
    supramarginal g.
habenula
Haenel symptom
Haller (von Haller)
    line
Hallervorden-Spatz
    syndrome
Hallgren syndrome
hallucination
    See in *Psychiatry* section.
halo
    h.-pelvic traction
    h. traction
Halstead-Reitan
    battery
    test
hammer
    h. palsy
Hammond
    syndrome

Hammond (continued)
    disease
handshaking
hangman's fracture
Harris
    migrainous neuralgia
Hartnup
    disease
    syndrome
Haven syndrome
Hawes-Pallister-Landor syndrome
Haynes
    operation
head
    classification
    zones
headache
    cluster h.
    exertional h.
    Horton h.
    jolt h.
    meningeal h.
    migraine h.
    muscle contraction h.
    neuralgic h.
    nitroglycerin h.
    orgasmic h.
    paraplegic h.
    postconcussional h.
    pressor h.
    spinal fluid loss h.
    tension h.
    thunderclap h.
    traction h.
    traumatic h.
    vascular h.
Head-Holmes syndrome
head nodding, head-nodding
Heine-Medin disease
helicopod
    h. gait
Helweg
    bundle
    tract
hemangioblastoma
hemangiomatosis
hematoma
    epidural h.

hematoma (continued)
    extradural h.
    intracerebral h.
    intramural h.
    subdural h.
hematomyelia
hemianencephaly
hemianesthesia
    bulbar h.
    peduncular h.
hemiballismus
hemichorea
    paralytic h.
    posthemiplegic h.
    preparalytic h.
hemicorticectomy
hemicrania
hemicraniectomy
hemifacial microsomia
hemigastrectomy
    h. and vagotomy (H&V)
hemihypesthesia
hemihypoplasia
hemiplegia
    See also *paraplegia, palsy,*
    and *paralysis.*
    Avellis h.
    bulbar h.
    cerebellar h.
    collateral h.
    congenital h.
    functional h.
    hysterical h.
    organic h.
    pontine h.
hemisection
    h. of spinal cord
hemisphere
    cerebellar h.
    cerebral h.
    nondominant h.
hemispherectomy
hemispherium (hemispheria)
    h. cerebelli
hemorrhage
    cerebellar h.
    Duret h.
    epidural h.

hemorrhage (continued)
    intracerebral h.
    intracranial h.
    intradural h.
    intraparenchymal h.
    intraventricular h.
    meningeal h.
    neonatal subdural h.
    pontine h.
    putaminal h.
    subarachnoid h.
    subdural h.
    subgaleal h.
    thalamic h.
hemorrhagic
Henneberg disease
Henoch
    chorea
Henoch-Schönlein
    purpura
    syndrome
hepatic
    h. coma
    h. encephalopathy
heredoataxia
hernia
    h. of brain
herniated
herniation
    disk h.
    h. of intervertebral disk
    h. of nucleus pulposus
    tentorial h.
    tonsillar h. of nucleus pulposus
    transtentorial h.
    uncal h.
herpes
    h. meningoencephalitis
    neuralgic h.
herpesencephalitis
Hertwig-Magendie
    phenomenon
    sign
    syndrome
hertz (Hz)
Heschl convolution
heterotonic

Heubner
    artery
    disease
Hibbs
    operation
highly selective vagotomy
hilum (hila)
    h. of caudal olivary nucleus
    h. of dentate nucleus
    h. of inferior olivary nucleus
    h. nuclei olivaris caudalis
    h. nuclei olivaris inferioris
    h. nuclei dentati
hilus (hili). See *hilum.*
hindbrain
"hipnahgojik" Phonetic for hypnagogic.
"hipno–" Phonetic for words beginning hypno–.
"hipo–" Phonetic for words beginning hypo–.
Hippel-Lindau. See *von Hippel-Lindau.*
hippocampal
hippocampus
    h. leonis
    h. nudus
Hirschberg reflex
His [eponym]
    isthmus
    space
HMSN—hereditary motor and sensory neuropathy
HNP—herniated nucleus pulposus
hodology
Hoffmann
    atrophy
    phenomenon
    reflex
    sign
Hoffmann-Werdnig syndrome
Holmes
    ataxia
    degeneration
    phenomenon
    sign
Holmes-Adie
    syndrome

Holmes-Stewart phenomenon
holorachischisis
Homén syndrome
homolateral
homonymous
    h. hemianopia
horn
    Ammon h.
Horner
    syndrome
Hortega cell
Horton
    arteritis
    cephalalgia
    disease
    headache
    syndrome
H-reflex
HSV encephalopathy
Huguenin edema
Hunt
    atrophy
    disease
    neuralgia
    paradoxical phenomenon
    paralysis
    striatal syndrome
    syndrome
    tremor
Huntington
    chorea
    disease
    sign
Hurler-Scheie
    compound
    syndrome
Hurst disease
Huschke
    auditory teeth
Hutchinson
    facies
    mask
H&V—hemigastrectomy and vagotomy
hydantoins [a class of drugs]
hydrocele
    h. colli
hydrocephalic

hydrocephalocele
hydrocephaloid
hydrocephalus
    communicating h.
    h. ex vacuo
    low-pressure h.
    noncommunicating h.
    obstructive h.
    otitic h.
    postmeningitic h.
    post traumatic h.
hydromeningitis
hydromeningocele
hydromicrocephaly
hydromyelia
hydromyelocele
hydromyelomeningocele
hygroma
    subdural h.
hypalgesia
hypencephalon
hyperalgesia
hyperalgesic
hyperammonemia
hyperaphia
hyperaphic
hyperarousal
hyperbilirubinemia
    congenital h.
    conjugated h.
    constitutional h.
    hereditary nonhemolytic h.
    neonatal h.
    unconjugated h.
hyperbilirubinemic
hyperbrachycephalic
hyperbrachycephaly
hypercryalgesia
hypercryesthesia
hyperequilibrium
hyperesthesia
    cerebral h.
    muscular h.
    oneiric h.
    tactile h.
hyperesthetic
hyperexplexia
hypergeusesthesia

hypergeusia
hyperglycerolemia
    infantile-type h.
    juvenile-type h.
    microdeletion-type h.
hyperglycinemia
    ketotic h.
    nonketotic h.
hyperinnervation
hyperkinesia
hyperkinesis
hyperkinetic
hypermetria
hypermyotonia
hyperosmia
hyperosmolar
hyperosphresia
hyperostosis
    calvarial h.
    h. cranii
    h. frontalis interna
    Morgagni h.
hyperpallesthesia
hyperpathia
hyperphonia
hyperphosphatasemia
hyperpipecolatemia
hyperplasia
hyperplastic
hyperponesis
hyperponctic
hyperpraxia
hyperpselaphesia
hyperreactive
hyperreflexia
hyperresponsive
hyperresponsiveness
hypersensibility
hypersensitive
hypersensitivity
    carotid sinus h.
hypersensitization
hyperserotonemia
hypersomnia
    continuous h.
    paroxysmal h.
    periodic h.
hypersomnolence

hyperspongiosis
hyperstimulation
hypersympathicotonus
hypertarachia
hypertensive
       h. encephalopathy
hyperthermalgesia
hyperthermesthesia
hypertonia
hypertonic
hypertonicity
hyperventilation
hypervigilance
hypesthesia
hypnagogic
hypnagogue
hypnoanesthesia
hypnogenic
hypnoid
hypnoidal
hypnology
hypnonarcosis
hypnopompic
hypnosis
hypnotics [a class of drugs]
hypoactive
       h. deep tendon reflexes
hypoactivity
hypoalphalipoproteinemia
hypocalcemia
hypocalcemic
hypochordal
hypodynamia
hypoequilibrium
hypoesthesia
       acoustic h.
       gustatory h.
       olfactory h.
       tactile h.
hypoesthetic
hypoexcitability
hypoexcitable
hypogeusia
hypoglycorrhachia
hypohypnotic
hypoisotonic
hypokinesia
hypokinesis

hypokinetic
hypolemmal
hypometria
hypomyotonia
hypopallesthesia
hypophonia
hypophosphatasia
hypophosphatemia
       hereditary h.
       X-linked h.
hypophosphatemic
hypophysectomize
hypophysectomy
       transsphenoidal h.
hypophysial
hypophysioportal
hypophysioprivic
hypophysis
       accessory h.
       h. cerebri
hypophysitis
hypophysoma
hypopinealism
hypopituitary
hypoplasia
hypoponesis
hypopotentia
hypopraxia
hypopselaphesia
hyporeactive
hyporeflexia
hyposensitive
hyposensitivity
hyposmia
hyposomnia
hyposthenia
hypostheniant
hyposthenic
hyposympathicotonus
hyposynergia
hypotaxia
hypotelorism
       orbital h.
hypotension
       chronic idiopathic orthostat-
         ic h.
       chronic orthostatic h.
       familial orthostatic h.

hypotension (continued)
  idiopathic orthostatic h.
  intracranial h.
  orthostatic h.
  postural h.
  vascular h.
hypothalamic
hypothalamotomy
hypothalamus
hypothermia
hypothermic
hypotonia
  benign congenital h.
  infantile h.
hypotonic
hypotrophy
hypoxemia
hypoxemic
hypoxia
hypoxic
  h. insult
hypsarrhythmia
hysteroneurasthenia
Hz—hertz
IASP—International Association
  for the Study of Pain
iatrogenic
IC—intracerebral
  intracranial
ICA—internal carotid artery
  intracranial aneurysm
ICAO—internal carotid artery
  occlusion
ICP—intracranial pressure
ictal
ictus
  i. epilepticus
  i. paralyticus
  i. sanguinis
ideokinetic
ideomotion
ideomotor
idiomuscular
idioneural
idiopathic
idioretinal
idiospasm
IEMG—integrated electromyogram

IJP—internal jugular [vein] pressure
IJV—internal jugular vein
"iktus" Phonetic for ictus.
illness
  debilitating i.
imaging
  See in *Radiology, Nuclear
    Medicine, and Other
    Imaging* section.
impulse
  proprioceptive i.'s
inactivity
  electrocerebral i.
incisura (incisurae)
  i. angularis ventriculi
  i. cerebelli
  i. clavicularis sterni
  i. frontalis
  i. pterygoidea
  i. temporalis
  i. tentorii cerebelli
incisural
incisure
incoherent
incontinentia
  i. pigmenti
incoordination
index (indexes, indices)
  See also *classification.*
  i. of mental deterioration
indusium griseum
"ineon" Phonetic for inion.
infarction
  brain stem i.
  cerebral i.
  lacunar i.
  pituitary i.
  watershed i.
infection
  cysticercosis i.
infraorbital
  i. suture
infundibulum (infundibula)
  i. hypothalami
inhibitor
  acetylcholinesterase (AChE)
    inhibitors [a class of drugs]

inhibitor (continued)
    cholinesterase i.'s [a class of drugs]
    COMT i.'s [a class of drugs]
inion
innervated
insensible
insomnia
insomniac
insomnic
insula (insulae)
    i. of Reil
insult
    cerebellar i.
    cerebral i.
    hypoxic i.
intellect
interictal
interneuron
interparietal
    i. suture
interpediculate
interpeduncular
interspinous
interval
    lucid i.
intervertebral
intracephalic
intracerebellar
intracerebral
intracisternal
intracranial
    i. pressure (IP)
intralobar
intramedullary
    i. tractotomy
intraparietal
intraspinal
intravascular
    i. coagulation
ipsiversion
    ocular i.
IPSP—inhibitory postsynaptic potential
irritation
    cerebral i.
    meningeal i.
    spinal i.

irritation (continued)
    sympathetic i.
ischemia
    brain stem i.
    transient carotid i.
    transient cerebral i.
    vasospastic cerebral i.
ischogyria
island
    i.'s of Calleja
    olfactory i.'s
    i. of Reil
"is-mus" Phonetic for isthmus.
isotope
    i. ventriculography
isthmectomy
isthmi (plural of isthmus)
isthmic
isthmus (isthmi)
    i. of cingulate gyrus
    gyral i.
    i. gyri fornicati
    i. hippocampi
IT—intrathecal
IV—intravenous
IVD—intervertebral disk
IVH—intraventricular hemorrhage
Jackson
    epilepsy
    law
    paralysis
    rule
    sign
    syndrome
    theory
jacksonian
    j. epilepsy
    j. march
jacksonism
Jacod
    syndrome
Jacod-Negri
    syndrome
Jakob
    disease
    pseudosclerosis
Jakob-Creutzfeldt
    disease

Jakob-Creutzfeldt (continued)
    syndrome
Janet
    disease
    test
Japanese B encephalitis
jargonaphasia
"jeel duh lah too-ret" Phonetic for
    Gilles de la Tourette.
Jendrassik maneuver
"jibberish" Phonetic for gibberish.
Joffroy
    reflex
    sign
joint
    atlantoaxial j.
    j. position sense
    suture j.
    temporomandibular j. (TMJ)
Jolly
    reaction
    sign
    test
Joseph
    syndrome
juga (plural of jugum)
jugal
    j. suture
jugular
jugum (juga)
Kaes
    feltwork
    line
Kaes-Bekhterev
    band
    layer
    stripe
Kahler
    law
Kalischer
    disease
Kaplan test
Katayama
    disease
    syndrome
Kearns-Sayer syndrome
Keen
    operation

Kehrer
    reflex
Kehrer-Adie
    syndrome
Kennedy
    disease
    syndrome
Kerr
    sign
Kiloh-Nevin
    myopathy
kinanesthesia
kinesia
    paradoxical k.
kinesiesthesiometer
kinesiology
kinesioneurosis
kinesis
kinesitherapy
kinesodic
kinesthesia
kinesthetic
kinetic
Kinsbourne syndrome
Klippel disease
Klippel-Feil
    malformation
    sign
    syndrome
Klumpke
    palsy
    paralysis
Klumpke-Dejerine
    paralysis
    syndrome
Klüver-Bucy
    syndrome
Koerber-Salus-Elschnig syndrome
Kohnstamm phenomenon
koilorrhachic
"kolee–" Phonetic for words begin-
    ning chole–, choli–, coli–.
"kolesteatoma" Phonetic for
    cholesteatoma.
"ko-mees" Phonetic for comes.
"kon-tre-koo" Phonetic for contre-
    coup.

"kor–" Phonetic for words begin-
    ning cor– and chor–.
Korsakoff (Korsakov)
    amnesia
    disease
    syndrome
Koschewnikow, Kozhevnikov. Vari-
    ants of *Koshevnikoff.*
Koshevnikoff
    disease
    epilepsy
Krabbe
    disease
    hypoplasia
    leukodystrophy
    sclerosis
    syndrome
Krause
    ventricle
"krus" Phonetic for crus.
Kufs disease
Kugelberg-Welander disease
Kuhne
    muscular phenomenon
Kümmell
    disease
    spondylitis
Kümmell-Verneuil disease
Kussmaul-Landry paralysis
"kvos-tek" Phonetic for Chvostek.
KW—Kugelberg-Welander [syn-
    drome]
L1 through L5—lumbar vertebrae
    1–5
LA—local anesthesia
labia (plural of labium)
labial
labialism
labiochorea
labium (labia)
        See *border, limbus,* and *mar-
            gin.*
laceration
    brain l.
lactulose
lacuna (lacunae)
    cerebral lacunae
    lateral lacunae

lacunar
    l. infarct
lacunula (lacunulae)
lacunule
Lafora
    disease
    epilepsy
    sign
laloplegia
lambda
lambdoid, lambdoidal
    l. suture
Lambert-Eaton myasthenic syndrome
lamina (laminae)
    l. dura
    inferior l. of sphenoid bone
    medullary laminae of thala-
        mus
    medullary l., external
    medullary l., internal
    medullary l. of corpus stria-
        tum, external
    medullary l. of lentiform
        nucleus
    Rexed laminae
    l. of septum pellucidum
    l. of vertebra
    l. of vertebral arch
    white laminae of cerebellum
laminagram
laminar
laminectomy
    cervical l.
    decompressive l.
    lumbar l.
    thoracic l.
laminitis
laminotomy
Landouzy
    disease
    dystrophy
Landouzy-Dejerine
    atrophy
    dystrophy
    type
Landry
    disease
    paralysis

Landry (continued)
    syndrome
Landry-Guillain-Barré
    syndrome
Lasègue
    maneuver
    sign
    test
latency
    absolute l.
    distal l.
    motor l.
    proximal l.
    reducible l.
    REM (rapid eye movement) l.
    residual l.
    sensory l.
    sleep l.
    terminal l.
    total reflex l.
laterality
    crossed l.
    dominant l.
    mixed l.
lateralization
laterodeviation
lateroflexion
lateroposition
lateropulsion
lathyrism
lathyritic
lathyrogen
lathyrogenic
Laumonier ganglion
Laurence-Biedl
    syndrome
Laurence-Moon
    syndrome
Laurence-Moon-Biedl
    law
    syndrome
Lauth ligament
law
    See also *rule.*
    Aran l.
    Babinski l.
    Bastian l.
    Bastian-Bruns l.

law (continued)
    Bell l.
    Bell-Magendie l.
    Cushing l.
    Flatau l.
    Jackson l.
    Magendie l.
    Meyer l.
    Waller l.
    wallerian l.
layer
    See *line* and *stria.*
LCA—left carotid artery
lead ["leed"]
    See also *electrode.*
    black EEG l.
    dual electrode l.
    EEG (electroencephalo-
        gram) l.
    grid l.
    left-sided l.
    multi-electrode l.
    right-sided EEG l.
    sphenoid fossa l.
    white EEG l.
"lee" Phonetic for Leigh.
Leichtenstern sign
Leigh
    disease
    encephalopathy
    syndrome
lemniscus (lemnisci)
    See *bundle, fasciculus,* and
        tract.
Lennox
    syndrome
Lennox-Gastaut
    syndrome
lenticulo-optic
lenticulostriate
lenticulothalamic
lentivirus
Leão spreading depression
Lépine-Froin syndrome
leptocephalia
leptocephalic
leptomeningeal
leptomeninges

leptomeningioma
leptomeningitis
    l. interna
    sarcomatous l.
leptomeningopathy
leptomeninx
Léri
    sign
Leriche
    disease
    operation
    syndrome
lesion
    Brown-Séquard l.
    central l.
    dendritic l.
    DREZ (dorsal root entry
      zone) l.
    Duret l.
    functional l.
    irritative l.
    lower motor neuron l.
    organic l.
    peripheral l.
    primary l.
    ring-wall l.
    space-occupying intracranial
      l.
    structural l.
lethargy
    induced l.
    lucid l.
lethologica
lethonomia
leukodystrophia cerebri progressiva
leukodystrophy
    cerebral l.
    demyelinogenic l.
    globoid l.
    globoid cell l.
    hereditary cerebral l.
    Krabbe l.
    melanodermic l.
    metachromatic l.
    progressive cerebral l.
    spongiform l.
    sudanophilic l.

leukoencephalitis
    acute hemorrhagic l.
    concentric periaxial l.
    l. periaxialis concentrica
    Scholz metachromatic l.
    subacute sclerosing l.
    van Bogaert sclerosing l.
leukoencephalopathy
    acute hemorrhagic l.
    acute necrotizing hemor-
      rhagic l.
    metachromatic l.
    multifocal progressive l.
    progressive multifocal l.
    subacute sclerosing l.
leukomyelitis
leukomyelopathy
leukotomy
    transorbital l.
Lévy-Roussy syndrome
Leyden
    ataxia
    disease
Leyden-Möbius
    dystrophy
    syndrome
    type
Lhermitte sign
Lichtheim
    aphasia
    disease
    plaques
    sign
lidocaine HCl [anesthetic agent]
Liepmann apraxia
ligamentum (ligamenta)
    ligamenta flava, l. flavum
"likenshadel" Phonetic for lücken-
    schädel.
limb
limbal
    l. suture
limbic
limbous
    l. suture
limbus (limbi)
    See also *border* and *margin*.
    l. of sphenoid bone

limen (limina)
    l. of insula
    l. insulae
liminal
Lindau-von Hippel. See *von Hippel-Lindau.*
line
    See also *stria.*
    base l.
    base-apex l.
    l. of Gennari
    Rolando l.
    suture l.
linea (lineae)
linguistic deficit
lingula (lingulae)
    l. cerebelli
    l. of cerebellum
    l. of sphenoid
    sphenoidal l.
    l. of sphenoidalis
lingular
lipohyalinosis
liquid
    See *fluid* and *liquor.*
liquor (liquors, liquores)
    See also *fluid.*
    l. cerebrospinalis
Lissauer
    column
    marginal zone
    paralysis
    tract
Little [eponym]
    disease
    paralysis
lobe
    caudate l. of cerebrum
    crescentic l. of cerebellum
    flocculonodular l.
    limbic l.
    occipital l.
    parietal l.
    quadrangular l. of cerebellum
    quadrate l. of cerebral hemisphere
    temporal l.

lobe (continued)
    temporosphenoidal l. of cerebral hemisphere
lobectomy
    occipital l.
    temporal l.
lobi (plural of lobus)
lobotomy
    frontal l.
    prefrontal l.
    transorbital l.
lobulated
lobulation
lobule
    l. of cerebellum
    posteromedian l.
lobuli (plural of lobulus)
lobulization
lobulose
lobulus (lobuli)
    l. semilunaris
lobus (lobi)
    l. frontalis
    l. occipitalis
    l. parietalis
    l. temporalis
locus (loci)
    l. cinereus
logagnosia
logagraphia
logamnesia
logaphasia
logasthenia
logoclonia
logogram
logopathy
logoplegia
logoscopy
longitudinal
    l. suture
    l. suture of palate
long tract signs
"loop" Phonetic for loupe.
Louis-Bar
    disease
    syndrome
Löwe
    disease

Löwe (continued)
    syndrome
LP—lumbar puncture
LS—lumbosacral
Lucas
    groove
lucid
lucidity
lückenschädel
"luko–" Phonetic for words begin-
    ning leuko–.
lumbar
    l. sympathectomy
lumbodorsal
    l. splanchnicectomy
    l. sympathectomy
Luschka
    foramen
    joints
Lust
    phenomenon
    reflex
Luys
    body
    body syndrome
    nucleus
Lyle syndrome
μ—micro- [prefix; alphabetized as
    m]
mA—milliampere(s)
Machado-Joseph disease
MacKay-Marg electronic tonometer
Mackenzie
    syndrome
macrencephaly
macrocephalous
macrocephaly
macrocrania
macroesthesia
macrogenitosomia
    m. praecox
macrography
macrogyria
macromelia
    m. paresthetica
macula (maculae)
    See also *macule* and *spot.*
    cerebral m.

macular
macule
    See also *macula* and *spot.*
    ash-leaf m.
    lance-ovate m.
maculocerebral
Magendie
    foramen
    law
    sign
    space
    symptom
Magendie-Hertwig sign
mAh, mA-h—milliampere-hour
mal
    grand m.
    haut m.
    petit m.
maladie
    m. des tics ["da teek']
malformation
    Arnold-Chiari. m.
    arteriovenous m. (AVM)
    Chiari-type m.
malleation
mAm, mA-m—milliampere-minute
maneuver
    See also *method.*
    Adson m.
    cross-leg Patrick m.
    doll's head m.
    Valsalva m.
mania
    epileptic m.
mannerism
MAP—muscle action potential
Marcaine HCl [anesthetic agent]
marche à petits pas [small steps]
Marchiafava-Bignami disease
margin
    See also *border* and *limbus.*
    coronal m. of frontal bone
    coronal m. of parietal bone
margo (margines)
Marie
    ataxia
    sclerosis
    syndrome (I, II)

Marinesco
    sign
Marinesco-Radovici
    reflex
Marinesco-Sjögren
    syndrome
Marinesco-Sjögren-Garland
    syndrome
"marsh ah peh-tee pah" Phonetic
    for marche à petits pas.
Marshall Hall facies
mAs, mA-s—milliampere-second
Matson
    operation
Mauchart ligament
Mayer
    reflex
MBD—minimal brain damage
    minimal brain dysfunction
MBP—myelin basic protein
MCA—middle cerebral artery
McArdle
    disease
    syndrome
McCarthy
    reflex
McKenzie
    See *Mackenzie.*
MD—movement disorder
    muscular dystrophy
Meckel
    cavity
    ganglion
    plane
    space
    syndrome
mecocephalic
medical
    m. vagotomy
Medin
    disease
    poliomyelitis
medulla (medullae)
    m. oblongata
    spinal m.
    m. spinalis
medullary
medullated

medullation
medullispinal
medullitis
medulloblast
medulloblastoma
    Cushing m.
    desmoplastic m.
medulloencephalic
medulloepithelioma
megalocephalic
megalocephaly
megaloceros
Melkersson
    syndrome
membranate
membrane
    arachnoid m.
    Schwann m.
memory
Mendel
    reflex
    test
Mendel-Bekhterev
    reflex
    sign
Ménière
    disease
    syndrome
meningeal
meningematoma
meningeocortical
meningeoma
meningeorrhaphy
meninges (plural of meninx)
meninghematoma
meningina
meningioma
    anaplastic m.
    angioblastic m.
    angiomatous m.
    arachnotheliomatous m.
    endotheliomatous m.
    fibrous m.
    hemangioblastic m.
    hemangiopericytic m.
    meningothelial m.
    meningotheliomatous m.
    mesodermal m.

meningioma (continued)
    mixed m.
    myxomatous m.
    m. of olfactory groove
    olfactory groove m.
    parasagittal m.
    psammomatous m.
    syncytial m.
    transitional m.
meningiomatosis
meningism
meningismus
meningitic
meningitis (meningitides)
    acute aseptic m.
    acute septic m.
    African m.
    aseptic m.
    Bacteroides m.
    basal m.
    m. of the base, basilar m.
    benign lymphocytic m.
    benign recurrent endotheli-
      oleukocytic m.
    brucellar m.
    m. carcinomatosa
    cerebral m.
    cerebrospinal m.
    chemical m.
    chronic posterior basic m.
    m. circumscripta spinalis
    cryptococcal m.
    curable serous m.
    eosinophilic m.
    epidemic cerebrospinal m.
    external m.
    gonococcal m.
    granulomatous m.
    gummatous m.
    herpetic m.
    influenzal m.
    internal m.
    leptospiral m.
    localized tuberculous m.
    lymphocytic m.
    meningococcal m.
    meningococcic m.
    metastatic m.

meningitis (meningitides) (continued)
    Mollaret m.
    mumps m.
    mycobacterial m.
    mycotic m.
    m. necrotoxica reactiva
    neonatal m.
    occlusive m.
    m. ossificans
    otitic m.
    otogenic m.
    parameningococcus m.
    plague m.
    plasmodial m.
    pneumococcal m.
    posterior m.
    posterior basic m.
    post-traumatic m.
    purulent m.
    pyogenic m.
    Quincke m.
    rheumatic m.
    sarcoid m.
    septicemic m.
    m. serosa
    m. serosa circumscripta
    m. serosa circumscripta cys-
      tica
    serous m.
    serum m.
    simple m.
    spinal m.
    staphylococcal m.
    sterile m.
    streptococcal m.
    suppurative m.
    m. sympathica
    syphilitic m.
    torula m., torular m.
    trypanosomal m.
    tubercular m., tuberculous m.
    typhoid m.
    viral m.
    Wallgren aseptic m.
    yeast m.
meningoarteritis
meningoblastoma
meningocele

meningocephalitis
meningocerebritis
meningococcemia
    acute fulminating m.
    chronic m.
meningococci (plural of meningo-
    coccus)
meningococcidal
meningococcin
meningococcosis
meningococcus (meningococci)
meningocortical
meningoencephalitis
    biundulant m.
    chronic m.
    eosinophilic m.
    mumps m.
    primary amebic m.
    syphilitic m.
    trypanosomal m.
    Tüga m.
meningoencephalocele
meningoencephalomyelitis
meningoencephalomyelopathy
meningoencephalo-myeloradiculitis
meningoencephalopathy
meningoexothelioma
meningofibroblastoma
meningogenic
meningoma
meningomalacia
meningomyelitis
    blastomycotic m.
    sporotrichotic m.
    torular m.
meningomyelocele
meningomyeloencephalitis
meningomyeloradiculitis
meningomyelorrhaphy
meningo-osteophlebitis
meningopathy
meningopneumonitis
meningorachidian
meningoradicular
meningoradiculitis
meningorecurrence
meningorrhagia
meningorrhea

meningothelioma
meningotyphoid
meningovascular
meninguria
meninx (meninges)
    m. fibrosa
    m. serosa
    m. tenuis
    m. vasculosa
Menkes disease
mentation
MEP—motor evoked potential
    multimodality evoked poten-
    tial
MEPP—miniature end-plate potential
meralgia
    m. paresthetica
merorachischisis
Merzbacher-Pelizaeus
    disease
    sclerosis
mesencephalic
    m. tractotomy
mesencephalitis
mesencephalohypophysial
mesencephalon
mesencephalotomy
mesoglia
metacoele
metastasis (metastases)
metathalamus
metencephalic
metencephalon
metencephalospinal
methemoglobinemia
    acquired m.
    congenital m.
    hereditary m.
    toxic m.
methemoglobinemic
methemoglobinuria
method
    See also *maneuver.*
    Dubois m.
metopic
    m. suture
metrizamide
    m. cisternography

Meyer
  law
  theory
Meyerding
  gouge
  mallet
Meynert
  bundle
  cells
  commissure
  decussation
  fasciculus
  fibers
  layer
  tract
MG—muscle group
  myasthenia gravis
mHz—milliherz
microaneurysm
microcalcification
microcephalus
microcephaly
  encephaloclastic m.
  schizencephalic m.
microcirculation
microcirculatory
microcrania
microemboli (plural of microembolus)
microembolization
microembolus (microemboli)
  showers of microemboli
microglial
microglioma
microgliomatosis
  m. cerebri
microgliosis
micrographia
microgyri (plural of microgyrus)
microgyria
microgyrus (microgyri)
microinfarct
microneurosurgery
microplethysmography
microthrombi (plural of microthrombus)
microthrombosis
microthrombus (microthrombi)

microvasculature
midbrain
midline
  m. myelotomy
"miel–" Phonetic for words beginning myel–.
migraine
  abdominal m.
  acute confusional m.
  m. without aura
  m. with aura
  basilar m., basilar artery m.
  Bickerstaff m.
  classic m.
  common m.
  complicated m.
  epileptic m.
  familial hemiplegic m.
  fulgurating m.
  hemiplegic m.
  hormonal m.
  menstrual m.
  neurologic m.
  ocular m.
  ophthalmic m.
  ophthalmoplegic m.
  retinal m.
migraineur
migrainoid
migrainous
migratory
  m. neuralgias
Millard-Gubler
  paralysis
  syndrome
milliammeter
milliampere(s) (mA)
milliampere-hour (mAh, mA-h)
milliampere-minute (mAm, mA-m)
milliampere-second (mAs, mA-s)
milliherz (mHz)
millijoule(s) (mJ)
Millikan rays
millisecond(s) (ms, msec)
millivolt(s) (mV)
Mills
  disease
  test

Minamata
    disease
    syndrome
minimum (minima)
    m. sensibile
Minor [eponym]
    disease
    sign
    syndrome
"mio–" Phonetic for words begin-
    ning myo–.
miopragia
miosis
    spinal m.
Mitchell
    disease
mJ—millijoule(s)
MNCV—motor nerve conduction
    velocity
Möbius
    disease
    sign
    syndrome (I, II)
Moersch-Woltman syndrome
Mollaret meningitis
Monakow (von Monakow)
    fasciculus aberrans (fascicu-
        lus aberrans of Monakow)
    syndrome
    tract
Mönckeberg
    sclerosis
monitor
    apnea m.
    ICP (intracranial pressure) m.
monodiplopia
monomyoplegia
monomyositis
mononeuritis
    m. multiplex
mononeuropathy
    cranial m.
    m. multiplex
monoparesis
monoparesthesia
monophasic
monoplegia
monosyllabic

Monro
    fissure
    foramen (foramen of Monro)
    sulcus
monticulus
    m. cerebelli
Moore
    syndrome
Morgagni
    disease
    hyperostosis
    syndrome
Morgagni-Adams-Stokes syndrome
Morquio
    sign
Morvan
    chorea
    disease
    syndrome
motoneuron
motor
motorium
    m. commune
Mouchet disease
Mount-Reback syndrome
Moynahan
    syndrome (I, II)
MRF—mesencephalic reticular for-
    mation
μs—microsecond(s)
ms, msec—millisecond(s)
MS—mental status
    morphine sulfate
    multiple sclerosis
multi-infarct
    m. dementia
multiple sclerosis (MS)
mumps
    m. meningoencephalitis
MUP—motor unit potential
Murray Valley
    disease
    encephalitis
Murri
    disease
    syndrome
muscarinic
    m. agonists [a class of drugs]

muscle
> See also in *Orthopedics and Sports Medicine* section.
> epicranial m.
> frontal m.
> inferior oblique m. of head
> Jung m.
> long m. of head
> longissimus m. of head
> longissimus m. of neck
> long m. of neck
> occipital m.
> occipitofrontal m.
> sternocleidomastoid m.
> temporoparietal m.
> tonic m.
> trachelomastoid m.

musculus (musculi)
> See in *Orthopedics and Sports Medicine* section.

μV [microV]—microvolt(s)
myalgia
myasthenia
> m. gravis
> m. gravis pseudoparalytica

myatonia
mydriasis
> alternating m.
> bounding m.
> paralytic m.
> spasmodic m., spastic m.
> spinal m.
> springing m.

myelalgia
myelanalosis
myelapoplexy
myelasthenia
myelatelia
myelatrophy
myelauxe
myelencephalitis
myelencephalon
myelencephalospinal
myelencephalous
myeleterosis
myelic
myelin
myelinated

myelinic
myelinization
> dystopic cortical m.

myelinoclasis
> acute perivascular m.
> postinfection perivenous m.

myelinolysin
myelinolysis
> central pontine m.

myelinopathy
myelinosis
> pontine m.

myelinotoxic
myelinotoxicity
myelitic
myelitis
> acute m.
> acute syphilitic m.
> amyotrophic syphilitic m.
> angiohypertrophic spinal m.
> apoplectiform m.
> ascending m.
> bulbar m.
> cavitary m.
> central m.
> chronic m.
> compression m.
> concussion m.
> cornual m.
> descending m.
> diffuse m.
> disseminated m.
> focal m.
> funicular m.
> hemorrhagic m.
> interstitial m.
> metastatic m.
> neuro-optic m.
> parenchymatous m.
> periependymal m.
> postvaccinal m.
> pressure m.
> pseudotumoral m.
> radiation m.
> sclerosing m.
> subacute necrotic m.
> systemic m.
> transverse m.

myelitis (continued)
    traumatic m.
    tuberculous m.
    m. vaccinia
myeloarchitecture
myelobrachium
myelocele
myelocisternoencephalography
myelocoele
myelocone
myelocyst
myelocystic
myelocystocele
myelocystomeningocele
myelodysplasia
myeloencephalic
myeloencephalitis
    eosinophilic m.
myelofibrosis
    osteosclerosis m.
myelofugal
myelogenesis
myelogeny
myelogram
myelography
    air m.
    computer-assisted m. (CAM)
    opaque m.
    oxygen m.
myeloid
myclolysis
myelolytic
myeloma
    Bence Jones m.
    endothelial m.
    extramedullary m.
    giant cell m.
    indolent m.
    localized m.
    multiple m.
    plasma cell m.
    solitary m.
myelomalacia
myelomatosis
myelomenia
myelomeningitis
myelomeningocele
myelon

myeloneuritis
myelo-opticoneuropathy
    subacute m.
myeloparalysis
myelopathic
myelopathy
    apoplectiform m.
    ascending m.
    cervical m.
    compression m.
    concussion m.
    descending m.
    focal m.
    funicular m.
    hemorrhagic m.
    interstitial m.
    ischemic m.
    necrotic m.
    parenchymatous m.
    radiation m.
    sclerosing m.
    spondylotic cervical m.
    subacute necrotic m.
    systemic m.
    toxic m.
    transverse m.
    traumatic m.
myelophthisis
myeloplegia
myeloradiculitis
myeloradiculodysplasia
myeloradiculopathy
myelorrhagia
myelorrhaphy
    commissural m.
myelosarcoma
myelosarcomatosis
myeloschisis
myeloscintogram
myelosclerosis
myelosis
myelospasm
myelospongium
myelosyphilis
myelosyphilosis
myelotomy
    Bischof m.
    commissural m.

myelotomy (continued)
    midline m.
Myerson
    sign
MyG—myasthenia gravis
myoclonia
    m. epileptica
    m. fibrillaris multiplex
    fibrillary m.
    pseudoglottic m.
    Unverricht m.
myoclonic
myoclonus
    action m.
    epileptic m.
    hereditary essential m.
    intention m.
    massive epileptic m.
    m. multiplex
    nocturnal m.
    ocular m.
    palatal m.
    petit mal m.
    postural m.
    spinal m.
    startle m.
myodynamic
myodynamics
myodynia
myodystonia
myodystrophia
    m. fetalis
myofascial
myogram
myograph
myography
myohypertrophia
    m. kymoparalytica
myokymia
    facial m.
    hereditary m.
myoneural
myoneuralgia
myoneurasthenia
myoparalysis
myoparesis
myopathia
myopathic

myopathy
    alcoholic m.
    centronuclear m.
    corticosteroid-induced m.
    Cushing disease m.
    endocrine m.
    glucocorticoid-induced m.
    hypertrophic branchial m.
    hypothyroid m.
    infiltrative m.
    late distal hereditary m.
    mitochondrial m.
    myotubular m.
    myxedematous m.
    nemaline m.
    nemaline (rod) m.
    ocular m.
    primary progressive m.
    progressive atrophic m.
    rod m.
    slow hereditary distal m.
    steroid m.
    thyrotoxic m.
    Welander m., Welander distal m.
myophagism
myositis
    m. ossificans
myotactic
myotomic
myotonia
    m. congenita
    m. congenita intermittens
    congenital m.
    m. hereditaria
    m. neonatorum
Nadbath
    akinesia
Naffziger
    syndrome
    test
"nay-gro" Phonetic for Negro
    [eponym].
napex
narcolepsy
narcoleptic
narcose

narcosis
> basal n., basis n.
> carbon dioxide n.
> insufflation n.
> nitrogen n.
> prolonged n.

narcotic
narcotic agonist-antagonists [a class of drugs]
narcotics; narcotic agonists [a class of drugs]
NCA—neurocirculatory asthenia
NCV—nerve conduction velocity
necrencephalus
necrosis (necroses)
> cerebrocortical n.
> postpartum pituitary n.
> n. ustilaginea

necrotic
needle
> n. electromyography

Negro [eponym]
> phenomenon
> sign

Nelson
> syndrome

Nembutal [anesthetic agent]
neocerebellum
neocortex
neokinetic
neopallium
neostigmine
> n. bromide

neostriatum
neothalamus
nerve
> abducens n.
> accessory n.
> acoustic n.
> afferent n.
> autonomic n.
> Bell n.
> n. conduction study
> cranial n.'s (I–XII)
> efferent n.
> facial n.
> glossopharyngeal n.
> great sciatic n.

nerve (continued)
> intermediate n.
> oculomotor n.
> olfactory n.'s
> ophthalmic n.
> ophthalmic n. of Willis
> optic n.
> orbital n.'s
> parasympathetic n.
> recurrent n., ophthalmic
> sciatic n.
> sensorimotor n.
> sensory n.
> spinal n.'s
> splanchnic n.'s
> supraorbital n.
> sympathetic n.
> thoracodorsal n.
> trigeminal n.
> trochlear n.
> vagus n.

nerve block
nervi (plural of nervus)
nervous
> central n. system
> peripheral n. system

nervus (nervi)
> n. abducens

net
> See *plexus* and *rete*.

network
> See *plexus* and *rete*.

"neu–" Phonetic for words beginning pneu–.
neuradynamia
neuragmia
neural
> n. pathway

neuralgia
> atypical facial n.
> brachial n.
> cervical n.
> cervicobrachial n.
> cranial n.
> Fothergill n.
> glossopharyngeal n.
> hallucinatory n.
> Harris migrainous n.

neuralgia (continued)
    Hunt n.
    mandibular joint n.
    migrainous n.
    Parsonage and Turner amyo-
        trophic n.
    postherpetic n.
    sciatic n.
    stump n.
    trigeminal n.
    vidian n.
    Wartenberg paresthetic n.
neuralgic
neuralgiform
neuranagenesis
neurangiosis
neurapophysis
neurapraxia
neurarchy
neurasthenia
neurastheniac
neurasthenic
neurataxia
neurataxy
neuratrophia
neuratrophic
neuratrophy
neuraxial
neuraxis
neuraxitis
    epidemic n.
    multilocular n.
neuraxon
neure
neurectasia
neurectomy
    Abbe n.
    gastric n.
    opticociliary n.
    presacral n.
    retrogasserian n.
    tympanic n.
neurectopia
neurergic
neurexeresis
neuriatry
neurilemma
neurilemmal

neurilemmitis
neurilemoma
    acoustic n.
    malignant n.
    trigeminal n.
neurility
neurinoma
    acoustic n.
    malignant n.
neuritic
neuritis
    adventitial n.
    alcoholic n.
    amyloid n.
    arsenical n.
    ascending n.
    brachial n.
    central n.
    compression n.
    degenerative n.
    descending n.
    dietetic n.
    diphtheric n.
    disseminated n.
    endemic n.
    femoral n.
    Gombault n.
    influenzal n.
    interstitial n.
    interstitial hypertrophic n.
    intraocular n.
    ischemic n.
    latent n.
    lead n.
    leprous n.
    malarial n.
    malarial multiple n.
    n. migrans, migrating n.
    multiple n.
    n. multiplex endemica
    n. nodosa
    optic n.
    orbital optic n.
    paralytic brachial n.
    parenchymatous n.
    periaxial n.
    peripheral n.
    porphyric n.

neuritis (continued)
    postfebrile n.
    postocular n.
    pressure n.
    radiation n.
    radicular n.
    retrobulbar n.
    rheumatic n.
    n. saturnina
    sciatic n.
    segmental n.
    senile n.
    serum n.
    shoulder-girdle n.
    syphilitic n.
    tabetic n.
    toxic n.
    traumatic n.
neuro—neurologic
neuroactive
neuroallergy
neuroamebiasis
neuroanastomosis
neuroanatomy
neuroarthropathy
neuroastrocytoma
neurobehavioral
neuroblastoma
    olfactory n.
neuroborreliosis
neurocanal
neurocardiac
neurocentrum
neuroceptor
neurochemistry
neurocirculatory
neurocladism
neurocommunications
neurocranial
neurocranium
neurocristopathy
neurocutaneous
neurocytoma
    olfactory n.
neurodegenerative
neurodiagnosis
neurodynia
neuroelectricity

neuroelectrotherapeutics
neuroencephalomyelopathy
    optic n.
neuroendocrine
neuroendocrinology
neuroepidermal
neuroepithelial
neuroepithelioma
neuroepithelium
    n. of ampullary crest
    n. cristae ampullaris
    n. of maculae
    n. macularum
neurofiber
neurofibra (neurofibrae)
neurofibril
neurofibrilla (neurofibrillae)
neurofibrillar
neurofibroma
    acoustic n.
neurofibromatosis
neurofibrosarcoma
neurofibrositis
neurofilament
neurogangliitis
neuroganglioma
neuroganglion
neurogen
neurogenesis
neurogenic
neurogenous
neuroglia
    fascicular n.
    interfascicular n.
    peripheral n.
    protoplasmic n.
neuroglial, neurogliar
neurogliocytoma
neuroglioma
    n. ganglionare
neurogliosis
neuroglycopenia
neurogram
neurography
neurohormonal
neurohormone
neurohypophysectomy
neurohypophysial

neurohypophysis
neuroimaging
neuroimmunologic
neuroimmunology
neurolabyrinthitis
    viral n.
neurolathyrism
neuroleptanalgesia
neuroleptanalgesic
neuroleptanesthesia
neuroleptanesthetic
neuroleptic
neurolinguistics
neurolipomatosis
    n. dolorosa
neurologic, neurological
neurologist
neurology
    clinical n.
neurolues
neurolymphomatosis
    n. gallinarum
    peripheral n.
neurolysis
    alcohol n.
    chemical n.
    intramuscular n.
    intrathecal n.
    phenol n.
    trigeminal n.
neurolytic
neuroma
    acoustic n.
    amyelinic n.
    false n.
    ganglionar n., ganglionated
      n., ganglionic n.
    medullated n.
    multiple n.'s
    myelinic n.
    nevoid n.
    plexiform n.
    post-traumatic n.
    n. telangiectodes
    traumatic n.
    true n.
    Verneuil n.
neuromalacia

neuromatosis
neuromatous
neuromechanism
neuromeningeal
neuromere
neuromimetic
neuromodulation
neuromotor
neuromyasthenia
    epidemic n.
neuromyelitis
    n. optica
neuromyopathic
neuromyopathy
    carcinomatous n.
neuromyositis
neuromyotonia
neuronal
neuronephric
neuronitis
    myoclonic spinal n.
    vestibular n.
neuro-ophthalmology. See in *Ophthalmology* section.
neuro-otology
neuroparalysis
neuroparalytic
neuropathic
neuropathic joint disease
neuropathogenesis
neuropathogenicity
neuropathology
neuropathy
    alcoholic n.
    alcohol-nutritional n.
    amyloid n.
    Andrade-type amyloid n.
    ascending n.
    axonal n.
    brachial plexus n.
    compression-entrapment n.
    descending n.
    diabetic n.
    entrapment n.
    focal n.
    giant axonal n.
    granulomatous n.

neuropathy (continued)
    hereditary hypertrophic
      interstitial n.
    hereditary sensorimotor n.
      (types I–III)
    hereditary sensory radicular n.
    hypertrophic n.
    infectious n.
    intercostal n.
    ischemic n.
    isoniazid n.
    lead n.
    multifocal n.
    myxedematous n.
    optic n.
    periaxial n.
    peripheral n.
    pressure n.
    progressive hypertrophic
      interstitial n.
    radiation n.
    segmental (demyelination) n.
    selective autonomic n.
    sensorimotor n.
    sensory n.
    serum n., serum sickness n.
    trigeminal n.
neuropharmacology
neurophonia
neurophysiology
neuroplasty
neuroplexus
neuropodion
neuropodium (neuropodia)
neuroradiology
neuroregulation
neuroretinopathy
    hypertensive n.
neuroroentgenography
neurorrhaphy
neurosarcocleisis
neurosarcoma
neuroscience
neurosclerosis
neurosecretion
neurosegmental
neurosensory
neuroskeletal

neuroskeleton
neurosome
neurospasm
neurosplanchnic
neurospongioma
neurospongium
neurostatus
neurostimulator
neurosurgeon
neurosurgery
    functional n.
    microvascular n.
    stereotaxic n.
neurosuture
neurosyphilis
    asymptomatic n.
    congenital n.
    ectodermogenic n.
    juvenile n.
    latent n.
    meningeal n.
    meningovascular n.
    mesodermogenic n.
    parenchymatous s.
    paretic n.
    tabetic n.
neurotabes
    n. diabetica
neurotendinous
neurotherapy
neurotization
neurotmesis
neurotomography
neurotomy
    opticociliary n.
    radio frequency n. [also:
      radiofrequency]
    retrogasserian n.
neurotony
neurotoxic
neurotoxicity
neurotoxin
neurotransducer
neurotransmission
neurotransmitter
    false n.
neurotrauma
neurotropic

neurotropism
neurovaricosis
neurovascular
neurovegetative
neurovirulence
neurovirulent
neurovisceral
"new–" Phonetic for words beginning pneu–.
NICU—neurological intensive care unit
nidus (nidi)
   n. avis
Niemann-Pick
   cells
   disease
   lipid
NINDB—National Institute of Neurologic Diseases and Blindness
Nissl bodies
"nistagmus" Phonetic for nystagmus.
NM—neuromuscular
nocturnal
   n. polysomnography
nod
   bishop's n.
node
   Heberden n.
nodi (plural of nodus)
nodule
   Schmorl n.
noduli (plural of nodulus)
nodulous [adj.]
nodulus (noduli)
nodus (nodi)
Nonne
   syndrome
   test
non-REM—non–rapid eye movement
nonsteroidal anti-inflammatory drugs (NSAIDs) [a class of drugs]
"noo–" Phonetic for words beginning pneu–.
Norman-Wood syndrome
notch
notencephalocele
notencephalus

Nothnagel
   acroparesthesia
   bodies
   sign
   syndrome, II syndrome
   type
notomyelitis
noxious
   n. stimuli
NP—neuropsychiatric
NPH—normal-pressure hydrocephalus
NREM—non–rapid eye movement
NS—neurosurgery
NSAIA—nonsteroidal anti-inflammatory agent
NSAID, NSAIDs—nonsteroidal anti-inflammatory drug(s) [a class of drugs]
"nu–" Phonetic for words beginning pneu–.
nuclei (genitive and plural of nucleus)
nucleiform
nucleus (nuclei)
   n. accumbens
   n. ambiguus
   n. arcuati
   n. basalis
   cuneate n.
   Darkschewitsch n.
   n. gracilis
   hypoglossal n.
   n. lateralis medullae oblongatae
   n. pulposus
   n. pulposus disci intervertebralis
   pulpy n.
   red n.
   reticular n.
   vestibular n.
Nupercaine HCl [anesthetic agent]
"nur–" Phonetic for words beginning neur–.
Nussbaum
   narcosis
nvCJD—new variant Creutzfeldt-Jakob disease

nystagmus
    ataxic n.
    Baer n.
    Bekhterev n.
    benign positional n.
    central n.
    Cheyne n.
    Cheyne-Stokes n.
    congenital n., congenital
      hereditary n.
    convergence n.
    disjunctive n.
    dissociated n.
    downbeat n.
    electrical n.
    end-point n.
    end position n.
    fixation n.
    galvanic n.
    jerk n., jerky n.
    labyrinthine n.
    latent n.
    lateral n.
    miner's n.
    n.-myoclonus
    ocular n.
    opticokinetic n., optokinetic
      n. (OKN)
    oscillating n.
    palatal n.
    paretic n.
    pendular n.
    periodic alternating n.
    positional n.
    railroad n.
    rebound n.
    resilient n.
    retraction n., n. retractorius
    rhythmical n.
    rotatory n.
    secondary n.
    see-saw n.
    spontaneous n.
    undulatory n.
    unilateral n.
    upbeat n.
    vertical n.
    vestibular n.

nystagmus (continued)
    vibratory n.
    visual n.
    voluntary n.
OA—occipital artery
Obersteiner-Redlich area
obex
obliteration
    cortical o.
obnubilation
OBS—organic brain syndrome
obstructive
    o. sleep apnea (OSA)
obtund
obtundation
obtundent
occipital
    o. lobectomy
    o. suture
occipitalis
occipitalization
occipitoatloid
occipitoaxoid
occipitobasilar
occipitobregmatic
occipitocalcarine
occipitocervical
occipitofacial
occipitofrontal
occipitomastoid
    o. suture
occipitomental
occipitoparietal
    o. suture
occipitosphenoidal
    o. suture
occipitotemporal
occipitothalamic
occiput
oculocephalic
oculogyric
oculospinal
Oehler
    symptom
"ofthal–" Phonetic for words begin-
    ning ophthal–.
OKN—opticokinetic nystagmus
"oksesefale" Phonetic for oxycephaly.

olfactory
oligoclonal bands, banding
oligodendrocyte
oligodendroglia
oligodendroglioma
oligophrenia
    phenylpyruvic o.
    o. phenylpyruvica
oligophrenic
oliva (olivae)
olivary
olive
    inferior o.
    spurge o.
    superior o.
olivifugal
olivipetal
olivopontocerebellar
OP—opening pressure
opaque
    o. myelography
operation
    See also in *General Surgical Terms.*
    Bischof o.
    Cloward o.
    Cotte o.
    Dana o.
    Förster-Penfield o.
    Frazier-Spiller o.
    Gardner o.
    Gill o.
    Haynes o.
    Hibbs o.
    Keen o.
    Leriche o.
    Matson o.
    Pancoast o.
    Puusepp o.
    Ramadier o.
    Royle o.
    saccus o.
    Sjöqvist o.
    Smith-Robinson o.
    Smithwick o.
    Sonneberg o.
    Stookey-Scarff o.
    Taarnhøj o.

operation (continued)
    tack o.
    Torkildsen o.
opercula (plural of operculum)
opercular
operculate
operculum (opercula)
    frontal o., o. frontale
    frontoparietal o., o. frontoparietale
    o. insulae
    occipital o.
    opercula of insula
    parietal o.
    temporal o., o. temporale
ophthalmencephalon
ophthalmoplegia
    diabetic o.
opiate
opioid
opisthion
opisthotonoid
opisthotonos
Oppenheim
    amyotonia
    disease
    gait
    reflex
    sign
    syndrome
opsoclonus
opticociliary
    o. neurectomy
    o. neurotomy
organic
    o. brain syndrome (OBS)
orientation
oriented
    alert and o. (AO)
    o. to time, place, and person (OTPP)
    o. to time, place, person, and situation [or circumstance]
    o. times three, o. x3
orthosis (orthoses)
    halo o.
    poster o.

os (ossa) [bone]
See in *Orthopedics and Sports Medicine* section.
OSA—obstructive sleep apnea
OSAS—obstructive sleep apnea syndrome
oscillation
oscillopsia
osteoma
o. spongiosum
osteotomy
OT—occupational therapy
otohemineurasthenia
otomastoiditis
otorrhea
cerebrospinal fluid o.
oxazolidinediones [a class of drugs]
oxycephalic
oxycephaly
oxygen (O)
o. cisternography
o. myelography
moyamoya disease
PA—paralysis agitans
PAC—phenacetin, aspirin, caffeine
Pacchioni
foramen
fossae
granulations
pacchionian
p. corpuscles
p. depressions
p. foramen
p. glands
p. granula, p. granulations
pachycephalia
pachyleptomeningitis
pachymeningitis
cerebral p.
circumscribed p.
external p.
hemorrhagic internal p.
internal p.
p. intralamellaris
purulent p.
serous internal p.
spinal p.
syphilitic p.

pachymeninx (pachymeninges)
"pakeonean" Phonetic for pacchionian.
paleencephalon
paleocerebellar
paleocerebellum
paleocortex
paleophrenia
paleothalamus
paligraphia
palikinesia
palinphrasia
pallesthesia
pallidal
pallidectomy
pallidoansection
pallidoansotomy
pallidofugal
pallidotomy
pallidum
p. I
p. II
pallium
palsy
See also *hemiplegia, paralysis,* and *paraplegia.*
acute thyrotoxic bulbar p.
atonic cerebral p.
Bell p.
bilateral cord p.
birth p.
brachial p.
brachial plexus p.
bulbar p.
cerebral p.
cranial nerve p.
creeping p.
crossed leg p.
diver's p.
epidemic infantile p.
Erb p.
facial p.
hammer p.
hypotonic cerebral p.
infantile cerebral p.
infantile progressive bulbar p.
inherited bulbar p.
ischemic p.

palsy (continued)
    Klumpke p.
    Landry p.
    lateral popliteal p.
    minimal cerebral p.
    night p.
    ocular p.
    painter's p.
    posticus p.
    pressure p.
    printer's p.
    progressive supranuclear p.
    pseudobulbar p.
    radial p.
    Saturday night p.
    scrivener's p.
    shaking p.
    spastic bulbar p.
    supranuclear p.
    tardy median p.
    tardy ulnar p.
    Todd p.
    transverse p.
    ulnar p.
    unilateral cord p.
    wasting p.
PAN—periarteritis nodosa
    periodic alternating nystag-
      mus
    polyarteritis nodosa
Pancoast
    operation
    syndrome
    tumor
panencephalitis
    Pette-Döring p.
    subacute sclerosing p.
Pansch
    fissure
papilloma
    p. of choroid plexus
    p. neuroticum
paradoxic, paradoxical
parafascicular
    p. thalamotomy (PFT)
paraganglioma
    medullary p.
    nonchromaffin p.

paralexia
paralysis (paralyses)
    See also *hemiplegia, palsy,*
      and *paraplegia.*
    abducens p.
    abducens-facial p., congenital
    p. of accommodation
    acoustic p.
    acute ascending spinal p.
    acute atrophic p.
    acute bulbar p.
    acute spinal p.
    p. agitans
    p. agitans, juvenile (of Hunt)
    alcoholic p.
    alternate p., alternating p.
    ambiguo-accessorius p.
    ambiguo-accessorius-
      hypoglossal p.
    ambiguohypoglossal p.
    ambiguospinothalamic p.
    anesthesia p.
    anterior spinal p.
    arsenical p.
    ascending p.
    ascending tick p.
    association p.
    asthenic bulbar p.
    asthenobulbospinal p.
    atrophic muscular p.
    atrophic spinal p.
    Avellis p.
    axillary nerve p.
    basal-ganglionic p.
    Bell p.
    bifacial p.
    bilateral p.
    bilateral laryngeal abductor p.
    birth p.
    brachial p.
    brachial plexus p.
    brachiofacial p.
    Brown-Séquard p.
    bulbar p.
    bulbospinal p.
    central p.
    central facial p.
    centrocapsular p.

paralysis (paralyses) (continued)
    cerebral p.
    cerebral spastic infantile p.
    cerebral sympathetic p.
    circumflex p.
    common peroneal nerve p.
    complete p.
    compression p.
    congenital abducens-facial p.
    congenital oculofacial p.
    congenital p. of horizontal
      gaze
    conjugate p.
    cortical p.
    creeping p.
    crossed p.
    crossed hypoglossal p.
    crural p.
    crutch p.
    Cruveilhier p.
    cubital p.
    decubitus p.
    Dejerine-Klumpke p.
    diaphragmatic p.
    diphtheric p., diphtheritic p.
    diver's p.
    Duchenne p.
    Duchenne-Erb p.
    epidemic infantile p.
    epidural ascending spinal p.
    Erb p.
    Erb-Duchenne p.
    Erb syphilitic spinal p.
    esophageal p.
    essential p.
    extraocular p.
    facial p.
    false p.
    familial hyperkalemic peri-
      odic p.
    familial hypokalemic peri-
      odic p.
    familial infantile bulbar p.
    familial periodic p.
    familial recurrent p.
    familial spastic p.
    faucial p.
    femoral nerve p.

paralysis (paralyses) (continued)
    flaccid p.
    functional p.
    p. of gaze
    general p.
    general p. of the insane
    glossolabial p., glos-
      sopharyngolabial p.
    Gubler p.
    Gubler-Millard p.
    hereditary cerebrospinal p.
    histrionic p.
    hyperkalemic periodic p.
    hypoglossal p.
    hypokalemic periodic p.
    hysterical p.
    idiopathic facial p.
    incomplete p.
    Indian bow p.
    infantile p.
    infantile cerebral ataxic p.
    infantile cerebrocerebellar
      diplegic p.
    infantile flaccid and atrophic
      spinal p.
    infantile spastic p.
    infantile spinal p.
    inferior alternate p.
    infranuclear p.
    internuclear p.
    ischemic p.
    Jackson p.
    juvenile p.
    juvenile p. agitans (of Hunt)
    juvenile distal atrophic p.
    Klumpke p.
    Klumpke-Dejerine p.
    Kussmaul p., Kussmaul-
      Landry p.
    labial p., labioglossolaryn-
      geal p., labioglossopha-
      ryngeal p.
    Landry p.
    laryngeal p.
    laryngeal abductor p.
    lead p.
    lingual p.
    Lissauer p.

paralysis (paralyses) (continued)
Little p.
local p.
masticatory p.
medial popliteal nerve p.
median p.
medullary tegmental p.'s
mesencephalic p.
Millard-Gubler p.
mimetic p.
mixed p.
morning p.
motor p.
motor trigeminal p.
musculocutaneous nerve p.
musculospiral p.
myogenic p.
myopathic p.
narcosis p.
neurogenic p.
normokalemic periodic p.
p. notariorum
nuclear p.
obstetric p.
obturator nerve p.
occupational p.
ocular p.
oculofacial p., congenital
oculomotor p.
organic p.
palatal p.
parotitic p.
parturient p.
cruciate p.
periodic p., thyrotoxic
peripheral p.
peripheral facial p.
peroneal p.
pharyngeal p.
phonetic p.
phrenic p.
postdiphtheric p.
postdormital p.
postepileptic p.
posthemiplegic p.
posticus p.
Pott p.
pressure p.

paralysis (paralyses) (continued)
progressive bulbar p.
pseudobulbar p.
pseudohypertrophic muscu-
lar p.
psychic gaze p.
radial p.
Ramsay Hunt p.
recurrent laryngeal nerve p.
reflex p.
Remak p., Remak-type p.
Rieder p.
rucksack p.
Saturday night p.
sensory p.
serratus anterior p.
serum p.
sleep p.
sodium-responsive periodic p.
spastic p.
spastic spinal p.
spinal accessory nerve p.
spinomuscular p.
Sunday morning p.
superior laryngeal nerve p.
syphilitic spastic spinal p.
tegmental mesencephalic p.
tick p.
Todd p.
tourniquet p.
trigeminal p.
trigeminal masticator p.
trochlear p.
ulnar nerve p.
unilateral p.
unilateral vocal cord p.
p. vacillans
vagal p.
vagoaccessory hypoglossal p.
vasomotor p.
Vernet p.
vestibular p.
vocal cord p.
Volkmann ischemic p.
waking p.
wasting p.
Weber p.
Werdnig-Hoffmann p.

paralysis (paralyses) (continued)
    writer's p.
    Zenker p.
paramedian
parameningeal
paramyoclonus
paramyotonia
    p. congenita
    symptomatic p.
paraparesis
    spastic p.
paraparetic
paraplegia
    See also *hemiplegia, palsy,*
      and *paralysis.*
    alcoholic p.
    ataxic p.
    cerebral p.
    cervical p.
    Erb spastic p.
    Erb syphilitic spastic p.
    familial spastic p.
    flaccid p.
    functional p.
    hereditary spastic p.
    hysterical p.
    peripheral p.
    Pott p.
    reflex p.
    senile p.
    spastic p.
    spastic p., congenital
    spastic p., infantile
    spastic p., primary
    p. superior
    syphilitic p.
    toxic p.
paraplegic
parapraxia
parapraxis
parapyramidal
parasellar
parasite
    See specific parasites in
      Laboratory, Pathology,
      and Chemistry Terms.
parasympathin
parasympatholytic

parasympathomimetics [a class of
    drugs]
paratonia
paratonic
paratrophy
para-Wernicke encephalopathy
paresis
    general p.
    parturient p.
paresthesia
    Bernhardt p.
    visceral p.
parietal
    p. cell vagotomy
    p. suture
parietofrontal
parietomastoid
    p. suture
parieto-occipital
    p.-o. suture
parietosphenoid
parietotemporal
    p. suture
Parinaud
    ophthalmoplegia
    syndrome
Parkinson
    complex
    crisis
    disease
    facies
    mask
    rigidity
    sign
    syndrome
parkinsonian
parkinsonism
    drug-induced p.
    postencephalitic p.
    postencephalitis p.
    primary p.
    secondary p.
    vascular p.
parkinsonism-plus
Parrot [eponym]
    pseudoparalysis
Parry-Romberg
    syndrome

pars (partes)
    p. anterior
    p. distalis
    p. interarticularis
    p. intermedia
patch
    blood p.
Paterson-Brown-Kelly
    syndrome
pathogen
    See specific pathogens in
    Laboratory, Pathology,
    and Chemistry Terms.
pathognomonic
pathologic, pathological
pathway
    dopaminergic nigrostriatal p.
Patrick
    cross-leg maneuver
    sign
    test
    trigger areas
Patterson
    See *Paterson.*
paucity
    p. of speech
PB—phenobarbital
PBN—paralytic brachial neuritis
PCA—patient-controlled analgesia
PCB—paracervical block
PD—Parkinson disease
peak
    Bragg p.
peduncle
    cerebellar p.
    cerebral p.
    p. of flocculus
    p. of hypophysis
    olfactory p.
    olivary p. of Schwalbe
    pineal p.
    p. of pineal body
    p. of thalamus, inferior
pedunculi (plural of pedunculus)
pedunculotomy
pedunculus (pedunculi)
PEG—pneumoencephalogram
"peh-tee mahl" Phonetic for petit mal.

"peh-tee pah" Phonetic for petit pas.
Pelizaeus-Merzbacher disease
Penfield
    epilepsy
    syndrome
perception
    extrasensory p. (ESP)
perceptorium
perceptual
perforans (perforantes)
periarterial
    p. sympathectomy
pericranitis
pericranium
periodic lateralized epileptiform
    discharge (PLED)
peripheral
    p. angiography
central nervous system (CNS)
peripheral nervous system (PNS)
peronarthrosis
perseverate
perseveration
pes (pedes)
    p. cerebri
    p. hippocampi
    p. hippocampi major
    p. hippocampi minor
    p. pedunculi
PET—positron emission tomogra-
    phy [scan]
petit mal
petit pas
petrobasilar
    p. suture
petroclinoid
petrosal
petrosphenobasilar
    p. suture
petrosphenoid
petrosphenooccipital
    p. suture of Gruber
petrosquamosal
    p. suture
"pettee mahl" Phonetic for petit mal.
"pettee pah" Phonetic for petit pas.
PFT—parafascicular thalamotomy
phakoma

phakomatosis (phakomatoses)
phalanx (phalanges)
    Deiters phalanges
phantom
    p. limb pain
pharmacopsychosis
phenomenology
phenomenon (phenomena)
    arm p.
    autokinetic visible light p.
    Babinski p.
    Bell p.
    Bowditch staircase p.
    brake p.
    break-off p.
    cheek p.
    clasp-knife p.
    cogwheel p.
    Cushing p.
    Dejerine-Lichtheim p.
    doll's head p.
    Duckworth p.
    Erben p.
    escape p.
    extinction p.
    face p., facialis p.
    finger p.
    Gowers p.
    Grasset p.
    Grasset-Gaussel p.
    Hertwig-Magendie p.
    hip-flexion p.
    Hochsinger p.
    Hoffmann p.
    Holmes p., Holmes-Stewart p.
    Hunt paradoxical p.
    intercritical epileptic p.
    interictal epileptic p.
    Kienböck p.
    Kleist opposition motor p.
    Kohnstamm p.
    Kühne muscular p.
    Leichtenstern p.
    Lust p.
    Negro p.
    Orbeli p.
    paradoxical diaphragm p.
    paradoxical p. of dystonia

phenomenon (phenomena) (continued)
    peroneal-nerve p.
    Pool p.
    Porret p.
    pronation p.
    Queckensteds p.
    radial p.
    rebound p.
    release p.
    Riddoch p.
    Rieger p.
    Rust p.
    Schlesinger p.
    Souques p.
    springlike p.
    staircase p.
    toe p.
    Trousseau p.
    Tullio p.
    Wedensky p.
    Westphal p.
phenylketonuria (PKU)
    p. II
    p. III
    atypical p.
    maternal p.
phenylpyruvic
    p. oligophrenia
phenyltriazines [a class of drugs]
pheochromocytoma
phlebitis
photophobia
phycomycosis
    cerebral p.
physiologic, physiological
physiology
physiopathologic
physiopathology
pia
    p. mater
pia-arachnitis
pia-arachnoid
pia-glia
pial
pia mater
    p.m. encephali
    p.m. spinalis

piamatral
piarachnitis
piarachnoid
PICA—posterior inferior cerebellar
artery
PICA aneurysm
Pick [eponym]
 atrophy
 bodies
 convolutional atrophy
 disease
 syndrome
"pikno–" Phonetic for words beginning pykno–.
pill-rolling
pineal
pinealectomy
pinealoma
 ectopic p.
pink disease
Piotrowski sign
"pira–" Phonetic for words beginning pyra–.
PKU—phenylketonuria
plagiocephalic
plagiocephaly
plane
 axial p.
 coronal p.
 sagittal p.
planum (plana)
plaque
 Lichtheim p.'s
 Redlich-Fisher miliary p.'s
 senile p.'s
plate
 basal p. of cranium
 cribriform p.
 cribriform p. of ethmoid bone
 end p.
 pterygoid p., lateral
 pterygoid p., medial
 quadrigeminal p.
 wing p.
platybasia
PLED—periodic lateralized epileptiform discharge

plethysmograph
 body p.
plexectomy
plexus (plexus, plexuses)
 brachial p.
 carotid p.
 cervical p.
 p. cervicobrachialis
 choroid p.
 p. choroideus ventriculi lateralis
 p. choroideus ventriculi quarti
 p. choroideus ventriculi tertii
 lumbosacral p.
 Remak p.
 p. vertebralis
PM—physical medicine
PMA—progressive muscular atrophy
PMD—progressive muscular dystrophy
PML—progressive multifocal
leukoencephalopathy
PMR—physical medicine and rehabilitation
PN—periarteritis nodosa
peripheral neuropathy
pneumatocele
 p. cranii
 extracranial p.
 intracranial p.
pneumocephalon
 p. artificiale
pneumocephalus
pneumococcal
 p. meningitis
pneumoencephalogram
pneumoencephalography (PEG)
 cerebral p.
 fractional p.
pneumoencephalomyelogram
pneumoencephalomyelography
pneumoencephalos
pneumography
 cerebral p.
pneumomyelography
pneumophonia
pneumorachicentesis
pneumorachis

poikilothermia
point
    Valleix p.'s
poison
    narcotic p.'s
    sedative p.'s
pole
    frontal p. of hemisphere of
      cerebrum
    occipital p. of hemisphere of
      cerebrum
    temporal p. of hemisphere
      of cerebrum
poli (genitive and plural of polus)
poliencephalomyelitis
polio—poliomyelitis
polioclastic
poliodystrophia
poliodystrophy
polioencephalitis
polioencephalomeningomyelitis
polioencephalomyelitis
polioencephalopathy
poliomyelencephalitis
poliomyelitis
    bulbar p.
    cerebral p.
    spinal paralytic p.
poliomyelopathy
polioneuromere
poliovirus
polus (poli)
    p. frontalis hemispherii cere-
      bri
    p. occipitalis hemispherii
      cerebri
    p. temporalis hemispherii
      cerebri
polyarteritis
    p. nodosa
polyclonia
polyneural
polyneuralgia
polyneuritic
polyneuritis
    acute febrile p.
    acute idiopathic p.
    acute infective p.

polyneuritis (continued)
    acute postinfectious p.
    alcoholic p.
    anemic p.
    ascending p.
    p. cerebralis menieriformis
    cranial p.
    diabetic p.
    endemic p., p. endemica
    p. gallinarum
    Guillain-Barré p.
    infectious p.
    Jamaica ginger p.
    postinfectious p.
    p. potatorum
    progressive hypertrophic p.
    triorthocresyl phosphate p.
polyneuromyositis
polyneuropathy
    symmetrical p.
    uremic p.
polyneuroradiculitis
polysomnography
    nocturnal p.
polytomography
pons (pontes)
    p. cerebelli
    p. et cerebellum
    p. oblongata
pontibrachium
ponticulus (ponticuli)
pontile
pontine
    p. lesion
pontobulbia
Pontocaine [anesthetic agent]
pontocerebellar
    p. angle tumor
Pool
    phenomenon
position
    See in *General Surgical*
      Terms.
positive
    p. contrast encephalography
positron
    p. emission tomography
      (PET)

postanoxic
posterior
    p. rhizotomy
postictal
postsynaptic
potential
    action p. (AP)
    after-p. [pref: afterpotential]
    average evoked p.
    brain stem auditory evoked
      p. (BAEP)
    compound action p.
    evoked p. (EP)
    evoked cortical p.'s
    excitatory postsynaptic p.
      (EPSP)
    fasciculation p.
    fibrillation p.'s
    inhibitory postsynaptic p.
    injury p.
    late vertex p.
    motor unit p. (MUP)
    motor unit action p. (MUAP)
    nerve p.
    polyphasic p.
    polyspike p.
    postsynaptic p.'s
    sensory p.
    sensory nerve action p.
      (SNAP)
    serrated action p.
    somatosensory evoked p.
      (SEP)
    spike p.
    visual evoked p. (VEP)
    visual evoked cortical p.
Pott
    paralysis
    paraplegia
    puffy tumor
pouch
    Rathke p.
    Seessel p.
preconvulsant
preconvulsive
precuneus
predisposition
    convulsive p.

predisposition (continued)
    epileptic p.
prefrontal
    p. lobotomy
preganglionic
presacral
    p. neurectomy
pressure
    brain p.
principal [primary, main]
principle [rule]
    See *law* and *rule.*
procedure
    See *maneuver, method,* and
      operation.
process
    See also *apophysis* and *pro-*
      tuberance.
    conoid p.
    sphenoidal p.
processus (processus)
    p. clinoideus anterior
    p. clinoideus medius
    p. clinoideus posterior
prodroma (plural of prodromon)
prodromal
prodromata [incorrect term for pro-
    droma, plural of prodromon]
prodrome
    epileptic p.
prodromic
projection
    eccentric p.
    erroneous p.
prominence
    See *apophysis, process,* and
      protuberance.
prominentia (prominentiae)
proprioceptor
prosencephalon
prosopagnosia
proton
    p. beam (Bragg peak)
protuberance
    See also *apophysis* and
      process.
    occipital p.
psalterium

pseudo-Argyll Robertson
    See also *Argyll Robertson.*
    pupil
    syndrome
pseudo-Babinski sign
pseudocele, pseudocoele
pseudocoma
pseudodelirium
pseudodementia
pseudohypertrophy
pseudoincontinence
pseudopapilledema
pseudoparalysis
    Parrot p.
    syphilitic p.
pseudosclerosis
    spastic p.
    p. spastica
    Strümpell-Westphal p.
    Westphal-Strümpell p.
pseudosyncope
pseudotabes
    pupillotonic p.
pseudotumor
    p. cerebri
    orbital p.
pseudo-Turner syndrome
PSP—progressive supranuclear palsy
psychalgia
psychalgic
psychobiological
psychobiology
psychocortical
psychodometer
psychodometry
psychoepilepsy
psychogalvanometer
psychogenic
psycholinguistics
psychologic, psychological
psychomotor
psychonomy
psychophysical
psychophysics
psychophysiology
psychoplegia
psychoplegic
psychosurgery

PT—physical therapist
    physical therapy
PTA—post-traumatic amnesia
pterion
pulvinar
punctum (puncta)
    puncta vasculosa
puncture
    bone marrow p.
    cisternal p.
    Corning p.
    cranial p.
    lumbar p. (LP)
    Quincke p.
    spinal p.
    subdural p.
    suboccipital p.
    thecal p.
    ventricular p.
purpura
    brain p.
putamen
Putnam-Dana syndrome
Putti
    syndrome
Puusepp
    operation
    reflex
P&V—pyloroplasty and vagotomy
pyknophrasia
pyloroplasty
    vagotomy and p. (V&P)
    p. and vagotomy (P&V)
pyramidal
    p. tractotomy
pyramidalis
pyramidotomy
    spinal p.
pyramis (pyramides)
pyrazolopyrimidines [a class of
    drugs]
quadrantanopia
quadriplegia
Queckenstedt
    maneuver
    phenomenon
    sign
    test

Queckenstedt-Stookey test
Quincke
    meningitis
    puncture
Quinquaud
    sign
"rabdo–" Phonetic for words begin-
    ning rhabdo–.
raccoon eyes
rachialgia
rachicentesis
rachidial
rachidian
rachigraph
rachiocampsis
rachiocentesis
rachiochysis
rachiodynia
rachiomyelitis
rachioscoliosis
rachiotomy
rachischisis
    r. partialis
    r. posterior
    r. totalis
radiatio (radiationes)
radiation
    r. myelitis
radices (plural of radix)
radiciform
radicis (genitive of radix)
radicle [noun: branch of nerve or
    vessel]
radicotomy
radiculectomy
radiculitis
radiculoganglionitis
radiculomedullary
radiculomeningomyelitis
radiculomyelopathy
radiculoneuritis
radiculoneuropathy
radiculopathy
    brachial r.
    cervical r.
    spinal r.
    spondylotic caudal r.
radii (genitive and plural of radius)

radioactive
    r. brain scan
radioencephalogram
radioencephalography
radio frequency, radiofrequency
    r.f. neurotomy
radionuclide
    r. cisternography
    r. ventriculography
radius (radii)
    r. fixus
radix (radices)
Raeder syndrome
"ra-fee" Phonetic for raphe.
"rakeal–" Phonetic for words begin-
    ning rachial–.
"rakee–" Phonetic for words begin-
    ning rachi–.
Ramadier
    operation
rami (genitive and plural of ramus)
ramicotomy
ramisection
ramisectomy
ramitis
ramose
Ramsay Hunt
    disease
    syndrome
ramulus (ramuli)
ramus (rami)
Ranawat sign
raphe (raphae)
    r. corporis callosi
    median r. of medulla oblon-
      gata, r. mediana medullae
      oblongatae
    median r. of neck, posterior
    median r. of pons, r. medi-
      ana pontina
    r. of medulla oblongata, r.
      medullae oblongatae
    r. mesencephali
    r. of pons, r. pontis
raphes (genitive of raphe)
Rathke
    cyst
    pocket

Rathke (continued)
    pouch
    tumor
Raymond
    apoplexy
Raymond-Cestan syndrome
reaction
    See also *phenomenon, reflex, sign,* and *test.*
    alarm r. (AR)
    Bekhterev r.
    Cushing r.
    fight-or-flight r.
    graft-versus-host r. (GVHR)
    hemianopic pupillary r.
    Jolly r.
    paradoxical pupillary r.
    startle r.
    Wernicke r.
    Wernicke hemianopic r.
receptaculum (receptacula)
    r. ganglii petrosi
receptor
    central r.'s
    cholinergic r.'s
    contact r.
    equilibratory r.'s
    muscarinic r.'s
    muscle r.
    nicotinic r.'s
    N_1 r.'s [N1]
    N_2 r.'s [N2]
    pain r.
    pressure r.
recess
    Tröltsch r.'s, r.'s of Tröltsch
recessus (recessus)
    r. pinealis
    r. suprapinealis
    r. triangularis
reciprocal
Recklinghausen (von Recklinghausen)
    disease
recrudescent
    r. pain
red herring
Redlich-Fisher miliary plaques

reflex
    See also *phenomenon, reaction, sign,* and *test.*
    Achilles tendon r.
    ankle r.
    antagonistic r.'s
    aponeurotic r.
    Aschner r.
    autonomic r.
    axon r.
    Babinski r.
    Babkin r.
    Barkman r.
    Bekhterev r.
    Bekhterev deep r.
    Bekhterev-Mendel r.
    Bezold r.
    biceps r.
    Bing r.
    blink r.
    brachioradialis r.
    Brain [eponym] r.
    Brain [eponym] quadrupedal r.
    Brissaud r.
    Brudzinski r.
    bulbocavernous r.
    carotid sinus r.
    cerebral cortex r.
    Chaddock r.
    chin r.
    ciliospinal r.
    clasping r.
    clasp-knife r.
    contralateral r.
    coordinated r.
    crossed r.
    crossed adductor r.
    crossed extensor r.
    crossed flexor r.
    dartos r.
    deep tendon r.'s (DTRs)
    defense r.
    deglutition r.
    delayed r.
    deltoid r.
    depressor r.
    digital r.

reflex (continued)

- diving r.
- doll's eye r.
- embrace r.
- Escherich r.
- extensor r.
- external hamstring r.
- external oblique r.
- femoral r.
- finger-thumb r.
- flexor r., paradoxical
- flexor withdrawal r.
- fusion r.
- gag r.
- galvanic skin r.
- Gault cochleopalpebral r.
- Geigel r.
- glabellar tap r.
- gluteal r.
- Gordon r.
- Gower-Henry r.
- grasp r., grasping r.
- great toe r.
- gripping r.
- H-r.
- Haab r.
- hamstring r.
- heel-tap r.
- Hirschberg r.
- Hoffmann r.
- Hughes r.
- hypogastric r.
- hypothenar r.
- inguinal r.
- interscapular r.
- iris contraction r.
- jaw r., jaw jerk r.
- Joffroy r.
- Juster r.
- Kehrer r.
- Kisch r.
- knee flexion r.
- knee jerk r.
- Kocher r.
- Landau r.
- latent r.
- laughter r.
- Liddell and Sherrington r.

reflex (continued)

- Lovén r.
- lumbar r.
- Lust r.
- Marinesco-Radovici r.
- mass r.
- Mayer r.
- McCarthy r.
- McCormac r.
- menace r.
- Mendel r., Mendel dorsal r. of foot
- Mendel-Bekhterev r.
- Mondonesi r.
- Morley peritoneocutaneous r.
- motor r.
- muscular r.
- myotatic r.
- nasal r.
- nasolabial r.
- nasomental r.
- neck-righting r.
- nociceptive r. of Riddoch and Buzzard
- nociceptive r.'s
- obliquus r.
- oculocephalogyric r.
- oculopharyngeal r.
- oculopupillary r.
- oculovagal r.
- oculovestibular r.
- Oppenheim r.
- opticofacial winking r.
- orbicularis r.
- orbicularis oculi r.
- orbicularis pupillary r.
- orbiculopupillary r.
- pain r.
- palatal r., palatine r.
- palmar r.
- palm-chin r.
- palmomental r.
- paradoxical r.
- paradoxical ankle r.
- paradoxical extensor r.
- paradoxical flexor r.
- paradoxical patellar r.
- paradoxical pupillary r.

reflex (continued)
    paradoxical triceps r.
    patellar r.
    patelloadductor r.
    pathologic r.'s
    pectoral r.
    pharyngeal r.
    phasic r.
    Philippson r.
    Piltz r.
    Piotrowski r.
    placing r.
    plantar r.
    plantar flexor r.
    platysmal r.
    postural r.
    pressor r.
    Preyer r.
    pronator r.
    proprioceptive r.
    psychic r.
    psychogalvanic r.
    pupillary r.
    Puusepp r.
    quadriceps r.
    quadrupedal extensor r.
    radial r.
    rectus abdominis r.
    regional r.
    Remak r.
    resistance r.
    retrobulbar pupillary r.
    reversed pupillary r.
    Riddoch mass r.
    righting r.
    Roger r.
    Romberg r.
    rooting r.
    Rossolimo r.
    Ruggeri r.
    Saenger r.
    scapular r.
    scapulohumeral r.
    Schaeffer (Schäffer) r.
    scrotal r.
    segmental r.
    senile r.
    simple r.

reflex (continued)
    skin r.
    skin pupillary r.
    sneezing r.
    Snellen r.
    sole r.
    sole-tap r.
    somatointestinal r.
    spinal r.
    stapedial r.
    startle r.
    static r.
    statotonic r.'s
    stepping r.
    Stookey r.
    stretch r.
    Strümpell r.
    sucking r.
    superficial r.
    supinator jerk r.
    supinator longus r.
    supraorbital r.
    suprapatellar r.
    suprapubic r.
    supraumbilical r.
    swallowing r.
    tarsophalangeal r.
    tendon r.
    tensor fasciae latae r.
    threat r.
    Throckmorton r.
    tibioadductor r.
    toe r.
    tonic r.
    tonic neck r.
    triceps r.
    triceps surae r.
    trigeminus r.
    ulnar r.
    vagovagal r.
    vagus r.
    vascular r.
    vasomotor r.
    vasopressor r.'s
    vasovagal r.
    vertebra prominens r.
    vesical r.
    vestibular r.'s

reflex (continued)
    vestibulo-ocular r.
    visceral r.
    visceromotor r.
    viscerosensory r.
    viscerotrophic r.
    von Mering r.
    Wartenberg r.
    Weingrow r.
    Westphal-Piltz r.
    Westphal pupillary r.
    withdrawal r.
    wrist clonus r.
    wrist flexion r.
    zygomatic r.
refractory
    r. pain
Refsum
    disease
    syndrome
region
    anterior hypothalamic r.
    anterior r. of neck
    basilar r.
    Broca r.
    cervical r.
    cingulate r.
    intermediate hypothalamic r.
    lateral r. of neck
    limbic r.
    motor r.
    r. of nape
    nuchal r.
    occipital r.
    opticostriate r.
    parietal r.
    parietotemporal r.
    posterior hypothalamic r.
    posterior r. of neck
    prefrontal r.
    pterygomaxillary r.
    rolandic r.
    sensory r.
    subthalamic r.
    temporal r.
rehab—rehabilitation
Reil
    island (island of Reil)

reinnervation
Reitan-Indiana aphasic screening test
REM—rapid eye movement
Remak
    reflex
Rendu tremor
repertoire
repetition
respiration
    Biot r.
response
    brain stem evoked r. (BSER)
restibrachium
restiform
rete (retia)
    See also *plexus.*
    r. canalis hypoglossi
retial
retrobulbar
retrocollis
retrogasserian
    r. neurectomy
    r. neurotomy
    r. rhizotomy
retropulsion
Rett
    syndrome
rhabdoid
    r. suture
rhabdomyoma
rhinencephalon
rhinocoele
rhinorrhea
    cerebrospinal fluid (CSF) r.
rhizolysis
rhizomeningomyelitis
rhizotomy
    anterior r.
    dorsal r.
    posterior r.
    retrogasserian r.
    trigeminal r.
rhombencephalon
rhombocoele
rhomboid
rhythm
    alpha r.
    Berger r.

rhythm (continued)
    beta r.
    delta r.
    gamma r.
    theta r.
rhythmic, rhythmical
rhythmicity
Ribes ganglion
Richards-Rundle syndrome
Riddoch
    mass reflex
    phenomenon
rider's
Ridley sinus
Rieder
    paralysis
    syndrome
rigidity
    alpha-r.
    cerebellar r.
    clasp-knife r.
    cogwheel r.
    decerebrate r.
    extrapyramidal r.
    hemiplegic r.
    hysterical r.
    lead-pipe r.
    muscular r.
    mydriatic r.
    nuchal r.
    paratonic r.
    parkinsonian r.
    pathologic r.
    spasmodic r.
    spastic r.
rigor
    r. nervorum
    r. tremens
Riley-Day
    syndrome
Riley-Shwachman
    syndrome
Rimbaud-Passouant-Vallat syndrome
rimula
RIND—reversible ischemic neurologic disability
RINE—reversible ischemic neurologic event

"rinensefalon" Phonetic for rhinencephalon.
ring
    fibrous r. of intervertebral disk
"rino–" Phonetic for words beginning rhino–.
risus
    r. caninus
    r. sardonicus
"rithm" Phonetic for rhythm.
"rizo–" Phonetic for words beginning rhizo–.
Roger
    reaction
    symptom
Rolandi
    substantia r.
rolandic fissure
Rolando
    fasciculus (fasciculus of Rolando)
    tubercle (tubercle of Rolando)
rolandometer
Roller nucleus
ROM—range of motion
"rombensefalon" Phonetic for rhombencephalon.
Romberg
    disease
    facial hemiatrophy
    sign
    spasm
    station
    syndrome
    test
    trophoneurosis
Romberg-Howship syndrome
rombergism
"rombosel" Phonetic for rhombocoele.
Rosenbach
    law
Rosenthal
    syndrome
Roser-Braun sign
Rossolimo
    reflex
    sign

rostra (plural of rostrum)
rostrad
rostral
rostralis
rostrate
rostriform
rostrum (rostrums, rostra)
    r. corporis callosi
    r. of corpus callosum
    r. of sphenoid
    sphenoidal r.
    r. sphenoidale
Roth
    disease
    syndrome
Roth-Bernhardt
    disease
    syndrome
Roussy-Cornil syndrome
Roussy-Dejérine syndrome
Roussy-Lévy
    disease
    hereditary ataxic dystasia
    syndrome
Rovsing sign
Royle
    operation
Rubinstein syndrome
Rubinstein-Taybi syndrome
rubrospinal
Rud
    syndrome
rudiment
    r. of corpus striatum
    hippocampal r.
Ruggeri
    reflex
    sign
rule
    See also *law.*
    Jackson r.
Rumpf sign
Russell
    syndrome
Russian
    spring-summer encephalitis
S1 through S5—sacral vertebrae 1–5

Sachs
    disease
sacrospinal
sacrovertebral
Saenger
    reflex
    sign
Saenger-Brown ataxia
Saethre-Chotzen syndrome
sagittal
    s. suture
SAH—subarachnoid hemorrhage
"sal–" Phonetic for words begin-
    ning psal–.
salaam
    s. activity
    s. convulsion
    s. spasm
salicylates [a class of drugs]
saltation
sand
    brain s.
Sänger. See *Saenger.*
Sarbó sign
sarcoma (sarcomas, sarcomata)
    See also in *Oncology and*
        Hematology section.
    cerebral reticulum cell s.
    circumscribed cerebellar
        arachnoid s.
    meningeal s.
    neurogenic s.
    s. of peripheral nerve
satellitosis
Saunders
    disease
    sign
scale
    Cattell Infant Intelligence S.
    Glasgow Coma S.
    Minnesota preschool s.
scalene
scalenus anticus syndrome
scan
    See also in *Radiology,*
        Nuclear Medicine, and
        Other Imaging section.
    bone marrow s.

scan (continued)
  brain s.
scanning
  radioisotope s.
scansion
scaphocephalia
Schaeffer (Schäffer)
  reflex
Schäffer (Schaeffer)
  reflex
Schilder
  disease
  encephalitis
schizocephalia
schizogyria
Schlesinger
  rongeur
Schmidt
  syndrome
Schmorl
  body
  disease
  furrow
  nodule
Scholz
  disease
  sclerosis
Scholz-Greenfield disease
Schrötter chorea
Schüller
  phenomenon
Schultze
  acroparesthesia
  sign
Schultze-Chvostek
  sign
Schultze-type acroparesthesia
Schutz
  bundle
  tract
Schwalbe
  olivary peduncle of s.
Schwann
  sheath
  white substance
schwannoma
  granular cell s.
  malignant s.

Schwartz-Jampel
  myotonia
  syndrome
scintillating scotoma
scissors
  s. gait
scleromeninx
sclérose en plaques
sclerosis
  acute diffuse familial infan-
    tile cerebral s.
  Alzheimer s.
  amyotrophic lateral s. (ALS)
  annular s.
  anterolateral s.
  arterial s.
  arteriolar s.
  arteriopapillary s.
  Baló concentric s.
  benign s.
  bulbar s.
  Canavan diffuse s.
  cerebellar s.
  cerebral s.
  cerebrospinal s.
  cervical s.
  combined s.
  diffuse s.
  diffuse cerebral s.
  diffuse cortical s.
  diffuse systemic s.
  disseminated s.
  Erb s.
  familial centrolobar s.
  focal s.
  hereditary spinal s.
  hyperplastic s.
  insular s.
  Krabbe s.
  Krabbe-type diffuse s.
  lateral s.
  lateral spinal s.
  lenticular nuclear s.
  lobar s.
  Marie s.
  mesial temporal s.
  miliary s.
  Mönckeberg s.

sclerosis (continued)
    multiple s. (MS)
    nodular s.
    nuclear s.
    Pelizaeus-Merzbacher s.
    posterior s., posterior spinal s.
    posterolateral s.
    presenile s.
    primary lateral s.
    progressive lateral s.
    s. redux
    renal arteriolar s.
    Scholz-Bielschowsky-Hen-
      neberg diffuse cerebral s.
    Scholz cerebral s.
    transitional s.
    s. tuberosa
    tuberous s.
    unicellular s.
    vascular s.
    ventrolateral s.
score
    Dubowitz s.
    Glasgow [coma] s.
scotoma (scotomata)
Scribner shunt
second (s, sec.)
    milliampere s. (mAs)
sectio (sectiones)
section
    pituitary stalk s.
    trigeminal root s.
sedation
sedatives [a class of drugs]
    cerebral s.
    nerve trunk s.
    spinal s.
"sefal–" Phonetic for words begin-
    ning cephal–.
segmenta (plural of segmentum)
segmental
segmentum (segmenta)
Seguin signal symptom
Seitelberger
    disease
    dystrophy
    syndrome

seizure
    absence s.
    akinetic s.
    atonic s.
    audiogenic s.
    autonomic s.
    cerebral s.
    complex partial s.
    febrile s.
    generalized s.
    hysterical s.
    infantile myoclonic s.
    jackknife s.
    jacksonian s.
    lightning s.
    major motor s.
    minor motor s.
    myoclonic s.
    neonatal s.
    partial s.
    photogenic s.
    psychic s.
    psychomotor s.
    reflex anoxic s.
    sylvian s.
    tonic-clonic s.
    traumatic s.
    uncinate s.
    versive s.
    vertiginous s.
selective
    highly s. vagotomy
    s. vagotomy
self-suspension
sella (sellae)
    empty s. (syndrome)
    s. turcica
sellar
semicoma
semicomatose
seminarcosis
"seng-ker" Phonetic for Zenker.
sensorial
sensorineural
sensorium
    general s.
sensory
    s. deficit

SEP—sensory evoked potential
  somatosensory evoked
   potential
septa (plural of septum)
septal
  s. nuclei
septum (septa)
  cervical s., intermediate
  s. lucidum
  median s. of spinal cord
  pellucid s., s. pellucidum
  precommissural s., s. pre-
   commissurale
  transverse s. of ampulla
  true s.
  s. verum
sequela (sequelae)
SER—somatosensory evoked
  response
serotonin
serrated
  s. suture
SFEMG—single-fiber electromyogram
"sfeno–" Phonetic for words beginning spheno–.
sheath
  arachnoid s.
  carotid s.
  dural s.
  endoneurial s.
  medullary s.
  myelin s.
  Schwann s., s. of Schwann
shingles
shock
  neurogenic s.
"shogren" Phonetic for Sjögren.
"shok-vist" Phonetic for Sjöqvist.
"shov-stek," "shvo-stek" Phonetic
  for Chvostek.
shunt
  Holter s.
  peritoneosubarachnoid s.
  Ramirez s.
  Silastic ventriculoperitoneal s.
  Torkildsen s.
  ventriculoatrial s.

shunt (continued)
  ventriculoperitoneal s.
  ventriculopleural s.
  ventriculovenous s.
"shwah-no-mah" Phonetic for
  schwannoma.
Shy-Drager syndrome
"siatik" Phonetic for sciatic.
Sicard syndrome
Siegert sign
Siemerling nucleus
"sifilis" Phonetic for syphilis.
"sifilo–" Phonetic for words begin-
  ning syphilo–.
sign
  See also *phenomenon, reac-
   tion, reflex,* and *test.*
  Abadie s.
  Achilles tendon s.
  André Thomas s.
  anterior drawer s.
  anterior tibial s.
  anticus s.
  Apley s.
  Argyll Robertson pupillary s.
  Babinski s.
  Babinski toe s.
  Baillarger s.
  Bamberger s.
  banana s.
  Bard s.
  Barré s.
  Barré pyramidal s.
  Bastian-Bruns s.
  Battle s.
  Beevor s.
  Bekhterev s.
  Bell s.
  Berger s.
  Biernacki s.
  Biot s.
  Bordier-Fränkel s.
  Bragard s.
  Brown-Séquard s.
  Brudzinski s.
  Bruns s.
  Cantelli s.
  Cestan s.

sign (continued)
    Chaddock s.
    Charcot s.
    Cheyne-Stokes s.
    Chvostek s.
    Chvostek-Weiss s.
    Claude hyperkinesis s.
    cogwheel s.
    complementary opposition s.
    contralateral s.
    coughing s.
    Crichton-Browne s.
    Crowe s.
    Dejerine s.
    de la Camp s.
    distal tingling on pressure
        (DTP) s.
    doll's eye s.
    DTP (distal tingling on pres-
        sure) s.
    Duckworth s.
    echo s.
    Escherich s.
    external malleolar s.
    facial s.
    Fajersztajn crossed sciatic s.
    fan s.
    forearm s.
    formication s.
    Fränkel s.
    glabellar tap s.
    Gordon s.
    Gowers s.
    Grasset s.
    Grasset-Bychowski s.
    Grasset-Gaussel-Hoover s.
    Guilland s.
    Hahn s.
    Heilbronner s.
    Hennebert s.
    Hochsinger s.
    Hoffmann s.
    Holmes s.
    Hoover s.
    Horsley s.
    Hoyne s.
    Huntington s.
    hyperkinesis s.

sign (continued)
    interossei s.
    jugular s.
    Kernig s.
    Kerr s.
    Kleist s.
    Klippel-Weil s.
    Lafora s.
    Lasègue s.
    leg s.
    Leichtenstern s.
    Leri s.
    Lhermitte s.
    Lichtheim s.
    Linder s.
    long tract s.
    Lust s.
    Macewen s.
    Magendie s.
    Magendie-Hertwig s.
    Mannkopf s.
    Marcus Gunn pupillary s.
    Marie-Foix s.
    Marinesco s.
    Minor s.
    Morquio s.
    Myerson s.
    neck s.
    Negro s.
    Neri s.
    Nothnagel s.
    Oppenheim s.
    orbicularis s.
    Parkinson s.
    Parrot s.
    Patrick s.
    Pende s.
    peroneal s.
    Piotrowski s.
    Pitres s.
    Plummer s.
    Pool-Schlesinger s.
    Prévost s.
    pronation s.
    pseudo-Babinski s.
    pyramid s., pyramidal s.
    pyramidal tract s. of lower
        extremities

sign (continued)
    Queckenstedt s.
    Quinquaud s.
    Radovici s.
    Remak s.
    reservoir s.
    Romberg s.
    rope s.
    Rosenbach s.
    Rossolimo s.
    Ruggeri s.
    Rumpf s.
    Rust s.
    Saenger s.
    Sarbó s.
    Schepelmann s.
    Schultze s.
    Schultze-Chvostek s.
    Séguin s.
    setting-sun s.
    Siegert s.
    Signorelli s.
    Simon s.
    Soto-Hall s.
    Souques s.
    spine s.
    stairs s.
    Stewart-Holmes s.
    Stokes s.
    Strümpell s.
    swinging flashlight s.
    Tay s.
    Theimich lip s.
    Thomas s.
    Throckmorton s.
    tibialis s.
    Tinel s.
    toe s.
    Trendelenburg s.
    Trousseau s.
    Turyn s.
    Valleix s.
    Vanzetti s.
    von Strümpell s.
    Wartenberg s.
    Weber s.
    Westphal s.
Signorelli sign

"sike–" Phonetic for words beginning psych–.
silence
    electrical s.
    electrocerebral s.
siliqua
    s. olivae
Simmonds
    disease
    syndrome
Simon
    position
sin–. See also words beginning cin–, syn–.
sinciput
"sinerea" Phonetic for cinerea.
"singul–" Phonetic for words beginning cingul–.
sinistrocerebral
sinus (sinus, sinuses)
    articular s. of atlas
    articular s. of atlas, superior
    articular s. of axis, anterior
    articular s. of vertebrae, inferior
    s. of atlas, anterior
    Breschet s.
    carotid s.
    s. cavernosus, cavernous s.
    cerebral s.
    circular s.
    s. of corpus callosum
    cranial s.'s
    dermal s.
    dural s.
    s.'s of dura mater
    intercavernous s.'s
    s. of internal jugular vein, inferior
    s. of internal jugular vein, superior
    lateral s.
    marginal s., s. marginalis
    middle s. of atlas
    petrosal s., inferior
    petrosal s., superior
    rhomboid s.
    rhomboid s. of Henle

sinus (sinus, sinuses) (continued)
 Ridley s.
 sagittal s., inferior
 sagittal s., superior
 sigmoid s.
 sphenoparietal s.
 straight s.
 subarachnoidal s.'s
 subcapsular s.'s
 subpetrosal s.
 superpetrosal s.
 transverse s. of dura mater
 venous s.
 venous s.'s of dura mater
sinusography
 cerebral s.
Sipple syndrome
"siringo–" Phonetic for words
 beginning syringo–.
Sjögren
 disease
 syndrome
Sjögren-Larsson
 syndrome
Sjöqvist
 operation
 tractotomy
"skafo–" Phonetic for words beginning scapho–.
skeletization
skeletonize
"sklero–" Phonetic for words beginning sclero–.
skull
 cloverleaf s.
 hot-cross-bun s.
 lacuna s.
 maplike s.
 natiform s.
 steeple s.
 sutures of s.
 tower s.
 West-Engstler s.
 West lacuna s.
sleep
 fast-wave s.
 non–rapid eye movement
 (NREM) s.

sleep (continued)
 rapid eye movement (REM)
 s.
 rolandic s.
 slow-wave s.
sleep apnea
 obstructive s.a. (OSA)
 s.a. syndrome
SLR—straight leg raising
SLRT—straight leg-raising test
SMA—supplementary motor area
small-vessel disease
Smith-Robinson
 operation
Smithwick
 operation
SMON—subacute myelo-opti-
 coneuropathy
SNS—sympathetic nervous system
SOA-MCA—superficial occipital
 artery to middle cerebral artery
softening
 s. of the brain
solanine
solanism
solution
 See *fluid* and *liquor.*
somatomotor
somatopsychic
somatosensory
 s. evoked potential (SEP)
 s. evoked response (SER)
somatotopic
somnambulism
somniloquism
somnipathy
somnolentia
Sonneberg
 operation
Soto-Hall sign
Sottas disease
sound
 cracked-pot s., cranial
space
 arachnoid s.
 Broca s.
 epidural s.
 extradural s.

space (continued)
    Magendie s.'s
    pia-arachnoid s.
    subarachnoid s.
    subdural s.
spasm
    athetoid s.
    cerebral s.
    clonic s.
    facial s.
    intention s.
    Romberg s.
    salaam s.
    saltatory s.
    tetanic s., tonic s.
spectrum (spectra)
    fortification s.
Spens syndrome
sphenion (sphenia)
sphenoethmoid, sphenoethmoidal
    s. suture
sphenofrontal
    s. suture
sphenoidal
sphenoidostomy
sphenoidotomy
spheno-occipital
    s. suture
sphenoparietal
    s. suture
sphenopetrosal
    s. suture
sphenosquamous
    s. suture
sphenotemporal
    s. suture
sphingolipidosis
    cerebral s.
    late-onset cerebral s.
Spielmeyer-Vogt
    disease
Spiller syndrome
spina (spinae)
    s. bifida
    s. bifida anterior
    s. bifida aperta
    s. bifida cystica
    s. bifida manifesta

spina (spinae) (continued)
    s. bifida occulta
    s. bifida posterior
spinal
    s. arteriography
    s. pyramidotomy
spinal cord
    s.c. angiography
spinant
spine
    alar s.
    angular s.
    cervical s.
    Civinini s.
    cleft s.
    ethmoidal s. of Macalister
    lumbar s.
    lumbosacral (LS) s.
    posterior inferior iliac s.
    posterior superior iliac s.
    sphenoidal s.
    s. of sphenoid bone
    thoracic s.
    typhoid s.
    s. of vertebra
    vertebral s.
spinobulbar
spinocerebellar
spinogalvanization
spinogram
spinothalamic
    s. tractotomy
spinous
spiral
    Herxheimer s.'s
splanchnicectomy
    lumbodorsal s.
splanchnicotomy
"splank–" Phonetic for words
    beginning splanch–.
splenium
    s. corporis callosi
spondylodesis
spondylolysis
spondylomalacia
spondylopathy
spondylopyosis
spondyloschisis

spondylosis
> cervical s.
> s. chronica ankylopoietica
> degenerative s.
> hyperostotic s.
> lumbar s.
> rhizomelic s.
> s. uncovertebralis

spondylosyndesis
spondylotomy
spongioblast
spongioblastoma
> s. multiforme
> s. unipolare

spot
> See also *macula* and *macule*.
> café au lait s.
> hypnogenetic s.
> pain s.
> temperature s.
> Trousseau s.

squamomastoid
> s. suture

squamoparietal
> s. suture

squamosphenoid
> s. suture

squamous
> s. suture
> s. suture of cranium

SSP, SSPE—subacute sclerosing panencephalitis
Staderini nucleus
staircase phenomenon
STA-MCA—superficial temporal artery to middle cerebral artery
St. Anthony's
> disease
> fire

status
> absence s.
> s. choreicus
> s. convulsivus
> s. cribalis
> s. cribrosus
> s. criticus
> s. dysgraphicus
> s. dysmyelinatus

status (continued)
> s. dysmyelinisatus
> s. dysraphicus
> s. epilepticus
> s. hemicranicus
> s. lacunaris
> s. lacunosus
> s. marmoratus
> mental s.
> petit mal s.
> s. post [event]
> psychomotor s.
> s. spongiosus
> s. verrucosus
> s. vertiginosus

Steele-Richardson-Olszewski
> disease
> syndrome

"stefaneon" Phonetic for stephanion.
Steinert
> disease
> myotonic dystrophy
> syndrome

stellate
stem
> brain s.

stenion
stenosis (stenoses)
> spinal s.

stephanion
stereoanesthesia
stereoencephalotomy
stereognosis
stereotactic
stereotaxis
Stewart-Holmes sign
Stewart-Morel
> syndrome

stimulants [a class of drugs]
stimulate
stimulus (stimuli)
stimulus-response (S-R)
St. Louis encephalitis
Stock-Spielmeyer-Vogt syndrome
Stokes
> law
> sign
> syndrome

Stokes-Adams
    disease
    syndrome
Stookey-Scarff
    operation
Strachan
    disease
    syndrome
Strachan-Scott syndrome
strata (plural of stratum)
stratiform
stratum (strata)
    deep white s. of quadrigemi-
      nal body
    white s. of quadrigeminal
      body, deep
streak
    See *line* and *stria.*
strephosymbolia
stria (striae)
    See also *line.*
    Francke s.
    habenular s.
    s. of Lanci
    medullary s. of corpus stria-
      tum, medial
    medullary striae of fourth
      ventricle
    medullary striae of rhom-
      boid fossa
    medullary s. of corpus stria-
      tum, external
    medullary s. of thalamus
    meningitic s.
    olfactory s.
    olfactory s., intermediate
striatal
striatonigral
striatum
stroke
    atherothrombotic s.
    cardioembolic s.
    cerebral s.
    completed s.
    embolic s.
    s. in evolution
    ischemic s.
    lacunar s.

stroke (continued)
    light s.
    lightning s.
    paralytic s.
    progressive s.
Stromeyer cephalhematocele
Strümpell
    disease
    reflex
    sign
Strümpell-Leichtenstern
    disease
    encephalitis
    hemorrhagic encephalitis
stupor
    anergic s.
    benign s.
    Cairns s.
    catatonic s.
    delusion s.
    depressive s.
    epileptic s.
    lethargic s.
    postconvulsive s.
    spike-wave s.
    s. vigilans
stuporous
Sturge
    disease
    syndrome
Sturge-Weber
    disease
    encephalotrigeminal
      angiomatosis
    syndrome
Sturge-Weber-Dimitri disease
stuttering
    labiochoreic s.
St. Vitus dance
subarachnoid
    s. hemorrhage
subarachnoiditis
subconscious
subconsciousness
subcortical
subdural
    s. hematoma
subependymal

subgaleal
subjective
subpial
subpontine
substance
  white s. of Schwann
substantia (substantiae)
  s. alba
  s. cinerea
  s. grisea
  s. nigra
subthalamus
succinimides [a class of drugs]
"sudo–" Phonetic for words beginning pseudo–.
sulci (plural of sulcus)
sulciform
sulculus (sulculi)
sulcus (sulci)
  anterolateral s. of medulla oblongata
  anterolateral s. of spinal cord
  basilar s. of pons
  bulbopontine s., s. bulbopontinus
  bulboventricular s.
  calcarine s.
  callosal s.
  callosomarginal s.
  central s. of cerebrum
  cerebral s., lateral
  sulci of cerebrum
  chiasmatic s.
  cingulate s.
  s. of cingulum
  circular s. of insula
  collateral s.
  s. of corpus callosum
  s. of sigmoid sinus
  s. of greater petrosal nerve
  hemispheric s.
  hypothalamic s.
  interparietal s.
  intraparietal s.
  lateral s.
  lateral occipital s.
  lunate s.
  s. lunatus

sulcus (sulci) (continued)
  median s.
  meningeal sulci
  s. of Monro
  oculomotor s.
  paramedial s.
  parietooccipital s.
  petrobasilar s.
  pontobulbar s.
  pontopeduncular s.
  postolivary s.
  postpyramidal s.
  prepyramidal s.
  prerolandic s.
  s. of pterygoid hamulus
  rolandic s.
  s. of spinal nerve
  subparietal s.
  supraorbital s.
  suprasylvian s.
  s. Sylvii
  temporal s.
  Turner s.
  s. of vertebral artery of atlas
sulfamates [a class of drugs]
Sunday morning paralysis
supination
  s. of foot
supratentorial
surgery
  See also *maneuver, method, operation, procedure,* and *technique.*
  stereotactic s., stereotaxic s.
surgical
  s. vagotomy
surgical procedure
  See *operation.*
sutura (suturae)
sutural
suture [anatomy]
  bony s.
  coronal s.
  cranial s.'s
  dentate s.
  ethmoidolacrimal s.
  ethmoidomaxillary s.
  frontal s.

suture [anatomy] (continued)
    frontolacrimal s.
    frontoparietal s.
    frontosphenoid s.
    frontozygomatic s.
    infraorbital s.
    interparietal s.
    jugal s.
    lambdoid s., lambdoidal s.
    limbal s.
    limbous s.
    longitudinal s.
    metopic s.
    occipital s.
    occipitomastoid s.
    occipitoparietal s.
    occipitosphenoidal s.
    parietal s.
    parietomastoid s.
    parieto-occipital s.
    parietotemporal s.
    petrobasilar s.
    petrosphenobasilar s.
    petrospheno-occipital s. of
      Gruber
    petrosquamosal s.
    rhabdoid s.
    sagittal s.
    serrated s.
    s.'s of skull
    sphenoethmoidal s.
    sphenofrontal s.
    spheno-occipital s.
    sphenoparietal s.
    sphenopetrosal s.
    sphenosquamous s.
    sphenotemporal s.
    squamomastoid s.
    squamoparietal s.
    squamosphenoid s.
    squamous s.
    squamous s. of cranium
    temporal s.
    temporomalar s.
    temporozygomatic s.
    transverse s. of Krause
    true s.
    zygomaticofrontal s.

suture [anatomy] (continued)
    zygomaticosphenoid s.
    zygomaticotemporal s.
suture [material]
    See in *General Surgical*
      Terms.
suture [technique]
    See in *General Surgical*
      Terms.
swelling
    See *apophysis, process,* and
      protuberance.
    brain s.
SWS—slow-wave sleep
Sydenham chorea
sylvian
    s. aqueduct syndrome
    s. fissure
Sylvii
    cisterna fossae S.
Sylvius
    aqueduct (aqueduct of
      Sylvius)
    cistern (cistern of Sylvius)
    fissure (fissure of Sylvius)
    ventricle of S.
symmetric, symmetrical
sympathectomy
    cervical s.
    chemical s.
    lumbar s.
    lumbodorsal s.
    periarterial s.
sympathicoblastoma
sympathicogonioma
sympathicopathy
sympathicotherapy
sympathicotripsy
sympatholytic
sympathomimetic
symptom
    See also in *General Medical*
      Terms.
    Bonhoeffer s.
    Brauch-Romberg s.
    Buerger s.
    Castellani-Low s.
    Chvostek s.

symptom (continued)
    Colliver s.
    dissociation s.
    Ganser s.
    Gordon s.
    Haenel s.
    localizing s.'s
    Magendie s.
    Oehler s.
    premonitory s.
    prodromal s.
    prodromal epileptic s.
    Remak s.
    Roger s.
    Romberg-Howship s.
    Seguin signal s.
    signal s.
    Trendelenburg s.
    Wernicke s.
syn–. See also words beginning
    cin–, sin–.
synapse
    axodendritic s.
    axodendrosomatic s.
    axosomatic s.
    en passant s. [ahn pah-sahn]
    loop s.
synchondrosis (synchondroses)
synclonus
    s. beriberica
syncope
    cardiac s.
    carotid s.
    carotid sinus s.
    cough s.
    defecation s.
    micturition s.
    orthostatic s.
    postural s.
    tussive s.
    vasodepressor s.
    vasovagal s.
syndrome
    See also *disease.*
    acute brain s.
    acute organic brain s.
    Adie s.
    Alzheimer s.

syndrome (continued)
    amnesic s.
    amnestic s.
    amnestic-confabulatory s.
    Apert s.
    aqueduct of Sylvius s.
    Arnold-Chiari s.
    ataxia-telangiectasia s.
    Baastrup s.
    Babinski s.
    Babinski-Nageotte s., s. of
        Babinski-Nageotte
    Babinski-Vaquez s.
    Balint s.
    Bárány s.
    Barré-Liéou s.
    Bärtschi-Rochain s.
    Beard s.
    Beck s.
    Blackfan-Diamond s.
    Bonnet s.
    Bonnet sphenoidal foramen s.
    Bourneville s.
    Bourneville-Pringle s.
    boxer's s.
    brachial s.
    brain s.
    Brissaud-Sicard s.
    Bristowe s.
    Brown-Séquard s.
    Bruns s.
    Brushfield-Wyatt s.
    burning feet s.
    callosal s.
    capsular thrombosis s.
    capsulothalamic s.
    carotid sinus s.
    carpal tunnel s. (CTS)
    cavernous sinus s.
    cerebellar s.
    cervical disk s.
    cervical rib s.
    cervicobrachial s.
    Cestan s.
    Cestan-Chenais s., s. of Ces-
        tan-Chenais
    Cestan-Raymond s.
    Charcot s.

syndrome (continued)
- Charcot-Marie-Tooth-Hoffmann s.
- Chinese restaurant s. (CRS)
- chorea s.
- chronic brain s.
- chronic organic brain s.
- Churg-Strauss s.
- Claude s.
- Claude Bernard-Horner s.
- Claude-Lhermitte s.
- closed head s.
- cloverleaf skull deformity s.
- Collet s.
- Collet-Sicard s.
- concussion s.
- contracture s.
- Creutzfeldt-Jakob s.
- cri-du-chat s.
- cubital s.
- cubital tunnel s.
- Cushing s.
- Cushing s. medicamentosus
- Dandy-Walker s.
- Dejerine s.
- Dejerine anterior bulbar s.
- Dejerine interolivary s.
- Dejerine-Klumpke s.
- Dejerine-Roussy s., s. of Dejerine-Roussy
- Dejerine-Sottas s.
- de Morsier s.
- de Morsier-Gauthier s.
- Dennie-Marfan s.
- Denny-Brown s.
- De Sanctis-Cacchione s.
- Devic s.
- disk s.
- Down s.
- Duchenne s.
- Duchenne-Erb s.
- Eaton-Lambert s.
- effort s.
- empty sella s.
- Erb s.
- Erb-Goldflam s.
- Erb-Oppenheim-Goldflam s.
- facet s.

syndrome (continued)
- Foix-Alajouanine s.
- Foix paramedian s.
- fourth ventricle s.
- Foville s.
- Friderichsen-Waterhouse s.
- Friedmann vasomotor s.
- Fröhlich s.
- Froin s.
- Garcin s.
- Gélineau s.
- Gerstmann s.
- Gilles de la Tourette s.
- Gowers s.
- Gradenigo s.
- Gradenigo-Lannois s.
- Guillain-Barré s.
- Hakim s.
- Hallervorden-Spatz s.
- Hartnup s.
- hemiplegia, hemiconvulsions, and epilepsy (HHE) s.
- herniated disk s.
- Holmes-Adie
- Homén s.
- Horner s.
- Horner-Bernard s.
- Horton s.
- Hunt striatal s.
- Hurler s.
- Hutchison s.
- internal carotid artery s.
- Jackson s.
- Jacod s.
- Jacod-Negri s.
- Jakob-Creutzfeldt s.
- Kearns-Sayre s.
- Kehrer-Adie s.
- Kiloh-Nevin s.
- kleeblattschädel (cloverleaf skull) s.
- Kleine-Levin s.
- Klippel-Feil s.
- Klippel-Feldstein s.
- Klumpke-Dejerine s.
- Klüver-Bucy s.
- Korsakoff s.
- Kugelberg-Welander s.

syndrome (continued)
 Lambert-Eaton myasthenic s.
 Laurence-Biedl s.
 Laurence-Moon s.
 Lennox s.
 Lennox-Gastaut s.
 Lesch-Nyhan s.
 Lévy-Roussy s.
 Leyden-Möbius s.
 locked-in s.
 loculation s.
 Louis-Bar s.
 Mackenzie s.
 Marcus Gunn s.
 Marcus Gunn inverse s.
 Marcus Gunn jaw-winking s.
 Marie s. (I, II)
 Marinesco-Sjögren s.
 Marinesco-Sjögren-Garland s.
 Melkersson s.
 Ménière s.
 Millard-Gubler s.
 minimal brain dysfunction
  (MBD) s.
 Möbius s.
 Morgagni s.
 Morgagni-Stewart-Morel s.
 myasthenia gravis s.
 Naffziger s.
 Nelson s.
 neuroleptic malignant s.
 nonpsychotic organic brain s.
 Nothnagel s.
 organic brain s.
 Parinaud s.
 Parkinson s.
 parkinsonian s.
 Parry-Romberg s.
 Paterson-Brown-Kelly s.
 pickwickian s.
 postconcussional s.
 post-lumbar puncture s.
 post-traumatic brain s.
 pseudo-Turner s.
 Putti s.
 Raeder s.
 Raeder paratrigeminal s.
 Ramsay Hunt s.

syndrome (continued)
 restless legs s.
 Rett s.
 Reye s.
 Riley-Day s.
 Riley-Shwachman s.
 Rimbaud-Passouant-Vallat s.
 Roth s.
 Roth-Bernhardt s.
 Roussy-Cornil s.
 Roussy-Lévy s.
 Rud s.
 scalenus s.
 scalenus anticus s.
 Schwartz-Jampel s.
 shaken baby s.
 Shy-Drager s.
 Sjögren s.
 Sjögren-Larsson s.
 sleep apnea s.
 Spielmeyer-Sjögren s.
 Stewart-Morel s.
 stroke s.
 Sturge-Weber s.
 subclavian steal s.
 temporomandibular dysfunc-
  tion s.
 temporomandibular joint
  (TMJ) s.
 thoracic outlet s.
 Tourette s.
 trisomy 21 s.
 trisomy D s.
 trisomy E s.
 Vernet s.
 Vogt s.
 Vogt-Koyanagi-Harada s.
 Wallenberg s.
 Waterhouse-Friderichsen s.
 Weill-Reys s.
 Weill-Reys-Adie s.
 Wernicke s.
 Wernicke-Korsakoff s.
 West s.
synesthesia
 s. algica
synesthesialgia
synreflexia

syntactic
syntaxis
syntonic
syphilis
>   cerebrospinal s.
>   meningovascular s.
syphilitic
syphilopsychosis
syringobulbia
syringocele
syringocoele
syringoencephalia
syringoencephalomyelia
syringomeningocele
syringomyelia
>   s. atrophica
>   traumatic s.
syringomyelitis
syringomyelocele
syringomyelus
syringopontia
syrinx
system
>   autonomic nervous s.
>   central nervous s. (CNS)
>   Conolly s.
>   peripheral nervous s.
>   Pinel s.
T1 through T12—thoracic vertebrae 1–12
Taarnhøj
>   operation
tabes
>   cerebral t.
>   diabetic t.
>   t. dorsalis
>   t. ergotica
>   Friedreich t.
>   t. spinalis
>   vessel t.
tabetic
taboparesis
tabula (tabulae)
>   t. externa ossis cranii
>   t. interna ossis cranii
>   t. vitrea
tabular

tache ["tahsh"]
>   t. cérébrale ["say-ray-brahl"]
>   t. méningéale ["may-na-zha-ahl"]
>   t. motrice ["mo-trees"]
>   t. spinale ["spe-nahl"]
tack operation
taenia (taeniae) [anatomy: flat band]
>   t. cinerea
>   t. of fornix
>   t. of fourth ventricle
>   medullary t. of thalamus
>   t. pontis
>   t. tectae
>   t. telae
>   t. of thalamus
>   t. of third ventricle
taeniacides [a class of drugs]
"tahsh" Phonetic for tache.
Talma disease
tapeinocephaly
tapeta (plural of tapetum)
tapetal
tapetum (tapeta)
>   t. corporis callosi
>   t. ventriculi
tardive
>   t. akathisia
>   t. dyskinesia (TD)
>   t. dystonia
Tay-Sachs disease
TCI—transient cerebral ischemia
TCIE—transient cerebral ischemic episode
TD—tardive dyskinesia
>   tic douloureux
technique
>   See maneuver and method.
tectospinal
"tedeum" Phonetic for taedium.
tegmen (tegmina)
>   t. ventriculi quarti
tegmenta (plural of tegmentum)
tegmental
tegmentum (tegmenta)
>   hypothalamic t.
>   t. mesencephali, t. of mesencephalon

tegmentum (tegmenta) (continued)
    t. of pons
    pontile t.
    t. pontis
    t. rhombencephali
    subthalamic t.
tegmina (plural of tegmen)
"te-kur" Phonetic for tiqueur.
tela (telae)
    t. choroidea inferior
    t. choroidea of fourth ventricle
    t. choroidea of third ventricle
    t. choroidea superior
telangiectasis (telangiectases)
telar
telencephalon
tempora (plural of tempus)
temporal
    t. lobectomy
    t. suture
temporalis
temporoauricular
temporofacial
temporofrontal
temporohyoid
temporomalar
    t. suture
temporomandibular
temporomaxillary
temporo-occipital
temporoparietal
temporopontile
temporosphenoid
temporozygomatic
    t. suture
tenia (teniae)
    See also *taenia [flat band].*
    t. choroidea
    t. telae
tenial
TENS—transcutaneous electrical nerve stimulator
Tensilon [anesthetic agent]
tentorium (tentoria)
    t. cerebelli
    t. of cerebellum
    t. of hypophysis

tephromalacia
tephromyelitis
"tere–" Phonetic for words beginning pteri–, ptery–.
termini (plural of terminus)
terminus (termini)
test
    See also *phenomenon, reaction, reflex,* and *sign.*
    See also in *Laboratory, Pathology, and Chemistry Terms.*
    Apley t.
    apprehension t.
    Babinski t.
    balance t.
    Bárány pointing t.
    Benton t. for visual retention
    Bielschowsky head-tilting t.
    carotid sinus t.
    Chvostek t.
    contralateral straight leg raising t.
    dexamethasone suppression t.
    Dix-Hallpike t.
    doll's eye t.
    duck waddle t.
    edrophonium t.
    finger-to-finger t.
    finger-to-nose t.
    Hallpike t.
    Halstead-Reitan t.
    heel-to-knee t.
    heel-to-shin t.
    heel-tap t.
    Janet t.
    labyrinthine t.
    Lasègue t.
    orientation t.
    Pandy t.
    Patrick t.
    pendular eye-tracking t. (PETT)
    Phalen t.
    pointing t.
    postauricular myogenic (PAM) reflex t.
    recruitment t.

test (continued)
> Reitan-Indiana aphasic
> > screening t.
> Romberg t.
> squatting t.
> station t.
> straight leg raising t. (SLRT)
> Tobey-Ayer t.
> Valsalva t.
> Wada t.
> Walter bromide t.
> Wernicke t.
> Yerkes-Bridges t.

tethered cord syndrome
tetraplegia
textus (textus)
TGA—transient global amnesia
thalamectomy
thalamencephalic
thalamencephalon
thalami (genitive and plural of thal-
> amus)
thalamic
thalamocele
thalamocortical
thalamolenticular
thalamomamillary
thalamotegmental
thalamotomy
> anterior t.
> dorsomedial t.
> parafascicular t. (PFT)

thalamus (thalami)
> dorsal t., t. dorsalis
> optic t.
> t. ventralis

theca (thecae)
> t. medullare spinalis
> t. vertebralis

thecal
theory
> Meyer t.

therapy
> anticoagulant t.
> anticonvulsant t.
> antiplatelet t.
> beam t.
> carbon dioxide t.

therapy (continued)
> intrathecal t.
> sleep t.
> thrombolytic t.

third ventriculostomy
Thomas sign
Thomayer sign
Thomsen
> disease

thoracic
> t. laminectomy
> t. outlet syndrome

threshold
> t. of consciousness
> convulsant t.
> differential sensory t.
> t. of discomfort
> epileptic t.
> t. for two-point discrimination
> myoclonic t.
> pain t.

Throckmorton reflex
thrombi (plural of thrombus)
thromboangiitis
> t. obliterans

thrombosis
> See also *thrombus*.
> See also in *Cardiology* sec-
> > tion.
> arterial t.
> cavernous sinus t.
> cerebellar t.
> cerebral t.
> marantic t., marasmic t.

thrombus (thrombi)
> See also *thrombosis*.
> marantic t., marasmic t.

thunderclap headache
TIA—transient ischemic attack
tic
> blinking t.
> bowing t.
> convulsive t.
> degenerative t.
> t. de Guinon
> t. de pensée ["da pon-say"]
> t. de sommeil ["da soma"]
> t. douloureux ["doo-loo-roo"]

tic (continued)
  facial t.
  gesticulatory t.
  laryngeal t.
  mimic t.
  motor t.
  t. nondouloureux
  progressive choreic t.
  rotatory t.
  saltatory t.
  spasmodic t.
  winking t.
tick paralysis
TIE—transient ischemic episode
time (T)
  Achilles tendon reflex t.
  apex t.
  conduction t.
  deep tendon reflex relax-
    ation t.
  inertia t.
  reaction t.
  recognition t.
  relaxation t.
  stimulus-response t.
tinnitus
  t. aurium
  clicking t.
  Leudet t.
  nervous t.
  nonvibratory t.
  objective t.
  vibratory t.
tiqueur
titubation
  lingual t.
TM—temporomandibular
TMJ—temporomandibular joint
TMJ syndrome
Tobey-Ayer
  test
Todd
  palsy
  paralysis
tolerance
  drug t.
Toma
  sign

tomography
  computed t. (CT)
  computerized axial t. (CAT)
  cranial computed t. (CCT)
  positron emission t. (PET)
tongue
  choreic t.
  t. of sphenoid bone
tonography
  carotid compression t.
tonsil
  t. of cerebellum
tonsilla (tonsillae)
  t. cerebelli
  t. cerebelli, t. of cerebellum
  t. of cerebellum
tonsillar
tonus
  neurogenic t.
"too-mur" Phonetic for tumeur.
"too-ret" Phonetic for Tourette.
tooth (teeth)
  auditory teeth of Corti
  auditory teeth of Huschke
  t. of axis
  Corti auditory teeth
  t. of epistropheus
  Huschke auditory teeth
Tooth [eponym]
  atrophy
  disease
  type
topagnosis
topectomy
Torkildsen
  operation
torticollis
  acute t.
  congenital t.
  dermatogenic t.
  fixed t.
  hysterical t.
  infantile t.
  intermittent t.
  labyrinthine t.
  mental t.
  myogenic t.
  neurogenic t.

torticollis (continued)
    ocular t.
    paralytic t.
    reflex t.
    rheumatoid t.
    spasmodic t.
    spastic t.
    spurious t.
    symptomatic t.
tortipelvis
"tosh" Phonetic for tache.
Tourette (Gilles de la Tourette)
    disease
    syndrome
tourniquet
    t. paralysis
trabecula (trabeculae)
    arachnoid trabeculae
    t. cerebri
    t. cinerea
    t. cranii
trabecularism
trabeculate
trabeculation
trachelism
trachelismus
tract
    See also *bundle* and *fasciculus.*
    bulbospinal t.
    Burdach t.
    cerebellorubral t.
    cerebellorubrospinal t.
    cerebellospinal t.
    corticospinal t.
    extrapyramidal t.
    Foville t.
    Goll t.
    Gowers t.
    Helweg t.
    Lissauer t.
    Meynert t.
    neospinothalamic t.
    paleospinothalamic t.
    pyramidal t.
    spinocerebellar t.
    spinothalamic t.
    sympathetic t.

tract (continued)
    tectospinal t.
    Türck t.
traction
    halo t.
    halo-pelvic t.
tractotomy
    descending root t.
    intramedullary t.
    mesencephalic t.
    pyramidal t.
    Sjöqvist t.
    spinothalamic t.
    trigeminal t.
tractus (tractus)
    See *bundle, fasciculus,* and
       tract.
transcortical
transection
    spinal t.
transorbital
    t. leukotomy
    t. lobotomy
transsphenoidal
    t. hypophysectomy
transverse
    t. suture of Krause
trauma (traumas, traumata)
traumasthenia
treatment
    Frenkel t.
    Weir Michell t.
tremor
    action t.
    alternating t.
    benign familial t.
    bread-crumbing t.
    coarse t.
    continuous t.
    effort t.
    epileptoid t.
    essential t.
    familial t.
    fine t.
    flapping t.
    Hunt t.
    intention t.
    intermittent t.

tremor (continued)
    kinetic t.
    t. linguae
    motofacient t.
    motor t.
    muscular t.
    nonintention t.
    parkinsonian t.
    passive t.
    persistent t.
    physiologic t.
    pill-rolling t.
    t. potatorum
    purring t.
    Rendu t.
    rest t.
    resting t.
    senile t.
    static t.
    striocerebellar t.
    titubating t.
    toxic t.
    trombone t. of tongue
    volitional t.
Trendelenburg
    symptom
trephination
trephinement
trichion (trichia)
trifurcation
trigeminal
    t. neuralgia
    t. rhizotomy
    t. tractotomy
trigonal
trigonocephaly
trigonum (trigona)
    t. acustici
    t. cerebrale
    t. collaterale
    t. habenulae
    t. lemnisci
    t. nervi hypoglossi
    t. olfactorium
triplegia
trismus
Trousseau
    phenomenon

Trousseau (continued)
    sign
    spot
    twitching
true suture
truncal
    t. vagotomy
truncate
truncus (trunci)
    t. corporis callosi
    t. lumbosacralis
    t. sympathicus
"tseng-ker" Phonetic for Zenker.
tuber (tubers, tubera)
    t. annulare
    t. anterius hypothalami
    t. cinereum
    t. corporis callosi
    frontal t., t. frontale
    t. vermis
tubercle
    Babès t.
    t. of Rolando
tubercula (plural of tuberculum)
tuberculate, tuberculated
tuberculation
tuberculitis
tuberculization
tuberculoid
tuberculoma
    t. en plaque
tuberculosis (TB)
    cerebral t.
    meningeal t.
    spinal t., t. of spine
tuberculous
    t. meningitis
tuberculum (tubercula)
    t. caroticum
    t. cuneiforme, t. cuneiforme
      (Wrisbergi)
    t. gracile
    t. sellae turcicae
    t. trigeminale
tuberosis
tuberositas (tuberositates)
tuberosity
    frontal t.

tubocurarine
  t. chloride
tubulization
Tuerck. See *Türck*.
Tuffier
  retractor
Tullio phenomenon
tumeur
  t. perlée
tumor
  acoustic nerve t.
  cerebellopontine angle t.
  Cushing t.
  extramedullary t.
  intramedullary t.
  parasagittal t.
  parasellar t.
  paravertebral t.
  Rathke t.
  Rathke pouch t.
  sellar t.
  supratentorial t.
Türck
  bundle
  column
  degeneration
  fasciculus
Turner
  familial syndrome
  male syndrome
  phenotype with normal
    karyotype
  sulcus
  syndrome
  syndrome in females with
    normal X chromosome
Turyn sign
tutamen (tutamina)
  t. cerebri
twitching
  fascicular t.
  fibrillar t.
  Trousseau t.
tympanic
  t. neurectomy
type
  Charcot-Marie t., Charcot-
    Marie-Tooth t.

type (continued)
  Dejerine t.
  Dejerine-Landouzy t.
  Duchenne-Aran t.
  Duchenne-Landouzy t.
  Duchenne-t. muscular dys-
    trophy
  Kretschmer t.'s
  Landouzy t.
  Landouzy-Dejerine t.
  Leyden-Möbius t.
  Wernicke-Mann t.
  Zimmerlin t.
"u–" Phonetic for words beginning
    eu–.
ulegyria
Ullrich
    syndrome
unarousable
uncal
unci (genitive and plural of uncus)
unciform
unciforme ["un-si-for-mee"]
uncinate
uncinatum
unconditioned
unconsciousness
uncus (unci)
    u. corporis vertebrae cervi-
      calis
    u. gyri fornicati
    u. gyri hippocampi
    u. gyri parahippocampalis
underhorn
"ung-kus" Phonetic for uncus.
unguis (ungues)
    u. ventriculi lateralis cerebri
unit
    See also in *General Medical
      Terms* and *Laboratory,
      Pathology, and Chemistry
      Terms*.
    motor u.
    muscle u.
    nerve u.
    neurological intensive care
      u. (NICU)
    slow-motor u.

unresponsive
"unsi–" Phonetic for words begin-
    ning unci–.
Unverricht
    disease
    myoclonia
    syndrome
Unverricht-Lundborg type of epilepsy
UR—unconditioned response
uvula (uvulae)
        u. cerebelli, u. of cerebellum
        u. vermis
uvular
uvularis
VA—vertebral artery
vadum
vagal
vagina (vaginae)
        v. externa nervi optici
        v. interna nervi optici
        vaginae nervi optici
vaginate
vagotomy
        bilateral v.
        hemigastrectomy and v.
            (H&V)
        highly selective v.
        medical v.
        parietal cell v.
        pyloroplasty and v. (P&V)
        selective v.
        surgical v.
        truncal v.
vagotonia
vagus
vallate
vallecula (valleculae)
        v. cerebelli
        v. sylvii
vallecular
Valleix
        points
        sign
Valsalva
        maneuver
valve
        v. of Sylvius
van Bogaert-Bertrand disease

van Bogaert-Divry syndrome
van Bogaert-Nyssen-Peiffer disease
van Bogaert-Scherer-Epstein syn-
    drome
Van Lint
        akinesia
Vanzetti sign
variant
        petit mal v.
variation
varicella
        v.-zoster virus
varix (varices)
        aneurysmal v., aneurysmoid v.
varolian
vascular serotonin 5-HT$_1$ [5-HT1]
    receptor agonists [a class of
    drugs]
vasculopathy
vasoactive
        v. amines
vasoconstrictive
vasoconstrictors [a class of drugs]
vasodilatation
vasoneuropathy
vasovagal
VEE—Venezuelan equine encepha-
    lomyelitis
vegetative
velamenta cerebri
velamentum (velamenta)
        velamenta cerebri
velum (vela)
        medullary v., anterior
        medullary v., cranial
        medullary v., inferior
        medullary v., posterior
        medullary v., rostral
        medullary v., superior
        v. of Tarinus
venereal
Venezuelan equine encephalitis
Venezuelan equine encephalomyeli-
    tis
venography
        extradural v.
        vertebral v.

ventricle
    v. of Arantius
    v.'s of the brain
    cerebral v.
    v. of cerebrum
    v. of cord
    Duncan v.
    fifth v.
    first v. of cerebrum
    fourth v. of cerebrum
    Krause v.
    lateral v. of cerebrum
    v. of myelon
    second v. of cerebrum
    v. of spinal cord
    v. of Sylvius
    terminal v. of spinal cord
    third v. of cerebrum
    Verga v.
    Vieussens v.
ventricornu
ventricornual
ventricose
ventriculi (plural of ventriculus)
ventriculitis
ventriculoatriostomy
ventriculocisternostomy
ventriculogram
ventriculography
    bubble v.
    cerebral v.
    contrast v.
    isotope v.
    radionuclide v.
ventriculomegaly
ventriculometry
ventriculoperitoneal
ventriculoscopy
ventriculostium
ventriculostomy
    third v.
ventriculosubarachnoid
ventriculus (ventriculi)
    v. dexter cerebri
    v. lateralis cerebri
    v. quartus cerebri
    v. sinister cerebri
    v. terminalis medullae spinalis

ventriculus (ventriculi) (continued)
    v. tertius cerebri
ventromedial
VEP—visual evoked potential
VER—visual evoked response
Veraguth fold
Verbiest syndrome
Verga
    ventricle
vermis
    v. cerebelli
Vernet
    paralysis (paralyses)
    syndrome
Verneuil
    neuroma
vertebra (vertebrae)
    See also in *Orthopedics and*
        Sports Medicine section.
    cervical v. (C1–C7)
    vertebrae colli
    cranial v.
    v. dentata
    odontoid v.
    vertebrae spuriae
vertebral
    v. angiography
    v. arteriography
    v. venography
vertebrobasilar
vertex (vertices)
    v. of bony cranium
    v. cranii
    v. cranii ossei
vertiginous
vertigo
    benign paroxysmal position-
        al v.
    benign paroxysmal postural v.
    central v.
    disabling positional v.
    encephalic v.
    epileptic v.
    essential v.
    height v.
    horizontal v.
    hysterical v.
    labyrinthine v.

vertigo (continued)
   neurasthenic v.
   ocular v.
   organic v.
   paralytic v.
   paralyzing v.
   paroxysmal positional v.
   positional v., postural v.
   pressure v.
   primary v.
   residual v.
   rider's v.
   rotary v., rotatory v.
   subjective v.
   toxemic v., toxic v.
   vestibular v.
vestibular
vestibulocerebellar
vestibulocerebellum
vestibulo-ocular reflex
vestibulopathy
vestige
vibration
vibratory
vidian
   v. artery
   v. canal
   v. nerve
Vieussens
   ansa
   ventricle
Villaret syndrome
vinculum (vincula)
   See also *frenulum.*
   vincula lingulae cerebelli
virus
   See also in *Laboratory,
      Pathology, and Chemistry
      Terms.*
   herpes zoster v.
   LCM (lymphocytic chori-
      omeninigitis) v.
   lymphocytic choriomeningi-
      tis v. (LCM)
   poliomyelitis v.
   Powassan v.
   St. Louis encephalitis v.
visuopsychic

"vitselzookt" Phonetic for witzelsucht.
Vogt
   disease
   point
   syndrome
Vogt-Hueter
   point
Voit nucleus
volition
volitional
Volkmann
   paralysis
Volkovitsch sign
von Economo
   disease
   encephalitis
von Haller. See *Haller.*
von Hippel-Lindau
   disease
   syndrome
von Leyden. See *Leyden.*
von Monakow. See *Monakow.*
von Recklinghausen. See *Recklinghausen.*
"vos-tek" Phonetic for *Chvostek.*
V&P—vagotomy and pyloroplasty
Vulpian atrophy
Waardenburg
   disease
   syndrome
Wachenheim-Reder
   sign
Wada
   test
Wallenberg
   syndrome
wallerian
   degeneration
   law
Wallgren aseptic meningitis
Walter bromide test
Wartenberg
   disease
   neuralgia
   phenomenon
   sign
   symptom

wave
  alpha w.
  beta w.
  brain w.
  delta w.'s
  electroencephalographic w.'s
  plateau w.
  random w.
  sharp w.
  slow occipital w.'s
  slow posterior w.'s
  theta w.'s
waveform
Weber
  disease
  paralysis
  sign
  syndrome
WEE—western equine encephalo-
    myelitis
Weill-Reys
  syndrome
Weill-Reys-Adie
  syndrome
Weir Mitchell
  disease
  treatment
Werdnig-Hoffmann
  atrophy
  disease
  paralysis
  syndrome
  type
Wernicke
  aphasia
  area
  campus
  disease
  encephalopathy
  encephalopathy (para-Wer-
    nicke encephalopathy)
  reaction
  sign
  syndrome
Wernicke-Korsakoff
  psychosis
  syndrome

West
  skull
  spasm
  syndrome
western equine encephalitis (WEE)
Westphal
  sign
Westphal-Strümpell
  disease
  pseudosclerosis
white matter disease
Whitnall tubercle
Whytt disease
Wilks
  symptom complex
  syndrome
Willis
  circle (circle of Willis)
Wilson
  degeneration
  disease
  pronator sign
  syndrome
wing
  w.'s of sphenoid bone
  sphenoid w.
Winkelman
  disease
withdrawal
  w. reflex
Wright
  syndrome
xanthochromia
xanthochromic
xanthoma (xanthomas, xanthomata)
  disseminated x., x. dissemi-
    natum
  x. multiplex
Xylocaine with epinephrine [anes-
    thetic agent]
"yoo–" Phonetic for words begin-
    ning eu–.
Zenker
  paralysis
"zheel duh lah too-ret" Phonetic for
    Gilles de la Tourette.
Ziehen-Oppenheim
  disease

Ziemssen motor points
Zimmerlin atrophy
zona (zonae)
    z. reticularis
    z. rolandica
    z. spongiosa
zonal
zonary
zone
    dolorogenic z.
    entry z.
    epileptogenic z., epileptoge-
        nous z.
    z. of exclusion
    Golgi z.
    Kambin triangular working z.
    language z.
    median root z.
    medullary z.
    motor z.
    Rolando z.

zone (continued)
    root z.
    trigger z.
    Wernicke z.
zonesthesia
Zuckerkandl convolution
zygapophyseal
zygion
zygoma
zygomatic
zygomaticofacial
zygomaticofrontal
    z. suture
zygomaticomaxillary
zygomatico-orbital
zygomaticosphenoid
    z. suture
zygomaticotemporal
    z. suture
zygomaxillary

Obstetrics and Gynecology

Ab, ab—abortion
abdominal
    a. gestation
    a. hysterectomy
    a. hysterotomy
    a. myomectomy
    a. ovariotomy
    total a. hysterectomy (TAH)
abdominogenital
abdominohysterectomy
abdominohysterotomy
abdominouterotomy
abdominovaginal
    a. hysterectomy
abdominovesical
Abell
    operation
abembryonic
ablactation
ablatio
    a. placentae
ABO
    compatibility
    incompatibility
abort
aborticide
abortient
abortifacients [a class of drugs]
abortigenic
abortion
    afebrile a.
    ampullar a.
    cervical a.
    complete a.
    contagious a.
    criminal a.
    elective a.
    epizootic a.
    habitual a.
    imminent a.
    incomplete a.

abortion (continued)
    induced a.
    inevitable a.
    infectious a.
    justifiable a.
    late a.
    missed a.
    natural a.
    nontherapeutic a.
    partial a.
    partial birth a.
    saline a.
    septic a.
    spontaneous a.
    therapeutic a.
    threatened a.
    tubal a.
    vibrio a.
abortionist
abortive
abortus
ABR—absolute bed rest
abruptio
    a. placentae
    a. placentae marginalis
abruption
    a. of placenta
abscess
    Bartholin a., bartholinian a.
    breast a.
    broad ligament a.
    canalicular a.
    central mammary a.
    chronic a.
    diverticular a.
    interlobular a.
    interlobular mammary a.
    mammary a.
    milk a.
    parametrial a., parametric a.
    parametritic a.

abscess (continued)
    pelvic a.
    periductal a.
    periductal mammary a.
    premammary a.
    retromammary a.
    subareolar a.
    submammary a.
    tubo-ovarian a.
Aburel
    operation
AC—anterior colporrhaphy
acanthosis
    malignant a. nigricans
    a. nigricans
accommodation
    obstetric a.
accouchement
    a. forcé
accoucheur
accoucheuse
acephalia
acephalic
acephalobrachia
acephalobrachius
acephalocardia
acephalocardius
acephalochiria
acephalochirus
acephalogaster
acephalogastria
acephalopodia
acephalopodius
acephalorhachia
acephalostomia
acephalostomus
acephalothoracia
acephalothorus
acephalous
acephalus
    a. dibrachius
    a. dipus
    a. monobrachius
    a. monopus
    a. paracephalus
    a. sympus
acetrizoate sodium
Achard-Thiers syndrome

acid
    folic a.
acme
    a. of contraction
    a. of disease
ACNM—American College of
    Nurse-Midwives
ACOG—American College of
    Obstetricians and Gynecologists
acrocyanosis
acrohysterosalpingectomy
acromastitis
action
    See *effect* and *phenomenon.*
acuminatum (acuminata, acuminatae)
    condyloma acuminatum,
        condylomata acuminata
    verruca acuminata, verrucae
        acuminatae
Acuson
    transvaginal sonography
acyesis
adenitis
    Bartholin a.
    syphilitic inguinal a.
    vestibular a.
adenocarcinoma
    clear cell a.
    follicular a.
    mammary a.
adenocele
adenofibroma
    a. of ovary
adenofibrosis
adenoleiomyofibroma
adenoma
    adnexal a.
    embryonal a.
    a. endometrioides ovarii
    endometroid a.
    fibroid a.
    a. ovarii testiculare
    trabecular a.
    a. tubulare testiculare ovarii
    tubulovillous a.
adenomatosis
    erosive a. of nipple
adenomyometritis

adenomyositis
adenosalpingitis
adenosis
    blunt duct a.
    mammary sclerosing a.
    sclerosing a. of breast
    a. vaginae, vaginal a.
adhesion
    amniotic a.
    fibrinous a.'s
    fibromembranous a.'s
    filamentous a.'s
    periadnexal a.
    traumatic uterine a.
aditus
    a. ad pelvem
    a. vaginae
adnexa [grammatically plural, no
    singular form]
    a. uteri
adnexal
adnexectomy
adnexitis
adnexogenesis
adnexopexy
adnexorganogenic
adrenocorticoid
ADS—anonymous donor sperm
aerocolpos
aeroperitonia
AF—amniotic fluid
afetal
afibrinogenemia
AFP—alpha-fetoprotein
AFS—American Fertility Society
afterbirth
after-coming head [of infant]
aftercontraction
afterpains
AFV—amniotic fluid volume
AGA—appropriate for gestational
    age
age
      childbearing a.
      coital a.
      fertilization a.
      fetal a.
      gestational a.

age (continued)
    a. of menarche, menarcheal a.
    menstrual a.
    ovulational a.
    postovulatory a.
    reproductive a.
agenesis
    müllerian a.
    ovarian a.
    vaginal a.
agenitalism
AGH—amenorrhea-galactorrhea
    hypothyroidism
agonist
    beta-adrenergic a.
AH—abdominal hysterectomy
A&H—amenorrhea and hirsutism
Ahlfeld sign
Ahumada-del Castillo syndrome
AI—artificial insemination
AID—artificial insemination by
    donor
AIDS—acquired immunodeficiency
    syndrome
AIH—artificial insemination by
    husband
albuginea
    a. ovarii
alcohol
    fetal a. syndrome
Aldridge
    operation
Alexander
    operation
Alexander-Adams
    operation
algomenorrhea
algorithm
allantoamnion
allantochorion
allantoenteric
allantogenesis
allantoic
allantoid
allantoidoangiopagous
allantoidoangiopagus
allantoinuria
allantois

Allen-Masters syndrome
All-Flex diaphragm
allosensitization
alochia
alopecia
>   postpartum a.
alpha
>   a.-fetoprotein (AFP)
Alport
>   syndrome
amastia
amazia
amenia
amenorrhea
>   absolute a.
>   dysponderal a.
>   functional a.
>   hypothalamic a.
>   lactation a.
>   ovarian a.
>   pathologic a.
>   physiologic a.
>   pituitary a.
>   post-pill a.
>   premenopausal a.
>   primary a.
>   relative a.
>   secondary a.
amenorrheal
ametria
aminoglycosides [a class of drugs]
amniocentesis
amniochorial
amniogenesis
amniogram
amniography
amnioma
amnion
>   anterior cul-de-sac a.
>   caudal cul-de-sac a.
>   ectoplacental a.
amnionic
amnionitis
amniorrhea
amniorrhexis
amnioscopy
Amniostat-FLM (fetal lung maturity) test

amniotic
>   a. fluid
amniotomy
ampullary
analgesia
>   obstetric a.
anastomosis (anastomoses)
>   See also *operation* and *procedure.*
>   ureterotubal a.
androgenic
androgenization
androgenized
androgenous
androgens [a class of drugs]
androstenedione
anencephalia
anencephalic
anencephalohemia
anencephalous
anencephaly
anesthesia
>   See in *General Surgical Terms.*
angiokeratoma
>   a. of Fordyce
>   scrotal a., a. of scrotum
>   vulvar a., a. of vulva
angioma
>   spider a.
angiomatoid
angiomatosis
"angkilo–" Phonetic for words beginning ankylo–.
angle
>   costovertebral a.
>   uterine a.
ankylocolpos
ankylosed
ankylotic
anogenital
anomaly
anopelvic
anoperineal
anorexigenic
anorgasmy
anotus
anovaginal

CES—clitoral engorgement syndrome
cesarean
    c. hysterectomy
cesarean section
    cervical c.s.
    classic c.s.
    corporeal c.s.
    extraperitoneal c.s.
    Kerr c.s.
    Krönig c.s.
    Latzko c.s.
    low c.s.
    low-cervical c.s.
    lower segment c.s.
    Munro-Kerr c.s.
    Porro c.s.
    radical c.s.
    transperitoneal c.s.
    transverse c.s.
    Waters c.s.
CG—chorionic gonadotropin
CGT—chorionic gonadotropin
CH—crown-heel (length)
Chadwick sign
chair
    birthing c.
challenge
    oxytocin c. test (OCT)
Champetier de Ribes bag
chandelier sign
chart
    Liley c.
chemical
    c. hysterectomy
Chiari-Frommel
    disease
    syndrome
Chlamydia sepsis
Chlamydiazyme test
chloasma
    c. gravidarum
    c. uterinum
chlorosis
    c. vulvae
chondromalacia
    c. fetalis

chorea
    c. gravidarum
    c. gravis
    Sydenham c.
choreal
chorioadenoma
    c. destruens
chorioamnionic
chorioangiofibroma
chorioangioma
chorioangiopagus parasiticus
chorioblastosis
choriocarcinoma
chorioepithelioma
    c. malignum
chorion
    c. avillosum
    c. frondosum
    c. villosum
chorionic
    c. gonadotropin
    c. villi
    c. villus biopsy (CVB)
chorionic gonadotropin (CG)
    human c.g. (hCG)
chorioplacental
chromohydrotubation
chromosomal
cicatrix (cicatrices)
cin–. See also words beginning
    sin–, syn–.
CIN—cervical intraepithelial neoplasia
circulation
    chorionic c.
    embryonic c.
circumoral
CIS—carcinoma in situ
Clado
    anastomosis
    band
clamp
    Bonney c.
classification
    See also *index.*
    Berman c. of pelves
    Caldwell-Moloy c.

classification (continued)
    FIGO c. of endometrial car-
        cinoma (stages 0–IV)
    Papanicolaou c.
    White c. (classes A–H, R, T)
Claudius fossa
clean-catch urine specimen
cleidotomy
cleidotomy (fetal)
cleidotripsy
climacteric
climacterium
        c. praecox
clitoral
clitoralgia
clitoridauxe
clitoridean
clitoridectomy
clitoriditis
clitoridotomy
clitoris
        bifid c.
        crura of c.
        prepuce of c.
clitorism
clitoritis
clitoritomy
clitoromegaly
clitorotomy
cloaca (cloacae)
        congenital c.
        persistent c.
cloacal
Cloquet node
closure
        Latzko c.
clunis (clunes)
CMB—carbolic methylene blue
CNM—Certified Nurse-Midwife
coagulation
        diffuse intravascular c. (DIC)
coagulopathy
        disseminated intravascular c.
            (DIC)
coccygeal
Coffey
        operation

coitus
        c. à la vache
        c. incompletus
        c. interruptus
        c. reservatus
coleocele
coleocystitis
coleoptosis
coleospastia
coleotomy
Colles fascia
colliculi (plural of colliculus)
colliculitis
colliculus (colliculi)
        c. of Barkow
        cervical c. of female urethra
Collin
        pelvimeter
        test
Collyer
        pelvimeter
colostrum
        c. gravidarum
        c. puerperarum
colovaginal
colpalgia
colpatresia
colpectasia
colpectasis
colpectomy
colpeurysis
colpismus
colpitic
colpitis
        c. emphysematosa
        emphysematous c.
        c. granulosa
        c. mycotica
"colpo" Slang for colposcopy.
colpocele
colpoceliocentesis
colpoceliotomy
colpocleisis
colpocystitis
colpocystocele
colpocystoplasty
colpocystotomy
colpocystoureterocystotomy

colpocystourethropexy
colpocytogram
colpocytology
colpodynia
colpoepisiorrhaphy
colpohyperplasia
colpohysterectomy
colpohysteropexy
colpohysterorrhaphy
colpohysterotomy
colpolaparotomy
colpomicroscopic
colpomicroscopy
colpomycosis
colpomyomectomy
colpomyomotomy
colpoperineoplasty
colpoperineorrhaphy
colpopexy
colpoplasty
colpopoiesis
colpopolypus
colpoptosis
colporectopexy
colporrhagia
colporrhaphy
colporrhexis
colposcopy
colpospasm
colpostat
colpostenosis
colpostenotomy
colpotherm
colpotomy
colpoureterocystotomy
colpoureterotomy
colpoxerosis
columnar
comedomastitis
commissura (commissurae)
    c. labiorum anterior
    c. labiorum posterior
    c. labiorum pudendi
commissural
commissure
    anterior c. of labia
    posterior c. of labia

complete
    See also *total.*
    c. hysterectomy
conception
conceptus
condom
conduplicato
    c. corpore
condyloma (condylomata)
    flat c.
    giant c.
    c. latum, condylomata lata
    pointed c.
    c. subcutaneum
condylomatoid
condylomatosis
condylomatous
condylotomy
cone biopsy
configuration
    arcuate c.
confinement
conglutinatio
    c. orificii externi
conization
    cold knife c.
conjugata
    c. vera obstetrica
conjugate
    diagonal c.
    obstetric c.
contraception
contraceptive
contraction
    Braxton-Hicks c.
    false uterine c.
    premonitory c.
convulsion
    puerperal c.
Coombs
    serum
    test
Cooper
    neuralgia
copious
copulation
cord
    c. blood

cord (continued)
    c. compression
    medullary c.
    ovigerous c.
    umbilical c.
Corner-Allen
    test
cornu (cornua)
    cornua of the uterus
cornual
cornuate
corporis (genitive of corpus)
corpus (corpora)
    c. atretica
    corpora cavernosa
    c. clitoridis
    c. hemorrhagicum
    c. luteum
    corpora uteri
    uterine c.
costovertebral
cotyledon
Couvelaire uterus
COX-2 (cyclooxygenase-2) inhibitors [a class of drugs]
CPD—cephalopelvic disproportion
CPID—chronic pelvic inflammatory disease
CR—crown-rump (length)
crab louse
cranioclasis (fetal)
cranioclast
    Auvard c.
    Braun c.
    Zweifel-DeLee c.
craniotomy (fetal)
CRD—crown-rump distance
Credé method
crista (cristae)
    c. urethralis femininae
    c. urethralis muliebris
cristal
cristate
criterion (criteria)
    Spiegelberg criteria for ovarian pregnancy
CRL—crown-rump length

Crohn
    disease
crown-heel (length of fetus)
crowning
crura (plural of crus)
crural
crus (crura)
    c. clitoridis
    c. of clitoris
    c. glandis clitoridis
cryptomenorrhea
crystalline
CS—cesarean section
C-section—cesarean section
cuboidal
cul-de-sac
    Douglas c.d.s.
culdocentesis
culdoscopy
culdotomy
Cullen sign
cumulus (cumuli)
    c. oophorus
    ovarian c.
    c. ovaricus
cuneihysterectomy
cunnilingus
cup
    Silastic c.
curettage
    fractional c.
    gentle c.
    sharp c.
    suction c.
curettement
Curtis–Fitz-Hugh syndrome
Curtius syndrome
curve
    oxygen dissociation c.
CV—conjugata vera
CVB—chorionic villus biopsy
CVO—conjugate diameter of pelvic inlet (L. conjugata vera obstetrica)
CWP—childbirth without pain
cx—cervix
CxMT—cervical motion tenderness
cyanotic

cycle
    aberrant c.
    anovulatory c.
    endometrial c.
    genesial c.
    gonadotropic c.
    menstrual c.
    myometrial c.
    oogenetic c.
    ovarian c.
    reproductive c.
    sexual c.
cyclooxygenase-2 (COX-2) inhibitors [a class of drugs]
cyema
cyesedema
cyesiognosis
cyesiology
cyesis
cyestein
cyogenic
cyonin
cyophoria
cyophoric
cyotrophy
cyst
    adnexal c.
    atheromatous c.
    Bartholin c.
    blue dome c.
    chocolate c.
    chorionic c.
    corpus luteum c.
    dermoid c.
    embryonal c.
    endometrial c.
    epoophoron c.
    follicular c.
    gartnerian c.
    granulosa lutein c.
    hemorrhagic c.
    hymenal c.
    inclusion c.
    inflammatory c.
    lutein c.
    c. of Morgagni
    morgagnian c.
    Naboth c.

cyst (continued)
    nabothian c.
    oophoritic c.
    ovarian c.
    paroophoritic c.
    parovarian c.
    pedicled c.
    polycystic c.
    retention c.
    Sampson c.
    sebaceous c.
    theca-lutein c.
    tubo-ovarian c.
    vaginal inclusion c.
    wolffian c.
cystadenofibroma
cystadenoma
    mucinous c.
    pseudomucinous c.
    serous c.
cystic
    c. fibrosis
    c. mastitis
cystocele
cystoelytroplasty
cystolutein
cystoma
    myxoid c.
    c. serosum simplex
cystomatitis
cystomatous
cystometrogram
cystorectocele
cystosarcoma
    c. phylloides
cystoscopy
cystoureterocele
cystourethrocele
cystourethrogram
    bead-chain c.
cystourethroscopy
cytogenetic
cytogenic
cytomegalic inclusion disease (CID, CMID)
cytotrophoblast
Danforth
    method

Danforth (continued)
    sign
DAPT—direct agglutination pregnancy test
David
    disease
Davis
    operation
D&C—dilatation and curettage
    dilation and curettage
D&C, diagnostic
D&C, fractional
D&C, suction
D&E—dilatation and evacuation
    dilation and evacuation
debris
    clots and d.
"decels" Slang for decelerations of fetal heart rate.
decidua
    basal d.
    d. basalis
    capsular d.
    d. capsularis
    menstrual d.
    d. menstrualis
    parietal d.
    d. parietalis
    reflex d.
    d. reflexa
    d. serotina
    d. vera
decidual
decidualitis
deciduate
deciduation
deciduitis
deciduoma
deciduomatosis
decipara
Decker
    operation
defervesced
deficiency
    21-hydroxylase enzyme d.
deflection
    vesicouterine d.
defundation

defundectomy
degeneration
    cerebellar d.
DeLee
    pelvimeter
"DeLee'd" Slang for DeLee suction was performed.
DeLee-Hillis
    obstetric stethoscope
delivery
    breech d.
    low-forceps d.
    mid forceps d.
    spontaneous d.
denidation
depression
    postpartum d.
    reactive d.
dermatosis (dermatoses)
    menstrual d.
dermoid
Dermoplast
DES—diethylstilbestrol
DES daughter
descensus
    d. uteri
    uterine d.
desensin
desultory
    d. labor
detachment
    annular d.
detrusor
Deventer
    diameter
    pelvis
device
    Fletcher-Suit afterloading d.
Dewees sign
DEXA—dual energy x-ray absorptiometry [scan]
dextroposition
dextrorotation
Dextrostix
dextroverted
DFU—dead fetus in utero
DHT—dihydrotachysterol

diabetes
    class A d.
    d. mellitus
    pregnancy d., d. of pregnancy
diagnostic
    d. dilatation and curettage
       (D&C)
diameter
    Deventer d.
    Löhlein d.
diaphanography
diaphragm
    All-Flex d.
    Ramses d.
    urogenital d.
    vaginal d.
diastasis
    d. recti abdominis
DIC—diffuse intravascular coagulation
    disseminated intravascular
      coagulation
Diday law
didelphia
didelphic
Dienst test
diethylstilbestrol (DES)
dihysteria
dilatation
    d. and curettage (D&C)
    d. and evacuation (D&E)
dilatation and curettage (D&C)
    diagnostic d. and c.
    fractional d. and c.
    suction d. and c.
dilated
dilation and curettage (D&C)
dimer
    D-d.
diovulatory
diphasia
dis–. See also words beginning dys–.
disease
    See also *syndrome.*
    autoimmune d. (AID)
    Basedow d.
    Behçet d.
    Bowen d.

disease (continued)
    Breisky d.
    Crohn d.
    cytomegalic inclusion d.
      (CID, CMID)
    David d.
    extramammary Paget d.
    fibrocystic d.
    Fox-Fordyce d.
    Frommel d.
    Graves d.
    Halban d.
    Keshan d.
    mammary Paget d.
    Neumann d.
    Niemann-Pick d.
    Paget d.
    Paget d. of the nipple
    pelvic inflammatory d.
    Phocas d.
    Schimmelbusch d.
    Schroeder d.
    Sheehan d.
    Tay-Sachs d.
    Tillaux d.
    Valsuani d.
    von Willebrand d.
disproportion
    cephalopelvic d.
DMPA—depomedroxyprogesterone
   acetate
Döderlein
    bacilli
    operation
Döhle
    inclusion bodies
Doléris
    operation
Donald
    operation
Donald-Fothergill
    operation
Donovan body
"doosh" Phonetic for douche.
doptone
douche
    Betadine d.
    vinegar d.

Douglas
    cul-de-sac
    fold
    line
    method
    pouch
douglascele
douglasitis
dowager's hump
Dow-Corning implant
Down [eponym]
    syndrome
Doyen
    operation
    vaginal hysterectomy
DPG—displacement placentogram
dressing
    See in *General Surgical*
        Terms.
drip
    pitocin d.
DUB—dysfunctional uterine bleeding
Dubowitz
    evaluation
    examination
    infant maturity scale
    Neurological Assessment
    score
duct
    Gartner d.
    mesonephric d.
    müllerian d.
    omphalomesenteric d.
    ovarian d.
    paramesonephric d.
    Reichel cloacal d.
    Skene d.
    vitelline d.
    wolffian d.
ductulus (ductuli)
    ductuli transversi epoophori
ductus (ductus)
    d. arteriosus
    d. epoophori
    d. longitudinalis
    d. venosus
Dudley
    operation

Dührssen
    operation
    tampon
duipara
Duncan mechanism
dye
    indigo carmine d.
dys–. See also words beginning dis–.
dysfunctional
    d. uterine bleeding (DUB)
dysgenesis
    gonadal d.
    mosaic gonadal d.
dyskinesia
    uterine d.
dysmaturity
dysmenorrhea
    d. intermenstrualis
    plethoric d.
    psychogenic d.
dyspareunia
dysponderal
dystocia
dystrophy
    hyperplastic d.
EAb, EAB—elective abortion
easy-pulls
EBL—estimated blood loss
ECC—endocervical curettage
ECE—endocervical ecchymosis
echo time (TE)
ectasia
    mammary duct e.
ectocervix
ectoderm
    dorsal e.
EDC—estimated date of confinement
    expected date of confinement
EDD—expected date of delivery
edema
    gestational e.
effaced
effacement
effect [noun: result, outcome]
    Arias-Stella e.
    estrogen e., estrogenic e.
    Poseiro e.
EGA—estimated gestational age

"eko–" Phonetic for words beginning echo–.
electrocardiography (ECG)
 fetal e.
electrohysterogram
electrohysterography
electrometrogram
elephantiasis
 e. of vulva
ELITT—endometrial laser
 intrauterine thermotherapy
Elliott
 treatment
Ellis-van Creveld syndrome
emansio mensium
embolism
embolus (emboli)
embryectomy
embryoctony
embryogenesis
embryogenetic
embryogenic
embryology
embryonal
embryonate
embryonic
 e. fallopian tube
embryoniform
embryonism
embryonization
embryonoid
embryopathia
 e. rubeolaris
embryopathology
embryotocia
embryotome
embryotomy
emesis
 e. gravidarum
emmenagogic
emmenagogue
emmenia
emmenic
emmeniopathy
emmenology
Emmet
 operation
Emmet-Gellhorn pessary

Emmet-Studdiford
 method
 perineorrhaphy
encephalopathy
 bilirubin e.
endocervical
 e. canal
 e. mucosa
 e. polyp
endocervicitis
endocervix
endocolpitis
endoderm
 ventral e.
endodermal
endolymphatic
endometrectomy
endometria
endometrial
 e. laser intrauterine thermotherapy (ELITT)
endometrioid
endometriosis
 e. externa
 e. interna
 ovarian e.
 e. ovarii
 e. uterina
 e. vesicae
endometriotic
endometritis
 bacteriotoxic e.
 decidual e.
 e. dissecans
 exfoliative e.
 glandular e.
 membranous e.
 postpartum e.
 puerperal e.
 syncytial e.
endometrium
 hyperplastic e.
 secretory e.
 Swiss-cheese e.
endomyoparametritis
endosalpingitis
endosalpingoma
endosalpingosis

endosalpinx
endothelioma
endouterine
engorge
enucleated
EP—ectopic pregnancy
epichorion
epimenorrhagia
epimenorrhea
episioclisia
episioelytrorrhaphy
episioperineoplasty
episioperineorrhaphy
episioplasty
episiorrhaphy
episiostenosis
episiotomy
    central e. and repair (CER)
    Matsner e.
    Matsner median e. and repair
    median e.
    mediolateral e.
epistasis
epistatic
epithelia (plural of epithelium)
epithelialization
epithelialize, epithelialized
epitheliitis
epithelioma
    e. of Malherbe
epithelium (epithelia)
    dysplastic e.
    follicular e.
    e. superficiale ovarii
    surface e.
    visceral e.
epoophorectomy
epoophoron
ER—estrogen receptor
ERA—estrogen receptor assay
eroded
erosion
erythroblastosis
    e. fetalis
    e. neonatorum
erythroplasia
    e. of Queyrat
escutcheon

esophagitis
    reflux e.
Estes
    operation
β-estradiol [now: estradiol 17β (17-beta)]
estradiol
    e.-17α [e.-17-alpha]
    e.-17β [e.-17-beta]
estrogen
    e. effect
estrogens [a class of drugs]
etrohysterectomy
EUA—examination under anesthesia
eumenorrhea
eumetria
eunuchoid
eutocia
evaluation
    Dubowitz e.
EWB—estrogen withdrawal bleeding
examination
    bimanual e.
    Dubowitz e.
    gynecologic e.
    hanging-drop e.
    postpartal e.
    speculum e.
    vaginorectal e.
excavatio (excavationes)
    e. rectouterina
    e. vesicouterina
excavation
    rectouterine e.
    vesicouterine e.
exercise
    Kegel e.'s
exfetation
exometritis
exophytic
expectant
exploratory
    e. laparotomy
expression
    manual e. of placenta
expulsion
extended radical mastectomy
external os

extraction
 breech e.
 vacuum e.
extraembryonic
 e. celom
extrafascial
 e. hysterectomy
extragenital
extramammary Paget disease
extraperitoneal
extrauterine
extravaginal
extremitas (extremitates)
extremity
 tubal e. of ovary
FACOG—Fellow of the American College of Obstetricians and Gynecologists
factor
 rhesus (Rh) f.
failed forceps delivery
Falk
 operation
Falk-Shukuris
 operation
fallopian
 f. arch
 embryonic f. tube
 f. ligament
 f. pregnancy
 f. tube
Falope ring
Family APGAR Questionnaire
"fanenstel" Phonetic for Pfannenstiel.
Farre line
Farris test
fascia (fasciae)
 Camper f.
 cervical f.
 cervical visceral f.
 Colles f.
 deep cervical f.
 endopelvic f.
 f. lata, fasciae latae
 pubovesicocervical f.
 rectovaginal f.
 Scarpa f.
 subvesical f.

fascia (fasciae) (continued)
 f. transversalis
FDP—frontodextra posterior
Fe—iron
FECG—fetal electrocardiogram
FEKG—fetal electrocardiogram
femur length
fenestrate
"fenil–" Phonetic for words beginning phenyl–.
"fenomenon" Phonetic for phenomenon.
Ferguson
 reflex
ferning
fertile
fertility
fertilization
fetal
 f. alcohol syndrome
 f. allograft
 f. asphyxia
 f. breathing
 f. circulation
 f. distress
 f. electrocardiography
 f. head
 f. heart sound
 f. heart tone
 f. hemolysis
 f. hydantoin syndrome
 f. hydrops
 f. monitor
 f. oophoritis
 f. oxygenation
 f. postmaturity syndrome
 f. skull
 f. structure
 f. tachycardia
 f.-to-maternal ratio
 f. warfarin syndrome
 f. weight
 f. well-being
fetal position
 LFA—left frontoanterior
 LFP—left frontoposterior
 LFT—left frontotransverse
 LMA—left mentoanterior

fetal position (continued)
>LMP—left mentoposterior
>LMT—left mentotransverse
>LOA—left occipitoanterior
>LOP—left occipitoposterior
>LOT—left occipitotransverse
>LSA—left sacroanterior
>LScA.—left scapuloanterior
>LScP.—left scapuloposterior
>LSP—left sacroposterior
>LST—left sacrotransverse
>RFA—right frontoanterior
>RFP—right frontoposterior
>RFT—right frontotransverse
>RMA—right mentoanterior
>RMP—right mentoposterior
>RMT—right mentotransverse
>ROA—right occipitoanterior
>ROP—right occipitoposterior
>ROT—right occipitotrans-
>verse
>RSA—right sacroanterior
>RScA.—right scapuloanterior
>RScP.—right scapuloposterior
>RSP—right sacroposterior
>RST—right sacrotransverse

fetation
feticide
feticulture
fetogram
fetography
fetomaternal
fetometry
fetoplacental
α-fetoprotein (AFP) [alpha-]
fetus
>f. acardiacus
>f. amorphus
>calcified f.
>f. compressus
>harlequin f.
>f. in fetu
>macerated f.
>mummified f.
>paper-doll f.
>papyraceous f.
>f. papyraceus
>parasitic f.

fetus (continued)
>f. sanguinolentis
>sireniform f.

Feulgen stain
FHR—fetal heart rate
FHS—fetal heart sound(s)
FHT—fetal heart tone(s)
Fibrindex test
fibroadenoma
fibrocystadenoma
fibrocystic
fibrocystic disease
fibroid
fibroidectomy
fibroleiomyomatosis
fibroma
>calcified f.
>submucous f.

fibromatogenic
fibromatoid
fibromatosis
fibromatous
fibromectomy
fibromembranous
>f. adhesions

fibromyoma
fibromyomata
fibromyomectomy
fibrothecoma
FIGO—Federation of International
Gynecology and Obstetrics
FIGO
>classification of endometrial
>carcinoma
>nomenclature
>staging

filamentous
>f. adhesions

fimbria (fimbriae)
>fimbriae of fallopian tube
>ovarian f.
>f. ovarica
>fimbriae tubae uterinae

fimbrial
fimbriated
fimbriation
fimbriatum
fimbriectomy

fimbriocele
fingerbreadth (fingerbreadths)
fishmouth
    f. laceration
fistula (fistulas, fistulae)
    enterovaginal f.
    rectolabial f.
    rectovaginal f.
    ureterocervical f.
    ureterovaginal f.
    urinary f.
    uterovesical f.
    vaginoperineal f.
    vesicocervical f.
    vesicovaginal f.
    vulvorectal f.
Fitz-Hugh
    syndrome
Fitz-Hugh–Curtis
    syndrome
FLA—left frontoanterior (L. fronto-
    laeva anterior)
"flebitis" Phonetic for phlebitis.
"flebo–" Phonetic for words begin-
    ning phlebo–.
"fleg–" Phonetic for words begin-
    ning phleg–.
Fleming
    operation
Fletcher-Suit afterloading device
FLP—left frontoposterior (L. fron-
    tolaeva posterior)
FLT—left frontotransverse (L. fron-
    tolaeva transversa)
fluffs [fluffy dressing]
fluid
    amniotic f.
    crystalline f.
fluor
    f. albus
FMR—fetal-to-maternal ratio
Foerster. See *Förster.*
fold
    Douglas f.
    Pawlik f.'s
    rectouterine f.
    vesicouterine f.
"folee" Phonetic for Foley.

follicle
    graafian f.
    Naboth f.
    nabothian f.
    ovarian f.
    polyovular ovarian f.
    primordial f.
    secondary f.
folliculoma
    f. lipidique
fontanelle
    See also in *Neurology and
       Pain Management* section.
    anterior f.
forceps
    Bonney f.
    failed f. delivery
forewaters
fornix (fornices)
fossa (fossae)
    Claudius f.
    navicular f.
    f. navicularis
    obturator f.
    ovarian f.
    f. ovarica
    f. of vestibule of vagina
    f. vestibuli vaginae
    f. of Waldeyer
Fothergill
    operation
    suture
Fothergill-Donald
    operation
fourchette
Fox-Fordyce disease
fractional
    f. curettage
    f. dilatation and curettage
       (D&C)
Frangenheim-Goebell-Stoeckel
    operation
Frank
    operation
frena (plural of frenum)
frenal
frenectomy
frenoplasty

frenulum (frenula)
>See also *band* and *frenum.*
>f. of clitoris
>f. labiorum pudendi

frenum (frena)
>See also *band* and *frenulum.*
>f. of labia, labial f.
>f. labiorum

fretum (freta)
>f. halleri

Freund
>law
>operation

Friedman
>test

Friedman-Lapham test
frigid
frigidity
Fritsch
>operation

Fritsch-Asherman syndrome
Frommel
>disease
>operation

Frommel-Chiari
>syndrome

frozen pelvis
FSH—follicle-stimulating hormone
FT—full term
FTLB—full-term live birth
FTND—full-term normal delivery
fulcrum
fulguration
functionalis
fundal
fundectomy
fundus (fundus)
>f. uteri
>f. of uterus
>f. of vagina
>f. vaginae

fungus (fungi)
>See specific fungi in *Laboratory, Pathology, and Chemistry Terms.*

funicular
funiculate

funiculus (funiculi)
>f. umbilicalis

funis
g—gram(s)
G—gravida
GA—gestational age
Gabastou hydraulic method
galactacrasia
galactagogues [a class of drugs]
galactemia
galactic
galactischia
galactocele
galactogenous
galactoma
galactometastasis
galactophlebitis
galactophore
galactophoritis
galactophorous
galactophygous
galactoplania
galactopoiesis
galactopoietic
galactopyra
galactosis
galactostasis
galactotrophy
galacturia
Galli-Mainini test
gamete
gametic
gametocidal
gametocide
gametocyst
ganglion (ganglia, ganglions)
>cervical ganglia of uterus

Gartner duct
gastrocolpotomy
gastrointestinal (GI)
>g. bypass

Gauss sign
GC—gonococcus
Gellhorn
>pessary

geminus (gemini)
>gemini aequales

generation time

genesial
genital
  g. ridge
  g. tract
genitalia [grammatically plural; no
  singular form]
gentle curettage
Genupak tampon
gestation
gestational
  g. age
  g. sac
  g. trophoblastic neoplasia
gestosis
Gigli
  operation
Gilliam
  operation
Gilliam-Doleris
  operation
Giordano
  operation
gland
  adrenal g.
  Bartholin g.
  BUS (Bartholin, urethral,
    and Skene) g.'s
  endometrial g.'s
  Littre g.
  Naboth g., nabothian g.
  Skene g.
  thyroid g.
  urethral g.
  vestibular g.
glandula (glandulae)
glandular
glandule
glandulous [adj.]
glans
  g. clitoridis
  g. of clitoris
glomerular
  g. filtration rate
GM—grand multiparity
Goebel-Stoeckel
  operation
Goffe
  operation

Golden sign
gonad
gonadal
  g. dysgenesis
gonadogenesis
gonadotropic
gonadotropin
  chorionic g.
gonadotropins [a class of drugs]
gonorrhea
Goodall-Power
  operation
Goodell
  law
  sign
Gordan-Overstreet
  syndrome
Gottschalk
  operation
graafian
  g. follicle
  g. ovules
  g. vesicles
grandmother theory
Grant-Ward
  operation
granuloma
  g. inguinale
  pyogenic g.
granulosa
  g. lutein
  g.-theca cell tumor
Graves
  disease
gravid
gravida (0, 1, 2, etc.) [number of
  pregnancies]
gravidarum
gravidic
gravidism
graviditas
  g. examnialis
  g. exochorialis
gravidity
gravidocardiac
gravidopuerperal
Green-Armytage
  operation

grip, grippe
    Pawlik g.
GTN—gestational trophoblastic
    neoplasia
GTT—glucose tolerance test
gyn, GYN—gynecology
gynandrism
gynandroblastoma
gynatresia
gynecogen
gynecography
gynecoid
gynecologic, gynecological
gynecologist
gynecomastia
gynecopathy
gynecotokology
gyneduct
gynogamon
gynomerogon
gynomerogony
gynopathic
gynopathy
gynoplastics
gynoplasty
Haase
    rule
Haemophilus
Halban
    disease
    sign
Halsted
    radical mastectomy
hamartoma
    leiomyomatous h.
Hamilton
    method
hanging
    h.-drop test
Harrison
    method
Haultaim
    operation
HB—hepatitis B
HBV—hepatitis B virus
HBW—high birthweight
hCG—human chorionic gonadotropin
β-hCG [beta hCG]

hCS, hCSM—human chorionic
    somatomammotropin
healing
    h. by first intention
    h. by granulation
    h. by second intention
    h. per primam intentionem
        (L. by first intention)
Heaney
    vaginal hysterectomy
heaves
    dry h.
Hegar
    operation
HELLP syndrome [hemolysis, ele-
    vated liver enzymes, and low
    platelet count occurring in
    association with preeclampsia]
hematocele
    parametric h.
    pudendal h.
    retrouterine h.
    vaginal h.
hematochlorine
hematocolpometra
hematocolpos
hematoma
    puerperal h.
hematome
hematometra
hematosalpinx
hemoglobinopathy
hemolytic
hemophilus
    See in *Laboratory, Patholo-
        gy, and Chemistry Terms.*
hemorrhage
    accidental antepartum h.
hemorrhagic
hepatitis B
hermaphroditism
herpes
    genital h.
    h. genitalis
    h. gestationis
    menstrual h.
    h. menstrualis
    h. progenitalis

Hicks
  contractions
  sign
  version
hidradenitis
  h. axillaris
  h. suppurativa
  suppurative h.
hilum (hila)
  h. ovarii
  h. of ovary
hilus (hili). See *hilum.*
"hipo–" Phonetic for words beginning hypo–.
Hirst
  operation
hirsutism
  idiopathic h.
His [eponym]
  rule
histocompatibility
HIV—human immunodeficiency
  virus
hLH—human luteinizing hormone
HM—hydatidiform mole
hMG—human menopausal gonadotropin
Hodge
  maneuver
Hoehne sign
hood
  Rock-Mulligan h.
hormonal
hormone
  luteinizing h.
  thyrotropin-releasing h.
hormonotherapy
horn
  h. of clitoris
  uterine h.
  h. of uterus
Horrocks maieutic
HPV—human papillomavirus
H&R—hysterectomy and radiation
  [therapy]
HSG—hysterosalpingogram
Huhner test

Hunter
  ligament
Huntington
  operation
Hyams
  operation
hydatid
  h. of Morgagni
hydatidostomy
hydramnios
hydrocele
  h. feminae
  h. muliebris
  Nuck h.
hydrocolpos
hydroparasalpinx
hydrops
  h. fetalis
  h. folliculi
hydrorrhea
  h. gravidarum
hydrosalpinx
  h. follicularis
  intermittent h.
  h. simplex
hydrotubation
hydroureter
hydrovarium
hydroxylase
  11β-h. [11-beta-]
  17α-h. [17-beta-]
  21-h.
hydroxysteroid
  3β-h. [3-beta-]
  17-h.
hymen
  annular h.
  h. bifenestratus
  h. biforis
  circular h.
  cribriform h.
  denticular h.
  falciform h.
  fenestrated h.
  imperforate h.
  infundibuliform h.
  lunar h.
  septate h.

hymen (continued)
   h. septus
   h. subseptus
hymenal
   h. band
   h. ring
hymenectomy
hymenitis
hymenorrhaphy
hymenotome
hymenotomy
hyperandrogenism
hypercyesis
hyperdynamia
   h. uteri
hyperechoic
hyperemesis
   h. gravidarum
hyperemetic
hyperestrogenemia
hyperestrogenism
hyperestrogenosis
hyperflexion
hypergalactia
hypergalactous
hyperinvolution
hyperlactation
hyperluteinization
hypermastia
hypermenorrhea
hyperovaria
hyperovarianism
hyperovarism
hyperphenylalaninemia
   maternal h.
hyperpituitarism
hyperplasia
   adenomatous h.
   adrenal h.
   cystic-glandular h. of
      endometrium
   cystic h. of breasts
   endometrial h., h. endometrii
   hilus cell h.
   ovarian stromal h.
   postmenopausal h.
   proliferative h.
   stromal h.

hyperplastic
   h. endometrium
hyperprogesteronemia
hyperprolactinemic
hyperprolactinism
hyperstimulation
hyperthecosis
   testoid h.
hyperthelia
hypoechoic
hypoestrogenemism
hypofertile
hypofertility
hypofunction
hypogalactia
hypogalactous
hypohormonal
hypomastia
hypomenorrhea
hypo-ovaria
hypo-ovarianism
hypopituitarism
   postpartum hemorrhagic h.
hypoplasia
hypospadias
   female h.
hypotonia
hypotonic
hypotony
hypovaria
hypovarianism
hysteralgia
hysteratresia
hysterectomy
   abdominal h.
   abdominovaginal h.
   Bonney h.
   cesarean h.
   chemical h.
   complete h.
   Doyen vaginal h.
   extrafascial h.
   Heaney vaginal h.
   intrafascial h.
   Lash h.
   Latzko radical h.
   Mayo-Ward vaginal h.
   paravaginal h.

hysterectomy (continued)
    partial h.
    Porro h.
    radical h.
    Ries-Wertheim h.
    Schauta-Amreich vaginal h.
    Schauta radical vaginal h.
    Spalding-Richardson h.
    subtotal h.
    supracervical h.
    supravaginal h.
    total h.
    total abdominal h. (TAH)
    total vaginal h. (TVH)
    vaginal h. (VH)
    Ward-Mayo vaginal h.
    Wertheim radical h.
hystereeuryntcr
hystereurysis
hysterobubonocelc
hysterocarcinoma
hysterocele
hysterocervicotomy
hysterocleisis
hysterocolpectomy
hysterocystic
hysterocystocleisis
hysterocystopexy
hysterodynia
hysteroedema
hysterogram
hysterograph
hysterography
hysterolith
hysterolysis
hysterometer
hysterometry
hysteromyoma
hysteromyomectomy
hysteromyotomy
hystero-oophorectomy
hystero-ovariotomy
hysteropathy
hysteropexy
hysteroplasty
hysteroptosia
hysteroptosis
hysterorrhaphy

hysterorrhexis
hysterosalpingectomy
hysterosalpingogram
hysterosalpingography
hysterosalpingo-oophorectomy
hysterosalpingostomy
hysterosalpinx
hysteroscopic
hysteroscopy
    laparoscopic-assisted vagi-
      nal h. (LAVH)
hysterospasm
hysterostomatomy
hysterothermometry
hysterotomy
    abdominal h.
    vaginal h.
hysterotrachelectasia
hysterotrachelectomy
hysterotracheloplasty
hysterotrachelorrhaphy
hysterotrachelotomy
hysterotubography
hysterovaginoenterocele
IAS—intra-amniotic saline
IAS infusion
ICD—intrauterine contraceptive
    device
ichthyosis
    i. intrauterina
    i. uteri
idiometritis
IH—idiopathic hyperprolactinemia
"ikthe–" Phonetic for words begin-
    ning ichthy–.
ILB, ILBW—infant of low birth-
    weight
imaging
    See in *Radiology, Nuclear*
      Medicine, and Other
      Imaging section.
IMB—intermenstrual bleeding
IMC—irregular menstrual cycle
IM cocktail—intramuscular cocktail
Imlach
    fat pad
    fat plug
    ring

implant
  Dow-Corning i.
implantation
incision
  Bar i.
  Munro Kerr i.
  smile i., smiling i.
  Willy Meyer i.
incompatibility
incontinence
  overflow i.
  stress i.
  urge i.
  urinary i.
incontinent
incoordination
  first-degree uterine i.
  second-degree uterine i.
index (indexes, indices)
  See also *classification.*
  Broders i. (1–4)
  Mengert i.
indigo carmine dye
indirect
  i. placentography
induction
inertia
  primary uterine i.
  secondary uterine i.
  uterine i.
infection
  ascending i.
  perinatal i.
  puerperal i.
  toxoplasmosis, other agents,
    rubella, cytomegalovirus,
    herpes simplex (TORCH) i.
  transcervical i.
  transplacental i.
Infectious Disease Society for
  Obstetrics and Gynecology
infertilitas
  i. feminis
inframamillary
infundibula (plural of infundibulum)
infundibuliform
infundibulopelvic

infundibulum (infundibula)
  i. of fallopian tube
  i. tubae uterinae
  i. of uterine tube
inhibitor
  COX-2 (cyclooxygenase-2)
    i.'s [a class of drugs]
inlet
  pelvic i.
inoperable
insemination
  artificial i. donor
  heterologous i.
  homologous i.
insufficiency
  uteroplacental i.
insufflation
  methylene blue i.
  tubal i.
intercalary
intercourse
intermenstrual
intermural
internal os
interphase
interposition
  i. operation
intersexual
intracavitary
intracervical
intracranial
intrafascial
  i. hysterectomy
intrafetation
intraligamentous
intranatal
intraovarian
intrapartum
intraplacental
intratubal
intrauterine
  endometrial laser i. ther-
    motherapy (ELITT)
  i. fetal death
  i. growth retardation
intrauterine device (IUD)
  Mirena
  Progestasert

intravaginal
introitus
  marital i.
  parous i.
  i. vaginae
inversion
  forced i.
  spontaneous i.
  i. of uterus
involution
involutional
IO—internal os
IPPI—interruption of pregnancy for psychiatric indication
irritability
  uterine i.
Irving
  operation
Isaac differential distortion divergent method
ischiopubic
ischiopubiotomy
ischiovaginal
island
  Wolff i.
"is-mus" Phonetic for isthmus.
isoimmunization
  rhesus i.
isthmectomy
isthmi (plural of isthmus)
isthmic
isthmica nodosa
isthmic-cornual
isthmus (isthmi)
  i. of fallopian tube
  i. tubae uterinae
  tubal i.
  i. uteri
  i. of uterus
IU—intrauterine
IUCD—intrauterine contraceptive device
IUD—intrauterine death
  intrauterine device
IUGR—intrauterine growth rate
  intrauterine growth retardation
IUT—intrauterine transfusion

IV—intravenous
Jacquemier sign
Jarcho
  pressometer
Jarjavay
  ligaments
  muscle
Jobst
  stockings
Johanson-Blizzard syndrome
joint
  See in *Orthopedics and Sports Medicine* section.
Jones
  operation
Jungbluth
  vasa propria (vasa propria of Jungbluth)
  vessels
Kanter sign
Kapeller-Adler test
Kegel exercises
Kelly
  operation
  sign
Kennedy
  operation
keratinized
keratoderma
  k. climactericum
Kergaradec sign
Kerr
  cesarean section
Keshan disease
kg—kilogram(s)
Kleihauer-Betke test
Kline flocculation test
"kloasma" Phonetic for cloasma.
Klotz syndrome
Kluge method
kocherization
kocherized
Kocks
  operation for uterine prolapse
"koleo–" Phonetic for words beginning coleo–.
"kolp–, kolpo–" Phonetic for words beginning colp–, colpo–.

"kondilo–" Phonetic for words beginning condylo–.
"kor–" Phonetic for words beginning cor– and chor–.
"kotiledon" Phonetic for cotyledon.
kraurosis
    k. vulva
Krause
    ligament
Kristeller method
Kroener
    operation
Krönig
    cesarean section
    technique
Krukenberg tumor
"krus" Phonetic for crus.
"kryo–" Phonetic for words beginning cryo–.
Kuhne
    methylene blue
"kuldo–" Phonetic for words beginning culdo–.
Kupperman test
Küstner
    law
    operation
    sign
kyphosis
    dorsal k.
kyphotic
labia (plural of labium)
labial
labium (labia)
    See also *margin.*
    labia majora (plural of l. majus)
    l. majus pudendi (labia majora pudendi)
    labia minora (plural of l. minus)
    l. minus pudendi (labia minora pudendi)
    l. posterius ostii uteri
labor
    active l.
    arrested l.
    artificial l.

labor (continued)
    atonic l.
    complicated l.
    delayed l.
    desultory l.
    dry l.
    dyskinetic l.
    false l.
    habitual l.
    habitual premature l.
    immature l.
    induced l.
    instrumental l.
    mimetic l.
    missed l.
    multiple l.
    obstructed l.
    postmature l.
    postponed l.
    precipitate l.
    premature l.
    prodromal l.
    prolonged l.
    protracted l.
    spontaneous l.
    spurious l.
    stages of l.
    trial of l.
laboratory
    clinical l.
Laborde
    method
    sign
    test
laborious
    l. detail
    l. workup
lac (lacta)
    l. femininum
laceration
    first-degree obstetric l.
    fishmouth l.
    fourth-degree obstetric l.
    perianal l.
    second-degree obstetric l.
    third-degree obstetric l.
lactation
lactational

lacteal
lactiferous
lactifuge
lactigenous
lactigerous
lactogen
      human placental l. (hPL)
lactogenesis
lactogenic
lactogenic hormone
lactosuria
lacuna (lacunae)
      intervillous l.
lacunar
lacunula (lacunulae)
lacunule
Ladin sign
Laminaria tent
Landou sign
Langhan
    cell
    stria
LAO—left anterior oblique [projection]
laparocolpohysterotomy
laparocystotomy
laparohysterectomy
laparohystero-oophorectomy
laparohysterosalpingo-oophorectomy
laparohysterotomy
laparomonodidymus
laparomyomectomy
laparosalpingectomy
laparosalpingo-oophorectomy
laparosalpingotomy
laparoscopic
    l.-assisted vaginal hysteroscopy (LAVH)
laparoscopy
laparotomy
    exploratory l.
    second-look l.
    staging l.
laparouterotomy
laser
    endometrial l. intrauterine thermotherapy (ELITT)

Lash
    hysterectomy
    operation
    technique
latent
    l. phase
    l.-phase endometrium
    l. phase of labor
lateroversion
Latzko
    cesarean section
    closure
    operation
    radical hysterectomy
Launois-Cléret
    syndrome
law
    See also *rule*.
    Diday l.
    Freund l.
    Goodell l.
    Küstner l.
    Leopold l.
    Levret l.
    Pajot l.
layer
    See also *band, line, streak,* and *stria*.
    muscular l. of fallopian tube
    Nitabuch l.
LB—live birth(s)
LBWI—low-birthweight infant
LC—living children
LDA—left dorsoanterior [position]
Le Fort
    operation
Le Fort-Neugebauer
    operation
leiomyoma (leiomyomas, leiomyomata)
    l. uteri
leiomyomatosis
leiomyomatous
Leopold
    law
    maneuver
    operation
Lerous method

lesion
    precancerous l.
leukokraurosis
leukophlegmasia
leukoplakia
    l. vulvae
leukorrhagia
leukorrhea
    menstrual l.
    periodic l.
leukorrheal
levator (levatores)
    l. ani
level
    pregnanediol l.
Levret
    law
Leydig cell
LFA—left frontoanterior [position]
LFP—left frontoposterior [position]
LFT—left frontotransverse [position]
LH—luteinizing hormone
LHRF—luteinizing
    hormone–releasing factor
LHRH—luteinizing
    hormone–releasing hormone
libidinal
libido (libidines)
lice (plural of louse)
lichen
    l. sclerosis
ligament
    anterior l.
    broad l.
    cardinal l.
    fallopian l.
    Hunter l.
    infundibulopelvic l.
    Jarjavay l.
    keystone l.
    lacunar l.
    lateral l.
    Mackenrodt l.
    ovarian l.
    posterior l.
    pubic l. of Cowper
    pubocervical l.
    rectouterine l.

ligament (continued)
    round l.
    sacrogenital l.
    sacrouterine l.
    suspensory l.
    uterosacral l.
    vesicouterine l.
ligamentum (ligamenta)
ligation
    tubal l.
Liley chart
line
    See also *band, layer, streak,*
    and *stria.*
    Douglas l.
    Farre white l.
linea (lineae)
    l. alba
    l. nigra
"lio–" Phonetic for words beginning
    leio–.
Lipschütz
    disease
    ulcer
liquor (liquors, liquores)
    l. amnii
    l. chorii
    l. folliculi
lithopedion
Littre glands
littritis
Litzmann obliquity
LMA—left mentoanterior [position]
LMP—last menstrual period
    left mentoposterior [position]
LMT—left mentotransverse [posi-
    tion]
LNMP—last normal menstrual peri-
    od
LOA—left occipitoanterior [position]
lobi (plural of lobus)
lobulation
    fetal l.
lobus (lobi)
lochia
    l. alba
    l. cruenta
    l. purulenta

lochia (continued)
 l. rubra
 l. sanguinolenta
lochial
lochiocolpos
lochiocyte
lochiometra
lochiometritis
lochiopyra
lochiorrhagia
lochiorrhea
lochioschesis
lochiostasis
lochometritis
lochoperitonitis
Löhlein diameter
LOP—left occipitoposterior [position]
LOT—left occipitotransverse [position]
louse (lice)
 crab l.
 pubic l.
Lovset maneuver
LOWBI—low-birthweight infant
low-cervical
 l.-c. cesarean section
LPO—left posterior oblique [projection]
L/S—lecithin-sphingomyelin [ratio]
LSA—left sacroanterior [position]
LScA—left scapuloanterior [position]
LScP—left scapuloposterior [position]
LSCS—lower segment cesarean section
LSP—left sacroposterior [position]
LST—left sacrotransverse [position]
Lugol stain
lumen (lumina)
 uterine l.
 vaginal l.
lumpectomy
luteal
luteectomy
luteinic
luteinization
luteinizing hormone (LH)

luteoid
luteoma
luteum
lying-in
lymphatic
lymphogranuloma
 l. benignum
 Schaumann benign l.
 venereal l.
 l. venereum
"lyo–" Phonetic for words beginning leio–.
lyra
 l. uteri
 l. uterina
 l. vaginae
lyre
 l. of uterus
 l. of vagina
maceration
Mackenrodt
 ligament
 operation
macroclitoris
macrogenitosomia
macroscopic
macrosomia
macula (maculae)
 m. folliculi
 m. gonorrhoeica
 Saenger m.
macular
macule
Madlener
 operation
maieutic
 Horrocks m.
main ["mah"]
 m. d'accoucheur ["dah koo-shoor"]
Malherbe
 epithelioma (epithelioma of Malherbe)
malposition
malpresentation
mamma (mammae)
 m. accessoria
 accessory mammae

mamma (mammae) (continued)
  m. areolata
  m. masculina
  supernumerary mammae
  m. virilis
mammary
mammary Paget disease
mammiform
mammilla (mammillae)
mammillary
mammogram
mammography
mammoplasia
mammose
Manchester
  operation
  ovoid
maneuver
  See also *method* and *technique.*
  Bracht m.
  Brandt-Andrews m.
  DeLee m.
  Hodge m.
  Leopold m.
  Lovset m.
  Massini m.
  Mauriceau m.
  Mauriceau-Smellie m.
  Mauriceau-Smellie-Veit m.
  McDonald m.
  Müller-Hillis m.
  Munro-Kerr m.
  Phaneuf m.
  Pinard m.
  Prague m.
  Ritgen m.
  Saxtorph m.
  Scanzoni m.
  Schatz m.
  Smellie-Veit m.
  van Horne m.
  Wigand m.
mania
  puerperal m.
Marañon
  syndrome (I, II, III)
Marchetti test

Marckwald
  operation
margin
  See also *labium.*
  cervical m.
  free m. of ovary
  mesovarial m. of ovary
margo (margines)
Marshall-Marchetti
  operation
  test
Marshall-Marchetti-Birch
  operation
Marshall-Marchetti-Krantz (MMK)
  operation
Marshall and Tanner pubertal staging
marsupial
Martin
  operation
Martius
  operation
masculinization
masculinize
masculinizing
masculinovoblastoma
Massini maneuver
mastadenitis
mastectomy
  Auchincloss modified radical m.
  extended radical m.
  Halsted radical m.
  Meyer m.
  modified m.
  modified radical m.
  partial m.
  radical m. (RM)
  segmental m.
  simple m. (SM)
  subcutaneous m.
  total m.
  Willy Meyer radical m.
masthelcosis
mastitis
  chronic cystic m.
  cystic m.
  gargantuan m.
  glandular m.

mastitis (continued)
>   interstitial m.
>   parenchymatous m.
>   periductal m.
>   phlegmonous m.
>   plasma cell m.
>   puerperal m.
>   retromammary m.
>   stagnation m.
>   submammary m.
>   suppurative m.

mastodynia
mastomenia
mastopathia
>   m. cystica

mastopathy
>   cystic m.

mastoptosis
mastorrhagia
mastoscirrhus
matrix (matrices)
>   intercellular m.

Matsner
>   episiotomy
>   median episiotomy and repair

maturation
>   ovarian follicular m.

mature, matured
Mauriceau maneuver
Mauriceau-Smellie maneuver
Mauriceau-Smellie-Veit maneuver
Mayer-Rokitansky-Kustner syndrome
Mayor sign
Mayo-Ward
>   vaginal hysterectomy

Mazlin spring IUD
MB—methylene blue
MBAS—methylene blue active sub-
>   stance

MBD—methylene blue dye
McCall
>   operation

McCall-Schuman
>   operation

McCune-Albright syndrome
McDonald
>   maneuver
>   operation

McDowell operation
McIndoe
>   operation

MDA—right mentoanterior (L. men-
>   todextra anterior) [position]

MDP—right mentoposterior (L. men-
>   todextra posterior) [position]

MDT—right mentotransverse (L.
>   mentodextra transversa) [posi-
>   tion]

meatal
meati [incorrect word for plural of
>   meatus]

meatus (meatus)
>   fish-mouth m.
>   m. of urethra
>   m. urinarius
>   urinary m.

mechanism
>   Duncan m.
>   m. of labor
>   Schultze m.
>   suspensory m.

median
>   m. episiotomy

medicine
>   fetal-maternal m.
>   neonatal m.
>   perinatal m.

mediolateral
>   m. episiotomy

medulla (medullae)
>   m. ovarii
>   m. of ovary

medullated
medullation
megaloclitoris
megavoltage
Meigs-Cass syndrome
melasma
>   m. gravidarum

membranate
membrane
>   birth m.'s
>   endoneural m.
>   hymenal m.
>   mucous m.
>   virginal

membrum (membra)
    m. muliebre
menalgia
menarchal
menarche
    delayed m.
menarcheal
menarchial
Mendelson
    syndrome
Menge
    operation
Mengert index
menhidrosis
meningocele
menolipsis
menometrorrhagia
menopausal
menopause
menophania
menoplania
menorrhagia
menorrhalgia
menorrhea
menorrheal
menoschesis
menosepsis
menostasis
menostaxis
menotoxic
menotoxin
menoxenia
menses
menstrual
menstruant
menstruate
menstruation
    anovular m.
    anovulatory m.
    nonovulational m.
    ovulatory m.
    regurgitant m.
    retrograde m.
    scanty m.
    supplementary m.
    suppressed m.
    vicarious m.
menstruous

menstruum
mesenchyma
mesenchymal
mesoderm
mesometritis
mesometrium
mesonephric
mesonephroi (plural of mesonephros)
mesonephroma
mesonephros (mesonephroi)
    caudal m.
    cranial m.
    genital m.
mesosalpinx
mesothelial
mesovarium
metacyesis
metaplasia
    squamous m.
metastasis (metastases)
method
    See also *maneuver* and *technique.*
    Beuttner m.
    Bonnaire m.
    Credé m. of expressing placenta
    Danforth m.
    Douglas m.
    Emmet-Studdiford m.
    Gabastou hydraulic m.
    Hamilton m.
    Harrison m.
    Isaac differential distortion divergent m.
    Kluge m.
    Kristeller m.
    Lerous m.
    Mauriceau-Smellie-Veit m.
    Pajot m.
    Pomeroy m.
    Puzo m.
    rhythm m.
    Schultze m.
    Schuman m.
    Smellie m.
    Smellie-Veit m.
    Watson m.

methylene blue insufflation
metra
metralgia
metratonia
metratrophia
metrechoscopy
metrectasia
metrectomy
metrectopia
metreurynter
metreurysis
metria
metritis
    m. dissecans
    dissecting m.
    puerperal m.
metrocampsis
metrocarcinoma
metrocele
metrocolpocele
metrocystosis
metrocyte
metrodynia
metroendometritis
metrofibroma
metrogenous
metrogonorrhea
metrography
metroleukorrhea
metromalacia
metromalacoma
metromenorrhagia
metroparalysis
metropathia
    m. haemorrhagica
metropathic
metropathy
metroperitoneal
metroperitonitis
metrophlebitis
metroplasty
metroptosis
metrorrhagia
    m. myopathica
metrorrhea
metrorrhexis
metrosalpingitis
metrosalpingogram

metrosalpingography
metrostaxis
metrostenosis
metrotome
metrotomy
metrotoxin
metrotubography
Meyer
    mastectomy
MFD—midforceps delivery
microinvasive
micromastia
microsomia
    m. fetalis
microtransducer
microvillus (microvilli)
    placental m.
"middle-shmertz" Phonetic for mit-
    telschmerz.
midsegment
migration
    external m.
    internal m.
    m. of ovum
    transperitoneal m.
Miller
    operation
Millin-Read
    operation
minilaparotomy
"mio–" Phonetic for words begin-
    ning myo–.
Mirena (IUD)
mittelschmerz [pain with ovulation]
MLA—left mentoanterior (L. men-
    tolaeva anterior) [position]
MLP—left mentoposterior (L. men-
    tolaeva posterior) [position]
MLT—left mentotransverse (L. men-
    tolaeva transverse) [position]
MM—Marshall-Marchetti
MM operation
MMK—Marshall-Marchetti-Krantz
    [operation]
modified
    m. mastectomy
    m. radical mastectomy

mole
    Breu m.
    hydatidiform m.
molimen (molimina)
    menstrual m.
molluscum
    m. contagiosum
monitor
    ICP (intracranial pressure) m.
monitoring
    fetal m.
monoamniotic
monochorionic
monocyclic
monocyesis
monospermy
monovular
monovulatory
monozygosity
monozygotic
    m. twins
mons
    m. pubis
    m. ureteris
    m. veneris
monstrum (monstra)
    m. abundans
    m. deficiens
    m. per defectum
    m. per excessum
    m. per fabricam alienam
    m. sirenoforme
Montgomery strap
morcellement
    m. operation
Morel
    syndrome
Morel-Wildi syndrome
Morgagni
    cyst of M.
    hydatid
morgagnian
    m. cyst
Morris syndrome
"mor-sel-maw" Phonetic for mor-
    cellement.
morula

motility
    altered sperm m.
MP—menstrual period
    multiparous
MPA—medroxyprogesterone acetate
MT—malignant teratoma
MTI—malignant teratoma, interme-
    diate
MTT—malignant teratoma, tro-
    phoblastic
MTX—methotrexate
mucocolpos
mucosa
    endocervical m.
mucosal
mucosanguineous
mucoserous
mucous [adj.]
    m. plug
mucus [noun]
Müller
    operation
    tubercle
Müller-Hillis
    maneuver
müllerian
    m. agenesis
    m. duct
    m. mixed tumor
    m. tubercle
müllerianoma
müllerianosis
mülleriosis
multigravida
multiloculated
"multip" Slang for multiparous.
multipara
multiparity
multiparous
multiphasic
mummification
Munnell
    operation
Munro Kerr
    cesarean section
    incision
    maneuver

muscle
    See also in *Orthopedics and*
       Sports Medicine section.
    Braune m.
    bulbocavernous m.
    external oblique m.
    iliopsoas m.
    interfoveolar m.
    internal oblique m.
    ischiocavernous m.
    Jarjavay m.
    levator ani m.
    oblique m. of abdomen
      (external, internal)
    obturator m. (external, inter-
      nal)
    organic m.
    m.'s of pelvic diaphragm
    perineal m.'s, m.'s of per-
      ineum
    pubicoperitoneal m.
    pubococcygeal m.
    puborectal m.
    pubovaginal m.
    pubovesical m.
    pyramidal m.
    rectouterine m.
    rectus m.
    Ruysch m.
    transverse m. of abdomen
    transverse perineal m. (deep,
      superficial)
    transverse m. of perineum
      (deep, superficial)
    visceral m.
musculus (musculi)
    See also *muscle.*
    See also in *Orthopedics and*
      Sports Medicine section.
    m. pubococcygeus
    m. rectus abdominis
    m. transversus abdominis
mycoplasmal
myelocele
myocolpitis
myoma (myomas, myomata)
    m. previum
    m. uteri, uterine m.

myomagenesis
myomata (plural of myoma)
myomatectomy
myomatosis
myomatous
myomectomy
    abdominal m.
    vaginal m.
myometrial
myometritis
myometrium
myomohysterectomy
myomotomy
myosalpingitis
myosalpinx
myosarcoma
MZ—monozygotic
Naboth
    cysts
    follicles
    glands
    ovules
    vesicles
nabothian
Nägele
    obliquity
    pelvis
    rule
natis (nates)
    See *breech.*
nausea
    n. gravidarum
nauseated
nauseous
navel
    blue n.
navicular
NB—newborn
NBW—normal birthweight
ND—neonatal death
    normal delivery
necrosis (necroses)
    peripheral n.
    postpartum pituitary n.
necrospermia
necrospermic
necrotic
necrozoospermia

neogala

neonate

neonatologist

neonatology

neoplasia

    gestational trophoblastic n.

    intraepithelial n.

    multiple endocrine n. (MEN)

neoplasm

    adrenal n.

    stromal cell n.

    trophoblastic n.

    vascular n.

neoplastic

neosalpingostomy

neovagina

nerve

    cavernous n.'s of clitoris

    dorsal n. of clitoris

    ilioinguinal n.

    pudendal n.

    uterine n.'s

    vaginal n.'s

net

    See *plexus* and *rete.*

network

    See *plexus* and *rete.*

"neu–" Phonetic for words beginning pneu–.

Neumann

    disease

neuralgia

    pudendal plexus n.

neuralgic

neurectomy

    presacral n.

neuritic

neuritis

    fallopian n.

    n. puerperalis traumatica

neuropeptide

nevus (nevi)

    See in *Dermatology* section.

"new–" Phonetic for words beginning pneu–.

newborn

NFTD—normal full-term delivery

NHC—neonatal hypocalcemia

Nickerson medium smear

NICU—neonatal intensive care unit

Nitabuch layer

NMP—normal menstrual period

NND—neonatal death

node

    Cloquet n., n. of Cloquet

    iliac n.

    obturator n.

    para-aortic lymph n.

nodule

    discrete n.

noma

    n. pudendi

    n. vulvae

nonviable

    n. fetus

"noo–" Phonetic for words beginning pneu–.

norethindrone test

norethynodrel test

NR—nonreactive

NSD—normal spontaneous delivery

NST—nonstress test

NSVD—normal spontaneous vaginal delivery

"nu–" Phonetic for words beginning pneu–.

Nuck

    canal, canal of N.

    diverticulum

    hydrocele, hydrocele of N.

nulligravida

nullipara

nulliparity

nulliparous

"nur–" Phonetic for words beginning neur–.

nympha (nymphae)

    n. of Krause

nymphectomy

nymphitis

nymphocaruncular

nymphohymeneal

nymphoncus

nymphotomy

OA—occiput anterior

OB—obstetrics

OBG, OB-GYN—obstetrics and
gynecology·
obliquity
Litzmann o.
Nägele o.
Roederer o.
obstetrician
obstetrics
OC—oral contraceptive
OCA—oral contraceptive agent
occipitoanterior
occipitoposterior
occlusion
fimbrial o.
isthmic cornual o.
midsegment o.
tubal o.
OCT—oxytocin challenge test
octigravida
octipara
ODA—right occipitoanterior (L.
occipitodextra anterior) [posi-
tion]
ODP—right occipitoposterior (L.
occipitodextra posterior) [posi-
tion]
ODT—right occipitotransverse (L.
occipitodextra transversa)
[position]
OG, O&G—obstetrics and gynecology
OLA—left occipitoanterior (L.
occipitolaeva anterior) [position]
oligoamnios
oligogalactia
oligohydramnios
oligohypermenorrhea
oligohypomenorrhea
oligo-ovulation
oligospermatic
oligospermatism
oligozoospermatism
oligozoospermia
OLP—left occipitoposterior (L.
occipitolaeva posterior) [posi-
tion]
Olshausen
operation

Olshausen (continued)
sign
OLT—left occipitotransverse (L.
occipitolaeva transversa) [posi-
tion]
Ombrédanne
operation
oocyesis
oocyte
oocytin
oogenesis
oogenetic
oogonia
oophoralgia
oophorectomize
oophorectomy
oophoritis
oophorocystectomy
oophorocystosis
oophorogenous
oophorohysterectomy
oophoroma
oophoron
oophoropathy
oophoropeliopexy
oophoropexy
oophoroplasty
oophororrhaphy
oophorosalpingectomy
oophorosalpingitis
oophorostomy
oophorotomy
oophorrhagia
operation
See also in *General Surgical
Terms.*
Abell o.
Aburel o.
Aldridge o.
Alexander o.
Alexander-Adams o.
Baldwin o.
Ball o.
Basset o.
Baudelocque o.
Beatson o.
Bissell o.
Bouilly o.

operation (continued)

Bozeman o.
Bricker o.
Brunschwig o.
Burch o.
Coffey o.
Davis o.
Decker o.
Döderlein o.
Doléris o.
Donald o.
Donald-Fothergill o.
Doyen o.
Dudley o.
Dührssen o.
Emmet o.
Estes o.
Falk o.
Falk-Shukuris o.
Fleming o.
Fothergill o.
Fothergill-Donald o.
Frangenheim-Goebell-
Stoeckel o.
Frank o.
Freund o.
Fritsch o.
Frommel o.
Gigli o.
Gilliam o.
Gilliam-Doleris o.
Giordano o.
Goebel-Stoeckel o.
Goffe o.
Goodall-Power o.
Gottschalk o.
Grant-Ward o.
Green-Armytage o.
Haultaim o.
Hegar o.
Hirst o.
Huntington o.
Hyams o.
interposition o.
Irving o.
Jones o.
Kelly o.
Kennedy o.

operation (continued)

Kocks o. for uterine prolapse
Kroener o.
Küstner o.
Lash o.
Latzko o.
Le Fort o.
Le Fort-Neugebauer o.
Leopold o.
Mackenrodt o.
Madlener o.
Manchester o.
Marckwald o.
Marshall-Marchetti o.
Marshall-Marchetti-Birch o.
Marshall-Marchetti-Krantz
(MMK) o.
Martin o.
Martius o.
McCall o.
McCall-Schuman o.
McDonald o.
McDowell o.
McIndoe o.
Menge o.
Miller o.
Millin-Read o.
Müller o.
Munnell o.
Olshausen o.
Ombrédanne o.
O'Sullivan o.
Oxford o.
Péan o.
Pomeroy o.
Porro o.
Porro-Veit o.
Pozzi o.
Récamier o.
Ries-Wertheim o.
Rizzoli o.
Rubin o.
Saenger o.
Scanzoni o.
Schauffler o.
Schauta o.
Schauta-Amreich vaginal o.
Schauta-Wertheim o.

operation (continued)
    Schröder o.
    Schuchardt o.
    Shirodkar o.
    Simon o.
    Spalding-Richardson o.
    Spinelli o.
    Strassman-Jones o.
    Sturmdorf o.
    TeLinde o.
    Torpin o.
    Tuffier o.
    Twombly o.
    Twombly-Ulfelder o.
    Uchida o.
    uterine suspension o.
    vacuum extraction o.
    Vernon-David o.
    Warren o.
    Waters o.
    Watkins transposition o. for
        uterine prolapse
    Watkins-Wertheim o.
    Webster o.
    Wertheim o.
    Wertheim-Schauta o.
    Wharton o.
    Whitacre o.
    Williams o.
    Williams-Richardson o.
    Wylie o.
opercula (plural of operculum)
opercular
operculate
operculum (opercula)
    trophoblastic o.
orifice
    abdominal o. of uterine tube
    external urethral o.
    hymenal o.
    o. of uterus
    vaginal o.
orificia (plural of orificium)
orificial
orificium (orificia)
    o. urethrae externum
        muliebris
    o. vaginae

os (ora) [opening, mouth]
    o. externum uteri
    incompetent cervical o.
    Scanzoni second o.
    o. of uterus, external
Osiander sign
osteomalacia
    puerperal o.
osteoporosis
osteoporotic
ostia (plural of ostium)
ostial [pertaining to opening, aper-
    ture, orifice]
ostium (ostia)
    o. uteri
    o. vaginae
O'Sullivan
    operation
OTR—Ovarian Tumor Registry
outlet
    marital o.
ovaria (plural of ovarium)
ovarian
ovariectomy [pref: oophorectomy]
ovaries (plural of ovary)
ovarin
ovariocele
ovariocentesis
ovariocyesis
ovariodysneuria
ovariogenic
ovariohysterectomy [pref: oophoro-
    hysterectomy]
ovariopexy
ovariorrhexis
ovariosalpingectomy [pref: salpingo-
    oophorectomy]
ovariosteresis
ovariotomy
    abdominal o.
    Beatson o.
    vaginal o.
ovariotubal [pref: tubo-ovarian]
ovaritis [pref: oophoritis]
ovarium (ovaria)
    o. bipartitum
    o. gyratum
    o. lobatum

ovary (ovaries)
 adenocystic o.
 embryonic o.
 oyster o.'s
 polycystic o.
overgrowth
 candidal o.
 fungal o.
 yeast o.
ovi (genitive of ovum)
oviduct
ovoid
 Manchester o.
ovotestis
ovotherapy
ovula
ovulate
ovulation
ovulatory
ovule
 graafian o.'s
 Naboth o.
 primitive o.
 primordial o.
ovulogenous
ovum (ova)
 blighted o.
 fertilized o.
 permanent o.
 unfertilized o.
Oxford
 operation
oxytocia
oxytocics [a class of drugs]
oxytocin
 o. challenge test (OCT)
P—para
 postpartum
PA—primary amenorrhea
pack
 Bellow p.
Pagano-Levin medium smear
Paget
 disease
 disease, mammary
 disease of the nipple
 syndrome (I)
 test

pagetoid
Pajot
 law
 method
palma (palmae)
 palmae plicatae
palpation
panel
 urine drug p. (UDP)
panhysterectomy
panhysterocolpectomy
panhystero-oophorectomy
panhysterosalpingectomy
panhysterosalpingo-oophorectomy
Pap—Papanicolaou
Papanicolaou (Pap)
 smear
 stain
 test
papilla (papillae)
 p. mammae, mammary p.
 p. mammaria
papillate
papillation
papilliferous
papilliform
papilloma
 cockscomb p.
 ductal p.
 intraductal p.
 p. venereum
papule
 moist p., mucous p.
papulosis
 bowenoid p.
papyraceous
para (0, 1, 2, etc.) [number of deliveries]
paracervical
paracolic
paracolpitis
paracolpium
paracyesis
paragomphosis
paralysis (paralyses)
 obstetric p.
 parturient p.
parametria

parametrial
parametric image
parametritic
parametritis
parametrium
paraovarian
para-primipara
pararectal
parasalpingeal
parasalpingitis
parasite
 See specific parasites in
 Laboratory, Pathology,
 and Chemistry Terms.
parasitic
paratubal
parauterine
paravaginal
 p. hysterectomy
 p. incision
paravaginitis
paravesical
parenchymatous
paresis
 parturient p.
paries (parietes)
parietitis
parietosplanchnic
parietovisceral
parity
paroöphoric
paroöphoritis
paroöphoron
parous
parovarian
parovariotomy
parovaritis
parovarium
Parrot [eponym]
 atrophy of the newborn
 disease
 pseudoparalysis
 sign
 syndrome (I, II)
 syphilitic osteochondritis
pars (partes)
 p. fetalis placentae
 p. uterina placentae

partial
 p. hysterectomy
 p. mastectomy
parturient
parturifacient
parturiometer
parturition
partus
 p. agrippinus
 p. caesareus
 p. immaturus
 p. maturus
 p. precipitatus
 p. prematurus
 p. serotinus
 p. siccus
path—pathology
pathogen
 See specific pathogens in
 Laboratory, Pathology,
 and Chemistry Terms.
pattern
 rugal p.
pavilion
 p. of the oviduct
Pawlik
 fold
 grip
 triangle
PCO—polycystic ovary
Péan
 operation
peau
 p. d'orange (Fr. orange peel
  skin)
pelves (plural of pelvis)
pelvic
 p. congestion syndrome
 p. exenteration
 p. inflammatory disease (PID)
 p. inlet
 p. outlet
 p. plane diameter
 p. thrombophlebitis
pelvicellulitis
pelvicephalography
pelvicephalometry
pelvifixation

pelvigraph
pelvimeter
    Breisky p.
    Collin p.
    Collyer p.
    DeLee p.
    Thoms p.
pelvimetry
pelvis (pelves)
    See also in *Orthopedics and Sports Medicine* section.
    android p.
    anthropoid p.
    beaked p.
    bony p.
    brachypellic p.
    contracted p.
    Deventer p.
    dolichopellic p.
    flat p.
    frozen p.
    funnel-shaped p.
    generally contracted p.
    generally enlarged p.
    giant p.
    gynecoid p.
    infantile p.
    p. justo major
    p. justo minor
    juvenile p.
    large p.
    p. major
    mesatipellic p.
    p. minor
    Nägele p.
    oblique p.
    obliquely contracted p.
    pithecoid p.
    p. plana
    platypellic p.
    platypelloid p.
    Robert p.
    rostrate p.
    p. rotunda
    round p.
    simple flat p.
    small p.
    triangular p.

pelvis (pelves) (continued)
    true p.
pendulous
Pereyra
    procedure
pericolpitis
perimetric
perimetrium
perimetrosalpingitis
perineal
    p. body
    p. pad
    p. sensation
perineauxesis
perineocele
perineocolporectomyomectomy
perineometer
perineoplasty
perineorrhaphy
    Emmet-Studdiford p.
perineosynthesis
perineotomy
perineovaginal
perineovaginorectal
perineovulvar
perineum
    anterior p.
    posterior p.
    watering-can p.
period
    child-bearing p.
    p. of gestation, gestational period
perioophoritis
perioophorosalpingitis
perioothecitis
perioothecosalpingitis
perisalpingitis
perisalpingo-ovaritis
perisalpinx
peritonealize
peritoneopexy
peritoneum
    parietal p.
periumbilical
periuterine
perivaginal
perivaginitis

per vaginam
pessary
    contraceptive p.
    cup p.
    diaphragm p.
    doughnut p.
    Emmet-Gellhorn p.
    Gariel p.
    Gehrung p.
    Gellhorn p.
    gynefold p.
    Hodge p.
    lever p.
    ring p.
    Smith p.
    Smith-Hodge p.
    stem p.
    Thomas p.
    Wylie p.
    Zwanck p.
PET—pre-eclamptic toxemia
PG—prostaglandin
$PGF_{2\alpha}$ [PGF2-alpha]—prostaglandin $F_{2\alpha}$ [F2-alpha]
pH—hydrogen ion concentration
Phaneuf
    maneuver
phantom
    Schultze p.
phase
    luteal p.
    menstrual p.
    proliferative p.
    secretory p.
phenomenon (phenomena)
    Arias-Stella p.
    fern p.
phenylketonuria (PKU)
    p. II
    p. III
    atypical p.
    maternal p.
Phenylstix
phimosis
    p. vaginalis
phlebitis
phlebometritis

phlegmasia
    p. alba dolens
    p. alba dolens puerperarum
    cellulitic p.
    thrombotic p.
Phocas disease
phototherapy
PID—pelvic inflammatory disease
"pielo–" Phonetic for words beginning pyelo–.
PIF—prolactin-inhibiting factor
pileus
pill
Pinard
    maneuver
    sign
"pio–" Phonetic for words beginning pyo–.
Piskacek sign
pithecoid
pitocin drip
pituitary
    p. disease
    p. gland
    p.-hypothalamus
placenta (placentas, placentae)
    ablatio placentae
    abruptio placentae
    accessory p.
    p. accreta
    adherent p.
    allantoic p.
    annular p.
    battledore p.
    bidiscoidal p.
    bilobate p., bilobed p.
    p. bipartita, bipartite p.
    central p. previa
    chorioallantoic p.
    choriovitelline p.
    p. circumvallata
    circumvallate p.
    p. cirsoides
    cirsoid p., p. cirsoides
    complete p. previa
    deciduate p., deciduous p.
    p. diffusa
    p. dimidiata, dimidiate p.

placenta (placentas, placentae)
(continued)
   discoid p., p. discoidea
   Duncan p.
   duplex p.
   endotheliochorial p.
   epitheliochorial p.
   p. febrilis
   p. fenestrata
   fenestrated p.
   fetal p., p. foetalis
   first-degree p. previa
   fundal p.
   furcate p.
   hemochorial p.
   hemodichorial p.
   hemoendothelial p.
   hemomonochorial p.
   hemotrichorial p.
   horseshoe p.
   incarcerated p.
   incomplete p. previa
   p. increta
   labyrinthine p.
   lobed p.
   marginal p. previa
   p. marginata
   maternal p.
   p. membranacea
   monochorionic monoamni-
      otic p.
   multilobate p., multilobed
      p., p. multipartita
   p. multipartita
   p. nappiformis
   nondeciduate p., nondecidu-
      ous p.
   p. obsoleta
   panduriform p., p. panduri-
      formis
   p. panduriformis
   partial p. previa
   p. percreta
   p. previa
   p. previa centralis
   p. previa marginalis
   p. previa partialis
   p. reflexa

placenta (placentas, placentae)
(continued)
   reniform p.
   p. reniformis
   retained p.
   Schultze p.
   second-degree p. previa
   p. spuria
   stone p.
   p. succenturiata
   succenturiate p.
   syndesmochorial p.
   third-degree p. previa
   total p. previa
   trapped p.
   p. triloba, trilobate p.
   p. tripartita, tripartite p.
   p. triplex
   p. truffée
   tubal-cornual p.
   p. uterina, uterine p.
   varicose p.
   velamentous p.
   villous p.
   yolk-sac p.
   zonary p., zonular p.
placental
   p. abruption
   p. barrier
   p. tissue
   p. vascular anastomosis
placentitis
placentocytotoxin
placentogenesis
placentogram
placentography
      indirect p.
placentoid
placentologist
placentology
placentoma
placentopathy
placentotherapy
plate
      chorionic p.
platypellic
platypelloid

plexus (plexus, plexuses)
    See also *rete.*
    Auerbach p.
    p. cavernosus clitoridis
    cavernous p. of clitoris
    ovarian p.
    p. ovaricus
    pampiniform p.
    p. pampiniformis
    utcrinc p.
    uterovaginal p.
    p. uterovaginalis
    vaginal p.
    p. venosus vaginalis
    venous p.
plica (plicae)
    p. pubovesicalis
    p. rectouterina
    plicae vaginae
plug
    cervical p.
PMB—postmenopausal bleeding
PMP—past menstrual period
    previous menstrual period
PMS—premenstrual syndrome
PMT—premenstrual tension
pneumoamnios
pneumogynecogram
pneumohydrometra
pneumonia
    neonatal p.
"po-do-rahnj" Phonetic for peau
    d'orange.
pole
    placental p.
polycyesis
polycystoma
polyhydramnios
polyhypermenorrhea
polyhypomenorrhea
polymenorrhea
polyostotic
polyp
    cervical p.
    endocervical p.
    endometrial p.
    inflammatory p.
    leiomyomatous p.

polyp (continued)
    myomatous p.
    neoplastic p.
    non-neoplastic p.
    pedunculated p.
    sessile p.
Pomeroy
    method
    operation
Porro
    cesarean section
    hysterectomy
    operation
Porro-Veit
    operation
portio (portiones)
    p. supravaginalis cervicis
    p. vaginalis cervicis
Poseiro effect
position
    See *fetal position* and *pre-sentation.*
    semi-Fowler p.
postabortal
postacrosomal
postcoital
post coitum
postmastectomy
postmenopausal
postmenstrua
postpartum
    p. blues
    p. depression
    p. hemorrhage
Potter
    version
pouch
    p. of Douglas
    perineal p., deep
    perineal p., superficial
    rectouterine p.
    rectovaginal p.
    uterovesical p.
    vesicouterine p.
Pozzi
    operation
PP—postpartum
PPH—postpartum hemorrhage

Prague maneuver
PRBV—placental residual blood
    volume
precipitate
        p. labor
precocity
pregnancy
        abdominal p.
        afetal p.
        bigeminal p.
        cornual p.
        ectopic p.
        entopic p.
        exochorial p.
        extrauterine p.
        fallopian p.
        gemellary p.
        heterotopic p.
        hydatid p.
        hysterical p.
        interstitial p.
        intraligamentary p.
        intramural p.
        intraperitoneal p.
        intrauterine p.
        mesenteric p.
        molar p.
        mural p.
        ovarioabdominal p.
        oviductal p.
        parietal p.
        post-term p.
        sacrofetal p.
        sacrohysteric p.
        spurious p.
        stump p.
        term p.
        tubal p.
        tuboabdominal p.
        tuboligamentary p.
        tubo-ovarian p.
        tubouterine p.
        uteroabdominal p.
        utero-ovarian p.
        uterotubal p.
pregnanediol level
pregnant
Pregnosticon test

premenarchal
premenopausal
premenstrua
premenstruum
prenatal
prepuce
preputial
preputium
        p. clitoridis
presacral
        p. neurectomy
presentation
        See also *fetal position.*
        arm p.
        breech p.
        breech p., complete
        breech p., double
        breech p., frank
        breech p., incomplete
        breech p., single
        brow p.
        cephalic p.
        compound p.
        p. of the cord
        double-footling p.
        face p.
        footling p.
        footling breech p.
        frank breech p.
        full breech p.
        funic p.
        funis p.
        hand and head p.
        knee breech p.
        longitudinal p.
        mentoanterior face p.
        oblique p.
        parietal p.
        pelvic p.
        placental p.
        polar p.
        shoulder p.
        single footling p.
        torso p.
        transverse p.
        trunk p.
        vertex p.
        vertex-vertex p.

previable
PRF—prolactin-releasing factor
PRFM—prolonged rupture of fetal
    membranes
PRH—prolactin-releasing hormone
primigravid
primigravida
primip—primipara [woman bearing
    first child]
primipara
primiparity
primiparous
primitiae
primordia (plural of primordium)
primordial
    p. follicle
    p. germ cells
primordium (primordia)
    genital p.
    lens p.
    uterovaginal p.
principle [rule]
    See *law* and *rule.*
procedure
    See also *maneuver, method,*
        operation, and *technique.*
    Pereyra p.
    Shirodkar p.
    Stamey p.
    Strap p.
    Temple p.
process
procidentia
    p. uteri
progenital
Progestasert IUD
progestational
progesteroid
progestins [a class of drugs]
progestogen
progestomimetic
progravid
projection
    left anterior oblique (LAO) p.
    left posterior oblique (LPO)
        p.
    right anterior oblique (RAO)
        p.

projection (continued)
    right posterior oblique
        (RPO) p.
prolactin
prolapse
    uterine p.
    vaginal p.
prolapsus
    p. uteri
PROM—premature rupture of
    membranes
    prolonged rupture of mem-
        branes
prominence
prostaglandin (PG)
    See also in *Laboratory,*
        Pathology, and Chemistry
        Terms.
    p. $F_{2\alpha}$ [F2-alpha] $(PGF_{2\alpha})$
    p. $F_{2\alpha}$ tromethamine [F2-
        alpha]
prostaglandins [a class of drugs]
protuberance
prurigo
    Besnier p. of pregnancy
    p. gestationis of Besnier
pruritus
    p. vulvae
psammoma bodies
pseudocorpus luteum
pseudocyesis
pseudoendometritis
pseudoerosion
pseudohermaphroditism
pseudomamma
pseudomenopause
pseudomenstruation
pseudomucin
pseudomucinous
pseudomyxoma
    p. peritonei
pseudopregnancy
ptosis
pubarche
puberty
    delayed p.
    precocious p.
    pseudoprecocious p.

pubic
> inferior p. ligament
> p. lice
> p. ligament of Cowper
> p. region
> superior p. ligament
> p. symphysis

pubocervical
pubovesicocervical
pudenda (plural of pudendum)
pudendal
pudendum (pudenda)
> female p.
> p. femininum
> p. muliebre

puerpera
puerperal
puerperalism
puerperant
puerperium
puerperous
pulmonary
> p. embolism
> p. maturity

pump
> breast p.

purpura
Puzo method
PV—through the vagina (L. per vaginam)
pyelitis
> p. gravidarum

pyelocystitis
pyelonephritis
> p. of pregnancy

pyocolpocele
pyocolpos
pyometra
pyometritis
pyometrium
pyo-ovarium
pyosalpingitis
pyosalpingo-oophoritis
pyosalpingo-oothecitis
pyosalpinx
Q-tip test
quadripara
quadruplets

quintipara
rachitic
Racine syndrome
radiation
> hysterectomy and r. (H&R)

radical [adj.]
> Auchincloss modified r. mastectomy
> extended r. mastectomy
> Halsted r. mastectomy
> r. hysterectomy
> Latzko r. hysterectomy
> r. mastectomy (RM)
> modified r. mastectomy
> Schauta r. vaginal hysterectomy
> Wertheim r. hysterectomy
> Willy Meyer r. mastectomy

radioreceptor assay
"ra-fee" Phonetic for raphe.
"rakitic" Phonetic for rachitic.
ramus (rami)
> ischiopubic r.

Randall
> sign

RAO—right anterior oblique [projection]
raphe (raphae)
> amniotic r.

raphes (genitive of raphe)
Rasch sign
rating
> Apgar r.

ratio
> lecithin-sphingomyelin (L/S) r.

RDA—right dorsoanterior [position]
RDI—rupture-delivery interval
RDP—right dorsoposterior [position]
reaction
> acrosome r.
> depressive r.

Récamier
> operation

receptor
> estrogen r.
> progesterone r.

recombinant
  r. DNA
rectocele
rectolabial
rectouterine
rectovaginal
rectum
reflex
  Ferguson r.
  milk ejection r., milk let-
    down r.
region
  genitourinary r.
  pelvic r.
  perineal r.
  pubic r.
  suprapubic r.
  umbilical r.
  urogenital r.
Reichel cloacal duct
renal
  r. function
renin
  r. angiotensin system
repair
  central episiotomy and r.
    (CER)
  Matsner median episiotomy
    and r.
reperitonealize
reproductive
respiration
  fetal r.
resuscitation
rete (retia)
  See also *plexus.*
  r. ovarii
retia (plural of rete)
retial
retraction
  uterine r.
retrocervical
retrocessed
retrocession
retrodisplacement
retroplacental
retroposition
retrouterine

retroversion
retroverted
Retzius
  space
Reusner sign
RFA—right frontoanterior [position]
RFP—right frontoposterior [position]
RFT—right frontotransverse [posi-
  tion]
Rh—Rhesus
Rh
  antibody
  blood group
  factor
  immunization
  incompatibility
  isoantigen
rhesus (Rh)
  r. factor
  r. isoimmunization
Rh neg—Rhesus factor–negative
RhoGAM test
Rh pos—Rhesus factor–positive
Rh sensitization
Richardson
  technique
Ries-Wertheim
  hysterectomy
  operation
rima (rimae)
  r. pudendi
  r. vulvae
rimal
ring
  Bandl r.
  Falope r.
  hymenal r.
Rinman sign
Ritgen maneuver
Rizzoli
  operation
RLQ—right lower quadrant
RMA—right mentoanterior [position]
RMP—right mentoposterior [posi-
  tion]
RMT—right mentotransverse [posi-
  tion]

ROA—right occipitoanterior [position]
Robert pelvis
Rock-Mulligan
    hood
Roederer obliquity
roentgentherapy
    intravaginal r.
Rohr stria
Rokitansky-Küster-Hauser syndrome
ROM—rupture of membranes
rooming-in
ROP—right occipitoposterior [position]
ROT—right occipitotransverse [position]
rotation
    internal r.
    manual r.
Rotunda treatment
RPO—right posterior oblique [projection]
RPR—rapid plasma reagin (test)
RSA—right sacroanterior [position]
RScA—right scapuloanterior [position]
RScP—right scapuloposterior [position]
RSP—right sacroposterior [position]
RST—right sacrotransverse [position]
rubella
rubeola
Rubin
    operation
    test
rudiment
    r. of vaginal process
rudimentum (rudimenta)
    r. processus vaginalis
ruga (rugae)
    rugae of vagina, rugae vaginales
rugal pattern
rugate
rule
    See also *law.*
    Arey r.
    Haase r.

rule (continued)
    His r.
    Nägele r.
rump
rupture
    artificial r. of membranes (AROM)
    r. of gravid uterus
    r. of membranes (ROM)
    premature r. of membranes (PROM)
    prolonged r. of membranes (PROM)
    spontaneous r.
Ruysch
    muscle
SA—secondary amenorrhea
Sabin-Feldman test
sacciform
sacculation
    uterine s.
sacrouterine
sactosalpinx
Saenger
    macula
    operation
saline
Salmon sign
salpingectomy
salpinges (plural of salpinx)
salpingian
salpingitic
salpingitis
    chronic interstitial s.
    chronic vegetating s.
    hemorrhagic s.
    hypertrophic s.
    s. isthmica nodosa
    mural s. nodular s.
    parenchymatous s.
    s. profluens
    pseudofollicular s.
    purulent s.
    tuberculous s.
salpingocele
salpingocyesis
salpingogram
salpingography

salpingolithiasis
salpingolysis
salpingo-oophorectomy
salpingo-oophoritis
salpingo-oophorocele
salpingo-ovariectomy
salpingo-ovariotomy
salpingoperitonitis
salpingopexy
salpingoplasty
salpingorrhaphy
salpingosalpingostomy
salpingoscopy
salpingostomatoplasty
salpingostomy
salpingotomy
salpinx (salpinges)
    s. uterina
Sampson cyst
Sänger. See *Saenger.*
sanguineous
sarcoidosis
    Boeck s.
sarcoma (sarcomas, sarcomata)
    See also in *Oncology and
       Hematology* section.
    botryoid s., s. botryoides
    endometrial stromal s.
sarcomatous
Saxtorph maneuver
SB—stillbirth
scale
    Apgar s.
    Dubowitz infant maturity s.
scan
    See in *Radiology, Nuclear
       Medicine, and Other
       Imaging* section.
Scanzoni
    maneuver
    operation
scapuloanterior
scapuloposterior
Scardino
    uteropelvioplasty
scarification
    chemical s.

Scarpa
    fascia
ScDA—right anterior scapular (L.
    scapulodextra anterior) [posi-
    tion]
ScDP—right posterior scapular (L.
    scapulodextra posterior) [posi-
    tion]
Schatz maneuver
Schauffler
    operation
Schaumann benign lymphogranuloma
Schauta
    operation
    radical vaginal hysterectomy
Schauta-Amreich
    vaginal hysterectomy
    vaginal operation
Schauta-Wertheim
    operation
Schiller test
Schimmelbusch disease
Schroeder
    disease
    operation
    syndrome
Schuchardt
    operation
Schüller stain
Schultze
    mechanism
    method
    placenta
Schuman method
ScLA—left anterior scapular (L.
    scapulolaeva anterior) [position]
sclerocystic
sclero-oophoritis
sclero-oothecitis
ScLP—left posterior scapular (L.
    scapulolaeva posterior) [posi-
    tion]
"scopes" See under full name.
    stethoscope
score
    Apgar s.
    Bishop s.
    Dubowitz s.

score (continued)
    Silverman s.
screen
    urine drug s. (UDS)
screening
    neonatal s.
    prenatal s.
Scully tumor
SD—spontaneous delivery
SDA—right anterior sacral (L. sacrodextra anterior) [position]
SDP—right posterior sacral (L. sacrodextra posterior) [position]
SDT—right transverse sacral (L. sacrodextra transversa) [position]
second-look laparotomy
section
    See also *cesarean section.*
    frozen s.
secundigravida
secundina (secundinae)
    s. uteri
secundine
secundipara
secundiparity
secundiparous
"sefal–" Phonetic for words beginning cephal–.
segment
    equatorial s.
    lower uterine s.
segmenta (plural of segmentum)
segmental
    s. mastectomy
segmentum (segmenta)
seizures
semen
semi-Fowler position
seminoma
    ovarian s.
separation
    s. of placenta
sepsis
    puerperal s.
septa (plural of septum)
septate
septation

septigravida
septimetritis
septipara
septum (septa)
    interplacental s.
    longitudinal s.
    placental s.
    rectovaginal s.
    rectovesical s.
    urogenital s.
septuplet
SERMs—selective estrogen receptor modulators [a class of drugs]
serocystoma
serous
Sertoli-Leydig cell tumor
serum (serums, sera)
    s. alpha-fetoprotein (AFP)
    pregnancy s.
"serviko–" Phonetic for words beginning cervico–.
sex cords
sextigravida
sextipara
SGA—small for gestational age
"shan-deh-lir" Phonetic for chandelier.
sharp curettage
Sheehan
    disease
    syndrome
shield
    Dalkon s.
Shirodkar
    operation
    procedure
shock
    obstetric s.
    toxic s.
Shorr stain
show
    bloody
sibling
sickness
    morning s.
"sifilis" Phonetic for syphilis.
"sifilo–" Phonetic for words beginning syphilo–.

sign

See also *phenomenon, reflex,*
and *test.*
Ahlfeld s.
Arnoux s.
Beccaria s.
Beclard s.
Bolt s.
Braun-Fernwald s., Braun-
von Fernwald s.
Braxton-Hicks s.
Chadwick s.
chandelier s.
Cullen s.
Danforth s.
Dubois s.
Gauss s.
Golden s.
Goodell s.
Halban s.
halo s.
Hegar s.
Hicks s.
Hoehne s.
Horner s.
Jacquemier s.
Kanter s.
Kelly s.
Kergaradec s.
Küstner s.
Ladin s.
Landou s.
lemon s.
Mayor s.
Olshausen s.
Osiander s.
Pinard s.
Piskacek s.
placental s.
Randall s.
Rasch s.
Reusner s.
Rinman s.
Salmon s.
Spalding s.
Sumner s.
Tarnier s.
twin peak s.

sign (continued)
Von Fernwald s.
Silverman
score
Simon
operation
"simphysis" Phonetic for symphysis.
simple
s. mastectomy (SM)
Simpson
sound
Sims
sound
sin–. See also words beginning
cin–, syn–.
Sinografin
sinus (sinus, sinuses)
lacteal s.'s, actiferi
lactiferous s.'s
urogenital s.
uterine s.'s
uteroplacental s.
situs (situs)
s. perversus
s. transversus
Skene
ducts
glands
Skene gland
SLA—left anterior sacral (L. sacrolaeva anterior) [position]
SLP—left posterior sacral (L.
sacrolaeva posterior)
sacrolaeva posterior [position]
SLT—left transverse sacral (L.
sacrolaeva transversa) [position]
SM—simple mastectomy
smear
buccal s.
Nickerson medium s.
Pagano-Levin medium s.
Papanicolaou (Pap) s.
smegma
s. clitoridis
s. embryonum
Smellie
method
Smellie-Veit maneuver

smile, smiling
    s. incision
SO—salpingo-oophorectomy
"so-as" Phonetic for psoas.
"so-is" Phonetic for psoas.
solution
somatotropin release-inhibiting factor
sonogram
sonography
    Acuson transvaginal s.
"soo-fl," "soo-flay" Phonetic for
    souffle.
sore
    venereal s.
souffle
    fetal s.
    funic s., funicular s.
    placental s.
    umbilical s.
    uterine s.
space
    Colles s.
    Douglas s.
    pararectal s.
    paravesical s.
    perineal s., deep
    perineal s., superficial
    presacral s.
    prevesical s.
    Retzius s., s. of Retzius
    suprapubic s.
Spalding
    sign
Spalding-Richardson
    hysterectomy
    operation
spermatogenesis
spermicidal
    s. sponge
spermicides [a class of drugs]
sphincter
    anal s.
    s. vaginae
Spinelli
    operation
spinnbarkeit
sponge
    s. biopsy

sponge (continued)
    spermicidal s.
spot
    pelvic s.
spray
    Dermoplast s.
squamocolumnar
stage
    first s. of labor
    fourth s. of labor
    premenstrual s.
    prodromal s. of labor
    rotation s. of labor
    second s. of labor
    s.'s of labor (1−4)
    Tanner s.
    third s. of labor
staging
    s. laparotomy
stain
    Feulgen s.
    Lugol s.
    Papanicolaou s.
    Schüller s.
    Shorr s.
Stamey procedure
Stein-Leventhal syndrome
stellate
stenosis (stenoses)
stent
    foam rubber vaginal s.
sterility
    absolute s.
    female s.
    primary s.
    relative s.
    secondary s.
sterilization
sterilize
Steri-Strip
stethoscope
    DeLee-Hillis obstetric s.
stigma (stigmas, stigmata)
    follicular s.
    syphilitic s.'s
stigmatic
stigmatism
stigmatization

stillbirth
stillborn
Stockholm box
stocking
> Jobst s.
> thromboembolic s.

stomatomy
strap
> Montgomery s.

Strap procedure
Strassman
> metroplasty
> phenomenon
> technique
> transverse fundal incision

Strassman-Jones
> operation

strata (plural of stratum)
stratiform
stratum (strata)
> s. spongiosum

strawberry cervix
streak
> See *band, layer, line,* and
> *stria.*
> germinal s.
> primitive s.

stress
> s. incontinence

stria (striae)
> See also *band, layer, line,*
> and *streak.*
> striae albicantes
> s. albicantes gravidarum
> striae atrophicae
> striae gravidarum
> Langhans s.
> Rohr s.

striatal
stripe
> endometrial s. [on sonogram
> of uterus]

Stroganoff (Stroganov) treatment
stroma (stromata)
> ovarian s.
> s. ovarii, s. of ovary

stromal

stromatosis
> endometrial s.

STS—serologic test for syphilis
study
> air s.
> cytogenetic s.

Sturmdorf
> operation

subareolar
subcutaneous
> s. mastectomy

subinvolution
submucous
> s. fibroma

subperitoneal
subserous
subtotal hysterectomy
subumbilical
subvesical
suction
> s. curettage
> s. dilatation and curettage
> (D&C)

"sudo–" Phonetic for words begin-
> ning pseudo–.

sulci (plural of sulcus)
sulciform
sulcus (sulci)
Sulkowich test
superfecundation
supracervical
> s. hysterectomy

suprapubic
supravaginal
> s. hysterectomy

surfactant
surgical procedure
> See *operation, procedure,*
> and *technique.*

surrogate
suture [material]
> See in *General Surgical
> Terms.*

suture [technique]
> See also in *General Surgical
> Terms.*
> Fothergill s.

SVD—spontaneous vaginal delivery

swelling
    labial s.
    premenstrual s.
Swiss-cheese endometrium
Swyer
    syndrome
Syed-Nesbit template
symphyseal
symphysis (symphyses)
    s. ossium pubis
    pubic s.
    s. pubica, s. pubis
symptom
    See also in *General Medical Terms.*
    deficiency s.
symptothermal
syn–. See also words beginning cin–, sin–.
synclitism
syncytioma
syncytiotoxin
syndrome
    See also *disease.*
    abruptio placentae s.
    Achard-Thiers s.
    acid aspiration s.
    Ahumada-del Castillo s.
    Allen-Masters s.
    amniotic infection s. of Blane
    androgen insensitivity s.
    Asherman s.
    bacterial overgrowth s.
    Ballantyne s.
    Brentano s.
    Chiari-Frommel s.
    Curtis–Fitz-Hugh s.
    Curtius s.
    Cushing s.
    Cushing s. medicamentosus
    DES (diethylstilbestrol) s.
    Down s.
    Ellis-van Creveld s.
    fetal alcohol s.
    fetal hydantoin s.
    fetal postmaturity s.
    fetal warfarin s.
    Fitz-Hugh s.

syndrome (continued)
    Fitz-Hugh–Curtis s.
    Fritsch-Asherman s.
    Frommel-Chiari s.
    galactorrhea-amenorrhea s.
    Gordan-Overstreet s.
    HELLP s. [hemolysis, elevated liver enzymes, and low platelet count occurring in association with preeclampsia]
    Kallmann s.
    Klinefelter s.
    Klotz s.
    Launois-Cléret s.
    Mayer-Rokitansky-Küster s.
    McCune-Albright s.
    Meigs s.
    Meigs-Cass s.
    Mendelson s.
    Paget s. (I)
    pelvic congestion s.
    polycystic ovary s.
    premenstrual s. (PMS)
    Rokitansky-Küster-Hauser s.
    Schroeder s.
    Sheehan s.
    Stein-Leventhal s.
    Swyer s.
    testicular feminization s.
    TORCH (toxoplasmosis, other agents, rubella, cytomegalovirus, herpes simplex) s.
    toxoplasmosis, other agents, rubella, cytomegalovirus, herpes simplex (TORCH) s.
    Turner s.
    Young s.
    Youssef s.
synechia (synechiae)
    s. vulvae
"syo–" Phonetic for words beginning cyo–.
syphilis
    prenatal s.
syphilitic

TA—therapeutic abortion
tachycardia
    fetal t.
TADAC—therapeutic abortion,
    dilation, aspiration, curettage
taenia (taeniae) [anatomy: flat band]
    t. tubae
TAH—total abdominal hysterectomy
tandem
Tarnier
    sign
Tatum-T IUD
Tay-Sachs disease
TD—transverse diameter
technique
    See also *maneuver* and
       method.
    Scc also in *General Surgical*
       Terms.
    Brandt t.
    hanging-drop t.
    Krönig t.
    Richardson t.
TED, T.E.D. (thromboembolic dis-
    ease) [T.E.D. is trademark form]
    hose
    stockings
tela (telae)
    t. submucosa tubae uterinae
    t. submucosa vesicae urinar-
      iae
    t. subserosa tubae uterinae
    t. subserosa uteri
telar
TeLinde
    operation
temperature (T, temp)
    body t., basal
template
    Syed-Nesbit t.
Temple procedure
tent
    Laminaria t.
teratoblastoma
teratogen
teratogenesis
teratogenetic
teratogenic

teratogenicity
teratogenous
teratoid
teratologist
teratology
teratoma (teratomas, teratomata)
    adult t.
    anaplastic malignant t.
    benign cystic t.
    cystic t.
    differentiated t.
    immature t.
    malignant t.
    mature t.
    solid t.
    tropoblastic malignant t.
    undifferentiated malignant t.
teratomatous
teratospermia
tertigravida
tertipara
test
    See also in *Laboratory,*
      Pathology, and Chemistry
      Terms.
    agglutination inhibition t.
    alpha-fetoprotein (AFP) t.
    Apgar t.
    Aschheim-Zondek (AZ) t.
    benzidine t.
    beta-hCG t.
    Biocept-G t.
    Bonney t.
    Brouha t.
    chorionic gonadotropin t.
    Collin t.
    contraction stress t.
    Coombs t.
    Corner-Allen t.
    cotton-tip applicator t.
    cross-matching t.
    D-dimer t.
    dexamethasone suppression t.
    Dienst t.
    early pregnancy t.
    estrogen receptor assay
      (ERA) t.
    Farris t.

test (continued)
    fern t.
    fetal electrocardiogram t.
    Fibrindex t.
    foam stability t.
    Friedman t.
    Friedman-Lapham t.
    frog t.
    Galli-Mainini t.
    gonadotropin-releasing hormone stimulation t.
    Gravindex t.
    hanging-drop t.
    Hogben t.
    Huhner t.
    immunologic t.
    immunologic pregnancy t.
    Kapeller-Adler t.
    Kleihauer-Betke t.
    Kline flocculation t.
    Kupperman t.
    t. of labor
    male frog t., male toad t.
    Marchetti t.
    Marshall-Marchetti t.
    methylene blue t.
    nitrazine t.
    nonstress t.
    norethindrone t.
    norethynodrel t.
    oxytocin challenge t.
    oxytocin sensitivity t.
    Paget t.
    Papanicolaou (Pap) t.
    pregnancy t.
    Pregnosticon t.
    progesterone withdrawal t.
    prolactin t.
    provocative t.
    Q-tip t.
    RhoGAM t.
    RPR (rapid plasma reagin) t.
    Rubin t.
    Sabin-Feldman t.
    Schiller t.
    serologic t. for syphilis (STS)
    Sims-Huhner t.

test (continued)
    smear t.
    stimulation t.
    stress t.
    Sulkowitch t.
    syphilis t.
    Thorn t.
    thymol turbidity t.
    toad t.
    ultrasound t.
    VDRL (Venereal Disease Research Laboratories) t. [abbreviation not expanded]
    Visscher-Bowman t.
    von Poehl t.
    Wampole t.
    whiff t,
    Wilson t.
    Xenopus t., *Xenopus laevis* t.
testiculoma
    t. ovarii
theca (thecae)
    t. cell
    t. externa
    t. of follicle
    t. of follicle of von Baer
    t. folliculi
    t. interna
    t. lutein
thecal
thecoma
thecomatosis
thecosis
thelalgia
thelarche
theleplasty
thelerethism
thelia (plural of thelium)
thelitis
thelium (thelia)
thelorrhagia
thelygenic
therapy
    endocrine t.
    hormonal t., hormone t.
thermography

thermotherapy
    endometrial laser intrauter-
       ine t. (ELITT)
Thomas
    pessary
Thoms
    test
thrombi (plural of thrombus)
thrombocytopenia
    thrombotic t.
thrombocytopenic
    t. purpura
thrombophlebitis
    iliofemoral t., postpartum
thrombose, thrombosed
thrombosis
    See also *thrombus.*
    See also in *Cardiology* sec-
       tion.
    placental t.
    puerperal t.
    venous t.
thrombus (thrombi)
    See also *thrombosis.*
    milk t.
Tillaux disease
time (T)
    doubling t.
    echo t. (TE)
    generation t.
tissue
    endometrial t.
    interstitial t.
titer
    rubella t.
    toxoplasmosis, other agents,
      rubella, cytomegalovirus,
      herpes simplex (TORCH)
      t.
TL—tubal ligation
TND—term normal delivery
TOA—tubo-ovarian abscess
tocograph
tocography
tocology
tocolysis
tocolytic
tocolytics [a class of drugs]

toluidine blue
tophus (tophi)
    t. syphiliticus
topography
TORCH—toxoplasmosis, other
    agents, rubella, cytomegalovi-
    rus, herpes simplex [syndrome]
TORCH
    infection
    titer
Torpin
    operation
torsion
total
    See also *complete.*
    t. abdominal hysterectomy
      (TAH)
    t. hysterectomy
    t. mastectomy
    t. vaginal hysterectomy
      (TVH)
toxic shock
    t.s. syndrome (TSS)
TPG—transplacental gradient
TPH—transplacental hemorrhage
trachelectomy
trachelitis
tracheloplasty
trachelorrhaphy
trachelosyringorrhaphy
trachelotomy
traction handle
    Barton t.h.
    Bill t.h.
    Luikart-Bill t.h.
transvaginal
trauma (traumas, traumata)
    birth t.
    perinatal t.
treatment
    Brandt t.
    Elliott t.
    Rotunda t.
    Stroganoff (Stroganov) t.
Trendelenburg
    position
triangle
    Pawlik t.

trimester
triphasic
triple test
Tri-screen
TRNG—tetracycline-resistant *Neisseria gonorrhoeae*
trophoblast
trophospongium (trophospongia)
tuba (tubae)
    t. uterina, t. uterina (Falloppii)
tubal
    t. ligation
    t. occlusion
    t. pregnancy
    t. sterilization
tubatorsion
tube
    embryonic fallopian t.
    fallopian t.
    uterine t.
tuber (tubers, tubera)
tubercle
    Müller t.
    müllerian t.
tuberculate, tuberculated
tuberculation
tuberculitis
tuberculization
tuberculoid
tuberculosis (TB)
    chronic fibroid t.
    genital t.
    genitourinary t.
tuboabdominal
tuboadnexopexy
tuboligamentous
tubo-ovarian
tubo-ovariotomy
tubo-ovaritis
tuboperitoneal
tuboplasty
tubouterine
tubovaginal
Tuffier
    operation
tumor
    Brenner t.
    corticoadrenal t.

tumor (continued)
    cystic t.
    dermoid t.
    endodermal sinus t.
    fibroid t.
    germ cell t.
    gonadal-stromal t.
    granulosa-theca cell t.
    Grawitz t.
    hilus cell t.
    hypernephroid t.
    Krukenberg t.
    lipid cell t.
    lipoid cell t.
    luteinized granulosa-theca cell t.
    mesenchymal t.
    müllerian mixed t.
    Scully t.
    Sertoli-Leydig cell t.
    theca cell t.
    Wilms t.
tunic
    fibrous t. of liver
    mucous t.
    muscular t.
tunica (tunicae)
    t. adventitia
    t. albuginea
    t. albuginea ovarii
    t. fibrosa
    t. mucosa
    t. mucosa uteri
    t. mucosa vaginae
    t. muscularis
    t. serosa
    t. spongiosa urethrae femininae
    t. spongiosa vaginae
    t. submucosa urethrae muliebris
tunicate
TVC—transvaginal cone
TVH—total vaginal hysterectomy
twin
    acardiac t.
    allantoidoangiopagous t.'s
    binovular t.'s

twin (continued)
    conjoined t.
    dichorial t.'s
    dichorionic t.'s
    dissimilar t.'s
    dizygotic t.
    enzygotic t.'s
    false t.'s
    fraternal t.
    heterologous t.'s
    hetero-ovular t.'s
    identical t.
    impacted t.'s
    monoamniotic t.'s
    monochorial t.'s
    monochorionic t.'s
    mono-ovular t.'s, monovular
      t.'s
    monozygotic t.
    omphaloangiopagous t.'s
    one-egg t.'s
    parabiotic t.'s
    parasitic t.
    placental parasitic t.
    Siamese t.'s
    similar t.'s
    true t.'s
    two-egg t.'s
    uniovular t.'s
    unlike t.'s
twinning
Twombly
    operation
Twombly-Ulfelder
    operation
tympanites
    uterine t.
"u–" Phonetic for words beginning
    eu–.
UA—uterine aspiration
UAP—uterine arterial pressure
UC—uterine contraction
UCG—urinary chorionic gonado-
    tropin
Uchida
    operation
UDP—urine drug panel
UDS—urine drug screen

ulcera (plural of ulcus)
ulcus (ulcera)
    u. penetrans
    u. phagedaenicum corrodens
    u. vulvae acutum
umbilical cord
umbilicus
    amniotic u.
    decidual u.
unengaged
unicollis
unicornate
unicornis
unit
    See also in *General Medical
      Terms* and *Laboratory,
      Pathology, and Chemistry
      Terms.*
    Corner-Allen u.
    corpus luteum hormone u.
    estrone u.
    Felton u.
    international u. of estrogenic
      activity
    international estrone u.
    international u. of
      gonadotrophic activity
    international u. of luteiniz-
      ing activity
    international u. of progesta-
      tional activity
    international progesterone u.
    international prolactin u.
    mouse u.
    u. of oxytocin
    progesterone u.
    prolactin u.
UPI—uteroplacental insufficiency
UPP—uterine perfusion pressure
uremia
    puerperal u.
ureteroneocystostomy
ureterouterine
ureterovaginal
urethra
    u. feminina
    u. muliebris

urethral
> u. caruncle
> u. diverticulum
> u. syndrome

urethrocele
urethrocystocele
urethrocystography
urethrocystometry
urethrocystoscopy
urethropexy
urethroscopy
urethrovaginal
urethrovesical
urinary
> u. diversion
> u. fistula
> u. frequency
> u. incontinence
> u. sodium
> u. tract

urine
> clean-catch u. specimen
> u. drug panel (UDP)
> u. drug screen (UDS)

uroflowmetry
urogenital
> u. diaphragm
> u. ridge
> u. sinus

USO—unilateral salpingo-
> oophorectomy

uteralgia [pref: hysteralgia]
uteri (plural of uterus)
uterine
> u. tube
> u. venography

uteroabdominal
uterocentesis
uterocervical
uterodynia
uterofixation
uterogestation
uterography
uterolith
uterometer
uterometry
utero-ovarian

uteropelvioplasty
> Scardino u.

uteropexy
uteroplacental
> u. insufficiency
> u. ischemia

uteroplasty
uterorectal
uterosacral
uterosalpingogram
uterosalpingography
uterosclerosis
uterothermometry
uterotomy
uterotonic
uterotropic
uterotubal
uterotubography
uterovaginal
uteroventral
uterovesical
uterus (uteri)
> u. acollis
> arcuate u.
> u. arcuatus
> u. bicameratus vetularum
> u. bicornis
> u. bicornis bicollis
> u. bicornis unicollis
> bicornuate u.
> bifid u.
> u. biforis
> u. bilocularis
> bipartite u.
> u. bipartitus
> bosselated u.
> capped u.
> cochleate u.
> u. cordiformis
> Couvelaire u.
> u. didelphys
> double-mouthed u.
> u. duplex
> duplex u., u. duplex
> embryonic u.
> fetal u.
> fibroid u.
> fibromyomata uteri

uterus (uteri) (continued)
    gravid u.
    u. incudiformis
    infantile u.
    ovoid u.
    u. parvicollis
    Piskacek u.
    u. planifundalis
    pubescent u.
    ribbon u.
    u. rudimentarius
    sacculated u.
    saddle-shaped u.
    scarred u.
    u. septus
    u. simplex
    subseptate u.
    u. subscptus
    u. triangularis
    u. unicornis
    unicornuate u.
    unscarred u.
utriculoplasty
UV—umbilical vein
UVA—urethrovesical angle
UVP—uterine venous pressure
VA—vacuum aspiration
vacuum
    v. extraction operation
vagina (vaginae)
    v. muliebris
vaginal
    v. celiotomy
    Doyen v. hysterectomy
    Heaney v. hysterectomy
    v. hysterectomy (VH)
    v. hysterotomy
    laparoscopic-assisted v. hysteroscopy (LAVH)
    Mayo-Ward v. hysterectomy
    v. myomectomy
    v. ovariotomy
    v. plate
    Schauta-Amreich v. hysterectomy
    Schauta radical v. hysterectomy

vaginal (continued)
    v. septum
    total v. hysterectomy (TVH)
    v. vault
vaginalis
    processus v.
vaginapexy
vaginate
vaginectomy
vaginicoline
vaginiperineotomy
vaginismus
vaginitis
    v. adhaesiva
    atrophic v.
    catarrhal v.
    diphtheritic v.
    emphysematous v.
    glandular v.
    granular v.
    monilial v.
    papulous v.
    senile v.
    Trichomonas v.
vaginoabdominal
vaginocele
vaginocutaneous
vaginodynia
vaginofixation
vaginogenic
vaginogram
vaginography
vaginolabial
vaginometer
vaginomycosis
vaginopathy
vaginoperineal
vaginoperineorrhaphy
vaginoperineotomy
vaginoperitoneal
vaginopexy
vaginoplasty
vaginoscopy
vaginotome
vaginotomy
vaginovesical
vaginovulvar

vagitus
    v. uterinus
    v. vaginalis
Valsuani disease
van Horne (van Hoorn, van Hoorne)
    maneuver
varicocele
       ovarian v.
       utero-ovarian v.
varicosity
vas (vasa)
       vasa praevia
       vasa propria of Jungbluth
vault
       vaginal v.
VB—viable birth
vectis
VEE—vagina ectocervix and endo-
    cervix
VEE smear
vein
       ovarian v.
velamen (velamina)
    v. vulvae
velamentous
venereal
    v. disease (VD)
venography
       uterine v.
venter (ventres)
ventrofixation
ventrohysteropexy
ventrosuspension
ventrovesicofixation
vernix
Vernon-David
    operation
verruca (verrucae)
    v. acuminata, verrucae
       acuminatae
verrucous
version
       bipolar v.
       Braxton-Hicks v.
       cephalic v.
       Hicks v.
       podalic v.
       Potter v.

version (continued)
    Wigand v.
    Wright v.
vesical [adj.: pertaining to the blad-
    der]
vesicle [noun: blister, small sac]
    Baer v.
    chorionic v.
    graafian v.'s
    Naboth v.'s
vesicocervical
vesicouterine
vesicouterovaginal
vesicovaginal
vesicovaginorectal
vesicula (vesiculae)
    vesiculae graafianae
    vesiculae nabothi
    v. serosa
vessel
    Jungbluth v.'s
    pudendal v.
vestibula (plural of vestibulum)
vestibular
    v. bulb
vestibule
    urogenital v.
    v. of vagina
vestibulourethral
vestibulum (vestibula)
    v. vaginae
vestigial
vestigium (vestigia)
VH—vaginal hysterectomy
viability
viable
    v. birth
    v. fetus
villi (plural of villus)
villiferous
villitis
villose, villous [adj.]
    v. placenta
villositis
villosity
villus (villi)
    amniotic v.
    anchoring v.

villus (villi) (continued)
  chorionic v.
  free v.
  primary v.
  secondary v.
  tertiary v.
vinculum (vincula)
  See *band, frenulum,* and
   frenum.
VIP—voluntary interruption of
 pregnancy
virilism
virus
  See also in *Laboratory,*
   Pathology, and Chemistry
   Terms.
  human papilloma v. (papillomavirus)
  papilloma v.
  rubella v.
visceralgia
Visscher-Bowman test
vomiting
  morning v.
  v. of pregnancy
vomitus
  v. gravidarum
von Baer. See *Baer.*
von Fernwald
  sign
von Poehl
  test
von Willebrand (Willebrand)
  disease
  syndrome
vulva
  v. clausa
  v. conivens
  fused v.
  v. hians
vulvae
  kraurosis v.
  noma v.
vulval
vulvar
vulvectomy
vulvismus

vulvitis
  v. blenorrhagica
  creamy v.
  diabetic v.
  diphtheric v.
  diphtheritic v.
  eczematiform v.
  follicular v.
  irritative leukoplakic v.
  monilial v.
  phlegmonous v.
  plasma cell v.
  pseudoleukoplakic v.
  ulcerative v.
vulvocrural
vulvopathy
vulvorectal
vulvouterine
vulvovaginal
Waldeyer fossa
Walthard cell
Wampole test
Ward-Mayo
  vaginal hysterectomy
Warren
  operation
wart
  venereal w.
waters
  bag of w.
Waters [eponym]
  cesarean section
  operation
Watkins
  transposition operation for
   uterine prolapse
  uterine prolapse
Watkins-Wertheim
  operation
Watson
  method
Webster
  operation
weight
  birth w. [pref: birthweight]
Wertheim
  operation
  radical hysterectomy

Wertheim-Schauta
    operation
wet mount
Wharton
    gelatin
    jelly
    operation
whiff test
Whitacre
    operation
White [eponym]
    classification
Wiedemann syndrome
Wigand
    maneuver
    version
Willebrand. See *von Willebrand.*
Willebrand-Jürgens
    syndrome
Williams
    operation
Williams-Richardson
    operation
Willy Meyer
    incision
    radical mastectomy
Wilms tumor
Wilson test
wolffian
    w. cyst
    w. duct

Wright
    version
Wylie
    operation
    pessary
Xenopus laevis test
xerogram
xerography
xeromammogram
xeromammography
xeromenia
yolk sac
"yoo–" Phonetic for words beginning eu–.
Young
    syndrome
Youssef syndrome
"zero–" Phonetic for words beginning xero–.
zona (zonae)
    z. pellucida
zonal
zonary
zone
    erogenous z., erotogenic z.
    perifollicular z.
    placental z.
zygosity
zygote

Oncology and Hematology

AAA—acquired aplastic anemia
ABC—Adriamycin, bleomycin, cis-
    platin
Abernethy
        sarcoma
ABMT—autologous bone marrow
    transplantation
ABO
        blood groups
Abrikosov (Abrikossoff) tumor
abscess
        Pautrier a.
ABV—Adriamycin, bleomycin,
    vinblastine
ACA—adenocarcinoma
acanthosis
        malignant a. nigricans
ACC—adenoid cystic carcinoma
        alveolar cell carcinoma
achrestic
acrolein
acrospiroma
        eccrine a.
ACS—American Cancer Society
ACT—activated coagulation time
action
activated coagulation time (ACT)
activated partial thromboplastin
        time (APTT, aPTT)
activator
        plasminogen a.
        single-chain urokinase-type
            plasminogen (scu-PA) a.
            (prourokinase)
        tissue plasminogen a. (t-PA,
            tPA, TPA)
        urinary plasminogen a., u-
            plasminogen a. (urokinase)
activity
        leukemia-associated inhibi-
            tory a. (LIA)

adamantinoma
        a. of long bones
        pituitary a.
        tibial a.
addisin
Addison
        anemia
Addison-Biermer anemia
addisonian
        a. anemia
adenocarcinoma
        acinar a.
        acinic cell a.
        acinous a.
        alveolar a.
        bronchioalveolar a.
        bronchiolar a.
        bronchioloalveolar a.
        bronchoalveolar a.
        bronchogenic a.
        clear cell a.
        ductal a. of prostate
        follicular a.
        gastric a.
        a. of infantile testis
        a. of kidney
        a. of lung
        mammary a.
        mucinous a.
        papillary a.
        polymorphous low-grade a.
        polypoid a.
        renal a.
        scirrhous a.
        sebaceous a.
        terminal duct a.
        testicular a. of infancy
        urachal a.
adenoepithelioma
adenosquamous
adjunct

adjunctive
adjuvant
    a. chemotherapy
    a. therapy
agent
    chemotherapeutic a.
aggregation
    platelet a.
AGL—acute granulocytic leukemia
agranulocytosis
AHA—acquired hemolytic anemia
    autoimmune hemolytic anemia
AHD—autoimmune hemolytic disease
AILD—angioimmunoblastic lymphadenopathy with dysproteinemia
aleukemic
aleukocytic
alpha
    a.-thalassemia
AMBL—acute myeloblastic leukemia
ameloblastoma
    malignant a.
    pituitary a.
o-aminoazotoluene [o-, ortho-]
p-aminobenzoate (PAB) [p-, para-]
p-aminobenzoic acid (PABA) [p-, para-]
ε-aminocaproic acid [epsilon-]
ammonemia
AML—acute myelogenous leukemia
amyloidosis
    a. of multiple myeloma
ancillary
    a. measures
    a. therapy
anemia
    achlorhydric a.
    achrestic a.
    acquired sideroblastic a.
    ancylostome a.
    aplastic a.
    arctic a.
    asiderotic a.
    atrophic a.

anemia (continued)
    autoimmune hemolytic a.
    Baghdad spring a.
    Banti a.
    Biermer-Ehrlich a.
    breast a.
    a. of chronic disease
    Chvostek a.
    congenital a. of newborn
    congenital dyserythropoietic a.
    congenital nonspherocytic hemolytic a.
    constitutional aplastic a.
    Cooley a.
    Coombs-negative immune hemolytic a.
    crescent cell a.
    Czerny a.
    Diamond-Blackfan a.
    Dresbach a.
    Edelmann a.
    enzyme deficiency hemolytic a.
    erythroblastic a. of childhood
    Faber a.
    familial erythroblastic a.
    Fanconi a.
    febrile pleiochromic a.
    fish tapeworm a.
    fragmentation hemolytic a.
    globe cell a.
    glucose-6-phosphate dehydrogenase deficiency a.
    hemolytic a.
    Herrick a.
    hyperchromic a.
    hypochromic a.
    a. hypochromica siderochrestica hereditaria
    hypoplastic a.
    hypoplastic a., congenital
    icterohemolytic a.
    immunohemolytic a.
    Israels-Wilkinson a.
    Jaksch a.
    Larzel a.
    lead a.

anemia (continued)
Lederer a.
Leishman a.
leukoerythroblastic a.
lysolecithin hemolytic a.
macrocytic a.
malignant a.
Mediterranean a.
megaloblastic a.
meniscocytic a.
microcytic a.
microdrepanocytic a.
microelliptopoikilocytic a. of
Rietti, Greppi, and Micheli
myelophthisic a.
myelosclerotic a.
a. neonatorum
normochromic a.
normocytic a.
ovalocytary a.
pernicious a.
pernicious a., juvenile
physiologic a.
a. pseudoleukemica infantum
pyridoxine-responsive a.
pyruvate-kinase deficiency a.
radiation a.
sex-linked hypochromatic a.
of Rundles and Falls
sickle cell a.
sideremic a.
sideroblastic a.
sideropenic a.
spherocytic a.
target cell a.
thrombopenic a.
thrombotic microangiopathic
hemolytic a.
toxic a.
traumatic a.
triose-phosphate isomerase
deficiency a.
tunnel a.
unstable hemoglobin
hemolytic a.
von Jaksch a.
Wills a.
x-ray a.

angioimmunoblastic
a. lymphadenopathy
a. lymphadenopathy with
dysproteinemia (AILD)
aniline
a. fuchsin
a. gentian violet
a. red
anomaly
Chédiak-Higashi a.
Chédiak-Steinbrinck-
Higashi a.
Chiari a.
Hegglin a.
Huët-Pelger nuclear a.
May-Hegglin a.
Pelger-Huët a.
Pelger-Huët nuclear a.
Steinbrinck a.
anorexigenic
Ansbacher unit
anthracyclines [a class of drugs]
antiandrogens [a class of drugs]
antibody (antibodies)
See also in *Laboratory,
Pathology, and Chemistry
Terms.*
ABO a.
anti-Rh (Rhesus) a.
maternal a.
O a.
anticholinergics [a class of drugs]
anticoagulant
circulating a.
anticoagulants [a class of drugs]
anticoagulated
antidopaminergics [a class of drugs]
antiemetics [a class of drugs]
antiestrogens [a class of drugs]
antigen (Ag)
See also in *Laboratory,
Pathology, and Chemistry
Terms.*
ABO a.
Rh (Rhesus) factor a.
tumor-associated a.
tumor-specific a.
antinauseants [a class of drugs]

antineoplastics [a class of drugs]
antineoplastons [a class of drugs]
antisense drugs [a class of drugs]
Antoni
    neurilemoma, type A, type B
APA—aldosterone-producing ade-
    noma
aplastic
    a. anemia
    a. crisis
    a. pancytopenia
APTT, aPTT—activated partial
    thromboplastin time
area (areae, areas)
    body surface a. (BSA)
armamentarium
aromatase
    a. inhibitors
arrested
arthropathy
    hemophilic a.
ASCO—American Society of Clini-
    cal Oncology
ASH—American Society of Hema-
    tology
assay
    cancer antigen 125 (CA
        125) a.
    D-dimer a.
    estrogen receptor a. (ERA)
Astler-Coller
    modification of Dukes clas-
        sification
    staging system
atrophy
    paraneoplastic cerebellar a.
Auer
    bodies
    rods
AUL—acute undifferentiated leuke-
    mia
autologous
    a. transfusion
AVM—Adriamycin, vincristine,
    methotrexate
bacille Calmette-Guérin (BCG) vac-
    cine

bacillus (bacilli)
    See in *Laboratory, Patholo-
        gy, and Chemistry Terms.*
Bacillus
    See in *Laboratory, Patholo-
        gy, and Chemistry Terms.*
Bamberger
    hematogenic albuminuria
Banti
    splenic anemia
Bard
    syndrome
baseline
    b. film
basophilia
    pituitary b.
    punctate b.
basophilism
    Cushing b.
    pituitary b.
Bassen-Kornzweig
    disease
    syndrome
Bateman
    disease
    purpura
    syndrome
B cell [noun]
B-cell [adj.]
    B-c. lymphoma
BCG (bacille Calmette-Guérin) vac-
    cine
BCNU—bis-chloroethyl-nitrosourea
Béguez César
    disease
benefited
benignant
Bennett
    disease
    leukemia
benzo[a]pyrene
Bernard-Soulier syndrome
Biermer
    anemia
    disease
Billroth
    disease
bioavailability

biopsy
>bone marrow b.
>scalene lymph node b.

Biörck
>syndrome

Biörck-Axén-Thorson syndrome

Biörck-Thorson syndrome

Bizzozero
>cells
>corpuscles
>platelets

Blackfan-Diamond
>anemia
>syndrome

blastoma
>pulmonary b.

bleeder

bleeding
>postmenopausal b.
>punctate b.

blocker
>selective serotonin 5-HT$_3$
>(hydroxytryptamine) b.'s
>[a class of drugs]

blood
>occult b.
>whole b.

blood groups
>ABO
>Rh

blood volume expanders [a class of drugs]

BM—bone marrow

body (bodies)
>embryoid b.
>fuchsin b.
>Gamna-Gandy b.
>Howell b.
>Howell-Jolly b.
>Jolly b.
>psammoma b.
>Russell b.

bone marrow
>b.m. transplant

borderline

Borrmann gastric cancer typing system (types I–IV)

bowenoid

brachytherapy
>interstitial b.
>intracavitary application b.
>remote afterloading b.

braking radiation

Breslow
>classification
>thickness

Broders
>classification
>index (1–4)

Brompton
>cocktail

BT—bladder tumor
>brain tumor

BUDR—bromodeoxyuridine [now: broxuridine]

Burkitt
>lymphoma
>tumor

Ca, CA—cancer
>carcinoma

cachexia

CAF—cyclophosphamide, Adriamycin, fluorouracil

calcification
>conjunctival metastatic c.

CALLA—common acute lymphoblastic leukemia antigen

Calmette
>vaccine

cancer
>See also *carcinoma*.
>acinous c.
>adenoid c.
>arsenic c.
>asbestos c.
>c. atrophicans
>3,4-benzpyrene c.
>cellular c.
>cerebriform c.
>chromate c.
>chutta c.
>colorectal c.
>dendritic c.
>dermoid c.
>endothelial c.
>epidermal c.

cancer (continued)
    epithelial c.
    fungous c.
    glandular c.
    hematoid c.
    c. in situ
    Lobstein c.
    medullary c.
    melanotic c.
    metastatic c.
    mineral oil c.
    multicentric c.
    nickel c.
    osteoblastic c.
    osteolytic c.
    radiologist's c.
    radium c.
    retrograde c.
    Schneeberg c.
    scirrhous c.
    shale oil c.
    shale-worker's c.
    smoker's c.
    solanoid c.
    spider c.
    testicular c.
    tubular c.
    ulcer c.
    ulcerated c.
    villous duct c.
    vinyl chloride c.
    withering c.
    x-ray c.
canceration
canceremia
cancericidal
cancerigenic
carbonemia
γ-carboxyglutamate [gamma-]
carboxyhemoglobinemia
carcinoembryonic antigen (CEA)
carcinogen
carcinogenesis
carcinogenicity
carcinoid
    bronchial c.
    c. tumor

carcinoma (carcinomas, carcinomata)
    See also *cancer.*
    acinic cell c.
    acinous c.
    adenocystic c.
    adenoid cystic c.
    c. adenomatosum
    adenosquamous c.
    adrenal c.
    alveolar c.
    alveolar cell c.
    ampullary c.
    anaplastic c.
    apocrine c.
    argentaffin c.
    c. asbolicum
    basal cell c.
    c. basocellulare
    basosquamous cell c.
    betel-nut c.
    bile duct c.
    biliary c.
    brachiogenic c.
    bronchioalveolar c.
    bronchiolar c.
    bronchogenic c.
    burn scar c.
    cavitated c.
    cerebriform c.
    chorionic c.
    clear cell c.
    cloacogenic c.
    colloid c.
    colorectal c.
    comedo c.
    corpus c.
    cribriform c.
    c. cuniculatum
    c. cutaneum
    cylindrical c.
    cylindrical cell c.
    cylindromatous c.
    desmoplastic c.
    ductal c.
    ductal papillary c.
    c. durum
    embryonal c.
    embryonal c. of testis

carcinoma (carcinomas, carcinomata)
  (continued)
    encephaloid c.
    c. en cuirasse
    endometrioid c.
    epibulbar c.
    epidermoid c.
    epithelial c.
    c. epitheliale adenoides
    erectile c.
    erysipeloid c.
    c. erysipeloides
    esophageal c.
    exophytic c.
    c. exulcere
    fibrosing basal cell c.
    c. fibrosum
    follicular c.
    fungating c.
    gelatiniform c.
    gelatinous c.
    giant cell c.
    c. gigantocellulare
    glandular c.
    glottic c.
    granular cell c.
    granulosa cell c.
    gyriform c.
    hair-matrix c.
    hematoid c.
    hepatocellular c.
    hilar c.
    Hürthle cell c.
    hyaline c.
    hypernephroid c.
    infiltrating c.
    infiltrating ductal cell c.
    inflammatory c.
    c. in situ
    intermediary c.
    intermediate cell c.
    intraepidermal c.
    intraepithelial c.
    intrahepatic bile duct c.
    invasive c.
    islet cell c.
    Kulchitzky cell c.
    laryngeal c.

carcinoma (carcinomas, carcinomata)
  (continued)
    lenticular c.
    c. lenticulare
    lipomatous c.
    liver cell c.
    lobular c.
    macrofolliculoid c.
    c. mastitoides
    medullary c.
    c. melanodes
    melanotic c.
    Merkel cell c.
    metastatic c.
    metatypical c.
    microfolliculoid c.
    c. molle
    morphea-type basal cell c.
    mucinous c.
    c. muciparum
    c. mucocellulare
    mucoepidermoid c.
    mucoid c.
    c. mucosum
    c. myxomatodes
    nasopharyngeal c.
    nevoid basal cell c.
    c. nigrum
    nonencapsulated sclerosing c.
    oat cell c.
    occult c.
    oncocytic c.
    c. ossificans
    osteoid c.
    oxyphilic c.
    pancreatic c.
    papillary c.
    papillary serous c.
    parafollicular thyroid c.
    parenchymatous c.
    periportal c.
    peritoneal c.
    polypoid c.
    postcricoid c.
    preinvasive c.
    prickle cell c.
    pseudomucinous c.
    pultaceous c.

carcinoma (carcinomas, carcinomata)
(continued)
    pyriform fossa c.
    radiogenic c.
    renal cell c.
    c. sarcomatodes
    schneiderian c.
    scirrhous c.
    c. scroti
    sebaceous c.
    seminal c.
    signet-ring cell c.
    c. simplex
    solanoid c.
    spheroidal cell c.
    spindle cell c.
    spinous cell c.
    c. spongiosum
    squamous c.
    squamous cell c.
    string c.
    sweat gland c.
    c. telangiectaticum
    c. telangiectodes
    teratoid c.
    tonsillar c.
    trabecular c.
    transitional cell c.
    c. tuberosum
    tuberous c.
    undifferentiated c.
    V2 c.
    verrucous c.
    c. villosum
    VX2 c.
    c. with productive fibrosis
carcinomatoid
carcinomatosis
    meningeal c.
    c. of meninges
    c. peritonei
    c. pleurae
carcinomatous
carcinophilia
carcinophilic
carcinosarcoma
    Flexner-Jobling c.
    Walker c. 256

carrier
    hemophilia c.
cascade
    extrinsic coagulation c.
    intrinsic coagulation c.
Cassidy
    syndrome
Cassidy-Scholte
    syndrome
castration
    radiologic c.
CAV—cyclophosphamide, Adria-
    mycin, vincristine
CBC—complete blood count
CCT—composite cyclic therapy
CEA—carcinoembryonic antigen
cell
    See also in *Laboratory,*
        Pathology, and Chemistry
        Terms.
    bone marrow c.
    Paget c.
    red c.'s, red blood c.'s (RBCs)
    sickle c.
    white c.'s, white blood c.'s
        (WBCs)
cerebellopontine angle tumor
CF—Christmas factor
    citrovorum factor
CGL—chronic granulocytic leukemia
CHA—chronic hemolytic anemia
    congenital hypoplastic anemia
Chaussier
    areola
    line
    sign
Chédiak-Higashi
    disease
    syndrome
Chédiak-Steinbrinck-Higashi anom-
    aly
"chemo" Slang for chemotherapy.
chemistry (chemistries)
    blood c. studies
chemosuppression
chemotherapeutics
chemotherapy
    combination c.

chimera
    radiation c.
chimerism
    blood group c.
cholangiocarcinoma
chondrosarcoma
    juxtacortical c.
CHOP—cyclophosphamide,
    hydroxydaunomycin, Oncovin,
    prednisone
chordoma
choriocarcinoma
Christmas
    disease
    factor
Chvostek
    anemia
cin–. See also words beginning
    sin–, syn–.
CIS—carcinoma in situ
Clark
    classification of malignant
      melanoma (levels I–V)
    levels (I–V)
classification
    See also *index.*
    Astler-Coller modification
      of Dukes c.
    Borrmann c.
    Breslow c.
    Broders c.
    Clark c. of malignant mela-
      noma (levels I–V)
    Dukes c. (A, B, B_2, C_1, C_2)
      [B2, C1, C2]
    FIGO c. of endometrial car-
      cinoma (stages 0–IV)
    French-American-British
      (FAB) c.
    Jewett c. of bladder carcino-
      ma (stages 0, A–D)
    Jewett and Strong c. of
      bladder carcinoma (stages
      0, A–D)
    Kiel c. of non-Hodgkin lym-
      phoma
    Lennert c. of non-Hodgkin
      lymphoma

classification (continued)
    Lukes-Butler c.
    Lukes-Collins c. of non-
      Hodgkin lymphoma
    Marshall-Jewett-Strong c.
    McNeer c.
    REAL (Revised European
      American Lymphoma) c.
    Rye histopathologic c. of
      Hodgkin disease
    TNM (tumor, node, metasta-
      sis) c.
CLL—chronic lymphocytic leukemia
Cloudman melanoma
CMF—cyclophosphamide, metho-
    trexate, 5-fluorouracil
CML—chronic myelocytic leukemia
    chronic myelogenous leuke-
      mia
    chronic myeloid leukemia
CMM—cutaneous malignant mela-
    noma
C-MOPP—cyclophosphamide,
    mechlorethamine, Oncovin,
    procarbazine, prednisone
coagulant effect
coagulants [a class of drugs]
coagulation
    diffuse intravascular c. (DIC)
coagulopathy
    disseminated intravascular c.
      (DIC)
comedocarcinoma
concomitant
    c. chemotherapy
    c. radiation therapy
Cooley
    anemia
    disease
Coombs
    serum
    test
COP—cyclophosphamide, Oncovin,
    prednisone
coumarins [a class of drugs]
Cowden
    disease
    syndrome

CR—complete remission
crisis (crises)
 hemolytic c.
 sickle cell c.
cross-fire
 c-f. radiation therapy
 c-f. treatment
CTx—chemotherapy
culprit
 c. lesion
CVP—cyclophosphamide, vincristine, prednisone
cyclo—cyclophosphamide
cystocarcinoma
cytoprotective agents [a class of drugs]
Czerny anemia
DDAVP—desmopressin acetate [trademarked name]
Debré-de Toni-Fanconi syndrome
deficiency
 factor VIII d.
 fibrinogen d.
degeneration
 cerebellar d.
dehydroepiandrosterone (DHEA)
deleterious
 d. effects
Denny-Brown syndrome
dermatitis (dermatitides)
 carcinomatous d.
dermatosis (dermatoses)
 precancerous d.
 radiation d.
de Toni-Debré-Fanconi
 syndrome
de Toni-Fanconi
 syndrome
de Toni-Fanconi-Debré
 syndrome
DHL—diffuse histiocytic lymphoma
Diamond-Blackfan
 anemia
 syndrome
DIC—diffuse intravascular coagulation
 disseminated intravascular coagulation

Di Guglielmo
 disease
 syndrome
dimer
 D-d.
7,12-dimethylbenz[a]anthracene (DMBA)
dis–. See also words beginning dys–.
discrete
 d. lesion
 d. nodule
disease
 See also syndrome.
 Béguez César d.
 extramammary Paget d.
 Franklin d.
 Gaisböck d.
 graft-versus-host d. (GVHD)
 mammary Paget d.
 Paget d.
 Paget d. of bone
 Paget d. of the nipple
 Paget d. of penis
 Reed-Hodgkin d.
 sickle cell d.
 sickle cell–hemoglobin C d.
 sickle cell–hemoglobin D d.
 sickle cell–thalassemia d.
 Stuart-Prower factor deficiency d.
 Symmers d.
 Valsuani d.
 Vaquez d.
 Vaquez-Osler d.
 Werlhof d.
DL—Donath-Landsteiner (test)
DMBA—dimethylbenzanthracene
dose
 loading d.
DPDL—diffuse poorly differentiated lymphoma
Dresbach
 anemia
drip
 heparin d.
DTIC—dacarbazine
Dubreuilh precancerous melanosis

Dukes
  classification (A, B, B$_2$, C$_1$, C$_2$ [B2, C1, C2])
Dutcher body
Dyke-Young syndrome
dys–. See also words beginning dis–.
dyscrasia
  blood d.
EAC—Ehrlich ascites carcinoma
EBF—erythroblastosis fetalis
Edelmann
  anemia
  cell
effect [noun: result, outcome]
  additive e.
  adverse e.
  Deelman e.
  deleterious e.'s
  estrogen e., estrogenic e.
  mass e.
  side e.'s
efficacious
efficacy
Ehlers-Danlos
  disease
  syndrome
encased
ependymoma
epithelioma
  basal cell e.
epsilon
  e.-aminocaproic acid
ER—estrogen receptor
ERA—estrogen receptor assay
Erdheim
  tumor
"erithro–" Phonetic for words beginning erythro–.
erythremia
  high-altitude e.
erythroblastemia
erythroblastopenia
erythrocytapheresis
erythrocythemia
erythrocytic
erythrocytolysis
erythrocytophagous
erythrocytophagy

erythrocytorrhexis
erythrocytoschisis
erythrocytosis
erythrodegenerative
erythroid
erythroleukothrombocythemia
erythromyeloblastosis
erythroneocytosis
erythropenia
erythroplakia
erythrose
  e. péribuccale pigmentaire
    of Brocq
erythrosis
  e. of Bechterew
Estren-Dameshek syndrome
estrogen
  e. effect
Ewing
  sarcoma
  tumor
extramammary Paget disease
FAB—French-American-British
  [classification]
Faber
  anemia
  syndrome
factor
  f. I
  f. II
  f. III
  f. IV
  f. V
  f. VI
  f. XII
  f. VIII
  f. VIII:c
  f. VIII:CAg
  f. VIIIR:Ag
  f. VIII T
  f. IX
  f. X
  f. XI
  f. XII
  f. XIII
  activated clotting f.'s
  coagulation f.'s I–V, VII–XII
  f. D

factor (continued)
  f. H
  platelet-activating f.
  rhesus (Rh) f.
  tissue plasminogen f.
  von Willebrand f.
"fago–" Phonetic for words begin-
    ning phago–.
Fanconi
  anemia
  disease
  pancytopenia
  syndrome
FAP—familial adenomatous poly-
    posis
Felty syndrome
"fenomenon" Phonetic for phenom-
    enon.
FFP—fresh frozen plasma
fibroma
  desmoplastic f.
fibromatogenic
fibromatoid
fibromatosis
fibromatous
FIGO—Federation of International
    Gynecology and Obstetrics
FIGO
  classification of endometrial
    carcinoma
  nomenclature
  staging
Finzi-Harmer
  operation
Flexner-Jobling carcinosarcoma
FLSA—follicular lymphosarcoma
Fowler
  solution
FPC—familial polyposis coli
fraction
  blood plasma f.
Franklin disease
Froin syndrome
FU—fluorouracil
FUDR, FUdR—5-fluorouracil
    deoxyribonucleoside [now:
    floxuridine]

Gaisböck
  disease
  syndrome
galactemia
gamma
  g.-carboxyglutamate
  g.-glutamylcysteine syn-
    thetase (deficiency)
ganglial
ganglion (ganglia, ganglions)
  Troisier g.
Garcin syndrome
Gasser
  syndrome
Glanzmann
  disease
  thrombasthenia
Gleason
  grading score
  score on prostate carcinoma
γ-glutamylcysteine synthetase defi-
    ciency [gamma-]
glycopeptides [a class of drugs]
Goldstein
  disease
  hematemesis
  hemoptysis
Gorlin
  syndrome
Gross leukemia
GVHD—graft-versus-host disease
GVHR—graft-versus-host reaction
hairy cell leukemia
Halbrecht syndrome
Hare syndrome
Hb, Hgb—hemoglobin
HCC—hepatocellular carcinoma
Hct, hct—hematocrit
Hedinger syndrome
HELLP syndrome [hemolysis, ele-
    vated liver enzymes, and low
    platelet count occurring in
    association with preeclampsia]
hemangioma
  h.-thrombocytopenia syn-
    drome
hemangiosarcoma
hematinics [a class of drugs]

hematocrit (Hct, hct)
hematologic, hematological
hematology
hematopoietics [a class of drugs]
heme
hemoglobin (Hb, Hgb)
   sickle h.
   unstable h.
hemoglobin C-thalassemia disease
hemoglobinemia
hemoglobin E-thalassemia disease
hemoglobinopathy
hemoglobinuria
   intermittent h.
hemolytic
   h. anemia
   h. disease
hemophilia
   h. A
   h. B
   h. C
   Leyden h. B
   h. neonatorum
   vascular h.
hemosiderosis
   transfusional h.
hemostatics [a class of drugs]
heparin
   low-molecular-weight h.'s [a
     class of drugs]
hepatocarcinogenesis
hepatocarcinogenic
hepatocarcinoma
hepatocholangiocarcinoma
Herrick anemia
HF—Hageman factor
Hgb, Hb—hemoglobin
5-HIAA—hydroxyindoleacetic acid
"hipo–" Phonetic for words beginning hypo–.
histiocytosis
   malignant h.
HN—nitrogen mustard, mechloreth-
   amine
Hodgkin
   disease
   lymphoma

Hodgkin (continued)
   Rye classification of H. dis-
     ease
   sarcoma
Howel-Evans
   syndrome
Howell
   bodies
HS—hereditary spherocytosis
Huët-Pelger nuclear anomaly
Hürthle
   cell
   cell adenoma
   cell carcinoma
   cell tumor
Hutchinson
   lentigo
Hutchinson-Boeck
   disease
   syndrome
hyperalbuminemia
hyperalbuminosis
hypercellular
hypercellularity
hypercoagulability
hypercoagulable
hypercythemia
hypererythrocythemia
hyperhemoglobinemia
hyperhemolytic
hyperheparinemia
hypermetaplasia
hypernephroma
hyperplasia
   C-cell h.
   follicular h.
   giant follicular h.
   giant lymph node h.
   pseudoepitheliomatous h.
   Schwann h.
   thymic medullary h.
hyperplastic
hyperpyremia
hypersegmentation
   hereditary h. of neutrophils
hyperthrombinemia
hypertransfusion
hypervolemia

hypervolemic
hypochromatism
hypochromatosis
hypochromia
    idiopathic h.
hypocoagulability
hypocoagulable
hypocythemia
hypocytosis
hypoeosinophilia
hypoferremia
hypo-orthocytosis
hypoprothrombinemia
hyposarca
hypothrombinemia
IDU—idoxuridine
IH—idiopathic hyperprolactinemia
IHA—indirect hemagglutination
IL—interleukin [IL-1, IL-2, IL-3]
IL-2R—interleukin-2 receptor
Imerslund
    syndrome
Imerslund-Graesbeck
    syndrome
Imerslund-Najman-Graesbeck
    syndrome
immune
    i. neutropenia
immunosuppressants [a class of
    drugs]
immunosuppression
immunosuppressive
immunotherapy
incipient
    i. tumor
indanediones [a class of drugs]
index (indexes, indices)
    See also *classification.*
    Broders i. (1–4)
    hematopneic i.
    hemolytic i.
    maturation i.
    red blood cell indices, red
        cell indices
indolent
    i. lesion
    i. tumor

infection
    metastatic i.
    opportunistic i.
    secondary i.
    subclinical i.
inhibitor
    factor VIII i.
    matrix metalloproteinase
        (MMP) i.'s [a class of
        drugs]
    MMP i.'s [a class of drugs]
    phosphodiesterase III (PDE
        III) i.'s [a class of drugs]
    thymidylate synthase (TS)
        i.'s [a class of drugs]
    topoisomerase I i.'s [a class
        of drugs]
inoperable
insult
    hemorrhagic i.
interleukin
    i. 1 (IL-1)
    i. 2 (IL-2)
    i. 2R (IL-2R)
    i. 3 (IL-3)
irradiation
ITP—idiopathic thrombocytopenic
    purpura
IV—intravenous
Ivy
    bleeding time test
    method
Jaksch (von Jaksch)
    anemia
Jansky classification
Job syndrome
Joseph
    See *Sister Joseph.*
Josephs-Diamond-Blackfan syn-
    drome
"kahk–," "kak–" Phonetic for words
    beginning cac–, cach–.
Kahler
    disease
Kaplan-Meier survival curves
Kaposi
    sarcoma

Karnofsky
    rating scale
    status
    tumor grading
Kast syndrome
Kaznelson syndrome
"kemo–" Phonetic for words beginning chemo–.
Kiel classification
"kor–" Phonetic for words beginning cor– and chor–.
Kostmann
    disease
    syndrome
Krompecher
    carcinoma
Kulchitsky
    carcinoid
Kveim
    test
"kvos-tek" Phonetic for Chvostek.
Lambert-Eaton myasthenic syndrome
Larzel anemia
Launois-Cléret
    syndrome
lazy leukocyte syndrome (LLS)
LCL—lymphocytic lymphosarcoma
Leede-Rumpel phenomenon
Leishman
    anemia
Lennert classification
lentigo (lentigines)
    l. maligna
lesion
    cold l.
    destructive l.
    hot l.
    mass l.
    primary l.
    ring-wall l.
leukapheresis
leukemia
    acute lymphoblastic l. (ALL)
    acute nonlymphocytic l. (ANLL)
    acute promyelocytic l.
    adult T-cell l.
    aleukemic l.

leukemia (continued)
    aleukocythemic l.
    aplastic l.
    basophilic l.
    blast cell l.
    blastic l.
    Burkitt-type acute lymphoblastic l.
    chronic granulocytic l.
    chronic lymphocytic l. (CLL)
    chronic myelocytic l. (CML)
    embryonal l.
    eosinophilic l.
    granulocytic l.
    Gross l.
    hairy cell l.
    hemoblastic l.
    hemocystoblastic l.
    hemocytoblastic l.
    histiocytic l.
    leukopenic l.
    lymphatic l.
    lymphoblastic l.
    lymphocytic l.
    lymphogenous l.
    lymphoid l.
    lymphoidocytic l.
    lymphosarcoma cell l.
    mast cell l.
    megakaryocytic l.
    micromyeloblastic l.
    monocytic l.
    myeloblastic l.
    myelocytic l.
    myelogenous l.
    myeloid l.
    myeloid granulocytic l.
    myelomonocytic l.
    Naegeli l.
    nonlymphocytic l.
    plasma cell l.
    plasmacytic l.
    prolymphocytic l.
    promyelocytic l.
    reticuloendothelial cell l.
    Rieder cell l.
    Schilling l.
    smoldering l.

leukemia (continued)
    splenomedullary l.
    splenomyelogenous l.
    stem cell l.
    subleukemic l.
    testicular l.
    undifferentiated cell l.
leukocyte
    l.-poor red blood cells
leukocythemia
leukocytosis
    absolute l.
    agonal l.
    basophilic l.
    mononuclear l.
    neutrophilic l.
    pathologic l.
    physiologic l.
    pure l.
    relative l.
    terminal l.
    toxic l.
leukoerythroblastosis
leukopenia
    basophil l.
    basophilic l.
    congenital l.
    eosinophilic l.
    lymphocytic l.
    malignant l.
    monocytic l.
    neutrophilic l.
    pernicious l.
leukosarcoma
Leyden
    hemophilia B
Lloyd syndrome
LLS—lazy leukocyte syndrome
loading dose
low-molecular-weight heparins [a
    class of drugs]
Lukes-Collins classification
lymphangitis
    l. carcinomatosa
    carcinomatous l.
lymphocytosis
    acute infectious l.

lymphoma
    adult T-cell leukemia l.
    African l.
    B-cell l.
    Burkitt l.
    Burkitt-like l.
    clasmocytic l.
    cutaneous T-cell l.
    l. cutis
    diffuse l.
    follicular l.
    follicular center cell l.
    giant follicle l.
    giant follicular l.
    granulomatous l.
    histiocytic l.
    Hodgkin l.
    large cell l.
    Lennert l.
    lymphoblastic l.
    lymphocytic l.
    lymphocytic l., poorly dif-
        ferentiated
    lymphocytic l., well-differ-
        entiated
    malignant l.
    Mediterranean l.
    mixed lymphocytic-histio-
        cytic l.
    nodular l.
    non-Hodgkin l.
    null-type non-Hodgkin's l.
    pleomorphic l.
    sclerosing l.
    signet-ring cell l.
    small B-cell l.
    stem cell l.
    T-cell l.'s.
    T-cell l., convoluted
    T-cell l., cutaneous
    T-cell l., small lymphocytic
    testicular l.
    U-cell (undefined) l.
    undifferentiated l.
lymphomatous
lymphosarcoma
    fascicular l.
    sclerosing l.

MA—moderately advanced
MACC—methotrexate, Adriamycin, cyclophosphamide, CCNU (lomustine)
macrocythemia
malignancy
malignant
mammary Paget disease
marrow
    bone m.
    depressed m.
Marshall-Jewett-Strong classification
Mary Joseph
    See *Sister Joseph.*
mass
    m. effect
matrix metalloproteinase (MMP) inhibitors [a class of drugs]
MC, MTC—mytomycin C
MCH—mean corpuscular hemoglobin
MCHC—mean corpuscular hemoglobin concentration
MCHg—mean corpuscular hemoglobin
MCT—medullary carcinoma of thyroid
MCV—mean corpuscular volume
M/E—myeloid-erythroid [ratio]
medicine
    nuclear m.
melanoma
    lentigo maligna m.
    malignant m.
    nodular m.
    superficial spreading m.
melanotic [pertaining to melanin]
melenic [pertaining to melena, blood in the stool]
Merkel
    cell carcinoma
mesenchymoma
    benign m.
    malignant m.
metastasis (metastases)
    biochemical m.
    cannonball m.
    contact m.

metastasis (metastases) (continued)
    cotton-ball m.
    crossed m.
    direct m.
    hematogenous m.
    implantation m.
    lymphangitic m.
    mediastinal m.
    miliary m.
    nodular m.
    osteoblastic m.
    osteolytic m.
    osteoplastic m.
    paradoxical m.
    pleural m.
    retrograde m.
    transplantation m.
metastasize
metastatic
methemoglobinemia
    acquired m.
    congenital m.
    hereditary m.
    toxic m.
methemoglobinemic
methemoglobinuria
methylene blue
mets—metastases
MHB—methemoglobin
microabscess
    Pautrier m.
microadenoma
microinvasion
microinvasive
microlesion
micrometastasis
micronodular
"miel–" Phonetic for words beginning myel–.
migratory
    m. tumor
Mikulicz (von Mikulicz)
    syndrome
Mikulicz-Radecki
    syndrome
Mikulicz-Sjögren
    syndrome

mitotic
    m. inhibitors [a class of drugs]
M/L—monocyte-lymphocyte [ratio]
MLA—monocytic leukemia, acute
MLC—myelomonocytic leukemia, chronic
MLD—median lethal dose
MLS—myelomonocytic leukemia, subacute
MM—malignant melanoma
    multiple myeloma
MMP—matrix metalloproteinase
MMP inhibitors [a class of drugs]
monocyte
monocytic
monotherapy
MOPP—nitrogen mustard, Oncovin, prednisone, procarbazine
Moschcowitz
    disease
Mosse syndrome
MPD—maximum permissible dose
MS—morphine sulfate
MT—malignant teratoma
MTC—mytomycin C
MTI—malignant teratoma, intermediate
MTT—malignant teratoma, trophoblastic
MTX—methotrexate
müllerian
    m. mixed tumor
mumps
    metastatic m.
mustard
    L-phenylalanine m. (L-PAM)
    nitrogen m.
    uracil m.
myasthenia
    carcinomatous m.
myelitis
    metastatic m.
myelocytic
myelocytosis
myelodysplasia
myeloid
    m. metaplasia

myeloidosis
myeloma
    Bence Jones m.
    endothelial m.
    extramedullary m.
    giant cell m.
    indolent m.
    localized m.
    multiple m.
    plasma cell m.
    solitary m.
myelomatosis
myelopathy
myelopoiesis
myelosarcoma
myelosarcomatosis
myelosis
    aleukemic m.
    aplastic m.
    chronic nonleukemic m.
    erythremic m.
    funicular m.
    nonleukemic m.
myelosuppression
myelosuppressive
myelotherapy
myelotoxic
myelotoxicity
myopathy
    carcinomatous m.
"mytotic" Phonetic for mitotic.
myxocystoma
Naegeli
    leukemia
    syndrome
narcotic
National Cancer Institute (NCI)
National Prostatic Cancer Treatment Group (NPCTG)
NCI—National Cancer Institute
necrosis (necroses)
    radiation n.
    radium n.
necrotic
Nelson
    syndrome
neoadjuvant
    n. therapy

neoplasia
>gestational trophoblastic n.
>intraepithelial n.
>multiple endocrine n. (MEN)

neoplasm
>adrenal n.
>malignant n.
>metastatic n.
>stromal cell n.
>trophoblastic n.
>vascular n.

neoplastic

NER—no evidence of recurrence

NERD—no evidence of recurrent disease

Neumann
>syndrome

neurilemoma
>malignant n.

neurinoma
>malignant n.

neuritic

neuritis
>radiation n.

neuroblastoma
>olfactory n.

neuromyopathy
>carcinomatous n.

neuropathy
>carcinomatous n.
>radiation n.

neutropenia
>chronic benign n. of childhood
>chronic hypoplastic n.
>congenital n.
>cyclic n.
>familial benign chronic n.
>hypersplenic n.
>idiopathic n.
>Kostmann n.
>malignant n.
>neonatal n., transitory
>periodic n.
>peripheral n.
>primary splenic n.
>transitory neonatal n.

nitrogen mustards [a class of drugs]

nitrosoureas [a class of drugs]

NM—nuclear medicine

node
>Sister Mary Joseph n.

nodule
>Sister Mary Joseph n.

noninvasive

nonlymphocytic

NPCTG—National Prostatic Cancer Treatment Group

NSHD—nodular sclerosing Hodgkin disease

nuclear
>n. medicine

null
>n. cell lymphoblastic leukemia

"nur–" Phonetic for words beginning neur–.

occult

oligodendroglioma

operable

operation
>See in *General Surgical Terms.*

optimal

ortho
>o.-aminoazotoluene

Osler
>disease
>triad

osteopenia

osteopenic

osteoradionecrosis

osteosarcoma

osteosarcomatous

OTD—organ tolerance dose

OTR—Ovarian Tumor Registry

overtransfusion

Owren
>deficiency
>disease

PAB—*p*-aminobenzoate [p-, para-]

PABA—*p*-aminobenzoic acid [p-, para-]

PAF—platelet-activating factor

Paget
>cell

Paget (continued)
    disease
    disease, mammary
    disease of bone
    disease of the nipple
    disease of penis
    syndrome (I)
    test
pagetoid
Pancoast
    syndrome
    tumor
pancytopenia
    congenital p.
    Fanconi p.
panhematopenia
    primary splenic p.
papillomatosis
    malignant p. of Degos
para
    p.-aminobenzoate (PAB)
    p.-aminobenzoic acid (PABA)
Paterson
    syndrome
Paterson-Brown-Kelly
    syndrome
Paterson-Kelly
    syndrome
pathema (pathemas, pathemata)
pathogenic
pathognomonic
pathologic, pathological
PCV—packed cell volume
    polycythemia vera
PCV-M—polycythemia vera with
    myeloid metaplasia
PDE III (phosphodiesterase III)
    inhibitors [a class of drugs]
PDLL—poorly differentiated lym-
    phocytic lymphoma
pearl
    epidermic p.'s
    epithelial p.'s
Pel-Ebstein
    disease
    fever
    pyrexia
    symptom

Pelger nuclear anomaly
Pepper [eponym]
    neuroblastoma
    syndrome
pericarditis
    carcinomatous p.
petechia (petechiae)
phagocytosis
phagocytotic
phenomenon (phenomena)
    See also *sign.*
    Hecht p.
    Herendeen p.
    irradiation p.
    Leede-Rumpel p.
    Rumpel-Leede p.
phosphodiesterase III (PDE III)
    inhibitors [a class of drugs]
piggyback
piggybacking
"pikno–" Phonetic for words begin-
    ning pykno–.
plasma
    blood p.
plasma expanders [a class of drugs]
plasma protein fractions [a class of
    drugs]
Plummer-Vinson
    syndrome
pneumonitis
    irradiation p. and fibrosis
podophyllotoxins [a class of drugs]
polioencephalomyelopathy
    carcinomatous p.
polycythemia
    absolute p.
    appropriate p.
    benign p.
    chronic splenomegalic p.
    compensatory p.
    p. hypertonica
    inappropriate p.
    myelopathic p.
    primary p.
    relative p.
    p. rubra
    p. rubra vera
    secondary p.

polycythemia (continued)
    splenomegalic p.
    spurious p.
    stress p.
    p. vera
polyemia
polyneuropathy
    carcinomatous p.
POMP—prednisone, Oncovin,
    methotrexate, 6-mercaptopurine
postmastectomy
PPB—platelet-poor blood
PPTT—prepubertal testicular tumor
PRCs—packed red cells
PRD—postradiation dysplasia
precipitous
    p. drop [in blood pressure or
      laboratory indices]
    p. rise [in blood pressure or
      laboratory indices]
pro—prothrombin
profound
    p. anemia
protein-glutamine γ-glutamyltrans-
    ferase [gamma-]
pseudoanemia
    p. angiospastica
pseudoleukemia
PT—prothrombin time
pterins [a class of drugs]
PTT—partial thromboplastin time
pulmonary
    p. neoplasm
    p. sarcoidosis
purpura
    autoimmune thrombocytope-
      nic p.
    benign hyperglobulinemic p.
    cocktail p.
    dependent nonthrombocy-
      topenic p.
    fibrinolytic p.
    fibrinolytica
    hemogenic p.
    p. hemorrhagica
    hypergammaglobulinemic p.
    hyperglobulinemic p.
    p. hyperglobulinemica

purpura (continued)
    idiopathic p.
    idiopathic thrombocytopenic
      p. (ITP)
    malignant p.
    nonthrombocytopenic p.
    secondary thrombocytopenic
      p.
    thrombocytopenic p. (TP)
    p. thrombolytica
    thrombopenic p.
    thrombotic p.
    thrombotic thrombocytope-
      nic p.
    thrombotic thrombohemolyt-
      ic p.
    vascular p.
    Waldenström hyperglobu-
      linemic p.
PV—polycythemia vera
pyknocytosis
radiation
    r. dermatitis
    r. necrosis
    r. oncology
    r. sickness
    r. syndrome
    r. therapy
radiation therapy
    See *Radiology, Nuclear Med-*
      icine, and Other Imaging.
radiotherapy
    See *Radiology, Nuclear Med-*
      icine, and Other Imaging.
ratio
    myeloid-erythroid (M/E) r.
Rauscher leukemia virus
RBC—red blood cell(s)
    red blood [cell] count
RCA—red cell aplasia
RCV—red cell volume
RDW—red blood cell distribution
    width index
reaction
    graft-versus-host r. (GVHR)
reagent
    Sickledex r.

receptor
    estrogen r.
Recklinghausen-Appelbaum
    disease
Reed-Hodgkin disease
refractory
    r. anemia
regimen
    chemotherapeutic r.
registry
    cancer r.
renal
    r. cell carcinoma
"retic" Slang for reticulocyte (count).
reticulum (reticula)
    r. cell carcinoma
retinoids [a class of drugs]
Rh—Rhesus
Rh
    antibody
    blood group
    factor
    immunization
    incompatibility
    isoantigen
rhesus (Rh)
    r. factor
Rh neg—Rhesus factor–negative
Rh pos—Rhesus factor–positive
Rieder
    cell
    cell leukemia
roentgentherapy
    intraoral r.
    intravaginal r.
RT—radiation therapy, radiotherapy
Rumpel-Leede
    phenomenon
    sign
    test
Rundles-Falls
    anemia
Runeberg
    anemia
    disease
Rust [eponym]
    phenomenon
    sign

Rye classification of Hodgkin disease
SA—sarcoma
SAA—severe aplastic anemia
sarcocarcinoma
sarcocystosis
sarcoid
    Boeck s., s. of Boeck
    Darier-Roussy s.
    Schaumann s.
    Spiegler-Fendt s.
sarcoidosis
    beryllium s.
    Boeck s.
    s. cordis
    muscular s.
    myocardial s.
sarcoma (sarcomas, sarcomata)
    Abernethy s.
    adipose s.
    alveolar soft part s.
    ameloblastic s.
    botryoid s., s. botryoides
    cerebral reticulum cell s.
    chloromatous s.
    chondroblastic s.
    circumscribed cerebellar
        arachnoid s.
    clear cell s.
    deciduocellular s.
    embryonal s.
    endometrial stromal s.
    epithelioid s.
    Ewing s.
    fascial s.
    fibroblastic s.
    giant cell s.
    glandular s.
    granulocytic s.
    histiocytic s.
    Hodgkin s.
    idiopathic multiple pigment-
        ed hemorrhagic s.
    immunoblastic s. of B cells
    immunoblastic s. of T cells
    intracanalicular s.
    Kaposi s.
    Kupffer cell s.
    leukocytic s.

sarcoma (sarcomas, sarcomata)
(continued)
    lymphangioendothelial s.
    lymphatic s.
    melanotic s.
    meningeal s.
    mixed cell s.
    multiple idiopathic hemor-
       rhagic s.
    myeloid s.
    neurogenic s.
    osteoblastic s.
    osteogenic s.
    osteoid s.
    osteolytic s.
    parosteal s.
    periosteal s.
    s. of peripheral nerve
    polymorphous s.
    pseudo-Kaposi s.
    reticulum cell s.
    serocystic s.
    soft tissue s.
    spindle cell s.
    synovial s.
    telangiectatic s.
    s. of testis
sarcomatoid
sarcomatous
satellite lesion
SC—sickle cell
scale
    Karnofsky s.
scan
    See in *Radiology, Nuclear*
    Medicine, and Other
    Imaging section.
SCAT—sickle cell anemia test
Schaumann
    bodies
    disease
    sarcoid, sarcoidosis
    syndrome
Schilling
    leukemia
Schüller
    disease
    syndrome

Schüller-Christian
    disease
    syndrome
schwannoma
    malignant s.
scirrhoid
scirrhoma
    s. caminianorum
scirrhophthalmia
scirrhous [adj.]
scirrhus [noun]
score
    Gleason grading s.
section
    frozen s.
selective serotonin 5-HT_3 (hydroxy-
    tryptamine) blockers [a class
    of drugs]
seminome
Sertoli
    cell
    column
    tumor
Sertoli cell–only syndrome
Sertoli-Leydig cell tumor
shelf
    rectal s.
"shov-stek," "shvo-stek" Phonetic
    for Chvostek.
"shwah-no-mah" Phonetic for
    schwannoma.
sickle cell
    s.c. anemia
    s.c. disease
    s.c.–hemoglobin C disease
    s.c.–hemoglobin D disease
    s.c. hemoglobinopathy
    s.c.–thalassemia disease
    s.c. trait
sicklemia
sicklemic
sickler
side effect
sign
    See also *phenomenon.*
    Leser-Trélat s.
    Mosler s.
    Rommelaere s.

signature
  tumor s.
sin–. See also words beginning
  cin–, syn–.
Sipple syndrome
Sister Joseph, Sister Mary Joseph
  node
  nodule
SMA—sequential multiple analyzer
  [SMA 6/60, SMA 12/60, SMA
  20/60]
SMAC ["smack"]—sequential multiple analyzer plus computer
  [SMAC 7, SMAC 12, SMAC
  20]
solanine
solanism
spherocytosis
  hereditary s.
squamatization
squamous cell
ST—survival time
stab [German word for band, immature neutrophil]
stadium (stadia)
  s. acmes
  s. augmenti
  s. caloris
  s. decrementi
  s. defervescentiae
  s. fluorescentiae
  s. frigoris
  s. incrementi
  s. invasionis
  s. sudoris
staging
  clinical s. of cancer
  TNM (tumor, node, metasta-
    sis) s.
Steinbrinck anomaly
Sternberg
  disease
  giant cells
Stokvis
  disease
Stokvis-Talma syndrome
stool
  s. guaiac

Stuart-Prower factor deficiency disease
substitute
  blood s., plasma s.
Symmers
  disease
sympexion (sympexia)
syn–. See also words beginning
  cin–, sin–.
syndrome
  See also disease.
  Bazex s.
  Biörck-Axén-Thorson s.
  Biörck s.
  Biörck-Thorson s.
  carcinoid s.
  Cassidy s.
  Cassidy-Scholte s.
  Debré-de Toni-Fanconi s.
  Degos s.
  de Toni-Debré-Fanconi s.
  de Toni-Fanconi s.
  de Toni-Fanconi-Debré s.
  Gaisböck s.
  Gasser s.
  gasserian s.
  giant platelet s.
  HELLP s. [hemolysis, ele-
    vated liver enzymes, and
    low platelet count occur-
    ring in association with
    preeclampsia]
  hemangioma-thrombocyto-
    penia s.
  hemolytic-uremic s.
  Hutchison s.
  Imerslund s.
  Imerslund-Graesbeck s.
  Imerslund-Najman-Graes-
    beck s.
  Launois-Cléret s.
  lazy leukocyte s. (LLS)
  metastatic carcinoid s.
  Mikulicz-Radecki s.
  Mikulicz-Sjögren s.
  Nelson s.
  Neumann s.
  nevoid basal cell carcinoma s.

syndrome (continued)
    Paget s. (I)
    Paterson s.
    Paterson-Brown-Kelly s.
    Paterson-Kelly s.
    post-transfusion s.
    Rh-null s.
    runting s.
    s. of sea-blue histiocytes
    Sertoli-cell-only s.
    thrombocytopenia-absent radius (TAR) s.
    transfusion s.
synovial
    s. chondrosarcoma
    s. sarcoma
synovioma
    malignant s.
system
    ABO blood group s.
    TNM (tumor, node, metastasis) staging s.
T—tumor
TAT—thromboplastin activation test
taxanes, taxoids [a class of drugs]
TBSA—total body surface area
T cell [noun]
T-cell [adj.]
teratocarcinoma
teratologic, teratological
teratologist
teratoma (teratomas, teratomata)
    anaplastic malignant t.
    malignant t.
    tropoblastic malignant t.
    undifferentiated malignant t.
test
    See also in *Laboratory, Pathology, and Chemistry Terms.*
    CEA (carcinoembryonic antigen) t.
    D-dimer t.
    estrogen receptor assay (ERA) t.
    Kveim t.
    Paget t.

test (continued)
    partial thromboplastin time (PTT) t.
    platelet aggregation t.
    prothrombin t. (PT)
    Quick tourniquet t. (for prothrombin time)
    sickle cell t.
    thromboplastin generation t. (TGT)
thalassemia
    α-t. [alpha-]
    β-t. [beta-]
    δ-t. [delta-]
    δ β-t. [delta beta-]
    hemoglobin C-t.
    hemoglobin E-t.
    hemoglobin S-t.
    t. intermedia
    t. major
    t. minor
    sickle cell t.
theory
    somatic mutation t. of cancer
theraccines [a class of drugs]
therapy
    adjuvant t.
    anticoagulant t.
    antiplatelet t.
    combined-modality t.
    contact radiation t.
    hormonal t., hormone t.
    immunosuppressive t.
    neoadjuvant t.
    vaccine t.
threshold
thrombi (plural of thrombus)
thrombin
thrombocythemia
    essential t.
    hemorrhagic t.
    idiopathic t., primary t.
thrombocytopathic
thrombocytopathy
thrombocytopenia
    essential t.
    HIV-associated t.
    idiopathic t.

thrombocytopenia (continued)
    immune t.
    malignant t.
    thrombotic t.
thrombocytopenic
thrombocytopenic purpura (TP)
thrombocytosis
thrombogenic
thromboid
thrombolytics [a class of drugs]
thrombopenia
    essential t.
thrombosis
    See also *thrombus.*
    See also in *Cardiology* sec-
        tion.
thrombus (thrombi)
    See also *thrombosis.*
    agglutinative t.
    currant jelly t.
    fibrin t.
    hyaline t.
    laminated t.
    plate t., platelet t.
thrush
thymidylate synthase (TS) inhibi-
    tors [a class of drugs]
time (T)
    median survival t.
TIS—tumor in situ
TLD—tumor lethal dose
TMIF—tumor-cell migration–inhi-
    bition factor
TNF—tumor necrosis factor
TNM—tumor, nodes, metastases
    [tumor staging system]
topoisomerase I inhibitors [a class
    of drugs]
trait
    sickle cell t.
    thalassemia t.
transfusion
    bone marrow t.
transplantation
    allogeneic marrow t.
    bone marrow t.
treatment
    Minot-Murphy t.

treatment (continued)
    palliative t.
Troisier
    ganglion
    node
    sign
    syndrome
TSA—tumor-specific antigen
TSPAP—total serum prostatic acid
    phosphatase
TTP—thrombotic thrombocytope-
    nic purpura
tube
    Wintrobe t.
tumor
    argentaffin carcinoid t.
    Burkitt t.
    carcinoid t. of bronchus
    Hürthle cell t.
    migrated t.
    migratory t.
    müllerian mixed t.
    oat cell t.
    villous t.
type
    blood t.'s
UM—uracil mustard
unit
    See also in *General Medical
        Terms* and *Laboratory,
        Pathology, and Chemistry
        Terms.*
    Ansbacher u.
Valsuani
    disease
VAMP—vincristine, amethopterine,
    6-mercaptopurine, prednisone
vascular
    v. hemophilia
    v. tumor
VB, VBL—vinblastine
VC, VCR—vincristine
VDP—vincristine, daunorubicin,
    prednisone
vertebra (vertebrae)
    ivory v.
vertebral

villose, villous [adj.]
    v. duct cancer
    v. tumor
vinca alkaloids [a class of drugs]
Virchow-Hassall body
virus
    See also in *Laboratory,*
       Pathology, and Chemistry
       Terms.
    cancer-inducing v.
    human T-cell leukemia/lym-
       phoma v. (HTLV) [now:
       HIV]
    human T-cell lymphotrophic
       v., (HTLV) [now: HIV]
    papilloma v.
von Jaksch. See *Jaksch.*
von Willebrand (Willebrand)
    disease
    factor
    factor deficiency
    syndrome
"vos-tek" Phonetic for *Chvostek.*
VPC—volume of packed cells
Waldenström
    macroglobulinemia
    syndrome

Walker carcinoma 256
Wartenberg
    disease
wasting
    w. syndrome
WBC—white blood cell
    white blood [cell] count
WBR—whole-body radiation [ther-
    apy]
WDLL—well-diffcrentiated lym-
    phocytic lymphoma
Werlhof
    disease
Willebrand. See *von Willebrand.*
Willebrand-Jürgens
    syndrome
Wills
    anemia
Wintrobe
    tube
Witts anemia
WRCs—washed red cells
xanthoma (xanthomas, xanthomata)
    generalized plane x.
    planar x., plane x., x. planum
xanthosarcoma

Ophthalmology

A—amplitude of accommodation
    atropine
AAO—American Academy of Oph-
    thalmology
Abadie sign
Abbe
    condenser
abducens
    a. nerve
    nervus a.
    a. palsy
abducent
    a. muscle
    a. nerve
abductor
aberrant
    a. regeneration
abetalipoproteinemia
abient
abiotrophy
    retinal a.
ablatio
    a. retinae
ablation
ablepharia
ablepharon
ablepharous
ablephary
ablepsia
ablepsy
abradant
abrade
abrasio
    a. corneae
abrasion
    marginal a.
abrasor
abscess
    infraorbital space a.
    lacrimal a.
    orbital a.

abscess (continued)
    prelacrimal a.
    ring a.
    vitreous a.
abscessus
abscissa
abscission
    corneal a.
absinthe
absolute
    a. glaucoma
    a. hyperopia
    a. scotoma
abtorsion
AC—anterior chamber
acanthamebiasis
acanthocytosis
accommodate
accommodation
    absolute a.
    amplitude of a.
    binocular a.
    excessive a.
    negative a.
    positive a.
    range of a.
    relative a.
    subnormal a.
accommodative
    a. convergence
    a. convergence-accommoda-
      tion ratio
    a. effort syndrome
    a. esotropia
    a. iridoplegia
    a. palsy
    a. spasm
    a. target
accommodometer
ACG—angle closure glaucoma
achromocytosis

achromat
achromate
achromatic
    a. lens
    a. perimetry
achromatism
achromatopia
achromatopic
achromatopsia
acid
    boric a.
aclastic
acne
    a. ciliaris
acorea
acrocephalosyndactyly
    a. of Apert
action
acuity
    Vernier a.
    visual a.
acute angle closure glaucoma
adaptation
    chromatic a.
    color a.
    dark a.
    light a.
    photopic a.
    retinal a.
    scotopic a.
adaptometer
adduct
adduction
adductor
adenocarcinoma
adenologaditis
adenoma
    basophilic a.
    chromophobe a.
adenophthalmia
adherence
    a. syndrome
adhesive
    a. syndrome
Adie
    pupil
    syndrome

aditus
    a. orbitae, a. orbitalis
adnexa [grammatically plural, no singular form]
    a. oculi
adnexal
adumbration
aerial
    a. haze
"a-fak-e-a" Phonetic for aphakia.
afferent
    a. defect
    a. nerve
afferentiation
aftercataract
afterimage
    negative a.
    positive a.
    Purkinje a.
afterperception
Agnew
    operation
agnosia
    chromatic a.
    visual a.
    visual-spatial a., visuospatial a.
agonist
    prostaglandin a.'s [a class of drugs]
Ah—hypermetropic astigmatism
Aicardi syndrome
akinesia
    O'Brien a.
    Van Lint a.
aknephascopia
alacrima
albedo
    a. retinae
albinism
    a. I, a. II
    acquired a.
    Amish a.
    autosomal dominant oculo-cutaneous a.
    autosomal recessive ocular a. (AROA)
    brown a.

albinism (continued)
    complete imperfect a.
    complete perfect a.
    Forsius-Eriksson–type ocular a.
    localized a.
    Nettleship-Falls–type ocular a.
    ocular a. (OA)
    oculocutaneous a. (OCA)
    partial a.
    piebald a.
    red a.
    tyrosinase-negative (ty-neg) oculocutaneous a.
    tyrosinase-positive (ty-pos) oculocutaneous a.
    xanthous a.
    X-linked ocular a. (Nettleship) (XOAN)
    yellow mutant (ym) a.
Albright
    disease
albuginea
    a. oculi
albugo
albuminuric
    a. retinitis
Alcon cryophake
Alexander
    law
alexia
    optical a.
alexic
Alezzandrini syndrome
Allen
    cyclodialysis
    operation
allesthesia
    visual a.
allokeratoplasty
alopecia
    a. orbicularis
alpha
    a.-galactosidase A
Alport
    syndrome

Alström
    disease
    syndrome
Alström-Olsen syndrome
alternating
    a. esotropia
    a. strabismus
    a. sursumduction
AM—myopic astigmatism
amacrine
    a. cells
amaurosis
    albuminuric a.
    Burns a.
    cat-eye s., cat's eye a.
    central a.
    a. centralis
    cerebral a.
    compression a.
    congenital a.
    diabetic a.
    a. fugax
    hysterical a.
    intoxication a.
    Leber a.
    saburral a.
    uremic a.
amaurotic
    a. familial idiocy (AFI)
    a. nystagmus
    a. pupil
ambiopia
amblyope
amblyopia
    a. alcoholica
    ametropic a.
    arsenic a.
    astigmatic a.
    a. crapulosa
    crossed a.
    a. cruciata
    deprivation a.
    eclipse a.
    a. ex anopsia
    nocturnal a.
    postmarital a.
    quinine a.
    receptor a.

amblyopia (continued)
    reflex a.
    strabismic a.
    suppression a.
    tobacco a.
    toxic a.
    traumatic a.
    uremic a.
    West Indian a.
amblyopiatrics
American Hydron
Ames test
ametrometer
ametropia
    axial a.
    curvature a.
    index a.
    position a.
    refractive a.
ametropic
Ammon
    blepharoplasty
    canthoplasty
    dacryocystotomy
    filaments
    fissure
    operation
amotio
    a. retinae
amphamphoterodiplopia
amplitude
    a. of accommodation
    a. of convergence
AMPPE—acute multifocal placoid
    pigment epitheliopathy
ampulla (ampullae)
    a. canaliculi lacrimalis
    a. ductus lacrimalis
Amsler
    chart
    corneal graft operation
    grid
    marker
    test
anaglyph
Anagnostakis
    operation
anaphoria

anatomic equator
Andogsky syndrome
Anel
    lacrimal duct dilation
    operation
anesthesia
    See in *General Surgical
      Terms.*
Angelucci
    syndrome
angiogram
    fluorescein a.
angiography
    fluorescein a.
    orbital a.
angiokeratoma
    a. corporis diffusum
    a. corporis diffusum univer-
      sale
    diffuse a.
angiomatosis
    a. of retina
    a. retinae
angiopathia retinae juvenilis
angiophakomatosis
angioscotoma
angle
    alpha a.
    a. of anomaly
    anterior chamber a.
    a. closure glaucoma
    a. of deviation
    a. gamma
    a. of incidence
    inner a. of eye
    a. kappa
    a. lambda
    a. of minimum deviation
    nasal a. of eye
    outer a. of eye
    prism a.
    a. of refraction
angor
    a. ocularis
angular blepharitis
angulus
    a. iridocornealis
    a. oculi lateralis

angulus (continued)
    a. oculi medialis
anicteric
aniseikonia
aniseikonic
anisoaccommodation
anisocoria
anisometrope
anisometropia
anisometropic
anisophoria
anisopia
ankyloblepharon
    a. filiforme adnatum
annular
    a. plexus
    a. scotomo
annulus (annuli) [compare: anulus]
    a. ciliaris
    a. of Zinn
anomalopia
anomalous
    a. retinal correspondence
    a. trichromatism
anomaly
    Axenfeld a.
    Chédiak-Higashi a.
    Chédiak-Steinbrinck-
      Higashi a.
    Peters a.
    Rieger a.
    Steinbrinck a.
anophoria
anophthalmia
anopia
anopsia
anorthopia
anotropia
antagonist
    contralateral a.
    ipsilateral a.
anterior
    a. chamber
    a. chamber angle
    a. chamber cleavage
    a. chamber top
    a. ciliary arteries
    a. corneal staphyloma

anterior (continued)
    a. focal point
    a. hyaloid membrane
    a. megalophthalmos
    a. pole
    a. sclerotomy
    a. segment
    a. synechia
    a. uveitis
Anthony
    compressor
antimetropia
antimongoloid slant
antireflective coating
antisuppression exercise
Anton
    symptom
    syndrome
Anton-Babinski syndrome
anulus (anuli) [compare: annulus]
    a. of conjunctiva, a. con-
      junctivae
    a. iridis major
    a. iridis minor
    a. tendineus communis
AOA—American Optometric Asso-
    ciation
A pattern
Apert
    disease
    syndrome
aperture
apex (apices, apexes)
aphake
aphakia
aphakic
aphasia
    visual a.
apical
    a. clearance
    a. radius
    a. zone
apices (plural of apex)
apicitis
    orbital a.
aplasia
    retinal a.
aponeurosis (aponeuroses)

apparatus
    electro-oculogram a.
    Howard-Dolman a.
appearance
    beaten-silver a.
    cushingoid a.
applanation
    a. tonometry
applanometer
apprehension
    a. test
aqueous
    a. flare
    a. humor
    a. outflow
ARC—abnormal retinal correspon-
    dence
arch
    inferior palpebral a.
    marginal a. of eyelid
    Salus a.
arcuate
    a. scotoma
arcuation
arcus
    corneal a.
    a. juvenilis
    a. lipoides corneae
    a. palpebralis inferior
    a. palpebralis superior
    a. parieto-occipitalis
    a. senilis
    a. superciliaris
area (areae, areas)
    Broadmann a.
    a. choroidea
    cortical oculomotor a.
    cortico-oculocephalogyric a.
    fusion a.
    optic a.
    Panum a.
argamblyopia
argema
argon laser trabeculoplasty
Argyll Robertson
    See also *pseudo-Argyll*
      Robertson.
    pupil

Argyll Robertson (continued)
    sign
argyrosis
Arlt (von Arlt)
    disease
    line
    operation
    recess
    sinus
    trachoma
Arlt-Jaesche
    operation
Arroyo sign
arteriola (arteriolae)
    a. macularis inferior
    a. macularis superior
    a. medialis retinae
    a. nasalis retinae inferior
    a. nasalis retinae superior
    a. temporalis retinae inferior
    a. temporalis retinae superior
arteriole
    medial a. of retina
    nasal a. of retina
    temporal a. of retina
arteriosclerosis
    retinal a.
arteritis (arteritides)
artery
    cilioretinal a.
    hyaloid a.
    long posterior ciliary a.
    posterior conjunctival a.
    retinal a.
    short posterior ciliary a.
arthritis (arthritides)
Artificial Tears wetting drops
ARVD—Association for Research
    in Vision and Ophthalmology
AS—arteriosclerosis
A-scan
Ascher
    aqueous influx phenomenon
    negative glass rod phenome-
      non
    positive glass rod phenome-
      non

Aschner
>phenomenon
>reflex
>sign
>test
ASCO—American Society of Contemporary Ophthalmology
Aseptron II
AsH—hyperopic astigmatism
aspheric
>a. lenticular spectacles
asteroid hyalosis
asthenocoria
asthenometer
asthenope
asthenopia
>accommodative a.
>muscular a.
>nervous a.
>retinal a.
>tarsal a.
asthenopic
astigmagraph
astigmatic
>a. axis
>a. clock
>a. dial
astigmatism
>a. against the rule
>compound a.
>corneal a.
>hypermetropic a.
>hyperopic a.
>lenticular a.
>mixed a.
>myopic a.
>oblique a.
>retinal a.
>simple a.
>a. with the rule
astigmatometer
astigmatoscopy
astigmia
astigmic
astigmometer
astigmometry
asymmetric, asymmetrical
asymmetry

Atkinson
>technique
Atkinson-type lid block
atopic
atresia
>a. iridis
atrophia
>a. choroideae et retinae
>a. dolorosa
>a. gyrata of choroid
>a. striata et maculosa
atrophy
>Behr a.
>circumpapillary chorioretinal a.
>Fuchs a.
>optic a.
>Schnabel a.
>Schweninger-Buzzi macular a.
>senile a.
atropinism
atropinization
atypical
>a. monochromacy
>a. monochromat
Aubert
>phenomenon
autokeratoplasty
auto-ophthalmoscope
auto-ophthalmoscopy
Auto-Plot
axanthopsia
Axenfeld
>anomaly
>loop
>suture
>syndrome
Axenfeld-Crukenberg spindle
axial
>a. hyperopia
>a. length
>a. myopia
axis (axes)
>a. of Fick
>optic a.
>visual a.

bacillus (bacilli)
See in *Laboratory, Pathology, and Chemistry Terms.*
Bacillus
See in *Laboratory, Pathology, and Chemistry Terms.*
bacterium (bacteria)
See specific bacteria in *Laboratory, Pathology, and Chemistry Terms.*
Badal
operation
Baer
nystagmus
Bálint syndrome
Ballet
disease
sign
Bamatter syndrome
band
See also *layer, line, streak, and stria.*
b. keratopathy
silicone b.
bandage
See in *General Surgical Terms.*
Bárány
positional vertigo
Bard
sign
Bardelli
operation
Bardet-Biedl syndrome
Barkan
operation
Barraquer
method
operation
suture
Barraquer-Krumeich-Swinger
refractive set
bar reader
barrel
b. distortion
Barrio
operation

basal
b. iridectomy
b. lamina
base
b. of iris
Basedow
disease
triad
Bassen-Kornzweig
disease
syndrome
Basterra
operation
Batten
disease
Batten-Mayou
disease
Baumgarten
glands
Bausch & Lomb
cleaner
lubricant
solution
bay
lacrimal b.
Béal
conjunctivitis
syndrome
bear tracks
Becker
astigmatism test
phenomenon
sign
bedewing
Beer
collyrium
operation
Behr
atrophy
disease
pupil
syndrome
Bekhterev (Bechterew)
nystagmus
Bell
phenomenon
sign

Bence Jones
    test
Benedikt syndrome
Benson
    disease
Béraud valve
Berens
    3-character test
    operation
Berger
    sign
    space
    symptom
Bergmeister papilla
Berke
    operation
Berlin
    disease
    edema
Bernard
    syndrome
Bernard-Horner syndrome
Berneheimer fibers
Best
    disease
    macular degeneration
beta
    b. blockers [a class of drugs]
    b.-galactosidase
Biber-Haab-Dimmer
    degeneration
biconcave
biconvex
Biedl
    disease
Bielschowsky
    disease
    operation
    sign
    test
Bielschowsky-Jansky
    disease
Bielschowsky-Lutz-Cogan syndrome
Biemond
    syndrome (type I, type II)
Bietti
    dystrophy
    syndrome

bifixation
bifocal
bifocals
bifoveal
binasal
binocular
    b. indirect ophthalmoscopy
binocularity
binoculus
biomicroscopy
    slit lamp b.
bioptic
biorbital
biprism
Birch-Hirschfeld
    entropion operation
birdshot chorioretinopathy
birefractive
birefringence
birefringent
bitemporal
Bitot
    spots
bizygomatic
Bjerrum
    scotoma
    scotometer
    screen
    sign
black sunburst
Blair
    operation
Blasius
    operation
Blaskovics
    operation
Blatt
    operation
bleb
    filtering b.
    nuclear b.
"blef–" Phonetic for words beginning bleph–.
blennorrhagic
blennorrhea
    b. adultorum
    inclusion b.
    b. neonatorum

blennorrheal
blepharadenitis
blepharal
blepharectomy
blepharelosis
blepharism
blepharitis
    b. angularis
    b. ciliaris
    b. marginalis
    nonulcerative b.
    seborrheic b.
    b. squamosa
    b. ulcerosa
blepharoadenoma
blepharoatheroma
blepharochalasis
blepharochromidrosis
blepharoclonus
blepharocoloboma
blepharodiastasis
blepharoncus
blepharopachynsis
blepharophimosis
blepharoplast
blepharoplasty
    Ammon b.
blepharoplegia
blepharoptosis
blepharopyorrhea
blepharorrhaphy
blepharospasm
blepharosphincterectomy
blepharostat
blepharostenosis
blepharosynechia
blepharotomy
blepharoxysis
Blessig
    cysts
    lacunae
    spaces
Blessig-Iwanoff
    cysts
blind
blindness
    amnesic color b.
    apperceptive b.

blindness (continued)
    Bright b.
    central b.
    color b.
    cortical psychic b.
    eclipse b.
    flash b.
    letter b.
    night b.
    sign b.
    snow b.
    solar b.
    twilight b.
blink reflex
Bloch-Stauffer
    syndrome
Bloch-Sulzberger
    syndrome
block
    O'Brien b.
    retrobulbar b.
    Van Lint b.
blocker
    beta b.'s (β-blockers) [a
        class of drugs]
blow-in fracture
blown pupil
blow-out fracture
blue sclera
bobbing
Bochdalek
    valve
body (bodies)
    ciliary b.
    cytoid b.
    cytomegalic inclusion b.
    Elschnig b.'s
    fatty b. of orbit
    geniculate b.
    Hollenhorst b.
    Lipschütz b.
    Prowazek-Greeff b.
    trachoma b.'s
Böhm
    operation
Bonaccolto-Flieringa
    operation

Bonnet
    capsule
    syndrome
Bonnet-Dechaume-Blanc syndrome
Bonnier syndrome
Bonzel
    operation
border
    See also *limbus* and *margin*.
    lacrimal b.
Bordier-Fränkel sign
Borthen
    operation
Bossalino
    operation
Bourneville
    phakomatosis
Bourneville-Brissaud
    disease
Bowen
    disease
Bowman
    membrane
    muscle
    operation
    tubes
boxcarring
Braid
    strabismus
Brailey
    operation
braille
branch vein occlusion
Briggs
    law
    operation
Bright
    blindness
    disease
    eye
Brodmann areas
Brown-Kelly
    sign
Bruch
    gland
    layer
    membrane
Bruchner test

Brücke
    fibers
    lens
    lines
    muscle
    reagent
    tunic, tunica nervea
brunescent
Brushfield spots
B scan ultrasonogram
BSS—buffered saline solution
BSV—binocular single vision
BU—base (of prism) up
buckle
    scleral b.
Budinger
    operation
bufilcon A
bulb
bulbus
    b. oculi
Bumke pupil
bundle
    b. of Drualt
    papillomacular b.
Bunker implant
buphthalmia
buphthalmos
buphthalmus
Burch
    operation
burn
    corneal b.
Burns amaurosis
Burow
    operation
Busacca nodule
buttonhole
    b. iridectomy
Buzzi
    operation
BVA—best corrected visual acuity
b-wave
"byerrum" Phonetic for Bjerrum.
CA—corneal abrasion
Cairns
    operation
calcarine fissure

calcification
    conjunctival metastatic c.
caliculus (caliculi)
    c. ophthalmicus
caligo
    c. corneae
    c. lentis
    c. pupillae
Callahan
    operation
Calmette
    conjunctival reaction
    ophthalmic reaction
    ophthalmoreaction
caloric
    c. nystagmus
    c. testing
camera (camerae)
    c. anterior bulbi
    c. oculi
    c. oculi anterior
    c. oculi posterior
    c. posterior bulbi
    c. pulpi
    c. vitrea bulbi
campimeter
campimetry
canal
    Cloquet c.
    collateral pulp c.
    corneal c.
    Ferrein c.
    hyaloid c.
    Petit c.
    c. of Schlemm
    Sondermann c
    zygomatico-orbital c.
canaliculi (plural of canaliculus)
canaliculitis
canaliculization
canaliculodacryocystostomy
canaliculorhinostomy
canaliculus (canaliculi)
    c. lacrimalis
cancer
candela (cd)
candle-guttering
candle power

candlewax drippings
Cantelli sign
canthal
canthectomy
canthi (plural of canthus)
canthitis
cantholysis
canthoplasty
    Ammon c.
canthorrhaphy
canthotomy
canthus (canthi)
    inner c.
    c. inversus
    lateral c.
    medial c.
    nasal c.
    outer c.
    temporal c.
capillary (capillaries)
    c. hemangioma
capsitis
capsula (capsulae)
    c. lentis
capsulation
capsule
    c. of Tenon
capsulectomy
capsulolenticular
capsulotomy
carbonic anhydrase inhibitors [a
    class of drugs]
carcinoma (carcinomas, carcinomata)
    See also in *Oncology and*
        Hematology section.
    epidermoid c.
cardinal
    c. movements
    c. points
carotid
    c. artery
    c. cavernous fistula
Carter
    operation
caruncle
    c. epicanthus
    lacrimal c.

caruncula (carunculae)
    c. lacrimalis
caruncular
Casanellas
    operation
caseous
Caspar ring opacity
Castroviejo
    operation
cataphoria
cataphoric
cataract
    adherent c.
    adolescent c.
    after c.
    arborescent c.
    aridosiliculose c.
    aridosiliquate c.
    axial c.
    axillary c.
    black c.
    blood c.
    blue dot c.
    bony c.
    bottlemaker's c.
    brunescent c.
    calcareous c.
    capsular c.
    capsulolenticular c.
    caseous c.
    cerulean c.
    cheesy c.
    choroidal c.
    concussion c.
    congenital c.
    contusion c.
    coralliform c.
    coronary c.
    cortical c.
    cupuliform c.
    cystic c.
    diabetic c.
    discission c.
    dry-shelled c.
    embryonal nuclear c.
    extracapsular c.
    fibroid c.
    floriform c.

cataract (continued)
    fusiform c.
    glass blower's c.
    glaucomatous c.
    gray c.
    hard c.
    heat-ray c.
    hedger c.
    heterochromic c.
    hypermature c.
    immature c.
    incipient c.
    infantile c.
    intracapsular c.
    intumescent c.
    irradiation c.
    juvenile c.
    Koby c.
    lacteal c.
    lamellar c.
    lenticular c.
    lightning c.
    mature c.
    membranous c.
    milky c.
    morgagnian c.
    myotonic c.
    naphthalinic c.
    nuclear c.
    O'Brien c.
    occupational c.
    overripe c.
    perinuclear c.
    peripheral c.
    polar c.
    primary c.
    progressive c.
    puddler's c.
    punctate c.
    pyramidal c.
    reduplication c.
    ripe c.
    sanguineous c.
    secondary c.
    sedimentary c.
    senile c.
    siliculose c.
    siliquose c.

cataract (continued)
    snowflake c.
    snowstorm c.
    spindle c.
    stationary c.
    stellate c.
    subcapsular c.
    subtotal c.
    sunflower c.
    sutural c.
    syphilitic c.
    total c.
    toxic c.
    traumatic c.
    tremulous c.
    unripe c.
    Vogt c.
    zonular c.
cataracta
    c. accreta
    c. aridosiliquata
    c. brunescens
    c. cerulea
    c. complicata
    c. congenita membranacea
    c. coronaria
    c. electrica
    c. membranacea accreta
    c. neurodermatica
    c. nigra
    c. ossea
    c. syndermotica
cataractogenic
cataractous
catarrh
    vernal c.
cat-eye, cat's eye
    c-e. amaurosis
    c-e. pupil
    c-e. reflex
    c-e. syndrome
cautery
    Graefe c. (von Graefe c.)
    Hildreth c.
    Mueller c.
    Rommel c.
    Rommel-Hildreth c.
    Scheie c.

cautery (continued)
    Wadsworth-Todd c.
    wetfield c.
    Ziegler c.
cavernous
    c. hemangioma
    c. sinus
CDR—cup-to-disk ratio
cecocentral
cell
    See also in *Laboratory,*
        Pathology, and Chemistry
        Terms.
    activated reticular c.
    amacrine c.
    c. and flare
cellophane
    c. retinopathy
cellulose
    c. acetate butyrate
Celsus operation
center of rotation
centrage
central
    c. fixation
    c. fusion
    c. retinal artery
    c. retinal artery occlusion
    c. retinal vein
    c. retinal vein occlusion
    c. scotoma
    c. serous chorioretinopathy
    c. suppression
    c. visual acuity
centralis
centraphose
centraxonial
centric
centrocecal
centrophose
cerclage
cerebellopontine angle tumor
cerebral
    c. dyschromatopsia
cerebro-ocular
Cestan
    sign
    syndrome

Cestan-Chenais
   syndrome
Cestan-Raymond
   syndrome
CF—count fingers
CFF—critical flicker fusion test
CG—Cardio-Green
c̄ gl—correction with glasses
chalcosis
   c. lentis
   c. oculi
chamber
   anterior c.
   aqueous c.
   posterior c.
   vitreous c.
Chandler
   syndrome
Charcot
   triad
chart
   Donder c.
   Duane accommodative c.
   E-type c.
   Landolt c.
   Landolt ring c.
   Lebensohn c.
   pseudoisochromatic c.
   Reuss color c.
   Snellen c.
Chédiak-Steinbrinck-Higashi anomaly
chemosis
Cheyne
   nystagmus
chiasm
   optic c.
chiasma (chiasmata)
   See also *commissura.*
   c. arachnoiditis
   c. opticum
   c. syndrome
chiasmal
chiasmatic
Chievitz
   layer
chlorolabe
chloropsia

choke
   ophthalmovascular c.
choked disk
choriocapillaris
choriocele
chorioid
chorioidea
chorioretinal
chorioretinopathy
   birdshot c.
choroid
choroidal
   c. detachment
   c. flush
   c. hemorrhage
   c. hyperfluorescence
   c. nevus
choroidea
choroideremia
choroiditis
   areolar c.
   Doyne c.
   Förster c.
   c. guttata senilis
   Jensen c.
   juxtapapillitic c.
   c. myopica
   c. serosa
   syphilitic c.
   Tay c.
   toxoplasmic c.
choroidocyclitis
choroidoiritis
choroidopathy
   areolar c.
   guttate c.
choroidoretinitis
Choyce
   implant
   Mark VIII lens
chromatic
   c. aberration
   c. dispersion
   c. perimetry
chromatopsia
chromatoptometer
chromophobe
chromostereopsis

chymotrypsin
CI—complete iridectomy
Cibasoft
cibisotome
cicatrices (plural of cicatrix)
cicatricial
cicatrix (cicatrices)
    filtering c.
CICE—combined intracapsular cataract extraction
cilia
ciliarotomy
ciliary
    c. arteries
    c. body
    c. flush
    c. ganglion
    c. hyperemia
    c. muscle
    c. nerve
    c. process
    c. spasm
    c. vein
    c. zonule
ciliectomy
cilioretinal
    c. artery
    c. vein
cilioscleral
ciliotomy
cilium
cillosis
cin–. See also words beginning sin–, syn–.
cinching
circadian
    c. heterotropia
circinate
    c. exudate
    c. retinopathy
circlet
    Zinn c.
circumduction
cirsophthalmia
classification
    See also *index.*
    Duane c. of strabismus

classification (continued)
    Keith-Wagener-Barker c. (groups 1–4)
    Reese-Ellsworth c. of retinoblastoma
    van Heuven anatomical c. of diabetic retinopathy
Claude
    syndrome
Claude-Lhermitte syndrome
cleft
    corneal c.
Clens
Clerz
clinometer
clock dial
Cloquet canal
CME—cystoid macular edema
CMV—cytomegalovirus
co—contraction [syndrome]
CO—corneal opacity
COAG—chronic open-angle glaucoma
Coats
    disease
    retinitis
    ring
cobblestones
Cockayne
    disease
    syndrome
COG—closed angle glaucoma
Cogan
    disease
    dystrophy
    syndrome
cogwheel
    c. phenomenon
cogwheeling
Collier sign
Collin-Beard
    operation
collyrium
    Beer c.
coloboma
    c. of choroid
    Fuchs c.
    c. iridis

coloboma (continued)
    c. of iris
    c. lentis
    c. lobuli
    c. of optic nerve
    c. palpebrale
    c. retinae
    c. of vitreous
colorblind, color-blind
comitant
commissura (commissurae)
    See also *chiasma.*
    c. palpebrarum lateralis
    c. palpebrarum medialis
    c. supraopticae
commissural
commissure
    arcuate c.
    chiasmatic posterior c.
    Gudden c., c. of Gudden
    interthalamic c.
    lateral (palpebral c.
    medial palpebral c.
    Meynert c.
    optic c.
    palpebral c.
    supraoptic
commotio
    c. retinae
complementary
    c. afterimage
    c. chromaticities
    c. colors
complete
    c. iridectomy (CI)
compressor
    Anthony c.
conclination
concomitant
cone
    c. dystrophy
    c. monochromacy
    c. monochromat
    ocular c.
    retinal c.
    twin c.
    visual c.

conformer
    Fox c.
confrontation fields
congruence
congruent
congruous
conjunctiva (conjunctivae)
    c. adnata
    c. arida
    bulbar c.
    corncal c.
    fornix c.
    injected conjunctivae
    irritation of conjunctivae
    limbal c.
    marginal c.
    ocular c.
    orbital c.
    pale conjunctivae
    pallor of conjunctivae
    palpebral c.
    pink conjunctivae
    scleral c.
    tarsal c.
    tunica c.
conjunctivitis
    acne rosacea c.
    actinic c.
    allergic c.
    anaphylactic c.
    arc-flash c.
    atopic c.
    atropine c.
    bacterial c.
    Beal c.
    blennorrheal c.
    calcareous c.
    catarrhal c.
    chemical c.
    chronic c.
    contact c.
    croupous c.
    diphtheritic c.
    diplobacillary c.
    eczematous c.
    Egyptian c.
    Elschnig c.
    follicular c.

conjunctivitis (continued)
    gonococcal c.
    gonorrheal c.
    granular c.
    inclusion c.
    larval c.
    c. medicamentosa
    membranous c.
    meningococcus c.
    molluscum c.
    Morax-Axenfeld c.
    c. necroticans infectiosus
    neonatal c.
    parasitic c.
    Parinaud c.
    Pascheff c.
    c. petrificans
    phlyctenular c.
    prairie c.
    pseudomembranous c.
    purulent c.
    Samoan c.
    Sanyal c.
    scrofular c.
    squirrel plague c.
    trachomatous c.
    c. tularensis
    uratic c.
    vernal c.
    viral c.
    welder c.
    Widmark c.
    Wucherer c.
conjunctivodacryocystostomy
conjunctivoma
conjunctivoplasty
conjunctivorhinostomy
conoid
    Sturm c.
conophthalmus
consensual
constricted
Contino
    epithelioma
    glaucoma
Contique
contralateral
    c. antagonist

contralateral (continued)
    c. synergist
convergence
    accommodative c.
    c. amplitudes
    fusional c.
    c. insufficiency
    proximal c.
    relative c.
    c. spasm
    voluntary c.
convergent
convergiometer
convex
convexity
convexoconcave
    c. lens
convexoconvex
Copeland
    implant
copiopia
copper
    c. wire effect
    c. wiring
Corbett spud
coreclisis
corectasis
corectome
corectomedialysis
corectomy
corectopia
coredialysis
corediastasis
corelysis
coremorphosis
corenclisis
coreometer
coreometry
coreoplasty
corestenoma
coretomedialysis
coretomy
cornea
    conical c.
    c. farinata
    c. globosa
    c. guttata
    c. opaca

cornea (continued)
    c. plana
    sugar-loaf c.
    Vogt c.
corneal
    c. abrasion
    c. apex
    c. astigmatism
    c. bedewing
    c. button
    c. cap
    c. dellen
    c. dystrophy
    c. erosion
    c. lens
    c. reflex
    c. scraping
    c. transplant
    c. tubes
    c. ulcer
corneal graft
    lamellar c.g.
    mushroom c.g.
    penetrating c.g.
corneitis
corneoblepharon
corneoiritis
corneosclera
corona (coronae)
    c. ciliaris
    Zinn c.
coronal
coroparelcysis
coroplasty
coroscopy
corotomy
corporis (genitive of corpus)
corpus (corpora)
    c. vitreum
correspondence
    anomalous retinal c.
    harmonious retinal c.
    retinal c.
cortex (cortices)
    c. lentis
    occipital c.
corticis (genitive of cortex)

cotton-wool
    c.-w. exudates
    c.-w. patches
    c.-w. spots
couching
CPEO—chronic progressive external ophthalmoplegia
CR—corneal reflex
cramosynostosis
cranial [adj.]
craniofacial
craniophyaryngioma
CRAO—central retinal artery occlusion
Credé prophylaxis
cribriform
    c. ligament
    c. plate
cribrum (cribra)
crisis (crises)
    Pel crises
Critchett
    operation
crocodile tears
Crouzon
    disease
    syndrome
CRV—central retinal vein
CRVO—central retinal vein occlusion
cryodestruction
cryoextraction
cryoextractor
    Amoils c.
    Bellows c.
cryogenic
cryopexy
cryophake
    Alcon c.
    Keeler c.
cryoprobe
    Amoils c.
cryoptor
    Thomas c.
crypt
    c.'s of Fuchs
    c.'s of iris
cryptophthalmos
crystalline

C&S—conjunctiva and sclera
cuff
    Honan c.
cul-de-sac
    conjunctival c.
cupped disk
cupping
cup-to-disk ratio
cupuliform
curettement
Custodis
    operation
Cutler-Beard
    operation
Cutlet implant
CV—color vision
CVF—central visual field
CWS—cotton-wool spot
cx—convex
cyanolabe
cyanosis
    c. bulbi
    c. retinae
cyclectomy
cyclicotomy
cyclitic
cyclitis
    heterochromic c.
    purulent c.
    serous c.
cycloanemization
cycloceratitis
cyclochoroiditis
cyclocryopexy
cyclocryotherapy
cyclodamia
cyclodeviation
cyclodialysis
cyclodiathermy
cycloduction
cycloelectrolysis
cyclogram
cyclokeratitis
cyclophoria
cyclophorometer
cyclopia
cycloplegia
cycloplegics [a class of drugs]

cyclops
cyclospasm
cyclotomy
cyclotorsion
cyclotropia
cycloversion
cylindrical
cyst
    Blessig c.
    Blessig-Iwanoff c.
    meibomian c.
cystitomy
cystoid macular edema
cytomegalic inclusion disease (CID,
    CMID)
cytomegalovirus (CMV)
Czermak
    operation
D—diopter
dacryadenalgia
dacryadenoscirrhus
dacryagogatresia
dacryagogic
dacryagogue
dacrycystalgia
dacrycystitis
dacryelcosis
dacryoadenalgia
dacryoadenectomy
dacryoblennorrhea
dacryocanaliculitis
dacryocele
dacryocyst
dacryocystalgia
dacryocystectasia
dacryocystectomy
dacryocystis
    phlegmonous d.
    syphilitic d.
    trachomatous d.
    tuberculous d.
dacryocystitome
dacryocystoblennorrhea
dacryocystocele
dacryocystogram
dacryocystography
dacryocystoptosis
dacryocystorhinostenosis

dacryocystorhinostomy
dacryocystorhinotomy
dacryocystostenosis
dacryocystostomy
dacryocystosyringotomy
dacryocystotome
dacryocystotomy
    Ammon d.
dacryogenic
dacryohelcosis
dacryohemorrhea
dacryolin
dacryolith
    Desmarres d.
dacryolithiasis
dacryoma
dacryon
dacryops
dacryopyorrhea
dacryopyosis
dacryorhinocystotomy
dacryorrhea
dacryosinusitis
dacryosolenitis
dacryostenosis
dacryostomy
dacryosyrinx
Dalen-Fuchs nodule
Dalrymple
    disease
    sign
darkfield
    d. examination
Daviel
    operation
Davis
    spud
DCC—double concave
DCx—double convex
DD—disk diameter
DDH—dissociated double hyper-
    tropia
debrider
    Sauer d.
decentration
declination
decompression
    Naffziger orbital d.

decussatio (decussationes)
    See *chiasma* and *commissura.*
degeneration
    Best macular d.
    Biber-Haab-Dimmer d.
    cerebromacular d.
    congenital macular d.
    hyaline d.
    Kozlowski d.
    lattice d.
    macular d.
    retinal lattice d.
    vitelliform d.
    Vogt d.
de Grandmont
    operation
dehiscence
    iris d.
Dejean syndrome
delacrimation
delimiting keratotomy
dellen
Del Toro
    operation
de Morsier
    syndrome
de Morsier-Gauthier
    syndrome
Demours membrane
demyelinate
demyelinization
dendrite
deorsumduction
deorsumvergence
deorsumversion
deprimens oculi
depth of perception
dermoid cyst
Descartes law
Descemet
    membrane
descemetitis
descemetocele
Desmarres
    dacryolith
    law
    scarifier

detachment
  d. of retina
  retinal d.
  rhegmatogenous d.
  d. of vitreous
deterioration
deutan
deuteranomalopia
deuteranomaly
deuteranopia
deviation
  primary d.
  secondary d.
  skew d.
Devic
  disease
  syndrome
DeWecker
  operation
dextroclination
dextrocular
dextrocularity
dextrocycloduction
dextrocycloversion
dextroduction
dextrotorsion
D-film
DFP—diisopropyl fluorophosphate
diabetic retinopathy
dial
  clock d.
  fan d.
  Lancaster Regan d.
  sunburst d.
dialysis
  d. retinae
diastasis
  iris d.
dichromatism
dichromatopsia
diffraction
diktyoma
dilator
  d. muscle
  d. pupillae
Dimitri
  disease
Dimmer keratitis

DIMOAD—diabetes insipidus, diabetes mellitus, optic atrophy, deafness [syndrome]
dimple
  Fuchs d.
diopsimeter
diopter
  prism d.
dioptometer
dioptometry
dioptoscopy
dioptre
dioptric
dioptrics
dioptrometer
dioptrometry
dioptroscopy
dioptry
diplopia
  binocular d.
  crossed d.
  heteronymous d.
  homonymous d.
  monocular d.
  paradoxical d.
  pathologic d.
  physiologic d.
  torsional d.
diplopiometer
direct
  d. ophthalmoscopy
dis–. See also words beginning dys–.
disc
  See *disk.*
disci (genitive and plural of discus)
disciform ["disiform"]
discission
  d. of lens
discitis [pref: diskitis]
disclination
disconjugate
discus (disci)
disease
  See also *syndrome.*
  Albright d.
  Arlt d.
  Ballet d.
  Basedow d.

disease (continued)
  Batten d.
  Batten-Mayou d.
  Behr d.
  Benson d.
  Berlin d.
  Best d.
  Biedl d.
  Bielschowsky d.
  Bielschowsky-Jansky d.
  Bourneville-Brissaud d.
  Bowen d.
  Coats d.
  Crouzon d.
  cytomegalic inclusion d.
    (CID, CMID)
  Dalrymple d.
  Devic d.
  Dimitri d.
  Eales d.
  Flatau-Schilder d.
  Franceschetti d.
  Gaucher d.
  Goldflam d.
  Goldflam-Erb d.
  Graefe d.
  Graves d.
  Hand-Schüller-Christian d.
  Harada d.
  Heerfordt d.
  Hippel d.
  Hünermann d.
  Jensen d.
  Kalischer d.
  Kimmelstiel-Wilson d.
  Koeppe d.
  Kuhnt-Junius d.
  Lauber d.
  Leber d.
  Lindau d.
  Lindau-von Hippel d.
  Marsh d.
  Masuda-Kitahara d.
  Mikulicz d.
  Möbius d.
  Niemann-Pick d.
  Norrie d.
  Oguchi d.

disease (continued)
  Purtscher d.
  Recklinghausen d.
  Reis-Bücklers d.
  Reiter d.
  Schilder d.
  Sichel d.
  Sjögren d.
  Sneddon-Wilkinson d.
  Steinert d.
  Vogt d.
  Vogt-Spielmeyer d.
  von Hippel-Lindau d.
  von Recklinghausen d.
  Wagner d.
  Weil d.
  Westphal-Strümpell d.
  Wilson d.
"disiform" Phonetic for disciform.
disinsertion
disjugate
disk
    *Note: Some specialists and
      references prefer* disc.
  anangioid d.
  ciliary d.
  d. diameter
  d. drusen
  optic d.
  Placido d.
  Rekoss d.
  stroboscopic d.
diskiform
dissociated
  d. nystagmus
  d. position
  d. vertical deviation
distichiasis
distometer
divergence
  d. amplitudes
  d. excess
  d. insufficiency
Dix spud
D&N—distance and near [vision]
Doherty implant
doll's head
    phenomenon

dominance
Donders
    chart
    glaucoma
    law
    line
dot
    See also *disk, macula, macule,* and *spot.*
    Gunn d.
    Mittendorf d.
    Trantas d.
Dougherty irrigator
Douvas rotoextractor
downbeat nystagmus
down-gaze
Doyne
    choroiditis
    colloid degeneration
    familial honeycombed
        choroiditis
    iritis
DR—diabetic retinopathy
Draeger tonometer
dressing
    See in *General Surgical Terms.*
dropper
    Undine d.
Drualt
    bundle (bundle of Drualt)
dry eye syndrome
Duane
    accommodative chart
    syndrome
Duchenne-Erb
    paralysis
duct
    lacrimal d.
    lacrimonasal d.
    nasolacrimal d.
    tear d.
duction
ductus (ductus)
    d. lacrimales
Duddell membrane
Duke-Elder lamp
duochrome test

Dupuy-Dutemps
    operation
Durr
    operation
DUSN—diffuse unilateral subacute
    neuroretinitis
DV—double vision
DVA—distance visual acuity
DVD—dissociated vertical deviation
    dissociated vertical diver-
        gence
dys–. See also words beginning dis–.
dyschromatopsia
dyscoria
dysmegalopsia
dysmetria
    ocular motor d.
dysopia
    d. algera
dysopsia
dysplastic coloboma
dystrophy
    Bietti d.
    Cogan d.
    corneal d.
    Fehr d.
    Fleischer d.
    Franceschetti d.
    Francois d.
    Fuchs d.
    Groenouw d.
    Maeder-Danis d.
    Meesmann d.
    oculocerebrorenal d.
    Pillat d.
    Salzmann d.
    Schlichting d.
    Schnyder d.
    vitelliform macular d.
E—electron emmetropia
    esophoria
    esotropia
Eales
    disease
ECC—extracapsular cataract
ECCE—extracapsular cataract
    extraction

eccentric
    e. fixation
ECD—endothelial corneal dystrophy
ECF—epicanthic fold
echinophthalmia
echography
echo-ophthalmography
ectasia
    e. iridis
ectiris
ectochoroidea
ectocornea
ectopia
    e. lentis
    e. pupillae congenita
ectropion
    e. cicatriceum
    cicatricial e.
    flaccid e.
    e. luxurians
    e. paralyticum
    e. sarcomatosum
    e. senilis
    e. spasticum
    e. uveae
ectropium
edema
    Berlin e.
    Iwanoff retinal e.
    Stellwag brawny e.
Edinger-Westphal nucleus
effect [noun: result, outcome]
    See also *phenomenon, reflex,*
      and *sign.*
    copper wire e.
    McCollough e.
    Purkinje e.
    silver wire e.
efferent
egilops
Egyptian
    conjunctivitis
    ophthalmia
eightball hyphema
eikonometer
EKC—epidemic keratoconjunctivitis
"eko–" Phonetic for words begin-
    ning echo–.

elastosis
    e. dystrophica
Eldridge-Green lamp
electrode
    Gradle e.
    Kronfeld e.
    Pischel e.
    Weve e.
electromagnetic
    e. spectrum
electronystagmogram (ENG)
electronystagmography
electro-oculogram (EOG)
electro-oculography
electroparacentesis
electroperimetry
electroretinogram (ERG)
electroretinograph
electroretinography
Elliot
    corneal trephination
    operation
Elschnig
    conjunctivitis
    operation
    spots
    syndrome
Ely
    operation
Em—emmetropia
embolism
    retinal e.
embolus (emboli)
embryotoxon
emergent ray
emmetrope
emmetropia
emmetropic
endophthalmitis
    e. phakoanaphylactica
endothelia (plural of endothelium)
endothelialization
endothelioid
endothelioma
    Sidler-Huguenin e.
endothelium (endothelia)
    e. camerae anterioris oculi
    corneal e.

endpoint nystagmus
ENG—electronystagmogram
    electronystagmography
enophthalmos
enstrophe
entoptic
entoptoscopy
entoretina
entropion
    e. cicatriceum
    cicatricial e.
    e. spasticum
    e. uveae
entropium
EOG—electro-oculogram
EOM—extraocular movement(s)
    extraocular muscle(s)
EOMI—extraocular muscles intact
epiblepharon
epibulbar
epicanthal
epicanthus
epicapsular
epicauma
epiphora
episclera
episcleral
episcleritis
    gouty e.
    e. partialis fugax
episclerotitis
epitarsus
epithelia (plural of epithelium)
epithelial
    e. downgrowth
epitheliitis
epithelioma
    Contino e.
epitheliopathy
    acute multifocal placoid pigment e.
epitheliosis
    e. desquamativa conjunctivae
epithelium (epithelia)
    e. anterius corneae
    e. corneae
    corneal e.
    e. of lens

epithelium (epithelia) (continued)
    e. lentis
    e. pigmentosum partis ciliaris retinae
    e. posterius pigmentosum partis iridicae retinae
    retinal pigment e.
equator
    e. bulbi oculi
    e. of crystalline lens
    e. of eyeball
    e. of lens
    e. lentis
equatorial
    e. degeneration
    e. meridian
equilibrating
    e. operation
Erb-Duchenne paralysis
ERG—electroretinogram
erosion
erythrolabe
erythropia
erythropsia
esodeviation
esophoria
esophoric
esotropia
esotropic
ET—esotropia
E test
ethmoid bone
E trisomy
euchromatopsy
euryopia
euthyphoria
Eversbusch
    operation
evulsio
    e. nervi optici
Ewald
    law
ex—exophthalmos
examination
    darkfield e.
excavatio (excavationes)
    e. disci
    e. papillae nervi optici

excavation
    atrophic e.
    glaucomatous e.
    e. of optic disk
    physiologic e.
excycloduction
excyclophoria
excyclotropia
excyclovergence
exodeviation
exophoria
exophoric
exophthalmic
exophthalmogenic
exophthalmometer
    Hertel e.
    Luedde e.
exophthalmometric
exophthalmos
    endocrine e.
    pulsating e.
exorbitism
exotropia
exotropic
expressor
    Arruga e.
    Heath e.
    Smith e.
expulsive
externus
extinction
extorsion
extracapsular
extraction
    roto e.
exudative
    e. retinitis
eye
    blear e.
    Bright e.
    cinema e.
    dark-adapted e.
    doll's e.'s
    epiphyseal e.
    exciting e.
    hare e.
    Klieg e.
    lazy e.

eye (continued)
    light-adapted e.
    monochromatic e.
    Nairobi e.
    parietal e.
    pineal e.
    pink e. [also: pinkeye, pink-
        eye]
    schematic e.
    Snellen reform e.
    squinting e.
    sympathizing e.
eyeball
eyebrow
eyecup
eyeground
eyelash
eyelid
eyespot, eye spot
eyestrain
F—field of vision
facies (facies)
    Hutchinson f.
facultative
    f. hyperopia
    f. suppression
Faden procedure
"fako–" Phonetic for words begin-
    ning phaco–.
falciform fold
Farnsworth
    D-100 test
farsighted
farsightedness
Fasanella-Servat
    operation
fascia (fasciae)
    f. bulbi
    lacrimal f.
    muscular f. of eye
    Tenon f.
fasciculus (fasciculi)
FD—focal distance
Federov implant
Fehr dystrophy
"fenomenon" Phonetic for phenom-
    enon.
FER—familial exudative retinopathy

Ferree-Rand
    perimeter
Ferrein canal
FEV—familial exudative vitreo-
    retinopathy
FFF—flicker, fusion, frequency (test)
FFT—flicker fusion threshold
fiber
    Berneheimer f.
    Brücke f.
    Monakow f.'s
    Muller f.
    optic nerve f.
    Sappey f.
fiberoptics
fibroplasia
    retrolental f.
fibrosis
Fick
    axis
    halo
field
Fiessinger-Leroy-Reiter
    syndrome
figure
    achromatic f.
    chromatic f.
    fortification f
    Purkinje f.
    Stifel f.
    Zollner f
filament
filamentary
Filatov
    operation
Filatov-Marzinkowsky
    operation
Finnoff transilluminator
Fisher
    syndrome
fishmouth
    f. tear
fissura (fissurae)
fissure
    corneal f.
    palpebral f.
fistula (fistulas, fistulae)

fixation
    f. axis
    binocular f.
    f. reflex
Flajani
    operation
Flatau-Schilder
    disease
Fleischer
    dystrophy
    ring
Flexlens
Flieringa ring
"flikt–" Phonetic for words begin-
    ning phlyct–.
floater
flock of floaters
"flor–" Phonetic for words begin-
    ning fluor–.
Florentine iris
Flouren law
fluctuation
fluid
    intraocular f.
fluorescein
    f. angiography
    f. dye disappearance test
    f. fundus photography
    f. sodium
fluorescence
    f. retinal photography
fluorophotometry
"flur–" Phonetic for words begin-
    ning fluor–.
focimeter
focus (foci)
    aplanatic f.
    conjugate f.
    principal foci
    real f.
Foerster. See *Förster.*
fogging
Foix
    syndrome
"fokt" Phonetic for Vogt.
fold
    epicanthal f.
    falciform f.

fold (continued)
    semilunar f. of conjunctiva
Fontana
    spaces
foot-candle
foramen (foramina)
    infraorbital f., f. infraorbitale
    optic f. of sclera
foraminal
foreign body (FB)
    retained f.b. (RFB)
fornix (fornices)
    f. approach
    f.-based flap
    f. conjunctivae
    inferior f.
    f. of lacrimal sac
"foro–" Phonetic for words beginning phoro–.
Förster (Foerster)
    choroiditis
    disease
    operation
    sign
    uveitis
Förster-Fuchs black spot
fortification
    f. spectrum
fossa (fossae)
    orbital f.
    suborbital f.
fossette
Foster-Kennedy syndrome
four diopter base-out prism test
fovea (fovea)
    f. centralis
    f. trochlearis
foveal
foveate
foveation
foveola (foveolae)
    f. retinae
foveolar
foveolate
Foville
    syndrome
Foville-Wilson
    syndrome

Fox
    conformer
    implant
    irrigator
    operation
    shield
fracture
    blow-out f.
framing
Franceschetti
    disease
    dystrophy
    operation
    syndrome
Francis spud
François dystrophy
Franklin glasses
Fraser syndrome
Fresnel
    lens
Frey
    implant
Fricke
    operation
Friede
    operation
Friedenwald
    operation
    syndrome
frontozygomatic
    f. suture
Frost-Lang
    operation
Fuchs
    atrophy
    coloboma
    crypts
    dimples
    dystrophy
    heterochromia
    heterochromic cyclitis
    keratitis
    operation
    sign
    spot
    syndrome
Fuchs-Kraupa
    syndrome

Fukala
    operation
fundus (fundus)
    albinotic f.
    f. albipunctatus
    f. camera
    f. flavimaculatus
    fluorescein f. photography
    f. microscopy
    f. oculi
    tessellated f.
    f. tigroid
funduscopic
"fwah" Phonetic for Foix.
galactitol
α-galactosidase A [alpha-]
β-galactosidase [beta-]
ganglion cell layer
ganglionitis
    gasserian g.
Gartner
    canal
    cyst
    duct
    phenomenon
    tonometer
Gaucher
    disease
Gaule spots
Gayet
    operation
gaze
    conjugate g.
    g. movement
    g. palsy
    g. paretic nystagmus
geniculate body
geniculocalcarine tract
geometric
    g. axis
    g. equator
    g. perspective
Gerlach
    network
gerontotoxon, gerontoxon
    g. lentis
Gerstmann syndrome
Gibson irrigator

Gifford
    operation
    reflex
    sign
Gifford-Galassi reflex
Gilbert-Behçet syndrome
Gillies
    flap
    operation
Girard
    operation
    procedure
    treatment
Giraud-Teulon law
glabella
gland
    inferior lacrimal g.
    Krause g.
    lacrimal g.
    Manz g.
    meibomian g.
    Moll g.
    Rosenmüller g.
    superior lacrimal g.
    tarsal g.
    Wolfring g.
    g. of Zeis, zeisian g.
glare
glasses
    Franklin g.
    Hallauer g
glassy
glaucoma
    g. absolutum
    acute angle closure g.
    air block g.
    angle-recession g.
    aphakic g.
    apoplectic g.
    auricular g.
    capsular g.
    chronic narrow-angle g.
    chronic open-angle g.
    closed angle g.
    g. consummatum
    Contino g.
    Donders g.
    enzyme g.

glaucoma (continued)
    fulminant g.
    hemorrhagic g.
    g. imminens
    infantile g.
    inflammatory g.
    juvenile g.
    lenticular g.
    malignant g.
    narrow-angle g.
    neovascular g.
    noncongestive g.
    obstructive g.
    open-angle g.
    phakogenic g.
    phakolytic g.
    pigmentary g.
    primary open-angle g.
    g. simplex
    traumatic g.
    vitreous-block g.
    wide-angle g.
glaucomato-cyclitic crisis
glaucomatous
glaucosis
glioma
    g. endophytum
    g. exophytum
    g. retinae
globe
globus (globi)
Goldflam disease
Goldflam-Erb disease
Gomez-Marquez
    operation
Gonin
    operation
Gonin-Amsler marker
goniodysgenesis
goniolens
goniophotocoagulation
goniophotography
gonioprism
goniopuncture
gonioscopy
goniosynechia
goniotomy
gonoblennorrhea

Gowers
    sign
GPC—giant papillary conjunctivitis
Gradenigo
    syndrome
Gradle
    electrode
    operation
Graefe (von Graefe)
    cautery
    disease
    operation
    sign
    syndrome
graft
    corneal g.
granuloma
    g. iridis
granulomatous
    g. uveitis
Graves
    disease, ophthalmic
gray
    line
gray-out
Green [eponym]
    replacer
Gregg syndrome
Greig syndrome
grid
    Amsler g.
Grieshaber
    trephine
Groenouw
    corneal dystrophy
Grönblad-Strandberg
    syndrome
Grossmann
    operation
Gruning magnet
Gudden commissure
Guist implant
Gullstrand
    law
    slit lamp
gumma (gummas, gummata)
gummate

gummatous
    g. meningitis
Gunn
    dots
    law
    pupillary phenomenon
    sign
    syndrome
Gutzeit
    operation
Guyton
    operation
gyrate atrophy
H—hypermetropia
Haab
    magnet
    striae
Haag-Streit slit lamp
Haik implant
Hallauer glasses
Haller (von Haller)
    circle
    layer
    ring
Hallermann-Streiff
    syndrome
Hallgren syndrome
halo
    Fick h.
    h. glaucomatosus
    glaucomatous h.
    h. saturninus
Halpin
    operation
handle
    Beaver h.
Hand-Schüller-Christian
    disease
    syndrome
Hannover canal
haptic
Harada
    disease
    syndrome
Hardy-Rand-Ritter plates
Hasner
    operation
    valve

Hassall-Henle warts
Hawes-Pallister-Landor syndrome
head-tilt test
Heath
    expressor
Heerfordt
    disease
    syndrome
Heine
    operation
hemangioblastoma
    h. retinae
hemangiomatosis
    h. retinae
hematoma
hemeralopia
hemiachromatopsia
hemianopia
    absolute h.
    altitudinal h.
    binasal h.
    bitemporal h.
    h. bitemporalis fugax
    congruous h.
    equilateral h.
    heteronymous h.
    homonymous h.
    incongruous h.
    nasal h.
    quadrantic h.
    temporal h.
    unilateral h.
    uniocular h.
hemianopic
hemianoptic
hemianosmia
hemifacial microsomia
hemiopalgia
hemiopia
hemiopic
hemophthalmos
hemorrhage
    blot h.
    dot h.
    salmon-patch h.
    subconjunctival h.
hemorrhagic
Henle fiber layer

hepatolenticular degeneration
Herbert
    operation
    pits
heredoretinopathia congenita
Hering
    law
    test
    theory
herpes
    h. corneae
    h. iridis
    ocular h.
    h. ophthalmicus
Hertel exophthalmometer
Hertwig-Magendie
    phenomenon
    sign
    syndrome
Hess
    operation
Hess-Lees screen
heterochromia
    Fuchs h.
    h. iridis
heterochromic
heteronymous
heterophoralgia
heterophoria
heterophoric
heterophthalmia
heteropsia
heteroptics
heteroscopy
heterotropia
hexachromic
high
    h. hyperopia
"hipo–" Phonetic for words beginning hypo–.
Hippel-Lindau. See *von Hippel-Lindau.*
hippus
Hirschberg
    magnet
    method
histo spots
HL—hypermetropia, latent

HM—manifest hyperopia
Hogan
    operation
Hollenhorst plaque
Holmes-Adie
    syndrome
Holmgren test
Holth
    operation
    punch
Homer
    law
    muscle
    ptosis
    pupil
    syndrome
Homer-Trantas spots
homokeratoplasty
homonymous
    h. diplopia
    h. hemianopia
Honan cuff
horizontal
    h. gaze
    h. meridian
    h. nystagmus
    h. raphe
Horner
    law
    muscle
    ptosis
    pupil
    syndrome
Horner-Bernard syndrome
horopter
    Vieth-Muller h.
horror
    h. fusionis
Horvath
    operation
Hosford spud
Hotz
    operation
HRR—Hardy-Rand-Ritter (plates)
HRR plates
HSV—herpes simplex virus
HT—hypermetropia, total
Ht—total hyperopia

Hudson
    line
Hudson-Stähli line
Hueck
    ligament
Hughes
    implant
    operation
Hummelsheim procedure
humor
    aqueous h.
    h. aquosus
    h. cristallinus
    crystalline h.
    ocular h.
    vitreous h.
    h. vitreus
Hünermann
    disease
Hurler-Scheie
    compound
    syndrome
Hutchinson
    disease
    facies
    patch
    pupil
Hy—hypermetropia
hyalitis
    asteroid h.
    h. punctata
    h. suppurativa
hyaloid
    h. canal
    h. membrane
hyalomucoid
hyalonyxis
hydrophthalmos
hyperemia
    conjunctival h.
hyperemic
hyperesophoria
hyperesthesia
    optic h.
hyperesthetic
hypereuryopia
hyperexophoria
hyperfluorescence

hyperkeratosis
hypermature
    h. cataract
hypermetrope
hypermetropia
hypermetropic
hyperope
hyperopia
    facultative h.
    manifest h.
hyperopic
hyperornithemia
hyperphoria
hyperpresbyopia
hypertelorism
    ocular h.
    orbital h.
hypertonia
    h. oculi
hypertonic
    h. saline
hypertonicity
hypertropia
hyphema
hypoalphalipoproteinemia
hypocyclosis
hypoesophoria
hypoexophoria
hypofluorescence
hypofunction
    convergence h.
    divergence h.
hypometropia
hypophoria
hypoplasia
hypopyon
hyposcleral
hypotonia
    ocular h.
    h. oculi
hypotonic
hypotony
hypotropia
hyptertensive
    h. retinopathy
hysterical
    h. amblyopia
    h. field

ianthinopsia
ICE—iridocorneal-endothelial [syndrome]
icteric
icterus
idioretinal
IDU—idoxuridine
Iliff
    operation
illusion
    Kuhnt i.
image
    i. displacement
    double i.
    i. jump
    i. point
    Purkinje i.'s
    Purkinje-Sanson mirror i.'s
    retinal i.
    Sanson i.
immature cataract
implant
    acorn-shaped i.
    acrylic i.
    Allen i.
    Alpar i.
    Arruga i.
    Berens i.
    Berens-Rosa i.
    Binkhorst i.
    Boyd i.
    Brown-Dohlman i.
    build-up i.
    Bunker i.
    Choyce i.
    Choyce Mark VIII i.
    conical i.
    Copeland i.
    corneal i.
    Cutler i.
    Doherty i.
    Federov i.
    Fox i.
    Frey i.
    glass sphere i.
    gold sphere i.
    Guist i.
    Haik i.

implant (continued)
    hemisphere i.
    Hughes i.
    Ivalon i.
    Levitt i.
    Lincoff i.
    lucite i.
    magnetic i.
    McGhan i.
    Mules i.
    plastic sphere i.
    Plexiglas i.
    polyethylene i.
    Rayner-Choyce i.
    reverse-shape i.
    scleral i.
    scleral buckler i.
    semishell i.
    shelf-type i.
    shell i.
    Silastic i.
    silicone i.
    Snellen i.
    sphere i.
    spherical i.
    Stone i.
    surface i.
    tantalum i.
    Teflon i.
    tire i.
    Troutman i.
    tunneled i.
    Vitallium i.
    Wheeler i.
implantation
Imre
    operation
    treatment
inclusion
    i. bodies
incomitant strabismus
incongruous
incycloduction
incyclophoria
incyclotropia
incyclovergence
indentation tonometry

index (indexes, indices)
    See also *classification.*
    absolute refractive i.
indirect
    binocular i. ophthalmoscopy
    i. ophthalmoscopy
infarct
infraduction
infranuclear
infraorbital
    i. suture
infraversion
inhibitor
    carbonic anhydrase i.'s [a
       class of drugs]
    matrix metalloproteinase
       (MMP) i.'s [a class of
       drugs]
    MMP i.'s [a class of drugs]
INO—internuclear ophthalmoplegia
insufficiency
    vascular i.
intercanthal
intercilium
internuclear
interpalpebral
interpupillary
intorsion
intracapsular
intracranial
intramarginal
    i. sulcus
intraretinal
intrascleral
intrasheath
    i. tenotomy
intrinsic
IO—intraocular
IOP—intraocular pressure
ipsiversion
    ocular i.
iridal
iridalgia
iridauxesis
iridectasis
iridectome
iridectomesodialysis
iridectomize

iridectomy
    basal i.
    buttonhole i.
    complete i. (CI)
    optic i.
    peripheral i. (PI)
    preparatory i.
    sector i.
    stenopeic i.
    therapeutic i.
iridectopia
iridectropium
iridemia
iridencleisis
iridentropium
irideremia
irides
iridesis
iridiagnosis
iridial
iridian
iridic
iridization
iridoavulsion
iridocapsulitis
iridocapsulotomy
iridocele
iridochoroiditis
iridocoloboma
iridoconstrictor
iridocorneal-endothelial (ICE) syn-
    drome
iridocorneosclerectomy
iridocyclectomy
iridocyclochoroiditis
iridocystectomy
iridodesis
iridodiagnosis
iridodialysis
iridodiastasis
iridodilator
iridodonesis
iridokeratitis
iridokinesia
iridokinesis
iridokinetic
iridoleptynsis
iridology

iridolysis
iridomalacia
iridomesodialysis
iridomotor
iridoncus
iridoparalysis
iridopathy
iridoperiphakitis
iridoplegia
iridoptosis
iridopupillary
iridorhexis
iridoschisis
iridosclerotomy
iridosteresis
iridotasis
iridotomy
iris
    bombé i.
    i. coloboma
    i. crypts
    Florentine i.
    i. inclusion operation
    i. pigment dispersion
    i. prolapse
    i. sphincter
    i. stroma
    tremulous i.
    umbrella i.
irisopsia
iritic
iritis
    i. blenorrhagique à rechutes
    i. catamenialis
    diabetic i.
    Doyne i.
    follicular i.
    gouty i.
    i. papulosa
    plastic i.
    purulent i.
    i. recidivans staphylococco-
      allergica
    serous i.
    spongy i.
    sympathetic i.
    tuberculous i.
    uratic i.

iritoectomy
iritomy
IRMA—intraretinal microvascular
    abnormalities
irradiance
irrigator
    DeVilbiss i.
    Dougherty i.
    Fox i.
    Gibson i.
    Sylva i.
Irvine-Gass syndrome
Irving
    operation
ischemia
    i. retinae
Ishihara
    plate
    test
isochromatic
isocoria
isoiconia
isoiconic lens
isophoria
isopia
isopter
Iwanoff (Iwanow)
    cysts
    retinal edema
Jacob
    membrane
    ulcer
Jacobson
    retinitis
Jacod
    syndrome
Jacod-Negri
    syndrome
Jadassohn
    macular atrophy
Jadassohn-Lewandowsky
    syndrome
Jaeger
    lid plate
    test
    test types
Jaesche-Arlt
    operation

Jameson
    operation
jaundice
Javal ophthalmometer
jaw-winking
Jellinek
    sign
    symptom
Jendrassik sign
Jensen
    choroiditis
    disease
    procedure
    retinitis
jerk nystagmus
Johnson
    syndrome
junction
    sclerocorneal j.
    j. scotoma
juvenile
    j. gangliosidosis
    j. retinoschisis
    j. xanthogranuloma
"kahla–" Phonetic for words beginning chala–.
Kalischer
    disease
"kalko–" Phonetic for words beginning chalco–.
Kandori flock retina
kappa angle
Kaufman vitrector
Kearns-Sayer syndrome
Keeler cryophake
Kehrer-Adie
    syndrome
Keith-Wagener-Barker classification (groups 1–4)
Kelman
    lens
    operation
"kemo–" Phonetic for words beginning chemo–.
Kennedy
    syndrome
keratalgia
keratectasia

keratectomy
keratic
keratitis
    acne rosacea k.
    actinic k.
    aerosol k.
    alphabet k.
    anaphylactic k.
    arborescens k.
    artificial silk k.
    band k.
    k. bandelette
    k. bullosa
    dendriform k.
    dendritic k.
    Dimmer k.
    k. disciformis
    epithelial k.
    exfoliative k.
    fascicular k.
    k. filamentosa
    Fuchs k.
    herpetic k.
    hypopyon k.
    interstitial k.
    lagophthalmic k.
    lattice k.
    marginal k.
    metaherpetic k.
    mycotic k.
    neuroparalytic k.
    neurotrophic k.
    k. nummularis
    oyster shucker's k.
    parenchymatous k.
    k. petrificans
    phlyctenular k.
    k. profunda
    k. punctata
    k. punctata subepithelialis
    purulent k.
    k. pustuliformis profunda
    k. ramificata superficialis
    reaper k.
    reticular k.
    ribbon-like k.
    rosacea k.
    Schmidt k.

keratitis (continued)
    sclerosing k.
    scrofulus k.
    serpiginous k.
    k. sicca
    striate k.
    stromal k.
    suppurative k.
    syphilitic k.
    Thygeson k.
    trachomatous k.
    trophic k.
    vascular k.
    vasculonebulous k.
    vesicular k.
    xerotic k.
keratocele
keratocentesis
keratoconjunctivitis
    epidemic k.
    epizootic k.
    flash k.
    limbic k.
    phlyctenular k.
    k. sicca
    viral k.
    welder's k.
keratoconus
keratocyte
keratoectasia
keratoglobus
keratohelcosis
keratohemia
keratoid
keratoiridocyclitis
keratoiritis
keratoleptynsis
keratoleukoma
keratomata
keratometer
keratometric
keratometry
keratomileusis
    laser-assisted in situ k.
    (LASIK)
    laser-assisted intrastromal k.
    (LASIK)
keratonosus

keratonyxis
keratopathy
    band k.
keratophakia
keratoplasty
    Hippel (von Hippel) k.
    lamellar k. (LKP)
    optic k.
    penetrating k. (PKP)
    tectonic k.
keratoprosthesis
keratorhexis
keratoscleritis
keratoscopy
keratotomy
    delimiting k.
    radial k. (RK)
keratotorus
keratouveitis
kerectasis
kerectomy
kernicterus
keroid
Kestenbaum
    procedure
    role
Key [eponym]
    operation
"kias–" Phonetic for words beginning chias–.
Kiloh-Nevin
    myopathy
Kimmelstiel-Wilson
    disease
kinetic perimetry
Kirby
    operation
    suture
kissing choroidals
Klieg eye
Kloepfer syndrome
Knapp
    operation
    procedure
    rule
    streaks
    striae

Knapp-Imre
    operation
Koby cataract
Koch-Weeks
    bacillus
    conjunctivitis
Koeppe
    disease
    nodule
Koerber-Salus-Elschnig
    syndrome
Koplik
    stigma
"kor–" Phonetic for words begin-
    ning cor– and chor–.
koroscopy
Kozlowski degeneration
KP—keratitis punctata
Kraupa
    operation
Krause
    syndrome
    valve
Kreiker
    operation
Kriebig
    operation
Krimsky
    method
Kronfeld
    electrode
Krönlein
    operation
Krönlein-Berke
    operation
Krukenberg spindle
Kuhnt
    illusion
    operation
Kuhnt-Szymanowski
    operation
Kurz syndrome
KW—Keith-Wagener [retinopathy]
    Kimmelstiel-Wilson [syn-
    drome]
KWB—Keith, Wagener, Barker
    [classification, groups 1–4]
L&A—light and accommodation

labium (labia)
    See *border, limbus,* and *mar-
    gin.*
labyrinthine
    l. nystagmus
LaCarrere
    operation
lacquer cracks
lacrima
lacrimal
    l. apparatus
    l. artery
    l. bone
    l. canaliculi
    l. duct
    l. gland
    l. lake
    l. nerve
    l. papilla
    l. sac
lacrimalin
lacrimase
lacrimation
lacrimator
lacrimatory
lacrimonasal
    l. duct
lacrimotomy
lacuna (lacunae)
    Blessig l.
lacunar
lacunula (lacunulae)
lacunule
lacus (lacus)
    l. lacrimalis
Lagleyze
    operation
lagophthalmos
Lagrange
    operation
lake
    lacrimal l.
lamella (lamellae)
    posterior border l. of Fuchs
    triangular l.
    vitreous l.
lamellar
    l. keratoplasty (LKP)

lamelliform
lamina (laminae)
    basal l. of choroid
    basal l. of ciliary body
    Bowman l.
    l. dots
    elastic l., external
    elastic l., internal
    episcleral l.
    limiting l., anterior
    limiting l., posterior
    orbital l.
    l. papyracea
    posterior limiting l.
    suprachoroid l.
    vascular l. of choroid
    vitreal l.
    vitreous l.
laminar
lamp
    Birch-Hirschfeld l.
    Duke-Elder l.
    Eldridge-Green l.
    Gullstrand slit l.
    Haag-Streit slit l.
    slit l.
Lancaster
    magnet
    red-green test
Lancaster Regan dial
lance
    Rolf l.
Landolt
    bodies
    chart
    operation
Landström muscle
Larcher sign
larva (larvae)
    ocular l. migrans
larval
laser
    l. trabeculoplasty
LASIK—laser-assisted in situ kera-
    tomileusis
        laser-assisted intrastromal
            keratomileusis
laterodeviation

lateroduction
laterotorsion
lattice
    l. degeneration
    space l.
Lauber disease
law
    See also *principle* and *rule.*
    Alexander l.
    Descartes l.
    Desmarres l.
    Donders l.
    Ewald l.
    Flouren l.
    Giraud-Teulon l.
    Gullstrand l.
    Hering l.
    Horner l.
    Listing l.
    Sherrington l.
    Snell l.
layer
    See also *band, line, streak,*
       and *stria.*
    Haller l.
    Henle fiber l.
lazy eye
LDD—light-dark discrimination
LE—left eye
Lebensohn chart
Leber
    amaurosis congenita (amau-
       rosis congenita of Leber)
    congenital amaurosis
    corpuscle
    disease
    hereditary optic atrophy
    idiopathic stellar neurore-
       tinitis
    plexus
leiomyoma (leiomyomas, leiomy-
    omata)
lemniscus (lemnisci)
lens
    absorptive l.
    achromatic l.
    acrylic l.
    adherent l.

lens (continued)
    anastigmatic l.
    aniseikonic l.
    anterior chamber intraocular l.
    AO soft l.
    aplanatic l.
    apochromatic l.
    Aquaflex l.
    aspheric l.
    astigmatic l.
    Bagolini l.
    baseball l.
    biconcave l.
    biconvex l.
    bicylindrical l.
    bifocal l.
    Binkhorst l.
    Binkhorst-Fyodorov l.
    bispherical l.
    bitoric contact l.
    Brücke l.
    cataract l.
    Comberg l.
    concave l.
    concavoconcave l.
    concavoconvex l.
    contact l.
    contact l., corneal
    contact l., gas-permeable
    contact l., hard
    contact l., scleral
    contact l., soft
    converging l.
    convex l.
    convexoconcave l.
    Coquille plano l.
    corneal l.
    Crookes l.
    l. crystallina
    crystalline l.
    cylindrical l.
    decentered l.
    dispersing l.
    Fresnel l.
    gas-permeable l.
    Gel Flex l.
    Hruby l.
    hydrophilic l.

lens (continued)
    immersion l.
    intraocular l. (IOL)
    iridocapsular/iris fixation l.
    iris plane l.
    isoiconic l.
    meniscus l.
    meniscus l., converging
    meniscus l., diverging
    meniscus l., negative
    meniscus l., positive
    meter l.
    minus l.
    multifocal introcular l.
    omnifocal l.
    orthoscopic l.
    periscopic l.
    periscopic concave l.
    periscopic convex l.
    piggyback l.
    plane l.
    plano l.
    planoconcave l.
    planoconvex l.
    plus l.
    posterior chamber intraocular l.
    progressive l.
    prosthetic l.
    punctal l.
    retinal laser l.
    retroscopic l.
    Shearing l.
    Sheets l.
    silicone l.
    Simcoe l.
    Sinskey l.
    size l.
    spherical l.
    spherocylindrical l.
    stigmatic l.
    Stokes l.
    toric l.
    trial l.
    trifocal l.
lensometer
Lensrins
lentectomize

lentectomy
lenticonus
lentiform
lentiglobus
leptotrichosis
    l. conjunctivae
lesion
    phlyctenule l.
    pinguecula l.
leukokoria
leukoma
    l. adhaerens
levator (levatores)
    l. muscle
Levitt implant
levoclination
levocycloduction
levocycloversion
levoduction
levotorsion
lid
    l. lag
    l. retraction
lid everter
    Walker l.e.
lid plate
    Jaeger l.p.
Liebreich symptom
ligament
    canthal l.
    ciliary l.
    l. of Lockwood
    pectinate l.
    suspensory l. of lens
    Zinn l.
light reflex
limbal
    l. groove
    l. vasculitis
limbic
limbus (limbi)
    See also *border* and *margin.*
    l. anterior palpebrae
    l. conjunctivae
    l. corneae
    l. luteus retinae
    limbi palpebrales anteriores
    limbi palpebrales posteriores

limbus (limbi) (continued)
    l. of sclera
limen (limina)
liminal
limulus lysate test
Lincoff
    implant
    operation
Lindau disease
Lindau-von Hippel. See *von Hippel-Lindau.*
Lindner
    operation
line
    See also *band, layer, streak,* and *stria.*
    Arlt l.
    Donders l.
    Helmholtz l.
    Hudson l.
    Hudson-Stähli l.
    Morgan l.
    pigmented l. of the cornea
    Schwalbe l.
    l. of sight
    Stähli pigment l.
    Zöllner l.'s.
linea (lineae)
lipemia
    l. retinalis
Listing law
lithiasis
    l. conjunctivae
LKP—lamellar keratoplasty
locator
    Berman l.
Lockwood
    ligament
    tendon
logadectomy
Löhlein
    operation
Londermann
    operation
"loop" Phonetic for loupe.
loop
    Axenfeld nerve l.
    Meyer l.

Lopez-Enriquez
    operation
louchettes
loupe [magnifying lens]
    corneal l.
Löwe
    disease
    ring
    syndrome
Löwenstein
    operation
LP—light perception
LPO—light perception only
Luedde
    exophthalmometer
luminance
luxation
Lyle syndrome
M—myopia
Machek
    operation
Machek-Blaskovics
    operation
Machek-Gifford
    operation
Mackay-Marg
    tonometer
macroblepharia
macrocornea
macrophthalmia
macrophthalmous
macropsia
macula (maculae)
    See also *disk, dot, macule,*
      and *spot.*
    m. corneae
    false m.
    m. flava retinae
    m. luteae, m. lutea retinae
    m. retinae
macular
    m. degeneration
    m. displacement
    m. edema
    m. pucker
    m. sparing
    m. splitting
    m. star

macule
    See also *disk, dot, macula,*
      and *spot.*
    ash-leaf m.
    lance-ovate m.
maculocerebral
maculopapular
maculopathy
    bull's eye m.
    ischemic m.
Maddox
    prism
    rod
    wing
Maeder-Danis
    dystrophy
Magitot
    operation
magnet
    Gruning m.
    Haab m.
    Hirschberg m.
    Lancaster m.
    Storz m.
magnification
Maier
    sinus (sinus of Maier)
Majewsky
    operation
malaise
M+Am—myopia plus astigmatism
maneuver
    See *method* and *technique.*
manifest
    m. hyperopia
    m. refraction
Mann
    sign
manner
    McLean m.
Manz glands
Marcus Gunn
    phenomenon
    pupillary syndrome
    sign
Marfan
    sign
    syndrome

margin
> See also *border* and *limbus*.
> ciliary m. of iris
> free m. of eyelid
> infraorbital m. of orbit
> lateral margin of orbit
> medial m. of orbit
> orbital m.
> pupillary m. of iris

margo (margines)
Marinesco-Sjögren
> syndrome
Marinesco-Sjögren-Garland
> syndrome
Mariotte spot
marker
> Gonin-Amsler m.
Marlow test
Marsh disease
Masselon spectacles
Masuda-Kitahara disease
matrix metalloproteinase (MMP)
> inhibitors [a class of drugs]
Mauksch
> operation
Mauthner test
Maxwell
> ring
> spot
May sign
McGavic
> operation
McGhan implant
McGuire
> operation
McLean
> manner
> tonometer
McReynolds
> operation
medical
> m. ophthalmoscopy
medium (media, mediums)
> refracting media
> transparent m. of eye
Meesmann dystrophy
megalocornea
megalophthalmos

meibomian
> m. cyst
> m. foramen
> m. froth
> m. gland
> m. stye
meibomianitis
meibomitis
melanocytoma
melanocytosis
> oculodermal m.
melanosis
> m. bulbi
> m. iridis, m. of iris
> m. oculi
> oculocutaneous m.
> m. sclerae
Meller
> operation
membrana (membranae)
> Bowman m.
> Bruch m.
> m. capsularis lentis posterior
> cyclitic m.
> Demours m.
> Descemet m.
> m. epipapillaris membrane
> hyaloid m.
> Jacob m.
membranate
membrane
> Bowman m.
> Bruch m.
> cyclitic m.
> Descemet m.
> Duddell m.
> Haller m.
> Jacob m.
> Ruysch m.
> ruyschian m.
> Tenon m.
> vitreous m.
> Zinn m.
membranectomy
meridianus (meridiani)
> meridiani bulbi oculi
mesiris
mesodermal

mesoretina
metaherpetic
metamorphopsia
    m. varians
method
    See also *technique.*
    Hirschberg m.
metric
    m. ophthalmoscopy
Meyer
    loop
Meynert
    commissure
microblepharia
microblepharon
microcoria
microcornea
microimmunofluorescent
microlesion
micronystagmus
microphakia
microphthalmic
micropsia
microptic
microsaccades
microscopy
    fundus m.
microstrabismus
migratory
    m. ophthalmia
Mikulicz (von Mikulicz)
    disease
    syndrome
Mikulicz-Radecki
    syndrome
Mikulicz-Sjögren
    syndrome
milium (milia)
Miller
    syndrome
miner's nystagmus
minimum (minima)
    m. cognoscibile
    m. legibile
    light m.
    m. visibile
Minsky
    operation

"mio–" Phonetic for words beginning myo–.
miosis
    endolymphatic stromal m.
    irritative m.
    paralytic m.
    spastic m.
    spinal m.
miotic effect
miotics [a class of drugs]
Mira
    photocoagulator
    unit
Mittendorf dot
MMP—matrix metalloproteinase
MMP inhibitors [a class of drugs]
Möbius
    disease
    sign
    syndrome (I, II)
Moll glands
molluscum
    m. contagiosum
Monakow (von Monakow)
    fibers
Moncrieff
    operation
monoblepsia
monochromacy
monochromatism
monocular
monoculus
monodiplopia
monofixation syndrome
Mooren ulcer
Morax
    operation
Morax-Axenfeld conjunctivitis
Morgagni
    cataract
    globules
    spheres
Mosher-Toti
    operation
Motais
    operation
Mount-Reback
    syndrome

movement
    conjugate m.'s
Mueller
    See *Müller.*
Mules
    implant
    operation
    scoop
Müller
    fibers
    muscle
    trigone
musca (muscae)
    muscae volitantes
muscle
    See also in *Orthopedics and
       Sports Medicine* section.
    abductor m
    Brücke m.
    ciliary m.
    depressor m., superciliary
    dilator m. of pupil
    Duverney m.
    extraocular m.'s (EOMs)
    m.'s of eye
    m. of Henle
    Horner m.
    inferior oblique m.
    inferior rectus m. of bulb
    intraocular m.'s
    iridic m.'s
    Landström m.
    lateral rectus m. of bulb
    levator m.
    levator m. of upper eyelid
    medial rectus m. of bulb
    Müller m.
    oblique m. of eyeball (inferi-
      or, superior)
    ocular m.'s, oculorotatory m.'s
    orbicular m. of eye
    orbital m.
    procerus m.
    Riolan m.
    Rouget m.
    sphincter m. of pupil
    superior oblique m.
    superior rectus m.

muscle (continued)
    tarsal m. (inferior, superior)
    zygomatic m. (greater, lesser)
musculus (musculi)
    See also *muscle.*
    See also in *Orthopedics and
       Sports Medicine* section.
    musculi bulbi
    m. orbicularis oculi
MVR—massive vitreous retraction
My—myopia
mydriasis
    alternating m.
    bounding m.
    paralytic m.
    spasmodic m., spastic m.
    spinal m.
    springing m.
mydriatic effect
mydriatics [a class of drugs]
myectomy
myiocephalon
myiodesopsia
myoclonus
    ocular m.
myodiopter
myopathy
    ocular m.
myope
myopia
    axial m.
    curvature m.
    index m.
    indicial m.
    malignant m., pernicious m.
    pernicious m.
    primary m.
    prodromal m.
    progressive m.
    simple m.
myopic
    m. crescent
    m. degeneration
myotomy
Naffziger
    decompression
    operation

Nagel
    anomaloscope
Nairobi eye
nanophthalmos
nasociliary
nasolacrimal
near-sight
nearsighted
nearsightedness
nebula (nebulae)
necrosis (necroses)
necrotic
neodymium (Nd)
    n.:yttrium-aluminum-garnet
      (Nd:YAG) laser
neostigmine
    n. bromide
neovascularization
nerve
    abducens n.
    infratrochlear n.
    optic n.
    orbital n.'s
    recurrent n., ophthalmic
    supraorbital n.
    trigeminal n.
    trochlear n.
    zygomatic n.
Nettleship-Falls–type ocular albinism
network
    Gerlach n.
neuralgia
neuralgic
neurapraxia
neurectomy
    opticociliary n.
neuritic
neuritis
    intraocular n.
    optic n.
    orbital optic n.
    postocular n.
    retrobulbar n.
neurochorioretinitis
neurochoroiditis
neurodealgia
neurodeatrophia
neuroepithelioma

neuroepithelium
    n. of maculae
    n. macularum
neuromyelitis
    n. optica
neuropathy
    optic n.
neuroretinal
neuroretinitis
neuroretinopathy
    hypertensive n.
neurotomy
    opticociliary n.
neurotrophic
    n. keratitis
nevus (nevi)
    See in *Dermatology* section.
nicking
Nida
    operation
NINDB—National Institute of Neu-
    rologic Diseases and Blindness
"nistagmus" Phonetic for nystagmus.
Nizetic
    operation
NLP—no light perception
NMG—no Marcus Gunn [phenom-
    enon]
nodal
nodularity
nodulated
nodulation
nodule
    Busacca n.'s
    Dalen-Fuchs n.'s
    Koeppe n.'s
Nonne
    syndrome
Norrie
    disease
    syndrome
NPC—near point of convergence
NRC—normal retinal correspondence
nuclear
    n. sclerosis
nucleus (nuclei)
    Edinger n.
    Edinger-Westphal n.

nucleus (nuclei) (continued)
    n. of lens
    n. lentiformis
    Perlia n.
"nur–" Phonetic for words begin-
    ning neur–.
Nv—naked vision
NVA—near visual acuity
nyctalopia
nystagmic
nystagmiform
nystagmograph
nystagmoid
nystagmus
    aural n.
    Baer n.
    Bekhterev n.
    benign positional n.
    central n.
    Cheyne n.
    Cheyne-Stokes n.
    convergence n.
    disjunctive n.
    dissociated n.
    downbeat n.
    electrical n.
    end-point n.
    end position n.
    fixation n.
    galvanic n.
    gaze n.
    gaze paretic n.
    jerk n., jerky n.
    labyrinthine n.
    lateral n.
    miner's n.
    n.-myoclonus
    ocular n.
    opticokinetic n., optokinetic
      n. (OKN)
    oscillating n.
    paretic n.
    pendular n.
    periodic alternating n.
    railroad n.
    rebound n.
    resilient n.
    retraction n., n. retractorius

nystagmus (continued)
    rhythmical n.
    rotary n.
    rotatory n.
    secondary n.
    see-saw n.
    spontaneous n.
    undulatory n.
    unilateral n.
    upbeat n.
    vertical n.
    vestibular n.
    vibratory n.
    visual n.
    voluntary n.
nystaxis
O—eye (L. oculus)
OAV—oculoauriculovertebral (dys-
    plasia)
O'Brien
    akinesia
    block
    cataract
occludable
occluder
occlusion
    branch retinal vein o.
O'Connor
    operation
O'Connor-Peter
    operation
ocular
    o. adnexa
    o. albinism
    o. aspergillosis
    o. bobbing
    o. dysmetria
    o. flutter
    o. histoplasmosis
    o. hypertelorism
    o. hypertension
    o. hypotony
    o. motility
    o. myoclonus
    o. myopathy
    o. pemphigus
    o. torticollis
oculentum

oculi (genitive and plural of oculus)
oculist
oculistics
oculocardiac reflex
oculocephalogyric
oculocutaneous
    o. albinism
oculofacial
oculogyration
oculogyria
oculogyric
oculomotor
oculomotorius
oculomycosis
oculonasal
oculopathy
    pituitarigenic o.
oculoplethysmography (OPG)
oculopneumoplethysmography
oculopupillary
oculoreaction
oculorespiratory reflex
oculospinal
oculozygomatic
oculus (oculi)
    o. caesius
    deprimens oculi
    o. dexter (OD) [L. right eye]
    fundus o.
    o. leporinus
    orbicularis oculi muscle
    o. sinister (OS) [L. left eye]
    o. uterque (OU) [L. each eye]
ocutome
OD—right eye (L. oculus dexter)
OD, O.D.—Doctor of Optometry
ODD—oculodentodigital
ODD dysplasia
"ofthal–" Phonetic for words beginning ophthal–.
Oguchi disease
OKN—opticokinetic nystagmus
onchocerciasis
    ocular o.
opacity
    Caspar ring o.
    snowball o.'s
open-angle glaucoma

open sky vitrectomy
operation
    See also in *General Surgical Terms.*
    Agnew o.
    Allen o.
    Ammon o.
    Amsler corneal graft o.
    Anagnostakis o.
    Anel o.
    Arlt (von Arlt) o.
    Arlt-Jaesche o.
    Arruga o.
    Badal o.
    Bardelli o.
    Barkan o.
    Barraquer o.
    Barrio o.
    Basterra o.
    Beer o.
    Berens o.
    Berke o.
    Bielschowsky o.
    Birch-Hirschfeld entropion o.
    Blair o.
    Blasius o.
    Blaskovics o.
    Blatt o.
    Böhm o.
    Bonaccolto-Flieringa o.
    Bonzel o.
    Borthen o.
    Bossalino o.
    Bowman o.
    Brailey o.
    Briggs o.
    Budinger o.
    Burch o.
    Burow o.
    Buzzi o.
    Cairns o.
    Callahan o.
    Carter o.
    Casanellas o.
    Castroviejo o.
    Celsus o.
    Collin-Beard o.
    Critchett o.

operation (continued)
    Custodis o.
    Cutler-Beard o.
    Czermak o.
    Daviel o.
    de Grandmont o.
    Del Toro o.
    DeWecker o.
    Dupuy-Dutemps o.
    Durr o.
    Elliott o.
    Elschnig o.
    Ely o.
    equilibrating o.
    Eversbusch o.
    Fasanella-Servat o.
    Filatov o.
    Filatov-Marzinkowsky o.
    Flajani o.
    Förster o.
    Fox o.
    Franceschetti o.
    Fricke o.
    Friede o.
    Friedenwald o.
    Frost-Lang o.
    Fuchs o.
    Fukala o.
    Gayet o.
    Gifford o.
    Gillies o.
    Girard o.
    Gomez-Marquez o.
    Gonin o.
    Gradle o.
    Graefe (von Graefe) o.
    Grossmann o.
    Gutzeit o.
    Guyton o.
    Halpin o.
    Hasner o.
    Heine o.
    Herbert o.
    Hess o.
    Hippel (von Hippel) o.
    Hogan o.
    Holth o.
    Horay o.

operation (continued)
    Horvath o.
    Hotz o.
    Hughes o.
    Iliff o.
    Imre o.
    iris inclusion o.
    Irving o.
    Jaesche-Arlt o.
    Jameson o.
    Kelman o.
    Key o.
    Kirby o.
    Knapp o.
    Knapp-Imre o.
    Kraupa o.
    Kreiker o.
    Kriebig o.
    Krönlein o.
    Krönlein-Berke o.
    Kuhnt o.
    Kuhnt-Szymanowski o.
    LaCarrere o.
    Lagleyze o.
    Lagrange o.
    Landolt o.
    Lincoff o.
    Lindner o.
    Löhlein o.
    Londermann o.
    Lopez-Enriquez o.
    Löwenstein o.
    Machek o.
    Machek-Blaskovics o.
    Machek-Gifford o.
    Magitot o.
    magnet o.
    Majewsky o.
    Mauksch o.
    McGavic o.
    McGuire o.
    McReynolds o.
    Meller o.
    Minsky o.
    Moncrieff o.
    Morax o.
    Mosher-Toti o.
    Motais o.

operation (continued)
    Mules o.
    Naffziger o.
    Nida o.
    Nizetic o.
    O'Connor o.
    O'Connor-Peter o.
    Panas o.
    Paufique o.
    Polyak o.
    Poulard o.
    Power o.
    Quaglino o.
    Richet o.
    Rowinski o.
    Rubbrecht o.
    Saemisch o.
    Scheie o.
    Schmalz o.
    Silva-Costa o.
    Smith o.
    Smith-Kuhnt o.
    Smith-Kuhnt-Szymanowski o.
    Snellen o.
    Soria o.
    Sourdille o.
    Spaeth o.
    Speas o.
    Spencer-Watson o.
    Stallard o.
    Stock o.
    Suarez-Villafranca o.
    Szymanowski o.
    Szymanowski-Kuhnt o.
    Tansley o.
    Terson o.
    Toti o.
    Toti-Mosher o.
    Trantas o.
    Troutman o.
    Verhoeff o.
    Verwey o.
    Waldhauer o.
    Weeks o.
    West o.
    Wheeler o.
    Wicherkiewicz o.
    Wiener o.

operation (continued)
    Wilmer o.
    Wolfe o.
    Worth o.
    Ziegler o.
opercula (plural of operculum)
opercular
operculate
operculum (opercula)
    o. orbitale
Ophthaine [anesthetic agent]
ophthalmagra
ophthalmalgia
ophthalmatrophia
ophthalmectomy
ophthalmencephalon
ophthalmia
    actinic ray o.
    catarrhal o.
    caterpillar o.
    o. eczematosa
    Egyptian o.
    electric o.
    o. electrica
    flash o.
    gonorrheal o.
    granular o.
    o. hivialis
    jequirity o.
    metastatic o.
    migratory o.
    mucous o.
    o. neonatorum
    neuroparalytic o.
    o. nodosa
    phlyctenular o.
    purulent o.
    scrofulous o.
    strumous o.
    sympathetic o.
    ultraviolet ray o.
    varicose o.
ophthalmiac
ophthalmiatrics
ophthalmic Graves disease
ophthalmitic
ophthalmitis
ophthalmoblennorrhea

ophthalmocarcinoma
ophthalmocele
ophthalmocopia
ophthalmodesmitis
ophthalmodiagnosis
ophthalmodiaphanoscope
ophthalmodiastimeter
ophthalmodonesis
ophthalmodynamometer
ophthalmodynamometry
ophthalmodynia
ophthalmoeikonometer
ophthalmograph
ophthalmography
ophthalmogyric
ophthalmolith
ophthalmologic, ophthalmological
ophthalmology
ophthalmomalacia
ophthalmometer
    Javal o.
ophthalmometry
ophthalmomycosis
ophthalmomyiasis
ophthalmomyitis
ophthalmomyositis
ophthalmomyotomy
ophthalmoneuritis
ophthalmoneuromyelitis
ophthalmoparalysis
ophthalmopathy
ophthalmophacometer
ophthalmophantom
ophthalmophlebotomy
ophthalmophthisis
ophthalmoplasty
ophthalmoplegia
    basal o.
    congenital o.
    diabetic o.
    exophthalmic o.
    o. externa
    external o.
    fascicular o.
    hyperthyroid o.
    o. interna
    internal o.
    internuclear o.

ophthalmoplegia (continued)
    nuclear o.
    orbital o.
    painful o.
    Parinaud o.
    partial o.
    o. partialis
    o. progressiva
    progressive external o.
    relapsing o.
    Sauvineau o.
    sensorimotor o.
    thyrotoxic o.
    total o.
    o. totalis
ophthalmoplegic
ophthalmoptosis
ophthalmoreaction
    Calmette o.
ophthalmorrhagia
ophthalmorrhea
ophthalmorrhexis
ophthalmoscopic
ophthalmoscopy
    binocular indirect o.
    direct o.
    indirect o.
    medical o.
    metric o.
ophthalmospectroscope
ophthalmospectroscopy
ophthalmostasis
ophthalmostat
ophthalmostatometer
ophthalmosteresis
ophthalmosynchysis
ophthalmothermometer
ophthalmotomy
ophthalmotonometer
ophthalmotonometry
ophthalmotoxin
ophthalmotrope
ophthalmotropometer
ophthalmovascular
ophthalmoxerosis
ophthalmoxyster
opportunistic
    o. infection

opsoclonia
optesthesia
optic
    o. atrophy
    o. axis
    o. chiasm
    o. cup
    o. disk
    o. foramen
    o. iridectomy
    o. keratoplasty
    o. nerve
    o. neuritis
    o. tract
    o. vesicle
optician
opticianry
opticist
opticociliary
    o. neurectomy
    o. neurotomy
opticocinerea
opticokinetic
opticonasion
opticopupillary
optics
optist
optoblast
optogram
optomeninx
optometer
optometrist
optometry
optomyometer
optophone
optostriate
optotype
ora
orbicular
orbicularis
    o. ciliaris muscle
    o. oculi muscle
orbiculus (orbiculi)
    o. ciliaris
orbita (orbitae)
orbital
    o. angiography
    o. apex

orbital (continued)
    o. cellulitis
    o. decompression
    o. fascia
    o. fat pads
    o. fissure
    o. floor fracture
    o. periosteum
    o. pseudotumor
    o. septum
orbitale
orbitalis
orbitonasal
orbitonometer
orbitonometry
orbitotemporal
orbitotomy
orthokeratology
orthometer
orthophoria
    asthenic o.
orthophoric
orthoptic
orthoptist
orthoptoscope
orthorater
orthoscopy
os (ora) [opening, mouth]
    ora serrata retinae
os (ossa) [bone]
    See in *Orthopedics and*
        Sports Medicine section.
OS—left eye (L. oculus sinister)
oscillation
oscillopsia
OU—each eye (L. oculus uterque)
outflow channels
overcorrection
P—presbyopia
    pupil
PA—phakic-aphakic
pachometer
pachyblepharon
pachyblepharosis
palinopsia
pallor
palpebra (palpebrae)
    p. inferior

palpebra (palpebrae) (continued)
    p. superior
    p. tertia
    tertius p.
palpebral
palpebralis
palpebrate
palpebration
palpebritis
palsy
    See also *paralysis.*
    acute thyrotoxic bulbar p.
    Bell p.
PAN—periodic alternating nystagmus
Panas
    operation
pannus
    degenerative p., p. degenera-
      tivus
    p. eczematosus
    glaucomatous p.
    phlyctenular p.
    p. siccus
    p. tenuis
    p. trachomatosus
panophthalmia
panophthalmitis
panoptic
panretinal photocoagulation
pantankyloblepharon
panuveitis
papilla (papillae)
    Bergmeister p.
    lacrimal p.
    p. nervi optici
    optic p.
papillary
papillate
papillation
papilledema
papilliferous
papilliform
papillomacular
    p. bundle
papilloretinitis
parafovea
parallax
parallel

paralysis (paralyses)
    See also *palsy.*
    abducens p.
    abducens-facial p., congenital
    p. of accommodation
    congenital p. of horizontal
      gaze
    conjugate p.
    Duchenne p.
    Duchenne-Erb p.
    Erb p.
    Erb-Duchenne p.
    extraocular p.
    familial infantile bulbar p.
    p. of gaze
    ocular p.
    oculofacial p., congenital
    oculomotor p.
    Weber p.
paramedian
parenchyma
    p. of lens
paresis
paretic
paries (parietes)
parietitis
Parinaud
    conjunctivitis
    ophthalmoplegia
    syndrome
parophthalmoncus
paropsis
pars (partes)
    p. caeca retinae
    p. ciliaris retinae
    p. optica retinae
    p. plana vitrectomy
    p. planitis
Pascheff conjunctivitis
PAT—prism adaption test
patch
    cotton-wool p.'s
Paterson-Brown-Kelly
    syndrome
pathogen
    See specific pathogens in
      Laboratory, Pathology,
      and Chemistry Terms.

Paufique
    operation
    trephine
PBC, PcB—point of basal convergence
PCD—posterior corneal deposits
PD—prism diopter
    pupillary distance
PDR—proliferative diabetic retinopathy
pearl
    Elschnig p.'s
"peh-tee" Phonetic for Petit.
Pel crises
Pel-Ebstein
    crisis
pemphigus
penalization
pendular
penetrating
    p. keratoplasty (PKP)
PEO—progressive external ophthalmoplegia
perception
    depth p.
    light and color p.
periarteritis
    p. nodosa
peribulbar
perichiasmal
perifoveal
perihilar
perikeratic
perilenticular
perimeter
    Ferree-Rand p.
perimetry
perineuritis
periocular
periophthalmitis
periorbita
periorbital
periorbititis
periphacitis
peripheral
    p. anterior synechia
    p. curve
    p. fusion

peripheral (continued)
    p. iridectomy (PI)
    p. retina
    p. uveitis
    p. vision
peripheraphose
periscleral
peritectomy
peritomize
peritomy
perivasculitis
Perkins tonometer
PERL—pupils equal, react to light
PERLA—pupils equal, react to light and accommodation
Perlia nucleus
PERRLA—pupils equal, round, react to light and accommodation
petechia (petechiae)
Peters
    anomaly
    syndrome
Petit
    canal
"pettee" Phonetic for Petit.
Petzetakis-Takos
    syndrome
phacocele
phacocyst
phacocystectomy
phacocystitis
phacodonesis
phacoemulsification
phacoerysis
phacoglaucoma
phacohymenitis
phacoiditis
phacolysis
phacolytic
phacomalacia
phacometachoresis
phacometer
phacopalingenesis
phacoplanesis
phacosclerosis
phacoscopy
phacoscotasmus
phacotoxic

phacozymase
phakitis
phakoma
    retinal p.
phakomatosis (phakomatoses)
    Bourneville p.
phenomenon (phenomena)
    See also *effect, reflex,* and
      sign.
    aqueous-influx p.
    Aubert p.
    Becker p.
    Bell p.
    blood-influx p.
    cogwheel p.
    doll's head p.
    Fick p.
    flicker p.
    Galassi pupillary p.
    glass-rod p., negative
    glass-rod p., positive
    Gunn p.
    Gunn pupillary p.
    Hertwig-Magendie p.
    inverse Marcus Gunn p.
    inverted Marcus Gunn p.
    jaw-winking p.
    Le Grand-Geblewics p.
    Marcus Gunn p.
    Marcus Gunn pupillary p.
    orbicularis p.
    paradoxical pupillary p.
    phi p.
    Piltz-Westphal p.
    Pullrich p.
    Purkinje p.
    shot-silk p.
    Westphal p.
    Westphal-Piltz p.
phlebophthalmotomy
phlyctena (phlyctenae)
phlyctenar
phlyctenoid
phlyctenosis
phlyctenula (phlyctenulae)
phlyctenular
phlyctenule

phlyctenulosis
    allergic p.
    tuberculous p.
phoria
phorometer
phorometry
phoroptor
phorotone
photism
photochemistry
photochromic
photocoagulator
    Mira p.
photography
    fluorescein fundus p.
    fluorescence retinal p.
photophobia
photophthalmia
photopia
photopic
photopsia
photoptometer
photoptometry
photoreceptor
phthisis
    p. bulbi
    p. corneae
    ocular p.
PI—peripheral iridectomy
Pick [eponym]
    retinitis
    vision
pie in the sky defect
pigmentosa
pigmentum
    p. nigrum
Pillat dystrophy
Piltz-Westphal phenomenon
pin
    Walker p.
pinguecula
pinhole
pinkeye, pink eye, pink-eye
Pischel
    electrode
    pin
PKP—penetrating keratoplasty
PL—light perception

Placido disk
pladarosis
plane
    Broca p.
planoconcave
planoconvex
planum (plana)
plaque
    Hollenhorst p.'s
plate
    Hardy-Rand-Ritter p
    Ishihara p.'s
    tarsal p.'s
plateau iris
pleoptics
Plexiglas implant
plexus (plexus, plexuses)
    annular p.
    intraepithelial p.
    ophthalmic p.
    p. ophthalmicus
    subepithelial p.
plica (plicae)
    plicae ciliares
    plicae iridis
    p. lacrimalis
PMMA—polymethyl methacrylate
    [usually not expanded]
pneumotonometer
point
    See *disk, dot, macula, mac-
    ule,* and *spot.*
    p. of basal convergence
    (PcB, PBC)
    p. of convergence
    convergence near p.
polarization
pole
    anterior p. of eyeball
    anterior p. of lens
    posterior p. of eyeball
    posterior p. of lens
polus (poli)
    p. anterior bulbi oculi
    p. anterior lentis
    p. posterior bulbi oculi
    p. posterior lentis

Polyak
    operation
polycoria
    p. spuria
    p. vera
polyopia, polyopsia
    binocular p.
    p. monophthalmica
pontine
    p. gaze
    p. lesion
porus (pori)
    p. opticus
Posner-Schlossman
    syndrome
posterior
    p. chamber
    p. sclerotomy
Poulard
    operation
power
Power [eponym]
    operation
Pr—presbyopia
preauricular
prechiasmal
precipitate
    keratic p.'s
    keratic p.'s, mutton-fat
    pigmented keratic p.'s
precorneal
preparatory iridectomy
preretinal
presbyope
presbyopia
presbyopic
presenile
    p. melanosis
principle [rule]
    See also *law* and *rule.*
    Huygens p.
    watermelon seed p.
prism
    p. diopter
    Maddox p.
    Risley p.
prismatic

procedure
> See also *maneuver, method, operation,* and *technique.*
>> Faden p.
>> Girard p.
>> Hummelsheim p.
>> Jensen p.
>> Kestenbaum p.
>> Knapp p.

processus (processus)

projection
> erroneous p.

prominence
> Ammon scleral p.

prophylaxis
> Credé p.

proptometer

prostaglandin (PG)
> p. agonists [a class of drugs]

prosthokeratoplasty

protanomalopia

protanomalous

protanomaly

protanopia

protanopic

protanopsia

protector
> Arruga p.

Prowazek-Greeff bodies

PRP—panretinal photocoagulation

pseudo-Argyll Robertson
> See also *Argyll Robertson.*
>> pupil
>> syndrome

pseudoexfoliation

pseudoglioma

pseudoisochromatic chart

pseudomembrane

pseudomyopia

pseudoneuritis

pseudonystagmus

pseudopapilledema

pseudophakia
> p. adiposa
> p. fibrosa

pseudopterygium

pseudoptosis

pseudoretinitis

pseudostrabismus

psorophthalmia

pterion

pterygium (pterygia)
> congenital p.

ptosis
> p. adiposa
> Horner p.
> p. lipomatosis
> morning p.
> p. sympathetica
> p. sympathica
> traumatic p.
> waking p.

ptotic

Pulfrich
> pendulum
> phenomenon

punctate

punctation

punctum (puncta)
> p. caecum
> lacrimal p.
> p. lacrimale
> p. luteum
> p. proximum
> p. remotum

punctumeter

pupil
> Adie p.
> Argyll Robertson p.
> Behr p.
> bounding p.
> Bumke p.
> cat-eyep., cat's eye p.
> cornpicker's p.
> fixed p.
> Horner p.
> Hutchinson p.
> keyhole p.
> pinhole p.
> skew p.
> stiff p.
> tonic p.

pupilla

pupillary

pupillatonia

pupillograph

pupillometer
pupillometry
pupillomotor
pupilloplegia
pupilloscopy
pupillostatometer
pupillotonia
Purkinje images
Purkinje-Sanson mirror images
Purtscher
 disease
 angipathic retinopathy
 syndrome
push plus
PVA—polyvinyl alcohol
pyophthalmia
quadrantanopia
quadrantanopsia
quadrantic
Quaglino
 operation
quiescent
"rabdo–" Phonetic for words beginning rhabdo–.
radial
 r. keratotomy (RK)
radius (radii)
 radii of lens, radii lentis
"ra-fee" Phonetic for raphe.
ramollitio
 r. retinae
ramus (rami)
raphe (raphae)
 horizontal r. of eye
 lateral r.
 palpebral r.
 r. palpebralis lateralis
raphes (genitive of raphe)
ratio
 cup-to-disk r.
Rayner-Choyce implant
RD—retinal detachment
reaction
 hemianopic pupillary r.
 indirect pupillary r.
 near-point r.
 paradoxical pupillary r.
 Wernicke r.

reaction (continued)
 Wernicke hemianopic r.
receptor
 contact r.
 distance r.
 sensory r.
 visual r.
recession
recessus (recessus)
 r. opticus
reciprocal
 r. innervation
Recklinghausen (von Recklinghausen)
 disease
reclination
Reese
 syndrome
Reese-Ellsworth retinoblastoma classification (I–V)
refixation
reflex
 See also *effect, phenomenon,* and *sign.*
 See also in *Neurology and Pain Management* section.
 blink r.
 cat-eye r., cat's eye r.
 consensual r.
 consensual light r.
 convergence r.
 corneal r.
 direct light r.
 fusion r.
 Gifford r.
 Gifford-Galassi r.
 iris contraction r.
 light r.
 myopic r.
 oculopupillary r.
 orbicularis r.
 orbicularis oculi r.
 orbicularis pupillary r.
 orbiculopupillary r.
 paradoxical pupillary r.
 pupillary r.
 red r.
 retrobulbar pupillary r.

reflex (continued)
  reversed pupillary r.
  shot-silk r.
  tapetal light r.
  watered-silk r.
  Weiss r.
  Westphal-Piltz r.
  Westphal pupillary r.
reflexion
refract
refraction
  double r.
  dynamic r.
  homatropine r.
  static r.
refractionist
refractive
refractometer
refractometry
refractor
Refsum
  disease
  syndrome
region
  r. of accommodation
  ciliary r.
  infraorbital r.
  ocular r.
  opticostriate r.
  orbital r.
  preoptic r.
  zygomatic r.
Reis-Bücklers
  disease
Reiter
  disease
  syndrome
Rekoss disk
Remy separator
replacer
  Green r.
rete (retia)
retial
retina
  coarctate r.
  leopard r.
  nasal r.
  physiologic r.

retina (continued)
  shot silk r.
  temporal r.
  tigroid r.
  watered-silk r.
retinal
  r. detachment
  fluorescence r. photography
  r. pigment epithelium
  r. tear
retinitis
  actinic r.
  r. albuminurica
  apoplectic r.
  central angiospastic r.
  r. centralis serosa
  r. circinata
  circinate r.
  Coats r.
  diabetic r.
  r. disciformans
  exudative r.
  r. gravidarum
  gravidic r.
  r. haemorrhagica
  hypertensive r.
  Jacobson r.
  Jensen r.
  leukemic r.
  metastatic r.
  r. nephritica
  Pick r.
  r. pigmentosa
  r. proliferans
  r. punctata albescens
  punctate r.
  renal r.
  serous r.
  solar r.
  splenic r.
  r. stellata
  striate r.
  suppurative r.
  r. syphilitica
  uremic r.
  Wagener r.
retinochoroid

retinochoroiditis
    birdshot r.
    r. juxtapapillaris
retinocytoma
retinodialysis
retinograph
retinography
retinoid
retinomalacia
retinopapillitis
retinopathy
    actinic r.
    arteriosclerotic r.
    background r.
    central disk-shaped r.
    central serous r.
    circinate r.
    diabetic r.
    exudative r.
    hemorrhagic r.
    hypertensive r.
    Keith-Wagener r.
    leukemic r.
    nonproliferative r.
    pigmentary r.
    Purtscher angiopathic r.
    renal r.
    stellate r.
retinopexy
    pneumatic r.
retinoschisis
retinoscopy
retinosis
retinotopic
retinotoxic
retraction
    lid r.
    massive vitreous r.
retrobulbar
retroillumination
retroiridian
retrolental
retrolenticular
retro-ocular
retro-orbital
retrotarsal
Reuss
    color charts

Reuss (continued)
    tables
RFB—retained foreign body
RGP—rigid gas-permeable (contact lens)
rhinommectomy
rhinoptia
rhytidosis
RI—recession index
Richet
    operation
Richner-Hanhart syndrome
Riddoch
    syndrome
Rieger
    anomaly
    dysgenesis
Rifkind sign
rigid gas-permeable (RGP) contact lens
rigidity
    mydriatic r.
Riley-Day
    syndrome
Riley-Smith
    syndrome
rima (rimae)
    r. palpebrarum
rimal
ring
    Bonaccolto scleral r.
    ciliary r. of iris
    Coats r.
    common tendinous r.
    conjunctival r.
    Fleischer keratoconus r.
    glaucomatous r.
    Kayser-Fleischer r.
    Löwe r.
    Maxwell r.
    r. scotoma
    Soemmering r.
    Vossius lenticular r.
Riolan muscle
ripe cataract
Risley prism
"riti–" Phonetic for words beginning rhyti–.

rivalry
>binocular r., retinal r.

rivus
>r. lacrimalis

RK—radial keratotomy

RLF—retrolental fibroplasia

Rochon-Duvigneaud syndrome

rod
>Maddox r.
>retinal r.

Rolf
>lance

Rollet
>syndrome

Romaña sign

Rönne nasal step

Rosenmüller
>gland

Roth
>spots

Roth-Bielschowsky syndrome

Rothmund
>syndrome

rotoextraction

rotoextractor
>Douvas r.

Rowinski
>operation

RP—retinitis pigmentosa

RPE—retinal pigment epithelium

Rubbrecht
>operation

rubeosis
>r. iridis
>r. retinae

Rubinstein syndrome

Rubinstein-Taybi syndrome

"ruby" Phonetic for Hruby.

rudiment
>lens r.

Ruggeri
>reflex
>sign

rule
>See also *law* and *principle*.
>Kestenbaum r.
>Knapp r.

rupture
>extracapsular r.
>intracapsular r.

Rutherfurd syndrome

Ruysch
>membrane
>tunic

ruyschian membrane

sac
>lacrimal s.
>tear s.

saccade

saccadic

sacci (genitive and plural of saccus)

sacciform

sacculated

sacculi (genitive and plural of sacculus)

sacculiform

sacculus (sacculi)
>s. lacrimalis

saccus (sacci)
>s. conjunctivalis
>s. lacrimalis

Saemisch
>operation
>ulcer

sagittal
>s. axis
>s. depth

Salus arch

Salzmann nodular corneal dystrophy

Samoan conjunctivitis

Sanders
>disease
>epidemic keratoconjunctivitis

Sanson images

Sanyal conjunctivitis

Sappey fibers

sarcoid
>Boeck s., s. of Boeck

sarcoma (sarcomas, sarcomata)
>See in *Oncology and Hematology* section.

satellite lesion

Sattler veil

Sauer
>débrider

Sauvineau ophthalmoplegia
s̄ c, s̄ gl—without correction (glass-
es) (L. sine correctione)
SC—scleral cautery
　　subconjunctival
scan
　　See also in *Radiology,*
　　Nuclear Medicine, and
　　Other Imaging section.
　　A s.
scarifier
　　Desmarres s.
Scarpa
　　staphyloma
Schäfer
　　syndrome
Scheie
　　cautery
　　ρperation
　　syndrome
schematic
Schilder
　　disease
　　encephalitis
Schiøtz tonometer
Schirmer test
Schlemm canal
Schlichting dystrophy
Schmalz
　　operation
Schmidt keratitis
Schnabel atrophy
Schnyder dystrophy
Schöbl scleritis
Schön theory
Schwalbe line
scimitar
scintillating scotoma
scirrhoblepharoncus
scirrhoid
scirrhophthalmia
scirrhous [adj.]
sclera (sclerae)
　　blue s.
scleral
　　s. buckle
　　s. crescent
　　s. icterus

scleral (continued)
　　s. lens
　　s. plexus
　　s. rigidity
　　s. spur
　　s. trabecula
scleratitis
sclerectasia
sclerectasis
sclerectoiridectomy
sclerectoiridodialysis
sclerectome
sclerectomy
scleriasis
scleriritomy
scleritis
　　Schöbl s.
sclerocataracta
sclerochoroiditis
scleroconjunctival
scleroconjunctivitis
sclerocornea
sclerocorneal
scleroiritis
sclerokeratitis
sclerokeratoiritis
sclerokeratosis
scleromalacia
　　s. perforans
scleronyxis
sclero-optic
sclerophthalmia
scleroplasty
sclerostomy
sclerotica
scleroticectomy
sclerotitis
sclerotomy
　　anterior s.
　　posterior s.
sclerous
"scopes" See under full name.
　　amblyoscope
　　anomaloscope
　　anorthoscope
　　astigmatoscope
　　binophthalmoscope
　　binoscope

"scopes" See under full name. (continued)
- cheiroscope
- ciliariscope
- clinoscope
- diploscope
- entoptoscope
- euthyscope
- fantascope
- funduscope
- gonioscope
- haploscope
- isoscope
- keratoiridoscope
- keratoscope
- kinescope
- leukoscope
- metronoscope
- microphthalmoscope
- microscope
- oculometroscope
- ophthalmofunduscope
- ophthalmoleukoscope
- ophthalmometroscope
- ophthalmoscope
- orthoptoscope
- orthoscope
- phacoidoscope
- phacoscope
- phoriascope
- phoroscope
- pupilloscope
- retinascope
- retinoscope
- stereophantoscope
- stereoscope
- stereostroboscope
- strobostereoscope
- synoptiscope
- troposcope
- visuoscope
- Visuscope

scotoma (scotomata)
- absolute s.
- annular s.
- arcuate s.
- Bjerrum s.
- cecocentral s.

scotoma (scotomata) (continued)
- central s.
- centrocecal s.
- color s.
- cuneate s.
- flittering s.
- hemianopic s.
- insular s.
- motile s.'s
- negative s.
- paracecal s.
- paracentral s.
- peripapillary s.
- peripheral s.
- physiologic s.
- positive s.
- relative s.
- ring s.
- scintillating s.
- Seidel s.
- suppression s.
- zonular s.

scotomagraph
scotomameter
scotomatous
scotometer
- Bjerrum s.

scotometry
scotopia
scotopic
screen
- Bjerrum s.
- Hess-Lees s.
- tangent s.

section
- Saemisch s.

sector
- s. iridectomy

Seidel scotoma
semilunar
senile
- s. cataract

septi (genitive of septum)
septum (septa)
- orbital s., s. orbitale

serous
serpiginous

s̄ gl, s̄ c—without glasses (correction) (L. sine correctione)
shadow
Purkinje s.'s
Shafer
sign
sheath
s. of eyeball
sheath syndrome
Sherrington law
shield
Buller s.
Fox s.
shingles
"shogren" Phonetic for Sjögren.
Sichel disease
siderosis
s. bulbi
s. conjunctivae
Sidler-Huguenin endothelioma
Siegrist-Hutchinson syndrome
Siemerling nucleus
sign
See also *effect, phenomenon,* and *reflex.*
Abadie s.
Argyll Robertson pupillary s.
Arroyo s.
Baillarger s.
Ballet s.
Bárány s.
Bard s.
Becker s.
Bekhterev s.
Bell s.
Berger s.
Bjerrum s.
Bordier-Fränkel s.
Boston s.
Brunati s.
Cantelli s.
Cestan s.
Collier s.
Cowen s.
Dalrymple s.
Dixon Mann s.
Elliot s.
Enroth s.

sign (continued)
Gianelli s.
Gifford s.
Gowers s.
Graefe (von Graefe) s.
Griffith s.
Gunn s.
Gunn crossing s.
Hennebert s.
Hutchinson s.
Jendrassik s.
Kestenbaum s.
Knies s.
Kocher s.
Larcher s.
Magendie s.
Magendie-Hertwig s.
Mann s.
Marcus Gunn pupillary s.
May s.
Means s.
Möbius s.
Munson s.
Piltz s.
pseudo-Graefe s.
Revilliod s.
Riesman s.
Rifkind s.
Seidel s.
Shafer s.
Snellen s.
Stellwag s.
Suker s.
swinging flashlight s.
Tay s.
Tournay s.
Weber s.
Wernicke s.
Widowitz s.
Wilder s.
Wood s.
siliquose
sillonneur
Silva-Costa
operation
silver wire
s.w. effect

sin–. See also words beginning
    cin–, syn–.
sinistrocular
sinistrocularity
sinistrogyration
sinistrotorsion
sinus (sinus, sinuses)
    s. of anterior chamber
    Arlt s.
    s. of Maier
    s. vcnosus sclerae
    venous s. of sclera
Sjögren
    disease
    syndrome
skew deviation
skiametry
skiascopy
Sklar-Schiøtz tonometer
sleeve
    Watzke s.
slit lamp
    s.l. biomicroscopy
    s.l. examination
SLKC—superior limbic keratocon-
    junctivitis
Smith
    operation
Smith-Kuhnt
    operation
Smith-Kuhnt-Szymanowski
    operation
Sneddon-Wilkinson disease
Snellen
    chart
    implant
    operation
    reform eye
Snell law
snowball opacities
snowballs
Soemmering
    ring
    spot
Sondermann canals
"sor–" Phonetic for words begin-
    ning psor–.

Soria
    operation
Sourdille
    operation
space
    Fontana s.
    periscleral s.
    retrobulbar s.
    Tenon s.
    zonular s.'s
Spaeth
    operation
Spanlang-Tappeiner syndrome
spatium (spatia)
    spatia anguli iridocornealis
    spatia anguli iridis (Fontanae)
    s. episclerale
    s. intervaginale
    spatia intervaginalia nervi
      optici
    s. perichorioideale, s. peri-
      choroideale
    spatia zonularia
Speas
    operation
spectacles
    aspheric lenticular s.
    Masselon s.
spectra (plural of spectrum)
spectral
spectrum (spectra)
    fortification s.
    ocular s.
    prismatic s.
    visible s.
Spencer-Watson
    operation
SPH—spherical lens
sphere
spherical
sphincter
    s. iridis
    s. oculi
    s. oris
    s. pupillae
sphincteric
sphincterismus
sphincteritis

sphincterolysis
spindle
    Krukenberg s.
sporotrichosis
sporotrichotic
spot
    See also *disk, dot, macula,*
      and *macule.*
    Bitot s.
    blind s.
    Brushfield s.
    cherry-red s.
    conjunctival s.
    cotton-wool s.'s
    Elschnig s.
    eye s.
    flame s.
    Forster-Fuchs black s.
    Fuchs s.
    Gaule s.
    histo s.
    Horner-Trantas s.
    interpalpebral s.
    lenticular s.
    Mariotte s.
    Maurer s.
    Maxwell s.
    Roth s.'s
    Soemmering s.
    Stephen s.
    Tay s.
    wet w.
spud
    Bahn s.
    Corbett s.
    Davis s.
    Dix s.
    Fisher s.
    Francis s.
    Hosford s.
    LaForce s.
    Walter s.
spur
    scleral s.
squid
squint
    comitant s., concomitant s.
    convergent s.

squint (continued)
    divergent s.
    noncomitant s.
    upward and downward s.
ST—esotropia
Stahli line
stain
    Giemsa s.
staining
    corneal s.
Stallard
    operation
staphyloma
    s. corneae
    s. cornea racemosum
    equatorial s.
    intercalary s.
    s. posticum
    Scarpa s.
    scleral s.
    uveal s.
staphylomatous
Stargardt
    disease
    syndrome
statometer
Steele-Richardson-Olszewski
    disease
    syndrome
Steinbrinck anomaly
stella (stellae)
    s. lentis hyaloidea
    s. lentis iridica
stellate
Stellwag
    brawny edema
    sign
stenocoriasis
stenopeic
    s. iridectomy
stenosis (stenoses)
step
    Rönne nasal s.
stereocampimeter
stereogram
stereo-ophthalmoscope
stereo-orthopter
stereopsis

Stifel
  figure
stigma (stigmas, stigmata)
  Koplik s. of degeneration
stigmatic
stigmatism
stigmatization
stigmatometer
Stilling
  syndrome
Stilling-Türk-Duane syndrome
Stock
  operation
Stokes
  lens
Stones implant
strabismic
strabismometer
strabismus
  Braid s.
  comitant s., concomitant s.
  concomitant s.
  s. deorsum vergens
  s. fixus
  kinetic s.
  noncomitant s.
  seesaw s.
  s. sursum vergens
strabometer
strabometry
strabotome
strabotomy
Strachan
  disease
  syndrome
Strachan-Scott
  syndrome
strata (plural of stratum)
stratiform
stratum (strata)
  ganglionic s. of optic nerve
  ganglionic s. of retina
  pigmented s. of ciliary body
  pigmented s. of iris
  pigmented s. of retina
streak
  See also *band, layer, line,*
    and *stria.*

streak (continued)
  angioid s.'s
  Knapp s.'s
stria (striae)
  See also *band, layer, line,*
    and *streak.*
  Haab s.
  Knapp s.
striatal
stroboscopic
  s. disk
stroma (stromata)
  s. of cornea
  s. iridis, s. of iris
  vitreous s., s. vitreum
stromal
Sturge
  disease
  syndrome
Sturge-Weber
  disease
  encephalotrigeminal
    angiomatosis
  syndrome
Sturm conoid
stye
  meibomian s.
  zeisian s.
Suarez-Villafranca
  operation
subcapsular
subconjunctival
subendothelial
subepithelial
  s. plexus
subhyaloid
sublatio
  s. retinae
subluxation
subretinal
substantia (substantiae)
"sudo–" Phonetic for words begin-
    ning pseudo–.
Suker
  sign
sulci (plural of sulcus)
sulciform

sulcus (sulci)
    chiasmatic s.
    infraorbital s. of maxilla
    infrapalpebral s.
    lacrimal s. of lacrimal bone
    lacrimal s. of maxilla
    oculomotor s.
    optic s.
    s. of optic chiasm
    scleral s.
    sclercorneal s.
    supraorbital s.
superciliary
supercilium
superimposition
suprachoroid
supraduction
supranuclear
supraocular
supraorbital
supratrochlear
surgical procedure
    See *operation, procedure,*
      and *technique.*
sursumduction
sursumvergence
sursumversion
suture [anatomy]
    frontozygomatic s.
    infraorbital s.
    transverse s. of Krause
    zygomaticofrontal s.
    zygomaticomaxillary s.
    zygomaticosphenoid s.
    zygomaticotemporal s.
suture [material]
    See in *General Surgical*
      Terms.
suture [technique]
    See also in *General Surgical*
      Terms.
    corneoscleral s.
    Kirby s.
Swan syndrome (I, II)
swelling
    blennorrhagic s.
Sylva irrigator
symblepharon

symblepharopterygium
symmetric, symmetrical
sympathetic
    s. nervous system
    s. ophthalmia
    s. uveitis
symptom
    See also in *General Medical*
      Terms.
    Anton s.
    halo s.
    Liebreich s.
    Magendie s.
    rainbow s.
syn–. See also words beginning
    cin–, sin–.
synathroisis
syncanthus
synchesis
synchysis
    s. scintillans
syndectomy
syndrome
    See also *disease.*
    Adie s.
    Alezzandrini s.
    Alport s.
    Alström s.
    Alström-Olsen s.
    Andogsky s.
    Angelucci s.
    Anton s.
    Anton-Babinski s.
    Axenfeld s.
    Balint s.
    Basmatter s.
    Bassen-Kornzweig s.
    Beal s.
    Behçet s.
    Behr s.
    Benedikt s., s. of Benedikt
    Bielschowsky-Lutz-Cogan s.
    Bietti s.
    Bloch-Stauffer s.
    Bloch-Sulzberger s.
    Bonnet-Dechaume-Blanc s.
    brittle cornea s.
    Brown s.

syndrome (continued)
    cat-eye s., cat's eye s.
    Cestan s.
    Cestan-Chenais s., s. of Cestan-Chenais
    Cestan-Raymond s.
    Chandler s.
    chiasma s.
    chorioretinopathy and pituitary dysfunction (CPD) s.
    Claude s.
    Claude Bernard-Horner s.
    Cogan s.
    CPD (chorioretinopathy and pituitary dysfunction) s.
    Dejean s.
    de Morsier s.
    de Morsier-Gauthier s.
    Duane s.
    Elschnig s.
    Fiessinger-Leroy-Reiter s.
    Foix s.
    Foster-Kennedy s.
    Foville s.
    Foville-Wilson s.
    Franceschetti s.
    Friedenwald s.
    Fuchs s.
    Fuchs-Kraupa s.
    Gerstmann s.
    Gradenigo s.
    Graefe s.
    Gregg s.
    Greig s.
    Grönblad-Strandberg s.
    Guillain-Barré s.
    Gunn s.
    Hallermann-Streiff s.
    Harada s.
    Hertwig-Magendie s.
    Hippel-Lindau s.
    Holmes-Adie
    Homer s.
    Horner s.
    Horner-Bernard s.
    Hutchinson s.
    ICE (iridocorneal-endothelial) s.

syndrome (continued)
    Irvine-Gass s.
    Jacod s.
    Jacod-Negri s.
    Jadassohn-Lewandowsky s.
    Johnson s.
    Kearns-Sayre s.
    Kehrer-Adie s.
    Kennedy s.
    keratitis-ichthyosis-deafness (KID) s.
    KID s.
    Kiloh-Nevin s.
    Kimmelstiel-Wilson s.
    Koerber-Salus-Elschnig s.
    Krause s.
    Kurz s.
    Laurence-Moon-Biedl s.
    Löwe s.
    Lyle s.
    Marcus Gunn s.
    Marfan s.
    Marinesco-Sjögren s.
    Marinesco-Sjögren-Garland s.
    Mikulicz s.
    Mikulicz-Radecki s.
    Mikulicz-Sjögren s.
    Millard-Gubler s.
    Miller s.
    Möbius s.
    morning glory s.
    Nothnagel s.
    Parinaud s.
    Paterson-Brown-Kelly s.
    Petzetakis-Takos s.
    pigment dispersion s.
    Posner-Schlossman s.
    Reese s.
    Reiter s.
    Riddoch s.
    Rieger s.
    Riley-Day s.
    Riley-Smith s.
    Rollet s.
    Rot-Bielschowsky s.
    Rothmund s.
    Rutherfurd s.
    Schäfer s.

syndrome (continued)
>Schaffer s.
>Siegrist-Hutchinson s.
>Sjögren s.
>Spanlang-Tappeiner s.
>Stargardt s.
>Stevens-Johnson s.
>Stilling-Türk-Duane s.
>Sturge-Weber s.
>Swan s. (I, II)
>Terry s.
>Thompson s.
>Tolosa-Hunt s.
>Touraine I s.
>Uyemura s.
>Vogt s.
>Vogt-Koyanagi s.
>Weber s., s. of Weber
>Weill-Marchesani s.
>Weill-Reys s.
>Weill-Reys-Adie s.
>Werner s.
>Wernicke s.
>Wolf s.
>Wolfram s.
synechia (synechiae)
>annular s.
>anterior s.
>circular s.
>posterior s.
>ring s.
>total anterior s.
>total posterior s.
synechotomy
synergist
synophrys
synophthalmia
synoptophore
syphilis
>s. of conjunctiva
>s. of iris
system
>McIntire aspiration-irriga-
>>tion s.
systemic
>s. lupus erythematosus (SLE)
>s. sclerosis

Szymanowski operation
Szymanowski-Kuhnt
>operation
T—tension (intraocular)
T− (T minus)—decreased tension
>(T−1, T−2)
T+ (T plus)—increased tension
>(T+1, T+2)
table
>Reuss t.
Tansley operation
TAP—tension by applanation
tapeta (plural of tapetum)
tapetal
tapetum (tapeta)
>t. choroideae
>t. lucidum
>t. nigrum
>t. oculi
tarsadenitis
tarsal
tarsectomy
tarsi
tarsitis
tarsocheiloplasty
tarsomalacia
tarsoplasty
tarsorrhaphy
tarsotomy
tarsus
>t. inferior palpebrae
>t. superior palpebrae
tattooing
>t. of cornea
Tay
>choroiditis
>disease
>sign
>spot
tear
>fishmouth t.
>retinal t.
tears
>crocodile t.
technique
>See also *method.*
>See also in *General Surgical
>>Terms.*

technique (continued)
    Atkinson t.
    Cutler-Beard t.
    Van Lint t.
tectonic
    t. keratoplasty
Teflon implant
teichopsia
telangiectasis (telangiectases)
telebinocular
telecanthus
temporal
    t. arteritis
    t. crescent
    t. loop
    t. pallor
tendo (tendines)
    t. oculi
    t. palpebrarum
tendon
    Lockwood t.
    superior oblique t.
    Zinn t.
tendotomy
tendovaginal
Tenon
    capsule
    fascia
    space
tenonitis
tenonometer
tenontotomy
tenotomist
tenotomize
tenotomy
    intrasheath t.
tension
    intraocular t.
"tere–" Phonetic for words begin-
    ning pteri–, ptery–.
Terrien ulcer
Terry syndrome
Terson
    operation
test
    See also in *Laboratory,*
       Pathology, and Chemistry
       Terms.

test (continued)
    Bielschowsky t.
    Bruchner t.
    color perception t.
    color vision t.
    complement fixation (CF) t.
    confrontation field t.
    cover t.
    duction t.
    duochrome t.
    E t.
    Farnsworth D-100 t.
    fluorescein dye disappear-
       ance t.
    forced duction t.
    four diopter base-out prism t.
    Frostig Developmental T. of
       Visual Perception
    Graefe t.
    head-tilt t.
    Hering t.
    Hirschberg t. for strabismus
    Holmgren t.
    Ishihara t.
    Jaeger t.
    Jones t.
    Lancaster red-green t.
    lantern t.
    limulus lysate t.
    Marlow t.
    Mauthner t.
    prism adaption t.
    red glass t.
    Schirmer t.
    shadow t.
    Snellen t.
    Titmus t.
    transillumination t.
    visual field t.
    visual-motor gestalt t.
    W4D (Worth four-dot) t.
    Wernicke t.
testing
    visual field t.
tetartanopia
tetartanopic
tetartanopsia
tetrastichiasis

theory
>Hering t.
>Schön t.
>Young-Helmholtz t.

therapeutic
>t. iridectomy

thermosector

"thi-sis" Phonetic for phthisis.

Thomas
>cryoptor

Thompson
>syndrome

threshold
>flicker fusion t.

Thygeson keratitis

thyrotrophic, thyrotropic

tic douloureux

"tikopseah" Phonetic for teichopsia.

time (T)
>fading t.

"ti-sis" Phonetic for phthisis.

Titmus stereo test

Tolosa-Hunt syndrome

tomography
>computed t. (CT)

tonogram

tonograph

tonographer

tonometer
>Draeger t.
>Goldmann applanation t.
>indentation t.
>Mackay-Marg t.
>McLean t.
>Perkins t.
>pneumatic t.
>Schiøtz t.
>Sklar-Schiøtz t.

tonometry
>applanation t.
>indentation t.

torpor
>t. retinae

torsion

tortuous

"tosis" Phonetic for ptosis.

Toti
>operation

"totic" Phonetic for ptotic.

Toti-Mosher
>operation

Touraine
>syndrome (I)

toxoplasmic

toxoplasmosis
>ocular t.

trabecularism

trabeculate

trabeculation

trabeculectomy

trabeculoplasty
>argon laser t.
>laser t.

trabeculotomy

trachoma (trachomata)
>Arlt t.
>brawny t.
>Türck t.

trachomatous

track
>bear t.'s

tractus (tractus)

transcorneal

transient
>t. ischemia
>t. obscuration

transilluminator
>Finnoff t.

transplant
>corneal t.

transplantation
>corneal t.

transposition

transverse
>t. suture of Krause

Trantas
>dots
>operation

trauma (traumas, traumata)

Treacher Collins
>syndrome

Treacher Collins-Franceschetti
>syndrome

treatment
>Imre t.

trepanation
    corneal t.
trephination
    corneoscleral t.
TRIC—trachoma-inclusion con-
    junctivitis
trichromat
trichromatopsia
trichromic
trifocal
trigeminal
    t. neuralgia
trigone
    Müller t.
triplokoria
triplopia
tritanopia
tritanopic
tritanopsia
trochlea (trochleae)
    t. of superior oblique muscle
trochleariform
trochlearis
tropia
tropometer
Troutman
    implant
    operation
tube
    Bowman t.'s
    corneal t.'s
tuber (tubers, tubera)
    t. zygomaticum
tubercula (plural of tuberculum)
tuberculoid
tuberculous
    t. keratoconjunctivitis
tuberculum (tubercula)
    t. articulare ossis temporalis
    t. marginale ossis zygomatici
tuberositas (tuberositates)
tuberosity
    malar t.
tuck
Tuerck. See *Türck.*
tunic
    Brücke t.
    fibrous t. of eyeball

tunic (continued)
    fibrous t. of liver
    mucous t.
    muscular t.
    proper t.
    Ruysch t.
tunica (tunicae)
    t. conjunctiva
    t. conjunctiva palpebrarum
    t. fibrosa
    t. fibrosa bulbi
    t. fibrosa oculi
    t. interna bulbi
    t. nervea of Brücke
    t. propria
    t. ruyschiana
    t. uvea
tunicary
tunicate
tunnel vision
Türck
    trachoma
tutamen (tutamina)
    tutamina oculi
Tyndall effect
"ty-sis" Phonetic for phthisis.
"u–" Phonetic for words beginning
    eu–.
ulcer
    Mooren u.
    Saemisch u.
    Terrien u.
ulcera (plural of ulcus)
ulcus (ulcera)
    u. serpens corneae
ulectomy
Ullrich-Feichtiger
    syndrome
ultrasonogram
    B scan u.
Undine dropper
unit
    See also in *General Medical*
        Terms and *Laboratory,*
        Pathology, and Chemistry
        Terms.
    Mira u.
up-gaze

Usher
 disease
 syndrome
uvea
uveitic
uveitis
 Förster u.
 heterochromic u.
 sympathetic u.
uveomeningitis
uveoparotid
uveoparotitis
uveoplasty
uveoscleritis
uviform
Uyemura syndrome
V—vision
 visual acuity
Va—visual acuity
vagina (vaginae)
 v. bulbi
 v. externa nervi optici
 v. interna nervi optici
 vaginae nervi optici
 v. oculi
vaginate
valve
 Foltz v.
 Hasner v.
 Rosenmüller v.
Van Lint
 akinesia
 block
 technique
variation
 diurnal v.
varicoblepharon
Varilux
vas (vasa)
 vasa sanguinea retinae
vascular
 v. insufficiency
vasoconstrictive
vasoconstrictors [a class of drugs]
vasodilatation
vasoinhibitory
VC—acuity of color vision
VDA—visual discriminatory acuity

VE—visual efficiency
vectograph
veil
 Sattler v.
vein
 ciliary v.
 cilioretinal v.
 posterior conjunctival v.
 retinal v.
 vorticose v.
vena (venae)
 venae centralis retinae
 venae vorticosae
ventriculi (plural of ventriculus)
venula (venulae)
 v. macularis inferior
 v. macularis superior
 v. medialis retinae
 v. nasalis retinae inferior
 v. nasalis retinae superior
 v. retinae medialis
 v. temporalis retinae inferior
 v. temporalis retinae superior
venular
venule
 medial v. of retina
 nasal v. of retina, inferior
  and superior
 temporal v. of retina, inferi-
  or and superior
Verga
 lacrimal groove
vergence
Verhoeff
 operation
vernal
 v. catarrh
 v. conjunctivitis
vernier [scale]
Vernier [eponym]
 acuity
version
vertebrobasilar
vertex (vertices)
 v. of cornea, v. corneae
vertigo
 rotary v., rotatory v.

Verwey
    operation
vesicle [noun: blister, small sac]
    ocular v.
    ophthalmic v.
    optic v.
vesicula (vesiculae)
    v. ophthalmica
vestibular
vestibulo-ocular
v.f.—visual field
VF—visual field
VH—vitreous hemorrhage
VHF—visual half-field
Vieth-Muller horopter
villi (plural of villus)
villiferous
villose, villous [adj.]
villosity
villus (villi)
    v. of choroid plexus
virus
    See also in *Laboratory,*
      Pathology, and Chemistry
      Terms.
viscous [adj.]
vision
    achromatic v.
    binocular v.
    chromatic v.
    color v.
    dichromatic v.
    foveal v.
    halo v.
    haploscopic v.
    iridescent v.
    monocular v.
    v. null
    oscillating v.
    peripheral v.
    photopic v.
    Pick v.
    pseudoscopic v.
    rod v.
    scoterythrous v.
    scotopic v.
    stereoscopic v.
    tunnel v.

visual
    v. acuity
    v. axis
    v. cortex
    v. evoked potential (VEP)
    v. field examination
    v. purple
visualization
visualize
visuometer
visuosensory
vitiligo (vitiligines)
    v. iridis
vitrectomy
    open sky v.
    pars plana v.
vitrector
    Kaufman v.
vitreocapsulitis
vitreoretinopathy
vitreous
    v. base
    v. body
    v. bulge
    detached v.
    v. floater
    v. hemorrhage
    v. humor
    v. opacity
    primary persistent hyper-
      plastic v.
    secondary v.
    v. tap
    tertiary v.
    v. touch
vitreum
vitritis
Vogt
    cataract
    cornea
    degeneration
    disease
    girdle
    syndrome
Vogt-Koyanagi
    syndrome
Vogt-Koyanagi-Harada
    syndrome

Vogt-Spielmeyer
  disease
von Haller. See *Haller.*
von Hippel (Hippel)
  disease
  keratoplasty
  operation
von Hippel-Lindau
  disease
  syndrome
von Monakow. See *Monakow.*
vortex (vortices)
  v. dystrophy
  Fleischer v.
  v. lentis
Vossius lenticular ring
VOU—vision, each eye (L. visio
  oculus uterque)
VS—without glasses
Wachendorf membrane
Wagener retinitis
Wagner
  disease
  line
  syndrome
Waldhauer
  operation
Walker
  lid everter
  pin
walleye
wart
  Hassall-Henle w.
Watzke sleeve
wavelength
W4D—Worth four-dot (test)
Weber
  paralysis
  sign
  syndrome
Weeks
  bacillus
  operation
Weil
  disease
Weill-Marchesani
  syndrome

Weill-Reys
  syndrome
Weill-Reys-Adie
  syndrome
Weiss reflex
Werner
  syndrome
Wernicke
  disease
  encephalopathy
  reaction
  sign
  syndrome
Wernicke-Korsakoff
  psychosis
  syndrome
West
  operation
Westphal-Strümpell
  disease
  pseudosclerosis
Weve
  electrode
Wheeler
  implant
  operation
Whitnall tubercle
Wicherkiewicz
  operation
Widmark conjunctivitis
Wiener
  operation
Wilder
  sign
Wildervanck syndrome
Wilmer
  operation
Wilson
  disease
wing
  Maddox w.
wipe-out syndrome
Wolf
  syndrome
Wolfe
  operation
Wolfram
  syndrome

Wolfring
  glands
Worth
  operation
Worth four-dot test
Wucherer
  conjunctivitis
xanthelasma
  x. palpebrarum
xanthelasmatosis
xanthism
xanthocyanopsia
xanthokyanopy
xanthoma (xanthomas, xanthomata)
  disseminated x., x. dissemi-
    natum
  x. multiplex
  x. palpebrarum
xanthomatosis
  x. bulbi
  x. iridis
xanthophane
xanthopsia
xenophthalmia
xeroma
xerosis
  x. conjunctivae
  conjunctival x.
  x. corneae
  corneal x.
  x. superficialis
XT—exotropia
"yoo–" Phonetic for words beginning eu–.
Young-Helmholtz
  theory
YS—yellow spot (of the retina)
Zeis
  glands, glands of Z.
zeisian gland
zeisian stye
Zeiss
  photocoagulator
"zero–" Phonetic for words beginning xero–.
"zheel-bare" Phonetic for Gilbert
  [Nicolas Augustin Gilbert].

Ziegler
  cautery
  operation
Zinn
  annulus
  circlet
  corona
  ligament
  tendon
  zonule
Zöllner
  figure
  lines
zone
  ciliary z.
  z.'s of discontinuity
  extravisual z.'s
  far z.
  focal z.
  interpalpebral z.
  near z.
  nuclear z.
  pupillary z.
  visual z.
  z. of Zinn
zonula (zonulae)
  z. ciliaris, z. ciliaris (Zinnii)
zonular
  z. fibers
  z. space
zonule
  ciliary z.
  z. of Zinn
zonulitis
zonulolysis
  enzymatic z.
zonulotomy
zygoma
zygomatic
zygomaticofrontal
  z. suture
zygomaticomaxillary
  z. suture
zygomaticosphenoid
  z. suture
zygomaticotemporal
  z. suture

Orthopedic and Sports Medicine

AAE—active assistive exercise
AAOS—American Academy of
    Orthopaedic Surgeons
AAPMR—American Academy of
    Physical Medicine and Reha-
    bilitation
AB—Ace bandage
abarthrosis
abarticular
abarticulation
abasic
Abbott
    method
    operation
Abbott-Lucas
    operation
abductor
ability
    general a.
ablation
abscess
    arthrifluent a.
    bone a.
    Brodie a.
    bursal a.
    hypostatic a.
    intramedullary a.
    ischiorectal a.
    lumbar a.
    ossifluent a.
    periarticular a.
    Pott a.
    sacrococcygeal a.
    serous a.
    subfascial a.
    subperiosteal a.
    supralevator a.
    syphilitic a.
    thecal a.

abscess (continued)
    traumatic a.
absconsio
AC—acromioclavicular
acampsia
acantha
accessiflexor
accident
    cerebrovascular a. (CVA)
acclimate, acclimated
acclimation
acclimatize
accommodation
    reflex a., a. reflex
accommodative
    a. equipment
acetabula (plural of acetabulum)
acetabular
    a. rim
acetabulectomy
acetabuloplasty
acetabulum (acetabula)
Achilles
    bursa
    bursitis
    jerk
    reflex
    tendon
achillobursitis
achillodynia
achillogram
achillorrhaphy
achillotenotomy
    plastic a.
achillotomy
achondrogenesis
achondroplasia
achondroplastic
achondroplasty

925

acidosis
  lactic a.
acidosteophyte
ACL—anterior cruciate ligament
aclasia
aclasis
  diaphyseal a.
  metaphyseal a.
  tarsoepiphyseal a.
aclastic
ACLF—adult congregate living
  facility
acnemia
acoustogram
ACPS—acrocephalopolysyndactyly
acral
ACRM—American College of
  Rehabilitation Medicine
acroarthritis
acrocontracture
acrocyanosis
acrodysplasia
acroesthesia
acromacria
acromegalic
acromegalogigantism
acromegaloidism
acromelia
acromelic
acrometagenesis
acromial
acromiale
  os a.
acromiocoracoid
acromiohumeral
acromion
acromionectomy
acromioneurosis
acromioscapular
acromiothoracic
acromyotonia
acromyotonus
acro-osteolysis
acropachia
acropachyderma
  a. with pachyperiostitis
acroparalysis

acroparesthesia
  Nothnagel-type a.
  Schultze-type a.
acropathology
acropathy
  amyotrophic a.
  ulcerative mutilating a.
acrostealgia
acrosyndactyly
ACSM—American College of
  Sports Medicine
action
active
  a. motion
  a. range of motion
activity
  a.'s of daily living (ADL,
    ADLs)
actomyosin
acupoint
acupressure
acute on chronic
  a.o.c. fracture
adactylous
adactyly
Adair-Dighton syndrome
Adamantiades-Behçet syndrome
adamantinoma
  a. of long bones
  tibial a.
Adams
  operation
adducent
adduct
adduction
adductor
Adelmann
  operation
adhesive
  methylmethacrylate a.
aditus
  a. ad pelvem
ADL, ADLs—activities of daily living
adminiculum (adminicula)
  a. lineae albae
adromia

advancement
    tendon a.
AE—above-elbow
AEA—above-elbow amputation
aerobic capacity
AFO—ankle-foot orthosis
aftercare
age
    bone a.
    skeletal a.
AGE—angle of greatest extension
AGF—angle of greatest flexion
"ah-mi-o–" Phonetic for words
    beginning amyo–.
aid
    prosthetic speech a.
    speech a.
    ultrasonic mobility a.
air
    a. arthrography
    a. bed
    laminar a. flow
    a. myelography
    a. splint
AirGEL
AK—above-knee, above-the-knee
AKA—above-knee amputation
"a-kil-ez" Phonetic for Achilles.
"a-kilo–" Phonetic for words begin-
    ning achillo–.
Akin
    bunionectomy
    operation
"a-kon-dro-plaz-ee-a" Phonetic for
    achondroplasia.
ala (alae)
    a. ilii
    a. ossis ilii
    a. ossis ilium
Alanson amputation
alar
Albee
    operation
Albee-Delbet
    operation
Albers-Schönberg
    disease
    syndrome

Albert
    disease
    operation
Albright
    disease
    dystrophy
    syndrome
algodystrophy
alignment
    anatomical a.
    optimal a.
Allen
    maneuver
Allis
    sign
alloarthroplasty
Alouette
    amputation
    operation
Alsberg
    angle
    triangle
alveolar
    segmental a. osteotomy
ambulation
amelia
    brachial a.
    complete a.
    unilateral a.
American Academy of Orthopaedic
    Surgeons (AAOS)
American College of Sports Medi-
    cine (ACSM)
American Physical Therapy Associ-
    ation (APTA)
Amoss sign
amphiarthrosis
amputation
    AK (above-knee) a.
    Alanson a.
    Alouette a.
    Anderson a.
    aperiosteal a.
    Béclard a.
    Berger a.
    Bier a.
    BK (below-knee) a.
    bloodless a.

amputation (continued)
>Bunge a.
Callander a.
Carden a.
cervix a.
chop a.
Chopart a.
cineplastic a.
circular a.
coat-sleeve a.
cutaneous a.
definitive a.
diaclastic a.
double-flap a.
Dupuytren a.
eccentric a.
elliptical a.
end-bearing a.
Forbes a.
forequarter a.
Gritti a.
Gritti-Stokes a.
guillotine a.
Guyon a.
Hancock a.
Hey a.
hindquarter a.
a. in contiguity
interilioabdominal a.
interinnominoabdominal a.
intermediary a.
interpelviabdominal a.
interscapulothoracic a.
intrapyretic a.
Jaboulay a.
Kirk a.
Langenbeck (von Langen-
beck) a.
Larrey a.
Le Fort a.
Lisfranc a.
Mackenzie a.
Maisonneuve a.
Malgaigne a.
mediotarsal a.
metacarpal a.
musculocutaneous a.
oblique a.

amputation (continued)
osteoplastic a.
pathologic a.
periosteoplastic a.
phalangophalangeal a.
Pirogoff a.
primary a.
provisional a.
pulp a.
racket a.
ray a.
rectangular a.
Ricard a.
secondary a.
semicircular flap a.
Stokes a.
subastragalar a.
submalleolar a.
subperiosteal a.
supracondylar a.
Syme a.
Teale a.
tertiary a.
through-the-knee a.
transfixation a.
transmetatarsal a.
traumatic a.
traverse a.
Tripier a.
Vladimiroff-Mikulicz a.
amyoplasia
a. congenita
amyotonia
a. congenita
Oppenheim a.
amyotrophia
neuralgic a.
a. spinalis progressiva
amyotrophic
amyotrophy
Aran-Duchenne a.
diabetic a.
neuralgic a.
neuritic a.
primary progressive a.
progressive nuclear a.
syphilitic a.
anabolic steroids [a class of drugs]

anapophysis
anarrhexis
anastomosis (anastomoses)
    See also *operation* and *pro-*
      cedure.
    nerve a.
anatomic, anatomical
anatomical snuffbox
ancillary
    a. therapy
anconeal
Anderson
    amputation
    operation
    pin fixation
    tibial lengthening
anesthesia
    See in *General Surgical*
      Terms.
Anghelescu sign
angiography
    peripheral a.
    spinal cord a.
    vertebral a.
angiokeratoma
    a. corporis diffusum
    a. corporis diffusum univer-
      sale
    diffuse a.
"angkilo–" Phonetic for words
    beginning ankylo–.
angle
    manubriosternal a.
    a. of supination
angulated
angulation
    a. osteotomy
ankle
    a. mortise
    tailor's a.
ankylodactyly
ankylopoietic
ankylosed
ankylosing
ankylosis (ankyloses)
    capsular a.
    extra-articular a.
    ligamentous a.

ankylosis (ankyloses) (continued)
    operative a.
    partial a.
    unsound a.
ankylotic
Annandale
    operation
annulus (annuli) [compare: anulus]
anomaly
    Poland a.
anosteoplasia
anostosis
antebrachium
antecubital
anteroinferior
anteroposterior
anterosuperior
anterosuperiorly
anteroventral
anthropokinetics
anti-inflammatory
anulus (anuli) [compare: annulus]
    a. of Zinn
AOTA—American Occupational
    Therapy Association
aperture
apex (apices, apexes)
    a. of arytenoid cartilage
    a. ossis sacralis, a. ossis sacri
    a. patellae
Apley
    grinding test
    knee test
    maneuver
    sign
    traction
apocope
apocoptic
"apofi–" Phonetic for words begin-
    ning apophy–.
aponeurectomy
aponeurorrhaphy
aponeurosis (aponeuroses)
    extensor a.
    a. of vastus muscles
aponeurotic
aponeurotomy
apophyseal

apophysis (apophyses)
    See also *process.*
    calcaneal a.
apophysitis
    a. tibialis adolescentium
apparatus
    Kirschner a.
    Sayre a.
    spine a.
appearance
    bone-within-bone a.
appliance
    See also *prosthesis.*
arachnoid
arachnoidal
arch
    cervical a.
    dorsal a. of wrist
    dorsal venous a. of hand
    fallen a.'s
    ischiopubic a.
    neural a.
    palmar carpal a.
    vertebral a.
arciform
arcuate
arcuation
area (areae, areas)
    donor a.
    Patrick trigger a.'s
    pericruciate a.
    thenar a.
areflexia
"areten–" Phonetic for words beginning aryten–.
Arnold-Chiari
    deformity
    malformation
    syndrome
arteriography
    peripheral a.
    spinal a.
    vertebral a.
artery
    basilic a.
    brachial a.
    cephalic a.
    femoral a.

artery (continued)
    genicular a.
    gluteal a.
    interosseous a.
    obturator a.
    peripheral a.
    peroneal a.
    popliteal a.
    princeps pollicis a.
    profunda brachii a.
    pudendal a.
    radial a.
    radialis indicis a.
    saphenous a.
    ulnar a.
    vesical a.
    volar a.
arthragra
arthralgia
    acromegalic a.
    nonspecific a.
    periodic a.
arthrectomy
arthrempyesis
arthritic
arthritis (arthritides)
    acromegalic a.
    Bekhterev a.
    chronic villous a.
    crystal a.
    degenerative a.
    erosive a.
    exudative a.
    gouty a.
    hypertrophic a.
    juvenile rheumatoid a.
    Lyme a.
    Marie-Strümpell a.
    monoarticular a.
    a. mutilans
    navicular a.
    nonarticular a.
    periosteal a.
    rheumatoid a.
    suppurative a.
    vertebral a.
arthritis arthrogram
arthrocele

arthrochalasis
arthrochondritis
arthroclasia
arthrodesis
    Charnley a.
    extra-articular a.
    Moberg a.
arthrodynia
arthrodysplasia
    hereditary a.
arthroempyesis
arthroereisis
arthrogenous
arthrogram
arthrography
    air a.
    double-contrast a.
    opaque a.
arthrokatadysis
arthrokleisis
arthrolith
arthrolithiasis
arthrology
arthrolysis
arthromeningitis
arthrometer
arthrometry
arthroncus
arthroneuralgia
arthronosos
arthro-onychodysplasia
arthro-osteo-onychodysplasia
arthropathia
arthropathic
arthropathology
arthropathy
    Charcot a.
    degenerative vertebral a.
    dislocating a.
    disuse a.
    gonococcal a.
    Heberden a.
    hemophilic a.
    ochronotic a.
    palindromic a.
    pyrophosphate a.
    stationary a.
arthrophyma

arthrophyte
arthroplasty
    Aufranc-Turner a.
    Bechtol a.
    cementless a.
    Charnley-Mueller a.
    Crawford-Adams a.
    Crawford-Adams cup a.
    Keller a.
    Lacey rotating-hinge a.
    Magnuson-Stack a.
    McAtee-Tharias-Blazina a.
    McKee-Farrar a.
    McKee-Farrar hip a.
    New England Baptist a.
    Putti-Platt a.
    Schlein-type elbow a.
    Stanmore shoulder a.
    total hip a.
    total knee a.
    Unipore hip a.
arthropneumoroentgenography
arthropyosis
arthrorheumatism
arthroscintigram
arthroscintigraphy
arthrosclerosis
arthroscopic meniscectomy
arthrosis
    Charcot a.
    a. deformans
arthrosteitis
arthrostomy
arthrosynovitis
arthrotomy
    Magnuson-Stack shoulder a.
arthroxerosis
arthroxesis
articular
articulate
articulated
articulatio
    a. coxae
    a. genu
    a. humeri
articulation
    carpal a.
    carpometacarpal a.

articulation (continued)
    chondrosternal a.
    congruent a.
    costocentral a.
    costochondral a.'s
    costosternal a
    costotransverse a.
    costovertebral a.
    coxal a.
    ellipsoidal a.
    false a.
    a.'s of free inferior limb
    a.'s of free inferior member
    freely movable a.
    a.'s of girdle of inferior
      member
    hinge a.
    humeroradial a.
    humeroulnar a.
    iliosacral a.
    immovable a.
    incongruent a.
    intermetacarpal a.
    intermetatarsal a.
    interphalangeal a.
    metacarpophalangeal a.
    metatarsophalangeal a.
    patellofemoral a.
    phalangeal a.
    radiocarpal a.
    reciprocal a.
    sacrococcygeal a.
    sacroiliac a.
    slightly movable a.
    sternochondral a.'s
    sternoclavicular a.
    talocalcaneonavicular a.
    talonavicular a.
    tarsometatarsal a
    tibiofibular a.
    trochoidal a.
articulatory
arytenoidectomy
arytenoiditis
arytenoidopexy
aspirate
aspiration
astragalar

astragalectomy
astragalocalcanean
astragalocrural
astragaloscaphoid
astragalotibial
astragalus
atelomyelia
atelopodia
atelorachidia
athlete
atlas [C1 vertebra]
atrophy
    Charcot-Marie-Tooth a.
    gauntlet a.
    inactivity a.
    Sudeck a.
    traction a.
    traumatic a.
attachment
    muscle-tendon a.
Aufranc-Turner
    arthroplasty
    operation
autologous
    a. transfusion
autonomy
autotransfusion
Avila
    operation
avulsion
Axer
    operation
axis [C2 vertebra]
axon
Baastrup
    disease
    syndrome
bacillus (bacilli)
    See in *Laboratory, Patholo-*
      gy, and Chemistry Terms.
Bacillus
    See in *Laboratory, Patholo-*
      gy, and Chemistry Terms.
back
    old man's b.
    static b.
    sway b. [pref: swayback]

bacterium (bacteria)
    See specific bacteria in *Laboratory, Pathology, and Chemistry Terms.*
Badgley
    operation
Baker
    cyst
Bakwin-Eiger syndrome
ball of foot
Bamberger-Marie
    disease
    syndrome
band
    See also *frenulum, frenum,* and *vinculum.*
    See also *line.*
    iliotibial b.
    Parham b.
    periosteal b.
bandage
    See also in *General Surgical Terms.*
Bankhart
    lesion
    operation
    reconstruction
Bardenheuer
    extension
    incision
Barker
    operation
Barkow
    ligaments
Barnes
    curve
Barsky
    operation
Bársony-Polgár syndrome
Bársony-Teschendorf syndrome
Barton
    fracture
Barwell
    operation
base
    b. of metatarsal
    b. of sacrum
basioccipital

basivertebral
Bateman
    operation
bath
    alternant-contrast b.
Baumann angle
BB—both bones
Beals syndrome
beanbag
Bechtol
    arthroplasty
Béclard
    amputation
Beevor sign
Bekhterev (Bechterew)
    arthritis
    disease
    rheumatoid spondylitis
    spondylitis
    test
Bekhterev-Strümpell spondylitis
belly
    muscle b.
Benedict-Roth
    apparatus
benefited
Bennett
    dislocation
    fracture
    posterior shoulder approach
Bent
    operation
Berger
    amputation
    operation
    paresthesia
Bertin
    ligament
Bertolotti syndrome
Besnier
    rheumatism
BG—bone graft
biarticular
biarticulate
bicapsular
biceps
    b. brachii
    b. femoris

Bichat
    ligament
bicipital
Bier
    amputation
    operation
Bigelow
    ligament
    septum
bi-ischial
bimalleolar
Biobrane
    adhesive
    glove
    synthetic skin substitute
biomechanics
bionics
biophysical
biopsy
    muscle b.
bipedal
bipennate, bipenniform
bisacromial
Bischof
    myelotomy
bisiliac
bisphosphonates [a class of drugs]
bitrochanteric
biventral
block
    articular b.
    ganglionic b.
    neuromuscular b.
    b. osteotomy
    parasacral b.
    paravertebral b.
    perineural b.
    presacral b.
    pudendal b.
    sacral b.
    stellate b.
    subarachnoid b.
    sympathetic b.
    transsacral b.
    vertebral b.
Blount
    disease
    operation

Blundell-Jones
    operation
board
    alphabet b.
    back b.
    spine b.
    transfer b.
Bobroff
    operation
body (bodies)
    fatty b. of acetabular fossa
    b. of ilium
    b. of ischium
    b. of radius
    b. of rib
    b. of talus
    b. of tibia
    b. of ulna
    vertebral b., body of vertebra
Böhler
    calcaneal angle
bone
    accessory b.
    acetabular b.
    acromial b.
    alar b.
    Albers-Schönberg b.
    alisphenoid b.
    ankle b.
    astragaloid b.
    astragaloscaphoid b.
    basihyal b.
    basilar b.
    Bertin b.
    breast b.
    bregmatic b.
    brittle b.
    calcaneal b.
    cancellated b.
    cancellous b.
    capitate b.
    carpal b.
    chalky b.
    coccygeal b.
    collar b.
    compact b.
    cortical b.
    costal b.

bone (continued)
    cranial b.
    cuneiform b.
    b. depression
    ectethmoid b.
    ectocuneiform b.
    endochondral b.
    entocuneiform b.
    epactal b.
    ethmoid b.
    exoccipital b.
    femoral b.
    fibular b.
    flank b.
    frontal b.
    hamate b.
    haunch b.
    b. head
    humeral b.
    hyoid b.
    iliac b.
    incarial b.
    intermaxillary b.
    interparietal b.
    intrachondrial b.
    ischial b.
    ivory b.
    lacrimal b.
    lenticular b.
    lunate b.
    maxillary b.
    mesocuneiform b.
    metacarpal b.
    metatarsal b.
    multangular b.
    nasal b.
    navicular b.
    occipital b.
    orbitosphenoidal b.
    parietal b.
    pelvic b.
    periosteal b.
    petrous b.
    phalangeal b.
    Pirie b.
    pisiform b.
    b. processes
    pubic b.

bone (continued)
    radial b.
    replacement b.
    rider's b.
    sacral b.
    scaphoid b.
    scapular b.
    sesamoid b.
    shin b.
    shoulder b.
    sphenoid b.
    spongy b.
    supernumerary b.
    tarsal b.
    temporal b.
    tibia b.
    trapezium b.
    trapezoid b.
    triangular b.
    triquetral b.
    turbinate b.
    ulna b.
    ulnar styloid b.
    unciform b.
    uncinate b.
    vesalian b.
    vomer b.
    b. wax
    whettle b.
    wormian b.
    xiphoid b.
    zygomatic b.
bone graft
    diamond inlay b.g.
    dual inlay b.g.
    hemicylindrical b.g.
    inlay b.g.
    intramedullary b.g.
    medullary b.g.
    onlay b.g.
    osteoperiosteal b.g.
    peg b.g.
    sliding inlay b.g.
bonelet
Bonnet
    sign
bony
    b. island

bony (continued)
    b. processes
    b. prominence
    b. suture
"boo-kay" Phonetic for bouquet.
"boor-zhe-ree(z)" Phonetic for
    Bourgery.
"boo-shahr(z)" Phonetic for
    Bouchard.
"boo-ton-year" Phonetic for bouton-
    nière.
border
    See also *limbus* and *margin.*
    interosseous b.
boss
    frontal b.
    parietal b.
bossing
    b. of cranium
Bosworth
    operation
    procedure
Bouchard
    disease
    nodes
    nodules
    sign
bouquet
Bourgery ligament
boutonnière
Bowen-Grover
    meniscotomy
bowleg, bowlegged
Boyd
    operation
brace
    See *appliance, orthosis,*
        prosthesis, and *splint.*
    See also *appliance, orthosis,*
        prosthesis, and *splint.*
bracelet
brachialgia
brachial plexus
brachiocrural
brachiocubital
brachiocyllosis
brachiocyrtosis
brachiogram

brachium (brachia)
brachymetapody
brachymetatarsia
brachyphalangia
brachyskelous
brachystasis
Bragard sign
branch
    thenar b. of median nerve
brawny
    b. edema
    b. induration
breach
Breschet
    bones
Brett
    operation
brevicollis
breviflexor
bridging osteophytes
brisement ["briz-mon"]
    b. forcé ["for-say"]
Brissaud
    scoliosis
Bristow
    operation
    procedure
Brittain
    operation
Brockman
    operation
Brodie
    abscess
    disease
    knee
    ligament
"broo-ee" Phonetic for bruit.
Bruck
    disease
Brudzinski
    reflex
    sign
bruit
    See in *Cardiology* and *Pul-*
        monary Medicine sections.
Bryant
    line
    sign

Bryant (continued)
    traction
    triangle
BSE—bilateral, symmetrical, and
    equal
Buck
    extension
    operation
    traction
buckle
    b. fracture
Büdinger-Ludloff-Laewen
    disease
Budin joint
BUE—both upper extremities
bundle
    cleidoepitrochlear b. of del-
      toid muscle
Bunge
    amputation
bunion
    tailor's b.
bunionectomy
    Akin b.
    Keller b.
    Mitchell b.
    Silver b.
    Stone b.
bunionette
Bunnell
    operation
    tendon transfer
Burns ligament
bursa (bursae)
    Achilles b.
    anserine b.
    b. of biceps brachii muscle
    epiploic b.
    b. of iliopsoas muscle
    ischiogluteal b.
    Monro b.
    olecranon b.
    patellar b.
    b. of pectoralis major muscle
    prepatellar b.
    radial b.
    radiohumeral b.
    retrocalcaneal b.

bursa (bursae) (continued)
    rider's b.
    sacral b.
    scapulohumeral b.
    subacromial b.
    subacromiodeltoid b.
    b. subcutanea sacralis
    b. subcutanea trochanterica
    subcutaneous calcaneal b.
    subcutaneous infrapatellar b.
    subcutaneous patellar b.
    subcutaneous synovial b.
    subcutaneous trochanteric b.
    subdeltoid b.
    subtendinous iliac b.
    subtendinous prepatellar b.
    b. of trapezius muscle
    ulnar b.
bursal
bursectomy
bursitis
    Achilles b.
    calcaneal b.
    Duplay b.
    ischial b.
    prepatellar b.
    radiohumeral b.
    subacromial b.
    subdeltoid b.
bursocentesis
bursolith
bursopathy
bursotomy
burst
Busquet
    disease
button
    bone b.
C1 through C7—cervical vertebrae
    1–7
Cabot
    splint
cachectic
cacomelia
CAD—computer-assisted design
Caffey
    syndrome

Caffey-Kenny
    disease
Caffey-Silverman syndrome
Caffey-Smyth-Roske syndrome
calcaneal
calcaneitis
calcaneoapophysitis
calcaneoastragaloid
calcaneocavus
calcaneocuboid
calcaneodynia
calcaneofibular
calcaneonavicular
calcaneoplantar
calcaneoscaphoid
calcaneotibial
calcaneovalgocavus
calcaneus
calcar
    c. femorale
    c. pedis
calcification
    periarticular c.
calcinosis
    c. intervertebralis
    tumoral c.
Caldani ligament
calisthenics
Callahan
    method
Callander amputation
Callaway test
callositas, callosity
callus [noun]
    definitive c.
    ensheathing c.
    intermediate c.
    medullary c.
    myelogenous c.
    permanent c.
    provisional c.
calvaria (calvariae)
calvarial
calvarium [incorrect term for cal-
    varia]
Calvé
    disease
Calvé-Legg-Perthes syndrome

Calvé-Perthes
    disease
calx
CAM—computer-assisted myelog-
    raphy
cambium
Campbell
    ligament
    operation
camptocormia
camptocormy
camptodactyly
camptomelia
camptospasm
Canadian crutch
canal
    Guyon c.
    haversian c.
    Hunter c.
    neural c.
    tarsal c.
canaliculus (canaliculi)
    bone canaliculi
    haversian c.
cancellated
cancelli (plural of cancellus)
cancellous [adj.]
cancellus (cancelli)
cancer
    See also in *Oncology and
        Hematology* section.
    osteoblastic c.
    osteolytic c.
cane
    adjustable c.
    broad-based c.
    English c.
    glider c.
    quadripod c.
    tripod c.
capeline
capita (plural of caput)
capitatum
capitellum
capitula (plural of capitulum)
capitular
capitulum (capitula)
capsula (capsulae)

capsular
capsulation
capsule
    articular c.
    articular c. of humerus
    articular c. of shoulder joint
    joint c.
capsulectomy
capsulitis
    adhesive c.
capsuloplasty
capsulorrhaphy
capsulotomy
caput (capita)
    c. ossis femoris
    c. radii
    c. tali
carcinoma (carcinomas, carcinomata)
    See *cancer*.
    See in *Oncology and Hema-*
       tology section.
Carden amputation
care
    custodial c.
    extended c.
    skilled nursing c.
Carleton spots
Carman
    meniscus sign
C-arm fluoroscopy
caro
    c. quadrata manus
    c. quadrata sylvii
carpal
    c. tunnel
    c. tunnel syndrome (CTS)
carpectomy
carpocarpal
carpopedal
carpophalangeal
carpoptosis
carpus
    c. curvus
Carrel
    method
    patch
    suture
    treatment

Carter
    mycetoma
cartilage
    articular c.
    condylar c.
    ensiform c.
    falciform c.
    floating c.
    interarticular c.
    interosseous c.
    intervertebral c.
    tendon c.
cast
    Cotrel c.
    Hexcelite c.
    long-arm c.
    long-leg c.
    Pietrie c.
    plaster of Paris c.
    Risser c.
    Risser localizer c.
    Sarmiento c.
    short-arm c.
    short-leg c.
    spica c.
cast room
catapophysis
cauda (caudae)
    c. equina
caudad [adv.]
caudal [adj.]
caudalward
caudate
caudectomy
caudocephalad
Cave
    operation
Cave-Rowe
    operation
cavitary
    c. lesion
cavitas (cavitates)
    c. medullaris
cavity
    joint c.
    medullary c.
    synovial c.
cavus

CCF—compound comminuted fracture
CDH—congenital dislocation of the hip
cement
    methylmethacrylate c.
cementation
cementless
    c. arthroplasty
center
    Béclard ossification c.
centra (plural of centrum)
centripetal
centrosclerosis
centrum (centra)
    c. medullare
cephalocaudad [adv.]
cephalocaudal [adj.]
ceramidase deficiency
cervical
    c. laminectomy
cervicalis
cervicoaxillary
cervicobrachial
cervicobrachialgia
cervicodorsal
cervicodynia
cervico-occipital
cervicoplasty
cervicoscapular
cervicothoracic
Chaddock
    reflex
    sign
Chance fracture
Chandler
    disease
Chaput method
Charcot
    arthropathy
    arthrosis
    foot
    gait
    joint
Charcot-Marie
    atrophy
    type

Charcot-Marie-Tooth
    atrophy
    disease
    type
charley horse
Charnley
    arthrodesis
Charnley-Mueller
    arthroplasty
Chassaignac tubercle
cheilectomy
cheiragra
cheiralgia
    c. paresthetica
cheirobrachialgia
cheiromegaly
cheiroplasty
cheiropodalgia
cheirospasm
chemonucleolysis
chevron
    c. osteotomy
CHH—cartilage-hair hypoplasia
chiasm
chiasma (chiasmata)
    c. tendinum digitorum manus
Chiene
    operation
    test
chondral
chondrectomy
chondric
chondrification
chondritis
    c. intervertebralis calcanea
chondroblast
chondroblastoma
chondrocarcinoma
chondroclast
chondrocostal
chondrodynia
chondrodysplasia
    genotypic c.
    hyperplastic c.
    McKusick-type metaphyseal c.
    c. punctata
    rhizomelic-type c.

chondrodystrophia
   c. calcificans congenita
   c. fetalis calcificans
chondrodystrophy
   c. malacia
chondroepiphyseal
chondroepiphysitis
chondrofibroma
chondrogenesis
chondrogenic
chondroglossus
chondroid
chondroitic
chondroitin sulfate
chondroitinuria
chondrolipoma
chondrolysis
chondroma
   medullary c.
chondromalacia
chondromatosis
   Reichel c.
   synovial c.
chondromatous
chondrometaplasia
   tenosynovial c.
chondromyoma
chondromyxofibroma
chondromyxoma
chondromyxosarcoma
chondronecrosis
chondro-osseous
chondro-osteodystrophy
chondropathia
chondropathology
chondropathy
chondrophyte
chondroplasia
chondroplastic
chondroplasty
chondroporosis
chondrosarcoma
chondrosarcomatosis
chondrosarcomatous
chondroskeleton
chondrosteoma
chondrosternal
chondrosternoplasty

chondrotome
chondrotomy
chondrotrophic
chondroxiphoid
chonechondrosternon
Chopart
   amputation
   articulation
   joint
   operation
chorda (chordae)
   c. dorsalis
   c. vertebralis
chordal
chordate
chordoma
cicatrix (cicatrices)
   vicious c.
CIL—center for independent living
cin–. See also words beginning
   sin–, syn–.
cineplasty
circumduction
Civinini
   canal
   ligament
   process
   spine
classification
   Frankel c. (groups A–E)
   Karnofsky status c. [score
      0–100]
   Neer c. of shoulder fracture
      (I–III)
   New York Heart Association
      (NYHA) c. (classes I–IV,
      A–D)
   Salter-Harris c. of epiphy-
      seal plate injuries
   Wiberg c. of patellar types
claudication
   intermittent c.
   venous c.
clavicle
clavicotomy
clavicula
clavicular
claviculus

clavipectoral
clawfoot
clawhand
clay shoveler's fracture
Cleeman sign
cleidagra
cleidal
cleidarthritis
cleidocostal
cleidocranial
clinodactyly
clinostatism
clinotherapy
Cloward
    back fusion
    drill
    operation
    rongeur
clubfoot
clubhand
cluneal
clunis (clunes)
Clutton joint
CMC—carpometacarpal (joint)
CMT—Charcot-Marie-Tooth [atrophy, disease, syndrome]
cnemial
cnemis [tibia]
cnemitis
Cobb
    gouge
coccygeal
coccygectomy
coccygerector
coccygeus
coccygotomy
Codivilla
    extension
    operation
Codman
    exercise
    sign
coenzyme
    c. Q 10 (CoQ 10)
cognitive
cogwheel
    c. gait
    c. rigidity

Coker technique
Cole
    operation
colla (plural of collum)
collar
    Thomas c.
Colles
    fascia
    fracture
    ligament
    splint
Collison screw
collum (colla)
    c. anatomicum humeri
    c. chirurgicum humeri
    c. cosine
    c. distortum
    c. femoris
    c. mallei
    c. processus condyloidei
        mandibulae
    c. radii
    c. scapulae
    c. tali
    c. valgum
Colonna
    operation
column
    spinal c.
    vertebral c.
comminuted
commissural
    c. myelotomy
Comolli sign
compact
compensatory
Compere
    operation
    pin
computer
    c.-assisted design (CAD)
concave
concavoconcave
concavoconvex
conditioning
condylar
condyle
condylectomy

condylion
condylotomy
condylus
congenerous
congruence
congruent
    c. articular surface
Conn
    operation
connective tissue disease
connexus
    c. intertendineus
Conradi
    disease
    syndrome
constitution
contractility
    idiomuscular c.
contracture
    Dupuytren c.
    ischemic c.
    Volkmann c.
contrecoup
contusion
conus
    c. medullaris
Cooper
    ligament
Coopernail sign
CoQ 10 (coenzyme Q 10)
coracoacromial
coracoclavicular
coracohumeral
coracoid
coracoiditis
coracoradialis
coracoulnaris
cornoid
cornu (cornua)
    cornua of spinal cord
cornual
cornuate
coronoid
corporis (genitive of corpus)
corpus (corpora)
cortex (cortices)
cortical
    c. hyperostosis

cortices (plural of cortex)
corticospinal
costa (costae)
    c. cervicalis
    c. fluctuans
    c. fluctuans decima
    costae fluitantes
    c. prima
    costae spuriae
    costae verae
costal
    c. margin
costalgia
costalis
costectomy
costicartilage
costicervical
costiform
costispinal
costocentral
costocervicalis
costochondral
costocoracoid
costogenic
costoinferior
costopleural
costoscapular
costoscapularis
costosternoplasty
costosuperior
costotomy
costotransverse
costotransversectomy
costovertebral
    c. angle (CVA)
    c. angle tenderness (CVAT)
costoxiphoid
Cotton fracture
cotyloid
cotylosacral
counterextension
counterirritants [a class of drugs]
countertraction
Coventry
    osteotomy
    screw
COX-2 (cyclooxygenase-2) inhibi-
    tors [a class of drugs]

coxa
    c. adducta
    c. flexa
    c. magna
    c. plana
    c. valga
    c. vara
    c. vara luxans
coxalgia
coxankylometer
coxarthria
coxarthritis
coxarthrocace
coxarthropathy
coxitis
    c. fugax
    senile c.
coxodynia
coxofemoral
coxotomy
coxotuberculosis
CPM—continuous passive motion
CPPD—calcium pyrophosphate
    dihydrate (crystals)
cramp
    tailor's c.
craniad [adv.]
cranial [adj.]
cranialis
cranioacromial
craniosacral
cranium
craterization
Crawford-Adams
    arthroplasty
    cup arthroplasty
Credo
    operation
crena
    c. ani
crepitation
crepitus
crest
cretinism
cricoid
cricoidectomy
crista (cristae)
cross-leg Patrick maneuver

cruciate
crura (plural of crus)
cruris (genitive of crus)
crus (crura)
crutch
    Canadian c.
    jocked stand c.
Crutchfield
    operation
Cruveilhier
    atrophy
    disease
    joint
    ligaments
    paralysis
cryptopodia
CS—chondroitin sulfate
CSA—chondroitin sulfate A
CSLR—crossed straight leg raising
    [test]
CSMT—capillary refill, sensation,
    motor function, temperature
CT—carpal tunnel
    computed tomography
CTD—carpal tunnel decompression
CTS—carpal tunnel syndrome
Cubbins
    operation
cubital
    c. tunnel syndrome
cubitocarpal
cubitoradial
cubitus
    c. valgus
    c. varus
cuboid
cuboidal
cue [signal, hint, suggestion]
    verbal c.'s
cuff
    musculotendinous c.
    rotator c.
cuneiform
    c. osteotomy
cuneocuboid
cuneonavicular
cuneoscaphoid
cup-and-ball osteotomy

curb tenotomy
curettement
curve
    stress-strain c.
cutis
    c. elastica
    c. hyperelastica
    c. laxa
CVA—costovertebral angle
CVAT—costovertebral angle tenderness
CVD—collagen vascular disease
cybernetics
Cybex test
cyclooxygenase-2 (COX-2) inhibitors [a class of drugs]
cyst
    Baker c.
Czerny
    disease
DA—degenerative arthritis
dactylospasm
Darrach
    operation
Davies-Colley
    operation
Dawbarn sign
DBM—demineralized bone matrix
DDD—degenerative disk disease
debilitated
    d. patient
    d. state
debilitating
    d. illness
debilitation
debilitative
    d. disease
debris
    loose d.
    tissue d.
decapitation
decompression
decompressive laminectomy
decortication
deformity
    Arnold-Chiari d.
    boutonnière d.
    buttonhole d.

deformity (continued)
    Ilfeld-Holder d.
    lobster-claw d.
    Madelung d.
    recurvatum d.
    seal-fin d.
    silver fork d.
    Sprengel d.
    swan neck d.
    ulnar drift d.
    valgus d.
    varus d.
    Velpeau d.
    Volkmann d.
Dega
    pelvic osteotomy
degeneration
    Zenker d.
degenerative joint disease
dehiscence
    Zuckerkandl d.
Dejerine
    sign
Delore method
delta
    d. mesoscapulae
Demianoff sign
demifacet
demigauntlet
Denucé
    quadrate ligament
deossification
DePuy
    splint
de Quervain
    disease
    fracture
    syndrome
    tenosynovitis
derangement
    Hey internal d.
DermaBond [topical adhesive]
Desault
    sign
desmalgia
desmectasis
desmodynia
desmology

desmoma
desmoneoplasm
desmopathy
desmoplasia
desmorrhexis
desmosis
desmotomy
Deutschländer
 disease
DEXA—dual energy x-ray absorptiometry [scan]
dextroverted
Deyerle
 plate
 punch
diaclasis
diadochokinesia
diaphyseal
diaphysectomy
diaphysis (diaphyses)
 proximal d.
diaphysitis
 tuberculous d.
diaplasis
diaplastic
diapophysis
diarthric
diarthrosis (diarthroses)
 planiform d.
 d. rotatoria
diastrophic
Dickson
 operation
Dickson-Diveley
 operation
Dieffenbach
 operation
digitation
digitus (digiti)
DIP—distal interphalangeal
DIPJ—distal interphalangeal joint
diploetic
diploic
dis–. See also words beginning dys–.
disarticulation
disc
 See *disk.*
discectomy [pref: diskectomy]

disci (genitive and plural of discus)
disciform ["disiform"]
discitis [pref: diskitis]
discogenic
discopathy
discus (disci)
disease
 See also *syndrome.*
 Albers-Schönberg d.
 Albright d.
 Blount d.
 Brodie d.
 Bruck d.
 Büdinger-Ludloff-Laewen d.
 Busquet d.
 Caffey-Kenny d.
 Calvé d.
 Calvé-Perthes d.
 Chandler d.
 Charcot-Marie-Tooth d.
 Czerny d.
 degenerative joint d.
 de Quervain d.
 Deutschländer d.
 Duplay d.
 Edsall d.
 Engelmann d.
 Engel-Recklinghausen d.
 Erb d.
 Erb-Goldflam d.
 Erichsen d.
 Freiberg d.
 Grisel d.
 Gumboro d.
 Haglund d.
 Hand-Schüller-Christian d.
 Henderson-Jones d.
 Hoffa-Kastert d.
 Hünermann d.
 Inman d.
 Jüngling d.
 Kashin-Bek d.
 Köhler bone d.
 Köhler-Pellegrini-Stieda d.
 König d.
 Kümmell d.
 Kümmell-Verneuil d.
 Larsen-Johansson d.

disease (continued)
    Legg d.
    Legg-Calvé-Perthes d.
    Legg-Calvé-Waldenström d.
    MacLean-Maxwell d.
    Marie-Bamberger d.
    Marie-Strümpell d.
    Marie-Tooth d.
    McArdle d.
    Moeller-Barlow d.
    Morquio d.
    Morton d.
    Mouchet d.
    Münchmeyer d.
    neuropathic joint d.
    Ollier d.
    Osgood-Schlatter d.
    Otto d.
    Paas d.
    Paget d. of bone
    Panner d.
    Pauzat d.
    Pellegrini d.
    Pellegrini-Stieda d.
    Perrin-Ferraton d.
    Perthes d.
    Poncet d.
    Pott d.
    Poulet d.
    Preiser d.
    pseudo-Pott d.
    Pyle d.
    Recklinghausen d.
    Rust d.
    Schanz d.
    Scheuermann d.
    Schlatter d.
    Schlatter-Osgood d.
    Schmorl d.
    Selter d.
    Sever d.
    Steinert d.
    Strümpell-Marie d.
    Swediaur d.
    Talma d.
    Thiemann d.
    Trevor d.
    Volkmann d.

disease (continued)
    von Recklinghausen d.
    Vrolik d.
    Waldenström d.
    Wartenberg d.
"disfajea" Phonetic for dysphagia.
"disfazea" Phonetic for dysphasia.
"disfonia" Phonetic for dysphonia.
"disfrasia" Phonetic for dysphrasia.
DISI—dorsiflexion intercalated seg-
    ment instability
"disiform" Phonetic for disciform.
disk
    Note: Some specialists and
        references prefer disc.
    acromioclavicular d.
    cartilaginous d.
    Engelmann d.
    herniated d.
    intervertebral d.
    protruded d.
    ruptured d.
    sternoclavicular d.
    triangular d. of wrist
diskectomy
diskiform
diskogram
dislocatio
    d. erecta
dislocation
    divergent d.
    Kienböck d.
    Monteggia d.
    Nélaton d.
    Smith d.
    subastragalar d.
    subcoracoid d.
    subglenoid d.
dismemberment
displacement
    d. osteotomy
distraction
diverticula (plural of diverticulum)
diverticulum (diverticula)
    supracondylar synovial d.
DJD—degenerative joint disease
doffing
    donning and d.

dolichostenomelia
dolor
    d. coxae
dome
    d. osteotomy
donning
    d. and doffing
dorsa (plural of dorsum)
dorsad [adv.]
dorsal [adj.]
dorsalgia
dorsalis
dorsi (genitive of dorsum)
dorsiduct
dorsiflex
dorsiflexion
dorsispinal
dorsolateral
dorsolumbar
dorsomedian
dorsomesial
dorsonuchal
dorsoradial
dorsoscapular
dorsoventrad
dorsoventral
dorsum (dorsa)
    d. of foot
    d. of hand
    d. manus
    d. pedis
    d. of scapula, d. scapulae
double-contrast
    d.-c. arthrography
dowager's hump
DPC—delayed primary closure
DPVNS—diffuse pigmented villo-
    nodular synovitis
drawer sign
drawn ankle clonus
dressing
    See in *General Surgical*
      Terms.
drilling
driver
    Küntscher d.
drop
    d. foot [also: footdrop]

drop (continued)
    d. phalangette
drop phalangette
DTP—distal tingling on pressure
Dugas test
Dunn-Brittain
    operation
Duplay
    bursitis
    disease
    syndrome
Dupuytren
    amputation
    contracture
    fascia
    fracture
    hydrocele
    operation
    sign
    splint
    suture
Durman
    operation
Duverney fracture
DuVries hammer toe repair
DVT—deep vein thrombosis
    deep venous thrombosis
dynamometer
    squeeze d.
dys–. See also words beginning dis–.
dysarthria
dysarthric
dysarthrosis
dyschondroplasia
    Ollier d.
dysphagia [difficulty swallowing]
dysphagic
dysphasia [difficulty with speech]
dysphonia
    d. clericorum
dysphonic
dysphrasia
dysplasia
    diaphyseal d.
    metaphyseal d.
dyspraxia
dystonia

dystrophy
    muscular d.
    scapulohumeral d.
    scapuloperoneal d.
EAST—external rotation and
    abduction stress test
ebonation
eccentro-osteochondrodysplasia
ecchondrotome
ECF—extended care facility
ectocondyle
ectromelia
ectromelus
ectrometacarpia
ectrometatarsia
ectrophalangia
ectrosyndactyly
Eddowes
    disease
    syndrome
Eden-Hybbinette
    operation
Edsall disease
effect [noun: result, outcome]
    See *phenomenon, reflex,* and
        sign.
Eggers
    operation
    plate
    screw
    splint
Ehlers-Danlos
    disease
    syndrome
EIP—extensor indicis proprius
elbow
    capped e.
    tennis e.
electroanalgesia
Ellis-Jones
    operation
Elmslie-Cholmeley
    operation
Ely test
embolism
embolus (emboli)
eminence
    thenar e.

eminentia
enarthrosis
enchondroma
enchondromatous
enchondrosarcoma
enchondrosis
endochondral
endoskeleton
endosteal
endosteitis
endosteoma
endosteum
Engelmann
    disease
    disk
Engel-Recklinghausen disease
English cane enostosis
"en-sed" Phonetic for NSAID (non-
    steroidal anti-inflammatory
    drug).
entepicondyle
epicondylalgia
epicondyle
epicondyli (plural of epicondylus)
epicondylian
epicondylic
epicondylitis
    external humeral e.
    lateral e.
    radiohumeral e.
epicondylus (epicondyli)
    e. lateralis femoris
    e. lateralis humeri
    e. medialis femoris
    e. medialis humeri
epicoracoid
"epifisis" Phonetic for epiphysis.
"epifizee–" Phonetic for words
    beginning epiphyse–.
epimysium
epiphyseal
epiphysectomy
epiphysiodesis
epiphysioid
epiphysiolysis
epiphysiometer
epiphysiopathy

epiphysis (epiphyses)
    capital e.
    e. cerebri
    slipped capital femoral e.
    stippled e.
epiphysitis
    vertebral e.
epipyramis
epirotulian
epispinal
epistropheus
epitendineum
epitenon
epithelia (plural of epithelium)
epitheliitis
epithelium (epithelia)
    muscle e.
    nerve e.
epitrochlea
epitrochlear
epitrochleitis
épluchage
equinovalgus
equinovarus
equinus
erasion
    e. of joint
Erb-Goldflam
    disease
Erdheim
    syndrome
ergogram
ergograph
    Mosso e.
ergometer
Erichsen
    disease
    sign
esquillectomy
Essex-Lopresti
    method
Evans
    operation
evertor
Ewing
    sarcoma
    tumor
exarticulation

exercise
    Codman e.
    Williams e.
exoskeleton
exostosectomy
exostosis (exostoses)
    e. bursata
    e. cartilaginea
    multiple e.'s
    osteocartilaginous e.
    subungual e.
extension
    Bardenheuer e.
    Buck e.
    Codivilla e.
extensor
extracarpal
extractor
    Jewett e.
    Moore e.
extradural
extraepiphyseal
extraligamentous
extramalleolus
extraosseous
extremital
extremitas (extremitates)
extremities
Eyler
    operation
fabella (fabellae)
fabere
    f. sign
    f. test [flexion, abduction,
        external rotation, exten-
        sion]
facet
facetectomy
facies (facies)
    acromegalic f.
facility
    acute care f. (ACF)
    adult congregate living f.
        (ACLF)
    extended care f. (ECF)
    intermediate care f. (ICF)
    skilled nursing f. (SNF)

FACSM—Fellow of the American College of Sports Medicine
Fahey
    operation
Fajersztajn
    sign
"falan–" Phonetic for words beginning phalan–.
"falanks" Phonetic for phalanx.
falx
    f. inguinalis
    f. ligamentosa
familial hypophosphatemic bone disease
Fanconi-Albertini-Zellweger syndrome
Farabeuf
    amputation
faradization
    galvanic f.
faradomuscular
fascia (fasciae)
    Dupuytren f.
    gluteal f.
    hypothenar f.
    f. lata femoris
    lumbar f.
    popliteal f.
    pubic f.
    f. of quadratus lumborum muscle
    Scarpa f.
    thenar f.
fasciaplasty
fascicle
fascicular
fasciculated
fasciculation
fasciculitis
fasciculus (fasciculi)
fasciectomy
fasciitis
    diffuse f.
    pseudosarcomatous f.
fasciodesis
fascioplasty
fasciorrhaphy
fasciotomy

Fazio-Londe
    atrophy
    disease
    syndrome
FDP—flexor digitorum profundus
FDS—flexor digitorum superficialis
feet (plural of foot)
female pseudo-Turner syndrome
femora (plural of femur)
femoral
    f. artery
femoroiliac
femorotibial
femur (femora, femurs)
fenestrated
    f. tenotomy
"fenomenon" Phonetic for phenomenon.
Fèvre-Languepin syndrome
fiber
    Sharpey f.
Fiberglas
fiberglass
fibril
    muscle f.
fibrocartilage
fibrocartilagines (plural of fibrocartilago)
fibrocartilaginous
fibrocartilago (fibrocartilagines)
    f. intervertebrales
    f. navicularis
fibroma
    chondromyxoid f.
    desmoplastic f.
    nonossifying f.
    nonosteogenic f.
    osteogenic f.
fibromatogenic
fibromatoid
fibromatosis
fibromatous
fibromectomy
fibromuscular
    f. disease
fibromyalgia
fibromyitis
fibromyositis

fibromyxolipoma
fibrosis
fibrotic
fibula
fibular
fibularis
fibulocalcaneal
"Fifer" Phonetic for Pfeiffer.
filum (fila)
    f. spinale
    f. terminale
finger
    baseball f.
    clubbed f.
    drumstick f.
    hammer f.
    hippocratic f.
    mallet f.
    trigger f.
    webbed f
Finkelstein
    test
fissure
fixation
    fracture f.
"fizeo–" Phonetic for words begin-
    ning physio–.
flail
flap
    f. operation
flatfoot
    spastic f.
flavectomy
flesh
    proud f.
flex
flexion
    plantar f.
flexor
    f. retinaculum
flexorplasty
Flood ligament
flow
    laminar air f.
Flower
    bone
    index
fluctuation

fluid
    synovial f.
focil, focile
"foke-mahn" Phonetic for Volkmann.
foot (feet)
    bifid f.
    broad f.
    cavus f.
    Charcot f.
    cleft f.
    club f. [pref: clubfoot
      (clubfeet)]
    congenital convex club f.
      [pref: clubfoot]
    dancer's f.
    dangle f.
    drop f. [also: footdrop]
    flatfoot
    Flex-F.
    forced f.
    Friedreich f.
    immersion f.
    Madura f.
    march f.
    Morand f.
    Morton f.
    mossy f.
    reel f.
    rocker-bottom f.
    SACH (solid-ankle, cush-
      ioned-heel) f.
    sag f.
    Seattle f.
    spatula f.
    splay f.
    split f.
    spread f.
    tabetic f.
    taut f.
    trench f.
    weak f.
footdrop
foramen (foramina)
    Hartigan f.
    ischiopubic f.
    f. magnum
    Weitbrecht f.
foraminal

foraminotomy
Forbes
    amputation
forearm
forefoot
formant
formation
    endochondral bone f.
    intracartilaginous bone f.
    intramembranous bone f.
formula
    digital f.
    vertebral f.
fossa (fossae)
    glenoid f. of scapula
    f. ischioanalis
    Jobert f.
    Mohrenheim f.
    supinator f.
    supraclavicular f.
Foster frame
fovea (fovea)
    f. capitis femoris
foveal
foveate
foveation
foveola (foveolae)
    f. coccygea
Fowler
    operation
fracture
    acute on chronic f.
    agenetic f.
    apophyseal f.
    articular f.
    atrophic f.
    avulsion f.
    Barton f.
    basal neck f.
    Bennett f.
    bimalleolar f.
    boxer f.
    bucket-handle f.
    bumper f.
    bursting f.
    butterfly f.
    buttonhole f.
    chip f.

fracture (continued)
    chisel f.
    clay shoveler's f.
    cleavage f.
    closed f.
    Colles f.
    comminuted f.
    compound f.
    compression f.
    condylar f.
    congenital f.
    cortical f.
    Cotton f.
    cough f.
    crush f.
    depressed f.
    de Quervain f.
    diacondylar f.
    displaced f.
    Dupuytren f.
    Duverney f.
    dyscrasic f.
    f. en coin ["ah kwa"]
    f. en rave ["ah rahv"]
    epiphyseal f.
    fatigue f.
    Galeazzi f.
    Gosselin f.
    greenstick f.
    Guérin f.
    hairline f.
    idiopathic f.
    impacted f.
    intercondylar f.
    intertrochanteric f.
    intra-articular f.
    intraperiosteal f.
    Jefferson f.
    lead pipe f.
    Le Fort f. (I–III)
    linear f.
    Lisfranc f.
    longitudinal f.
    mallet f.
    march f.
    Monteggia f.
    Moore f.

fracture (continued)
    neoplastic f.
    oblique f.
    occult f.
    open f.
    pathologic f.
    pertrochanteric f.
    pillion f.
    Pott f.
    reverse Colles f.
    Salter f. (I–VI)
    segmental f.
    shaft f.
    Shepherd f.
    silver fork f.
    Skillern f.
    Smith f.
    spiral f.
    splintered f.
    spontaneous f.
    sprinter f.
    stellate f.
    Stieda f.
    strain f.
    stress f.
    subcapital f.
    subperiosteal f.
    subtrochanteric f.
    supracondylar f.
    surgical neck f.
    tibial plateau f.
    torsion f.
    transcondylar f.
    transverse f.
    trimalleolar f.
    tuft f.
    ununited f.
    Wagstaffe f.
    willow f.
fracture-dislocation
    Monteggia f-d.
    posterior f-d.
fragilitas
    f. ossium
fragmentation
fraise
    diamond f.

Fränkel (Fraenkel)
    See also *Frenkel.*
    sign
Frankel
    classification (groups A–E)
Freeman-Sheldon syndrome
Freiberg
    disease
    infraction
frena (plural of frenum)
frenal
"freng-kuhl" Phonetic for Frankel
    and Frenkel.
Frenkel
    See also *Fränkel.*
    exercises
    movements
    tracks
    treatment
frenulum (frenula)
    See also *band, frenum,* and
        vinculum.
    f. of Macdowel (M'Dowel)
    f. synoviale
frenum (frena)
    See also *band, frenulum,*
        and *vinculum.*
    Macdowel (M'Dowel) f.
    synovial frena
freshen
freshened
Fritz-Lange
    operation
Fröhlich (Froehlich)
    dwarfism
FROM—full range of motion
Froment sign
functional
    f. status
funicular
funiculate
funiculus (funiculi)
    funiculi of spinal cord
funnel chest
fusimotor
fusion
    diaphyseal-epiphyseal f.
    spinal f.

fx—fracture
Gaenslen sign
gag reflex
gait
    antalgic g.
    ataxic g.
    calcaneous g.
    cerebellar g.
    Charcot g.
    cogwheel g.
    double-step g.
    drag-to g.
    drunken g.
    duck g.
    equine g.
    festinating g.
    footdrop g.
    four-point g.
    glue-footed g.
    gluteal g.
    gluteus maximus g.
    glutcus medius g.
    heel-toe g.
    helicopod g.
    hemiplegic g.
    listing g.
    myopathic g.
    Oppenheim g.
    paraparetic g.
    Petren g.
    reeling g.
    scissors g.
    skater's g.
    spastic equinus g.
    staggering g.
    stamping g.
    star g.
    steppage g.
    swing-through g.
    swing-to g.
    tabetic g.
    tandem g.
    three-point g.
    Todd g.
    Trendelenburg g.
    two-point g.
    waddling g.
gait and station

Galeazzi
    fracture
    sign
galvanization
gamekeeper's thumb
gampsodactylia
ganglia (plural of ganglion)
ganglial
ganglion (ganglia, ganglions)
    Acrel g.
ganglionectomy
ganglioneuroma
    dumbbell g.
    hourglass g.
ganglionic
ganglionitis
gangrene
    Pott g.
Gant
    operation
gargoylism
    X-linked recessive g.
Garré
    disease
    osteitis
    osteomyelitis
Gatellier
    operation
genicula (plural of geniculum)
genicular
geniculate
geniculum (genicula)
genu
    g. impressum
    g. recurvatum
    g. valgum
    g. varum
Ghormley
    operation
gibbosity
gibbous
gibbus
Gibney
    boot
    disease
    perispondylitis
Gibson
    operation

gigantism
  hyperpituitary g.
  pituitary g.
Gigli
  operation
Gill
  operation
Gillespie
  operation
ginglymoid
ginglymus
girdle
Girdlestone
  operation
glenohumeral
glenoid
globulus (globuli)
  globuli ossei
gluteal
gluteofemoral
gluteoinguinal
Goldthwait
  operation
  sign
gonarthritis
gonarthromeningitis
gonarthrosis
gonarthrotomy
gonatocele
gonial
gonitis
  fungous g.
  g. tuberculosa
gonocampsis
Gosselin fracture
goundou
GP—gutta-percha
Graber-Duvernay
  operation
gracilis muscle
graduated
  g. tenotomy
graft
  allogeneic g.
  autogenous g.
  autoplastic g.
  full-thickness g.
  heterogenous g.

graft (continued)
  homogenous g.
  homoplastic g.
  onlay bone g.
  Russe bone g.
  split-thickness g.
granulate
Graves
  scapula
Grice-Green
  operation
Grisel disease
Gritti
  amputation
  operation
Gritti-Stokes amputation
Guilland sign
Guleke-Stookey
  operation
Gumboro disease
Günz (Guenz) ligament
Guyon
  amputation
  canal
  operation
HA—hydroxyapatite
Haas
  operation
Hagie pin
Haglund
  deformity
  disease
Hallpike maneuver
hallux
  h. dolorosa
  h. flexus
  h. malleus
  h. rigidus
  h. valgus
  h. varus
halo
  h.-pelvic traction
  h. traction
hamartoma
  chondromatous h.
  leiomyomatous h.
  neuromuscular h.
hamate

hamatum
Hamilton test
hammer
    h. finger
    h. toe
hammock effect
Hammond
    operation
hamstring
hamulus
Hancock
    amputation
    operation
hand
    claw h.
    cleft h.
    club h. [pref: clubhand]
    Krukenberg h.
    lobster-claw h.
    mitten h.
    opera-glass h.
    trident h.
    writing h.
Hand [eponym]
    disease
    syndrome
handicap
handicapped
Hand-Schüller-Christian
    disease
    syndrome
Hark
    operation
Harrington
    nail
Harris-Beath
    operation
Hart
    splint
Hatcher pin
Hauser
    operation
haversian
    canal
    glands
    lamella
    spaces
    system

healing
    h. by first intention
    h. by granulation
    h. by second intention
    h. per primam intentionem
        (L. by first intention)
    h. per secundam intentionem
        [L. by second intention]
Heberden
    arthropathy
    disease
    nodes
    nodosities
    rheumatism
Hector tendon
Hefke-Turner sign
Heifitz
    operation
Helbing sign
helicopod
    h. gait
hemapophysis
hematoma
hemiarthrosis
hemimelia
hemipelvectomy
hemiphalangectomy
hemiplegia
    See in *Neurology and Pain*
        Management section.
hemivertebra
hemorrhage
    capsular h.
Henderson
    operation
Henderson-Jones disease
Hendry
    operation
Henry-Geist
    operation
herniated
herniation
    disk h.
    h. of intervertebral disk
    h. of nucleus pulposus
hetero-osteoplasty
Heuter
    operation

Hey
    amputation
    derangement
    internal derangement
    operation
Hey Groves
    clamp
Heyman
    operation
    technique
Hibbs
    operation
hindfoot
hinge osteotomy
hip
    snapping h.
    total h. arthroplasty
    Unipore h. arthroplasty
"hipo–" Phonetic for words begin-
    ning hypo–.
Hirschberg
    sign
HMP—hot moist pack
HNP—herniated nucleus pulposus
HOA—hypertrophic
    osteoarthroscopy
Hoffa
    disease
    operation
Hoffa-Kastert
    disease
Hoffa-Lorenz
    operation
Hohmann
    operation
Hoke
    operation
Holmes
    operation
Holmes-Stewart phenomenon
HOOD—hereditary osteo-onycho-
    dysplasia
Horwitz-Adams
    operation
Houston
    operation
Howship
    lacuna

H-shaped vertebra
Hubbard tank
Hueter
    line
    fracture sign
humeral
humeri (genitive and plural of
    humerus)
humeroradial
humeroscapular
humeroulnar
humerus (humeri)
    h. varus
humpback
Humphry ligament
Hünermann
    disease
Hurler
    disease
    polydystrophy
    syndrome
Hurler-Scheie
    compound
    syndrome
hydrocollator
hydromyelia
hyperbaric
    h. chamber
    h. oxygen
hyperbarism
hypercalcipexy
hyperchondroplasia
hyperesthesia
    muscular h.
hyperesthetic
hyperextension
hyperflexion
hypergenesis
hypergenetic
hyperkinesia
hyperkinesis
hyperkinetic
hyperlactacidemia
hyperlordosis
hypermetria
hypermineralization
hypermyotonia
hypermyotrophy

hyperosteogenesis
hyperosteogeny
hyperostosis
hyperostotic
hyperphalangia
hyperphosphatasemia
    chronic congenital idiopath-
        ic h.
    h. tarda
hyperplasia
    epiphyseal h.
    fibromuscular h.
hyperplastic
hyperprosody
hypersomatotropism
hypersomia
hypersthenia
hypersthenic
hypertrophy
    Marie h.
hyperuricemia
hyperuricemic
hypocalcemia
hypocalcemic
hypocalcification
hypochondroplasia
hypocondylar
hypodactyly
hypoevolutism
hypolemmal
hypomagnesemia
hypomineralization
hypophalangism
hypophosphatasia
hypophosphatemia
    hereditary h.
    X-linked h.
hypophosphatemic
hypoplasia
    congenital generalized mus-
        cular h.
hypoporosis
hypoprosody
hypostosis
hypothenar
    h. eminence
hypotrophy
IC—intermittent claudication

idiomuscular
IHO—idiopathic hypertrophic
    osteoarthropathy
ILD—ischemic leg disease
    ischemic limb disease
Ilfeld-Holder deformity
iliac [hip bone]
iliococcygeal
iliocostal
iliofemoral
iliofemoroplasty
ilioinguinal
iliolumbar
iliometer
iliopectineal
iliopelvic
iliopsoas
iliopubic
iliosacral
iliosciatic
iliospinal
iliotibial
iliotrochanteric
ilioxiphopagus
ilium (ilia) [hip bone]
illness
    debilitating i.
IM—intramuscularly
image
imagery
    guided i.
imaging
    See in *Radiology, Nuclear*
        Medicine, and Other
        Imaging section.
implant
    osseointegrated i.
incision
    Bardenheuer i.
    Langenbeck (von Langen-
        beck) i.
incisura (incisurae)
incisural
incisure
inclinatio (inclinationes)
    i. pelvis
inclination
incongruent

incontinentia
    i. pigmenti
induction
    spinal i.
infra-axillary
infraclavicular
infracostal
infraction
    Freiberg i.
infraglenoid
infrapatellar
infrascapular
infraspinous
infrasternal
infratrochlear
inhibitor
    COX-2 (cyclooxygenase-2)
        i.'s [a class of drugs]
Inman disease
innominate
    i. osteotomy
inochondritis
inotropism
inscriptio (inscriptiones)
inscription
inspiratory
instability
    lumbosacral i.
instep
insufficientia
    i. vertebrae
interarticular
intercarpal
intercartilaginous
interchondral
interclavicular
intercondylar
intercostohumeral
interdigital
interfemoral
intergluteal
intermetacarpal
interosseal
interpediculate
interphalangeal
interscapular
intersectio (intersectiones)

intersection
    aponeurotic i.
interspace
interspinal
interspinous
intertrochanteric
    i. osteotomy
intervertebral
intraosseous
    i. venography
intraspinal
involucrum
IP—interphalangeal
IPG—impedance plethysmography
ischialgia
ischiectomy
ischiocapsular
ischiococcygeal
ischiococcygeus
ischiofemoral
ischiofibular
ischiohebotomy
ischiopubic
ischiopubiotomy
ischiosacral
ischiovertebral
ischium
"iske–" Phonetic for words begin-
    ning ischi–.
island
    bone i.
    cartilage i.'s
isthmectomy
ithyokyphosis
IV—intervertebral
    intravenous
IVD—intervertebral disk
Jaboulay
    amputation
Jaccoud
    arthritis
    arthropathy
    syndrome
jacket
    Kydex body j.
    Minerva j.
    plaster-of-Paris j.
    Royalite body j.

jacket (continued)
  Sayre j.
Jansen
  test
Jeanselme nodules
Jefferson
  fracture
Jendrassik maneuver
jerk
  Achilles j.
  ankle j.
  quadriceps j.
  triceps surae j.
Jewett
  operation
Jobert fossa
Jobst
  boot
  stockings
Johanson-Blizzard syndrome
joint
  See also *articulation.*
  acromioclavicular (AC) j.
  amphidiarthrodial j.
  ankle j.
  apophyseal j.
  arthrodial j.
  atlantoaxial j.
  ball-and-socket j.
  biaxial j.
  bilocular j.
  Budin j.
  calcaneocuboid j.
  capitular j.
  carpometacarpal j.'s
  cartilaginous j.
  Charcot j.
  Chopart j.
  Clutton j.
  coccygeal j.
  composite j.
  compound j.
  condyloid j.
  costochondral j.'s
  costovertebral j.'s
  Cruveilhier j.
  cubital j.
  diarthrodial j.

joint (continued)
  dry j.
  elbow j.
  ellipsoidal j.
  enarthrodial j.
  false j.
  fibrocartilaginous j.
  fibrous j.
  flail j.
  freely movable j.
  fringe j.
  hinge j.
  hip j.
  immovable j.
  inferior radioulnar j.
  inferior tibiofibular j.
  interarticular j.'s
  intercarpal j.
  intercuneiform j.'s
  intermetacarpal j.'s
  interphalangeal j.'s
  irritable j.
  superior radioulnar j.
  knee j.
  ligamentous j.
  Lisfranc j.
  lumbosacral j.
  Luschka j.
  metacarpophalangeal
    (MCP) j.'s
  metatarsophalangeal (MTP)
    j.'s
  j. mice
  midcarpal j.
  midtarsal j.
  mixed j.
  mortise j.
  movable j.
  multiaxial j.
  pisotriquetral j.
  pivot j.
  plane j.
  polyaxial j.
  j. position sense
  radiocarpal j.
  rotary j.
  sacrococcygeal j.
  sacroiliac j.

joint (continued)
    saddle j.
    saddle-shaped j.
    scapuloclavicular j.
    shoulder j.
    simple j.
    slip j.
    spheroidal j.
    spiral j.
    sternoclavicular j.
    sternocostal j.'s
    stifle j.
    subtalar j.
    superior tibiofibular j.
    suture j.
    synarthrodial j.
    synovial j.
    tarsal j.
    tarsometatarsal j.'s
    trochoid j.
    uncovertebral j.
    uniaxial j.
    unilocular j.
    j.'s of vertebral column
    von Gies j.
    xiphisternal j.
    zygapophyseal j.'s
Jones
    fracture
    position
    splint
Joplin
    operation
Jung
    muscle
Jüngling disease
juxta-articular
juxtaepiphyseal
juxtaspinal
"kahk–," "kak–" Phonetic for words
    beginning cac–, cach–.
Kanavel
    canal
    sign
    triangle
Kapel
    operation
Kashin-Bek disease

Kast
    syndrome
Keen
    sign
Keller
    arthroplasty
    bunionectomy
    operation
Keller-Blake
    splint
Kellogg-Speed
    operation
Kenny-Caffey
    syndrome
Kerr
    sign
Kessler
    operation
Kidner
    operation
Kienböck
    disease
    dislocation
    phenomenon
"kifo–" Phonetic for words begin-
    ning kypho–.
Kiloh-Nevin
    myopathy
kineplasty
kinesalgia
kinesiology
kinesitherapy
King-Richards
    operation
Kirkaldy-Willis
    operation
Kirk amputation
Kirmisson
    operation
    raspatory
"kiro–" Phonetic for words begin-
    ning cheiro–.
Klippel-Feil
    malformation
    sign
    syndrome
Klippel-Trenaunay-Weber
    syndrome

knee
  Brodie k.
  conventional single-axis k.
  prosthesis
  total k. arthroplasty
  von Willebrandt k.
kneecap
knock-knee
Knowles pin
knuckle
Kocher
  operation
Kocher-Debré-Sémélaigne syndrome
Koenig-Wittek
  operation
Köhler
  bone disease
Köhler-Pellegrini-Stieda disease
"kokse–" Phonetic for words beginning coccy–.
Kolomnin
  operation
"kon–" Phonetic for words beginning chon–.
König
  disease
  operation
"kon-tre-koo" Phonetic for contrecoup.
"kor–" Phonetic for words beginning cor– and chor–.
Kraske
  operation
Kreuscher
  operation
Kristiansen screw
Krukenberg hand
"krus" Phonetic for crus.
Kümmell
  disease
  spondylitis
Kümmell-Verneuil disease
Küntscher
  driver
  nail
  reamer
Kydex body jacket
kyllosis

kyphos
kyphoscoliosis
kyphosis
  Scheuermann k.
kyphotic
kyrtorrhachic
L1 through L5—lumbar vertebrae
  1–5
labium (labia)
  See border and limbus.
labrum (labra)
  l. acetabulare
  l. articularis
  l. glenoidale
labyrinth
labyrinthus (labyrinthi)
lacerate, lacerated
lacertus
Lacey
  rotating-hinge arthroplasty
lactacidemia
lactaciduria
lactic
  l. acid
  l. acidosis
lacticacidemia
lacuna (lacunae)
  absorption l.
  bone l.
  cartilage l.
  Howship l.
  osseous l.
  resorption l.
lacunar
lacunula (lacunulae)
lacunule
LAF—laminar air flow
laloplegia
lambdacism
lambdacismus
Lambrinudi
  operation
lamella (lamellae)
  articular l.
  basic l.
  circumferential l.
  concentric l.
  endosteal l.

lamella (lamellae) (continued)
    ground l.
    haversian l.
    intermediate l.
    interstitial l.
    osseous l.
    periosteal l.
lamellar
lamelliform
lamina (laminae)
    l. of vertebra
    l. of vertebral arch
laminagram
laminar
    l. air flow
lamination
laminectomy
    cervical l.
    decompressive l.
    lumbar l.
    thoracic l.
laminitis
laminotomy
lancinating pain
Lane
    plate
Lange
    operation
Langenbeck (von Langenbeck)
    amputation
    flap
    incision
    operation
    triangle
Langer
    axillary arch
    muscle
Langoria sign
Lapidus
    operation
Laron
    syndrome
Larrey
    amputation
    operation
Larsen
    disease
    syndrome

Larsen-Johansson disease
latera (plural of latus)
lateral
lateralis
lateralization
lateroflexion
lateroposition
latissimus
    l. dorsi (muscle)
latus (latera)
Laugier sign
Laurence-Biedl
    syndrome
Laurence-Moon
    syndrome
Laurence-Moon-Biedl
    law
    syndrome
Lawrence-Seip syndrome
layer
    See *band* and *line*.
leech
    American l.
    artificial l.
    medicinal l.
leeching
Le Fort
    amputation
    fracture (I–III)
    osteotomy (I–III)
leg
    rider's l.
Legg
    disease
Legg-Calvé-Perthes
    disease
    syndrome
Legg-Calvé-Waldenström
    disease
Leichtenstern sign
Leinbach
    screw
leiomyoma (leiomyomas, leiomy-
    omata)
lemniscus (lemnisci)
L'Episcopo
    operation

Léri
- disease
- pleonosteosis
- sign
- syndrome

Léri-Weill syndrome

lesion
- compressive l. of lumbosacral region
- destructive l.
- impaction l.

levator (levatores)
- l. claviculae
- l. muscle

Levine
- operation

Lewin
- splint

Lhermitte sign

ligament
- accessory l.
- acromioclavicular l.
- acromiocoracoid l.
- adipose l.
- annular l.
- anterior l.
- arcuate l.
- Bertin l.
- Bigelow l.
- Brodie l.
- calcaneofibular l.
- calcaneonavicular l.
- Caldani l.
- Campbell l.
- capsular l.
- carpometacarpal l.
- collateral l.
- coracoacromial l.
- coracoclavicular l.
- coracohumeral l.
- costoclavicular l.
- cruciate l.
- crural l.
- cuboideonavicular l.
- cuneonavicular l.
- deltoid l.
- dentate l.
- fabellofibular l.

ligament (continued)
- falciform l.
- flaval l.
- hamatometacarpal l.
- iliofemoral l.
- iliotrochanteric l.
- inguinal l.
- laciniate l.
- lateral l.
- medial l.
- olecranon l.
- patellar l.
- pisohamate l.
- pisometacarpal l.
- plantar l.
- popliteal l.
- posterior l.
- pubocapsular l.
- pubofemoral l.
- quadrate l. of Denucé
- radiocarpal l.
- rhomboid l.
- sacrospinous l.
- sacrotuberous l.
- sternoclavicular l.
- sternocostal l.
- talocalcaneal l.
- talofibular l.
- talonavicular l.
- tendinotrochanteric l.
- transverse l.
- trapezoid l.
- ulnar l.
- ulnocarpal l.
- volar l.
- Wrisberg l.

ligamenta (plural of ligamentum)

ligamentous

ligamentum (ligamenta)
- ligamenta flava, l. flavum

limb

limbal

limbic

limbus (limbi)
- See also *border*.
- l. acetabuli

limen (limina)

liminal

Linder sign
line
> See also *band.*
> Bryant l.
> Duhot l.
> epiphyseal l.
> Feiss l.
> growth arrest l.
> Harris l.'s
> Hueter l.
> Kilian l.
> Meyer l.
> Moyer l.
> Nélaton l.
> Ogston l.
> posterior axillary l.
> Roser l.
> Schoemaker l.
> Shenton l.
> Skinner l.
> spiral l. of femur
> Trümmerfeld l.
> Ullmann l.
> Wagner l.

linea (lineae)
> l. glutea
linear
> l. osteotomy
lipomatous
lipomeningocele
Lisfranc
> amputation
> joint
> operation
Lissauer zone
Liston
> operation
> splint
Littler
> operation
Littlewood
> operation
LLC—long leg cast
LLE—left lower extremity
Lobstein
> disease
> syndrome

locomotion
locomotor
logogram
logopedics
logoscopy
LOM—limitation of motion
> loss of motion
longus
"loop" Phonetic for loupe.
Looser
> transformation zones
Looser-Milkman syndrome
lordoscoliosis
lordosis
> compensatory l.
> dorsal l.
lordotic
Lorenz
> operation
> osteotomy
> sign
Lottes
> nail
> operation
Lowman
> balance board
loxotomy
LS—lumbosacral
Lucas-Cottrell
> operation
Luck
> operation
Ludloff
> operation
> sign
LUE—left upper extremity
lumbago
lumbarization
lumbodorsal
lumbodynia
lumboiliac
lumbosacral
> l. kyphosis
> l. plexus
> l. radiculopathy
> l. spine
lumbrical
lumbus

lunare
lunate
    l. bone
lunatomalacia
Lund
    operation
lunula (lunulae)
    l. of scapula
Luschka
    joints
luxatio
    l. coxae congenita
    l. erecta
    l. imperfecta
    l. perinealis
luxation
    Malgaigne l.
Lyme
    arthritis
lytic
MacAusland
    operation
Macdowel (M'Dowel)
    frenulum
    frenum
Macewen
    osteotomy
Mackenzie
    amputation
MacLean-Maxwell
    disease
Macleod
    syndrome
macrobrachia
macrocheiria
macrocnemia
macrodactyly
Madelung
    deformity
    subluxation
Madura foot
Magnuson
    operation
Magnuson-Stack
    arthroplasty
    operation
    shoulder arthrotomy

Mahorner-Mead
    operation
main ["mah"]
    m. en crochet ["ah kroo-shay"]
    m. en griffe ["ah greef"]
    m. en lorgnette ["ah lor-nyet"]
    m. en pince ["ah pahs"]
    m. en squelette ["ah skeh-leht"]
    m. fourché ["foor-shay"]
    m. succulente ["soo-koo-laht"]
Maisonneuve
    amputation
    sign
maladjustment
malalignment
malformation
    Arnold-Chiari. m.
Malgaigne
    amputation
    luxation
malleolar
malleolus (malleoli)
    external m.
    m. externus
    m. fibulae
    fibular m.
    inner m.
    internal m.
    m. internus
    lateral m.
    m. lateralis
    m. lateralis fibulae
    lateral m. of fibula
    medial m.
    m. medialis
    m. medialis tibiae
    medial m. of tibia
    outer m.
    radial m.
    m. radialis
    m. tibiae
    tibial m.
    ulnar m.
    m. ulnaris
malleotomy

mallet
>m. finger
>m. toe

malum
>m. articulorum senilis
>m. coxae senilis

malunion
mandible
mandibular
maneuver
>See also *method.*
>Allen m.
>cross-leg Patrick m.
>Jendrassik m.

manubrium (manubria)
>m. sterni
>m. of sternum

manus
>m. cava
>m. extensa
>m. flexa
>m. plana
>m. superextensa
>m. valga
>m. vara

Marañon
>syndrome (I, II, III)

Marfan
>sign
>syndrome

margin
>m. of acetabulum
>axillary m. of scapula
>cartilaginous m. of acetabu-
>lum
>m. of fibula, anterior
>m. of fibula, posterior
>m. of foot, fibular
>m. of foot, lateral
>m. of foot, medial
>m. of humerus, lateral
>m. of humerus, medial
>interosseous m. of fibula
>interosseous m. of tibia
>interosseous m. of ulna

margo (margines)
Marie
>hypertrophy

Marie-Bamberger disease
Marie-Foix sign
Marie-Strümpell
>disease
>spondylitis
>syndrome

Marie-Tooth disease
Maroteaux-Lamy
>disease
>syndrome (I, II)

marrow
>red bone m.
>yellow bone m.

Marshall
>syndrome

marsupial
marsupium (marsupia)
>marsupia patellaris

Martin
>bandage
>disease

massage
>electrovibratory m.
>nerve-point m.
>trigger-point m.
>vibratory m.

Massie nail
matrix (matrices)
Mauck
>operation

maxillary
>total m. osteotomy

Mayer
>reflex

Mayo
>operation

Mazur
>operation

MBD—minimal brain damage
>minimal brain dysfunction

MC—metacarpal
McArdle
>disease
>syndrome

McAtee-Tharias-Blazina
>arthroplasty

McBride
>operation

McCarroll
    operation
McKee-Farrar
    arthroplasty
    hip arthroplasty
McKeever
    operation
McKenzie
    See *Mackenzie.*
McLaughlin
    operation
    plate
    screw
McMurray
    sign
    test
MCP—metacarpophalangeal
McReynolds adapter
MD—muscular dystrophy
M'Dowel. See *Macdowel.*
measurement
    skinfold m.'s
mechanoreceptor
medial
    m. meniscectomy
medicine
    occupational m.
    physical m.
    rehabilitation m.
    sports m.
medulla (medullae)
    m. of bone
    m. ossium
    m. ossium flava
    m. ossium rubra
    m. spinalis
medullated
medullation
medullitis
medullization
medulloarthritis
megalocheiria
megalodactyly
megalomelia
Melnick-Needles
    disease
    osteodysplasty
    syndrome

melorheostosis
melosalgia
membrane
    synovial m.
membranocartilaginous
membrum (membra)
    m. inferius
    m. superius
meninges (plural of meninx)
meningocele
meningomyelocele
meningosis
meninx (meninges)
meniscal
meniscectomy
    arthroscopic m.
    medial m.
menisci (plural of meniscus)
meniscitis
meniscopathy
meniscopexy
meniscosynovial
meniscotomy
    Bowen-Grover m.
    Smillie m.
meniscus (menisci)
    m. of acromioclavicular joint
    articular m., m. articularis
    converging m.
    discoid m.
    discoid lateral m.
    diverging m.
    m. of inferior radioulnar joint
    joint m.
    Kuhnt m.
    lateral m. of knee joint
    medial m. of knee joint
    negative m.
    positive m.
    m. of sternoclavicular joint
    tactile menisci
Mennell sign
meralgia
    m. paresthetica
merotomy
mesomelic
mesomorphic
mesomorphy

mesotendineum
metacarpal
metacarpectomy
metacarpophalangeal (MCP)
metacarpus
metaphyseal
metaphysis (metaphyses)
metaphysitis
metapodialia
metapophysis
metastasis (metastases)
    calcareous m.
metatarsal
metatarsalgia
metatarsectomy
metatarsophalangeal (MTP)
metatarsus
    m. adductocavus
    m. adductovarus
    m. adductus
    m. atavicus
    m. brevis
    m. latus
    m. primus varus
    m. varus
method
    See also *maneuver.*
    Abbott m.
    Chaput m.
    Delore m.
    Essex-Lopresti m.
    Hoffa tendon-shortening m.
    Lange tendon-lengthening m.
    Mosley anterior shoulder
       repair m.
    Stamm m.
methyl
    m. methacrylate
Meyer-Betz
    disease
    syndrome
Meyerding
    mallet
MG—muscle group
mice
    joint m.
Michaelis rhomboid
microanastomosis

microcalcificectomy
microcnemia
microdactyly
microemboli (plural of microembo-
    lus)
microembolization
microembolus (microemboli)
microfracture
micromelia
microthrombi (plural of
    microthrombus)
microthrombosis
microthrombus (microthrombi)
midcarpal
midfoot
midline
    m. myelotomy
midtarsal
"miel–" Phonetic for words begin-
    ning myel–.
"mik" Slang for Mikulicz.
Mikulicz (von Mikulicz)
    operation
    procedure
Milch
    operation
Milkman syndrome
Mills test
Minerva jacket
Minor sign
"mio–" Phonetic for words begin-
    ning myo–.
Mitchell
    bunionectomy
    operation
    osteotomy
mixed connective tissue disease
MM—medial malleolus
Moberg arthrodesis
mobilization
Moeller-Barlow
    disease
Mohrenheim
    fossa
    triangle
monarthritis
    m. deformans
monomyositis

monoplegia
    monostotic
Monro
    bursa
Monteggia
    dislocation
    fracture
Moore
    fracture
    template
Morand foot
Morestin
    operation
Morgagni
    hyperostosis
Morquio
    disease
    sign
    syndrome
Morquio-Brailsford syndrome
Morquio-Ullrich
    disease
    syndrome
Morton
    disease
    foot
    neuralgia
    neuroma
    test
    toe
Mosso ergograph
Mouchet disease
MP—metacarpophalangeal
MPJ—metacarpophalangeal joint
MS—musculoskeletal
MT—metatarsal
    music therapy
MTP—metatarsophalangeal
multifidus
multinodular
Mumford-Gurd
    operation
Münchmeyer disease
muscle
    abductor m. of great toe
    abductor m. of little finger
    abductor m. of little toe

muscle (continued)
    abductor m. of thumb (long, short)
    accessory flexor m.
    adductor m., great
    adductor m. (long, short)
    adductor m. of great toe
    adductor m., smallest
    adductor m. of thumb
    Aeby m.
    agonistic m.
    Albinus m.
    anconeus m. (lateral, medial)
    anconeus m., short
    antagonistic m.
    antigravity m.'s
    m. of antitragus
    appendicular m.'s
    arrector m.'s of hair
    articular m.
    articular m. of elbow
    articular m. of knee
    m.'s of auditory ossicles
    auricular m.'s (anterior, posterior, superior)
    axial m.
    biceps m. of arm
    biceps m. of thigh
    bicipital m.
    bipennate m.
    bipenniform m.
    Bowman m.
    brachial m.
    brachioradial m.
    bronchoesophageal m.
    buccopharyngeal m.
    Casser m., Casser perforated m., casserian m.
    ceratocricoid m.
    ceratopharyngeal m.
    Chassaignac axillary m.
    chondroglossus m.
    chondropharyngeal m.
    coccygeal m.'s
    congenerous m.'s
    coracobrachial m.
    cruciate m.
    deltoid m.

muscle (continued)
dorsal m.'s
Dupré m.
emergency m.'s
epimeric m.
epitrochleoanconeus m.
erector m. of spine
extensor m. of digits, common
extensor m. of fifth digit, proper
extensor m. of fingers
extensor m. of great toe (long, short)
extensor m. of index finger
extensor m. of little finger
extensor m. of thumb (long, short)
extensor m. of toes (long, short)
extrinsic m.
fast m.
femoral m.
fibular m. (long, short)
fibular m., third
fixation m.'s, fixator m.'s
flexor m., accessory
flexor m. of fingers (deep, superficial)
flexor m. of great toe (long, short)
flexor m. of little finger, short
flexor m. of little toe, short
flexor m. of thumb (long, short)
flexor m. of toes (long, short)
Folius m.
fusiform m.
gastrocnemius m. (lateral, medial)
gemellus m. (inferior, superior)
gluteal m.
gracilis m.
greater trochanter m.
hamstring m.'s
hypaxial m.'s
hypomeric m.

muscle (continued)
hypothenar m.'s
iliac m.
iliococcygeal m.
iliocostal m.'s
iliocostal m. of thorax
iliopsoas m.
infraspinous m.
intercostal m.'s (external, internal)
intercostal m.'s, innermost
interosseous m.
interosseous m.'s of foot, dorsal
interosseous m.'s of hand, dorsal
interosseous m.'s, palmar
interosseous m.'s, plantar
interosseous m.'s, volar
interspinal m.'s
interspinal m.'s of thorax
intertransverse m.'s
intertransverse m.'s, anterior
intertransverse m.'s of neck (anterior, posterior)
intertransverse m.'s of thorax
intrinsic m.
involuntary m.
Langer m.
lateral malleolus m.
latissimus dorsi m.
levator m.
levator m.'s of ribs (long, short)
levator m. of scapula
longissimus m.
longissimus m. of back
longissimus m. of head
longissimus m. of neck
longissimus m. of thorax
long m. of neck
lumbrical m.'s of foot
lumbrical m.'s of hand
Luschka m.'s
mesothenar m.
multifidus m.'s
multipennate m.
m.'s of neck

muscle (continued)

nonstriated m.
occipital m.
opposing m. of little finger
opposing m. of thumb
palmar m. (long, short)
paraspinal m.
pectineal m.
pectoral m. (greater, smaller)
m.'s of pelvic diaphragm
pennate m., penniform m.
peroneal m. (long, short)
peroneal m., third
Phillips m.
piriform m.
plantar m.
popliteal m.
postaxial m.
posterior intertransverse m.'s
    of neck
preaxial m.
pronator m., quadrate
pronator m., round
psoas m. (greater, smaller)
quadrate m.
quadrate m. of sole
quadrate m. of thigh
quadriceps m. of thigh
radial flexor m. of wrist
red m.
rhomboid m. (greater, lesser)
rider's m.'s
rotator m.'s (long, short)
rotator m.'s of neck
rotator m.'s of thorax
sacrococcygeal m. (anterior,
    posterior)
sacrococcygeal m. (dorsal,
    ventral)
sacrospinal m.
sartorius m.
scalene m. (anterior, middle,
    posterior)
scalene m., smallest
semimembranous m.
semispinal m.
semispinal m. of head
semispinal m. of neck

muscle (continued)

semispinal m. of thorax
semitendinous m.
serratus m., anterior
Sibson m.
skeletal m.'s
slow m.
smooth m.
soleus m.
somatic m.'s
sphincter m.
spinal m.
splenius m. of head
splenius m. of neck
sternal m.
sternocleidomastoid m.
sternomastoid m.
strap m.'s
striated m.
striped m.
subclavius m.
subcostal m.'s
suboccipital m.'s
subscapular m.
subvertebral m.'s
supinator m.
supraspinous m.
synergic m.'s, synergistic m.'s
tensor m. of fascia lata
teres major m.
teres minor m.
thenar m.'s
tibial m. (anterior, posterior)
tonic m.
trachelomastoid m.
transverse m. of neck
transverse m. of thorax
transversospinal m.
trapezius m.
triangular m.
triceps m. of arm
triceps m. of calf
tricipital m.
twitch m.
unipennate m.
unstriated m.
vestigial m.
voluntary m.

muscle (continued)
   white m.
   yoked m.'s
muscular
muscularity
musculature
musculoaponeurotic
musculocutaneous
musculoelastic
musculointestinal
musculoligamentous
musculomembranous
musculophrenic
musculospiral
musculotendinous
musculus (musculi)
   See also *muscle.*
   m. abductor digiti minimi
      manus
   m. abductor digiti minimi
      pedis
   m. abductor digiti quinti
      manus
   m. abductor digiti quinti pedis
   m. abductor hallucis
   m. abductor pollicis brevis
   m. abductor pollicis longus
   m. adductor brevis
   m. adductor minimus
   m. adductor pollicis
   m. biceps brachii
   m. biceps femoris
   m. brachialis
   m. brachioradialis
   m. coracobrachialis
   m. extensor carpi radialis
      brevis
   m. extensor carpi radialis
      longus
   m. extensor carpi ulnaris
   m. extensor digiti minimi
   m. extensor digiti quinti pro-
      prius
   m. extensor digitorum brevis
   m. extensor digitorum com-
      munis
   m. extensor digitorum longus
   m. extensor hallucis brevis

musculus (musculi) (continued)
   m. extensor hallucis longus
   m. extensor indicis proprius
   m. extensor pollicis brevis
   m. extensor pollicis longus
   m. flexor carpi radialis
   m. flexor carpi ulnaris
   m. flexor digitorum brevis
   m. flexor digitorum longus
   m. flexor digitorum profundus
   m. flexor digitorum sublimis
   m. flexor digitorum superfi-
      cialis
   m. flexor hallucis brevis
   m. flexor hallucis longus
   m. flexor pollicis brevis
   m. flexor pollicis longus
   m. gastrocnemius
   m. gluteus maximus
   m. gluteus medius
   m. gluteus minimus
   m. gracilis
   m. iliococcygeus
   m. iliopsoas
   m. infraspinatus
   musculi interspinales
   m. latissimus dorsi
   m. longissimus dorsi
   m. palmaris brevis
   m. palmaris longus
   m. pectoralis major
   m. pectoralis minor
   m. peroneus brevis
   m. peroneus longus
   m. peroneus tertius
   m. quadratus
   m. sacrospinalis
   m. sartorius
   m. scalenus anterior
   m. scalenus medius
   m. scalenus minimus
   m. scalenus posterior
   m. semitendinosus
   m. serratus anterior
   m. serratus posterior inferior
   m. serratus posterior superior
   m. spinalis
   m. spinalis dorsi

musculus (musculi) (continued)
    m. supinator
    m. supraspinatus
    m. tensor fasciae latae
    m. teres major
    m. teres minor
    m. trapezius
    m. triangularis
    m. triceps brachii
    m. triceps surae
    m. vastus latcralis
    m. vastus medialis
musicotherapy
myalgia
myectomy
myelocele
myelocystomeningocele
myelodysplasia
myelofugal
myelogenesis
myelogram
myelography
    air m.
    computer-assisted m. (CAM)
    opaque m.
    oxygen m.
myeloma
    See in *Oncology and Hematology* section.
myelomalacia
myelomatosis
myelomenia
myelomeningitis
myelon
myeloneuritis
myelo-opticoneuropathy
myeloparalysis
myelopathy
myelopetal
myelophthisis
myeloplegia
myelopoiesis
    ectopic m., extramedullary m.
myelopore
myeloradiculitis
myeloradiculodysplasia
myeloradiculopathy
myelorrhagia

myelosarcomatosis
myeloschisis
myelosclerosis
myelospasm
myelosyphilis
myelotomy
    Bischof m.
    commissural m.
    midline m.
myesthesia
myocele
myocerosis
myoclonia
myoclonic
myoclonus
    action m.
    epileptic m.
    hereditary essential m.
    intention m.
    massive epileptic m.
    m. multiplex
    nocturnal m.
    palatal m.
    spinal m.
myocrismus
myocutaneous
myocytoma
myodemia
myodiastasis
myodynamic
myodynamics
myodynia
myodystonia
myodystrophia
    m. fetalis
myoedema
myoelastic
myofascial
myofascitis
myofibril
myofibrillar
myofibroma
myofibrositis
myofilament
myogelosis
myogenic
myoglobinuria
    familial m.

myoglobinuria (continued)
    idiopathic m.
    paroxysmal m.
    traumatic m.
myoglobulinuria
myography
myohypertrophia
myoischemia
myokinesis
myokymia
myolipoma
myologia
myology
myolysis
myoma (myomas, myomata)
    m. striocellulare
myomatous
myomectomy
myomelanosis
myometer
myonecrosis
    clostridial m.
myoneural
myoneuralgia
myoneurasthenia
myoneurectomy
myonosus
myopachynsis
myoparalysis
myoparesis
myopathia
    m. infraspinata
myopathic
myopathy
    Welander m., Welander distal m.
myophagism
myoplastic
myoplasty
myorrhaphy
myorrhexis
myosarcoma
myoschwannoma
myosclerosis
myoseism
myoserum
myosin
myositic

myositis
    acute progressive m.
    m. fibrosa
    m. ossificans
    progressive ossifying m.
    rheumatoid m.
    m. serosa
    suppurative m.
myospasia
myospasm
myospasmia
myosteoma
myosthenic
myosthenometer
myosuture
myotactic
myotasis
myotatic
myotenontoplasty
myotenositis
myotenotomy
myotomic
myotomy
myotonia
    m. acquisita
    m. atrophica
    m. congenita
    m. congenita intermittens
    congenital m.
    m. dystrophica
    m. hereditaria
myotonoid
myotonometer
myotonus
myotrophic
myotrophy
myovascular
myxoma (myxomas, myxomata)
    enchondromatous m.
nailing
    intramedullary n.
    marrow n.
    medullary n.
navicula
navicular
nearthrosis
neck
    surgical n.

neck (continued)
 wry n.
necrosis (necroses)
 aseptic n.
 avascular n. of bone
 central n.
 coagulation n.
 coagulative n.
 dry n.
 epiphyseal ischemic n.
 gangrenous n.
 gummatous n.
 hyaline n.
 infectious bulbar n.
 ischemic n.
 mummification n.
 Paget quiet n.
 pressure n.
 septic n.
 superficial n.
 total n.
 n. ustilaginea
 Zenker n.
necrotic
necrotizing
 n. fasciitis
necrotomy
 osteoplastic n.
"neem–" Phonetic for words beginning cnem–.
Nélaton
 dislocation
 line
 operation
nerve
 cubital n.
 great sciatic n.
 peroneal n.
 sciatic n.
 sensorimotor n.
 somatic n.'s
 spinal n.'s
 thoracodorsal n.
 ulnar n.
 ulnar collateral n. of Krause
net
network

"neu–" Phonetic for words beginning pneu–.
Neufeld nail
Neumann
 syndrome
neuralgia
 brachial n.
 Morton n.
 sciatic n.
 stump n.
neuralgic
neurapraxia
neuritic
neuritis
 peripheral n.
 radicular n.
 sciatic n.
neuroanastomosis
neuroarthropathy
neurofibromatosis
neurofibrosarcoma
neurofibrositis
neurolysis
 alcohol n.
 chemical n.
 intrathecal n.
 phenol n.
neurolytic
neuroma
 amputation n.
 false n.
 Morton n.
 post-traumatic n.
 traumatic n.
neuromatosis
neuromatous
neuropathic joint disease
neuropathy
 peripheral n.
neuroplasty
neurorrhaphy
neuroskeletal
neurosuture
neurotendinous
Neviaser
 operation
"new–" Phonetic for words beginning pneu–.

New England Baptist
 arthroplasty
Nicola
 operation
Nicoll bone graft
NM—neuromuscular
nociceptor
 polymodal n.
node
 Bouchard n.
 Heberden n.
nodi (plural of nodus)
nodular
nodularity
nodulated
nodulation
nodule
 Schmorl n.
nodus (nodi)
nomogram
nonarticular
nonsteroidal anti-inflammatory drugs
 (NSAIDs) [a class of drugs]
nonunion
"noo–" Phonetic for words beginning pneu–.
notch
 acetabular n.
 clavicular n.
 coracoid n.
 interclavicular n.
 intercondylar n.
 intervertebral n.
 semilunar n.
 trochlear n.
 vertebral n.
NSAID, NSAIDs—nonsteroidal
 anti-inflammatory drug(s) [a
 class of drugs]
"nu–" Phonetic for words beginning
 pneu–.
nuchal
 n. rigidity
nucleus (nuclei)
 n. pulposus
 n. pulposus disci intervertebralis
 pulpy n.

"nur–" Phonetic for words beginning neur–.
NWB—nonweightbearing, non-
 weightbearing, non–weight-
 bearing, no weightbearing
NYHA (New York Heart Association) classification (I–IV)
OA—osteoarthritis
OAP—osteoarthropathy
OAV—oculoauriculovertebral (dysplasia)
Ober
 operation
 test
Ogston
 line
 operation
OI—osteogenesis imperfecta
olecranal
olecranarthritis
olecranarthrocace
olecranarthropathy
olecranoid
olecranon
olisthy
Ollier
 disease
 dyschondroplasia
 law
 layer
 operation
 osteochondromatosis
 syndrome
omoclavicular
omodynia
omohyoid
omoplata
omosternum
OMT—osteopathic manipulative
 therapy
opaque
 o. arthrography
 o. myelography
open
 o. tenotomy
operation
 See also in *General Surgical
  Terms.*

operation (continued)

    Abbott o.

    Abbott-Lucas o.

    Adams o.

    Adelmann o.

    Akin o.

    Albee o.

    Albee-Delbet o.

    Albert o.

    Alouette o.

    Anderson o.

    Annandale o.

    Aufranc-Turner o.

    Avila o.

    Axer o.

    Badgley o.

    Bankhart o.

    Barker o.

    Barsky o.

    Barton o.

    Barwell o.

    Bateman o.

    Bent o.

    Berger o.

    Bier o.

    Blount o.

    Blundell-Jones o.

    Bobroff o.

    Bosworth o.

    Boyd o.

    Brett o.

    Bristow o.

    Brittain o.

    Brockman o.

    Buck o.

    Bunnell o.

    Campbell o.

    Cave o.

    Cave-Rowe o.

    Chiene o.

    Chopart o.

    Cloward o.

    Codivilla o.

    Cole o.

    Colonna o.

    Compere o.

    Conn o.

    Credo o.

operation (continued)

    Crutchfield o.

    Cubbins o.

    Darrach o.

    Davies-Colley o.

    Dickson o.

    Dickson-Diveley o.

    Dieffenbach o.

    Dunn-Brittain o.

    Dupuytren o.

    Durman o.

    Eden-Hybbinette o.

    Eggers o.

    Ellis-Jones o.

    Elmslie-Cholmeley o.

    Evans o.

    Eyler o.

    Fahey o.

    flap o.

    Fowler o.

    Fritz-Lange o.

    Gant o.

    Gatellier o.

    Ghormley o.

    Gibson o.

    Gill o.

    Gillespie o.

    Girdlestone o.

    Goldthwait o.

    Graber-Duvernay o.

    Grice-Green o.

    Gritti o.

    Guleke-Stookey o.

    Guyon o.

    Haas o.

    Hammond o.

    Hancock o.

    Hark o.

    Harris-Beath o.

    Hauser o.

    Heifitz o.

    Henderson o.

    Hendry o.

    Henry-Geist o.

    Hey o.

    Heyman o.

    Hibbs o.

    Hoffa o.

operation (continued)

Hoffa-Lorenz o.
Hohmann o.
Hoke o.
Holmes o.
Horwitz-Adams o.
Houston o.
Jewett o.
Joplin o.
Kapel o.
Keller o.
Kellogg-Speed o.
Kessler o.
Kidner o.
King-Richards o.
Kirkaldy-Willis o.
Kirmisson o.
Kocher o.
Koenig-Wittek o.
Kolomnin o.
König o.
Kraske o.
Kreuscher o.
Lambrinudi o.
Lange o.
Langenbeck (von Langen-
  beck) o.
Lapidus o.
Larrey o.
L'Episcopo o.
Levine o.
Lisfranc o.
Liston o.
Littler o.
Littlewood o.
Lorenz o.
Lottes o.
Lucas-Cottrell o.
Luck o.
Ludloff o.
Lund o.
MacAusland o.
Magnuson o.
Magnuson-Stack o.
Mahorner-Mead o.
Mauck o.
Mayo o.
Mazur o.

operation (continued)

McBride o.
McCarroll o.
McKeever o.
McLaughlin o.
Mikulicz o.
Milch o.
Mitchell o.
Morestin o.
Mumford-Gurd o.
Nélaton o.
Neviaser o.
Nicola o.
Ober o.
Ogston o.
Ollier o.
Osborne o.
Osgood o.
Overholt o.
Paci o.
Palmer-Widen o.
Pauwels o.
Pheasant o.
Phelps o.
Phemister o.
Putti-Platt o.
Reichenheim-King o.
Reverdin o.
Ridlon o.
Routier o.
Roux-Goldthwait o.
Salter o.
Sayre o.
Schanz o.
Schede o.
shelf o.
shelving o.
Silver o.
Slocum o.
Smith-Petersen o.
Sofield o.
Speed-Boyd o.
Stamm o.
Steindler o.
Stokes o.
Swanson o.
Syme o.
Thompson o.

operation (continued)
  Turko o.
  van Gorder o.
  Vladimiroff o.
  Watson-Jones o.
  Whitman o.
  Wilson-McKeever o.
  Wyeth o.
  Yount o.
  Zahradnicek o.
  Zancolli o.
Oppenheim
  sign
opponens
ORIF—open reduction and internal
  fixation
orth, ortho—orthopedics
orthopaedic, orthopaedics [British
  spelling]
orthopedic
orthopedics
orthopedist
orthopercussion
orthopod [alternate term for ortho-
  pedist]
orthopraxy
orthosis (orthoses)
  ankle-foot o. (AFO)
  balanced forearm o.
  dynamic o.
  Engen extension o.
  flexor hinge o.
  functional o.
  halo o.
  hip-knee-ankle-foot o.
    (HKAFO)
  hyperextension o.
  ischial weightbearing
    (weight-bearing) o.
  knee-ankle-foot o. (KAFO)
  lumbosacral o. (LSO)
  opponens o.
  patellar tendon-bearing o.
  pneumatic o.
  poster o.
  resting o.
  serial stretch o.'s

orthosis (orthoses) (continued)
  SOMI o. [sternal-occipital-
    mandibular immobilizer]
  spinal o.
  standing o.
  static o.
  therapeutic o.
  thoracolumbosacral o.
    (TLSO)
orthotic
os (ossa) [bone]
  o. acetabuli
  o. acromiale
  o. calcis
  o. capitatum
  ossa carpi
  o. coxae
  ossa digitorum manus
  ossa digitorum pedis
  o. lunatum
  o. naviculare
  o. orbiculare
  os in os
  o. pisiforme
  o. pubis
  o. triquetrum
Osborne
  operation
oscillation
Osgood
  operation
Osgood-Schlatter
  disease
  syndrome
OSHA—Occupational Safety and
  Health Administration
osphyomyelitis
osphyotomy
ossa (plural of os) [bone]
ossature
ossein
osseoaponeurotic
osseocartilaginous
osseofibrous
osseointegrated implant
osseointegration
osseomucin
osseomucoid

ossicle
ossicula (plural of ossiculum)
ossicular
ossiculum (ossicula)
ossiferous
ossific
ossificans
ossification
    cartilaginous o.
    ectopic o.
    endochondral o.
    heterotopic o.
    intramembranous o.
    membranous o.
    metaplastic o.
    perichondral o.
    periosteal o.
ossifluence
ossiform
ossify
ossifying
osteal [bony, osseous]
ostealgia
osteanabrosis
osteanaphysis
ostearthrotomy
ostectomy
osteectopia
osteite
osteitic
osteitis
    alveolar o.
    o. condensans ilii
    o. deformans
    o. fibrosa cystica
    o. fibrosa osteoplastica
    o. fragilitans
    o. ossificans
    pagetoid o.
    o. pubis
ostempyesis
osteoanagenesis
osteoanesthesia
osteoaneurysm
osteoarthritis
    o. deformans
    o. deformans endemica
    endemic o.

osteoarthritis (continued)
    erosive o.
    hyperplastic o.
    hypertrophic o.
    interphalangeal o.
    primary generalized hyper-
      trophic o.
osteoarthropathy
    familial o. of fingers
    hypertrophic o., idiopathic
    hypertrophic o., primary
    hypertrophic pulmonary o.
    pneumogenic o.
    pulmonary o.
    secondary hypertrophic o.
    tabetic o.
osteoarthroscopy
osteoarthrosis
    o. juvenilis
osteoarticular
osteoblast
osteoblastic
osteoblastoma
osteocachectic
osteocachexia
osteocampsia
osteocartilaginous
osteochondral
osteochondritis
    o. deformans juvenilis
    o. dissecans
    o. ischiopubica
    o. necroticans
osteochondroarthropathy
osteochondrodysplasia
osteochondrodystrophia
    o. deformans
osteochondrodystrophy
    o. familial
osteochondrofibroma
osteochondrolysis
osteochondroma
osteochondromatosis
    synovial o.
osteochondromyxoma
osteochondropathy
osteochondrosarcoma
osteochondrosis

osteochondrous
osteoclasia
osteoclasis
osteoclast
    Collin o.
    Phelps-Gocht o.
    Rizzoli o.
osteoclastic
osteoclastoma
osteocomma
osteocope
osteocopic
osteocystoma
osteocyte
osteodesmosis
osteodiastasis
osteodynia
osteodysplasty
    o. of Melnick and Needles
osteodystrophia
    o. cystica
    o. fibrosa
osteodystrophy
    Albright hereditary o.
    azotemic o.
    parathyroid o.
    renal o.
osteoectasia
    familial o.
osteoepiphysis
osteofibrochondrosarcoma
osteofibroma
osteofibromatosis
osteofluorosis
osteogenesis
    endochondral o.
    o. imperfecta (OI), types I–IV
    o. imperfecta congenita (OIC)
    o. imperfecta cystica
    o. imperfecta tarda (OIT)
    periosteal o.
osteogenic
osteography
osteohalisteresis
osteohydatidosis
osteolipochondroma
osteolipoma
osteolysis

osteolytic
osteoma
    cavalryman's o.
    compact o.
    o. durum
    o. eburneum
    giant osteoid o.
    ivory o.
    o. medullare
    osteoid o.
    o. sarcomatosum
    o. spongiosum
osteomalacia
    osteogenic o.
    renal tubular o.
    senile o.
osteomalacic
osteomatoid
osteomatosis
osteometry
osteomiosis
osteomyelitic
osteomyelitis
    chronic hemorrhagic o.
    chronic sclerosing o.
    conchiolin o.
    Garré o.
    salmonella o.
    sclerosing nonsuppurative o.
    tuberculous spinal o.
    typhoid o.
    o. variolosa
osteomyelodysplasia
osteomyelography
osteon
osteonecrosis
osteoneuralgia
osteonosus
osteopathia
osteopathic
    o. manipulative therapy
      (OMT)
osteopathology
osteopathy
osteopenia
osteopenic
osteoperiosteal
osteoperiostitis

osteopetrosis
osteophlebitis
osteophore
osteophyma
osteophyte
osteophytosis
osteoplaque
osteoplastic
osteoplasty
osteopoikilosis
osteopoikilotic
osteoporosis
osteoporotic
osteopsathyrosis
osteoradionecrosis
osteorrhagia
osteorrhaphy
osteosarcoma
osteosarcomatous
osteosclerosis
osteosclerotic
osteosis
osteosuture
osteosynovitis
osteosynthesis
osteotelangiectasia
osteothrombophlebitis
osteothrombosis
osteotomy
    angulation o.
    block o.
    chevron o.
    Coventry o.
    cuneiform o.
    cup-and-ball o.
    Dega pelvic o.
    displacement o.
    dome o.
    hinge o.
    innominate o.
    intertrochanteric o.
    Le Fort o. (I–III)
    linear o.
    Lorenz o.
    Macewen o.
    Mitchell o.
    pelvic o.
    sagittal split o.

osteotomy (continued)
    Salter o.
    sandwich o.
    segmental alveolar o.
    Southwick o.
    step o.
    subtrochanteric o.
    total maxillary o.
    transtrochanteric o.
    visor o.
    visor/sandwich o.
osteotylus
osthexia, osthexy
ostosis
ostraceous
ostracosis
Ostrum-Furst syndrome
OT—occupational therapy
Otto
    disease
    pelvis
overextension
overflexion
overgrowth
    bony o.
Overholt
    operation
overriding
overstrain
oxygen (O)
    high-pressure o.
    hyperbaric o. (HBO)
    o. myelography
Paas disease
Paci
    operation
Paget
    disease of bone
    juvenile syndrome
    quiet necrosis
    syndrome (II)
    test
pagetoid
PAL—posterior axillary line
palm
palma (palmae)
    p. manus
palmar

palmaris
palmature
Palmer-Widen
    operation
palsy
    See in *Neurology and Pain*
      Management section.
panarthritis
Panner disease
panosteitis
papule
    painful piezogenic pedal p.'s
    piezogenic p.
paraganglioma
    medullary p.
parallagma
parallel
paralysis (paralyses)
    atrophic muscular p.
    common peroneal nerve p.
    compression p.
    crutch p.
    femoral nerve p.
    musculocutaneous nerve p.
    musculospiral p.
    myogenic p.
    myopathic p.
    p. notariorum
    peripheral p.
    peroneal p.
    Pott p.
    pressure p.
    Remak p., Remak-type p.
    rucksack p.
    serratus anterior p.
    spinomuscular p.
    tourniquet p.
    ulnar nerve p.
    writer's p.
parameniscus
paramyoclonus
    p. multiplex
paramyotonia
    ataxia p.
    p. congenita
paramyotonus
parapatellar
    p. incision

paraplegia
    See in *Neurology and Pain*
      Management section.
parapophysis
parasacrum
paraspinous
paratarsium
paratenon
paraxial
paresis
paresthesia
    Berger p.
Parham band
Parona space
paronychia
    p. tendinosa
parosteal
parosteitis
parosteosis
Parrot [eponym]
    syphilitic osteochondritis
pars (partes)
    p. interarticularis
patch
    Carrel p.
patella
    p. bipartita
    p. cubiti
    floating p.
    p. partita
    slipping p.
patellapexy
patellaplasty
patellar
patellectomy
patellofemoral
patellometer
pathogen
    See specific pathogens in
      Laboratory, Pathology,
      and Chemistry Terms.
Patrick
    cross-leg maneuver
    sign
    test
    trigger areas
Pauwels
    operation

Pauzat disease
PC—pubococcygeus
pecten (pectines)
    p. ossis pubis
pectineal
pectoral
pectoralis
pectus
    p. carinatum
    p. excavatum
    p. gallinatum
    p. recurvatum
pedicle
    p. of vertebral arch
pediculate
pediculus (pediculi) [anatomy]
    p. arcus vertebrae
Pellegrini disease
Pellegrini-Stieda disease
pelves (plural of pelvis)
pelvic
    p. osteotomy
pelvifemoral
pelvimetry
pelviotomy
pelvis (pelves)
    achondroplastic p.
    assimilation p.
    beaked p.
    bony p.
    cordate p., cordiform p.
    coxalgic p.
    dwarf p.
    false p.
    frozen p.
    greater p.
    high-assimilation p.
    kyphorachitic p.
    kyphoscoliorachitic p.
    kyphoscoliotic p.
    kyphotic p.
    lesser p.
    lordotic p.
    low-assimilation p.
    p. nana
    p. obtecta
    p. ossea
    osteomalacic p.

pelvis (pelves) (continued)
    Otto p.
    Prague p.
    pseudo-osteomalacic p.
    rachitic p.
    Rokitansky p.
    scoliotic p.
    p. spinosa
    split p.
    spondylolisthetic p.
    p. spuria
    stove-in p.
    true p.
pelvisacral
pelvisacrum
pelvisection
pelvisternum
pelvitrochanterian
pelvospondylitis
    p. ossificans
percuss
percussible
perforans (perforantes)
    p. manus
periarticular
peribursal
pericapsular
perichondrial
perichondritis
perichondrium
perichondroma
perichord
perichordal
pericoxitis
peridesmium
perimysia (plural of perimysium)
perimysial
perimysiitis
perimysium (perimysia)
    external p., p. externum
    internal p., p. internum
perineuritis
perineurium
periosteomyelitis
periosteophyte
periosteorrhaphy
periosteotomy
periostosis

peripatellar
peripheral
    p. angiography
    p. arteriography
perispondylitis
    Gibney p.
peritendineum
peritendinitis
    p. calcarea
    p. crepitans
peritenon
peritenoneum
peritenonitis
perivertebral
peronarthrosis
peroneal
    p. artery
    p. nerve
    p. vein
peroneotibial
per primam intentionem (L. by first intention)
Perrin-Ferraton disease
per secundam intentionem (L. by second intention)
perseverance
Perthes
    disease
    test
pes (pedes)
    p. abductus
    p. adductus
    p. anserinus
    p. calcaneus
    p. cavus
    congenital convex p. valgus
    p. equinovalgus
    equinovarus p.
    p. febricitans
    p. gigas
    p. planovalgus
    p. planus
    p. pronatus
    p. supinatus
    p. valgus
    p. varus
petechia (petechiae)
    calcaneal petechiae

Pfeiffer
    syndrome
PG—prostaglandin
PGE_2 [PGE2]—prostaglandin E_2
phalangeal
    p. articulation
    p. bone
    p. shaft
phalangectomy
phalanges (plural of phalanx)
phalangette
phalangitis
phalangization
phalangophalangeal
phalanx (phalanges)
    distal p.
    p. of finger, phalanges of fingers
    middle p. (of finger or toe)
    proximal p. (of finger or toe)
    p. of toe, phalanges of toes
    tufted p.
    ungual p. (of finger or toe)
Pheasant
    operation
Phelps
    operation
Phemister
    operation
phenomenon (phenomena)
    See also *reflex, sign,* and *test.*
    brake p.
    halisteresis p.
    Herendeen p.
    Holmes p., Holmes-Stewart p.
    Hunt paradoxical p.
    no-reflow p.
    pivot-shift p.
    pronation p.
    radial p.
    Raynaud p.
    Strümpell p.
    tibial p.
    toe p.
    Westphal p.
phocomelia
phonomyoclonus
phonomyogram

phonomyography
physeal
physiologist
physiology
physiotherapeutic
physiotherapist
physiotherapy
physis
piecemeal
"piknic" Phonetic for pyknic.
pillow
    Frejka p. splint
ping-pong fracture
Piotrowski sign
PIP—proximal interphalangeal
PIPJ—proximal interphalangeal joint
Pirie bone
piriform
Pirogoff
    amputation
pivot-shift
    p-s. phenomenon
    p-s. sign
    p-s. test
plantaris
plantigrade
planum (plana)
plastic
    p. achillotenotomy
plate
    alar p.
    Badgley p.
    Blount p.
    epiphyseal p.
    wing p.
platypodia
pleurapophysis
plexus (plexus, plexuses)
plombierung
PM—physical medicine
PMA—progressive muscular atrophy
PMMA—polymethyl methacrylate
    [usually not expanded]
PMR—physical medicine and reha-
    bilitation
        polymyalgia rheumatica
pneumarthrogram
pneumarthrography

pneumarthrosis
pneumatorrhachis
pneumoencephalogram
pneumoencephalomyelogram
pneumoencephalomyelography
poculum
    p. Diogenis
podagra
podagral
podiatric
podiatrist
podiatry
pododynia
point
    trigger p.
pointer
poker spine
Poland
    anomaly
    syndrome
pollex (pollices)
    p. extensus
    p. flexus
    p. valgus
    p. varus
pollicization
polyarthric
polyarthritis
polyarthropathy
polyarthrosis
polychondritis
polychondropathia
polychondropathy
polydactylia
polydactylism
polydysspondylism
polydystrophic
polydystrophy
polymetacarpia
polymetatarsia
polymyalgia
    p. rheumatica
polymyoclonus
polymyopathy
polymyositis
    trichinous p.
polyostotic
polyperiostitis

polyphalangia
polyphasic
polysyndactyly
polytendinitis
polytendinobursitis
Poncet
    disease
    rheumatism
POP—plaster of Paris
poples
popliteal
    p. artery
    p. fascia
    p. ligament
    p. muscle
    p. nerve
    p. region
    p. space
position
    See in *General Surgical Terms.*
Possum (Patient-Operated Selector Mechanism)
postminimus (postminimi)
Pott
    abscess
    curvature
    disease
    dwarfism
    fracture
    gangrene
    puffy tumor
    syndrome (I, II)
Poulet
    disease
PP—proximal phalanx
prehallux
Preiser disease
prepatellar
prescapular
prespondylolisthesis
presternum
pretarsal
pretibial
procedure
    See *maneuver, method, operation,* and *technique.*

process
    See also *apophysis.*
    acromion p.
    articular p.
    capitular p.
    condyloid p.
    conoid p.
    coracoid p.
    intercondylar p.
    mastoid p.
    maxillary p.
    odontoid p.
    olecranon p.
    spinous p.
    styloid p.
    ungual p.
processus (processus)
    p. spinosus vertebrarum
    p. transversus vertebrarum
Profichete
    disease
    syndrome
prominence
    See *apophysis* and *process.*
promontorium (promontoria)
    p. ossis sacri
pronate
pronation
pronatoflexor
pronator
pronator-supinator
propriospinal
prostaglandin (PG)
    See also in *Laboratory, Pathology, and Chemistry Terms.*
    p. E_2 [E2] (PGE_2)
prosthesis (prostheses)
    See also *appliance.*
    conventional single-axis knee p.
prosthetist
protovertebra
protuberance
    See *apophysis* and *process.*
proud flesh
pseudoarthrosis
pseudoarticulation

pseudo-Babinski sign
pseudoepiphysis
pseudofracture
pseudo-Hurler
  disease
  polydystrophy
pseudohypertrophic
pseudoluxation
pseudo-Pott disease
pseudo-Turner syndrome
psoas
  p. muscle
PT—physical therapist
  physical therapy
  physical training
PTD—permanent and total disability
pubic
  p. bone
  inferior p. ligament
  inferior p. ramus
  p. rami
  p. region
  superior p. ligament
  superior p. ramus
  p. symphysis
  p. tubercle
pubis (genitive of pubes; used alone
  for os pubis)
pubofemoral
pubotibial
Pugh nail
pull
pulley
pulseless
pulvinar
punctum (puncta)
  p. ossificationis
  p. ossificationis primarium
  p. ossificationis secundarium
puncture
  bone marrow p.
purchase
  p. point
Putti-Platt
  arthroplasty
  operation
PWB—partial weightbearing
  (weight-bearing)

PWC—physical work capacity
pyknic
Pyle disease
pylon
quadratipronator
quadriceps
quadricepsplasty
quadriplegia
Queckenstedt
  maneuver
  phenomenon
  sign
  test
Queckenstedt-Stookey test
Quervain. See *de Quervain.*
RA—rheumatoid arthritis
"rabdo–" Phonetic for words beginning rhabdo–.
rachialgia
rachidial
rachidian
rachigraph
rachilysis
rachiocampsis
rachiochysis
rachiodynia
rachiokyphosis
rachiometer
rachiomyelitis
rachiopathy
rachioscoliosis
rachiotome
rachiotomy
rachis
rachisagra
rachitic
rachitis
  r. fetalis annularis
  r. fetalis micromelica
  r. tarda
radiation
  r. osteitis
radices (plural of radix)
radiciform
radicis (genitive of radix)
radiculectomy
radiculitis
radiculoganglionitis

radiculomedullary
radiculomeningomyelitis
radiculomyelopathy
radiculoneuritis
radiculoneuropathy
radiculopathy
    brachial r.
    cervical r.
    spinal r.
    spondylotic caudal r.
radii (genitive and plural of radius)
radiobicipital
radiocarpal
radiocarpus
radiodigital
radiohumeral
radioisotope
    r. synovectomy
radiomuscular
radiopalmar
radioulnar
radius (radii)
    r. curvus
radix (radices)
"ra-fee" Phonetic for raphe.
ragocyte
"rakeal–" Phonetic for words beginning rachial–.
"rakee–" Phonetic for words beginning rachi–.
ramal
ramus (rami)
    inferior r.
    ischiopubic r.
    r. of ischium
    r. of pubis (ascending, descending)
range of motion
raphe (raphae)
    r. anococcygea, anococcygeal r.
raphes (genitive of raphe)
rarefaction
    bone r.
Rauchfuss
    sling
    triangle

ray
    digital r.
Raynaud
    disease
    gangrene
    phenomenon
    syndrome
reamer
    Küntscher r.
    Moore r.
    Rush r.
receptor
    stretch r.
recessus (recessus)
Recklinghausen (von Recklinghausen)
    canals
    disease
    disease of bone
recurvation
redislocation
redressement
reduction
    closed r.
    open r.
reef
reefing
reflex
    See also *phenomenon, sign, and test.*
    See also in *Neurology and Pain Management* section.
    Achilles tendon r.
    adductor r.
    ankle r.
    antagonistic r.'s
    aponeurotic r.
    Babinski r.
    Bekhterev deep r.
    Bekhterev-Mendel r.
    biceps r.
    brachioradialis r.
    Chaddock r.
    cremasteric r.
    crossed adductor r.
    crossed extensor r.
    crossed flexor r.
    deep tendon r.'s (DTRs)

reflex (continued)

> deltoid r.
> digital r.
> extensor r.
> external hamstring r.
> external oblique r.
> femoral r.
> finger-thumb r.
> flexor r., paradoxical
> flexor withdrawal r.
> gag r.
> gluteal r.
> great toe r.
> hamstring r.
> heel-tap r.
> hypothenar r.
> interscapular r.
> knee flexion r.
> knee jerk r.
> lumbar r.
> Mayer r.
> muscular r.
> myotatic r.
> palmar r.
> paradoxical r.
> paradoxical ankle r.
> paradoxical extensor r.
> paradoxical flexor r.
> paradoxical patellar r.
> paradoxical triceps r.
> patellar r.
> patelloadductor r.
> pectoral r.
> plantar r.
> plantar flexor r.
> platysmal r.
> pronator r.
> quadriceps r.
> radial r.
> Romberg r.
> scapular r.
> scapulohumeral r.
> sole r.
> sole-tap r.
> Stookey r.
> stretch r.
> Strümpell r.
> supinator jerk r.

reflex (continued)

> supinator longus r.
> suprapatellar r.
> swallowing r.
> tarsophalangeal r.
> tendon r.
> tensor fasciae latae r.
> tibioadductor r.
> toe r.
> triceps r.
> triceps surae r.
> ulnar r.
> wrist flexion r.

refracture

region

> antebrachial r., radial
> antebrachial r., ulnar
> antebrachial r., volar
> anterior antebrachial r.
> anterior brachial r.
> anterior crural r.
> anterior cubital r.
> anterior forearm r.
> anterior r. of neck
> anterior thigh r.
> axillary r.
> basilar r.
> calcaneal r.
> cervical r.
> deltoid r.
> elbow r.
> femoral r.
> gluteal r.
> iliac r.
> infraclavicular r.
> infrascapular r.
> infraspinous r.
> ischiorectal r.
> lateral r. of neck
> r.'s of leg, anterior and posterior
> lumbar r.
> r. of nape
> nuchal r.
> occipital r.
> olecranal r.
> olecranon r.
> patellar r.

region (continued)
    pectoral r.'s
    pelvic r.
    plantar r.'s of toes
    popliteal r.
    posterior antebrachial r.
    posterior brachial r.
    posterior crural r.
    posterior cubital r.
    posterior forearm r.
    posterior r. of neck
    posterior thigh r.
    pubic r.
    sacral r.
    sacrococcygeal r.
    scapular r.
    sternocleidomastoid r.
    subscapular r.
    supraclavicular r.
    suprapubic r.
    supraspinous r.
    trabecular r.
    vertebral r.
    volar r.'s of fingers
    volar r. of hand
rehab—rehabilitation
"reh-dres-maw" Phonetic for
    redressement.
Reichel
    chondromatosis
Reichenheim-King
    operation
repertoire
repetition
resonance
    hydatid r.
    osteal r.
rete (retia)
    r. articulare genus
    articular r. of knee
    r. calcaneum
    r. carpi dorsale
retial
reticulosis
    pagetoid r.
retinaculum (retinacula)
    Weitbrecht r.
retrocalcaneobursitis

retropatellar
retrosternal
Reverdin
    operation
rheumatism
    Besnier r.
    MacLeod capsular r.
    palindromic r.
    Poncet r.
rheumatologist
rhizomelic
rhomboid
    Michaelis r.
rib
    bicipital r.
    cervical r.
    false r.
    floating r.
    slipping r.
    spurious r.
    Stiller r.
    true r.
    vertebral r.
    vertebrocostal r.
    vertebrosternal r.
Ricard amputation
rickets
rider's
    r. bone
    r. bursa
    r. leg
    r. muscles
    r. sprain
    r. tendon
ridge
Ridlon
    operation
rigidity
    cogwheel r.
rigor
    acid r.
    heat r.
    water r.
Riley-Shwachman
    syndrome
RIND—reversible ischemic neuro-
    logic disability

ring
  fibrous r. of intervertebral disk
  periosteal bone r.
"rizo–" Phonetic for words beginning rhizo–.
RLE—right lower extremity
Robert ligament
rocker-bottom foot
rod
  Harrington r.
  Rush r.
Rokitansky
  pelvis
ROM—range of motion
Romberg sign
"romboid" Phonetic for rhomboid.
"rooma–" Phonetic for words
  beginning rheuma–.
Rosenbach
  disease
  syndrome
rotating
  r.-hinge arthroplasty
rotation
  external r.
  internal r.
  lateral r.
Routier
  operation
Roux-Goldthwait
  operation
Royalite body jacket
RP—rest pain
RT—recreational therapy
Rubinstein syndrome
Rubinstein-Taybi syndrome
RUE—right upper extremity
rupture
  extracapsular r.
  intracapsular r.
Russe bone graft
Russell
  traction
Rust [eponym]
  disease
  phenomenon
  sign
  syndrome

S1 through S5—sacral vertebrae 1–5
SA—salicylic acid
Sabolich Socket System
sacralgia
sacralization
sacrarthrogenic
sacrectomy
sacroanterior
sacrococcygeal
sacrococcyx
sacrocoxalgia
sacrocoxitis
sacrodynia
sacrolisthesis
sacrolumbar
sacroperineal
sacroposterior
sacropromontory
sacrosciatic
sacrospinal
sacrotomy
sacrovertebral
sacrum
  assimilation s.
  tilted s.
sagittal
  s. split osteotomy
Salter
  fracture (I–VI)
  operation
  osteotomy
sandwich
  s. osteotomy
  visor/s. osteotomy
Sarbó sign
sarcoblast
sarcoidosis
  muscular s.
sarcoma (sarcomas, sarcomata)
  See also in *Oncology and
    Hematology* section.
  alveolar soft part s.
  chondroblastic s.
  epithelioid s.
  Ewing s.
  fascial s.
  fibroblastic s.
  giant cell s.

sarcoma (sarcomas, sarcomata)
(continued)
    osteoblastic s.
    osteogenic s.
    osteoid s.
    osteolytic s.
    parosteal s.
    periosteal s.
sarcomatoid
sarcomatous
sarcoplasm
sarcoplast
Sayre
    apparatus
    jacket
    operation
    splint
SC—sacrococcygeal
    sternoclavicular (joint)
scale
    Karnofsky s.
scalene
scalenus
scan
    See also in *Radiology,*
    Nuclear Medicine, and
    Other Imaging section.
    bone s.
    bone marrow s.
    CT (computed tomography) s.
    isotope bone s.
scaphoiditis
    tarsal s.
scapula (scapulae)
    alar s., s. alata
    elevated s.
    Graves s.
    scaphoid s.
    winged s.
scapulalgia
scapular
scapulectomy
scapuloclavicular
scapulodynia
scapulohumeral
scapuloperoneal
scapulopexy

Scarpa
    fascia
Schanz
    disease
    operation
    syndrome
Schede
    operation
Scheuermann
    disease
    kyphosis
    syndrome
Scheuthauer-Marie-Sainton syndrome
Schlatter
    disease
    sprain
Schlatter-Osgood disease
Schlein-type elbow arthroplasty
Schlesinger
    phenomenon
    rongeur
    sign
Schmorl
    disease
    furrow
    nodule
Schneider nail
Schoemaker line
Schultze
    acroparesthesia
Schultze-type acroparesthesia
Schwartz-Jampel
    myotonia
    syndrome
sciatic
sclerodesmia
sclerogummatous
sclerosis
    bone s.
    diaphyseal s.
scleroskeleton
sclerozone
scoliokyphosis
scoliosis
    Brissaud s.
    cicatricial s.
    coxitic s.
    empyematic s.

scoliosis (continued)
    inflammatory s.
    ischiatic s.
    myopathic s.
    ocular s.
    ophthalmic s.
    osteopathic s.
    paralytic s.
    rachitic s.
    rheumatic s.
    sciatic s.
    static s.
scoliosometer
scoliotic
scoliotone
scolopsia
scurvy
section
    sagittal s.
SED—spondyloepiphyseal dysplasia
sedatives [a class of drugs]
    spinal s.
segmenta (plural of segmentum)
segmental
    s. alveolar osteotomy
segmentum (segmenta)
self-care
self-suspension
sella (sellae)
    s. turcica
sellar
Selter disease
semilunar
semilunare
semisulcus (semisulci)
"seng-ker" Phonetic for Zenker.
sensorimuscular
septa (plural of septum)
septic
    s. arthritis
septum (septa)
    Bigelow s.
    Cloquet s.
    crural s.
    femoral s., s. femorale, s.
      femorale (Cloqueti)
    iliopectineal s.
    intermuscular s.

sequestra (plural of sequestrum)
sequestral
sequestration
sequestrectomy
sequestrotomy
sequestrum (sequestra)
    primary s.
    secondary s.
    tertiary s.
serum (serums, sera)
    articular s.
"serviko–" Phonetic for words
    beginning cervico–.
sesamoid
sesamoiditis
Sever disease
SF—synovial fluid
"sfir–" Phonetic for words begin-
    ning sphyr–.
shaft
    s. of femur
    s. of fibula
    s. of humerus
    s. of metacarpal bone
    s. of metatarsal bone
    s. of phalanx (of finger or toe)
    s. of radius
    s. of tibia
    s. of ulna
Sharpey fibers
sheath
    femoral s.
    synovial s. of tendon
    tendinous s.
    tendon s.
shelf
    s. operation
shelving
    s. operation
Shenton
    line
Shepherd fracture
Sherman
    plate
    screw
SHO—secondary hypertrophic
    osteoarthropathy

shoulder
    s. blade
    bull's eye s.
    drop s.
    frozen s.
    knocked-down s.
    loose s.
    Magnuson-Stack s. arthroto-
      my
    round s.'s
    stubbed s.
Shwachman-Diamond
    syndrome
"siatik" Phonetic for sciatic.
sign
    See also *phenomenon, reflex,*
      and *test.*
    Achilles tendon s.
    Allis s.
    Amoss s.
    anatomical snuffbox s.
    Anghelescu s.
    anterior drawer s.
    Babinski s.
    Beevor s.
    Bonnet s.
    Bragard s.
    Bryant s.
    clavicular s.
    Cleeman s.
    Codman s.
    Comolli s.
    Coopernail s.
    Dawbarn s.
    Dejerine s.
    Delbet s.
    Demianoff s.
    Desault s.
    distal tingling on pressure
      (DTP) s.
    drawer s.
    DTP (distal tingling on pres-
      sure) s.
    Dugas s.
    Dupuytren s.
    Ely s.
    Erichsen s.

sign (continued)
    fabere (flexion, abduction,
      external rotation, exten-
      sion) s.
    fadir s.
    Fajersztajn crossed sciatic s.
    fat pad s.
    Fränkel s.
    Froment s., Froment paper s.
    Gaenslen s.
    Galeazzi s.
    Goldthwait s.
    Gorlin s.
    Gubler s.
    Hawkins s.
    Heberden s.'s
    Hefke-Turner s.
    Helbing s.
    Higouménaki s.
    Hirschberg s.
    Hoffmann s.
    Homans s.
    Howship-Romberg s.
    Hueter fracture s.
    Kanavel s.
    Keen s.
    Kernig s.
    Langoria s.
    Lasègue s.
    Laugier s.
    Leri s.
    Linder s.
    Lorenz s.
    Ludloff s.
    Lust s.
    Mahler s.
    Maisonneuve s.
    Marie-Foix s.
    McMurray s.
    Mendel-Bekhterev s.
    Mennell s.
    Minor s.
    Ober s.
    obturator s.
    Oppenheim s.
    Ortolani s.
    Patrick s.
    peroneal s.

sign (continued)
    pivot-shift s.
    posterior drawer s.
    pronation s.
    radialis s.
    Raynaud s.
    Romberg s.
    Rust s.
    sail s.
    Sarbó s.
    Schlesinger s.
    Soto-Hall s.
    Strümpell s.
    Strunsky s.
    Thomas s.
    Trendelenburg s.
    trepidation s.
    Turyn s.
    Unschuld s.
    Vanzetti s.
    von Strümpell s.
    Wartenberg s.
    Wimberger s.
SIJ—sacroiliac joint
Silver [eponym]
    bunionectomy
    operation
Silverskiöld
    syndrome
silver-spoon deformity
"simphysis" Phonetic for symphysis.
sin–. See also words beginning
    cin–, syn–.
sinew
"sino–" Phonetic for words begin-
    ning syno–.
sinus (sinus, sinuses)
    air s.
    coccygeal s.
    dermal s.
    lunate s. of radius
    lunate s. of ulna
    peroneal s. of tibia
    semilunar s. of tibia
    tarsal s.
    tentorial s.
    traumatic s.
skeletal

skeletization
skeletonize
skewfoot
Skillern
    fracture
SLE—systemic lupus erythematosus
sling
    Rauchfuss s.
    Teare s.
Slocum
    operation
SLR—straight leg raising
SLRT—straight leg-raising test
Smillie
    meniscotomy
    nail
Smith
    fracture
Smith-Petersen
    nail
    operation
snap
SNF ["sniff"]—skilled nursing
    facility
SOAP—Subjective, Objective,
    Assessment, Plan [format for
    medical reports]
"so-as" Phonetic for psoas.
Sofield
    operation
"so-is" Phonetic for psoas.
sore
    bed s.
    pressure s.
Soto-Hall sign
sound
    muscle s.
Southwick
    osteotomy
space
    antecubital s.
    palmar s.
    Parona s.
    popliteal s.
    thenar s.
    web s.
Spanish windlass

spasm
  muscle s.
  tailor's s.
spasmodic
spasmus
  s. nutans
spatium (spatia)
  spatia interossea metacarpi
  spatia interossea metatarsi
Speed-Boyd
  operation
sphyrectomy
sphyrotomy
spica
  hip s.
spicular
spiculated
spiculum
Spiller syndrome
spina (spinae)
  s. bifida occulta
spinal
  s. arteriography
spinal cord
  s.c. angiography
spinalgia
spinalis
spinant
spine
  alar s.
  angular s.
  anterior inferior iliac s.
  anterior superior iliac s.
  bamboo s.
  cervical s.
  dorsal s.
  s. of greater tubercle of
    humerus
  ischial s.
  s. of ischium
  kissing s.'s
  s. of lesser tubercle of
    humerus
  lumbar s.
  lumbosacral (LS) s.
  peroneal s. of os calcis
  posterior inferior iliac s.
  posterior superior iliac s.

spine (continued)
  s. of pubic bone
  railway s.
  rigid s.
  sacral s.
  s. of scapula
  thoracic s.
  s. of tibia
  tibial s.
  tibial s. of Macewen
  trochanteric s., greater
  trochanteric s., lesser
  typhoid s.
  s. of vertebra
  vertebral s.
spinifugal
spinipetal
spinobulbar
spinocerebellar
spinocostalis
spinogalvanization
spinoglenoid
spinous
spiral
  s. fracture
  Herxheimer s.'s
splayfoot
splint
  See also *appliance, brace,
    orthosis,* and *prosthesis.*
  Agnew s.
  airplane s.
  Anderson s.
  Angle s.
  Ashhurst s.
  Balkan s.
  banjo s.
  Baylor s.
  Böhler s.
  Böhler-Braun s.
  Bond s.
  Bowlby s.
  Brant s.
  Buck s.
  buddy s.
  Cabot s.
  Chandler s.
  coaptation s.

splint (continued)
    cock-up s.
    Colles s.
    Curry s.
    Davis s.
    Denis Browne clubfoot s.
    DePuy s.
    drop-foot s.
    Dupuytren s.
    Eggers s.
    Englemann s.
    Fox s.
    Frejka pillow s.
    Futura s.
    Hart s.
    Hodgen s.
    Jones s.
    Kanavel s.
    Kirschner wire s.
    Lewin s.
    Lewin-Stern s.
    Liston s.
    Lytle s.
    Mason-Allen s.
    opponens s.
    plaster s.
    Protecto s.
    Sayre s.
    Stader s.
    Taylor s.
    Thomas s.
    Tobruk s.
    Volkmann s.
    Wertheim s.
    Zimmer s.
splints
    shin s.
spondylalgia
spondylarthritis
    s. ankylopoietica
spondylarthrocace
spondylexarthrosis
spondylitic
spondylitis
    ankylosing s.
    Bekhterev s.
    s. deformans
    hypertrophic s.

spondylitis (continued)
    s. infectiosa
    Kümmell s.
    Marie-Strümpell s.
    rheumatoid s.
    rhizomelic s.
    tuberculous s.
    s. typhosa
spondylizema
spondylocace
spondylodesis
spondylodynia
spondylolisthesis
spondylolisthetic
spondylolysis
spondylomalacia
    s. traumatica
spondylopathy
    traumatic s.
spondylopyosis
spondyloschisis
spondylosis
    cervical s.
    s. chronica ankylopoietica
    degenerative s.
    hyperostotic s.
    lumbar s.
    rhizomelic s.
    s. uncovertebralis
spondylosyndesis
spondylotherapy
spondylotic
spondylotomy
spondylous
spongiosa
spongiosaplasty
spot
    Carleton s.
    pelvic s.
    trigger s.
sprain
    rider's s.
Sprengel deformity
spur
    calcaneal s.
    occipital s.
    olecranon s.
Spurling test

Spurway
    syndrome
stabilization
Stamm
    method
    operation
Stanmore
    shoulder arthroplasty
stapedial
    s. tenotomy
Steindler
    operation
Steinert disease
stellate
stenosed
stenosing
    s. tenosynovitis
stenosis (stenoses)
    spinal s.
step
    s. osteotomy
sternebra
sternoclavicular
sternocleidal
sternocleidomastoid
sternocostal
sternoscapular
sternoschisis
sternovertebral
sternum
Stieda
    disease
    fracture
Still
    disease
Stiller rib
stimulator
stocking
    Jobst s.
    thromboembolic s.
Stokes
    amputation
Stone [eponym]
    bunionectomy
Stookey
    reflex
strata (plural of stratum)
stratification

stratiform
stratum (strata)
streak
    See *band* and *line.*
Street pin
stress-strain
    s.-s. curve
stria (striae)
    See *band* and *line.*
Strümpell
    disease
    reflex
    sign
Strunsky sign
Struthers ligament
STSG—split-thickness skin graft
styloid
styloiditis
stylopodium
subacromial
subaponeurotic
subarachnoid
subastragalar
subcapsuloperiosteal
subchondral
subclavicular
subcostal
subcostalis (subcostales)
subdeltoid
subdural
subhumeral
subluxation
    Volkmann s.
submaxillary
subparietal
subperiosteal
subscapular
substantia (substantiae)
substitution
    creeping s. of bone
subsultus
    s. tendinum
subtalar
subtarsal
subtrochanteric
    s. osteotomy
subvertebral

Sudeck
    atrophy
    disease
    syndrome
Sudeck-Leriche syndrome
"sudo–" Phonetic for words begin-
    ning pseudo–.
sulci (plural of sulcus)
sulciform
sulcus (sulci)
    bicipital s.
    calcaneal s., s. calcanei
    carpal s., s. carpi
    costal s., inferior
    cuboid s.
    gluteal s.
    interarticular s. of calcaneus
    interarticular s. of talus
    intertubercular s. of humerus
    lateral bicipital s.
    malleolar s. of fibula
    malleolar s. of tibia
    medial bicipital s.
    obturator s. of pubis
    paraglenoid sulci of hip bone
    radial s. of humerus
    s. of radial nerve
    s. of semicanal of humerus
    semilunar s. of radius
    spiral s. of humerus
    supra-acetabular s.
    s. tali, s. of talus
    s. of ulnar nerve
    s. of wrist
supinate
supination
    s. of foot
supinator
supine
supracondylar
supracostal
supraepicondyle
supraepitrochlear
supraglenoid
supralumbar
supramalleolar
suprapatellar
suprapubic

suprascapular
supraspinal
supraspinous
suprasternal
supratrochlear
sura
sural
surgery
        See also *maneuver, method,*
            operation, and *procedure.*
    arthroscopic s.
    microvascular s.
    orthopedic s.
surgical procedure
        See *operation* and *procedure.*
suspensory
sustentacula (plural of sustentaculum)
sustentacular
sustentaculum (sustentacula)
    s. tali, s. of talus
suture [anatomy]
    bony s.
suture [material]
        See also in *General Surgical*
            Terms.
suture [technique]
        See in *General Surgical*
            Terms.
Swanson
    operation
swayback
Swediaur disease
swelling
        See *apophysis* and *process.*
symbrachydactyly
Syme
    amputation
    operation
symphalangia
symphyseal
symphysic
symphysiectomy
symphysiolysis
symphysiorrhaphy
symphysiotomy
symphysis (symphyses)
    s. ossium pubis
    pubic s.

symphysis (symphyses) (continued)
    s. pubica, s. pubis
symphysitis
symphysodactyly
symptom
    See also in *General Medical*
    Terms.
    Oehler s.
syn–. See also words beginning
    cin–, sin–.
synarthrophysis
synarthrosis
synchondrectomy
synchondroseotomy
synchondrosis (synchondroses)
    pubic s., s. pubis
    sacrococcygeal s.
    synchondroses of skull
    sternal s., s. sternalis
synchondrotomy
synclonus
syndactyly
syndesis
syndesmectomy
syndesmectopia
syndesmitis
    s. metatarsea
syndesmography
syndesmology
syndesmoma
syndesmo-odontoid
syndesmopexy
syndesmoplasty
syndesmorrhaphy
syndesmosis (syndesmoses)
    radioulnar s., s. radioulnaris
    tibiofibular s., s. tibiofibularis
syndesmotomy
syndrome
    See also *disease.*
    Albright s.
    Albright-McCune-Sternberg
    s.
    Arnold-Chiari s.
    Baastrup s.
    Bakwin-Eiger s.
    Barré-Liéou s.
    Bertolotti s.

syndrome (continued)
    brittle bone s.
    carpal tunnel s. (CTS)
    cervical s.
    cervical disk s.
    compartment s., compart-
      mental s.
    contracture s.
    cubital s.
    cubital tunnel s.
    de Quervain s.
    disk s.
    epiphyseal s.
    facet s.
    Fèvre-Languepin s.
    Guillain-Barré s.
    herniated disk s.
    Kiloh-Nevin s.
    Klippel-Feil s.
    Klippel-Trénaunay s.
    Klippel-Trénaunay-Weber s.
    knee pain s.
    Laron s.
    Laurence-Biedl s.
    Laurence-Moon s.
    Legg-Calvé-Perthes s.
    Looser-Milkman s.
    Macleod s.
    Marfan s.
    Milkman s.
    Naffziger s.
    Neumann s.
    Paget s. (II)
    Paget juvenile s.
    Poland s.
    pseudo-Turner s.
    Riley-Shwachman s.
    scalenus s.
    scalenus anticus s.
    Schanz s.
    Schwartz-Jampel s.
    Tietze s.
    Weill-Marchesani s.
synosteology
synosteotomy
synostosis (synostoses)
    radioulnar s.
    tarsal s.

synostosis (synostoses) (continued)
    transphalangeal s.
synovectomy
    radioisotope s.
synovia
synovial
    s. biopsy
    s. chondrosarcoma
    s. histopathology
    s. osteochondromatosis
    s. sarcoma
    s. stromal cells
synovialis
synovioma
    benign s.
    malignant s.
synoviorthesis
synoviosarcoma
synoviparous
synovitis
    bursal s.
    chronic purulent s.
    dendritic s.
    dry s.
    filiarial s.
    fungous s.
    s. hyperplastica
    localized nodular s.
    pigmented villonodular s.
    proliferative s.
    puerperal s.
    purulent s.
    scarlatinal s.
    serous s.
    s. sicca
    simple s.
    suppurative s.
    tendinous s.
    transient s.
    traumatic s.
    tuberculous s.
    vaginal s.
    vibration s.
    villonodular s.
syntenosis
synthesis
    s. of continuity
synthetism

syntripsis
syringocele
syringomyelitis
syringomyelocele
T1 through T12—thoracic vertebrae
    1–12
tabatière anatomique
tailbone
tailor's
    t.'s ankle
    t.'s bunion
    t.'s cramp
    t.'s spasm
TAL—tendo Achillis lengthening
talar
talectomy
taliped
talipes
    t. calcaneovalgus
    t. calcaneovarus
    t. calcaneus
    t. cavovalgus
    t. cavus
    t. equinovalgus
    t. equinovarus
    t. equinus
    t. planovalgus
    t. valgus
    t. varus
talipomanus
Talma disease
talocalcaneal
talocrural
talofibular
talonavicular
taloscaphoid
talotibial
talus
tank
    Hubbard t.
tarsal
tarsalgia
tarsectomy
tarsectopia
tarsoclasis
tarsomegaly
tarsometatarsal
tarsophalangeal

tarsoptosis
tarsotarsal
tarsotibial
tarsus
Teale
    amputation
tear
    bucket-handle t.
Teare sling
technique
    See *maneuver* and *method.*
TED, T.E.D. (thromboembolic disease) [T.E.D. is trademark form]
    hose
    stockings
"teerfo" Phonetic for tirefond.
template
    Moore t.
tendines (plural of tendo)
tendinitis
    bicipital t.
    calcific t.
    t. ossificans traumatica
    t. stenosans, stenosing t.
tendinoplasty
tendinosuture
tendinous
tendo (tendines)
    t. Achillis
    t. calcaneus
tendolysis
tendon
    Achilles t.
    calcaneal t.
    flexor carpi radialis t.
    flexor digitorum profundus t.
    flexor digitorum sublimis t.
    t. of Hector
    palmaris longus t.
    patellar t.
    rider's t.
tendoplasty
tendovaginal
tendovaginitis
tenodesis
tenodynia
tenolysis
tenomyotomy

tenonectomy
tenontagra
tenontitis
    t. prolifera calcarea
tenontodynia
tenontophyma
tenontothecitis
tenophyte
tenoplasty
tenorrhaphy
tenositis
tenostosis
tenosuspension
tenosynovectomy
tenosynovitis
    t. acuta purulenta
    adhesive t.
    t. crepitans
    de Quervain t.
    gonococcic t.
    gonorrheal t.
    granulomatous t.
    t. granulosa
    t. hypertrophica
    infectious t.
    nodular t.
    t. serosa chronica
    t. stenosans
    stenosing t.
    tuberculous t.
    villonodular t.
    villous t.
tenotomy
    curb t.
    fenestrated t.
    graduated t.
    open t.
    stapedial t.
tenovaginitis
TENS—transcutaneous electrical nerve stimulator
Tensilon test
tensor
teres
test
    See also in *Laboratory, Pathology, and Chemistry Terms.*

test (continued)
    apprehension t.
    Babinski t.
    Bekhterev t.
    Callaway t.
    Chiene t.
    contralateral straight leg
        raising t.
    Cybex t.
    Dix-Hallpike t.
    drawer t.
    Dugas t.
    Ely t.
    erythrocyte sedimentation
        rate (ESR) t.
    fabere (flexion, abduction,
        external rotation, exten-
        sion) t.
    femoral nerve stretch t.
    Finkelstein t.
    Flack t.
    Hallpike t.
    Hamilton t.
    Jansen t.
    knee dropping t.
    Lasègue t.
    latex fixation t.
    lupus erythematosus (LE)
        cell t.
    McMurray t.
    Mills t.
    Morton t.
    Ober t.
    Paget t.
    Patrick t.
    performance t.
    Phalen t.
    pivot-shift t.
    pronation-supination t.
    quadriceps t.
    rheumatoid factor (RF) t.
    Romberg t.
    ruler t.
    sciatic stretch t.
    serum calcium t.
    serum creatine kinase (CK) t.
    serum phosphorus t.
    Spurling t.

test (continued)
    squatting t.
    station t.
    straight leg raising t. (SLRT)
    Tensilon t.
    Thomas t.
    thumbnail t.
    Tinel t.
    traction t.
    trapeze t.
    Trendelenburg t.
    uric acid t.
textus (textus)
TFCC—triangular fibrocartilage
    complex
theca (thecae)
    t. medullare spinalis
    t. tendinis
    t. vertebralis
thecal
thecitis
thecostegnosis
thenar
    eminence
therapy
    art t.
    corrective t.
    hyperbaric oxygen t.
    intraosseous t.
    manipulative t.
    occupational t.
    physical t.
    relaxation t.
    speech t.
    ultrasonic t.
thermophore
Thibierge-Weissenbach syndrome
Thiele syndrome
Thiemann disease
Thomas
    collar
    sign
    splint
    test
Thompson
    operation
thoraces (plural of thorax)

thoracic
    t. laminectomy
thoracispinal
thoracolumbar
thorax (thoraces)
Thornton
    nail
    plate
    screw
threshold
    swallowing t.
thrombi (plural of thrombus)
thrombophlebitis
thrombose, thrombosed
thrombosis
    See also in *Cardiology* section.
    deep venous t. (DVT)
    venous t.
thrombus (thrombi)
    See *thrombosis.*
    See also in *Cardiology* section.
thrust
    paraspinal t.
thrypsis
thumb
    bifid t.
    tennis t.
    trigger t.
tibia
    saber t.
    t. valga
    t. vara
tibiad [adv.]
tibial [adj.]
tibialgia
tibialis
tibiocalcanean
tibiofemoral
tibiofibular
tibionavicular
tibioperoneal
tibioscaphoid
tibiotarsal
Tinel
    sign
    test

tirefond
tiring
tissue
    osseous t.
TLD—transcutaneous lumbar diskectomy
TLSO—thoracolumbosacral orthosis
TM—transmetatarsal
toe
    hammer t.
    Morton t.
tonoclonic
tonus
tophaceous
tophus (tophi)
    gouty tophi
torsion
torsionometer
torticollis
tortipelvis
total
    t. hip arthroplasty
    t. knee arthroplasty
    t. maxillary osteotomy
tourniquet
    t. paralysis
TPN—total parenteral nutrition
TPPN—total peripheral parenteral nutrition
trabecula (trabeculae)
    trabeculae of bone
trabecularism
trabeculate
trabeculation
tract
traction
    axis t.
    Bryant t.
    Buck t.
    Crutchfield skeletal t.
    external t.
    halo t.
    halo-pelvic t.
    halter t.
    Russell t.
    skeletal t.
    weight t.
tractus (tractus)

transfix
transfixion
transiliac
transischiac
translateral
transplantation
 tendon t.
transposition
transpubic
transsacral
transsection
transsternal
transtrochanteric
 t. osteotomy
transversalis
transverse
transversectomy
transversotomy
trapezial
trapeziform
trapeziometacarpal
trapezium
trapezoid
trauma (traumas, traumata)
treatment
 Carrel t.
 Frenkel t.
Trendelenburg
 gait
 test
Trevor disease
triangle
 Rauchfuss t.
 Ward t.
triceps
triphalangeal
triphasic
Tripier
 amputation
triquetrum
trochanter
trochanteric
trochanterplasty
trochlea (trochleae)
 t. humeri, t. of humerus
 muscular t., t. muscularis
 peroneal t. of calcaneus, t.
  peronealis calcanei

trochlea (trochleae) (continued)
 t. tali, t. of talus
trochleariform
trochlearis
"tseng-ker" Phonetic for Zenker.
tuber (tubers, tubera)
 t. calcanei
 iliopubic t.
 t. ischiadicum
 t. ischiale
 t. radii, t. of radius
tubercle
 pubic t.
tubercula (plural of tuberculum)
tuberculate, tuberculated
tuberculation
tuberculitis
tuberculization
tuberculoid
tuberculosis (TB)
 t. of bone
 t. of bones and joints
 cystic t. of bones
 skeletal t.
 spinal t., t. of spine
tuberculous
 t. spondylitis
tuberculum (tubercula)
 t. calcanei
 t. costae
tuberosis
tuberositas (tuberositates)
 t. sacralis
 t. tibiae
 t. ulnae
tuberosity
 bicipital t.
 t. of calcaneus
 t. of carpal bone
 t. of clavicle
 coracoid t.
 t. of cuboid bone
 distal t. of finger
 distal t. of toe
 t. of femur (external, internal, lateral, medial)
 gluteal t. of femur
 t. of greater multangular bone

tuberosity (continued)
    t.'s of humerus (greater, less-
      er)
    iliac t.
    infraglenoid t.
    ischial t., t. of ischium
    t. of metatarsal bone
    t. of navicular bone
    parietal t.
    patellar t.
    t. of pubic bone
    radial t., t of radius
    sacral t.
    t. of scaphoid bone
    scapular t. of Henle
    t. of second rib, t. for serra-
      tus anterior muscle
    supraglenoid t.
    t. of tarsal bone
    t. of tibia (external, internal)
    t. of trapezium
    t. of ulna
    ungual t., unguicular t.
tubiferous
tubulization
tumentia
tumor
    Ewing t.
    fibrous t.
    giant cell t.
    paravertebral t.
tumorous
tunic
    fibrous t. of liver
    muscular t.
tunicate
Turkel
    trephine
Turko
    operation
Turner
    familial syndrome
    male syndrome
    phenotype with normal
      karyotype
    syndrome
    syndrome in females with
      normal X chromosome

Turner-Keiser
    syndrome
Turyn sign
Tx—traction
UCTS—undifferentiated connective
    tissue syndrome
UE—upper extremity
ulcera (plural of ulcus)
ulcerate
ulcerating
ulceration
    ischemic u.
ulcerative
ulcus (ulcera)
    u. interdigitale
Ullmann line
Ullrich-Turner
    syndrome
ulna
ulnad [adv.]
ulnar [adj.]
    u. drift
    u. nerve
    u. tunnel syndrome
ulnare
ulnaris
ulnocarpal
ulnoradial
ultrasonics
uncal
uncarthrosis
unci (genitive and plural of uncus)
unciform
unciforme ["un-si-for-mee"]
uncinate
uncinatum
unconditioned
unco-ossified
uncotomy
uncovertebral
uncus (unci)
    u. corporis
    u. corporis vertebrae cervi-
      calis
    u. of hamate bone
"ung-kus" Phonetic for uncus.
uniarticular

Unipore
    hip arthroplasty
unmyelinated
Unna
    boot
"unsi–" Phonetic for words beginning unci–.
vaccine
    bursal disease v.
vagina (vaginae)
    v. femoris
    vaginae mucosae
    vaginae synoviales
    v. tendinis
vaginate
valgus
van Buchem
    disease
    syndrome
van der Hoeve
    syndrome
van der Hoeve-de Kleyn
    syndrome
van Gorder
    operation
Vanzetti sign
variation
varicosity
varus
vasculitic
vastus
vein
    antebrachial cephalic v.
    cephalic v.
    saphenous v.
Velpeau deformity
venography
    intraosseous v.
venter (ventres)
Verneuil
    disease
vertebra (vertebrae)
    abdominal vertebrae
    basilar v.
    butterfly v.
    caudal vertebrae, caudate vertebrae
    cervical v. (C1–C7)

vertebra (vertebrae) (continued)
    cleft v.
    vertebrae coccygeae, coccygeal vertebrae
    codfish v.
    vertebrae colli
    cranial v.
    v. dentata
    dorsal vertebrae
    false vertebrae
    hourglass v.
    H-shaped v.
    ivory v.
    vertebrae lumbales
    lumbar vertebrae (L1–L5)
    v. magnum
    movable v.
    odontoid v.
    picture frame v.
    v. plana
    primitive v.
    v. prominens, prominent v.
    sacral v., vertebrae sacrales (S1–S5)
    vertebrae spuriae
    sternal v.
    tail v.
    terminal v., great
    thoracic vertebrae (T1–T12)
    vertebrae thoracicae
    vertebrae thoracales
    toothed v.
    tricuspid v.
    true vertebrae
    v. vera
vertebral
    v. angiography
    v. arteriography
vertebrectomy
vertebrochondral
vertebrocostal
vertebrofemoral
vertebrogenic
vertebroiliac
vertebrosacral
vertebrosternal
vesalianum

vessel
 iliac v.
vibration
vibrator
villose, villous [adj.]
 v. tenosynovitis
villus (villi)
 synovial villi, villi synoviales
vinculum (vincula)
 See also *band, frenulum,*
 and *frenum.*
 v. breve
 v. longum
 vincula tendinum digitorum
 manus
 vincula of tendons of fingers
 vincula of tendons of toes
virus
 See specific viruses in *Labo-*
 ratory, Pathology, and
 Chemistry Terms.
visor
 v. osteotomy
 v./sandwich osteotomy
Vitallium
 screw
Vladimiroff
 operation
Vladimiroff-Mikulicz amputation
VNS—villonodular synovitis
vola (volae)
 v. manus
 v. pedis
volardorsal
volaris
Volkmann
 contracture
 deformity
 disease
 subluxation
vomer
von Gies
 joint
von Recklinghausen. See *Reckling-*
 hausen.
von Rokitansky. See *Rokitansky.*
vortex (vortices)
 coccygeal v., v. coccygeus

VR—vocational rehabilitation
VR&E—vocational rehabilitation
 and education
Vrolik disease
Waardenburg
 disease
 syndrome
Wagstaffe fracture
Waldenström
 disease
Ward triangle
Watson-Jones
 operation
WB—weightbearing (weight-bearing)
webbed
Wegner
 disease
 sign
Weill-Marchesani
 syndrome
Westphal
 sign
 zone
whitlow
 herpetic w.
 thecal w.
Whitman
 frame
 operation
Williams
 exercise
Wilson-McKeever
 operation
windlass
 Spanish w.
wing
 w. of ilium
wormian bones
wrench
 Wilson w.
Wrisberg
 ligament
wrist
wristdrop
wryneck
Wyeth
 operation

xanthoma (xanthomas, xanthomata)
    disseminated x., x. dissemi-
      natum
    synovial x.
    tendinous x., x. tendinosum
xanthosarcoma
xiphisternal
xiphisternum
xiphocostal
xiphoiditis
xiphopagotomy
Yount
    operation
Zahradnicek
    operation
Zancolli
    operation
Zenker
    degeneration
    necrosis
zenkerism
Zickel nail fixation

"zifisternum" Phonetic for xiphi-
    sternum.
"zifo–" Phonetic for words begin-
    ning xipho–.
"zifoid" Phonetic for xiphoid.
Zimmer
    pin
    screw
    splint
zonal
zonary
zone
    cornuradicular z.
    Kambin triangular working z.
    Lissauer z.
    Looser transformation z.'s
    orbicular z. of hip joint
    umbau z.'s
    Weber z.
    Westphal z.
Zuckerkandl dehiscence
zygapophysis (zygapophyses)

Otorhinolaryngology

AAO—American Academy of Otolaryngology
AAT—auditory apperception test
Abbe
    cheiloplasty (stage I, stage II)
Abbe-Estlander
    cheiloplasty
ablation
ABLB—alternate binaural loudness
balance (test)
abscess
    alveolar a.
    Bezold (von Bezold) a.
    circumtonsillar a.
    Dubois a.
    dural a.
    extradural a.
    intramastoid a.
    lacrimal a.
    masticator a.
    mastoid a.
    orbital a.
    otogenic a.
    parapharyngeal space a.
    parotid a.
    peritonsillar a.
    prelacrimal a.
    retropharyngeal a.
    retrotonsillar a.
    septal a.
    subdural a.
    sublingual space a.
    submandibular space a.
    submasseteric space a.
    submental space a.
    subperiosteal a.
    tonsillar a.
    Tornwaldt (Thornwaldt) a.
    tympanocervical a.
    tympanomastoid a.

absence
    congenital ossicular a.
AC—air conduction
acanthion
acinus (acini)
    thyroid acini
acouesthesia
acoumeter
acoumetry
acouophone
acouophonia
acoustic
    a. immitance
    a. neuroma
    a. reflex
    a. trauma
acousticofacial
acousticon
acoustics
acrocephalosyndactyly
action
acuity
    auditory a.
AD—right ear (L. auris dextra)
Adamantiades-Behçet syndrome
Adams
    operation
adenitis
    acute salivary a.
    cervical a.
adenocarcinoma
adenocele
adenofibroma
    a. edematodes
adenofibrosis
adenoid
    a. hypertrophy
adenoidectomy
    tonsillectomy and a. (T&A)
adenoidism
adenoiditis

adenoma
    ceruminous a.
    oxyphil a.
    pleomorphic a.
    serous cell a.
adenopathy
    cervical a.
adenopharyngitis
adenophlegmon
adenotomy
adenotonsillectomy
adequacy
    velopharyngeal a.
aditus
    a. ad antrum
    a. ad antrum mastoideum
    a. ad antrum tympanicum
    a. laryngis
adnexa [grammatically plural, no singular form]
    a. mastoidea
adnexal
Aeby
    muscle
    plane
aerosinusitis
aerotitis
aerotympanal
"a-fago-prak-sea" Phonetic for aphagopraxia.
"af-tha" Phonetic for aphtha.
"af-tho–" Phonetic for words beginning aphtho–.
agger
    a. nasi
    a. perpendicularis
agnosia
    acoustic a.
    auditory a.
aid
    air-conduction hearing a.
    binaural hearing a.
    body-worn hearing a.
    bone-conduction hearing a.
    contralateral routing of signals (CROS) a.
    electric hearing a.
    in-the-ear (ITE) hearing a.

aid (continued)
    mechanical hearing a.
air
    a. conduction
air-bone gap
airway
    endotracheal a.
    a. epithelium
    upper a.
ala (alae)
    a. auris
    a. nasi
alar
alaryngeal
Albers-Schönberg
    disease
Albert
    diphtheria stain
Albinus
    muscle
Albrecht
    bone
    suture
alinasal
allergic
    a. rhinitis
    a. salute
    a. shiner
allergy
    cold a.
    nasal a.
    seasonal a.
Almoor
    operation
Alport
    syndrome
Alström
    disease
    syndrome
alveoli (genitive and plural of alveolus)
alveololabial
alveololabialis
alveololingual
alveolomerotomy
alveolonasal
alveolopalatal

alveoloplasty
    interradicular a.
    intraseptal a.
alveolus (alveoli)
    alveoli dentales mandibulae
    alveoli dentales maxillae
Amberg lateral sinus line
ameloblastoma
    acanthomatous a.
    basal cell a.
    cystic a.
    extraosseous a.
    follicular a.
    granular cell a.
    malignant a.
    multicystic a.
    peripheral a.
    plexiform a.
    plexiform unicystic a.
    solid a.
    unicystic a.
amianthoid
amplification
amyloidosis
    a. of larynx
anaerobe
anakusis
anastomosis (anastomoses)
    Galen a.
    Jacobson a.
Andersch
    ganglion
    nerve
anesthesia
    See also in *General Surgical
        Terms.*
    olfactory a.
angina
    a. diphtheritica
    Ludwig a.
    Plaut-Vincent a.
anginal
angiofibroma
    intranasal a.
    juvenile nasopharyngeal a.
    nasopharyngeal a.
"angkilo–" Phonetic for words
    beginning ankylo–.

angle
    antegonial a.
    Frankfort-mandibular plane a.
    olfactive a.
    olfactory a.
    ophryospinal a.
    orificial a.
    Topinard a.
angulus
    a. mastoideus ossis parietalis
ankyloglossia
ankylosed
ankylosis (ankyloses)
    cricoarytenoid joint a.
    a. of stapes
ankylotic
ankylotomy
annulus (annuli) [compare: anulus]
    a. tracheae
    tympanic a.
    a. tympanicus
    Vieussens a.
anomalad
anomaly
    Pierre Robin a.
anosmatic
anosmia
    a. gustatoria
    preferential a.
    a. respiratoria
anosmic
anosphrasia
anotia
antagonist
    histamine H_1 a.'s [a class of
        drugs]
antegonial
    a. angle
    a. notch
anterior
    a. palatine suture
    a. pharyngotomy
    a. rhinoscopy
anthelix
anthracosis
    a. linguae
anthracotic
antihelix

antihistamines [a class of drugs]
antihistaminic
antitragus
antitussives [a class of drugs]
antra (plural of antrum)
antrectomy
antritis
antroatticotomy
antrocele
antronalgia
antronasal
antroscopy
antrostomy
    intranasal a.
    radical maxillary a.
antrotomy
    sublabial a.
antrotympanic
antrotympanitis
antrum (antra)
    attic-aditus a.
    a. auris
    ethmoid a.
    a. ethmoidale
    frontal a.
    a. of Highmore
    a. highmori
    mastoid a.
    a. mastoideum
    a. maxillare
    maxillary a.
    tympanic a.
    a. tympanicum
anulus (anuli) [compare: annulus]
    a. tympanicus
Apert
    disease
    syndrome
apertognathia
    Le Fort a. repair (I)
apertura (aperturae)
    a. chordae tympani
    a. externa aqueductus
        vestibuli
    a. sinus frontalis
    a. sinus sphenoidalis
    a. tympanica canaliculi

aperture
    bony anterior nasal a.
    a. of frontal sinus
    a. of larynx
    posterior nasal a.
    a. of sphenoid sinus
    tympanic a. of canaliculus
        of chorda tympani
apex (apices, apexes)
    a. of arytenoid cartilage
    a. auriculae, a. auriculare
    a. cartilaginis arytenoideae
    darwinian a.
    a. linguae, a. lingualis
    a. nasi
aphagopraxia
aphonia
    a. paralytica
    spastic a.
aphthosis
    Touraine a.
apices (plural of apex)
apnea
    sleep a.
aponeurosis (aponeuroses)
    See *process.*
apophysis (apophyses)
    See *process, prominence,*
        and *swelling.*
apparatus
    vestibular a.
    vocal a.
appearance
appliance
    See also *prosthesis.*
aqueduct
    a. of cochlea
    a. of Cotunnius
    fallopian a.
    a. of Fallopius
    a. of the vestibule
aqueductus
    a. endolymphaticus
    a. vestibuli
arachnorhinitis
arch
    auricular a.
    a. of Corti

arch (continued)
    palatine a.
arcus
    a. glossopalatinus
    a. lipoides myringis
    a. palatini
    a. palatoglossus
    a. palatopharyngeus
    a. pharyngopalatinus
area (areae, areas)
    auditory cortical a.
    auditory projection a.
    buccopharyngeal a.
    Kiesselbach a.
"areepi–" Phonetic for words beginning aryepi–.
"areten–" Phonetic for words beginning aryten–.
argyria
    a. nasalis
arhinia
"arjirea" Phonetic for argyria.
Arnold
    ganglion
    bodies
    bundle
    canal
    foramen (foramen of Arnold)
    nerve
    nerve reflex cough syndrome
    tract
Arslan
    operation
arteria (arteriae)
    a. nasales septi
arteritis (arteritides)
artery
    carotid a.
    occipital a.
    pharyngeal a.
    thyroid a.
arthritis (arthritides)
    cricoarytenoid a.
arthrosis
    temporomandibular a.
articulation
    a. of auditory ossicles
    cochlear a.

aryepiglottic
aryepiglotticus
aryepiglottidean
arytenoepiglottic
arytenoid
arytenoidectomy
arytenoideus
arytenoiditis
arytenoidopexy
AS—left ear (L. auris sinistra)
Asch
    operation
ASHA—American Speech and Hearing Association
asphyxia
aspiration
Assézat triangle
asterion
asthma
    Millar a. [stridorous laryngismus]
atelectasis
    a. of middle ear
atelectatic
atresia
    acquired a. of external auditory meatus
    a. of external auditory canal
atrium (atria)
    a. alveolare
    a. glottidis
    a. of glottis
    a. laryngis
    a. of larynx
    a. meatus medii
atrophy
    alveolar a.
    hypoglossal a.
attack
    apnea a.
attic
    a. disease
    tympanic a.
atticitis
atticoantrotomy
atticomastoid
atticotomy
    transmeatal a.

AU—each ear (L. auris utraque)
    [not: auris uterque]
audiogram
    Békésy a.
    pure tone a.
    self-recording a.
    serial a.
    speech a.
audiologist
audiology
audiometer
    Békésy a.
    evoked response a.
    Langenbeck (von Langen-
       beck) noise a.
    pure tone a.
    semiautomatic pure tone a.
audiometric
audiometrician
audiometry
    air-conduction a.
    bone-conduction a.
    brain stem evoked response
       (BSER) a.
    impedance a.
    industrial a.
    psychogalvanic skin-
       response a.
audiosurgery
audiphone
audition
auditive
auditognosis
auditory
    a. canal
    a. meatus
    a. tube
Aufrecht sign
augmentation
    a. rhinoplasty
aura
    a. asthmatica
auricle
auricular
auriculare
auricularis
auriculocranial
auriculotemporal

aurilave
aurinarium
aurinasal
auriphone
auripuncture
auris (aures)
    a. dextra (AD) (L. right ear)
    a. externa
    a. interna
    a. media
    a. sinistra (AS) (L. left ear)
    a. utraque (AU) (L. each ear)
aurist
auristics
aurogauge
aurometer
autophony
Avellis
    hemiplegia
    paralysis
    syndrome
Avellis-Longhi syndrome
axoneme
axonotmesis
axoplasm
bacillus (bacilli)
    See in *Laboratory, Patholo-
       gy, and Chemistry Terms.*
Bacillus
    See in *Laboratory, Patholo-
       gy, and Chemistry Terms.*
bacterium (bacteria)
    See specific bacteria in *Lab-
       oratory, Pathology, and
       Chemistry Terms.*
Baelz
    disease
    syndrome
bag
    Politzer b.
band
    See also *frenum* and *vincu-
       lum.*
    See also *line* and *stria.*
    Meckel b.
bandage
    See in *General Surgical
       Terms.*

Bárány
    drum
    noise apparatus whistle
    positional vertigo
    sign
    symptom
    syndrome
    test
barbula hirci
Barclay niche
barodontalgia
barosinusitis
barotitis
    b. media
barotrauma
    otic b., otitic b.
    sinus b.
base
    b. of stapes
basifacial
basihyoid
basioglossus
basipharyngeal
Bauhin
    gland
beak
    b. of sphenoid bone
Becker
    operation
Béclard
    anastomosis
    point
    triangle
Békésy
    audiometry
    calibration
Bell
    nerve
belly
    inferior b. of omohyoid
      muscle
bend
    labyrinthine b.'s
Berry
    ligament
Bertin
    bone
    ossicles

Bespaloff sign
Bezold (von Bezold)
    abscess
    mastoiditis
    perforation
    sign
    symptom
    triad
Bianchi
    valve
biauricular
Bichat
    fat pad
    fossa
    protuberance
Bickel ring
Biederman sign
Bieg sign
Biermer
    sign
bimastoid
bimaxillary
binaural
binauricular
Bing
    test
binotic
bipalatinoid
Björnstad syndrome
black hairy tongue
Blainville ears
Blandin
    ganglion
    glands
Blandin and Nuhn gland
Blasius
    duct
blennorrhagic
blennorrhea
    Stoerk b.
blennorrheal
blindness
    musical b.
BLM (buccal-lingual-masticatory)
    dyskinesia
block
    sphenopalatine b.

blocker
H₁ b.'s [a class of drugs]

Bochdalek
canal
duct
flower basket (flower basket
of Bochdalek)
ganglion
muscle
nerve

Bock
ganglion
nerve

body (bodies)
Bichat fatty b. of cheek
b. of hyoid bone
jugular b.
b. of mandible
b. of maxilla
b. of sphenoid
b. of tongue
turbinated b.
Virchow-Hassall b.

Boeck
See *Beck.*
See *Bock.*

Boettcher. See *Böttcher.*

boggy
b. mucous membranes

BOM—bilateral otitis media

Bondy
mastoidectomy
operation

bone
b. conduction
hyoid b.
petrous b.
squamosal b.
temporal b.
tympanic b.
zygomatic b.

"boo-kay" Phonetic for bouquet.
"boosh de tah-peer" Phonetic for
bouche de tapir.
"boo-zhe" Phonetic for bougie.

border
See also *labium, limbus,* and
margin.

border (continued)
mucocutaneous b.
vermilion b.

Bostock
catarrh
disease

Böttcher (Boettcher)
canal
cells
ganglion
space

bouche
b. de tapir

bouquet
b. of Riolan

bow
cupid's b.
labial b.

Bowman
glands

box
Bárány b.
voice b.

Boyer
bursa
cyst

Boyle
law

bradyglossia

brain stem
b.s. evoked response
(BSER) audiometry

branch
branches of vertebral artery

branchia

branchial
b. arch
b. cleft

branchiogenic
branchiogenous
branchioma
branchiomere
branchiomeric
branchiomerism
breathiness
breathing
glossopharyngeal b.

Breschet
    canals
    hiatus
    sinus
    veins
Breslow
Bretonneau
    angina
    disease
bridge
    malleus-footplate b.
    malleus-stapes b.
bridle
bronchi (plural of bronchus)
bronchitis
    acute laryngotracheal b.
bronchogram
bronchosinusitis
bronchus (bronchi)
    See in *Pulmonary Medicine*
    section.
Brunn (von Brunn)
    membrane
bruxism
BTE—behind the ear
bucca (buccae)
    b. cavi oris
buccal
    b. mucosa
    b. smear
buccally
buccoglossopharyngitis
buccolingually
buccomaxillary
buccopharyngeal
bulla (bullae)
    b. ethmoidalis cavi nasi
    b. ethmoidalis ossis eth-
      moidalis
    b. ossea
bullate
bullation
bursa (bursae)
    nasopharyngeal b.
    pharyngeal b.
    b. sublingualis
    Tornwaldt (Thornwaldt) b.
bursal

bursitis
    Tornwaldt (Thornwaldt) b.
cacogeusia
cacosmia
Caldwell-Luc
    operation
caliculus (caliculi)
    c. gustatorius
Calori bursa
caloric
    c. testing
calorics
canal
    alveolar c
    auditory c.
    auricular c.
    carotid c.
    c. of Corti
    eustachian c.
    external acoustic c.
    Huschke c.
    internal acoustic c.
    osseous cochlear c.
    osseous eustachian c.
    palatine c.
    pharyngotracheal c.
    pterygopalatine c.
    Scarpa c.
    semicircular c.
    spiral c. of Rosenthal
canaliculus (canaliculi)
    auricular c.
    canaliculi caroticotympanici
    c. chordae tympani, c. of
      chorda tympani
    c. of cochlea, cochlear c.
    canaliculi cochleae
    incisor c.
    mastoid c., mastoid c. for
      Arnold nerve
    c. mastoideus
    c. petrosus, petrous c.
    tympanic c. for Jacobson
      nerve
    c. tympanicus
canaloplasty
canal wall
    intact c.w. tympanoplasty

cancer
    See also *carcinoma.*
    See also in *Oncology and Hematology* section.
    adenoid c.
cancrum
    c. nasi
    c. oris
candidiasis
    oral c.
Canfield
    operation
cannulate
cannulation, cannulization [introduction of a cannula]
capita (plural of caput)
capitula (plural of capitulum)
capitular
capitulum (capitula)
    c. stapedis
capsule
    acoustic c.
    articular c.
    cartilaginous ear c.
    cricoarytenoid articular c.
    cricothyroid articular c.
    c. of labyrinth
    nasal c.
    olfactory c.
caput (capita)
    c. stapedis
carcinoma (carcinomas, carcinomata)
    See also *cancer.*
    See also in *Oncology and Hematology* section.
    acinic cell c.
    adenocystic c.
    basal cell c.
    epidermoid c.
    laryngeal c.
    mucoepidermoid c.
    nasopharyngeal c.
    schneiderian c.
    squamous cell c.
    tonsillar c.
Carhart notch
Carnochan
    operation

caroticotympanic
carotid
    c. artery
Carpue
    operation
    rhinoplasty
Carter
    operation
    splint
cartilage
    alar c.
    arytenoid c.
    corniculate c.
    cricoid c.
    cuneiform c.
    epiglottic c.
    hyaline c.
    intrathyroid c.
    laryngeal c. of Luschka
    paranasal c.
    paraseptal c.
    Santorini c.
    septal c.
    thyroid c.
    vomerian c. of Hirschfeld
    vomerian c. of Huschke
    vomerine c.
    vomeronasal c.
    Wrisberg c.
cartilago (cartilagines)
    cartilagines alares minores
    c. alaris major
    c. arytenoidea
    c. auriculae
    c. corniculata
    c. cricoidea
    c. cuneiformis
    c. epiglottica
    cartilagines laryngis
    c. meatus acustici
    cartilagines nasales accessoriae
    cartilagines nasi
    c. nasi lateralis
    c. septi nasi
    cartilagines sesamoideae nasi
    c. sesamoidea laryngis

cartilago (cartilagines) (continued)
   c. sesamoidea ligamenti
     vocalis
   c. thyroidea
   cartilagines tracheales
   c. triquetra
   c. tubae auditivae
   c. wrisbergi
caruncle
   salivary c.
   sublingual c.
caruncula (carunculae)
   c. salivaris
   c. sublingualis
caruncular
Cassel
   operation
Casser (Casserio, Casserius)
   fontanelle
   ligament
   muscle
catarrh
   autumnal c.
   Bostock c.
   epidemic c.
   spring c.
   summer c.
   vernal c.
catarrhal
catheterization
   eustachian c.
   laryngeal c.
   transseptal c.
cauda (caudae)
   c. helicis
cava (plural of cavum)
cavitas (cavitates)
   c. nasi ossea
cavity
   c. of middle ear
   tympanic c.
cavum (cava)
   c. conchae
   c. infraglotticum
   c. laryngis
   c. nasi
   c. nasi osseum
   c. oris

cavum (cava) (continued)
   c. oris externum
   c. oris proprium
   c. pharyngis
   c. tympani
Cawthorne maneuver
cecum
   cupular c. of cochlear duct
   c. cupulare ductus cochlearis
   vestibular c. of cochlear duct
   c. vestibulare ductus
     cochlearis
cellula (cellulae)
   c. anteriores ethmoidales
   cellulae ethmoidales osseae
   cellulae mastoideae
   c. medii ethmoidales
   cellulae pneumaticae tubae
     auditivae
   cellulae pneumaticae tubariae
   c. posteriores ethmoidales
   c. sensoria pilosa
   cellulae tympanicae
cellulitis
   cervical c.
   orbital c.
   peritonsillar c.
centrilobular
CEOM—chronic exudative otitis
   media
cephalalgia
   histamine c.
   pharyngotympanic c.
cephalgia
CERA—cortical evoked response
   audiometry
ceramidase deficiency
cerebellopontine
   c. angle
cerumen
   impacted c.
   inspissated c.
ceruminal
ceruminolysis
ceruminolytic
ceruminosis
ceruminous
CFA—craniofacial abnormality

chain
    ossicular c.
Charlin syndrome
Chausse
    III projection (third projec-
        tion of Chausse)
    view
Cheever
    operation
cheilectropion
cheilognathoprosoposchisis
cheilognathoschisis
cheilognathouranoschisis
cheiloplasty
    Abbe c. (stage I, stage II)
cheiloschisis
Chevalier Jackson
    operation
Cheyne
    nystagmus
Chievitz
    organ
choana (choanae)
    choanae osseae
choanal
    c. atresia
choanate
choanoid
cholesteatoma
    intracranial c.
    paranasal sinus c.
    primary acquired c.
    secondary acquired c.
    c. tympani
cholesteatomatous
cholesteatosis
chondroma
chondromalacia
    c. of larynx
chorda (chordae)
    c. tympani
chordal
chorditis
    c. cantorum
    c. fibrinosa
    c. nodosa
    c. tuberosa
    c. vocalis

chromorhinorrhea
cicatrices (plural of cicatrix)
cicatricial
cicatrix (cicatrices)
    manometric c.
cilia
cin–. See also words beginning
    sin–, syn–.
circular
    Livaditis c. myotomy
Citelli
    syndrome
classification
    See also *index.*
    Clark c. of malignant mela-
        noma (levels I–V)
    Tessier c. for clefts
    Wullstein c.
cleft
    laryngotracheoesophageal c.
    c. lip
    oblique facial c.
    orbitonasal c.
    c. palate
    pharyngeal c.
    submucous c.
    tubotympanic c.
clinoid
clinoid process
Cloquet ganglion
CM—cochlear microphonic [poten-
    tial]
Coakley
    operation
cochlea (cochleae)
cochlear
    c. duct
    c. implant
    c. nerve
cochleariform
cochleitis
cochleovestibular
cochlitis
Cody
    operation
Cogan
    disease
    syndrome

cog tooth of malleus
coil
    See also *helix* and *spiral.*
    helical c.
coldsore
cold water calorics
collum (colla)
collunarium
columella
    c. cochleae
    c. nasi
columna (columnae)
    c. nasi
combined approach
    c.a. mastoidectomy
    c.a. tympanoplasty
Commando
    operation
commissure
    laryngeal c.
commissurorrhaphy
complete
    See also *total.*
    c. laryngotomy
compliance
concha (conchae)
    c. of auricle
    c. auriculae
    c. bullosa
    ethmoidal c.
    c. nasalis inferior ossea
    c. nasalis media ossea
    c. nasalis superior ossea
    c. nasalis suprema ossea
    nasoturbinal c.
    Santorini c.
    sphenoidal c.
    c. sphenoidalis
conchiris
conchotomy
conduction
    air c.
    bone c.
congested
congestion
congestive
coniotomy
conjunctivorhinostomy

conservative
    c. mastoidectomy
conus
    c. elasticus laryngis
Converse [eponym]
    rongeur
COR—conditioned orientation
    response
CORA—conditioned orientation
    reflex audiometry
cord
    vocal c.
cordal
cordectomy
cordopexy
corniculate
cornu (cornua)
    ethmoid c.
cornual
cornuate
cornucommissural
corona (coronae)
coronal
coronale
coronalis
corone
coronion
coronoid
coronoidectomy
Corti
    arches
    canal
    organ
    rods
    tunnel
cortical
    c. mastoidectomy
coryza
    allergic c.
    c. oedematosa
cosmesis
Costen syndrome
Cotunnius
    aqueduct (aqueduct of
      Cotunnius)
cough
    aneurysmal c.
    ear c.

cough (continued)
    trigeminal c.
CP—cochlear potential
cranioaural
craniofacial
craniopharyngeal
cribra (plural of cribrum)
cribral
cribrate
cribration
cribriform
    c. spot
cribrum (cribra)
cricoarytenoid
cricoid
cricoidectomy
cricoidynia
cricopharyngeal
    c. myotomy
cricopharyngeus
cricothyreotomy
cricothyroid
cricothyroidotomy
cricothyrotomy
cricotomy
cricotracheotomy
Crikelair
    otoplasty
crista (cristae)
    c. ampullaris
    c. arcuata cartilaginis ary-
        tenoideae
    c. conchalis maxillae
    c. conchalis ossis palatini
    c. ethmoidalis maxillae
    c. ethmoidalis ossis palatini
    c. fenestrae cochleae
    c. frontalis
    c. galli
    c. nasalis maxillae
    c. nasalis ossis palatini
    c. tympanica
cristal
cristate
criterion (criteria)
    Hyams criteria
cross hearing

Crouzon
    disease
    syndrome
crura (plural of crus)
crurotomy
crus (crura)
    anterior c. of stapes
    c. anterius stapedis
    c. anthelicis
    c. of anthelix
    c. breve incudis
    c. helicis
    c. of helix
    posterior c. of stapes
    c. posterius stapedis
crypt
    lingual c.'s
crypta (cryptae)
cryptotia
CSF—cerebrospinal fluid
CSF rhinorrhea
culture
    sputum c.
    tracheal aspirate c.
cuneiform
cunicular
cuniculus (cuniculi)
    c. externus
    c. internus
    c. medius
cupula (cupulae)
    c. ampullaris
    c. of ampullary crest
    c. of cochlea
    c. cochleae
    c. cristae ampullaris
cupulolithiasis
curettement
CV—conversational voice
cymba (cymbae)
    c. conchae auriculae
cyst
    dermoid c.
    epidermoid c.
    Klestadt c.
    nasoalveolar c.
    nasopalatine c.
    odontogenic c.

cyst (continued)
 radicular c.
 retention c.
 sebaceous c.
 Tornwaldt (Thornwaldt) c.
cystic
 c. fibrosis
dacryocystorhinostenosis
dacryocystorhinostomy
dactylocostal
 d. rhinoplasty
Day
 operation
dB, db—decibel
deaf
deaf-mute
deaf-mutism
deafness
 acoustic trauma d.
 apoplectiform d.
 cerebral d.
 ceruminous d.
 conduction d.
 congenital d.
 cortical d.
 genetic d.
 labyrinthine d.
 Michel d.
 Mondini d.
 neural d.
 paradoxical d.
 perceptive d.
 Scheibe d.
 sensorineural d.
 toxic d.
 vascular d.
decibel (dB)
Deiters
 nucleus
 phalanges
Delphian node
Demarquay sign
demulcents [a class of drugs]
Denker
 operation
Derlacki
 gouge
 mobilizer

Derlacki (continued)
 operation
diapason
diastolization
DIMOAD—diabetes insipidus, diabetes mellitus, optic atrophy, deafness [syndrome]
diplacusis
 binaural d.
 d. binauralis dysharmonica
 d. binauralis echoica
 disharmonic d.
 echo d.
 monaural d.
direct
 d. laryngoscopy
dis–. See also words beginning dys–.
disc
 See *disk*.
discontinuity
discrimination
disease
 See also *syndrome*.
 Albers-Schönberg d.
 Alport d.
 Alström d.
 attic d.
 Fede d.
 Gerlier d.
 Hunt d.
 Legal d.
 Lyme d.
 Ménière d.
 Meyer d.
 Mikulicz d.
 Pendred d.
 Ramsay Hunt d.
 Refsum d.
 Sutton d.
 Takahara d.
 Tornwaldt (Thornwaldt) d.
 Usher d.
 von Recklinghausen d.
 Waardenburg d.
"disfajea" Phonetic for dysphagia.
"disfazea" Phonetic for dysphasia.
"disfonia" Phonetic for dysphonia.

disharmony
>maxillomandibular d.

disk
>*Note: Some specialists and references prefer* disc.
>mandibular d.

dissection
>d. tonsillectomy

Doerfler-Stewart test

"doosh" Phonetic for douche.

Dorello canal

dorsi (genitive of dorsum)

dorsum (dorsa)
>d. linguae
>d. nasi
>d. of tongue

dot
>See *disk, macula,* and *spot.*

Dott
>operation

douche
>air d.
>Bermingham nasal d.
>nasal d.

drainage
>d. headache

dressing
>See in *General Surgical Terms.*

drooling

drumhead

duct
>cochlear d.
>d. of Rivinus
>endolymphatic d.
>lacrimal d.
>lacrimonasal d.
>Stensen d.
>Walther d.
>Wharton d.

ductus (ductus)
>d. cochlearis
>d. endolymphaticus
>d. reuniens

dys–. See also words beginning dis–.

dysacousia

dysaudia

dysfluency

dysfunction
>temporomandibular joint d.

dysgeusia

dyskinesia
>BLM (buccal-lingual-masticatory) d.

dysosmia

dysostosis
>craniofacial d.
>mandibulofacial d.

dysphagia [difficulty swallowing]

dysphagic

dysphasia [difficulty with speech]

dysphonia
>d. plicae ventricularis
>dysplastic d.
>spasmodic d.
>d. clericorum
>d. spastica
>spastic d.

dysphonic

dysplasia
>fibrous d.

EAC—external auditory canal

EAHF—eczema, asthma, hay fever

EAM—external auditory meatus

earache

eardrum

echo
>cochlear e.

edema
>Reinke e.
>subglottic e.

edentulous

EEA—electroencephalic audiometry

effect [noun: result, outcome]
>See also *phenomenon.*
>Vulpian e.
>Wever-Bray e.

"eko–" Phonetic for words beginning echo–.

electrocochleogram

electrocochleograph

electrocochleographic

electrocochleography

electronystagmogram (ENG)

electronystagmography

electro-olfactogram (EOG)

electrosalivogram
eminence
    arytenoid e.
    nasal e.
    pyramidal e.
eminentia
    e. articularis ossis temporalis
    e. conchae
    e. fallopii
    e. fossae triangularis auriculae
emissarium
    e. mastoideum
encephalocele
enchondroma
endognathic
    e. suture
endolabyrinthitis
endolaryngeal
endolarynx
endolymph
endolympha
endolymphatic
    e. hydrops
endomastoiditis
endomesognathic
    e. suture
endonasal
endoscopy
    fiberoptic e.
    flexible e.
    lower gastrointestinal (LGI) e.
    peroral e.
    e. suite
    upper gastrointestinal
      (UGI) e.
endothelium (endothelia)
endotracheal (ET)
    e. intubation
ENG—electronystagmogram
    electronystagmography
English
    rhinoplasty
entacoustic
entotic
entotympanic
EOG—electro-olfactogram
epiglottectomy [pref: epiglottidecto-
    my]

epiglottic
epiglottidean
epiglottidectomy
epiglottiditis
epiglottis
epignathous [adj.]
epignathus [noun]
epimandibular
epiotic
epipharyngeal
epipharyngitis
epipharynx
epistaxis
epithelia (plural of epithelium)
epithelialize, epithelialized
epitheliitis
epithelium (epithelia)
    oral e.
epiturbinate
epitympanic
epitympanum
ER—evoked response
ERA—electric response audiometry
    evoked response audiometry
Erhard
    test
Erich
    splint
errhine
erythroplakia
    speckled e.
esophagectomy
esophagitis
    thrush e.
esophagolaryngectomy
esophagopharynx
esophagostomy
esophagotomy
esthesioneuroblastoma
Estren-Dameshek syndrome
ET—endotracheal
ethanolamines [a class of drugs]
ethmofrontal
ethmoid, ethmoidal
ethmoidectomy
    transantral e.
ethmoiditis

ethmoidolacrimal
    e. suture
ethmoidomaxillary
    e. suture
ethmoidotomy
ethmolacrimal
ethmomaxillary
ethmonasal
ethmopalatal
ethmosphenoid
ethmoturbinal
ethmovomerine
eustachian
    e. catheterization
    e. tube
    e. tuboplasty
eustachitis
eustachium
Ewing sign
excernent
excochleation
expectorants [a class of drugs]
expectorate
expectoration
    rusty e.
explorer
    Rosen e.
external
    e. frontoethmoidectomy
    e. pharyngotomy
extradural
facies (facies)
    adenoid f.
"fahringo–" Phonetic for words
    beginning pharyngo–.
fallopian
    f. aqueduct
    f. artery
    f. hiatus
    f. neuritis
Fallopius
    aqueduct of F.
"farin–" Phonetic for words begin-
    ning pharyn–.
"farinks" Phonetic for pharynx.
fascia (fasciae)
    alar f. of pharynx
    lacrimal f.

fascia (fasciae) (continued)
    pretracheal f.
fauces [grammatically plural; no
    singular form]
faucial
faucitis
Fede disease
fenestra (fenestrae)
    f. of cochlea
    f. cochleae
    f. nov-ovalis
    f. ovalis
    f. rotunda
    f. vestibuli
fenestrate
fenestrater
    Rosen f.
fenestration
    f. operation
"fenomenon" Phonetic for phenom-
    enon.
Fergusson
    incision
    operation
Ferris-Smith
    operation
fiber
    Prussak f.'s
fiberoptic
    f. laryngoscopy
fibroangioma
fibroma
    desmoplastic f.
    submucous f.
fibromatogenic
fibromatoid
fibromatosis
fibromatous
fibromectomy
Fick
    operation
"Fifer" Phonetic for Pfeiffer.
filtrum [part of larynx]
    See also *philtrum*.
    Merkel f. ventriculi
fimbria (fimbriae)
    fimbriae of tongue
fimbrial

fimbriated
Finzi-Harmer
    operation
fissula
    f. ante fenestrum
fissura (fissurae)
    f. antitragohelicina
fissure
    entorbital f.
    ethmoid f.
    glaserian f.
    petrotympanic f.
fistula (fistulas, fistulae)
    esophagotracheal f.
    frontal sinus f.
    f. of lip
    oroantral f.
    oronasal f.
    perilymph f.
    tracheal f.
    tracheoesophageal f.
flap
    tympanomeatal f.
"flebektazea" Phonetic for phlebec-
    tasia.
"flegmon" Phonetic for phlegmon.
Fleischman bursa
"flem" Phonetic for phlegm.
flower basket of Bochdalek
flu
fluid
    Scarpa f.
fold
    aryepiglottic f.
    salpingopharyngeal f.
folium (folia)
    lingual folia
fonticulus (fonticuli)
footplate
    floating f.
    stapedial f.
foramen (foramina)
    greater palatine f.
    Huschke f.
    Hyrtl f.
    f. incisivum
    jugular f.
    lesser palatine foramina

foramen (foramina) (continued)
    f. mastoideum
    f. ovale alae majoris
    foramina palatina minora
    f. of palatine tonsil
    rivinian f.
    Scarpa foramina
    f. sphenopalatinum
    Stensen f.
    f. stylomastoideum
    f. Vesalii, f. of Vesalius
foraminal
Forchheimer spots
foreign body (FB)
    retained f.b. (RFB)
formant
formula
    Seiler f.
fossa (fossae)
    conchal f.
    glossoepiglottic f.
    f. incudis
    lateral pharyngeal f.
    Merkel f.
    f. ovalis
    pharyngomaxillary f.
    postauditory f.
    Rosenmüller f.
    triangular f.
fossula (fossulae)
fossulate
foveola (foveolae)
    f. suprameatalis
    f. suprameatica
    triangular f.
foveolar
foveolate
fracture
    blow-out f.
    malar f.
    midfacial f.
    nasal f.
    nasomaxillary f.
    zygomaticomaxillary f.
Franke
    syndrome
    triad
frena (plural of frenum)

frenal
"freng-kuhl" Phonetic for Fränkel.
Frenkel
    See *Fränkel.*
frenotomy
frenulum (frenula)
    See *band, frenum,* and *vinculum.*
frenum (frena)
    See also *band* and *vinculum.*
    buccal f.
Frey
    syndrome
Frey-Baillarger syndrome
frontal
    f. bone
    f. lobe
frontoethmoidal
    f. sphenoidectomy
    f. suture
frontoethmoidectomy
    external f.
frontolacrimal
    f. suture
frontolateral
    f. partial laryngectomy
frontomalar
    f. suture
frontomaxillary
    f. suture
frontonasal
    f. suture
fronto-occipital
frontoparietal
    f. suture
frontosphenoid
    f. suture
frontotemporal
frontozygomatic
    f. suture
Fröschel symptom
fundus (fundus)
    f. meatus acustica interni
    f. tympani
fungus (fungi)
    See also specific fungi in
    Laboratory, Pathology,
    and Chemistry Terms.

fungus (fungi) (continued)
    thrush f.
furcula
gag
gag reflex
galea
    g. aponeurotica
    tendinous g.
Galen
    anastomosis
ganglial
ganglion (ganglia, ganglions)
    acoustic g.
    acousticofacial g.
    Cloquet g.
    geniculate g.
    g. geniculi nervi facialis
    nodose g.
    otic g.
    Scarpa g.
Garcin syndrome
Gasser
    ganglion
Gault test
Gellé test
geniohyoid
genioplasty
genyantralgia
genyantritis
genyantrum
genycheiloplasty
geographic tongue
Gerhardt
    sign
Gerlier disease
Gilbert-Behçet syndrome
Gillies
    operation
glabella
glabellad [adv.]
glabellar [adj.]
    g. frown line
    g. rotation flap
    g. wrinkle
gland
    lateral nasal g. of Stensen
    lingual g.
    Nuhn g.'s

gland (continued)
    palatine g.
    parotid g.
    Rivinus g.
    salivary g.
    Stahr g.
    sublingual g.
    submandibular salivary g.
    submaxillary g.
    Suzanne g.
    thyroid g.
glandula (glandulae)
glandular
glandule
glandulous [adj.]
glaserian fissure
glomera (plural of glomus)
glomerulus (glomeruli)
    olfactory g.
glomus (glomera)
    g. jugulare
    g. tympanicum
glossa
glossagra
glossal
glossalgia
glossanthrax
glossectomy
glossitis
    Moeller g.
    rhomboid g.
glossocele
glossocoma
glossodynamometer
glossoepiglottic
glossoepiglottidean
glossohyal
glossohyoidal
glossoncus
glossopalatinus
glossopathy
glossopexy
glossopharyngeal
glossopharyngeum
glossopharyngeus
glossoplasty
glossoplegia
glossoptosis

glossorrhaphy
glossoscopy
glossospasm
glossotomy
glottis (glottides)
gnathodynia
gnathoplasty
gnathoschisis
goiter
    adenomatous g.
    cabbage g.
    colloid g.
    cystic g.
    endemic g.
    exophthalmic g.
    familial g.
    fibrous g.
    follicular g.
    intrathoracic g.
    myxedematous g.
    nodular g.
    papillomatous g.
    parenchymatous g.
    substernal g.
    thoracic g.
    toxic g.
gonia (plural of gonion)
gonion (gonia)
gonorrhea
    oropharyngeal g.
    pharyngeal g.
Gottschalk
    aspirator
goundou
Gradenigo
    syndrome
grading system
    Hyams g.s.
granuloma
    Wegener g.
granulomatosis
    Wegener g.
Griesinger
    sign
    symptom
groove
    Verga lacrimal g.

Gross
    spud
Guérin
    fold
    fracture
    glands
    sinus
    valve
Guidi canal
Guilford
    stapedectomy
guillotine
    Sluder g. tonsillectomy
    g. tonsillectomy
H_1 blockers [a class of drugs]
Hajek
    operation
Hallgren syndrome
hammer
    Quisling h.
Harada
    disease
    syndrome
Hartmann
    rongeur
    tuning fork
Haverhill
    operation
hay fever
headache
    drainage h.
    hat band h.
    migraine h.
Heath
    operation
HEENT—head, eyes, ears, nose,
    and throat
Heerfordt
    disease
    syndrome
Heermann
    operation
helicine
helicoid
helicotrema
helix (helices, helixes)
    See also *coil* and *spiral.*
    h. of ear

Heller
    myotomy
hematoma
    h. auris
    sublingual h.
hemiglossal
hemiglossectomy
hemiglossitis
hemilaryngectomy
    horizontal h.
    vertical h.
hemimandibulectomy
hemimaxillectomy
hemorrhage
hemorrhagic
Henle spine
HEPA—high-efficiency particulate
    air [filter]
Herlitz
    disease
    syndrome
herpes
    buccal h.
    h. catarrhalis
    h. febrilis
    h. labialis
    lingual h.
    nasal h.
    orofacial h. simplex
    h. oticus
    pharyngeal h.
    h. pharyngitis
    h. zoster oticus
Heryng sign
HF—high frequency
hiatus
    Scarpa h.
    h. semilunaris
Highmore
    antrum
highmori
    sinus maxillaris h.
highmoritis
Hilger
    operation
"hipo–" Phonetic for words begin-
    ning hypo–.

histamine H$_1$ antagonists [a class of drugs]
Hitzig
    girdle
    syndrome
    test
HL—hearing loss
H$_2$O$_2$ [H2O2]—hydrogen peroxide
Hoffmann
    sign
Hopmann
    papilloma
    polyp
Horgan
    operation
horizontal
    h. hemilaryngectomy
Hough
    stapedectomy
House
    adaptor
    irrigator
    rod
    separator
    stapedectomy
Huguier sinus
Hunt
    disease
    syndrome
Hunter
    glossitis
Huschke
    auditory teeth
    canal
    foramen
    ligaments
    teeth
    valve
    vomerian cartilage
Hutchinson
    syndrome
    triad
Hyams
    criteria
    grading system
hydrocephalus
    otitic h.

hydrorrhea
    nasal h.
hydrotis
hydrotympanum
Hynes
    pharyngoplasty
hyothyroid
hypacusis
hyperacusis
hyperadenosis
hyperesthesia
    acoustic h.
    auditory h.
hyperesthetic
hypergeusesthesia
hypergeusia
hyperkeratosis
    h. lacunaris
hypernasal
hypernasality
hyperosmia
hyperosphresia
hyperphonesis
hyperphonia
hyperprosody
hyperptyalism
hyperventilation
hypesthesia
hypoacusis
hypoalphalipoproteinemia
hypobranchial
hypoesthesia
    acoustic h.
    olfactory h.
hypogeusia
hypoglossal
hypoglottis
hypognathous [adj.]
hypolarynx
hypomyxia
hyponasal
hyponasality
hypopharyngeal
hypopharyngectomy
hypopharyngoscopy
hypopharynx
hypophonesis

hypoplasia
 craniofacial h.
 nasomaxillary h.
hypopnea
hypoprosody
hypoptyalism
hyposalivation
hyposecretion
hyposialosis
hyposmia
hypostomia
hypotympanic
hypotympanotomy
hypotympanum
Hyrtl
 anastomosis
 loop
 recess
Hz—hertz
IA—internal auditory
IAC—internal auditory canal
IAM—internal auditory meatus
ichthyosis
 i. linguae
"ikthe–" Phonetic for words beginning ichthy–.
immune
 i. response
 i. system
impairment
 hearing i.
implant
 cochlear i.
incision
 myringotomy i.
incisura (incisurae)
 See also *incisure* and *notch*.
 i. anterior auris
 i. intertragica
 i. mastoidea ossis temporalis
 Santorini i.
 i. terminalis auris
 i. tympanica
incisural
incisure
 See also *incisura* and *notch*.
 Rivinus i.
incudopedial

incudal
incudectomy
incudomalleal
incudostapedial
incus
index (indexes, indices)
 See also *classification*.
 palatal i.
 palatal height i.
 palatine i.
 palatomaxillary i.
Indian
 operation
 rhinoplasty
indirect
 i. laryngoscopy
infection
 fungal i.
 upper respiratory i. (URI)
 upper respiratory tract i.
  (URTI)
 Vincent i.
inferior
 i. laryngotomy
 i. tracheotomy
influenza
 i. A
 i. B
 i. C
 clinical i.
 i. virus (A–C) [also: influen-
  zavirus]
influenzal
infrahyoid
 i. pharyngotomy
infraorbital
 i. suture
infundibula (plural of infundibulum)
infundibuliform
infundibulum (infundibula)
 ethmoidal i.
 i. of frontal sinus
 i. nasi
Ingrassia
 apophysis
 process
 wings

inlay
    i. myringoplasty
interarytenoid
intercricothyrotomy
interendognathic
    i. suture
intermaxillary
    i. suture
internal
    i. pharyngotomy
internarial
internasal
    i. suture
interpalatine
    i. suture
interradicular alveoloplasty
intralaryngeal
intramastoiditis
intranarial
intranasal
    i. antrostomy
intraseptal alveoloplasty
irrigation
    antral i.
irrigator
    House i.
    Shambaugh i.
    Shea i.
"is-mus" Phonetic for isthmus.
isthmectomy
isthmi (plural of isthmus)
isthmic
isthmitis
isthmoparalysis
isthmoplegia
isthmus (isthmi)
    i. of external auditory meatus
    i. faucium
Italian
    operation
    rhinoplasty
ITE—in the ear [hearing aid]
iter
Ivy
    rongeur
Jacob
    disease

Jacobson
    anastomosis
    canal
    cartilage
    nerve
    plexus
    ramus
Jansen
    operation
Jarvis
    operation
"jene–" Phonetic for words beginning geny–.
joint
    See also *articulation.*
    cochlear j.
    cricoarytenoid j.
    cricothyroid j.
    incudomalleolar j.
    incudostapedial j.
    temporomandibular j. (TMJ)
Joseph
    operation
    rhinoplasty
juga (plural of jugum)
jugale
jugate
jugomaxillary
jugular
jugulodigastric
jugum (juga)
Kartagener
    disease
    syndrome
    triad
Kawasaki
    disease
    syndrome
Kearns-Sayer syndrome
Keegan
    operation
keel
    k. operation
keratosis (keratoses)
    k. labialis
    k. linguae
    k. obturans
    k. pharyngea

keratosis (keratoses) (continued)
  wax k.
Kiesselbach
  area
  plexus
Killian
  operation
Killian-Freer
  operation
"kilo–" Phonetic for words beginning cheilo–.
King
  operation
Klestadt cyst
"koanah" Phonetic for choana.
"kokle–" Phonetic for words beginning cochle–.
"kolesteatoma" Phonetic for cholesteatoma.
König
  rods
Koplik
  spots
"kor–" Phonetic for words beginning cor– and chor–.
Körte-Ballance
  operation
Krause
  glands
"krus" Phonetic for crus.
Kuhnt
  operation
labia (plural of labium)
labial
labially
labium (labia)
  See also *border, limbus,* and *margin.*
  l. mandibulare
  l. maxillare
  labia oris
  l. vocale
labrale
labyrinth
  acoustic l.
  bony l.
  cochlear l.
  l. of ethmoid

labyrinth (continued)
  ethmoidal l.
  membranous l.
  nonacoustic l.
  olfactory l.
  osseous l.
  vestibular l.
  l. of vestibule
labyrinthectomy
  membranous l.
  transtympanic l.
  ultrasonic l.
labyrinthi (genitive and plural of labyrinthus)
labyrinthine
labyrinthitis
  circumscribed l.
  serous l.
  suppurative l.
  traumatic l.
labyrinthosis
labyrinthotomy
labyrinthus (labyrinthi)
  l. cochlearis
  l. ethmoidalis
  l. membranaceus
  l. osseus
  l. vestibularis
lacrimation
lacrimoconchal
  l. suture
lacrimoethmoidal
  l. suture
lacrimomaxillary
  l. suture
lacrimonasal
  l. duct
lacrimoturbinal
  l. suture
"lahringo–" Phonetic for words beginning laryngo–.
Lalouette pyramid
lamina (laminae)
  palatine l. of maxilla
  l. propria
  reticular l. of the cochlea
  reticular l. of the spiral organ
  spiral l., bony

lamina (laminae) (continued)
    vestibular l.
laminar
"laringo–" Phonetic for words
    beginning laryngo–.
laryngalgia
laryngeal
    l. catheterization
    l. stridor
    l. web
laryngectomee [person whose lar-
    ynx has been removed]
laryngectomy (LG)
    frontolateral partial l.
    lateral partial l.
    supraglottic l.
    total l.
laryngemphraxis
laryngismal
laryngismus
    l. paralyticus
    l. stridulus
laryngitic
laryngitis
    catarrhal l.
    croupous l.
    diphtheritic l.
    membranous l.
    phlegmonous l.
    l. sicca
    l. stridulosa
    subglottic l.
    syphilitic l.
    tuberculous l.
    vestibular l.
laryngocele
laryngocentesis
laryngofission
laryngofissure
laryngogram
laryngograph
laryngohypopharynx
laryngology
laryngomalacia
laryngometry
laryngoparalysis
laryngopathy
laryngophantom

laryngopharyngeal
laryngopharyngectomy
laryngopharyngeus
laryngopharyngitis
laryngopharyngography
laryngopharynx
laryngophony
laryngophthisis
laryngoplasty
laryngoplegia
laryngoptosis
laryngopyocele
laryngorhinology
laryngorrhagia
laryngorrhaphy
laryngorrhea
laryngoscleroma
laryngoscopic
laryngoscopist
laryngoscopy
    direct l.
    fiberoptic l.
    indirect l.
    mirror l.
    suspension l.
laryngospasm
laryngostasis
laryngostat
laryngostenosis
laryngotome
laryngotomy
    complete l.
    inferior l.
    median l.
    subhyoid l.
    superior l.
    thyrohyoid l.
laryngotracheal
laryngotracheitis
laryngotracheobronchitis
laryngotracheobronchoscopy
laryngotracheoesophageal
laryngotracheoscopy
laryngotracheotomy
laryngotyphoid
laryngovestibulitis
laryngoxerosis

larynx
     artificial l.
lateral
     l. partial laryngectomy
     l. pharyngotomy
     l. rhinotomy
Laurens
     operation
law
     Boyle l.
Law [eponym]
     position
     views
layer
     See *band, line,* and *stria.*
LDL—loudness discomfort level
Le Fort
     apertognathia repair (I)
Legal
     disease
leishmaniasis
     naso-oral l.
     nasopharyngeal l.
Lempert
     fenestration operation
Lermoyez
     syndrome
lesion
     retrocochlear l.
     Scheibe l.
leukoedema
leukokeratosis
     congenital oral l.
leukoplakia
     l. buccalis
     l. of larynx
     l. lingualis
     oral l.
     speckled l.
level
     bone-conduction hearing l.
Lewis
     snare
LG—laryngectomy
ligament
     annular l.
     axis l.
     cricoarytenoid l.

ligament (continued)
     cricopharyngeal l.
     cricothyroarytenoid l.
     cricothyroid l.
     cricotracheal l.
     hypoepiglottic l.
     posterior l.
     superior l.
     thyroepiglottic l.
     thyrohyoid l.
light reflex
limbal
limbic
limbus (limbi)
     See also *border, labium,* and
        margin.
     alveolar l. of mandible
     l. alveolaris mandibulae
     alveolar l. of maxilla
     l. alveolaris maxillae
     l. membranae tympani
limen (limina)
     l. nasi
liminal
line
     See also *band* and *stria.*
     cricoclavicular l.
     Topinard l.
linea (lineae)
lingua (linguae)
     l. frenata
     l. geographica
     l. nigra
     l. plicata
     l. villosa nigra
lingual
linguale
lingualis
lingually
linguatuliasis
lingula (lingulae)
     l. of lower jaw
     l. of mandible
     l. mandibulae
lingular
liquor (liquors, liquores)
     l. of Scarpa
     l. scarpae

Livaditis
    circular myotomy
lobe
    l.'s of thyroid gland
lobectomy
    thyroid l.
lobulated
lobulation
lobuli (plural of lobulus)
lobulization
lobulose
lobulus (lobuli)
logopedics
logoplegia
Lombard
    test
"loop" Phonetic for loupe.
loop
    Gerdy interauricular l.
    l. of hypoglossal nerve
    Hyrtl l.
    l. of recurrent laryngeal nerve
Love
    splint
Löwenberg
    canal
LTB—laryngotracheobronchitis
Ludwig
    angina
Luschka
    bursa
    cartilage
    gland
    laryngeal cartilage
    tonsil
Lyme
    disease
lymphatic
lymphoidectomy
lymphoma
    African l.
    Burkitt l.
    non-Hodgkin l.
lymphomatosum
    papillary adenocystoma l.
lymphomatous
lymphotism

MacFee
    neck flap
MacKenty
    choanal plug
macrocheilia
macrogenia
macroglossia
macrognathia
macrostomia
macrotia
macula (maculae)
    See also *disk* and *spot.*
    acoustic maculae
    maculae acusticae
    m. acustica sacculi
    m. acustica utriculi
    m. communis
    maculae cribrosae
    m. cribrosa inferior
    m. cribrosa media
    m. cribrosa superior
    m. flava laryngis
    maculae of membranous
        labyrinth
    m. sacculi
    m. utriculi
macular
macule
    See *disk, macula,* and *spot.*
malar
malformation
    arteriovenous m. (AVM)
malleoincudal
malleotomy
malleus
    cog tooth of m.
malocclusion
malomaxillary
    m. suture
mammillary
    m. suture
mandible
mandibula (mandibulae)
mandibular
mandibulectomy
mandibulofacial
mandibulopharyngeal
Mandl paint

maneuver
    See also *procedure, operation,* and *technique.*
    Heimlich m.
    Valsalva m.
manubrium (manubria)
    m. mallei
    m. of malleus
margin
    See also *border, labium,* and *limbus.*
    alveolar m. of mandible
    alveolar m. of maxilla
    infraorbital m. of maxilla
    infraorbital m. of orbit
    lacrimal m. of maxilla
    lateral margin of orbit
    malar m.
    medial m. of orbit
    orbital m.
margo (margines)
Martin
    syndrome
mastication
    muscles of m.
masticatory
mastoid
    m. obliteration operation
    m. operation
    m. suture
mastoidal
mastoidale
mastoidalgia
mastoidea
mastoidectomy
    Bondy m.
    combined approach m.
    conservative m.
    cortical m.
    modified radical m.
    radical m.
    Schwartze m.
    simple m.
mastoideocentesis
mastoideum
mastoiditis
    Bezold m.
    coalescent m.

mastoiditis (continued)
    m. externa
    m. interna
    sclerosing m.
    silent m.
mastoidotomy
mastoidotympanectomy
maxilla (maxillae, maxillas)
    frontal processes of maxillae
    inferior m.
maxillary
    radical m. antrostomy
maxillectomy
maxillitis
maxilloethmoidectomy
maxillolabial
maxillomandibular
maxillotomy
Mayer
    position
    splint
MBFLB—monaural bifrequency loudness balance
McGee
    operation
MCL—most comfortable loudness level
ME—middle ear
meatal
meati [incorrect word for plural of meatus]
meatoantrotomy
meatus (meatus)
    acoustic m.
    acoustic m., external
    acoustic m., external, bony
    acoustic m., external cartilaginous
    acoustic m., internal
    acoustic m., internal, bony
    m. acusticus externus
    m. acusticus externus cartilagineus
    m. acusticus externus osseus
    m. acusticus internus
    m. acusticus internus osseus
    m. auditorius externus

meatus (meatus) (continued)
    m. auditorius externus carti-
        lagineus
    m. auditorius externus osseus
    m. auditorius internus
    m. auditorius internus osseus
    auditory m.
    auditory m., external
    auditory m., external, bony
    auditory m., external, carti-
        laginous
    auditory m., internal
    auditory m., internal, bony
    m. conchae ethmoturbinalis
        minoris
    m. conchae maxilloturbinalis
    m. conchae turbinalis majoris
    external acoustic m.
    inferior m. of nose
    middle m. of nose
    nasal m., common, bony
    nasal m., inferior
    nasal m., inferior, bony
    nasal m., middle
    nasal m., middle, bony
    nasal m., superior
    nasal m., superior, bony
    m. nasi communis
    m. nasi communis osseus
    m. nasi inferior
    m. nasi inferior osseus
    m. nasi medius
    m. nasi medius osseus
    m. nasi superior
    m. nasi superior osseus
    nasopharyngeal m.
    m. nasopharyngeus
    m. nasopharyngeus osseus
    m. of nose, bony, common
    m. of nose, common
    m. of nose, inferior
    m. of nose, inferior, bony
    m. of nose, middle
    m. of nose, middle, osseous
    m. of nose, superior
    m. of nose, superior, osseous
    m. of nose
    superior m. of nose

Meckel
    band
    ligament
median
    m. laryngotomy
    m. palatine suture
    m. pharyngotomy
    m. rhinoscopy
    m. strumectomy
mediastinoscopy
medical
    m. thyroidectomy
Méglin
    point
melanoptysis
melanotrichia
    m. linguae
Meltzer
    punch
membrana (membranae)
    m. basilaris ductus cochlearis
    m. elastica laryngis
    m. fibroelastica laryngis
    m. mucosa nasi
    m. spiralis ductus cochlearis
    m. stapedis
    m. tympani secundaria
membranate
membrane
    Brunn m.
    buccopharyngeal m.
    Corti m.
    cricothyroid m.
    false m.
    hyothyroid m.
    hypoglossal m.
    mucous m.
    Reissner m.
    reticular m. of organ of Corti
    Rivinus m.
    Scarpa m.
    schneiderian m.
    Shrapnell m.
    tectorial m.
    tympanic m. (TM)
membranous
    m. labyrinthectomy

Ménière
    disease
    syndrome
meniscus (menisci)
    m. of temporomandibular
        joint
    m. of temporomaxillary joint
mentoplasty
Merkel
    fossa
mesocephalic
mesoturbinal
mesoturbinate
method
metopantralgia
metopantritis
Meyer
    disease
    sinus
MF—medium frequency
Michel
    deafness
    deformity
microglossia
microglossic
micrognathia
microlaryngoscopy
micromandible
micromaxilla
microphonia
microphonic
    cochlear m.'s
microphonograph
microrhinia
microscopy
microstomia
microsurgery
    laser m.
microtia
microtubule
middle
    m. palatine suture
Mikulicz (von Mikulicz)
    disease
    syndrome
Mikulicz-Radecki
    syndrome

Mikulicz-Sjögren
    syndrome
minimum (minima)
    m. audibile, m. audible
    m. separabile
"mio–" Phonetic for words begin-
    ning myo–.
mirror
    m. laryngoscopy
mobilization
    stapes m.
mobilizer
    Derlacki m.
modified
    m. radical mastoidectomy
modiolus
Moeller
    glossitis
    reaction
Mondini deafness
monitor
    apnea m.
monocorditis
Morel
    ear
Morgagni
    appendix
    cartilage
    concha
    prolapse
    sacculus
    sinus
    tubercle
    ventricle
Mosher
    punch
mouth gag
    Jennings m.g.
    Lane m.g.
    Roser m.g.
    Sluder-Jansen m.g.
MT—membrana tympani
MTDT—modified tone decay test
Muckle-Wells
    syndrome
mucocele
    ethmoid sinus m.
    frontal sinus m.

mucocele (continued)
    frontoethmoid m.
    lacrimal m.
    maxillary sinus m.
    paranasal sinus m.
    suppurating m.
mucociliary
mucogingival
mucoid
mucolytics [a class of drugs]
mucoperichondrial
mucoperichondrium
mucoperiosteal
mucoperiosteum
mucopurulent
mucopus
mucosa
mucosal
mucosanguineous
mucoserous
mucous [adj.]
    m. membrane
mucus [noun]
Mueller
    See *Müller.*
Müller
    sign
mumps
    iodine m.
    m. meningoencephalitis
muscle
    See also in *Orthopedics and
      Sports Medicine* section.
    aryepiglottic m.
    arytenoid m. (oblique, trans-
      verse)
    canine m.
    compressor m. of naris
    constrictor m. of pharynx
      (inferior, middle, superior)
    cricoarytenoid m. (lateral,
      posterior)
    cricopharyngeal m.
    cricothyroid m.
    depressor m. of angle of
      mouth
    depressor m. of lower lip

muscle (continued)
    depressor m. of septum of
      nose
    digastric m.
    dilator m. of naris
    eustachian m.
    facial m.'s, m.'s of facial
      expression
    facial and masticatory m.'s
    m.'s of fauces
    fixator m. of base of stapes
    genioglossus m.
    geniohyoid m.
    glossopalatine m.
    glossopharyngeal m.
    helicis m. (major, minor)
    m. of Henle
    Hilton m.
    hyoglossal m., hyoglossus m.
    m.'s of hyoid bone
    incisive m.'s of lip (inferior,
      lower, superior, upper)
    infrahyoid m.'s
    interarytenoid m.'s
    intraauricular m.'s
    intratympanic m.
    Jung m.
    m.'s of larynx
    levator m. of angle of mouth
    levator m. of palatine velum
    levator m. of thyroid gland
    levator m. of upper lip
    levator m. of upper lip and
      ala of nose
    levator m. of velum palatinum
    lingual m.'s
    longitudinal m. of tongue
      (inferior, superior)
    masseter m.
    m.'s of mastication
    masticatory m.
    Merkel m.
    mylohyoid m.
    mylopharyngeal m.
    nasal m.
    oblique m. of auricle
    omohyoid m.
    orbicular m. of mouth

muscle (continued)
    m.'s of ossicles
    m.'s of palate and fauces
    palatine m.'s
    palatoglossus m.
    palatopharyngeal m.
    pharyngeal constrictor m.
    pharyngopalatine m.
    platysma m.
    pterygoid m. (external, internal, lateral, medial)
    pterygopharyngeal m.
    pyramidal m. of auricle
    quadrate m. of lower lip
    quadrate m. of upper lip
    ribbon m.'s
    risorius m.
    salpingopharyngeal m.
    Santorini m.
    Soemmering m.
    stapedius m.
    sternocleidomastoid m.
    sternohyoid m.
    sternomastoid m.
    sternothyroid m.
    strap m.'s
    styloglossus m.
    stylohyoid m.
    stylopharyngeus m.
    suprahyoid m.'s
    temporal m.
    tensor m. of tympanic membrane
    tensor m. of tympanum
    tensor m. of velum palatinum
    thyroarytenoid m.
    thyroepiglottic m.
    thyrohyoid m.
    thyropharyngeal m.
    Tod m.
    m.'s of tongue
    tracheal m.
    m. of tragus
    transverse m. of auricle
    transverse m. of tongue
    m. of uvula
    Valsalva m.
    vertical m. of tongue

muscle (continued)
    vocal m.
musculoplasty
musculus (musculi)
    See also *muscle.*
    See also in *Orthopedics and Sports Medicine* section.
    m. aryepiglotticus
    m. orbicularis oris
    m. tensor veli palatini
Mustardé
    otoplasty
mute
mutism
    deaf-m.
myasthenia
    m. gravis
    m. gravis pseudoparalytica
    m. laryngis
mycosis (mycoses)
    m. leptothrica
Myles
    punch
    snare
mylohyoid
myoclonus
    jaw m.
    palatopharyngolaryngeal m.
myofascitis
myognathus
myotomy
    cricopharyngeal m.
    Heller m.
    Livaditis circular m.
myringa
myringectomy
myringitis
    m. bullosa
    bullous m.
myringodectomy
myringomycosis
    m. aspergillina
myringoplasty
    inlay m.
    onlay graft m.
    underlay m.
myringorupture
myringostapediopexy

myringotome
myringotomy
    m. incision
myrinx
myxoma (myxomas, myxomata)
    odontogenic m.
nare [incorrect term for naris, sin-
    gular of nares]
nares (plural of naris)
naris (nares)
    anterior n.
    external n.
    internal nares
    posterior nares
nasal
    n. allergy
    n. cavity
    n. congestion
    n. deformity
    n. filtration
    n. obstruction
    n. packing
    n. septum
    n. suture
    n. tampon
    n. turbinate
    n. vestibule
    n. vestibulitis
nasalis
nasality
nasioiniac
nasion
nasitis
nasoantral
nasoantritis
nasoantrostomy
nasobronchial
nasociliary
nasofrontal
    n. suture
nasograph
nasolabial
nasolacrimal
nasomanometer
nasomaxillary
    n. suture
nasonnement
naso-oral

nasopalatine
nasopharyngeal
    n. bursitis
nasopharyngitis
nasopharyngoscopy
nasopharynx
nasorostral
nasoseptal
nasoseptitis
nasosinusitis
nasospinale
nasoturbinal
nasus
    n. externus
"natho–" Phonetic for words begin-
    ning gnatho–.
Nebinger-Praun
    operation
neck flap
    MacFee n.f.
necrosis (necroses)
    diphtheritic n.
    exanthematous n.
    gummatous n.
    mandibular n.
    phosphorus n.
necrotic
necrotizing
    n. sialometaplasia
neoglottic
neoglottis
    phonatory n.
neomembrane
nerve
    abducens n.
    acoustic n.
    alveolar n.'s
    Arnold n.
    buccal n.
    buccinator n.
    chorda tympani n.
    cochlear n.
    ethmoidal n.
    facial n.
    glossopalatine n.
    glossopharyngeal n.
    hypoglossal n.
    infraorbital n.

nerve (continued)
   infratrochlear n.
   Jacobson n.
   laryngeal n.
   lingual n.
   mandibular n.
   masseteric n.
   maxillary n.
   mental n.
   nasopalatine n.
   olfactory n.'s
   palatine n.
   petrosal n.
   n. of pterygoid canal
   pterygopalatine n.'s
   recurrent n.
   stylohyoid n.
   stylopharyngeal n.
   sublingual n.
   submaxillary n.'s
   n. of tensor tympani
   trigeminal n.
   tympanic n. of Jacobson
   vagus n.
   vestibular n.
   vidian n.
"neu–" Phonetic for words beginning pneu–.
neuralgia
   glossopharyngeal n.
   mandibular joint n.
   retrobulbar n.
   trigeminal n.
neuralgic
neurapraxia
neurectomy
   tympanic n.
neurilemoma
   acoustic n.
neurinoma
   acoustic n.
neuritic
neuritis
   diphtheric n.
neuroblastoma
   olfactory n.
neurocytoma
   olfactory n.

neurofibroma
   acoustic n.
neuroma
   acoustic n.
"new–" Phonetic for words beginning pneu–.
"nistagmus" Phonetic for nystagmus.
node
   shotty n.
nodi (plural of nodus)
nodular
nodularity
nodulated
nodulation
nodule
noduli (plural of nodulus)
nodulous [adj.]
nodulus (noduli)
nodus (nodi)
"noo–" Phonetic for words beginning pneu–.
nose
   cleft n.
   potato n.
   saddle-back n.
   swayback n.
nosebleed
nostril
notch
   See also *incisura* and *incisure.*
   antegonial n.
   Carhart n.
   mandibular n.
   palatine n.
   rivinian n.
   n. of Rivinus
NP—nasopharyngeal
   nasopharynx
NT—nasotracheal
NTG—nontoxic goiter
"nu–" Phonetic for words beginning pneu–.
nuchal
nucleus (nuclei)
   Bekhterev n.
   Deiters n.
Nuhn glands

"nur–" Phonetic for words begin-
    ning neur–.
nystagmus
    aural n.
    caloric n.
    labyrinthine n.
    opticokinetic n., optokinetic
      n. (OKN)
    vestibular n.
OAV—oculoauriculovertebral (dys-
    plasia)
obstruction
    airway o.
obstructive
    o. sleep apnea (OSA)
occipitofrontal
occipitomastoid
    o. suture
occipitomental
occiput
OCV—ordinary conversational voice
OFD—oral-facial-digital
    orofaciodigital
OFD dysplasia
OFD syndrome (I, II)
"ofthal–" Phonetic for words begin-
    ning ophthal–.
ogo
Ogston-Luc
    operation
OKN—opticokinetic nystagmus
olfaction
olfactory
oligoptyalism
OM—otitis media
OMPA—otitis media, purulent, acute
onlay
    o. graft myringoplasty
operation
    See also in *General Surgical*
      Terms.
    Adams o.
    Almoor o.
    Arslan o.
    Asch o.
    Becker o.
    Bondy o.
    Caldwell-Luc o.

operation (continued)
    Canfield o.
    Carnochan o.
    Carpue o.
    Carter o.
    Cassel o.
    Cheever o.
    Chevalier Jackson o.
    Coakley o.
    Cody o.
    Commando o.
    Day o.
    Denker o.
    Derlacki o.
    Dott o.
    fenestration o.
    Fergusson o.
    Ferris-Smith o.
    Fick o.
    Finzi-Harmer o.
    Gillies o.
    Hajek o.
    Haverhill o.
    Heath o.
    Heermann o.
    Hilger o.
    Horgan o.
    Indian o.
    Italian o.
    Jansen o.
    Jarvis o.
    Joseph o.
    Keegan o.
    keel o.
    Killian o.
    Killian-Freer o.
    King o.
    Körte-Ballance o.
    Kuhnt o.
    Laurens o.
    Lempert fenestration o.
    mastoid o.
    mastoid obliteration o.
    McGee o.
    Nebinger-Praun o.
    Ogston-Luc o.
    osteoplastic frontal sinus o.
    palatal pushback o.

operation (continued)
    radical antrum o.
    Regnoli o.
    Ridell o.
    Roberts o.
    Rosen o.
    Rouge o.
    Schönbein o.
    Schuknecht o.
    Schwartze o.
    Shambaugh o.
    Sistrunk o.
    Sluder o.
    Socin o.
    Sonneberg o.
    Sourdille o.
    Stacke o.
    Stallard o.
    stapes mobilization o.
    Vicq d'Azyr o.
    West o.
    Wood o.
    Woodman o.
    Wullstein o.
    Yankauer o.
opercula (plural of operculum)
opercular
operculate
operculum (opercula)
    cartilaginous o.
opisthogenia
opisthognathism
opisthotic
oral
    o. mucosa
    o. tori
orbicular
orbicularis
    o. oris muscle
orbital
    o. cellulitis
    o. floor
orbitonasal
organ
    o. of Corti
organum (organa)
    o. spirale
    o. vestibulocochleare

orifice
    tympanic o.
orificial
    o. angle
oroantral
oronasal
os (ossa) [bone]
    See in *Orthopedics and*
        Sports Medicine section.
OSAS—obstructive sleep apnea
    syndrome
osmatic
osmesis
osmesthesia
osmics
osmology
osmoreceptor
osphresiology
osphresiometer
osphresis
osphretic
ossicle
    auditory o.
ossicula (plural of ossiculum)
ossicular
    o. chain
    o. disarticulation
    o. system
ossiculectomy
ossiculoplasty
ossiculotomy
ossiculum (ossicula)
    ossicula auditoria
    ossicula auditus
osteoacusis
osteoma
    ethmoid sinus o.
    frontal sinus o.
    maxillary o.
    sphenoidal sinus o.
osteomatoid
osteomatosis
osteopetrosis
osteophony
osteoplastic
    o. frontal sinus operation
osteoseptum
ostia (plural of ostium)

ostial [pertaining to opening, aperture, orifice]
ostium (ostia)
    o. maxillare
    o. pharyngeum tubae auditivae
    o. pharyngeum tubae auditoriae
    sphenoidal o.
    o. tympanicum tubae auditivae
OT—orotracheal
    otolaryngology
otacoustic
otagra
otalgia
    o. dentalis
    o. intermittens
    reflex o.
otalgic
otectomy
othelcosis
othematoma
othemorrhea
othygroma
otiatrics
otic capsule
oticodinia
otitic
    o. barotrauma
otitis
    adhesive o. media
    aviation o.
    barotraumatic o.
    catarrhal o.
    o. crouposa
    o. desquamativa
    o. diphtheritica
    secretory o. media
    o. externa
    o. externa circumscripta
    o. externa diffusa
    o. externa furunculosa
    o. externa hemorrhagica
    exudative o. media
    furuncular o.
    o. haemorrhagica
    influenzal o.

otitis (continued)
    o. interna
    o. labyrinthica
    malignant external o.
    malignant o. externa
    o. mastoidea
    o. media
    o. media, adhesive
    o. media catarrhalis acuta
    o. media catarrhalis chronica
    o. media purulenta acuta
    o. media purulenta chronica
    o. media sclerotica
    o. media, secretory
    o. media serosa
    o. media suppurativa
    o. media vasomotorica
    o. mycotica
    mycotic o. externa
    necrotizing external o.
    necrotizing o. externa
    necrotizing o. media
    parasitic o.
    pneumococcal o. media
    purulent o.
    o. sclerotica
    serous o. media
    traumatic o.
    tuberculous o. media
    suppurative o. media
otoantritis
otoblennorrhea
otocatarrh
otocephalus
otocerebritis
otocleisis
otoconia
otoconium
otocranial
otocranium
otocyst
otodynia
otoencephalitis
otoganglion
otogenic
otogenous
otography
otohemineurasthenia

otolaryngologist
otolaryngology
otolith
otolithiasis
otologic
otologist
otology
otomassage
otomastoiditis
otomicroscopy
otomucormycosis
otomyasthenia
otomycosis
    o. aspergillina
otomyiasis
otoncus
otonecrectomy
otoneuralgia
otoneurasthenia
otoneurology
otopharyngeal
    o. tube
otophone
otopiesis
otoplasty
    Crikelair o.
    Mustardé o.
otopolypus
otopyorrhea
otopyosis
otor
otorhinolaryngologist
otorhinolaryngology
otorhinology
otorrhagia
otorrhea
    cerebrospinal fluid o.
otosalpinx
otosclerectomy
otoscleronectomy
otosclerosis
otosclerotic
otoscopy
    pneumatic o.
otosis
otospongiosis
    o./otosclerosis syndrome

otosteal
otosteon
ototomy
ototoxic
ototoxicity
oulectomy
overjut
ozena
    o. laryngis
paint
    Mandl p.
palata (plural of palatum)
palatal
    p. height index
    p. index
palate
    cleft p.
    submucous cleft p.
palati (genitive of palatum)
palatine
    anterior p. suture
    p. bone
    p. index
    median p. suture
    middle p. suture
    posterior p. suture
    transverse p. suture
palatitis
palatoethmoidal
    p. suture
palatoglossal
palatognathous
palatograph
palatography
palatomaxillary
    p. index
    p. suture
palatomyograph
palatonasal
palatopharyngeal
palatoplasty
    Wardill p.
palatoplegia
palatoschisis
palatostaphylinus
palatouvularis
palatum (palata)
    p. durum

palatum (palata) (continued)
    p. durum osseum
    p. fissum
    p. molle
    p. ogivale
    p. osseum
palsy
    See also *paralysis.*
    Bell p.
PAN—periodic alternating nystagmus
panotitis
panseptum
pansinuitis
pansinusectomy
pansinusitis
panturbinate
papilla (papillae)
    acoustic p.
    arcuate papillae of tongue
    circumvallate papillae
    papillae conicae
    conical papillae
    conical papillae of tongue
    conoid papillae of tongue
    corolliform papillae of tongue
    filiform p.
    papillae filiformes
    papillae foliatae
    foliate p.
    fungiform p.
    papillae fungiformes
    gingival p., p. gingivalis
    gustatory papillae
    p. incisiva, incisive p.
    interproximal p.
    lenticular papillae, papillae
      lenticulares
    p. lentiformes
    lingual p.
    papillae linguales
    medial papillae of tongue
    obtuse papillae of tongue
    palatine p.
    parotid p., p. parotidea
    simple papillae of tongue
    small papillae of tongue
    sublingual p.

papilla (papillae) (continued)
    papillae vallatae, vallate
      papillae
    villous papillae of tongue
papillate
papillation
papilliferous
papilliform
papilloma
    inverted p.
    inverted nasal p.
    squamous p.
    squamous cell p.
paracusia
    p. acris
    p. duplicata
    p. loci
    p. willisiana
paraglottic
    p. space
paralysis (paralyses)
    See also *palsy.*
    acoustic p.
    acute bulbar p.
    ambiguo-accessorius-
      hypoglossal p.
    ambiguohypoglossal p.
    asthenic bulbar p.
    asthenobulbospinal p.
    bilateral laryngeal abductor p.
    bulbar p.
    crossed hypoglossal p.
    diphtheric p., diphtheritic p.
    faucial p.
    glossolabial p., glos-
      sopharyngolabial p.
    hypoglossal p.
    Jackson p.
    labial p., labioglossolaryn-
      geal p., labioglossopha-
      ryngeal p.
    laryngeal p.
    laryngeal abductor p.
    lingual p.
    masticatory p.
    palatal p.
    parotitic p.
    pharyngeal p.

paralysis (paralyses) (continued)
    phonetic p.
    postdiphtheric p.
    posticus p.
    progressive bulbar p.
    pseudobulbar p.
    recurrent laryngeal nerve p.
    superior laryngeal nerve p.
    trigeminal p.
    trigeminal masticator p.
    trochlear p.
    unilateral vocal cord p.
    vagoaccessory hypoglossal p.
    vestibular p.
    vocal cord p.
parapharyngeal
parathyroid
parathyroidectomy (PTX)
paries (parietes)
parietitis
parietofrontal
parietomastoid
parieto-occipital
parietosphenoid
parietosquamosal
parietotemporal
parosmia
parotidean
parotidectomy
pars (partes)
partial
    frontolateral p. laryngectomy
    lateral p. laryngectomy
    p. stapedectomy
patch
    Silastic p.
Paterson
    syndrome
Paterson-Brown-Kelly
    syndrome
Paterson-Kelly
    syndrome
pathogen
    See specific pathogens in
      Laboratory, Pathology,
      and Chemistry Terms.
pattern
    rugal p.

Patterson
    See *Paterson.*
PBZ—pyribenzamine
PE—pharyngoesophageal
    phenylephrine
pearl
    gouty p.
peenash
pemphigus
    p. vulgaris
Pendred
    disease
    syndrome
percervical tracheoscopy
perforation
    Bezold p.
    tympanic membrane p.
periadenitis
    p. mucosa necrotica recurrens
perichondritis
perichondrium
perilabyrinth
perilabyrinthitis
perilaryngeal
perilaryngitis
perilymph
perilymphatic
periodontitis
periorbital
periotic
perirhinal
perisinuous
perisinusitis
peritonsillar
peritonsillitis
peroral
    p. endoscopy
    p. tracheoscopy
perpendicular
petiolus
    p. epiglottidis
petromastoid
petro-occipital
petropharyngeus
petrosal
petrosectomy
petrositis
petrosphenoid

petrosquamosal
Pfeiffer
    disease
phalanx (phalanges)
    Deiters phalanges
pharyngalgia
pharyngeal
pharyngectasia
pharyngectomy
pharyngemphraxis
pharyngeus
pharyngism
pharyngismus
pharyngitic
pharyngitid
pharyngitis
    atrophic p.
    catarrhal p.
    croupous p.
    diphtheritic p.
    follicular p.
    gangrenous p.
    glandular p.
    granular p.
    p. herpetica
    hypertrophic p.
    p. keratosa
    membranous p.
    phlegmonous p.
    recurrent p.
    p. sicca
    p. ulcerosa
    viral p.
pharyngoamygdalitis
pharyngocele
pharyngoconjunctivitis
pharyngodynia
pharyngoepiglottic
pharyngoesophageal
pharyngoglossal
pharyngoglossus
pharyngokeratosis
pharyngolaryngeal
pharyngolaryngectomy
pharyngolaryngitis
pharyngolith
pharyngolysis
pharyngomaxillary

pharyngomycosis
pharyngonasal
pharyngo-oral
pharyngopalatine
pharyngoparalysis
pharyngopathy
pharyngoperistole
pharyngoplasty
    Hynes p.
pharyngoplegia
pharyngorhinitis
pharyngorhinoscopy
pharyngorrhagia
pharyngorrhea
pharyngosalpingitis
pharyngoscleroma
pharyngoscopy
pharyngospasm
pharyngostenosis
pharyngostomy
pharyngotherapy
pharyngotome
pharyngotomy
    anterior p.
    external p.
    infrahyoid p.
    internal p.
    lateral p.
    median p.
    subhyoid p.
    transhyoid p.
    translingual p.
    transthyroid p.
    transverse p.
pharyngotonsillitis
pharyngotympanic tube
pharyngotyphoid
phenomenon (phenomena)
    face p., facialis p.
    Hammerschlag p.
    mucus extravasation p.
    Tullio p.
    Wever-Bray p.
philtrum [vertical groove above
    upper lip; compare: filtrum]
phlebectasia
    p. laryngis
phlegm

phlegmon
phonatory
phonetic
phonetics
photophore
Pierre Robin syndrome
pillar
    p. of fauces, anterior
    p. of fauces, posterior
    p.'s of soft palate
pinna
pinnal
piperidines [a class of drugs]
piriform
piston
    stapedectomy p.
plate
    auditory p.
platinectomy
platysma
Plaut-Vincent angina
plegaphonia
plethysmography
    tympanic p.
plexus (plexus, plexuses)
    Kiesselbach p.
    laryngeal p.
    pharyngeal p.
    tympanic p.
plica (plicae)
    plicae alares
    p. nasi
    p. semilunaris
    p. triangularis
    p. vocalis
plicotomy
plug
    MacKenty choanal p.
Plummer-Vinson
    syndrome
PN—perceived noise
PND—postnasal drip, postnasal
  drainage
pneumatic
    p. otoscopy
pneumatization
pneumatocele
    parotid p.

pneumococcal
    p. meningitis
pneumomassage
pneumophonia
pneumotympanum
pocket
    Rathke p.
point
    See also *disk, macula,* and
      spot.
    p. Ba
Politzer
    bag
    test
    treatment
politzerization
pollen
pollination
pollinosis
pollution
polyp
    antrochoanal p.
    Hopmann p.
    inflammatory p.
    laryngeal p.
    p.'s of larynx
    nasal p.'s
    neoplastic p.
    non-neoplastic p.
    pedunculated p.
    sessile p.
polypiform
polysinusectomy
ponticular
ponticulus (ponticuli)
    p. auriculae
    p. promontorii
pori (genitive and plural of porus)
Porter sign
porus (pori)
    p. acusticus externus
    p. acusticus internus
    p. gustatorius
position
    See in *General Surgical*
      Terms.
positive Bing [test]
postaurale

postauricular
posterior
    p. palatine suture
    p. rhinoscopy
    p. tympanotomy
posturography
pouch
    anterior p. of Tröltsch
    laryngeal p.
    pharyngeal p.
    posterior p. of Tröltsch
    Prussak p.
    Rathke p.
    Seessel p.
PR—prosthion
preauricular
premaxillary
    p. suture
presbycusis
principle [rule]
    See *law.*
procedure
    See also *maneuver, operation,* and *technique.*
    obliteration p.
    Valsalva p.
process
    See also *prominence* and *swelling.*
    clinoid p.
    hamular p.
    mastoid p.
    maxillary p.
    styloid p.
    zygomatic p.
Proetz treatment
prognathism
prognathous
projection
    Chausse III p., third p. of Chausse
prominence
    See also *process* and *swelling.*
    laryngeal p.
    p. of lateral semicircular canal
    mallear p. of tympanic membrane
    spiral p.

prominentia (prominentiae)
    p. laryngea
    p. styloidea
promontorium (promontoria)
    p. tympani
protuberance
    See *process, prominence,* and *swelling.*
Prussak
    fibers
    pouch
    space
pseudocholesteatoma
pseudoglottis
pterygium (pterygia)
    p. colli
pterygomandibular
pterygomaxillary
pterygopalatine
PTFE—polytetrafluoroethylene
    [See *Teflon* in *General Surgical Terms.*]
PTX—parathyroidectomy
ptyalectasis
ptyalism
ptyalith
ptyalize
ptyalocele
ptyalolithiasis
ptyalolithotomy
ptyalorrhea
puncture
    tracheoesophageal p.
purulent
puruloid
pushback
    palatal p.
pyemia
    otogenous p.
pyocele
pyothorax
pyramid
    petrous p.
    p. of tympanum
pyramis (pyramides)
quinsy
    lingual q.
Quisling hammer

R—Rinne test
radical [adj.]
    r. antrum operation
    r. mastoidectomy
    r. maxillary antrostomy
    modified r. mastoidectomy
radices (plural of radix)
radiciform
radicis (genitive of radix)
radicle [noun: branch of nerve or
    vessel]
radioallergosorbent
radiosialographic
radix (radices)
"ra-fee" Phonetic for raphe.
Ramsay Hunt
    disease
    syndrome
ramus (rami)
    r. of jaw
ranula
raphe (raphae)
    buccal r.
    longitudinal r. of tongue
    r. pharyngis, r. of pharynx
raphes (genitive of raphe)
Rathke
    pocket
    pouch
    tumor
reaction
    See also *phenomenon, reflex,
    sign,* and *test.*
    Moeller r.
receptor
    contact r.
    distance r.
    equilibratory r.'s
    gustatory r.
    olfactory r.
    sensory r.
    taste r.
recess
    Hyrtl r.
    Tröltsch r.'s, r.'s of Tröltsch
recessus (recessus)
    r. piriformis
    r. pro utriculo

Recklinghausen (von Reckling-
    hausen)
    disease
reconstructive
    r. rhinoplasty
reflex
    See also *phenomenon, reac-
    tion, sign,* and *test.*
    See also in *Neurology and
    Pain Management* section.
    cough r.
    deglutition r.
    gag r.
    laryngeal r.
    light r.
    palatal r., palatine r.
    pharyngeal r.
    sneezing r.
    stapedial r.
    tympanic r.
Refsum
    disease
    syndrome
region
    anterior r. of neck
    buccal r.
    dorsal lip r.
    frontal r.
    lateral r. of neck
    mental r.
    mylohyoid r.
    nasal r.
    olfactory r.
    oral r.
    prefrontal r.
    pterygomaxillary r.
    respiratory r.
    retromaxillary r.
    subauricular r.
    submandibular r.
    submaxillary r.
    submental r.
    vestibular r.
    zygomatic r.
Regnoli
    operation
Reissner
    membrane

resection
    submucous r. (SMR)
    submucous r. and rhinoplasty (SMRR)
    submucous r. of nasal septum
    submucous r. of vocal cord
resonance
    nasal r.
respiratory
    r. system
    r. tract
    r. tract mucosa
reticulosis
    polymorphic r.
retroauricular
retrolabyrinthine
retromandibular
retromastoid
retronasal
retropharyngeal
retropharyngitis
retropharynx
RFB—retained foreign body
rhinal
rhinalgia
rhinallergosis
rhinectomy
    total r.
rhinedema
rhinenchysis
rhinesthesia
rhineurynter
rhinion
rhinism
rhinitis
    allergic r.
    anaphylactic r.
    atrophic r.
    r. caseosa
    catarrhal r.
    croupous r.
    dyscrinic r.
    fibrinous r.
    gangrenous r.
    hypertrophic r.
    infectious r.
    influenzal r.
    membranous r.

rhinitis (continued)
    perennial r.
    pseudomembranous r.
    purulent r.
    scrofulous r.
    r. sicca
    suppurative r.
    syphilitic r.
    tuberculous r.
    vasomotor r.
rhinoanemometer
rhinoantritis
rhinobyon
rhinocanthectomy
rhinocephalia
rhinocephalus
rhinocheiloplasty
rhinocleisis
rhinodacryolith
rhinodynia
rhinogenous
rhinokyphectomy
rhinokyphosis
rhinolalia
    r. aperta
    r. clausa
rhinolaryngitis
rhinolaryngology
rhinolith
rhinolithiasis
rhinologist
rhinology
rhinomanometer
rhinometer
rhinomiosis
rhinomycosis
rhinonecrosis
rhinonemmeter
rhinoneurosis
rhinopathia
    r. vasomotoria
rhinopathy
rhinopharyngeal
rhinopharyngitis
    r. mutilans
rhinopharyngocele
rhinopharyngolith
rhinopharynx

rhinophonia
rhinophore
rhinophycomycosis
rhinoplastic
rhinoplasty
    augmentation r.
    Carpue r.
    dactylocostal r.
    English r.
    Indian r.
    Italian r.
    Joseph r.
    reconstructive r.
    Tagliacozzi r.
rhinopneumonitis
rhinopolypus
rhinoreaction
rhinorrhagia
rhinorrhaphy
rhinorrhea
    cerebrospinal fluid (CSF) r.
rhinosalpingitis
rhinoscopic
rhinoscopy
    anterior r.
    median r.
    posterior r.
rhinosinusitis
rhinostegnosis
rhinostenosis
rhinotomy
    lateral r.
rhinotracheitis
rhinovaccination
rhomboid
rhonchal, rhonchial
rhonchus (rhonchi)
    See in the *Pulmonary Medicine* section.
RI—respiratory illness
Ridell
    operation
rima (rimae)
    r. glottidis
    r. glottidis cartilaginea
    r. glottidis membranacea
    intercartilaginous r.
    intermembranous r.

rima (rimae) (continued)
    r. oris
    r. vestibuli
    r. vocalis
rimal
ring
    fibrocartilaginous r. of tympanic membrane
    Waldeyer tonsillar r.
Ringer
    injection
    injection, lactated
    irrigation
    lactate
    mixture
    solution
    solution, lactated
Rinne test
"rino–" Phonetic for words beginning rhino–.
Rivinus
    ducts
    gland
    incisure
    membrane
    notch
RLN—recurrent laryngeal nerve
RND—radical neck dissection
Roberts
    operation
rod
    Corti r.
    House r.
    König r.'s
Roeder treatment
Roller nucleus
"rongk–" Phonetic for words beginning rhonch–.
Rose [eponym]
    position
Rosen
    explorer
    fenestrater
    operation
    separator
Rosenmüller
    fossa

Rouge
    operation
Rowland
    rongeur
ruga (rugae)
    rugae palatinae, palatine
        rugae
rugal pattern
rugate
rule
    See *law.*
rupture
    r. of tympanic membrane
RURTI—recurrent upper respiratory
    tract infection
Ruskin
    rongeur
Ruysch
    tube
sacciform
sacculated
saccule
    laryngeal s.
    s. of larynx
sacculi (genitive and plural of sac-
    culus)
sacculiform
sacculocochlear
sacculus (sacculi)
    s. communis
    s. lacrimalis
    s. laryngis
    s. morgagnii
    s. proprius
    s. rotundus
    s. sphaericus
    s. ventricularis
    s. vestibularis
saliva
salivant
salivary
salivation
salpingemphraxis
salpinges (plural of salpinx)
salpingian
salpingion
salpingitic

salpingitis
    eustachian s.
salpingopharyngeal
salpingoscopy
salpinx (salpinges)
    s. auditiva
Sandwith bald tongue
Santorini
    cartilage
    incisura
sarcoma (sarcomas, sarcomata)
    See also in *Oncology and
        Hematology* section.
    alveolar soft part s.
SC, S.C.—semilunar (valve) closure
scala (scalae)
    s. of Löwenberg
    s. media
    s. tympani
    s. vestibuli
scalariform
scan
    See also in *Radiology,
        Nuclear Medicine, and
        Other Imaging* section.
    See in *Radiology, Nuclear
        Medicine, and Other
        Imaging* section.
    salivary gland s.
scanning
    radiosialographic s.
scapha
Scarpa
    canals, canals of Scarpa
    fluid
    foramina
    ganglion
    hiatus
    liquor
    membrane
Scheibe deafness
Schick
    reaction
    sign
    test
Schmidt
    syndrome
Schmincke tumor

schneiderian membrane
Schönbein
    operation
Schuknecht
    excavator
    operation
    stapedectomy
Schüller
    position
    view
Schultz
    angina
    disease
    syndrome
Schwabach test
schwannoma
Schwartze
    mastoidectomy
    operation
    sign
scleroma
sclerosis
"scopes" See under full name.
    auriscope
    conchoscope
    microscope
    myringoscope
    otomicroscope
    otoscope
    rhinoscope
scotoma (scotomata)
    aural s., s. auris
scute
    tympanic s.
segmenta (plural of segmentum)
segmental
segmentum (segmenta)
Seiler
    formula
sella (sellae)
    s. turcica
sellar
semicanal
    s. of auditory tube
    s. of tensor tympani muscle
semicanalis (semicanales)
    s. musculi tensoris tympani
    s. tubae auditivae

semicrista (semicristae)
    s. incisiva
sensitized
sensorineural
    s. hearing loss
septa (plural of septum)
septal
    s. defect
    s. resection
septectomy
septi (genitive of septum)
septonasal
septoplasty
septostomy
septotomy
septum (septa)
    s. of auditory tube
    bony s. of eustachian canal
    bony s. of nose
    bucconasal s.
    deviated nasal s.
    dorsal median s.
    s. of frontal sinuses
    Körner s.
    s. linguae, lingual s.
    membranous s. of nose
    s. mobile nasi, mobile s. of
      nose
    s. of musculotubal canal
    nasal s., s. nasi
    osseous s. of nose
    pharyngeal s.
    sphenoidal s., s. of sphe-
      noidal sinuses
    s. of tongue
    tracheoesophageal s.
    transverse s. of ampulla
serum (serums, sera)
    antidiphtheria s.
"sfeno–" Phonetic for words begin-
    ning spheno–.
SH—sinus histiocytosis
shadow
    s. curve
Shambaugh
    headrest
    irrigator
    operation

Shea
    irrigator
    stapedectomy
Sheehy
    syndrome
Shrapnell membrane
"shwah-no-mah" Phonetic for
    schwannoma.
siagantritis
siagonagra
siagonantritis
sialaden
sialadenitis
sialadenography
sialadenoncus
sialagogic
sialagogue
sialaporia
sialectasia
sialectasis
sialitis
sialoadenectomy
sialoadenitis
sialoadenotomy
sialocele
sialodochiectasis
sialodochitis
sialodochoplasty
sialogram
sialography
sialolith
sialolithiasis
sialolithotomy
sialoma
sialorrhea
sialosis
sialostenosis
sialosyrinx
sialozemia
sign
    See also *phenomenon, reac-*
      tion, reflex, and *test.*
    Bárány s.
    Bespaloff s.
    Bezold s.
    Biederman s.
    Bieg s.
    Bozzolo s.

sign (continued)
    Brown s.
    Demarquay s.
    Ewing s.
    floating-tooth s.
    Granger s.
    Griesinger s.
    Hennebert s.
    Hutchinson s.
    reservoir s.
    rope s.
    Roux s.
    Schick s.
    Schwartze s.
    Widowitz s.
    Wreden s.
    Zaufal s.
simple
    s. mastoidectomy
sin–. See also words beginning
    cin–, syn–.
sinistraural
sinobronchitis
sinodural
sinography
sinus (sinus, sinuses)
    accessory s.'s of the nose
    anterior s.'s
    branchial s.
    s. cochleae
    ethmoidal s., s. ethmoidalis
    external branchial s.
    frontal s., s. frontalis
    frontal s., bony
    Huguier s.
    internal branchial s.
    laryngeal s.
    s. of larynx
    s. of Maier
    mastoid s.
    maxillary s.
    Meyer s., s. Meyeri
    middle s.'s
    s. of Morgagni
    nasal s.'s
    occipital s., s. occipitalis
    oral s.
    paranasal s.'s

sinus (sinus, sinuses) (continued)
    parasinoidal s.
    piriform s.
    posterior s.'s
    preauricular s.
    sphenoid s.
    sphenoidal s.
    sphenoidal s., bony
    thyroglossal s.
    tonsillar s.
    s. tympani, tympanic s.
    s. of tympanic cavity, posterior
sinusitis
    barotraumatic s.
    chronic caseous s.
    ethmoid s., ethmoidal s.
    frontal s.
    fungal s.
    hyperplastic s.
    intracranial s.
    maxillary s.
    orbital s.
    papillary s.
    sphenoid s.
    sphenoidal s.
    viral s.
sinusotomy
Sistrunk
    operation
"sklero–" Phonetic for words beginning sclero–.
sleep apnea
    obstructive s.a. (OSA)
    s.a. syndrome
SLN—superior laryngeal nerve
Sluder
    disease
    method
    neuralgia
    operation
    syndrome
    tonsillar guillotine
snare
    Bosworth s.
    Brown s.
    Bruening s.
    Krause s.

snare (continued)
    Lewis s.
    Myles s.
    Reiner-Beck s.
    Storz-Beck s.
    Stutsman s.
    Tydings s.
    Wilde-Bruening s.
    Wright s.
snoring
SOAP—Subjective, Objective, Assessment, Plan [format for medical reports]
Socin
    operation
solum (sola)
    s. tympani
solution
    Ringer s., lactated Ringer s.
SOM—secretory otitis media
    serous otitis media
Sonneberg
    operation
sore
    canker s.
    cold s. [pref: coldsore]
sore throat
    clergyman's s.t.
    epidemic streptococcal s.t.
    hospital s.t.
    putrid s.t.
    septic s.t.
    spotted s.t.
    streptococcal s.t.
    ulcerated s.t.
sound
    cavernous voice s.
Sourdille
    operation
space
    paraglottic s.
    poststyloid s.
    prestyloid s.
    Prussak s.
    pterygomandibular s.
    retropharyngeal s.
    Tröltsch s.'s

spasm
    glottic s.
spatium (spatia)
spatula
    s. mallei
speechreading
Spencer
    punch
sphenofrontal
sphenoidal
sphenoidectomy
    frontoethmoidal s.
sphenoiditis
sphenoidostomy
sphenoidotomy
sphenomalar
    s. suture
sphenomaxillary
    s. suture
spheno-orbital
    s. suture
sphenopalatine
sphenoparietal
sphenosquamous
sphenovomerine
    s. suture
sphenozygomatic
    s. suture
sphincter
    laryngeal s.
    palatopharyngeal s.
    pharyngoesophageal s.
spine
    s. of Henle
    s. of maxilla
    nasal s., anterior
    suprameatal s.
spiral
    See also *coil* and *helix.*
    s. canal of Rosenthal
    s. lamina
    lentula s.
    s. organ
    s. sulcus
splint
    Asch s.
    Carter s.
    Erich s.

splint (continued)
    Jones s.
    Kazanjian s.
    Love s.
    Mayer s.
spot
    acoustic s.
    cribriform s.
    deaf s.
    Forchheimer s.
    Koplik s.'s
    light s.
    spongy s.
spud
    Gross s.
squama (squamae)
squamomastoid
SRT—speech reception test
    speech reception threshold
Stacke
    operation
Stahr gland
Stallard
    operation
stapedectomy
    Guilford s.
    Hough s.
    House s.
    partial s.
    piston s.
    Schuknecht s.
    Shea s.
stapedial
stapediolysis
stapedioplasty
stapediotenotomy
stapediovestibular
stapes
    s. mobilization operation
staphylagra
staphylectomy
staphyledema
staphylematoma
staphyline
staphylinus
staphylion
staphylitis
staphyloangina

staphyloncus
staphylopharyngorrhaphy
staphyloplasty
staphyloptosia
staphyloptosis
staphylorrhaphy
staphyloschisis
staphylotome
staphylotomy
statoacoustic
statoconium (statoconia)
Stenger test
stenosis (stenoses)
    laryngeal s.
    nasal s.
    postdiphtheritic s.
    post-tracheostomy s.
    tracheal s.
Stensen
    duct
    foramen
Stenver
    position
stereocilium (stereocilia)
sternohyoid
sternomastoid
sternothyroid
sternotracheal
Stoerk blennorrhea
stomatitis (stomatitides)
    acute necrotizing s.
    allergic s.
    angular s.
    aphthobullous s.
    s. aphthosa
    aphthous s.
    s. arsenicalis
    bismuth s.
    catarrhal s.
    contact s.
    denture s.
    epidemic s.
    epizootic s.
    erythematopultaceous s.
    s. exanthematica
    fusospirochetal s.
    gangrenous s.
    gonococcal s.

stomatitis (stomatitides) (continued)
    gonorrheal s.
    herpetic s.
    infectious s.
    s. intertropica
    lead s.
    s. medicamentosa
    membranous s.
    mercurial s.
    mycotic s.
    necrotizing ulcerative s.
    s. nicotina
    nonspecific s.
    s. prosthetica
    recurrent aphthous s.
    s. scarlatina
    s. scorbutica
    syphilitic s.
    traumatic s.
    tropical s.
    ulcerative s.
    uremic s.
    s. venenata
    vesicular s.
    Vincent s.
    vulcanite s.
stomatomycosis
stomatoplasty
strata (plural of stratum)
stratiform
stratum (strata)
streak
    See *band, line,* and *stria.*
stria (striae)
    See also *band* and *line.*
    mallear s. of tympanic mem-
      brane
striatal
strumectomy
    median s.
stump
    tracheal s.
stuttering
stylohyal
stylohyoid
styloid
stylomandibular
stylomastoid

subarachnoid
subglossitis
subglottic
subhyoid
    s. laryngotomy
    s. pharyngotomy
sublabial
    s. antrotomy
sublingual
submandibular
submaxillary
submental
submucous
    s. cleft
    s. cleft palate
    s. fibroma
    s. resection (SMR)
    s. resection of nasal septum
    s. resection and rhinoplasty
      (SMRR)
    s. resection of vocal cord
succorrhea
suctioning
"sudo–" Phonetic for words beginning pseudo–.
sulci (plural of sulcus)
sulciform
sulculus (sulculi)
sulcus (sulci)
    s. of auditory tube
    buccal s.
    ethmoidal s. of nasal bone
    ethmoidal s. of Gegenbaur
    s. of eustachian tube
    greater palatine s. of maxilla
    greater palatine s. of palatine bone
    s. of greater petrosal nerve
    infraorbital s. of maxilla
    lacrimal s. of lacrimal bone
    lacrimal s. of maxilla
    mandibular s.
    median s. of tongue, s. medianus linguae
    mentolabial s.
    nasal s., posterior
    nasofrontal s.
    nasolabial s.

sulcus (sulci) (continued)
    olfactory s. of nose
    palatine sulci of maxilla
    s. of pharyngeal tonsil
    rhinal s., s. rhinalis
    sphenovomerian s.
    s. of tongue
    tympanic s.
    uvulonodular s.
    s. valleculae
    vomeral s.
summit
    s. of nose
superior
    s. laryngotomy
    s. tracheotomy
suppression
    otoacoustic s.
suppuration
suppurative
supraglottic
    s. laryngectomy
supraglottis
suprahyoid
supramandibular
supramastoid
supramaxillary
supramental
supranasal
supraorbital
suprastapedial
suprasternal
supratemporal
surgery
    See also *maneuver, method, operation, procedure,* and *technique.*
surgical procedure
    See *operation, procedure,* and *technique.*
suspension
    s. laryngoscopy
Sutton
    disease
suture [anatomy]
    anterior palatine s.
    endognathic s.
    endomesognathic s.

suture [anatomy] (continued)
    ethmoidolacrimal s.
    ethmoidomaxillary s.
    frontoethmoidal s.
    frontolacrimal s.
    frontomalar s.
    frontomaxillary s.
    frontonasal s.
    frontoparietal s.
    frontosphenoid s.
    frontozygomatic s.
    infraorbital s.
    interendognathic s.
    intermaxillary s.
    internasal s.
    interpalatine s.
    lacrimoconchal s.
    lacrimoethmoidal s.
    lacrimomaxillary s.
    lacrimoturbinal s.
    longitudinal s. of palate
    malomaxillary s.
    mammillary s.
    mastoid s.
    median palatine s.
    middle palatine s.
    nasal s.
    nasofrontal s.
    nasomaxillary s.
    occipitomastoid s.
    palatine s., anterior
    palatine s., median
    palatine s., middle
    palatine s., posterior
    palatine s., transverse
    palatoethmoidal s.
    palatomaxillary s.
    posterior palatine s.
    premaxillary s.
    sphenomalar s.
    sphenomaxillary s.
    spheno-orbital s.
    sphenovomerine s.
    sphenozygomatic s.
    temporomalar s.
    temporozygomatic s.
    transverse s. of Krause
    transverse palatine s.

suture [anatomy] (continued)
    tympanomastoid s.
    zygomaticofrontal s.
    zygomaticomaxillary s.
suture [material]
    See in *General Surgical Terms.*
suture [technique]
    See in *General Surgical Terms.*
Suzanne gland
swelling
    See also *process* and *prominence.*
    blennorrhagic s.
    lateral lingual s.'s
    tympanic s.
swimmer's
    s. ear
symptom
    See also in *General Medical Terms.*
    Bárány s.
    esophagosalivary s.'s
    Fröschel s.
    labyrinthine s.'s
syn–. See also words beginning cin–, sin–.
synchondrosis (synchondroses)
syndesmosis (syndesmoses)
    s. tympanostapedia, tympanostapedial s.
syndrome
    See also *disease.*
    Apert s.
    Avellis s.
    Avellis-Longhi s.
    BADS s.
    Baelz s.
    Bárány s.
    Bazex s.
    Costen s.
    Crouzon s.
    Gradenigo s.
    Heerfordt s.
    Homer s.
    Hurler s.
    Kartagener s.

syndrome (continued)
  keratitis-ichthyosis-deafness
    (KID) s.
  KID s.
  Klippel-Feil s.
  Lermoyez s.
  Ménière s.
  Mikulicz s.
  Mikulicz-Radecki s.
  Mikulicz-Sjögren s.
  Möbius s.
  Muckle-Wells s.
  Osler-Weber-Rendu s.
  Paterson s.
  Paterson-Brown-Kelly s.
  Paterson-Kelly s.
  Pierre Robin s.
  Plummer-Vinson s.
  Ramsay Hunt s.
  Richards-Rundle s.
  sleep apnea s.
  temporomandibular dysfunc-
    tion s.
  temporomandibular joint
    (TMJ) s.
  Tornwaldt (Thornwaldt) s.
  toxic shock s.
  Treacher Collins s.
  Treacher Collins-
    Franceschetti s.
  Wegener s.
  Wolfram s.
syringe
  irrigating s.
T&A—tonsillectomy and adenoid-
  ectomy
Tagliacozzi
  nasal reconstruction
  rhinoplasty
Takahara disease
Takahashi
  punch
tamponade
  nasal t.
  postnasal balloon t.
Tapia
  syndrome
  vagohypoglossal palsy

TB—tracheobronchitis
TD—tone decay
TDT—tone decay test
TE—tracheoesophageal
technique
    See also *maneuver, proce-
      dure,* and *operation.*
  guillotine t.
tectoria (plural of tectorium)
tectorial
tectorium (tectoria)
teeth (plural of tooth)
TEF—tracheoesophageal fistula
tegmen (tegmina)
  t. antri
  t. cellulae
  t. mastoideotympanicum
  t. mastoideum
  t. tympani
tegmenta (plural of tegmentum)
tegmental
tegmentum (tegmenta)
  t. auris
tegmina (plural of tegmen)
tela (telae)
  t. submucosa pharyngis
  t. submucosa tracheae
telar
temple
temporal
temporalis
temporoauricular
temporofacial
temporofrontal
temporohyoid
temporomalar
  t. suture
temporomandibular
temporomaxillary
temporo-occipital
temporoparietal
temporosphenoid
temporozygomatic
  t. suture
tendon
  stapedius t.
tentorial
tentorium (tentoria)

"tere–" Phonetic for words beginning pteri–, ptery–.

test

See also *phenomenon, reaction, reflex,* and *sign.*
See also in *Laboratory, Pathology, and Chemistry Terms.*
ABLB (alternate binaural loudness balance) t.
air-conduction t.
alternate binaural loudness balance (ABLB) t.
alternate loudness balance t.
auditory acuity t.
Bárány t.
binaural distorted speech t.'s
Bing t.
bone-conduction t.
caloric t.
clivogram t.
Doerfler-Stewart t.
Erhard t.
fistula t.
Fränkel t.
Gault t.
Gellé t.
impedance audiometry t.
labyrinthine t.
laryngeal mirror t.
Lombard t.
modified Rinne t.
monaural distorted speech t.'s
monaural loudness balance (MLB) t.
Monospot t.
Mono-Vac t.
Politzer t.
radioallergosorbent t. (RAST)
Rinne t.
rotation t.
Schick t.
Schwabach t.
short increment sensitivity index (SISI) t.
smear t.
Stenger t.
threshold tone decay t.

test (continued)
Tobey-Ayer t.
tone decay t.
torsion t.
tuning fork t.
watch t.
Weber t.
whisper t.
whistle t.
TG—toxic goiter
therapy
humidification t.
Thornwaldt. See *Tornwaldt.*
threshold
audiometric t.
auditory t.
speech reception t. (SRT)
thrush
thyrochondrotomy
thyrocricotomy
thyroglossal
thyrohyoid
t. laryngotomy
thyroid
t. cartilage
t. lobectomy
thyroidectomy
medical t.
thyroiditis
thyroidotomy
thyroparathyroidectomy
"tial–" Phonetic for words beginning ptyal–.
tic
t. douloureux ["doo-loo-roo"]
laryngeal t.
tinnitus
t. aurium
clicking t.
Leudet t.
nervous t.
nonvibratory t.
objective t.
vibratory t.
TM—temporomandibular
tympanic membrane
TMJ—temporomandibular joint
TMJ syndrome

Tobey-Ayer test
tongue
 adherent t.
 amyloid t.
 antibiotic t.
 baked t.
 bald t.
 beefy t.
 bifid t.
 black t.
 black hairy t.
 burning t.
 cardinal t.
 cerebriform t.
 choreic t.
 cleft t.
 coated t.
 cobble-stone t.
 crescent t.
 crocodile t.
 dotted t.
 double t.
 earthy t.
 encrusted t.
 fern leaf t.
 filmy t.
 fissured t.
 flat t.
 furred t.
 furrowed t.
 geographic t.
 glazed t.
 grooved t.
 hairy t.
 hobnail t.
 lobulated t.
 magenta t.
 mappy t.
 plicated t.
 raspberry t.
 raw-beef t.
 Sandwith bald t.
 scrotal t.
 smoker's t.
 smooth t.
 t. of sphenoid bone
 split t.
 stippled t.

tongue (continued)
 strawberry t.
 strawberry t., red
 strawberry t., white
 sulcated t.
 thrombone t.
 t.-tie, t.-tied
 white t.
tonsil
 adenoid t.
 buried t.
 eustachian t.
 faucial t.
 Gerlach t.
 hypertrophied t.
 lingual t.
 Luschka t.
 nasopharyngeal t.
 palatine t.
 pharyngeal t.
 submerged t.
 third t.
 t. of torus tubarius
 tubal t.'s
tonsilla (tonsillae)
 t. adenoidea
 t. lingualis
 t. palatina
 t. pharyngea
 t. pharyngealis
 t. tubaria
tonsillar
tonsillectomy
 t. and adenoidectomy (T&A)
 dissection t.
 guillotine t.
tonsillitic
tonsillitis
 caseous t.
 catarrhal t.
 diphtherial t.
 erythematous t.
 follicular t.
 herpetic t.
 lacunar t.
 t. lenta
 lingual t.
 mycotic t.

tonsillitis (continued)
    parenchymatous t.
    preglottic t.
    pustular t.
    streptococcal t.
    Vincent t.
tonsilloadenoidectomy
tonsillolith
tonsillopathy
tonsillopharyngitis
tonsilloscopy
tonsillotomy
"too-mur" Phonetic for tumeur.
tooth (teeth)
    auditory teeth of Corti
    auditory teeth of Huschke
    cog t. of malleus
    Corti auditory teeth
    Huschke auditory teeth
tophus (tophi)
    auricular t.
    t. of pinna
Topinard
    angle
    line
tori (plural of torus)
Tornwaldt (Thornwaldt)
    abscess
    bursa
    bursitis
    cyst
    disease
    syndrome
torus (tori)
    t. frontalis
    t. levatorius
    t. mandibulae
    t. mandibularis
    t. occipitalis
    palatine t.
    t. palatinus
    t. tubarius
total
    See also *complete.*
    t. laryngectomy
    t. rhinectomy
Touraine
    aphthosis

Towne
    view
trachea (tracheae)
    cervical t.
tracheaectasy
tracheal
    t. atresia
    t. cannula
trachealgia
tracheitis
tracheobronchial
tracheobronchitis
tracheocannula
    Montgomery t.
tracheocele
tracheofissure
tracheofistulization
tracheolaryngeal
tracheolaryngotomy
tracheomalacia
tracheopathia
tracheopharyngeal
tracheoplasty
tracheorrhaphy
tracheoscopy
    percervical t.
    peroral t.
tracheostenosis
tracheostomy
    post-t. stenosis
tracheotomy
    inferior t.
    superior t.
tract
    upper respiratory t.
traction
    intermaxillary t.
tragal
tragus
transantral
    t. ethmoidectomy
transhyoid
    t. pharyngotomy
translingual
    t. pharyngotomy
transmeatal
    t. atticotomy
    t. tympanotomy

transnasal
transseptal
    t. catheterization
transthyroid
    t. pharyngotomy
transtracheal
transtympanic
    t. labyrinthectomy
transverse
    t. palatine suture
    t. pharyngotomy
    t. suture of Krause
trauma (traumas, traumata)
    acoustic t.
Trautmann triangle
Treacher Collins
    syndrome
Treacher Collins-Franceschetti
    syndrome
treatment
    Politzer t.
    Proetz t.
    Roeder t.
trench mouth
triad
    Kartagener t.
triangle
    Trautmann t.
trigeminal
trismus
Tröltsch
    recesses
    spaces
Troutman
    gouge
tuba (tubae)
    t. acustica
    t. auditiva
    t. auditoria
tube
    auditory t.
    eustachian t.
    otopharyngeal t.
    pharyngotympanic t.
    Ruysch t.
tuber (tubers, tubera)
    t. cochleae
    eustachian t.

tuber (tubers, tubera) (continued)
    external t. of Henle
    t. maxillae
    t. maxillare
    maxillary t.
    mental t.
tubercle
    darwinian t., Darwin t.
tubercula (plural of tuberculum)
tuberculate, tuberculated
tuberculation
tuberculitis
tuberculization
tuberculoid
tuberculosis (TB)
    t. cutis orificialis
    laryngeal t.
    t. of larynx
    oral t.
    t. orificialis
    tracheobronchial t.
tuberculum (tubercula)
    t. articulare ossis temporalis
    t. auriculae, t. auriculae
      (Darwini)
    t. epiglotticum
    t. geniale
    t. labii superioris
    t. mentale mandibulae
    t. olfactorium
    t. pharyngeum
    t. septi
    t. supratragicum
    t. thyroideum inferius
    t. thyroideum superius
tuberositas (tuberositates)
    t. masseterica
    t. pterygoidea mandibulae
tuberosity
    malar t.
    masseteric t.
    t. of maxilla, maxillary t.
    pterygoid t. of mandible
    pyramidal t. of palatine bone
tuboplasty
    eustachian t.
tuborrhea
tubotorsion

tubotympanal
tubotympanic
    t. recess
tug, tugging
    tracheal t.
Tullio phenomenon
tumentia
tumeur
    t. perlée
tumor
    acoustic t.
    hypopharyngeal t.
    neuroectodermal t.
    neurogenic t.
    odontogenic t.
    Rathke t.
    Rathke pouch t.
    Schmincke t.
    Warthin t.
tunic
    fibrous t. of liver
    mucous t.
    pharyngeal t., pharyngobasi-
      lar t.
tunica (tunicae)
    t. mucosa
    t. muscularis
tuning fork
    Hartmann t.f.
tunnel
    t. of Corti
turbinate
    sphenoid t.
turbinectomy
turbinotome
turbinotomy
Tydings snare
tympanal
tympanectomy
tympanic
    t. neurectomy
    t. plethysmography
tympanichord
tympanichordal
tympanicity
tympanion
tympanitis
tympanoacryloplasty

tympanocentesis
tympanoeustachian
tympanogram
tympanolabyrinthopexy
tympanomalleal
tympanomandibular
tympanomastoid
    t. suture
tympanomastoiditis
tympanomeatal
tympanometry
tympano-ossicular system
tympanophonia
tympanoplasty
    t., types 2–5
    combined approach t.
    intact canal-wall t.
tympanosclerosis
tympanosquamosal
tympanostapedial
tympanosympathectomy
tympanotemporal
tympanotomy
    posterior t.
    transmeatal t.
tympanum
"u–" Phonetic for words beginning
    eu–.
ulcer
    contact u.
ulcerate
ulcerating
ulceration
    tracheal u.
ulcerative
uloglossitis
uloncus
ulotomy
ultrasonic
    u. labyrinthectomy
ultrasonogram
umbo (umbones)
    u. membranae tympani
    u. membranae tympanicae
    u. of tympanic membrane
umbonate
underlay myringoplasty
uniaural

unit
> See also in *General Medical Terms* and *Laboratory, Pathology, and Chemistry Terms.*
> Hertz u.

UR—upper respiratory [tract]
uraniscochasma
uraniscolalia
uranisconitis
uranoplasty
URD—upper respiratory disease
URI—upper respiratory infection
URTI—upper respiratory tract infection
Usher
> disease
> syndrome

utricle
uveoparotid
uveoparotitis
uvula (uvulae)
> bifid u.
> cleft u.
> u. fissura, forked u.
> u. palatina
> palatine u.
> split u.

uvular
uvularis
uvulectomy
uvulitis
uvulopalatopharyngoplasty (UPPP)
uvuloptosis
uvulotomy
V—voice volume
vallecula (valleculae)
> v. epiglottica

vallecular
Valsalva
> maneuver
> procedure

valve
> Huschke v.

vas (vasa)
> vasa auris internae
> vasa sanguinea integumenti communis

VASC—Verbal Auditory Screen for Children
vasoconstriction
vasoconstrictors [a class of drugs]
vasodilatation
vasomotoricity
vasoneuropathy
vault
> cartilaginous v.

"veek dah-zeer" Phonetic for Vicq d'Azyr.
velum (vela)
> Baker v.
> v. palati
> palatine v.
> v. palatinum
> pharyngeal v.

ventricle
> v. of larynx
> Morgagni v.

ventriculi (plural of ventriculus)
ventriculocordectomy
ventriculus (ventriculi)
> v. laryngis, v. laryngis (Morgagnii)

Verga
> lacrimal groove

vermilion
> v. border

vermilionectomy
vertical
> v. hemilaryngectomy

vertiginous
vertigo
> auditory v., aural v.
> labyrinthine v.
> paroxysmal positional v.
> positional v., postural v.
> rotary v., rotatory v.
> vestibular v.

vesiculotympanic
vestibula (plural of vestibulum)
vestibular
> v. nerve
> v. neuronitis
> v. reflex
> v. system

vestibulocochlear

vestibulo-ocular reflex
vestibulotomy
vestibulum (vestibula)
    v. auris
    v. glottidis
    v. laryngis
    v. nasale
    v. nasi
    v. oris
vibration
    bone-conduction v.
vibrator
vibrissa (vibrissae)
vibroacoustic
vibrometer
Vicq d'Azyr
    band
    body
    bundle
    fasciculus
    foramen
    operation
    stripe
    tract
vidian
    v. artery
    v. canal
    v. nerve
Vieussens
    annulus
view
    Chausse v.
    Law v.
    Owen v.
    Schüller v.
    Towne v.
    Waters v.
villi (plural of villus)
villiferous
villose, villous [adj.]
    v. papillae of tongue
villosity
villus (villi)
    lingual villi
Vincent
    infection
    tonsillitis

vinculum (vincula)
    See also *band* and *frenum.*
    v. linguae
virus
    See also in *Laboratory,*
        Pathology, and Chemistry
        Terms.
VMR—vasomotor rhinitis
vocal
voces (plural of vox)
vocis (genitive of vox)
voix
    v. de Polichinelle
Voltolini
    disease
vomer
vomeronasal
von Bezold. See *Bezold.*
von Brunn. See *Brunn.*
von Recklinghausen. See *Reckling-*
    hausen.
vox (voces)
VR—vocal resonance
VRI—viral respiratory infection
"vwah" Phonetic for voix.
W—Weber [test]
Waardenburg
    disease
    syndrome
Waldeyer ring
Walther
    ducts
Wardill
    palatoplasty
Wartenberg
    disease
    neuralgia
Warthin tumor
Waters [eponym]
    view
Watson-Williams
    punch
Wb—weber(s)
Weber
    test
Wegener
    granulomatosis
    syndrome

West
    operation
Wharton
    duct
wheezing
Whiting
    rongeur
Whitnall tubercle
whooping cough
Wilde
    punch
Wildervanck syndrome
Willis
    paracusis
window
    found w.
    oval w.
windowing
wing
    w. of vomer
Wolfram
    syndrome
Wood [eponym]
    operation
Woodman
    operation
Wreden sign
Wrisberg
    cartilage
Wullstein
    operation

WV—whispered voice
xanthoma (xanthomas, xanthomata)
    verruciform x.
xanthosis
    x. of septum nasi
xeromycteria
Yankauer
    operation
    punch
"yoo–" Phonetic for words begin-
    ning eu–.
"yulo–" Phonetic for words begin-
    ning ulo–.
Zaufal sign
"zheel-bare" Phonetic for Gilbert
    [Nicolas Augustin Gilbert].
zone
    Cozzolino z.
    dentofacial z.
    mesogastric z.
    z. of oval nuclei
    z. of round nuclei
zygoma
zygomatic
zygomaticofacial
zygomaticofrontal
    z. suture
zygomaticomaxillary
    z. suture
zygomaxillary

Pediatrics
Includes Genetic, Hereditary, and Congenital Diseases

AACP—American Academy of
    Child Psychiatry
AAP—American Academy of Pedi-
    atrics
Aarskog
    syndrome
Aarskog-Scott
    syndrome
Aase syndrome
ABC—apnea, bradycardia, cyanosis
    applesauce, bananas, cereal
    [diet]
abembryonic
aberration
    chromosome a.
    heterosomal a.
    intrachromosomal a.
abetalipoproteinemia
ability
abiotrophic
abiotrophy
ablactation
abnormity
ABO
    incompatibility
abrachia
abrachiatism
abrachius
abscess
    amebic a.
    Bezold (von Bezold) a.
    perinephric a.
    pyogenic a.
    retroesophageal a.
    retrotonsillar a.
absence
    atypical a. seizure

absence (continued)
    complex a. seizure
    congenital ossicular a.
    a. epilepsy
    a. seizure
    subclinical a. seizure
absentia
    a. epileptica
abuse
    child a.
    inhalant a.
    laxative a.
acanthocytosis
acanthosis
    congenital a.
    malignant a. nigricans
    a. nigricans
acardia
acardiac
acardius
acatalasemia
acatalasia
accident prone
acentric
acephalia
acephalic
acephalobrachia
acephalobrachius
acephalocardia
acephalocardius
acephalochiria
acephalochirus
acephalogaster
acephalogastria
acephalopodia
acephalopodius
acephalorhachia

acephalostomia
acephalostomus
acephalothoracia
acephalothorus
acephalous
acephalus
    a. dibrachius
    a. dipus
    a. monobrachius
    a. monopus
    a. paracephalus
    a. sympus
acetanilid
    a. poisoning
aceto-orcein
N-acetylgalactosamine-4-sulfatase
N-acetylgalactosamine-6-sulfatase
N-acetylgalactosamine-4-sulfatase
    deficiency
α-N-acetylgalactosaminidase [alpha-]
N-acetylglucosamine-6-sulfatase
α-N-acetylglucosaminidase [alpha-]
Achard syndrome
acheilia
acheilous
acheiria
acheiropodia
acheirus
achondrogenesis
achondroplasia
achondroplastic
achromia
    congenital a.
acidophilus [*Lactobacillus acido-philus*]
acidophilus milk
acidosis
    diabetic a.
    hyperchloremic renal a.
    metabolic a.
aciduric
aclasis
    diaphyseal a.
    metaphyseal a.
aclastic
acne
    adolescent a.
    a. conglobata, conglobate a.

acne (continued)
    halogen a.
    neonatal a., a. neonatorum
    a. vulgaris
acormia
acoustic
    a. reflex
    a. trauma
ACPS—acrocephalopolysyndactyly
acrania
acranial
acranius
acrobrachycephaly
acrocephalia
acrocephalic
acrocephalosyndactyly
    a. of Apert
acrocephalous
acrocephaly
acrocyanosis
acrodermatitis
    a. enteropathica
    infantile a.
    papular a.
    papular a. of childhood
acrodolichomelia
acrodynia
acrodysplasia
acromacria
acromegalic
acromegalogigantism
acromegaloidism
acromicria
acromphalus
acropigmentatio reticularis
acrosphenosyndactylia
acystia
adactylous
adactyly
Adair-Dighton syndrome
adaptation
    genetic a.
    phenotypic a.
ADD—attention deficit disorder
ADDH—a. deficit disorder with
    hyperactivity
Addison
    disease

adenine phosphoribosyl transferase
(APRT) deficiency
adenitis
cervical a.
mesenteric a.
adenocarcinoma
a. of infantile testis
testicular a. of infancy
adenoid
a. hypertrophy
adenoidectomy
adenoiditis
adenologaditis
adenoma
islet cell a.
a. sebaceum
ADHD—attention deficit hyperactivity disorder
Adie
pupil
syndrome
adiponecrosis
a. subcutanea neonatorum
adiposogenital dystrophy
adipsia
adipsous
adjuvant
pertussis a.
adrenal
a. cortex
a. crisis
a. gland
a. hyperplasia
a. medulla
adrenogenital
a. syndrome
adynamia
a. episodica hereditaria
AEq—age equivalent
aerophore
AFRD—acute febrile respiratory
disease
"af-tha" Phonetic for aphtha.
AGA—appropriate for gestational
age
aganglionic
agastria
agastric

age
achievement a.
bone a.
developmental a.
emotional a.
functional a.
gestational a.
a. of menarche, menarcheal a.
mental a.
physical a., physiologic a.
agenesia
a. corticalis
agenesis
anorectal a.
callosal a.
gonadal a.
nuclear a.
ovarian a.
renal a.
vaginal a.
agenitalism
agenosomia
agenosomus
agglutinin
cold a.
febrile a.
aggregation
familial a.
aglossia
aglossostomia
agnathia
agnathous
agnathus
agranulocytosis
infantile lethal a.
AGS—adrenogenital syndrome
AIDS—acquired immunodeficiency
syndrome
air
a. swallowing
akinesia
a. algera
"a-kon-dro-plaz-ee-a" Phonetic for
achondroplasia.
"ak-ro-brak-e-sef-al-e" Phonetic for
acrobrachycephaly.
alacrima

alalia
    developmental a.
Albini nodules
albinism
    a. I, a. II
    Amish a.
    autosomal dominant oculo-
        cutaneous a.
    autosomal recessive ocular
        a. (AROA)
    brown a.
    complete imperfect a.
    complete perfect a.
    Forsius-Eriksson–type ocu-
        lar a.
    localized a.
    Nettleship-Falls–type ocular
        a.
    ocular a. (OA)
    oculocutaneous a. (OCA)
    partial a.
    piebald a.
    red a.
    tyrosinase-negative (ty-neg)
        oculocutaneous a.
    tyrosinase-positive (ty-pos)
        oculocutaneous a.
    xanthous a.
    X-linked ocular a. (Nettle-
        ship) (XOAN)
    yellow mutant (ym) a.
albinoidism
albinotic
Albrecht
    bone
    suture
alcohol
    fetal a. syndrome
Alder anomaly
aldosteronism
    juvenile a.
aleukia
    congenital a.
Alexander
    disease
aleydigism
Alice in Wonderland syndrome
alkaptonuric

allele
allelism
allergic
    a. salute
    a. shiner
allergy
    hereditary a.
allotriophagy
alopecia
    a. areata
    congenital a.
    a. congenitalis
    congenital sutural a.
    congenital triangular a.
    a. triangularis congenitalis
Alpers
    disease
    polioencephalopathy
alpha
    a.-*N*-acetylgalactosaminidase
    a.-*N*-acetylglucosaminidase
    a.-L-fucosidase
    a.-galactosidase A
    1,4-a.-glucan branching
        enzyme
    a.-mannosidase
    a.-methylacetoacetyl CoA
        thiolase
amaurotic
    a. familial idiocy (AFI)
ambisexual
amelia
    brachial a.
    complete a.
    unilateral a.
amelus
aminoacidemia
aminoacidopathy
amniocele
amnionitis
amyloidosis
amylopectinosis
amyoplasia
    a. congenita
amyotonia
    a. congenita
analeptics [a class of drugs]
anasarca

ancylostomiasis
   cutaneous a.
   a. cutis
Andersen
   disease
   syndrome
   triad
androgenic
androgenization
androgenized
androgenous
anemia
   aplastic a.
   breast a.
   congenital a. of newborn
   congenital dyserythropoietic
      a.
   congenital nonspherocytic
      hemolytic a.
   Cooley a.
   Czerny a.
   erythroblastic a. of childhood
   familial erythroblastic a.
   Fanconi a.
   globe cell a.
   glucose-6-phosphate dehy-
      drogenase deficiency a.
   hemolytic a.
   a. hypochromica sidero-
      chrestica hereditaria
   hypoplastic a., congenital
   Jaksch a.
   Larzel a.
   Mediterranean a.
   megaloblastic a.
   microcytic a.
   a. neonatorum
   ovalocytary a.
   pernicious a., juvenile
   physiologic a.
   a. pseudoleukemica infantum
   pyridoxine-responsive a.
   sex-linked hypochromatic a.
      of Rundles and Falls
   sickle cell a.
   sideroblastic a.
   von Jaksch a.
anemic

anencephaly
angiofibroma
   juvenile nasopharyngeal a.
   nasopharyngeal a.
angiokeratoma
   a. circumscriptum
   a. of Mibelli
   solitary a.
angioma
   hereditary hemorrhagic a.
   spider a.
   strawberry a.
angiomatoid
angiomatosis
   Sturge-Weber a.
anomalad
anomaly
   Alder a.
   Alder-Reilly a.
   Alius-Grignaschi a.
   Chédiak-Higashi a.
   Chédiak-Steinbrinck-
      Higashi a.
   congenital a.
   fetal a.
   Huët-Pelger nuclear a.
   Pelger-Huët a.
   Pelger-Huët nuclear a.
   Peters a.
   Pierre Robin a.
   Poland a.
   Steinbrinck a.
   Uhl a.
   Undritz a.
anorchia
anorchism
anorexia
   a. nervosa
anorexigenic
anosmia
anotus
anoxia
   fetal a.
anthelmintics [a class of drugs]
antibody (antibodies)
      See also in *Laboratory,*
       Pathology, and Chemistry
       Terms.

antibody (antibodies) (continued)
    anti-Rh (Rhesus) a.
    maternal a.
anticonvulsants [a class of drugs]
antigen (Ag)
    See also in *Laboratory,*
       Pathology, and Chemistry
       Terms.
    Australia a.
    Rh (Rhesus) factor a.
anti–glomerular basement membrane
    (anti-GBM) antibody disease
antipyretics [a class of drugs]
antitussives [a class of drugs]
anus
    imperforate a.
aorta (aortae)
    dorsal embryonic a.
    double a.
Apert
    acrocephalosyndactyly
    disease
    hirsutism
    syndrome
Apert-Crouzon
    disease
Apgar
    rating
    scale
    score
    test
aphasia
    global a.
    Wernicke a.
aphtha (aphthae)
    Bednar a.
aplasia
    a. axialis extracorticalis con-
      genita
    a. cutis congenita
    gonadal a.
    Leydig cell a.
    nuclear a.
    retinal a.
    thymic a.
    thymic-parathyroid a.
aplastic
    a. anemia

aplastic (continued)
    a. crisis
    a. pancytopenia
apnea
    initial a.
    late a.
    a. neonatorum
apolipoprotein C-II (apo C-II) defi-
    ciency, familial
appearance
    hair-on-end a., hair-stand-
      ing-on-end a.
appendicitis
aqueductal
arachnidism
"arak–" Phonetic for words begin-
    ning arach–.
Aran-Duchenne
    disease
archenteronoma
Arnold-Chiari
    malformation
    syndrome
arrested
    a. growth and development
arrhenoblastoma
arrhinencephaly
arrhythmia
    sinus a.
arteriosclerosis
    infantile a.
arteritis (arteritides)
    a. umbilicalis
arthritis (arthritides)
    juvenile a.
    juvenile rheumatoid a.
    psoriatic a.
    septic a.
arthrodysplasia
    hereditary a.
arthrogryposis
    a. multiplex congenita
arthro-osteo-onychodysplasia
Ascher
    syndrome
ascites
    chylous a.

asphyxia
    a. neonatorum
assessment
    Dubowitz Neurological A.
asthma
    thymic a.
astigmatism
ataxia
    cerebellar a.
    Friedreich a.
    a.-telangiectasia
atelectasis
    congenital a.
    postnatal asphyxia a.
    primary a.
atelectatic
athetoid
athetosis
    congenital a.
atonia
atonic
atonicity
atopic
atopy
atresia
    biliary a.
    congenital a.
    esophageal a.
    ileal a.
    pyloric a.
    tricuspid a.
atrial
    a. septal defect (ASD)
atrophia
    a. bulborum hereditaria
atrophy
    Dejerine-Sottas a.
    Fazio-Londe a.
    infantile a.
    Parrot a. of the newborn
attack
attention
    a. deficit disorder (ADD)
    a. deficit disorder with
      hyperactivity (ADDH)
    a. deficit hyperactivity disor-
      der (ADHD)
audiogram

audiometry
aula.
aura
Australia antigen (Au)
autism
autistic
autosomal
    a. dominant
    a. recessive
"awla" Phonetic for aula.
Babinski-Fröhlich syndrome
baby
    test-tube b.
bacillus (bacilli)
    See in *Laboratory, Patholo-*
      gy, and Chemistry Terms.
Bacillus
    See in *Laboratory, Patholo-*
      gy, and Chemistry Terms.
bacterium (bacteria)
    See specific bacteria in *Lab-*
      oratory, Pathology, and
      Chemistry Terms.
bacteroidosis
Bakwin-Eiger syndrome
Ballantyne
    syndrome
Ballantyne-Runge syndrome
Ballard gestational assessment
Baller-Gerold syndrome
banana
    b. sign
band
    See also *line* and *stria.*
    belly b. [pref: bellyband]
Banti
    disease
    splenic anemia
    syndrome
Bardet-Biedl syndrome
Barlow
    disease
Barraquer
    disease
Barraquer-Simons syndrome
Bart syndrome
basiotic

Bassen-Kornzweig
    disease
    syndrome
Batten
    disease
Batten-Mayou
    disease
Bayley Scales of Infant Development
BBA—born before arrival [of doc-
    tor or midwife]
Beals syndrome
Beau
    lines
Beck
    disease
Becker
    dystrophy
Becker-type muscular dystrophy
Beckwith
    syndrome
Beckwith-Wiedemann
    syndrome
Bednar aphtha
bedwetting
Béguez César
    disease
Behçet
    disease
    syndrome
belly
    Delhi b.
    prune-b. syndrome
    spider b.
bellyache
bellyband
bellybutton
Berardinelli syndrome
Bergmeister papilla
Best
    disease
beta
    b.-galactosidase
    b.-glucuronidase
    b.-sitosterolemia
bezoar
Bezold (von Bezold)
    abscess

Biedl
    disease
Bielschowsky
    disease
    syndrome
Bielschowsky-Jansky
    . disease
Biemond
    syndrome (type I, type II)
bigeminum (bigemina)
biliary
    b. atresia
    b. hypoplasia
Bili mask
binge
bingeing and purging
birth
    breech b.
    immature b.
    live b.
    b. order
    b. palsy
    b. paralysis
    partial b.
    spontaneous breech b.
    b. trauma
    viable b.
birthmark
    port wine stain b.
    strawberry b.
birthweight
Björnstad syndrome
Blackfan-Diamond
    anemia
    syndrome
Blalock-Taussig
    operation
    shunt
blepharospasm
blister
    blood b.
    fever b.
    water b.
Bloch-Sulzberger
    syndrome
blood
    cord b.

Blount
    disease
blow-by oxygen
blue diaper syndrome
blue sclera
Bochdalek
    foramen
    foramen (of Bochdalek) her-
        nia
    hernia
Bodian-Schwachman syndrome
body (bodies)
    Alder-Reilly b.'s
Boeck
    See *Beck.*
BOM—bilateral otitis media
bone
    b. age
Bonnevie-Ullrich syndrome
Boo-Chai craniofacial cleft
Böök syndrome
Bornholm
    disease
Bouchut
    respiration
Bourneville
    disease
    syndrome
Bourneville-Brissaud
    disease
Bourneville-Pringle
    syndrome
bowleg, bowlegged
Brachmann-de Lange
    syndrome
brachycephalic
Brandt
    syndrome
brash
    water b.
    weaning b.
BRAT—bananas, rice cereal, apple-
    sauce, toast [diet]
breast
    supernumerary b.
breast-fed
breast-feed, breast-feeds
breast-feeding

breath
    lead b.
breath-holding
    blue b.
    white b.
breech
    complete b.
    b. delivery
    b. extraction
    frank b.
    incomplete b.
    b. presentation
    single footling b.
bregmatodymia
brephic
brephoplastic
brephotrophic
Brissaud
    dwarf
    infantilism
brittle diabetes
bronchiolectasia
bronchitis
    acute laryngotracheal b.
    arachidic b.
    asthmatic b.
    chronic obstructive b.
    croupous b.
    epidemic capillary b.
bronchogram
bronchospasm
bronchus (bronchi)
    See in *Pulmonary Medicine*
    section.
Brown-Symmers
    disease
Brudzinski
    reflex
    sign
Brushfield spots
Brushfield-Wyatt
    disease
    syndrome
Bruton
    agammaglobulinemia
    disease
bruxism

Budd-Chiari
>syndrome
Budin
>joint
>obstetric joint
Buhl
>desquamative pneumonia
>disease
bulimia
>b. nervosa
bullous
>b. congenital ichthyosiform
>>erythroderma
>b. dermatosis
>b. impetigo
>b. pemphigoid
Bürger-Grütz syndrome
burping
butt balm
butt butter
button
>belly b. [pref: bellybutton]
BW—birthweight
Byler
>disease
Byrd-Dew method
CA—croup-associated [virus]
Caffey
>disease
Caffey-Kenny
>disease
Caffey-Silverman syndrome
Caffey-Smyth-Roske syndrome
CAH—congenital adrenal hyperpla-
>sia
Cairns
>syndrome
calisthenics
Calvé
>disease
Calvé-Legg-Perthes syndrome
Calvé-Perthes
>disease
CA (cardiac-apnea) monitor
Camurati-Engelmann
>disease
>syndrome

Canavan
>disease
>sclerosis
>spongy degeneration
Canavan-van Bogaert-Bertrand
>disease
caput (capita)
>c. medusae
>c. quadratum
>c. succedaneum
carcinoma (carcinomas, carcinomata)
>See in *Oncology and Hema-*
>>*tology* section.
cardiomyopathy
cardiorespiratory
Caroli
>disease
Carpenter
>syndrome
carrier
>hemophilia c.
Casser (Casserio, Casserius)
>fontanelle
>ligament
>muscle
catarrhal
cat-scratch disease
cat's cry syndrome
Cattel Infant Intelligence Scale
CAV—congenital absence of vagina
>congenital adrenal virilism
>croup-associated virus
cavernous
>c. hemangioma
>c. sinus thrombosis
cavus foot
CC—cradle cap
CDH—congenital diaphragmatic
>hernia
>congenital dislocation of the
>>hip
celiac
>c. disease
>c. sprue
center
>poison control c.
cephalhematoma
cephalomegaly

cephalothoracopagus
    c. dibrachius
CERA—cortical evoked response
    audiometry
ceramidase deficiency
cereal
CF—cystic fibrosis
CF antibody titer
CFP—cystic fibrosis of pancreas
CHA—congenital hypoplastic ane-
    mia
Chagas
    disease
chalasia
Chapple syndrome
Charcot-Marie-Tooth
    syndrome
Charcot-Marie-Tooth-Hoffmann
    syndrome
CHD—childhood disease
    congenital heart disease
Cheadle
    disease
Chédiak-Higashi
    disease
    syndrome
Chédiak-Steinbrinck-Higashi anom-
    aly
CHH—cartilage-hair hypoplasia
chickenpox
Chievitz
    layer
chigger bite
Chilaiditi
    sign
    syndrome
chimerism
    blood group c.
cholera
    c. infantum
chondrodysplasia
    genotypic c.
    c. punctata
    rhizomelic-type c.
chondrodystrophia
    c. calcificans congenita
    c. fetalis calcificans

chondrodystrophy
    c. malacia
chondromalacia
chondro-osteodystrophy
chondrosarcoma
chondrosarcomatosis
chondrosarcomatous
chorea
    juvenile c.
    Sydenham c.
choreal
choreoathetosis
    paroxysmal familial c.
chorioepithelioma
choriomeningitis
    lymphocytic c.
Chotzen syndrome
Christensen-Krabbe
    disease
    poliodystrophy
Christ-Siemens-Touraine syndrome
chromaffinoma
chromosomal
chromosome
    c.-type aberration
cin–. See also words beginning
    sin–, syn–.
circulatory
    c. arrest
    c. failure
cirrhonosus
cirrhosis
    biliary c.
Citelli
    syndrome
citrullinuria
Clarke-Hadfield
    syndrome
CLAS—congenital localized
    absence of skin
classification
    Fredrickson and Lees c.
      (phenotypes I–V)
    Lund-Browder c.
cleft
    c. lip
    oblique facial c.
    orbitonasal c.

cleft (continued)
    c. palate
    pharyngeal c.
    submucous c.
    tubotympanic c.
clinodactyly
cloaca (cloacae)
    congenital c.
    persistent c.
cloacal
Clouston syndrome
clubfoot
clubhand
clunis (clunes)
CND—congenital neuromuscular
    disorder
CNSD—chronic nonspecific diarrhea
coarctation
    c. of the aorta
Coats
    disease
Cockayne
    disease
    syndrome
coeur en sabot
cold (frozen) breads for a teething
    infant
colic
colicky pain
colitis (colitides)
    granulomatous c.
    infectious c.
    tuberculous c.
collodion baby
coloboma
colostration
colostrum
coma
    diabetic c.
    hyperosmolar nonketotic c.
Comby sign
communicable disease
complex
    Eisenmenger c.
    Ghon c.
congested
congestion
congestive

Conradi
    disease
    syndrome
conversion
    hysterical c.
convulsion
    febrile c.
    infantile c.
Coombs
    serum
    test
cor
    c. biloculare
    c. triloculare biatriatum
Cori
    disease
Cornelia de Lange
    syndrome
Corrigan pulse
cortical
    c. hyperostosis
corticis (genitive of cortex)
coryza
cough
    habit c.
    psychogenic c.
Cowden
    disease
    syndrome
coxa
    c. vara
CP—cerebral palsy
CPD—congenital polycystic disease
craniopharyngioma
craniostenosis
crease
    simian c.
    sole c.
crepitation
cretin
cretinism
cretinistic
cretinoid
cretinous
crib
    clinical c.
    c. death
    tongue c.

cri du chat [cat's cry] syndrome
"kree doo shah" Phonetic for cri du
    chat.
cri-du-chat syndrome
Crigler-Najjar
    syndrome
crisis (crises)
    adrenal c.
criterion (criteria)
    Hyams criteria
    Jones criteria
Crohn
    disease
croupy
Crouzon
    disease
    syndrome
crural
crust
    milk c.
crusta (crustae)
    c. lactea
cryptocephalus
cryptomerorachischisis
cryptorchidism
cryptotia
cryptozygous
CTH—ceramide trihexoside
culture
    sputum c.
    tracheal aspirate c.
Curling ulcer
curse
    Ondine's c.
cutis
    c. elastica
    c. hyperelastica
    c. laxa
cyst
    choledochal c.
    colloid c.
    dermoid c.
    follicular c.
    hydatid c.
    inclusion c.
    omental c.
    popliteal c.
    porencephalic c.

cyst (continued)
    urachal c.
    vitelline duct c.
cystathionine γ-lyase [gamma-]
cystic
    c. fibrosis
    c. hygroma
cystitis
    c. cystica
    hemorrhagic c.
cytomegalic inclusion disease of the
    newborn
Czerny anemia
DA—developmental age
dacroadenitis
dacrostenosis
dacryocystostenosis
Dalrymple sign
dance
    St. Vitus d.
Dandy-Walker
    deformity
    syndrome
Darrow-Gamble syndrome
Debré-de Toni-Fanconi
    syndrome
Debré-Sémélaigne syndrome
defect
    atrial septal d.
    ventricular septal d.
deficiency
    disaccharidase d.
    erythrocyte glutathione per-
        oxidase d.
    factor VIII d.
    fibrinogen d.
    fructose d.
    galactokinase d.
    glucose-6-phosphate dehy-
        drogenase d.
    IgA d.
    IgM d.
    immunoglobulin d.
    pyruvate-kinase d.
    riboflavin d.
deformity
    cloverleaf skull d.
    Dandy-Walker d.

deformity (continued)
    Sprengel d.
    Volkmann d.
degeneration
    Best macular d.
    vitelliform d.
Dejerine
    disease
    syndrome
Dejerine-Klumpke
    palsy
    paralysis
    syndrome
Dejerine-Landouzy
    dystrophy
Dejerine-Sottas
    atrophy
    disease
    syndrome
de Lange
    syndrome
"DeLee'd" Slang for DeLee suction
    was performed.
delinquency
delinquent
    juvenile d.
de Morsier
    syndrome
de Morsier-Gauthier
    syndrome
Dennett diet
Dennie-Marfan syndrome
Denver Developmental Screening
    Test
dermatitis (dermatitides)
    ammonia d.
    atopic d.
    diaper d.
    d. gangrenosa infantum
    napkin d.
dermatosis (dermatoses)
    juvenile plantar d.
DES—diethylstilbestrol
DES daughter
De Sanctis-Cacchione syndrome
determination
    sweat chloride d.

de Toni-Debré-Fanconi
    syndrome
de Toni-Fanconi
    syndrome
de Toni-Fanconi-Debré
    syndrome
developmental
    d. milestones
Dextrostix
diabetes
    adult-onset d.
    brittle d.
    d. insipidus
    juvenile-onset d.
    maturity-onset d. of the
        young (MODY)
    d. mellitus
    type I d.
Diamond-Blackfan
    anemia
    syndrome
diaphysis (diaphyses)
diastasis
    d. recti
diencephalic syndrome
diet
    BRAT (bananas, rice cereal,
        applesauce, toast) d.
    Dennett d.
    Moro-Heisler d.
"difenilthiorea" Phonetic for
    diphenylthiourea.
"diftherea" Phonetic for diphtheria.
dilatation
    esophageal d.
diphenylthiourea
diplegia
    atonic-astatic d.
    facial d. congenital
    flaccid d.
    Förster d.
    infantile d.
    spastic d.
dis–. See also words beginning dys–.
disease
    See also *syndrome.*
    Addison d.
    Alexander d.

disease (continued)
    Alpers d.
    Andersen d.
    anti–glomerular basement
      membrane (anti-GBM)
      antibody d.
    Apert d.
    Apert-Crouzon d.
    Aran-Duchenne d.
    Barlow d.
    Batten d.
    Batten-Mayou d.
    Beck d.
    Béguez César d.
    Best d.
    Biedl d.
    Bielschowsky-Jansky d.
    Bornholm d.
    Bourneville d.
    Bourneville-Brissaud d.
    Brown-Symmers d.
    Brushfield-Wyatt d.
    Bruton d.
    Buhl d.
    Byler d.
    Caffey d.
    Caffey-Kenny d.
    Calvé d.
    Calvé-Perthes d.
    Canavan d.
    Canavan-van Bogaert-
      Bertrand d.
    Caroli d.
    cat-scratch d.
    celiac d.
    central nervous system d.
    Chagas d.
    Cheadle d.
    Christiansen-Krabbe d.
    Coats d.
    communicable d.
    congenital d.
    Conradi d.
    Cori d.
    Crohn d.
    Crouzon d.
    cytomegalic inclusion d.
      (CID, CMID)

disease (continued)
    cytomegalic inclusion d. of
      the newborn
    cytomegalovirus d.
    Dejerine d.
    Dejerine-Sottas d.
    Dukes d.
    Duroziez d.
    Fabry d.
    factor X deficiency d.
    Farber d.
    Fede d.
    Feer d.
    fibrocystic d.
    fifth d.
    Filatov-Dukes d.
    Fölling d.
    Forbes d.
    Fordyce d.
    ganglioside storage d.
    Gaucher d.
    Gee d.
    Gee-Herter d.
    Gee-Herter-Heubner d.
    Gee-Thaysen d.
    genetotrophic d.
    glycogen storage d.
    Goldstein d.
    Graves d.
    Guinon d.
    Hailey-Hailey d.
    Hartnup d.
    Heine-Medin d.
    helminthic d.
    hemoglobin C-thalassemia d.
    hemoglobin E-thalassemia d.
    hemolytic d. of the newborn
    Henoch d.
    hereditary d.
    heredoconstitutional d.
    heredodegenerative d.
    Hers d.
    Herter-Heubner d.
    Heubner-Herter d.
    Hirschsprung d.
    Hodgkin d.
    Hünermann d.
    Huntington d.

disease (continued)
  Hutinel d.
  hyaline membrane d.
  hydatid d.
  hydrocephaloid d.
  I-cell d.
  infantile celiac d.
  Kashin-Beck d.
  Kawasaki d.
  Keshan d.
  kinky hair d.
  Krabbe d.
  Kugelberg-Welander d.
  Langdon Down d.
  Leber d.
  Legg d.
  Legg-Calvé-Perthes d.
  Legg-Calvé-Waldenström d.
  legionnaires' d.
  Leigh d.
  Leiner d.
  Letterer-Siwe d.
  Lignac d.
  Lignac-Fanconi d.
  Lindau d.
  Little d.
  Luft d.
  Lyme d.
  maple syrup urine d. (MSUD)
  Marion d.
  McArdle d.
  Meige d.
  Melnick-Needles d.
  Milroy d.
  Moeller-Barlow d.
  Morquio d.
  Niemann-Pick d.
  Norrie d.
  Oguchi d.
  Oppenheim d.
  Osler-Weber-Rendu d.
  Owren d.
  Paas d.
  Pelizaeus-Merzbacher d.
  pelvic inflammatory d.
  phytanic acid storage d.
  pink d.
  Pompe d.

disease (continued)
  Potter d.
  pulseless d.
  Ramsay Hunt d.
  Recklinghausen d.
  Refsum d.
  renal cystic d.
  Riga-Fede d.
  Ritter d.
  Sachs d.
  Sandhoff d.
  Saunders d.
  Scheuermann d.
  Schilder d.
  Scholz d.
  Scholz-Greenfield d.
  sickle cell d.
  sickle cell–hemoglobin C d.
  sickle cell–hemoglobin D d.
  sickle cell–thalassemia d.
  Sjögren d.
  Sottas d.
  Spielmeyer-Vogt d.
  spinocerebellar degenerative d.
  Stargardt d.
  Sticker d.
  Still d.
  Stuart-Prower factor deficiency d.
  Sturge-Weber-Dimitri d.
  Swift d.
  Tangier d.
  Tay-Sachs d.
  Thiemann d.
  Thomsen d.
  Trevor d.
  Underwood d.
  Unverricht d.
  van Bogaert-Bertrand d.
  van Bogaert-Nyssen-Peiffer d.
  van Buchem d.
  Vogt-Spielmeyer d.
  Volkmann d.
  von Gierke d.
  von Hippel-Lindau d.
  von Recklinghausen d.
  von Willebrand d.

disease (continued)
>Vrolik d.
>Weil d.
>Werner d.
>Wilkins d.
>Wilson d.
>Witkop-Von Sallman d.
>Wolman d.
>wooly hair d.
>Ziehen-Oppenheim d.

"disfemia" Phonetic for dysphemia.
"disfonia" Phonetic for dysphonia.
"disjenisis" Phonetic for dysgenesis.
dislocation
disorder
>aggressive behavior d.
>attention deficit d. (ADD)
>attention deficit hyperactivity d. (ADHD)
>attention deficit d. with hyperactivity (ADDH)
>eating d.
>hereditary d.
>XXX d.
>XXXX d.
>XXXXY d.
>XXXY d.
>XXYY d.

distress
>idiopathic respiratory d. of newborn

diverticula (plural of diverticulum)
diverticulae [incorrect spelling/pronunciation of diverticula]
diverticuli [incorrect spelling/pronunciation of diverticula]
diverticulum (diverticula)
>congenital d.
>Meckel d.
>pharyngeal d.

doll's eye
>sign

doll's head
>maneuver

Donohue syndrome
dot
Down [eponym]
down [lanugo]

Down [eponym]
>disease
>syndrome

DPT—diphtheria, pertussis, tetanus
DPT vaccine
DQ—developmental quotient
Dresbach
>anemia
>syndrome

drooling
DT—diphtheria [vaccine] and tetanus toxoids [vaccine]
dT—diphtheria [booster] and tetanus toxoids [vaccine]
DTP—diphtheria and tetanus (toxoids) pertussis (vaccine)
Dubois
>abscesses
>disease
>sign

Dubowitz
>evaluation
>examination
>infant maturity scale
>Neurological Assessment
>score
>syndrome

Duchenne
>muscular dystrophy

Duchenne-type muscular dystrophy
duct
>müllerian d.
>omphalomesenteric d.
>Stensen d.
>vitelline d.

ductus (ductus)
>d. arteriosus

Dukes
>disease

duodenal
>d. ileus
>d. obstruction

duplication
>d. of colon
>d. cysts
>d. of duodenum
>d. of esophagus
>d. of ileum

duplication (continued)
    d. of rectum
    d. of stomach
Duroziez
    disease
dwarf
    achondroplastic d.
    hypopituitary d.
    Laron d.
    Paltauf d.
dwarfism
    pituitary d.
Dyggve-Melchior-Clausen syndrome
dys–. See also words beginning dis–.
dysautonomia
    familial d.
dysbetalipoproteinemia
dyschondroplasia
dysdiadochokinesis
dysfunction
    placental d.
dysgenesis
    gonadal d.
dyshepatia
    lipogenic d.
dyskeratosis
    d. congenita
dyslexia
dysmaturity
dysmorphology
dysnomia
dysostosis
    cleidocranial d.
    craniofacial d.
    mandibulofacial d.
    metaphyseal d.
    d. multiplex
    orodigitofacial d.
dysphemia
dysphonia
    d. puberum
dysphonic
dysplasia
    anhidrotic ectodermal d.
    arteriohepatic d.
    bronchopulmonary d.
    camptomelic d.
    chondroectodermal d.

dysplasia (continued)
    cleidocranial d.
    congenital alveolar d.
    craniodiaphyseal d.
    craniometaphyseal d.
    cretinoid d.
    diaphyseal d.
    diastrophic d.
    ectodermal d.
    d. epiphysealis hemimelica
    d. epiphysealis punctata
    frontometaphyseal d.
    hereditary bone d.
    hidrotic ectodermal d.
    Kniest d.
    metaphyseal d.
    metatropic d.
    oculoauriculovertebral
      (OAV) d.
    oculodentodigital (ODD) d.
    ophthalmomandibulomelic d.
    polyostotic fibrous d.
    punctate epiphyseal d.
    Robinow mesomelic d.
    spondyloepiphyseal d.
    spondylometaphyseal d.
    thanatophoric d.
    thymic d.
    trichorhinophalangeal d.
dyspraxia
dystaxia
    d. cerebralis infantilis
dystonia
    d. musculorum deformans
    torsion d.
dystrophy
    Becker d.
    Becker-type muscular d.
    Duchenne d.
    Duchenne muscular d.
    Duchenne-type muscular d.
    Fröhlich adiposogenital d.
    juvenile progressive muscu-
      lar d.
    limb-girdle d.
    Meesmann d.
    muscular d.
    myotonic d.

dystrophy (continued)
    oculocerebrorenal d.
    twenty-nail d.
    X-linked muscular d.
DZ—dizygous (twins)
Eagle-Barrett syndrome
EBF—erythroblastosis fetalis
eccentrochondroplasia
eccentro-osteochondrodysplasia
ectopia
    e. cordis
    e. lentis
eczema
    dyshidrotic e.
    e. herpeticum
    infantile e.
    e. marginatum
    e. neonatorum
    e. nummulare
    e. vaccinatum
Eddowes
    disease
    syndrome
edema
    angioneurotic e.
    hereditary angioneurotic e.
      (HANE)
    e. neonatorum
EEG—electroencephalogram
    electroencephalography
"efeb–" Phonetic for words begin-
    ning epheb–.
"efelidez" Phonetic for ephelides.
"efelis" Phonetic for ephelis.
effect [noun: result, outcome]
    Somogyi e.
effusion
EGA—estimated gestational age
"egzema" Phonetic for eczema.
Ehlers-Danlos
    disease
    syndrome
Eisenmenger complex
"eksan–" Phonetic for words begin-
    ning exan–.
"eksema" Phonetic for eczema.
elastosis
    e. performans serpiginosa

electroencephalography (EEG)
electroencephalograph
elephantiasis
    congenital e.
Ellis-van Creveld syndrome
embryoma
EMG—exophthalmos, macroglos-
    sia, gigantism
emphysema
    lobar e., infantile
emulsion
    Pusey e.
encephalitis (encephalitides)
    Dawson e.
    e. neonatorum
    Schilder e.
    St. Louis e.
encephalocele
encephalomyelitis
    eastern equine e. (EEE)
    western equine e. (WEE)
encephalopathy
    demyelinating e.
    spongiform e.
encephalotrigeminal
    e. angiomatosis
enchondroma
encopresis
endocarditis
    subacute bacterial e.
endocrinopathy
enteritis
    bacterial e.
    regional e.
enterocolitis
    necrotizing e.
enteroviral
enuresis [urinary incontinence, bed-
    wetting]
    nocturnal e.
ephebiatrics
ephebic
ephebogenesis
ephebogenic
ephebology
ephelides
ephelis
epicanthal

epicanthus
epidermolysis
    e. bullosa
epididymis
epididymitis
epidural
    e. abscess
    e. empyema
    e. hemorrhage
"epifisis" Phonetic for epiphysis.
"epifizee–" Phonetic for words
    beginning epiphyse–.
epilepsia
    e. partialis continua
epilepsy
    abdominal e.
    focal e.
    grand mal e.
    jacksonian e.
    myoclonus e.
    nocturnal e.
    petit mal e.
    photosensitive e.
    psychomotor e.
    rolandic e.
    temporal lobe e.
epileptic
epileptiform
epiphyseal
epiphysis (epiphyses)
epithelioma
    e. adenoides cysticum
Epstein
    pearls
    symptom
    syndrome
epulis (epulides)
    congenital e.
    e. of newborn
Erb-Duchenne
    paralysis
Erlacher-Blount
    syndrome
eruption
    Kaposi varicelliform e.
erythroblastosis
    e. fetalis
    e. neonatorum

erythroderma
    atopic e.
    e. desquamativum
erythroleukoblastosis
esophagitis
    reflux e.
esthesioneuroblastoma
Estren-Dameshek syndrome
état
    é. marbré
evaluation
    Dubowitz e.
Ewing
    sarcoma
    tumor
examination
    Dubowitz e.
exanthem
    e. subitum
exanthema (exanthemata)
    e. subitum
"exema" Phonetic for eczema.
exomphalos
Expanded Programme on Immun-
    nization
extragonadal
Fabry
    disease
    syndrome
facies (facies)
    adenoid f.
    f. bovina, bovine f.
    cow f.
    Marshall Hall f.
    Potter f.
factor
    f. VIII
    f. X deficiency disease
    f. D
    epithelial thymic-activating f.
    f. H
    Hageman f. inhibitor
    rhesus (Rh) f.
Fallot
    disease
    pentalogy of F.
    syndrome
    tetrad

Fallot (continued)
    tetralogy of F.
    triad
    trilogy of F.
familial
    f. osteochondrodystrophy
familial hypophosphatemic bone
    disease
Fanconi
    anemia
    disease
    pancytopenia
    syndrome
Fanconi-Albertini-Zellweger syn-
    drome
Fanconi-Petrassi syndrome
Farber
    disease
    syndrome
    test
fasciitis
    eosinophilic f.
fascioscapulohumeral
Fazio-Londe
    atrophy
    disease
    syndrome
FB—foreign body
fecalith
    appendiceal f.
Fede disease
Feer disease
female pseudo-Turner syndrome
"fenil–" Phonetic for words begin-
    ning phenyl–.
"fenomenon" Phonetic for phenom-
    enon.
fetal
    f. circulation
    f. crowding
    f. distress
    f. hydrops
    f. scalp blood sampling
fetus
    acardiac f.
    harlequin f.
    viable f.

fever
    cat-scratch f.
    Colorado tick f.
    Haverhill f.
    rat-bite f.
    rheumatic f.
    Rocky Mountain spotted f.
    scarlet f.
    typhoid f.
    undulant f.
    West Nile f.
    yellow f.
Fèvre-Languepin
    syndrome
fibrillation
    atrial f.
    ventricular f.
fibroadenoma
fibrocystic disease
fibroelastosis
    endocardial f.
fibroma
    nonossifying f.
    nonosteogenic f.
fibromatogenic
fibromatoid
fibromatosis
fibromatous
fibroplasia
    retrolental f.
fibrosis
    cystic f. (CF)
fibroxanthoma
"Fifer" Phonetic for Pfeiffer.
fifth disease
"fi-ko-mi-co-sis" Phonetic for phy-
    comycosis.
Filatov-Dukes
    disease
fissure
fistula (fistulas, fistulae)
    congenital coronary f.
    congenital urethrorectal f.
FJN—familial juvenile nephroph-
    thisis
flaring
    alar f.
    nasal f.

Flatau
> disease
> syndrome

Flexner
> dysentery
> serum

flukes

fluoridation

focus (foci)
> Ghon f.
> Simon foci

"foke-mahn" Phonetic for Volkmann.

"fokomelea" Phonetic for phocomelia.

"fokt" Phonetic for Vogt.

Fölling
> disease
> phenylketonuria

fontanelle
> See also in *Neurology and Pain Management* section.
> anterior f.

foot (feet)
> cleft f.
> congenital convex club f. [pref: clubfoot]

footprint

foramen (foramina)
> f. of Bochdalek
> f. of Bochdalek hernia
> f. ovale
> f. primum
> f. secundum

foraminal

Forbes
> disease

Forchheimer spots

Fordyce
> disease

foreign body (FB)
> retained f.b. (RFB)

formula
> Berkow f.
> Hardy-Weinberg f.

fragilitas
> f. ossium

Franceschetti
> syndrome

Fraser syndrome

Freeman-Sheldon syndrome

Freiberg infraction

fretum (freta)
> f. halleri

Friedreich
> ataxia

Fröhlich (Froehlich)
> dwarfism
> syndrome

FTT—failure to thrive

α-L-fucosidase [alpha-]

fulminant

fungus (fungi)
> See specific fungi in *Laboratory, Pathology, and Chemistry Terms.*

fungus balls

funicular

funiculate

funiculi (genitive and plural of funiculus)

funiculitis

funiculus (funiculi)
> f. umbilicalis

funis

funisitis

funnel chest

FUO—fever of undetermined origin
> fever of unknown origin

"fy-ko-my-co-sis" Phonetic for phycomycosis.

galactitol

galactopyra

α-galactosidase A [alpha-]

β-galactosidase [beta-]

gamma
> g.-glutamylcysteine synthetase (deficiency)
> g.-glutamyl transpeptidase

ganglioneuromatosis

ganglioside storage disease

gangliosidosis (gangliosidoses)
> generalized g.
> GM_1 g. [GM1]
> GM_2 g. [GM2]
> GM_2 g. (types I–III)
> GM_2 g., variant AB

gangliosidosis (gangliosidoses)
(continued)
GM_2 g., variant B
GM_2 g., variant O
gargoylism
X-linked recessive g.
gas
Gasser
syndrome
Gastaut
disease
syndrome
gastroenteritis
Gaucher
disease
gavage
g. feeding
Gee disease
Gee-Herter disease
Gee-Herter-Heubner
disease
"geel duh lah too-ret" Phonetic for
Gilles de la Tourette.
"gee-naw" Phonetic for Guinon.
Gee-Thaysen disease
geminus (gemini)
gemini aequales
gene
autosomal g.
g. bank
chimeric g.
g. code
codominant g.
dominant g.
complementary g.
g. complex
lethal g.
major g.
g. mapping
marker g.
mutant g.
recessive g.
reciprocal g.
regulator g., regulatory g.
repressor g.
sex-linked g.
silent g.
suicide g.

gene (continued)
supplementary g.
tumor-suppressor g.
X-linked g.
Y-linked g.
generation time
genetic
g. code
geneticist
genetotrophic disease
genitalia [grammatically plural; no
singular form]
genu
g. valgum
geophagia
Gerstmann syndrome
Gesell developmental schedule
gestation
gestational
GFD—gluten-free diet
GH—growth hormone
GHD—growth hormone deficiency
Ghon
complex
tubercle
GH-RF—growth hormone–releasing factor
giardiasis
intestinal g.
Gierke (von Gierke)
disease
gigantism
cerebral g.
eunuchoid g.
fetal g.
hyperpituitary g.
pituitary g.
gigantoblast
Gilbert-Dreyfus syndrome
Gilbert-Lereboullet syndrome
Gilles de la Tourette
disease
syndrome
gingivitis
herpetic g.
gingivostomatitis
herpetic g.

gland
Philip g.'s
glans
glioma
pontine g.
glomerular
g. filtration rate
1,4α-glucan branching enzyme [-alpha-]
glucan-1,4α-glucosidase [-alpha-]
glucoglycinuria
α-1,4-glucosidase deficiency [alpha-]
β-glucuronidase deficiency [beta-]
γ-glutamylcysteine synthetase deficiency [gamma-]
γ-glutamyl transpeptidase [gamma-]
γ-glutamyl transpeptidase deficiency [gamma-]
glutathione
glycinuria
glycogen storage disease
Goldenhar syndrome
Goldstein
disease
hematemesis
hemoptysis
toe sign
Goltz
syndrome
Goltz-Gorlin
syndrome
gonad
gonadarche
Gorlin
syndrome
Gorlin-Chaudhry-Moss
syndrome
Gorlin-Goltz
syndrome
Gorlin-Psaume
syndrome
Gowers
sign
GPA—grade-point average
Gradenigo
syndrome
grading system
Hyams g.s.

Graefe (von Graefe)
sign
Graham Steell
murmur
grand mal
g.m. epilepsy
g.m. seizure
Granger sign
granule
Fordyce g.
granuloma
g. annulare
telangiectatic g.
grasp reflex
Greither
syndrome
Greulich and Pyle
bone age staging
Griffith classification
Grünfelder reflex
grunting
GSH—growth-stimulating hormone
GTH—gonadotropic hormone
GTT—glucose tolerance test
Guinon
disease
Günther
syndrome
guttate
g. parapsoriasis
g. psoriasis
habituation
Hadfield-Clarke syndrome
HAE—hereditary angioneurotic edema
Haemophilus
Hailey-Hailey
disease
hairball
Halbrecht syndrome
Hallgren syndrome
Hall-Pallister syndrome
hallux
h. valgus
Hanhart syndrome
haptoglobin
Hardy-Weinberg formula
harlequin fetus

Hart
    syndrome
Hartnup
    disease
    syndrome
HBW—high birthweight
HCP—hereditary coproporphyria
HE—hereditary elliptocytosis
Head [eponym]
    reflex
heart block
    Wenckebach h.b.
hebetic
Hecht
    phenomenon
    pneumonia
heelstick hematocrit
Heine-Medin disease
heliotherapy
helix (helices, helixes)
    double h.
    Watson-Crick h.
helminthic disease
hemangioma
    cavernous h.
    macular h.
hematocrit (Hct, hct)
    heelstick h.
hematoma
    extradural h.
    subdural h.
    sublingual h.
    submental h.
hemiatrophy
hemifacial microsomia
hemivertebra
hemoglobin C-thalassemia disease
hemoglobin E-thalassemia disease
hemoglobinopathy
hemolytic
    h. disease of the newborn
hemophilus
    See in *Laboratory, Patholo-*
       gy, and Chemistry Terms.
hemopneumothorax
hemorrhage
    neonatal subdural h.
    sternocleidomastoid h.

hemorrhage (continued)
    subarachnoid h.
hemorrhagic
    h. disease of newborn
    h. fever
    h. telangiectasia
Henoch
    disease
heparan-α-glucosaminide *N*-acetyl-
    transferase [-alpha-]
hepatitis (hepatitides)
    h. A
    h. B
    fulminant h.
    giant cell h.
    neonatal h.
    non-A h.
    non-B h.
hepatoblastoma
hepatomegaly
hereditary
    h. disease
heredity
    autosomal h.
    dominant h.
    sex-linked h.
heredoataxia
heredobiologic
heredoconstitutional disease
heredodegeneration
heredodegenerative disease
heredodiathesis
heredoimmunity
heredoinfection
heredolues
heredoluetic
heredopathia
    h. atactica polyneuritiformis
heredoretinopathia congenita
heredosyphilis
heredosyphilitic
Hering-Breuer reflex
heritability
Hermansky-Pudlak syndrome
hermaphroditism
hernia
    Bochdalek h.
    congenital h.

hernia (continued)
    diaphragmatic h.
    hiatal h., hiatus h.
    incarcerated h.
    inguinal h.
    Morgagni h.
    paraduodenal h.
    peritoneopericardial h.
    pleuroperitoneal h.
    retrocecal h.
    retrosternal h.
    Richter h.
    transmesenteric h.
    umbilical h.
herpes
    h. labialis
    h. neonatalis
Hers disease
Herter
    infantilism
Herter-Heubner disease
Heubner-Herter
    disease
HFI—hereditary fructose intolerance
hGH—human growth hormone
HHT—hereditary hemorrhagic
    telangiectasia
hiatal, hiatus
    h. hernia
hiatus
HIB—*Haemophilus influenzae* type b
HIB disease
HIB polysaccharide vaccine
"hipo–" Phonetic for words begin-
    ning hypo–.
Hippel-Lindau. See *von Hippel-Lin-
    dau.*
"hipsarithmea" Phonetic for hypsar-
    rhythmia.
Hirschsprung disease
hirsutism
    Apert h.
histidinuria
histiocytosis
    h. X
HIV—human immunodeficiency
    virus

HMSN—hereditary motor and sen-
    sory neuropathy
Hodgkin
    disease
Hoffa
    operation
holoprosencephaly
homocystinemia
homunculus
HOOD—hereditary osteo-onycho-
    dysplasia
hookworm
Howel-Evans
    syndrome
HPP—hereditary pyropoikilocytosis
HPV—*Haemophilus pertussis* vac-
    cine
    human papillomavirus
HS—hereditary spherocytosis
Huët-Pelger nuclear anomaly
Hünermann
    disease
Hunt
    syndrome
Hurler
    disease
    polydystrophy
    syndrome
Hurler-Scheie
    compound
    syndrome
Hutchinson
    disease
    syndrome
    triad
Hutchinson-Gilford
    disease
    syndrome
Hutinel disease
hyaline membrane disease
Hyams
    criteria
    grading system
hydatid disease
hydroa
    h. aestivale
    h. puerorum
    h. vacciniforme

hydrocephalocele
hydrocephaloid
hydrocephaloid disease
hydrocolpos
hydrometrocolpos
hydronephrosis
hydrops
    h. fetalis
hymen
    imperforate h.
hyperacidity
hyperactive
hyperactivity
hyperalphalipoproteinemia
hyperammonemia
hyperandrogenism
hyperbilirubinemia
    congenital h.
    conjugated h.
    constitutional h.
    hereditary nonhemolytic h.
    h. I
    neonatal h.
    unconjugated h.
hyperbilirubinemic
hypercalcemia
    familial hypocalciuric h.
    idiopathic h.
hypercapnia
hypercapnic
hypercholesterolemia
    familial h.
hypercholesterolemic
hypercyanotic
hyperdactyly
hyperemesis
    h. lactentium
hyperemetic
hyperexplexia
hypergenitalism
hyperglycerolemia
    infantile-type h.
    juvenile-type h.
    microdeletion-type h.
hyperglycinemia
    ketotic h.
    nonketotic h.
hypergonadism

hypergonadotropic
hyperimmunoglobulin E
hyperirritability
hyperlacticacidemia
hyperlipemia
    essential familial h.
    familial fat-induced h.
hyperlipidemia
hyperlipidemic
hyperlipoproteinemia
    familial h. (types I–V, IIa, IIb)
hyperlycinemia
hyperopia
hyperornithemia
hyperosmolar
    h. coma
hyperostosis
    infantile conical h.
hyperphalangia
hyperphenylalaninemia
    malignant h.
    persistent h.
    transient h.
hyperphonia
hyperphosphatasemia
    chronic congenital idiopath-
      ic h.
hyperplasia
    adrenal cortical h., adreno-
      cortical h.
    congenital adrenal h. (CAH)
    congenital adrenocortical h.
    Leydig cell h.
    lipoid adrenal h.
    nodular adrenal h.
    lymphoid h.
    nodular adrenocortical h.
hyperplastic
hyperprolinemia
    h., type I, type II
    familial h.
hypersegmentation
    hereditary h. of neutrophils
hyperstimulation
hypertelorism
hyperthyroxinemia
hypertonia
hypertonic

hypertonicity
hypertransfusion
hypertrophy
    septal h.
hyperventilation
hypervigilance
hyphema
hypoallergenic
hypoalphalipoproteinemia
hypocalcemia
    neonatal h.
hypocalcemic
hypocalcification
hypocapnia
hypocapnic
hypochondroplasia
hypodactyly
hypogammaglobulinemia
    acquired h.
    congenital h.
    physiologic h.
    transient h.
hypogastropagus
hypogastroschisis
hypogenesis
hypogenetic
hypogenitalism
hypoglycemic
hypognathus [noun]
hypogonadism
    familial hypogonadotropic h.
hypoisotonic
hypomelanosis
    hereditary h.
    h. of Ito
hypomyotonia
hyponatremic
hypoparathyroidism
    familial h.
hypopharynx
hypophosphatasia
hypophosphatemia
    hereditary h.
    renal h.
    X-linked h.
hypophosphatemic
hypoplasia
    craniofacial h.

hypoplasia (continued)
    h. cutis congenita
    hereditary brown h. of enamel
hypoploid
hypopotassemia
hyporeactive
hyporeflexia
hyposegmentation
hyposomatotropism
hyposomia
hypostatic
hypotelorism
hypothermia
hypothermic
hypothyroidism
    familial goitrous h.
    infantile h.
hypotonia
    benign congenital h.
    infantile h.
hypotonic
hypotrichiasis
hypotrichosis
hypoventilation
hypovolemic
hypsarrhythmia
I-cell disease
ichthyosiform
    i. erythroderma
ichthyosis
    lamellar i.
    i. linearis circumflexa
    i. vulgaris
    X-linked i.
icterus
    i. gravis neonatorum
    i. melas
    i. neonatorum
idiopathic
α-L-iduronidase deficiency [alpha-]
IEM—inborn error of metabolism
IgA deficiency
IGDM—infant of gestational dia-
    betic mother
IgM deficiency
"ikthe–" Phonetic for words begin-
    ning ichthy–.

ILB, ILBW—infant of low birthweight
ileitis
   terminal i.
ileus
   adynamic i.
   meconium i.
   paralytic i.
Imerslund
   syndrome
Imerslund-Graesbeck
   syndrome
Imerslund-Najman-Graesbeck
   syndrome
iminoglycinuria
imitate
impaction
   fecal i.
impetigo
   bullous i.
   i. contagiosa
   i. neonatorum
incompatibility
   ABO i.
   Rh i.
incompetence
   gastroesophageal i.
incontinentia
   i. pigmenti
   i. pigmenti achromians
incubation
incubator
INE—infantile necrotizing
   encephalomyelopathy
infancy
infant
infantile
   i. celiac disease
infarct
   bilirubin i
   uric acid i.
infection
   toxoplasmosis, other agents,
      rubella, cytomegalovirus,
      herpes simplex (TORCH)
      i.
infraction
   Freiberg i.

inhibitor
   factor VIII i.
iniencephalus
iniencephaly
inoculate
inspiratory
   i. stridor
insufficiency
   adrenocortical i.
   aortic i.
   pyloric i.
intelligence
   i. quotient (IQ)
intertriginous
   i. candidosis
in-toeing
intracranial
intussusception
   cecocolic i.
   colocolic i.
   ileocolic i.
   ileoileal i.
intussusceptum
intussuscipiens
IPV—inactivated poliovirus vaccine
irritability
irritable
Isolette
isovalericacidemia
Ivemark syndrome
IVSD—interventricular septal defect
JA—juvenile arthritis
jacksonian
   j. epilepsy
Jacquet
   dermatitis
   erythema
Jadassohn-Lewandowsky
   syndrome
Jadelot
   furrows
   lines
Jaksch (von Jaksch)
   anemia
Jansen
   disease
   syndrome
Jansky-Bielschowsky syndrome

jaundice
  cholestatic j.
  congenital obliterative j.
  physiologic j.
"jeel duh lah too-ret" Phonetic for
  Gilles de la Tourette.
Jeune syndrome
jitteriness
jittery
Job syndrome
Johanson-Blizzard syndrome
Johnson
  syndrome
Joseph
  syndrome
Josephs-Diamond-Blackfan syndrome
JRA—juvenile rheumatoid arthritis
Juliusberg pustulosis vacciniformis
  acuta
juvenile
  j.-onset diabetes
  j. polyposis
  j. rheumatoid arthritis
juxtamedullary
JXG—juvenile xanthogranuloma
"kalazea," "ka-la-zhuh" Phonetic
  for chalasia.
Kandori flock retina
Kanner syndrome
Kaposi
  varicelliform eruption
"karnikterus" Phonetic for kernicterus.
Kartagener
  disease
  syndrome
  triad
karyotype
Kashin-Beck disease
Kaufman pneumonia
Kawasaki
  disease
  syndrome
Kearns-Sayer syndrome
Kenny-Caffey syndrome
keratitis
  interstitial k.

keratoconus
keratoderma
  k. palmare et plantare
keratolysis
  k. neonatorum
keratoma
  k. hereditarium mutilans
keratopathy
  band k.
keratosis (keratoses)
  k. diffusa fetalis
  k. follicularis contagiosa
  k. palmaris et plantaris
"ker on sa-bo" Phonetic for coeur
  en sabot.
Keshan disease
ketoacidosis
  diabetic k.
ketotic
kg—kilogram(s)
kidney
  congenital double k.
kinky hair disease
Kinsbourne syndrome
Klippel-Feil
  malformation
  syndrome
Klippel-Feldstein syndrome
Klippel-Trenaunay-Weber syndrome
Kloepfer syndrome
Klumpke
  paralysis
Klumpke-Dejerine
  paralysis
  syndrome
Kniest dysplasia
knock-knee, knock-kneed
Kobelt
  tubes
  tubules
Kocher-Debré-Sémélaigne syndrome
Koerber-Salus-Elschnig syndrome
koilonychia
Koplik
  sign
  spots
"kor–" Phonetic for words beginning cor– and chor–.

"koriza" Phonetic for coryza.

Koschewnikow, Kozhevnikov. Variants of *Koshevnikoff.*

Koshevnikoff
    disease
    epilepsy

Kostmann
    disease
    syndrome

Krabbe
    disease
    hypoplasia
    leukodystrophy
    syndrome

Kugelberg-Welander
    disease

Kurz syndrome

KW—Kugelberg-Welander [syndrome]

kwaski
    k. shakes

kyphosis
    k. dorsalis juvenilis

lac (lacta)
    l. femininum
    l. vaccinum

lactic
    l. acid
    l. acidosis

lacticacidemia

lactivorous

lactose
    l. intolerance

Lafora
    disease
    epilepsy

Landau
    reflex
    test

Langdon Down
    disease

Langer-Giedion
    syndrome

Langer-Saldino
    syndrome

"laringoskope" Phonetic for laryngoscope.

"larinks" Phonetic for larynx.

Laron
    dwarf
    syndrome

Larsen
    syndrome

larva (larvae)
    l. currens
    l. migrans

larval

laryngeal
    l. stridor

laryngospasm

laryngotracheobronchitis

laryngotracheoesophageal

Larzel anemia

Launois
    syndrome

Launois-Cléret
    syndrome

Laurence-Biedl
    syndrome

Laurence-Moon
    syndrome

Laurence-Moon-Biedl
    law
    syndrome

lavage
    gastric l.

layer
    See *line* and *stria.*

lazy leukocyte syndrome (LLS)

LBW—low birthweight

LBWI—low-birthweight infant

Leber
    amaurosis congenita (amaurosis congenita of Leber)
    congenital amaurosis
    disease
    hereditary optic atrophy

"lee" Phonetic for Leigh.

Legg
    disease

Legg-Calvé-Perthes
    disease
    syndrome

Legg-Calvé-Waldenström
    disease

legionnaires'
 l. disease
 l. pneumonia
Leigh
 disease
 encephalopathy
 syndrome
Leiner
 disease
leiomyoma (leiomyomas, leiomyomata)
leishmaniasis
Lejeune syndrome
Lennox
 syndrome
Lennox-Gastaut
lentigo (lentigines)
 nevoid lentigines
leptotrichosis
Leredde syndrome
Léri
 sign
 syndrome
Léri-Weill syndrome
lesion
 Ghon primary l.
lethargic
Letterer-Siwe
 disease
leukemia
 aplastic l.
 basophilic l.
 eosinophilic l.
 granulocytic l.
 hemoblastic l.
 leukopenic l.
 lymphocytic l.
 lymphosarcoma cell l.
 mast cell l.
 megakaryocytic l.
 micromyeloblastic l.
 myeloblastic l.
 myelogenous l.
 Schilling l.
leukocoria
leukodystrophy
 globoid cell l.

leukoencephalitis
 concentric periaxial l.
 l. periaxialis concentrica
leukoencephalopathy
 acute hemorrhagic l.
 acute necrotizing hemorrhagic l.
 metachromatic l.
 subacute sclerosing l.
Lévi-Lorain
 dwarfism
 infantilism
 syndrome
 type
Lévy-Roussy syndrome
lice (plural of louse)
lichen
 l. nitidus
 l. planus
 l. sclerosus et atrophicus
 l. scrofulosorum
 l. simplex chronicus
 l. spinulosus
 l. striatus
Lightwood-Albright syndrome
Lignac
 disease
 syndrome
Lignac-Fanconi
 disease
 syndrome
Lindau disease
Lindau-von Hippel. See *von Hippel-Lindau.*
line
 See also *stria.*
 Beau l.
 blue l.
 Burton l.
 De Salle l.
 Jadelot l.'s
 lead l.
 nasal l.
 Trümmerfeld l.
lipidosis
lipogranulomatosis
 l. subcutanea

lipoprotein lipase (LPL) deficiency,
    familial
lithiasis
LLS—lazy leukocyte syndrome
locus (loci)
    complex l.
    operator l.
Lorain
    disease
    infantilism
Lorain-Levi
    dwarf
Lorenz
    operation
Louis-Bar
    disease
    syndrome
louse (lice)
    head l.
LOWBI—low-birthweight infant
Löwe
    disease
    syndrome
L/S—lecithin-sphingomyelin [ratio]
Luft
    disease
lupus
    neonatal l.
    transient neonatal systemic
        l. erythematosus
Lutembacher
    complex
    disease
    syndrome
luteoma
Lyell
    disease
    syndrome
Lyme
    disease
lymphadenitis
    mesenteric l.
lymphangiectasis
    congenital pulmonary l.
lymphangioma
    l. circumscriptum
    l. cysticum

lymphogranuloma
    l. inguinale
    l. venereum
lymphoreticulosis
Macewen
    sign
macrocephalous
macrocephaly
macrogenitosomia
    m. praecox
macroglobulinemia
    Waldenström m.
macula (maculae)
    mongolian m.
macular
macule
    ash-leaf m.
    lance-ovate m.
Magnus and de Kleijn neck reflexes
MAI—*Mycobacterium avium-intra-*
    cellulare
Majewski syndrome
mal
    m. de Meleda
maladie
    m. des tics ["da teek']
malaise
malformation
    Arnold-Chiari. m.
    bronchopulmonary foregut m.
    vascular m.
malrotation
mammoplasia
    adolescent m.
maneuver
    doll's head m.
α-mannosidase [alpha-]
maple syrup urine disease (MSUD)
Marchesani syndrome
Marfan
    sign
    syndrome
Marie
    syndrome (I, II)
Marinesco-Sjögren
    syndrome
Marion disease

Maroteaux-Lamy
    disease
    syndrome (I, II)
Marshall
    syndrome
Marshall Hall facies
Marshall and Tanner pubertal staging
mastitis
    m. neonatorum
mastocytoma
    solitary m.
masturbation
maturity
    m.-onset diabetes of the
        young (MODY)
Mauriac
    syndrome
McCune-Albright syndrome
MD—maternal deprivation
measles
    German m.
    three-day m.
Meckel
    cartilage
    diverticulum
    syndrome
meconium
    m. ileus
    m. peritonitis
    m. plug
    m. staining
mediastinal
    m. collagenosis
    m. lymphadenitis
    m. teratoma
medicine
    adolescent m.
    neonatal m.
medullary
    m. tube
medusae
    caput m.
Meesmann dystrophy
megacolon
    congenital m.
    m. congenitum
megalencephaly
megalocephalic

megalocephaly
megaloceros
Meige disease
melanoma
    benign juvenile m.
    juvenile m.
melanotic [pertaining to melanin]
melena
    m. neonatorum
Melkersson-Rosenthal
    syndrome
mellitus
    diabetes m.
Melnick-Needles
    disease
    osteodysplasty
    syndrome
melorheostosis
membrane
    hyaline m.
    tympanic m. (TM)
menarche
    delayed m.
meningitic
meningitis (meningitides)
meningocele
meningococcemia
Menkes
    disease
    syndrome
menometrorrhagia
menstrual
mesoblastic
mesoblastoma
    m. ovarii
    m. vitellinum
metatarsus
    m. varus
methemoglobinemia
    congenital m.
    hereditary m.
methemoglobinemic
methemoglobinuria
method
    Byrd-Dew m.
α-methylacetoacetyl CoA thiolase
    [alpha-]
Metopirone test

Mibelli
    angiokeratoma
micrencephaly
microangiopathy
    thrombotic m.
microcephalus
microcephaly
    encephaloclastic m.
    schizencephalic m.
microcheilia
microcheiria
microcnemia
microcrania
microdactyly
microdontia
microgastria
microgenitalism
micrognathia-glossoptosis syndrome
microphallus
microsomia
    m. fetalis
"miel–" Phonetic for words begin-
    ning myel–.
migraine
    familial hemiplegic m.
"miksedema" Phonetic for myxede-
    ma.
milium (milia)
    multiple eruptive milia
    m. neonatorum
Milroy
    disease
    edema
"mio–" Phonetic for words begin-
    ning myo–.
miodidymus
miopus
mischievous
mitral
    m. insufficiency
    m. stenosis
    m. valve
MMR—measles, mumps, rubella
    [vaccine]
MODY—maturity-onset diabetes of
    the young
Moeller-Barlow
    disease

molluscum
    m. contagiosum
    m. fibrosum
mongolian
    m. macule
    m. spot
mongolism
    double-trisomy m.
    translocation m.
monitor
    apnea m.
mononeuropathy
mononucleosis
    infectious m.
monoplegia
monosomy
    m. 7 syndrome
monovular
monozygosity
monozygotic
    m. twins
Moro
    embrace reflex
    reflex
    test
Moro-Heisler diet
Morquio
    disease
    sign
    syndrome
Morquio-Brailsford syndrome
Morquio-Ullrich
    disease
    syndrome
Morris syndrome
mosaicism
    haploid-diploid m.
    Turner m.
    XO/XY m.
Mounier-Kuhn
    syndrome
Mount-Reback
    syndrome
Moynahan
    syndrome (I, II)
MPS—mucopolysaccharidosis
Muckle-Wells
    syndrome

mucocutaneous
    m. candidosis
    m. leishmaniasis
mucoid
mucolipid
mucolipidosis
mucopolysaccharidosis
    (mucopolysaccharidoses) (MPS)
    m. I–XIII (MPS I–XIII)
    m. IH (MPS I H)
    m. IH/S (MPS I H/S)
    m. IS (MPS I S)
mucoviscidosis
müllerian
    m. duct
mumps
    m. meningoencephalitis
Münchausen
    by proxy syndrome
    syndrome
murmur
    continuous m.
    diastolic m.
    functional m.
    Graham Steell m.
    holosystolic m.
    pansystolic m.
    Still m.
    systolic ejection m.
mute
myasthenia
    m. gravis
    m. gravis, familial infantile
    m. gravis pseudoparalytica
    neonatal m.
mycoplasmal
myelitis
    postvaccinal m.
    m. vaccinia
myelomeningocele
myelophthisis
myoclonic
myoclonus
    startle m.
myodystrophia
    m. fetalis
myoglobinuria
    familial m.

myognathus
myokymia
    hereditary m.
myopathy
    late distal hereditary m.
    mitochondrial m.
    slow hereditary distal m.
myositis
    m. ossificans circumscripta
    m. ossificans progressiva
myotonia
    m. congenita
    m. congenita intermittens
    congenital m.
    m. hereditaria
    m. neonatorum
myotonus
myringitis
    bullous m.
myxedema
    infantile m.
MZ—monozygotic
Nager
    acrofacial dysostosis
    syndrome
Nager-De Reynier
    syndrome
nasal
    n. flaring
    n. mastocytosis
    n. polyposis
    n. septal defect
nasojejunal
nasopharyngitis
natis (nates)
    See *breech.*
NB—newborn
NBW—normal birthweight
neck
    webbed n.
necrosis (necroses)
    exanthematous n.
    subcutaneous fat n.
necrotic
necrotizing
    n. enterocolitis (NEC)
neogala
"neogaster" Phonetic for pneogaster.

neonatal thymectomy syndrome
neonate
neonatologist
neonatology
nephroblastomatosis
nephronophthisis
    familial juvenile n.
nephropathy
    reflux n.
nephrophthisis
nepiology
nesidioblastosis
Netherton
    syndrome
Nettleship
    syndrome
Nettleship-Falls–type ocular albinism
"neu–" Phonetic for words begin-
    ning pneu–.
Neumann
    syndrome
neural
    n. tube
neuritic
neuritis
neuroblastoma
neurodermatitis
neurogenic
    n. tumor
neurosyphilis
    congenital n.
    juvenile n.
neutropenia
    chronic benign n. of child-
      hood
    congenital n.
    neonatal n., transitory
nevus (nevi)
    See in *Dermatology* section.
"new–" Phonetic for words begin-
    ning pneu–.
newborn
Nezelof
    syndrome
NFTD—normal full-term delivery
NHC—neonatal hypocalcemia
NICU—neonatal intensive care unit

Niemann
    disease
    splenomegaly
Niemann-Pick
    cells
    disease
    lipid
nil
    n. disease
NO—nitric oxide
nocturnal
    n. enuresis
nodule
    Bohn n.'s
noma
    n. pudendi
    n. vulvae
Nonne-Milroy-Meige syndrome
"noo–" Phonetic for words begin-
    ning pneu–.
Noonan syndrome
Norman-Wood syndrome
normocephalic
Norrie
    disease
    syndrome
"nu–" Phonetic for words beginning
    pneu–.
nuchal
    n. rigidity
"nur–" Phonetic for words begin-
    ning neur–.
nyctalopia
OAV—oculoauriculovertebral (dys-
    plasia)
ocular
    o. hypertelorism
    o. hypotony
    o. myopathy
oculocutaneous
    o. albinism
ODD—oculodentodigital
ODD dysplasia
OFD—oral-facial-digital
    orofaciodigital
OFD dysplasia
OFD syndrome (I, II)

"ofthal–" Phonetic for words begin-
      ning ophthal–.
Oguchi disease
OI—osteogenesis imperfecta
"oksesefale" Phonetic for oxycephaly.
Ollier
      syndrome
OM—otitis media
OMPA—otitis media, purulent, acute
omphalic
omphalitis
omphalocele
omphalus
"onik–" Phonetic for words begin-
      ning onych–.
onychia
onychophagy
onychotillomania
O&P—ova and parasites
operation
      See also in *General Surgical
         Terms.*
      Hoffa o.
      Lorenz o.
ophthalmia
      gonococcal o. of newborn
      o. neonatorum
ophthalmoplegia
      congenital o.
opisthotonos
      o. fetalis
Oppenheim
      amyotonia
      disease
      syndrome
opsomyoclonus
OPV—oral poliovirus vaccine
orchidoblastoma
orchitis
      mumps o.
      o. variolosa
"orkitis" Phonetic for orchitis.
orthomyxovirus
Ortolani test
Osgood-Schlatter
      disease
      syndrome

Osler-Weber-Rendu
      disease
      syndrome
osteitis
      o. condensans generalisata
      o. fibrosa
osteoarthrosis
      o. juvenilis
osteoblastoma
osteochondritis
      o. deformans juvenilis
      o. dissecans
      o. ischiopubica
osteochondroma
osteochondrosis
      o. deformans tibiae
osteodysplasty
      o. of Melnick and Needles
osteodystrophia
      o. juvenilis
osteodystrophy
      Albright hereditary o.
      renal o.
osteoectasia
      familial o.
osteogenesis
      endochondral o.
      o. imperfecta (OI), types I–IV
      o. imperfecta congenita (OIC)
      o. imperfecta cystica
      o. imperfecta tarda (OIT)
      periosteal o.
osteoma
osteomalacia
      infantile o.
      juvenile o.
osteopathia
      o. striata
osteopenia
osteopetrosis
      o. tarda
osteopoikilosis
osteoporosis
osteoporotic
osteopsathyrosis
osteosarcoma
osteotabes
ostia (plural of ostium)

ostial [pertaining to opening, aperture, orifice]
ostium (ostia)
    persistent o. primum
    o. primum defect
    o. secundum defect
Ostrum-Furst syndrome
otalgia
otitis
    adhesive o. media
    secretory o. media
    o. externa
    exudative o. media
    o. media
    o. media, adhesive
    o. media, secretory
    serous o. media
    suppurative o. media
otorrhea
otosclerosis
out-toeing
ovarian
    o. tubes
Owren
    deficiency
    disease
oxycephalic
oxycephaly
oxygen (O)
    blow-by o.
Paas
    disease
PAC—papular acrodermatitis of childhood
    pericarditis, arthropathy, camptodactyly (syndrome)
pachyonychia
    p. congenita
Paget
    juvenile syndrome
palate
    cleft p.
palatopharyngeal
    p. incompetence
pallor
palsy
    See also *paralysis.*
    birth p.

palsy (continued)
    brachial plexus p.
    cerebral p.
Paltauf dwarf
pancreatoblastoma
pancytopenia
    congenital p.
panniculalgia
papilloma
    p. of choroid plexus
Papillon-Lefèvre syndrome
parainfluenza
paralysis (paralyses)
    See also *palsy.*
    abducens-facial p., congenital
    p. agitans, juvenile (of Hunt)
    ascending tick p.
    birth p.
    congenital abducens-facial p.
    congenital oculofacial p.
    congenital p. of horizontal gaze
    diphtheric p., diphtheritic p.
    epidemic infantile p.
    familial hyperkalemic periodic p.
    familial hypokalemic periodic p.
    familial infantile bulbar p.
    familial periodic p.
    familial recurrent p.
    familial spastic p.
    hereditary cerebrospinal p.
    infantile p.
    infantile cerebral ataxic p.
    infantile cerebrocerebellar diplegic p.
    infantile flaccid and atrophic spinal p.
    infantile spastic p.
    infantile spinal p.
    juvenile p.
    juvenile p. agitans (of Hunt)
    juvenile distal atrophic p.
    Klumpke p.
    Klumpke-Dejerine p.
    obstetric p.
    parotitic p.

paralysis (paralyses) (continued)
    Ramsay Hunt p.
    rucksack p.
    tick p.
parapertussis
paraphimosis
parasite
    See specific parasites in
    *Laboratory, Pathology,
    and Chemistry Terms.*
paratesticular
parathyromatosis
Parenti-Fraccaro syndrome
paresis
paresthesia
    Berger p.
Parrot [eponym]
    atrophy of the newborn
    disease
    nodes
    pseudoparalysis
    sign
    syndrome (I, II)
    syphilitic osteochondritis
    ulcer
pasteurizer
Pastia sign
Patau syndrome
patch
    Peyer p.'s
    salmon p.
patent
    p. ductus arteriosus (PDA)
pathogen
    See specific pathogens in
    *Laboratory, Pathology,
    and Chemistry Terms.*
Paul-Bunnell-Davidsohn
    test
pavor
    p. diurnus
    p. nocturnus
PD—pediatrics
PDA—patent ductus arteriosus
pearl
    Bohn p.'s
    Epstein p.
    perineal p.'s

pectus
    p. excavatum
ped, peds—pediatrics
pedarthrocace
pediatrician
pedicterus
pediculicides
pediculosis
    p. capitis
    p. corporis
    p. pubis
pediculous
pedobaromacrometer
pedobarometer
pedologist
pedometer
"peh-tee mahl" Phonetic for petit mal.
Pelger nuclear anomaly
Pelizaeus-Merzbacher
    disease
pellagrous
Pellizzi syndrome
pelvis (pelves)
    dwarf p.
    p. nana
    split p.
pemphigoid
    bullous p.
pemphigus
    p. vulgaris
Pendred
    disease
    syndrome
Penfield
    epilepsy
    syndrome
periarteritis
    p. nodosa
pericardial
    p. tamponade
perineal
    p. pearls
perinephritis
peritoneum
peritonitis
    meconium p.
peroneal
pes (pedes)

Peters
    anomaly
    syndrome
petit mal
petrositis
"pettee mahl" Phonetic for petit mal.
Pfeiffer
    syndrome
Pflüger
    tubes
PG—prostaglandin
PGE$_1$ [PGE1]—prostaglandin E$_1$
pH—hydrogen ion concentration
phakomata
pharyngitis
    lymphonodular p.
    purulent p.
    streptococcal p.
    viral p.
phenomenon (phenomena)
    See also *reaction, reflex,*
      sign, and *test.*
    booster p.
    dawn p.
    Debré p.
    Rumpel-Leede p.
    Somogyi p.
phenylketonuria (PKU)
    p. II
    p. III
    atypical p.
    maternal p.
Philadelphia chromosome
Philip glands
phimosis
phocomelia
phycomycosis
phytanic acid α-hydroxylase [alpha-]
phytanic acid storage disease
phytobezoar
pica
PICU—pediatric intensive care unit
Pierre Robin syndrome
pigeon
    p. breast
    p. toe
"pikno–" Phonetic for words begin-
    ning pykno–.

pileus
"pilonephritis" Phonetic for
    pyelonephritis.
pilonidal
    p. cyst
    p. dimple
    p. sinus
pilus (pili)
    pili annulati
    pili canaliculi
    pili torti, p. tortus
pinealoma
pingueculum
pink disease
pinkeye, pink eye, pink-eye
pinna
pinworm
    human p.
pityriasis
    p. alba
    p. lichenoides chronica
    p. lichenoides et vario-
      liformis acuta
    p. rosea
    p. rubra pilaris
PKU—phenylketonuria
placentitis
plantar
    p. dermatosis, juvenile
    p. reflex
    p. wart
platybasia
pleuropulmonic
plumbism
pneogaster
pneumatocele
pneumatosis
    p. cystoides intestinorum
    intestinal p.
    p. intestinalis
pneumococcal
pneumonia
    adenoviral p.
    p. alba
    aspiration p.
    bacterial p.
    chemical p.
    chlamydial p.

pneumonia (continued)
  congenital p.
  congenital aspiration p.
  eosinophilic p.
  giant cell p.
  gram-negative p.
  Hecht p.
  hypostatic p.
  intrauterine p.
  Kaufman p.
  lipoid p.
  lobar p.
  neonatal p.
  plasma cell p.
  pneumococcal p.
  rheumatic p.
  staphylococcal p.
  streptococcal p.
  thrush p.
  viral p.
  white p.
pock
pockmark
point
poison
  p. ivy
  p. oak
  p. sumac
poison control center (PCC)
poisoning
  barbiturate p.
  lead p.
  petroleum distillate p.
  phenothiazine p.
  salicylate p.
  scopolamine p.
  strychnine p.
  thallium p.
Poland
  anomaly
  syndrome
polio—poliomyelitis
poliodystrophy
polioencephalitis
  bulbar p.
polyarteritis
  p. nodosa
polydactylia

polydipsia
polydysplasia
  hereditary ectodermal p.
polydysspondylism
polydystrophic
polydystrophy
  pseudo-Hurler p.
polymicrogyria
polyp
  juvenile p.'s
  pedunculated juvenile p.
polyposis
  colonic p.
polyserositis
  familial recurrent p.
  idiopathic p.
Pompe disease
porokeratosis [compare: parakerato-sis]
porphyria
  p. cutanea tarda
  p. variegata
port wine birthmark
potbelly
Potter
  disease
  facies
PPTT—prepubertal testicular tumor
Prader-Labhart-Willi
  syndrome
precocious
precocity
prenatal
prepubertal
prickly heat
prognathism
pronate
prostaglandin (PG)
  See also in *Laboratory,
  Pathology, and Chemistry
  Terms.*
  p. E_1 [E1] (PGE_1)
proteinuria
  orthostatic p.
  postural p.
prothrombokinase
prune-belly syndrome
pseudoachondroplasia

pseudohermaphroditism
pseudo-Hurler
      disease
      polydystrophy
pseudohypertrophic
pseudomenstruation
pseudoparalysis
pseudotumor
      p. cerebri
pseudo-Turner syndrome
psittacosis
pterygium (pterygia)
      p. colli
pubarche
pubertas
      p. praecox
puberty
      delayed p.
pubescence
pubescent
pulmonary
      p. agenesis
      p. atresia
      p. fibrosis
      p. gangrene
      p. maturity
      p. surfactant
pulmonic
      p. murmur
      p. plaque
pulseless
      p. disease
pump
      breast p.
purge
purging
      bingeing and p.
purpura
      anaphylactoid p.
      p. fulminans
      p. hemorrhagica
      p. of newborn
      thrombotic p.
pustulosis
      p. vacciniformis acuta
pyknocytosis
pyrexia (pyrexiae)

rachitic
      r. metaphysis
      r. rosary
Ramsay Hunt
      disease
      syndrome
rating
      Apgar r.
ratio
      lecithin-sphingomyelin (L/S)
         r.
RDS—respiratory distress syndrome
reaction
      See also *phenomenon, reflex,*
         sign, and *test.*
      startle r.
Recklinghausen (von Recklinghausen)
      disease
      disease, central, type II
reflex
      See also *phenomenon, reac-*
         tion, sign, and *test.*
      See also in *Neurology and*
         Pain Management section.
      body-righting r.
      defense r.
      embrace r.
      fontanel r.
      gagging r.
      grasp r., grasping r.
      gripping r.
      Grünfelder r.
      Head r.
      Hering-Breuer r.
      Landau r.
      Magnus and de Kleijn neck
         r.'s
      menace r.
      Moro r.
      Moro embrace r.
      neck-righting r.
      placing r.
      righting r.
      rooting r.
      snout r.
      startle r.
      stepping r.

reflex (continued)
    sucking r.
    threat r.
    walking r.
    withdrawal r.
reflux
    gastroesophageal r. (GER)
    intrarenal r.
    r. nephropathy
    vesicoureteral r. (VUR)
    vesicoureteric r.
Refsum
    disease
    syndrome
region
    umbilical r.
regurgitation
    vesicoureteral r.
renal
    r. agenesis
    r. dysgenesis
    r. dysplasia
    r. osteodystrophy
renal cystic disease
Rendu-Osler-Weber
    disease
    syndrome
respiration
    See also in the *Pulmonary Medicine* section.
    Bouchut r.
    Kussmaul r.
respiratory
    r. arrest
    r. distress
    r. distress syndrome (RDS)
    r. insufficiency
    r. paralysis
    r. scoring system
    r. syncytial virus (RSV)
resuscitation
retardation
    mental r.
retinitis
    r. pigmentosa
retinoschisis
retraction

Rett
    syndrome
Rh—Rhesus
Rh
    antibody
    blood group
    factor
    immunization
    incompatibility
    isoantigen
rhesus (Rh)
    r. factor
rheumatic
    r. fever
    r. heart disease
    r. pneumonia
rheumaticosis
rheumatoid
    r. arthritis
    r. factor
    r. nodules
rhinitis
    r. medicamentosa
rhizomelic
Rh neg—Rhesus factor–negative
rhonchus (rhonchi)
    See in the *Pulmonary Medicine* section.
Rh pos—Rhesus factor–positive
Richards-Rundle
    syndrome
Richner-Hanhart
    syndrome
Richter hernia
rickets
Rieger
    anomaly
    dysgenesis
Riga-Fede
    disease
Riley-Day
    syndrome
Riley-Shwachman
    syndrome
Riley-Smith
    syndrome
Ritter
    disease

Robin
   anomalad
   syndrome
rocker-bottom foot
Rokitansky-Küster-Hauser syndrome
Romaña sign
"rooma–" Phonetic for words
   beginning rheuma–.
roseola
   r. infantum
rotavirus
   r. gastroenteritis
Rothmann-Makai
   syndrome
Rothmund
   syndrome
Rothmund-Thomson
   syndrome
Rotor syndrome
Roussy-Lévy
   hereditary ataxic dystasia
   syndrome
RS—respiratory syncytial
RSV—respiratory syncytial virus
rubella
rubelliform
rubeola
Rubinstein syndrome
Rubinstein-Taybi syndrome
Rud
   syndrome
Rumpel-Leede
   phenomenon
   sign
   test
Russell
   syndrome
Ruysch
   disease
sacciform
Sachs
   disease
Saethre-Chotzen syndrome
Saldino-Noonan syndrome
salicylism
salmon patch
Sandhoff
   disease

Sanfilippo
   disease
   syndrome
sarcoma (sarcomas, sarcomata)
   See also in *Oncology and*
     Hematology section.
   botryoid s., s. botryoides
   Ewing s.
sarcomphalocele
sarcosinemia
SAT—Scholastic Aptitude Test
Saunders
   disease
   sign
scale
   Apgar s.
   Bayley s. of infant develop-
     ment
   Cattell Infant Intelligence S.
   developmental s.
   Dubowitz infant maturity s.
   Gesell developmental s.'s
   Minnesota preschool s.
   Tanner developmental s.
scan
   See in *Radiology, Nuclear*
     Medicine, and Other
     Imaging section.
scaphocephaly
scarlatina
Schäfer
   syndrome
Scheuermann
   disease
   kyphosis
   syndrome
Scheuthauer-Marie-Sainton syndrome
Schick
   reaction
   sign
   test
Schiller tumor
schistosomiasis
schizophrenia
   childhood s.
Scholz
   disease
   sclerosis

Scholz-Greenfield disease
Schüller
   disease
   syndrome
Schüller-Christian
   disease
   syndrome
Schwachman syndrome
Schwartz-Jampel
   myotonia
   syndrome
scissoring
sclera (sclerae)
   blue s.
scleredema
   s. neonatorum
sclerema
   s. neonatorum
sclerosis
   tuberous s.
score
   Apgar s.
   Dubowitz s.
   Silverman s.
screening
   neonatal s.
scrofula
sculptured nose
scurvy
   hemorrhagic s.
   infantile s.
sebaceous
   s. hyperplasia
Seckel
   dwarf
   syndrome
"sefa–" Phonetic for words beginning cepha–.
Seip-Lawrence syndrome
seizure
   atonic s.
   autonomic s.
   hysterical s.
   infantile myoclonic s.
   jackknife s.
   lightning s.
   myoclonic s.
   neonatal s.

seizure (continued)
   sylvian s.
   tonic-clonic s.
   versive s.
   vertiginous s.
self-esteem
seminoma
sensory
   s. deficit
   s. loss
   s. neuropathy
   s. stimulation
septa (plural of septum)
septic
   s. arthritis
   s. shock
septum (septa)
   Douglas s.
Sertoli
   tumor
Sertoli cell–only syndrome
"sfero–" Phonetic for words beginning sphero–.
SGA—small for gestational age
shock
   anaphylactic s.
   bacteremic s.
   cardiogenic s.
   endotoxic s.
   hypovolemic s.
   insulin s.
"shogren" Phonetic for Sjögren.
shunting
   left-to-right ductus s.
Shwachman-Diamond syndrome
sialidosis
sibling
sickle cell
   s.c. anemia
   s.c. dactylitis
   s.c. disease
   s.c.–hemoglobin C disease
   s.c.–hemoglobin D disease
   s.c. hemoglobulinopathy
   s.c. nephropathy
   s.c.–thalassemia disease
   s.c. trait
SID—sudden infant death

Sidbury syndrome
SIDS—sudden infant death syndrome
sign
    See also *phenomenon, reaction, reflex,* and *test.*
    banana s.
    Bard s.
    cardiorespiratory s.
    clavicular s.
    Comby s.
    Dalrymple s.
    doll's eye s.
    double-bubble s.
    Dubois s.
    flag s.
    Galeazzi s.
    Goldstein s.
    Gorlin s.
    Graefe (von Graefe) s.
    Granger s.
    Hahn s.
    harlequin s.
    Hatchcock s.
    Higouménaki s.
    Hutchinson s.
    Kernig s.
    Koplik s.
    Krisovski s.
    Lucas s.
    Macewen s.
    Mirchamp s.
    Parrot s.
    Pastia s.
    peroneal s.
    Quant s.
    Radovici s.
    Saunders s.
    Schick s.
    Siegert s.
    Sisto s.
    Tay s.
    Tresilian s.
    Weill s.
    Wimberger s.
    Wreden s.
silicosis
Silver [eponym]
    syndrome

Silverman
    score
Silver-Russell syndrome
Silverskiöld syndrome
Similac
sin–. See also words beginning cin–, syn–.
sinobronchitis
sinus (sinus, sinuses)
    omphalomesenteric s.
    s. venosus defect
"sironosus" Phonetic for cirrhonosus.
"sitakosis" Phonetic for psittacosis.
β-sitosterolemia [beta-]
situs (situs)
    s. inversus
    s. inversus viscerum
    s. perversus
    s. transversus
Sjögren
    disease
    syndrome
Sjögren-Larsson
    syndrome
"skafo–" Phonetic for words beginning scapho–.
skeletal
    s. dysplasia
"skizo–" Phonetic for words beginning schizo–.
"sklero–" Phonetic for words beginning sclero–.
skull
    cloverleaf s.
    hot-cross-bun s.
    maplike s.
    natiform s.
    steeple s.
    tower s.
sleep apnea
    s.a. syndrome
sleeptalking
sleepwalking
Smith-Lemli-Opitz syndrome
snuffles
SOAP—Subjective, Objective, Assessment, Plan [format for medical reports]

SOM—secretory otitis media
    serous otitis media
somnambulism
Somogyi
    effect
    phenomenon
"soo-fl," "soo-flay" Phonetic for
    souffle.
Sotos syndrome
Sottas disease
souffle
    fetal s.
    funic s., funicular s.
    umbilical s.
sound
    cracked-pot s., cranial
Spanlang-Tappeiner syndrome
spasm
    infantile massive s.'s
spasmus
    s. nutans
spasticity
spherocytosis
sphingolipidosis
    cerebral s.
    late-onset cerebral s.
Spielmeyer-Vogt disease
spina (spinae)
    s. bifida
    s. bifida anterior
    s. bifida aperta
    s. bifida cystica
    s. bifida manifesta
    s. bifida occulta
    s. bifida posterior
spinocerebellar degenerative disease
spirochetal
spleen
    accessory s.
spondylitis
    ankylosing s.
spongioblastoma
sporotrichosis
sporotrichotic
spot
    blue s.
    Brushfield s.
    Forchheimer s.

spot (continued)
    Fordyce s.
    Koplik s.'s
    mongolian s.
    sacral s.
Sprengel deformity
Spurway syndrome
squint
SSSS—staphylococcal scalded skin
    syndrome
staging
    Greulich and Pyle bone age s.
stammering
Stargardt
    disease
    syndrome
starvation
status
    s. asthmaticus
    s. epilepticus
    s. lymphaticus
    s. marmoratus
    s. thymicolymphaticus
    s. thymicus
steatorrhea
    idiopathic s.
Steinbrinck anomaly
Stein-Leventhal
    syndrome
Stellwag sign
stenosis (stenoses)
    anorectal s.
    antral s.
    aortic s. (AS)
    aqueductal s.
    congenital aortic s.
    congenital hypertrophic
        pyloric s.
    esophageal s.
    hypertrophic s.
    infundibular s.
    mitral s.
    postischemic s.
    pulmonic s.
    pyloric s.
    valvular pulmonic s.
Sticker
    disease

Still
   disease
   murmur
Still-Chauffard syndrome
Stilling
   syndrome
Stilling-Türk-Duane syndrome
stimulants [a class of drugs]
St. Louis encephalitis
Stock-Spielmeyer-Vogt syndrome
stomatocytosis
stool
   acholic s.
   currant jelly s.
"stooling" Slang for defecating.
"stooled" Slang for defecated.
strabismus
strawberry mark
streptococcal groups A, B, G
streptococcosis
stria (striae)
   See also *line*.
   striae albicantes
   striae atrophicae
striatal
stricture
   esophageal s.
stridor
   congenital laryngeal s.
   inspiratory s.
   laryngeal s.
strophulus
Stuart-Prower factor deficiency disease
Sturge
   disease
   syndrome
Sturge-Weber
   disease
   encephalotrigeminal
      angiomatosis
   syndrome
Sturge-Weber-Dimitri disease
stuttering
St. Vitus dance
submucous
   s. cleft
subphrenic

sucking reflex
"sudo–" Phonetic for words beginning pseudo–.
sulfhemoglobinemia
Sulzberger-Garbe syndrome
Sutton-Rendu-Osler-Weber
   syndrome
Swift disease
swimmer's
   s. ear
Swyer
   syndrome
Swyer-James
   syndrome
Swyer-James-Macleod
   syndrome
symptom
   Epstein s.
syn–. See also words beginning cin–, sin–.
synchondrosis (synchondroses)
   costoclavicular s.
   synchondroses of cranium
   pubic s., s. pubis
   sacrococcygeal s.
   synchondroses of skull
   sternal s., s. sternalis
syndactyly
syndrome
   See also *disease*.
   Aarskog s.
   Aarskog-Scott s.
   Abderhalden-Fanconi s.
   Abt-Letterer-Siwe s.
   Adie s.
   adrenogenital s.
   Albers-Schönberg s.
   Albright s.
   Aldrich s.
   Alice in Wonderland s.
   Alport s.
   Andogsky s.
   Arnold-Chiari s.
   asplenia s.
   BADS s.
   Ballantyne s.
   Ballantyne-Runge s.
   Banti s.

syndrome (continued)
    Bartter s.
    Bassen-Kornzweig s.
    battered child s.
    Beckwith s.
    Beckwith-Wiedemann s.
    Bielschowsky s.
    blind loop s.
    Bloch-Sulzberger s.
    Bloom s.
    blue diaper s.
    Bodian-Schwachman s.
    Bonnevie-Ullrich s.
    Bourneville s.
    Bourneville-Pringle s.
    Brachmann-de Lange s.
    Brandt s.
    bronze baby s.
    Brushfield-Wyatt s.
    Budd-Chiari s.
    Caffey-Silverman s.
    Caffey-Smyth-Roske s.
    Calve-Legg-Perthes s.
    Camurati-Engelmann s.
    carcinoid s.
    Carpenter s.
    cat's cry s.
    Chapple s.
    Charcot-Marie-Tooth-Hoff-
       mann s.
    Chédiak-Higashi s.
    Chilaiditi s.
    Christ-Siemens-Touraine s.
    Clarke-Hadfield s.
    cloverleaf skull deformity s.
    clumsy child s.
    Cockayne s.
    concussion s.
    Cornelia de Lange s.
    craniosynostosis-radial apla-
       sia s.
    cri-du-chat s.
    cri du chat [cat's cry] s.
    Crigler-Najjar s.
    cryptophthalmos s.
    cushingoid s.
    Dandy-Walker s.
    Danlos s.

syndrome (continued)
    Darrow-Gamble s.
    Debré-de Toni-Fanconi s.
    Debré-Semelaigne s.
    de Lange s.
    de Morsier s.
    de Morsier-Gauthier s.
    Dennie-Marfan s.
    Denny-Brown s.
    De Sanctis-Cacchione s.
    DES (diethylstilbestrol) s.
    de Toni-Debré-Fanconi s.
    de Toni-Fanconi s.
    de Toni-Fanconi-Debré s.
    Diamond-Blackfan s.
    diencephalic s.
    DiGeorge s.
    Donohue s.
    Down s.
    Duane s.
    Dubin-Johnson s.
    Dubowitz s.
    duplication-deficiency s.
    Dyggve-Melchior-Clausen s.
    dystocia-dystrophia s.
    Eagle-Barrett s.
    ectrodactyly-ectodermal dys-
       plasia-clefting (EEC) s.
    EEC s.
    Ehlers-Danlos s.
    elfin facies s.
    Ellis-van Creveld s.
    EMG s.
    empty sella s.
    epiphyseal s.
    Erlacher-Blount s.
    E_1 [E1] trisomy s.
    faciodigitogenital s.
    Fanconi s.
    Fanconi-Albertini-Zellweger
       s.
    Fanconi-Petrassi s.
    fetal alcohol s.
    fetal aspiration s.
    fetal distress s.
    Fèvre-Languepin s.
    floppy infant s.
    focal dermal hypoplasia s.

syndrome (continued)
    fragile X s.
    Franceschetti s.
    G s.
    Gardner s.
    Gasser s.
    gasserian s.
    Gee-Herter-Heubner s.
    Gerstmann s.
    Gianotti-Crosti s.
    Gilbert-Dreyfus s.
    Gilbert-Lereboullet s.
    Gilles de la Tourette s.
    Glanzmann s.
    Goltz s.
    Goltz-Gorlin s.
    gonadal agenesis s.
    Goodpasture s.
    Gorlin-Chaudhry-Moss s.
    Gorlin-Goltz s.
    Gorlin-Psaume s.
    Gradenigo s.
    gray s.
    gray baby s.
    Greither s.
    Guillain-Barré s.
    Günther s.
    Hakim s.
    Hallermann-Streiff s.
    Hallervorden-Spatz s.
    Hall-Pallister s.
    Hamman-Rich s.
    hand-foot s.
    Hand-Schüller-Christian s.
    Hanhart s.
    Hart s.
    Hartnup s.
    hemolytic-uremic s.
    hereditary benign intraep-
      ithelial dyskeratosis s.
    Hermansky-Pudlak s.
    Holt-Oram s.
    Hunter s.
    Hurler s.
    Hutchinson s.
    Hutchinson-Gilford s.
    17-hydroxylase deficiency s.
    hypoplastic left heart s.

syndrome (continued)
    hypotonic infant s.
    idiopathic respiratory dis-
      tress s.
    Imerslund s.
    Imerslund-Graesbeck s.
    Imerslund-Najman-Graes-
      beck s.
    inspissated milk s.
    Ivemark s.
    Jansen s.
    Jansky-Bielschowsky s.
    Jervell and Lange-Nielsen s.
    Job s.
    Johanson-Blizzard s.
    Joseph s.
    Kallmann s.
    Kanner s.
    Kartagener s.
    Kasabach-Mcrritt s.
    Kearns-Sayre s.
    Kenny-Caffey s.
    keratitis-ichthyosis-deafness
      (KID) s.
    KID s.
    kinky hair s.
    Kinsbourne s.
    kleeblattschädel (cloverleaf
      skull) s.
    Klinefelter s.
    Klippel-Feil s.
    Kloepfer s.
    Kocher-Debré-Sémélaigne s.
    Koerber-Salus-Elschnig s.
    Kugelberg-Welander s.
    Landry-Guillain-Barré s.
    Langer-Giedion s.
    Langer-Saldino s.
    Laron s.
    Larsen s.
    Launois s.
    Launois-Cléret s.
    Laurence-Biedl s.
    Laurence-Moon s.
    Laurence-Moon-Biedl s.
    Lennox s.
    Lennox-Gastaut s.
    leopard s., LEOPARD s,

syndrome (continued)
  Léri-Weill s.
  Lesch-Nyhan s.
  Lévy-Roussy s.
  Lightwood-Albright s.
  Lignac s.
  Lignac-Fanconi s.
  Löffler s.
  Louis-Bar s.
  Löwe s.
  Lutembacher s.
  Maffucci s.
  Majewski s.
  malabsorption s.
  Mallory-Weiss s.
  Marchesani s.
  Marfan s.
  Marie s. (I, II)
  Marinesco-Sjögren s.
  Maroteaux-Lamy s.
  maternal deprivation s.
    (MDS)
  Mauriac s.
  McCune-Albright s.
  meconium plug s.
  Melkersson-Rosenthal s.
  Menkes s.
  methionine malabsorption s.
  Minkowski-Chauffard s.
  Möbius s.
  Morquio s.
  Morquio-Ullrich s.
  Muckle-Wells s.
  multiple lentigines s.
  neonatal thymectomy s.
  nephrotic s.
  Netherton s.
  Nettleship s.
  Neumann s.
  Nezelof s.
  Noonan s.
  oculoauriculovertebral
    (OAV) s.
  oculodentodigital (ODD) s.
  ODD s.
  OFD s. (types I–III)
  Ollier s.
  OMM s.

syndrome (continued)
  OPD s.
  ophthalmomandibulomelic
    (OMM) s.
  oral-facial-digital, orofa-
    ciodigital (OFD) s. (types
    I–III)
  Osgood-Schlatter s.
  otopalatodigital s.
  Paget juvenile s.
  pancreatic insufficiency s.
  Papillon-Lefevre s.
  Parenti-Fraccaro s.
  Patau s.
  Pellizzi s.
  Pendred s.
  Peutz-Jeghers s.
  PHC s.
  pickwickian s.
  Pierre Robin s.
  placental dysfunction s.
  Poland s.
  postperfusion s.
  Prader-Willi s.
  prune-belly s.
  pseudo-Turner s.
  Ramsay Hunt s.
  Reifenstein s.
  Rendu-Osler-Weber s.
  respiratory distress s. (RDS)
  respiratory distress s. (RDS)
    of newborn
  Rett s.
  Reye s.
  Richner-Hanhart s.
  Riley-Day s.
  Riley-Shwachman s.
  Riley-Smith s.
  Rothmann-Makai s.
  Rothmund s.
  Rothmund-Thomson s.
  Rotor s.
  Roussy-Lévy s.
  Rubinstein s.
  Rubinstein-Taybi s.
  Rud s.
  Russell s.
  Saldino-Noonan s.

syndrome (continued)
Sanfilippo s.
scalded skin s., nonstaphylo-
coccal
scalded skin s., staphylococ-
cal
Schäfer s.
Scheie s.
Scheuthauer-Marie-Sainton s.
Schwartz-Jampel s.
sebaceous nevus s.
Seip-Lawrence s.
shaken baby s.
Shwachman s.
Shwachman-Diamond s.
sicca s.
sick cell s.
sick sinus s. (SSS)
Silver s.
Silver-Russell s.
Sipple s.
Sjögren s.
Sjögren-Larsson s.
sleep apnea s.
slick-gut s.
small left colon s.
Sotos s.
stagnant loop s.
Stargardt s.
Steinert myotonic dystrophy
s.
Stein-Leventhal s.
Stevens-Johnson s.
Still-Chauffard s.
Stilling-Türk-Duane s.
Stock-Spielmeyer-Vogt s.
Sturge-Weber s.
sudden infant death s. (SIDS)
Sutton-Rendu-Osler-Weber s.
Swyer s.
Swyer-James s.
testicular feminizing s.
thrombocytopenia-absent
radius (TAR) s.
TORCH (toxoplasmosis,
other agents, rubella,
cytomegalovirus, herpes
simplex) s.

syndrome (continued)
Tourette s.
toxoplasmosis, other agents,
rubella, cytomegalovirus,
herpes simplex (TORCH)
s.
Treacher Collins s.
Treacher Collins-
Franceschetti s.
trisomy 21 s.
trisomy C s.
trisomy D s.
trisomy E s.
Turner s.
Vogt s.
Waardenburg s.
Waterhouse-Friderichsen s.
Watson-Alagille s.
Weber-Christian s.
Weill-Marchesani s.
Werdnig-Hoffmann s.
Wermer s.
Werner s.
West s.
Whipple s.
Wiedemann s.
Willebrand-Jürgens s.
Williams s.
Wilson-Mikity s.
Wiskott-Aldrich s.
Wolff-Parkinson-White s.
(WPW)
Wolfram s.
X-linked lymphoprolifera-
tive s.
XXY s.
Young s.
Zellweger s.
Zinsser-Engman-Cole s.
Zollinger-Ellison s. (ZES)
synostosis (synostoses)
cranial s.
sagittal s.
tribasilar s.
syphilis
congenital s.
s. hereditaria tarda

tabes
    hereditary t.
    t. infantum
    t. mesaraica
    t. mesenterica
tabetic
tachycardia
    paroxysmal t.
taeniasis
"takekardea" Phonetic for tachycardia.
talcum
talipes
    t. calcaneovalgus
    t. cavus
    t. equinovarus
Tangier disease
Tanner
    developmental scale
    stages (I–V)
TAR—thrombocytopenia–absent
    radius [syndrome]
Taussig-Bing
    disease
    malformation
    syndrome
Tay-Sachs disease
TD—tetanus-diphtheria [vaccine—
    pediatric initial dose]
teething
Teilum tumor
telangiectasis (telangiectases)
teratic
teratism
teratoblastoma
teratocarcinoma
teratoma (teratomas, teratomata)
    sacrococcygeal t.
teratomatous
Terry syndrome
test
    See also *phenomenon, reaction, reflex,* and *sign.*
    See also in *Laboratory, Pathology, and Chemistry Terms.*
    Apgar t.
    Binet t.

test (continued)
    Binet-Simon t.
    Coombs t.
    Farber t.
    Frei t.
    Guthrie t.
    Landau t.
    leucine tolerance t.
    Metopirone t.
    Monospot t.
    Mono-Vac t.
    Moro t.
    mumps skin t.
    Ortolani t.
    Paul-Bunnell-Davidsohn t.
    Sabin-Feldman dye t.
    Schick t.
    Schilling t.
    sweat t.
    tine t., tine tuberculin t.
      (Rosenthal)
testes (plural of testis)
testicular
testis (testes)
    abdominal t.
    inguinal t.
    undescended t.
tetanus
    t. neonatorum
tetany
tetralogy
    t. of Fallot
tetraploidy
thalassemia
    t. intermedia
    t. major
    t. minor
thelalgia
thelarche
therapy
    aerosol t.
    gene t.
    light t.
    liquid air t.
    photodynamic t.
thermometer
    axilla t.
    infrared tympanic t.

thermometer (continued)
    oral t.
    rectal t.
    tympanic t.
Thiemann disease
Thompson
    syndrome
Thomsen
    disease
Thomson
    disease
    poikiloderma congenitale
thorax (thoraces)
thrombocytopenia
    idiopathic t.
thrush
thumbsucking
thymectomy
    neonatal t. syndrome
thyroglossal
thyroiditis
tic
tick paralysis
time (T)
    generation t.
    tincture of t.
tinea
    t. capitis
    t. corporis
    t. cruris
    t. nigra palmaris
    t. pedis
    t. unguium
    t. versicolor
tissue
    t. factor
titer
    antistreptolysin t.
    toxoplasmosis, other agents,
      rubella, cytomegalovirus,
      herpes simplex (TORCH)
      t.
toeing-in
toeing-out
toewalking
tongue
    lobulated t.
    t.-tie, t.-tied

tonsillar
tonsillectomy
tonsillitis
    white t.
tonsillopharyngitis
"too-mur" Phonetic for tumeur.
"too-ret" Phonetic for Tourette.
toothache
TOPV—trivalent oral poliovirus
    vaccine
TORCH—toxoplasmosis, other
    agents, rubella, cytomegalovi-
    rus, herpes simplex [syndrome]
TORCH
    infection
    titer
torticollis
    infantile t.
Tourette (Gilles de la Tourette)
    disease
    syndrome
tracheobronchial
tracheobronchitis
tracheobronchomegaly
tracheomalacia
trachoma (trachomata)
trait
    sickle cell t.
    thalassemia t.
transfusion
    exchange t.
translocation
    t. Down syndrome
transposition
    t. of great vessels
trauma (traumas, traumata)
    birth t.
    perinatal t.
Treacher Collins
    syndrome
Treacher Collins-Franceschetti
    syndrome
treatment
    light t.
treponematosis
Trevor
    disease
trichobezoar

trichorrhexis
    t. invaginata
    t. nodosa
trichuriasis
tricuspid
    t. atresia
    t. insufficiency
trigonocephaly
trismus
    t. nascentium
    t. neonatorum
trisomy
    t. 8 syndrome
    t. 9, 9p
    t. 11q syndrome
    t. 13 syndrome
    t. 13-15
    t. 13-15 D
    t. 16-18
    t. 18 E
    t. 18 syndrome
    t. 21 syndrome
    t. 22 syndrome
    t. C syndrome
    t. D syndrome
    t. E syndrome
truncate
truncus (trunci)
    t. arteriosus
tryptophanuria
tsp.—teaspoon(s), teaspoonful
tube
    cerebromedullary t.
    Kobelt t.'s
    medullary t.
    neural t.
    ovarian t.'s
    Pflüger t.'s
tuber (tubers, tubera)
tubercle
    Ghon t.
tuberculate, tuberculated
tuberculation
tuberculitis
tuberculization
tuberculoid
tuberculoma

tuberculosis (TB)
    abdominal t.
    childhood t.
    extrathoracic t.
    gastrointestinal t.
    intrathoracic t.
    miliary t.
    papulonecrotic t.
    t. papulonecrotica
    pulmonary t.
tuberculous
    t. dactylitis
    t. keratoconjunctivitis
    t. meningitis
    t. peritonitis
    t. spondylitis
tuberous
    t. sclerosis
tularemia
tumeur
    t. pileuse
tumor
    Ewing t.
    germ cell testicular t.
    granulosa cell t.
    Leydig cell t.
    pineal t.
    pontine t.
    Schiller t.
    Sertoli t.
    Teilum t.
    theca cell t.
    vitelline t.
    Wilms t.
    yolk sac t.
tunica (tunicae)
Turner
    familial syndrome
    male syndrome
    phenotype with normal
      karyotype
    syndrome
    syndrome in females with
      normal X chromosome
Turner-Keiser
    syndrome
twin
    acardiac t.

twin (continued)
    allantoidoangiopagous t.'s
    binovular t.'s
    conjoined t.
    dichorial t.'s
    dichorionic t.'s
    dissimilar t.'s
    dizygotic t.
    enzygotic t.'s
    false t.'s
    fraternal t.
    heterologous t.'s
    hetero-ovular t.'s
    identical t.
    impacted t.'s
    monoamniotic t.'s
    monochorial t.'s
    monochorionic t.'s
    mono-ovular t.'s, monovular
      t.'s
    monozygotic t.
    omphaloangiopagous t.'s
    one-egg t.'s
    parabiotic t.'s
    parasitic t.
    placental parasitic t.
    Siamese t.'s
    similar t.'s
    true t.'s
    two-egg t.'s
    uniovular t.'s
    unlike t.'s
twinship
tympanites
typhoid
tyrosinosis ulcer
    aphthous u.
    Curling u.
    Cushing-Rokitansky u.
    duodenal u.
    peptic u.
UCD, UChD—usual childhood dis-
    eases
Uhl anomaly
Ullrich
    syndrome
Ullrich-Feichtiger
    syndrome

Ullrich-Turner
    syndrome
umbilicus
Underwood disease
undescended testis
Undritz anomaly
unit
    See also in *General Medical*
      Terms and *Laboratory,*
      Pathology, and Chemistry
      Terms.
    map u.
    morgan u. (M)
    neonatal intensive care u.
      (NICU)
Unna
    disease
    syndrome
Unverricht
    disease
    myoclonia
    syndrome
urachal
urachus
    patent u.
ureterocele
ureteropelvic
urethra
urinary
    u. bladder
    u. tract infection
    u. voiding
urinoma
urolithiasis
urticaria
USN—ultrasonic nebulizer
uveitis
uveokeratitis
UVL—ultraviolet light
uvulitis
Uyemura syndrome
vaccines [a class of drugs]
van Bogaert-Bertrand disease
van Bogaert-Divry syndrome
van Bogaert-Nyssen-Peiffer disease
van Bogaert-Scherer-Epstein syn-
    drome

van Buchem
    disease
    syndrome
van der Hoeve
    syndrome
van der Hoeve-de Kleyn
    syndrome
varicella
    v. bullosa
    v. gangrenosa
    v. inoculata pustulosa
    vaccination v.
    v.-zoster immune globulin
      (VZIG)
varioliform
VASC—Verbal Auditory Screen for
    Children
venereal
ventricular
    v. septal defect
ventriculogram
vernix
    v. caseosa
verruca (verrucae)
    v. plana juvenilis
verrucous
vertebra (vertebrae)
vertebral
vesicobullous
vesicoureteral
    v. reflux (VUR)
    v. regurgitation
vestige
viable
    v. birth
    v. fetus
virus
    See also in *Laboratory,*
      Pathology, and Chemistry
      Terms.
    Coxsackie v. [now: coxsack-
      ievirus]
    ECHO 28 v.
    herpes simplex v. (HSV)
    influenza v.
    measles v.
    newborn pneumonitis v.
    respiratory syncytial v. (RSV)

virus (continued)
    RS (respiratory syncytial) v.
    rubella v.
vitreoretinopathy
    familial exudative v.
Vogt
    syndrome
Vogt-Spielmeyer
    disease
Vohwinkel syndrome
Volkmann
    deformity
    disease
Voltolini
    disease
volvulus
    v. of colon
    gastric v.
    v. neonatorum
vomiting
    projectile v.
von Bezold. See *Bezold.*
von Hippel-Lindau
    disease
    syndrome
von Jaksch. See *Jaksch.*
von Recklinghausen. See *Reckling-*
    hausen.
von Willebrand (Willebrand)
    disease
    syndrome
Vrolik disease
VZIG—varicella-zoster immune
    globulin
Waardenburg
    disease
    syndrome
wart
    plantar w.
Watson-Alagille syndrome
WC—whooping cough
weaning
webbing
    congenital w. of neck
weight
    birth w. [pref: birthweight]
Weil
    disease

Weill
   sign
Weill-Marchesani
   syndrome
Weinstein syndrome
Werdnig-Hoffmann
   atrophy
   disease
   paralysis
   syndrome
Werner
   disease
   syndrome
Wernicke aphasia
West
   skull
   spasm
   syndrome
wheezing
whooping cough
WIC—Women, Infants, and Children [a government assistance program]
Wiedemann syndrome
Wildervanck syndrome
Wilkins disease
Willebrand. See *von Willebrand.*
Willebrand-Jürgens
   syndrome
Williams
   syndrome
Williams-Campbell syndrome
Wilms tumor
Wilson-Mikity syndrome
Witkop-Von Sallman disease
Wolf
   syndrome
Wolfram
   syndrome
Wolman disease
wooly hair disease
Wreden sign
wryneck

xanthinuria
xanthinuric
xanthism
xanthochromia
xanthogranulomatosis
xanthogranulomatous
xanthoma (xanthomas, xanthomata)
   juvenile x.
xanthosis
   x. cutis
xanthurenic
   x. aciduria
X chromatin
xeroderma
   x. pigmentosum
xerography
xerosis
   x. conjunctiva
   x. corneae
X-linked
   X.-l. hypogammaglobulinemia
   X.-l. recessive inheritance
xylulose dehydrogenase deficiency
Y chromatin
yolk sac carcinoma
Young
   syndrome
"zero–" Phonetic for words beginning xero–.
"zheel-bare" Phonetic for Gilbert [Nicolas Augustin Gilbert].
"zheel duh lah too-ret" Phonetic for Gilles de la Tourette.
Ziehen-Oppenheim
   disease
Zinsser-Cole-Engman
   syndrome
Zinsser-Engman-Cole
   syndrome
zoster
zygodactyly
zygote

Plastic Surgery

AB—axiobuccal
Abbe
    cheiloplasty (stage I, stage II)
    lip flap
    operation
Abbe-Estlander
    cheiloplasty
    operation
ABC—axiobuccocervical
abdominoplasty
    Mladick a.
ABG—axiobuccogingival
ABL—axiobuccolingual
AC—axiocervical
AD—axiodistal
adamantoblastoma
Adams
    operation
ADC—axiodistocervical
ADG—axiodistogingival
adherence
    graft a.
adhesion
    sublabial a.
adhesive
    cyanoacrylate a.
adipectomy
adipocele
admaxillary
advancement
    a. flap
    maxillary a.
Aeby
    muscle
    plane
AG—axiogingival
agnathia
agnathous
agnathus
"ahn mahs" Phonetic for en masse.
AI—axioincisal

akinesia
    Van Lint a.
AL—axiolingual
ala (alae)
    a. nasi
alar
Albinus muscle
Albrecht
    bone
    suture
alloplastic
alloplasty
allotriodontia
Allport
    operation
Alsus-Knapp
    operation
alveolar
    a. arch
    a. ridge
alveolectomy
    transseptal a.
alveololabial
alveololabialis
alveololingual
alveolomerotomy
alveolonasal
alveolopalatal
alveoloplasty
    interradicular a.
    intraseptal a.
alveolotomy
alveolysis
Alvis
    operation
ameloblastoma
    acanthomatous a.
    basal cell a.
    cystic a.
    extraosseous a.
    follicular a.

ameloblastoma (continued)
    granular cell a.
    malignant a.
    multicystic a.
    peripheral a.
    plexiform a.
    plexiform unicystic a.
    solid a.
    unicystic a.
Ammon
    blepharoplasty
    canthoplasty
    dacryocystotomy
    filaments
    fissure
    operation
anaplasty
anaplerosis
Angelucci
    operation
angle
    antegonial a.
    Bennett a.
    cheilar a.
    conchal mastoid a.
    Frankfort-mandibular plane a.
    scaphoconchal a.
ankyloblepharon
ankylocheilia
ankylotomy
anomalad
anomaly
    Pierre Robin a.
antegonial
    a. angle
    a. notch
anterior
    a. palatine suture
anthelix
Antia-Busch chondrocutaneous flap
antitragus
antra (plural of antrum)
antrectomy
antrostomy
    intranasal a.
    radical maxillary a.
antrotomy
    sublabial a.

antrum (antra)
AP—axiopulpal
apertognathia
    Le Fort a. repair (I)
aperture
    pharyngeal a.
"aplooshahzh" Phonetic for
    épluchage.
approach
    transnasal a.
    transseptal a.
aqueduct
    fallopian a.
arch
    maxillary a.
    palatine a.
    zygomatic a.
area (areae, areas)
    donor a.
    Kiesselbach a.
Argamaso-Lewin composite flap
Aries-Pitanguy
    mammaplasty
    operation
    procedure
Arlt (von Arlt)
    operation
Ashford
    mamilliplasty
    mammaplasty
    retracted nipple operation
Assézat triangle
ATL—antitension line
Auchincloss
    modified radical mastectomy
augmentation
    a. mammaplasty
    a. rhinoplasty
autocystoplasty
autograft
autografting
avulsion
BAC—buccoaxiocervical
Bakamjian flap
Baker
    velum
bar
    fixation arch b.

Barsky operation
basifacial
basihyoid
Battle
    operation
B-B graft
BC—buccocervical
BD—buccodistal
beak
    b. of sphenoid bone
Beard-Cutler
    operation
Becker operation
Begg
    light-wire differential force
      technique
    paralleling
    torque
Bell
    nerve
    operation
Bennett
    angle
    movement
Berke
    operation
Berke-Motais
    operation
Bernard-Burrows
    operation
Bertin
    bone
    ossicles
BG—buccogingival
B graft
BI—burn index
Bichat
    fat pad
    protuberance
Biesenberger
    mammaplasty
    operation
Binnie
    operation
Biobrane
    adhesive
    glove
    synthetic skin substitute

Biograft
BL—buccolingual
Blair
    operation
Blair-Brown
    graft
    operation
Blaskovics
    operation
"blef–" Phonetic for words begin-
    ning bleph–.
blepharal
blepharectomy
blepharelosis
blepharism
blepharoatheroma
blepharochalasis
blepharoplasty
    Ammon b.
blepharoptosis
blepharorrhaphy
blepharostat
BM—buccomesial
Bochdalek
    ganglion
    muscle
body (bodies)
    b. of mandible
    b. of maxilla
    b. of sphenoid
Bondy
    mastoidectomy
bone
    malar b.
    maxillary b.
    sesamoid b.
Boo-Chai craniofacial cleft
border
    See also *margin.*
    mucocutaneous b.
    vermilion b.
Borges and Alexander line
bow
    cupid's b.
    labial b.
    Logan b.
bowl
    mastoid b.

Brauer
  operation
Braun
  graft
  operation
Braun-Wangensteen
  graft
  operation
breast
  supernumerary b.
Brent eyebrow reconstruction
bridge
  b. flap
Brophy
  operation
Brown
  operation
Brown-Blair
  operation
Bruner line
BSA—body surface area
BSB—body surface burned
buccal
  b. mucosa
  b. smear
buccally
buccolingually
bulla (bullae)
  b. ethmoidalis cavi nasi
  b. ethmoidalis ossis eth-
    moidalis
bullate
bullation
bundle
  neurovascular b.
Bunnell
  flap
burn
  chemical b.
  first-degree b.
  flash b.
  fourth-degree b.
  full-thickness b.
  high-tension b.
  immersion b.
  partial-thickness b.
  powder b.
  second-degree b.

burn (continued)
  third-degree b.
Burow
  See also *von Burow.*
  operation
  triangle
B-W graft
CA—cervicoaxial
canal
  pterygopalatine c.
  zygomatico-orbital c.
canine
canthoplasty
  Ammon c.
capillarectasia
capillaritis
capillaropathy
capsule
  cricoarytenoid articular c.
Carabelli
  cusp
  sign
  tubercle
carcinoma (carcinomas, carcinomata)
  See in *Oncology and Hema-
    tology* section.
cartilage
  alar c.
  septal c.
  sesamoid c.
  vomeronasal c.
cauda (caudae)
  c. helicis
center
  burn c.
centric
  power c.
  c. relation
  true c.
cephaloauricular angle
cephalocaudad [adv.]
cephalocaudal [adj.]
cervicoplasty
chalinoplasty
Charretera flap
cheilectomy
cheilectropion
cheilognathoprosoposchisis

cheilognathoschisis
cheilognathouranoschisis
cheiloplasty
     Abbe c. (stage I, stage II)
cheilorrhaphy
cheiloschisis
cheilostomatoplasty
cheilotomy
cheiroplasty
chemosurgery
     Mohs c.
Chopart
     operation
cin–. See also words beginning
     sin–, syn–.
CLAS—congenital localized
     absence of skin
classification
     See also *index.*
     Lund-Browder c.
     Tessier c. for clefts
cleft
     c. lip
     oblique facial c.
     orbitonasal c.
     c. palate
     pharyngeal c.
     submucous c.
     tubotympanic c.
clinoid process
columella
     c. cochleae
     c. nasi
columna (columnae)
combined approach
     c.a. mastoidectomy
conjunctivoplasty
conservative
     c. mastoidectomy
contouring
Converse [eponym]
     line
     operation
Conway
     mammaplasty
     operation
coronoidectomy

cortical
     c. mastoidectomy
cosmesis
cosmetic
     c. operation
Cox line
Crane
     flap
craniofacial cleft
     Boo-Chai c.c.
     Karfik c.c.
     Tessier c.c.
Crawford
     operation
cribra (plural of cribrum)
cribral
cribrate
cribration
cribriform
cribrum (cribra)
Crikelair
     otoplasty
Cronin
     operation
Cronin-Matthews cave flap
crura (plural of crus)
cruris (genitive of crus)
crus (crura)
     c. anthelicis
     c. laterale
     c. mediale
curettement
cushion
     Passavant c.
Cutler
     operation
cymba (cymbae)
     c. conchae auriculae
dacryocystotomy
     Ammon d.
Davis
     graft
     line
Davis-Kitlowski
     operation
DB—distobuccal
DC—distocervical

debris
    dermal d.
deformity
    trap door d.
de Grandmont
    operation
Demel-Ruttin
    operation
Denonvilliers
    operation
Derby
    operation
DermaBond [topical adhesive]
dermabraded
dermabrader
    Iverson d.
dermabrasion
dermatoplasty
    Thompson d.
Dermograft-TC
dermolipectomy
Dieffenbach
    operation
Dieffenbach-Warren
    operation
dis–. See also words beginning dys–.
disease
        See in medical specialty sections.
disharmony
        maxillomandibular d.
DLA—distolabial
Dorrance
    operation
Douglas
    graft
    operation
DPC—delayed primary closure
Dragstedt
    graft
    operation
duct
    lacrimal d.
    nasolacrimal d.
Duke-Elder
    operation
Dupuy-Dutemps
    operation

durum
    palatine d.
dys–. See also words beginning dis–.
EBF—elastic band fixation [of fracture]
EBF fixation of fracture
EBL—estimated blood loss
Eckstein-Kleinschmidt
    operation
Edgerton line
Eitner
    operation
ellipse
elliptic, elliptical
Elschnig
    operation
Ely
    operation
eminence
    malar e.
eminentia
    e. conchae
    e. triangularis
encompass, encompassed, encompassing
en masse
entirety
epicanthus
epidermatoplasty
epignathous [adj.]
epignathus [noun]
epimandibular
epithelialize, epithelialized
epithelioma
épluchage
Erich
    operation
eschar
    burn e.
escharotic
escharotomy
"eskar" Phonetic for eschar.
Esmarch
    operation
esophagoplasty
Esser
    graft
    operation

esthetic
Estlander
    operation
ethmofrontal
ethmoid, ethmoidal
Eversbusch
    operation
extended radical mastectomy
F, Fr—French [catheter gauge]
face-lift, face lift, facelift
    f.-l. operation
facioplasty
fallopian
    f. aqueduct
    f. artery
    f. hiatus
    f. neuritis
Fallopius
    aqueduct of F.
"farin–" Phonetic for words begin-
    ning pharyn–.
fascia (fasciae)
    f. lata femoris
fasciaplasty
fascioplasty
fasciorrhaphy
fauces [grammatically plural; no
    singular form]
Fergus
    operation
Fergusson
    incision
    operation
Fernandez
    operation
"Fifer" Phonetic for Pfeifer.
Filatov
    flap
Filatov-Gilles
    tubed pedicle
"fi-lay" Phonetic for fillet.
fillet, filleted, filleting
filtrum [part of larynx]
    See also *philtrum.*
    Merkel f. ventriculi
fissura (fissurae)
    f. antitragohelicina

fissure
    antitragohelicine f.
    palpebral f.
fistula (fistulas, fistulae)
    f. of lip
fixation
    arch bar f.
    elastic band f. (EBF) of
      fracture
    intermaxillary f.
flap
    Antia-Busch chondrocuta-
      neous f.
    Argamaso-Lewin f.
    artery island f.
    Bakamjian f.
    bilobed f.
    bipedicle f.
    Bunnell f.
    Charretera f.
    compound f.
    Crane f.
    Cronin-Matthews cave f.
    cross-lip f.
    delayed f.
    double-pedicle f.
    French sliding f.
    Fricke f.
    Gillies up-and-down f.
    Hodgson-Tuksu tumble f.
    Hueston spiral f.
    Indian rotation f.
    island leg f.
    Italian distant f.
    jump abdominal f.
    MacFee neck f.
    marsupial f.
    McGregor forehead f.
    Millard island f.
    Monks-Esser island f.
    Moore and Chong sandwich
      f.
    New sickle f.
    f. operation
    over-and-out cheek f.
    skin f.
    split-thickness f.
    Stein-Abbe lip f.

flap (continued)
    Stein-Kazanjian lower lip f.
    Stenstrom foot f.
    Tagliacozzi f.
    tumbler f.
    Wookey neck f.
    Zimany f.
    Zovickian f.
flesh
    proud f.
"flikt–" Phonetic for words beginning phlyct–.
fold
    salpingopalatine f.
    salpingopharyngeal f.
    semilunar f.
Fomon
    operation
foramen (foramina)
    greater palatine f.
    lesser palatine foramina
    mandibular f.
    mental f.
    f. ovale alae majoris
    foramina palatina minora
    Scarpa foramina
foraminal
formula
    Berkow f.
fornix (fornices)
    superior f.
fossa (fossae)
    Merkel f.
    Rosenmüller f.
    scaphoid f.
    f. triangularis auriculae
Fox
    operation
Fr, F—French [catheter gauge]
fracture
    blow-out f.
    comminuted f.
    malar f.
    midfacial f.
    nasal f.
    nasomaxillary f.
    zygomaticomaxillary f.

Franke
    syndrome
    triad
French
    method
    sliding flap
frenectomy
frenoplasty
freshen
freshened
Fricke
    flap
    operation
Friedenwald-Guyton
    operation
frontal
frontoethmoidal
    f. suture
frontomalar
    f. suture
frontomaxillary
    f. suture
frontonasal
    f. suture
frontosphenoid
    f. suture
frontozygomatic
    f. suture
furrow
    palpebral f.
GA—gingivoaxial
Gabarro
    graft
    operation
gag
Gaillard
    operation
ganglion (ganglia, ganglions)
    ganglia of facial nerve
Gavello
    operation
Gayet
    operation
genioplasty
genitoplasty
genycheiloplasty
Gersuny
    operation

Gibson-Stark and Kenedi line
Gifford
    operation
Gillies
    flap
    graft
    operation
    up-and-down flap
Gillies-Fry
    operation
Giralde
    operation
GLA—gingivolinguoaxial
glabellad [adv.]
glabellar [adj.]
    g. frown line
    g. rotation flap
    g. wrinkle
gland
    meibomian g.
    Stahr g.
    tarsal g.
glossectomy
glossoplasty
glossorrhaphy
glossotomy
gnathodynia
gnathoplasty
gnathoschisis
gonia (plural of gonion)
gonion (gonia)
Goulian
    mammaplasty
graft
    B g.
    B-B g.
    Blair-Brown g.
    bolus tie-over g.
    Braun g.
    Braun-Wangensteen g.
    B-W g.
    chessboard g.
    Davis g.
    Douglas g.
    Dragstedt g.
    Esser g.
    fascia lata g.
    free g.

graft (continued)
    full-thickness skin g.
    Gabarro g.
    Gillies g.
    Kebab g.
    König g.
    Ollier-Thiersch g.
    Padgett g.
    patch g.
    pedicle g.
    pinch g.
    Reverdin g.
    Seddon nerve g.
    split-thickness skin g.
    stent g.
    Tanner-Vanderput g.
    Thiersch g.
    Van Millingen g.
    Wolfe g.
    Wolfe-Krause g.
Grant
    operation
Grimsdale
    operation
groove
    sinus g.
Guérin
    fold
    fracture
    glands
    sinus
    valve
Guyton
    operation
gynecomastia
Hagedorn
    operation
Hagedorn-LeMesurier
    operation
Hagerty
    operation
Hajek
    operation
Haller (von Haller)
    ansa
Halsted
    radical mastectomy
hamular

hamulus
harelip
Harman
    operation
HBO—hyperbaric oxygen
healing
    h. by first intention
    h. by granulation
    h. by second intention
    h. per primam intentionem
        (L. by first intention)
    h. per secundam intentionem
        [L. by second intention]
Heath
    operation
hemimandibulectomy
hemimaxillectomy
hemisphincter
    pharyngeal h.
Hess
    operation
hiatus
    h. semilunaris
Hirschfeld
    canals
    disease
    method
Hodgson-Tuksu tumble flap
Holmes
    operation
homeotransplant
homograft
Hotchkiss
    operation
Hotz
    operation
Hueston spiral flap
Hughes
    operation
Hutchinson and Koop line
hyperbaric
    h. chamber
    h. oxygen
hyperbarism
hyperliposis
hypermastia
hyperthelia
hypoglossal

hypognathous [adj.]
hypopigmenter
hypoplasia
    craniofacial h.
    nasomaxillary h.
Iliff
    operation
IMPA—incisal mandibular plane
    angle
implant
    Silastic i.
incision
    Langenbeck (von Langen-
        beck) i.
    relaxing i.
    Risdon extraoral i.
    Willy Meyer i.
    Z-plasty i.
incisure
    See also *notch.*
index (indexes, indices)
    See also *classification.*
    palatal i.
    palatal height i.
    palatine i.
    palatomaxillary i.
Indian
    method
    operation
    rotation flap
infraorbital
infratrochlear
Ingrassia
    apophysis
    process
    wings
injection
    Silastic i.
intercartilaginous
intermaxillary
    i. suture
internasal
    i. suture
interpalatine
    i. suture
interradicular alveoloplasty
intranasal
    i. antrostomy

intraseptal alveoloplasty
Italian
    distant flap
    method
    operation
Jacobson
    cartilage
Jaesche
    operation
"jene–" Phonetic for words beginning geny–.
Johnson
    operation
joint
    temporomandibular j. (TMJ)
Jones
    operation
Joseph
    operation
juga (plural of jugum)
jugale
jugate
jugomaxillary
jugum (juga)
Kanavel
    line
Karfik craniofacial cleft
Kazanjian
    operation
Kazanjian and Converse line
Kebab graft
Kennedy
    classification
Kiesselbach
    area
    plexus
Killian
    operation
Killian-Freer
    operation
Kilner
    operation
"kilo–" Phonetic for words beginning cheilo–.
"kiro–" Phonetic for words beginning cheiro–.
Kitlowski
    operation

"koanah" Phonetic for choana.
Kocher
    line
Kolle-Lexer
    operation
König
    graft
    operation
Körte-Ballance
    operation
Krause
    graft
Krause-Wolfe
    graft
    operation
Krimer
    operation
Krönlein
    operation
"krus" Phonetic for crus.
Kuhnt-Szymanowski
    operation
LA—linguoaxial
labium (labia)
lacrimoconchal
    l. suture
lacrimoethmoidal
    l. suture
lacrimomaxillary
    l. suture
lacrimoturbinal
    l. suture
LAG—labiogingival
Lagleyze
    operation
lamina (laminae)
    palatine l. of maxilla
laminar
Lancaster
    operation
Landolt eyelid reconstruction
Langenbeck (von Langenbeck)
    flap
    incision
    triangle
Langer line
lateral
    l. rhinotomy

Laurens
>   operation

layer
>   submucous l.

LD—linguodistal

Leahey
>   operation

Le Fort
>   apertognathia repair (I)

LeMesurier
>   operation

Lewis line

Lexer
>   operation

ligament
>   medial palpebral l.

limbus (limbi)
>   See *border* and *margin.*

limen (limina)
>   l. nasi

line
>   Borges and Alexander l.
>   Bruner l.
>   cleavage l.'s
>   contour l.
>   Converse l.
>   Cox l.
>   crease l.
>   crinkle l.
>   Davis l.
>   dependency l.
>   division l.
>   dominant l.
>   dynamic facial l.
>   Edgerton l.
>   elastic l.
>   election l.
>   l.'s of expression
>   expression folds l.
>   facial l.
>   flexion l.
>   flexure l.
>   force l.
>   Gibson-Stark and Kenedi l.
>   grain l.
>   gravitational l.
>   Hutchinson and Koop l.
>   increased tension l.

line (continued)
>   junction l.
>   Kanavel l.
>   Kazanjian l.
>   Kazanjian and Converse l.
>   Kocher l.
>   Langer l.
>   Lewis l.
>   maximal tension l.
>   minimal tension l.
>   minimum extensibility l.
>   natural l.
>   orthostatic l.
>   relaxed skin tension l.'s
>   Stark l.
>   tension l.
>   Terry l.
>   Webster l.
>   wrinkle l.

Linton
>   lipectomy

lip
>   cleft l.

lipectomy
>   Linton l.
>   submental l.
>   suction l.

LM—linguomesial

Logan bow

Luc
>   operation

Luckett
>   operation

Lund-Browder burn scale

MacFee
>   neck flap

Machek
>   operation

macrocheilia

macromastia

macrostomia

macrostructural

macrotia

macula (maculae)

macule

Magnus
>   operation

Malbec
    operation
Malbran
    operation
malomaxillary
    m. suture
maloplasty
mamilliplasty
    Ashford m.
mammaplasty
    Aries-Pitanguy m.
    Ashford m.
    augmentation m.
    Biesenberger m.
    Conway m.
    Goulian m.
    reduction m.
    Strömbeck m.
mammary
mammillary
    m. suture
mandible
mandibula (mandibulae)
mandibular
    m. resection
mandibulectomy
maneuver
    See *method, operation, pro-*
       cedure, surgery, and *tech-*
       nique.
Marcks
    operation
margin
    See also *border.*
    alveolar m. of mandible
    alveolar m. of maxilla
    free m. of eyelid
    infraorbital m. of maxilla
    infraorbital m. of orbit
    lacrimal m. of maxilla
    lateral margin of orbit
    malar m.
    medial m. of orbit
    orbital m.
    m. of safety
marginoplasty
margo (margines)
marking pen

mastectomy
    Auchincloss modified radi-
       cal m.
    extended radical m.
    Halsted radical m.
    Meyer m.
    modified m.
    modified radical m.
    partial m.
    radical m. (RM)
    segmental m.
    simple m. (SM)
    subcutaneous m.
    total m.
    Willy Meyer radical m.
mastoid
    m. obliteration operation
    m. operation
    m. suture
mastoidectomy
    Bondy m.
    combined approach m.
    conservative m.
    cortical m.
    modified radical m.
    radical m.
    Schwartze m.
    simple m.
mastopexy
mastoptosis
mastostomy
mastotomy
maxilla (maxillae, maxillas)
maxillary
    radical m. antrostomy
    m. resection
maxillectomy
maxillotomy
McCash-Randall
    operation
McDowell
    operation
McGregor forehead flap
McKissock
    operation
measurement
    skinfold m.'s

median
> m. palatine suture

medium (media, mediums)
> marking m.

meloncus

meloplasty

membrane
> mucous m.

mental

mentalis

mentolabial

Merkel
> fossa

method
> See also *operation, proce-
> dure, surgery,* and *tech-
> nique.*
> French m.
> Indian m.
> Italian m.
> Thom flap m.
> triangle m.

metopoplasty

Meyer
> mastectomy

microanastomosis

micrognathia

micrognathism

microincision

micromastia

microstomia

microsurgery

microthelia

middle
> m. palatine suture

Millard
> island flap
> operation

Minsky
> operation

Mirault
> operation

Mirault-Brown-Blair
> operation

Mladick
> abdominoplasty
> ear reconstruction

modified
> m. mastectomy
> m. radical mastectomy
> m. radical mastoidectomy

Mohs
> chemosurgery
> procedure
> surgery
> technique

Monks
> operation

Monks-Esser island flap

Moore and Chong sandwich flap

Morestin
> operation

Motais
> operation

mouth gag
> Dott m.g.

mucocutaneous

mucogingival

mucomembranous

mucoperichondrial

mucoperichondrium

mucoperiosteal

mucoperiosteum

mucosa
> buccal m.

mucosal

mucosanguineous

mucoserous

Mueller
> See also *Müller.*
> operation

Mules
> operation

Müller
> See also *Mueller.*
> muscle

muscle
> See also in *Orthopedics and
> Sports Medicine* section.
> canine m.
> depressor m. of angle of
> mouth
> depressor m. of lower lip
> depressor m. of septum of
> nose

muscle (continued)
    depressor m., superciliary
    digastric m.
    facial m.'s, m.'s of facial
        expression
    facial and masticatory m.'s
    frontal m.
    glossopalatine m.
    glossopharyngeal m.
    incisive m.'s of lip (inferior,
        lower, superior, upper)
    Koyter m.
    levator m. of palatine velum
    levator m. of upper lip
    levator m. of upper lip and
        ala of nose
    levator m. of velum palatinum
    masseter m.
    m.'s of mastication
    masticatory m.
    Müller m.
    mylohyoid m.
    orbicular m. of eye
    orbicular m. of mouth
    palatine m.'s
    pharyngopalatine m.
    platysma m.
    procerus m.
    pterygoid m. (external, inter-
        nal, lateral, medial)
    quadrate m. of lower lip
    quadrate m. of upper lip
    Riolan m.
    risorius m.
    Santorini m.
    superior constrictor m.
    tarsal m. (inferior, superior)
    temporal m.
    tensor m. of velum palatinum
    transverse m. of chin
musculus (musculi)
    See also *muscle.*
    See also in *Orthopedics and*
        Sports Medicine section.
    m. orbicularis oculi
    m. orbicularis oris
Mustardé
    flap

Mustardé (continued)
    otoplasty
myognathus
myoplasty
nare [incorrect term for naris, sin-
    gular of nares]
naris (nares)
nasal
    n. suture
nasioiniac
nasion
nasoantral
nasociliary
nasofrontal
    n. suture
nasograph
nasolabial
nasolacrimal
nasomaxillary
    n. suture
naso-oral
nasopalatine
nasorostral
nasoseptal
nasoturbinal
nasus
    n. externus
"natho–" Phonetic for words begin-
    ning gnatho–.
neck
    turkey gobbler n.
neck flap
necrectomy
necrose, necrosed
necrosis (necroses)
necrotic
Nélaton
    operation
neodymium (Nd)
    n.:yttrium-aluminum-garnet
      (Nd:YAG) laser
neovagina
nerve
    buccal n.
    buccinator n.
    facial n.
    glossopalatine n.
    glossopharyngeal n.

nerve (continued)
    hypoglossal n.
    lingual n.
    mandibular n.
    masseteric n.
    maxillary n.
    mental n.
    palatine n.
    sublingual n.
    submaxillary n.'s
neuroanastomosis
neuroplasty
New [Eponym]
    sickle flap
nostril
notch
    antegonial n.
    intertragic n.
    mandibular n.
    palatine n.
oculus (oculi)
    orbicularis oculi muscle
OFD—oral-facial-digital
    orofaciodigital
OFD dysplasia
OFD syndrome (I, II)
"ofthal–" Phonetic for words begin-
    ning ophthal–.
Ogston-Luc
    operation
olfactory
Ollier-Thiersch
    graft
    operation
Ombrédanne
    operation
onlay
    o. graft
"on moss" Phonetic for en masse.
operation
    See also *method, procedure,*
    surgery, and *technique.*
    See also in *General Surgical*
    Terms.
    Abbe o.
    Abbe-Estlander o.
    Adams o.
    Allport o.

operation (continued)
    Alsus-Knapp o.
    Alvis o.
    Ammon o.
    Angelucci o.
    Aries-Pitanguy o.
    Arlt (von Arlt) o.
    Ashford retracted nipple o.
    Barsky o.
    Battle o.
    Beard-Cutler o.
    Becker o.
    Bell o.
    Berke o.
    Berke-Motais o.
    Bernard-Burrows o.
    Biesenberger o.
    Binnie o.
    Blair o.
    Blair-Brown o.
    Blaskovics o.
    Brauer o.
    Braun o.
    Braun-Wangensteen o.
    Brophy o.
    Brown o.
    Brown-Blair o.
    Burow o.
    Caldwell-Luc o.
    Chopart o.
    Commando o.
    Converse o.
    Conway o.
    cosmetic o.
    Crawford o.
    Cronin o.
    Cutler o.
    Davis-Kitlowski o.
    de Grandmont o.
    Demel-Ruttin o.
    Denonvilliers o.
    Derby o.
    Dieffenbach o.
    Dieffenbach-Warren o.
    Dorrance o.
    Douglas o.
    Dragstedt o.
    Duke-Elder o.

operation (continued)
    Dupuy-Dutemps o.
    Eckstein-Kleinschmidt o.
    Eitner o.
    Elschnig o.
    Ely o.
    Erich o.
    Esmarch o.
    Esser o.
    Estlander o.
    Eversbusch o.
    face-lift o.
    Fergus o.
    Fergusson o.
    Fernandez o.
    flap o.
    Fomon o.
    Fox o.
    Fricke o.
    Friedenwald-Guyton o.
    Gabarro o.
    Gaillard o.
    Gavello o.
    Gayet o.
    Gersuny o.
    Gifford o.
    Gillies o.
    Gillies-Fry o.
    Giralde o.
    Grant o.
    Grimsdale o.
    Guyton o.
    Hagedorn o.
    Hagedorn-LeMesurier o.
    Hagerty o.
    Hajek o.
    Harman o.
    Heath o.
    Hess o.
    Holmes o.
    Hotchkiss o.
    Hotz o.
    Hughes o.
    Iliff o.
    Indian o.
    Italian o.
    Jaesche o.
    Johnson o.

operation (continued)
    Jones o.
    Joseph o.
    Kazanjian o.
    Killian o.
    Killian-Freer o.
    Kilner o.
    Kitlowski o.
    Kolle-Lexer o.
    König o.
    Körte-Ballance o.
    Krause-Wolfe o.
    Krimer o.
    Krönlein o.
    Kuhnt-Szymanowski o.
    Lagleyze o.
    Lancaster o.
    Laurens o.
    Leahey o.
    LeMesurier o.
    Lexer o.
    Luc o.
    Luckett o.
    Machek o.
    Magnus o.
    Malbec o.
    Malbran o.
    Marcks o.
    mastoid o.
    mastoid obliteration o.
    McCash-Randall o.
    McDowell o.
    McKissock o.
    Millard o.
    Minsky o.
    Mirault o.
    Mirault-Brown-Blair o.
    Monks o.
    Morestin o.
    Motais o.
    Mueller o.
    Mules o.
    Nélaton o.
    Ogston-Luc o.
    Ollier-Thiersch o.
    Ombrédanne o.
    osteoplastic frontal sinus o.
    Pagenstecher o.

operation (continued)
 palatal pushback o.
 Panas o.
 Parkhill o.
 Partsch o.
 Pfeifer o.
 Pierce-O'Connor o.
 plastic o.
 radical antrum o.
 Randall o.
 Reese o.
 Regnoli o.
 Reverdin o.
 Rose o.
 Rosenburg o.
 Rose-Thompson o.
 Savin o.
 Sayoc o.
 Schimek o.
 Schuchardt-Pfeifer o.
 Sédillot o.
 Serre o.
 Simon o.
 Skoog o.
 Snellen o.
 Sourdille o.
 Spaeth o.
 Stallard o.
 Stein o.
 Straith o.
 Strömbeck o.
 Szymanowski o.
 Tansley o.
 Tanzer o.
 Teale o.
 Tennison o.
 Tennison-Randall o.
 Tessier o.
 Textor o.
 Thiersch graft o.
 Thiersch-Duplay o.
 Trainor-Nida o.
 Tripier o.
 Truc o.
 Ulloa o.
 van Millingen o.
 Veau o.
 Veau-Axhausen o.

operation (continued)
 Verhoeff o.
 Verwey o.
 Vogel o.
 von Burow (Burow) o.
 von Langenbeck o.
 V-Y o.
 Wardill-Kilner o.
 Wheeler o.
 Wicherkiewicz o.
 Wiener o.
 Wies o.
 Wolfe o.
 Worth o.
 Wright o.
 W-Y o.
 Z-plasty o.
opercula (plural of operculum)
opercular
operculate
operculum (opercula)
 cartilaginous o.
orbicularis
 o. oculi muscle
 o. oris muscle
orbital
orthopedics
 dentofacial o.
 functional jaw o.
osteoma
 ethmoid sinus o.
 frontal sinus o.
 maxillary o.
 sphenoidal sinus o.
osteoplastic
 o. frontal sinus operation
osteoplasty
osteoseptum
osteotomy
otoplasty
 Crikelair o.
 Mustardé o.
overgraft
overgrafting
oxygen (O)
 high-pressure o.
 hyperbaric o. (HBO)
 molecular o. (O_2) [O2])

oxygenation
    hyperbaric o.
Padgett
    graft
Pagenstecher
    operation
Paget
    See *Padgett.*
palata (plural of palatum)
palatal
    p. height index
    p. index
palate
    cleft p.
    submucous cleft p.
palati (genitive of palatum)
palatine
    anterior p. suture
    p. bone
    p. index
    median p. suture
    middle p. suture
    posterior p. suture
    transverse p. suture
palatoethmoidal
    p. suture
palatognathous
palatomaxillary
    p. index
    p. suture
palatonasal
palatoplasty
    Wardill p.
palatum (palata)
    p. durum
    p. durum osseum
    p. fissum
    p. molle
    p. ogivale
    p. osseum
palpebra (palpebrae)
palpebralis
Panas
    operation
Parkhill
    operation
partial
    p. mastectomy

Partsch
    operation
Passavant
    bar
    cushion
peau
    p. d'orange (Fr. orange peel skin)
per primam intentionem (L. by first intention)
per secundam intentionem (L. by second intention)
Pfeifer
    operation
pharyngoplasty
    Hynes p.
philtrum [vertical groove above upper lip; compare: filtrum]
phlyctena (phlyctenae)
phlyctenar
pie crusting
Pierce-O'Connor
    operation
pillar
    p.'s of soft palate
piriform
plane
    Baer p.
plastic
    p. operation
plate
    Brophy p.
    cortical p.
    perpendicular p. of ethmoid
    tarsal p.'s
platysma
pledget
plexus (plexus, plexuses)
    Kiesselbach p.
plica (plicae)
    p. nasi
    p. semilunaris
"po-do-rahnj" Phonetic for peau d'orange.
point
    p. Ba
polydactylism
polysinusectomy

ponticulus (ponticuli)
  p. auriculae
posterior
  p. palatine suture
PR—prosthion
preauricular
premaxillary
  p. suture
procedure
  See also *method, operation,
    surgery,* and *technique.*
  four-flap p.
  Mohs p.
  push-back p.
process
  clinoid p.
  hamular p.
  mastoid p.
  maxillary p.
  palatine p.
  uncinate p.
prognathism
prognathous
prosopoanoschisis
prosopodiplegia
prosopodysmorphia
prosoponeuralgia
prosopoplegia
prosopoplegic
prosoposchisis
prosopospasm
proud flesh
PS—plastic surgery
pterygium (pterygia)
  p. colli
pterygoid
pterygomandibular
pterygomaxillary
pterygopalatine
ptosis
pushback
  palatal p.
radical [adj.]
  r. antrum operation
  Auchincloss modified r.
    mastectomy
  extended r. mastectomy
  Halsted r. mastectomy

radical [adj.] (continued)
  r. mastectomy (RM)
  r. mastoidectomy
  r. maxillary antrostomy
  modified r. mastectomy
  modified r. mastoidectomy
  Willy Meyer r. mastectomy
"ra-fee" Phonetic for raphe.
Randall
  operation
raphe (raphae)
  lateral r.
  r. palati
  palatine r.
  palpebral r.
  r. palpebralis lateralis
  pterygomandibular r.
  r. pterygomandibularis
raphes (genitive of raphe)
reconstruction
  Brent eyebrow r.
  Landolt eyelid r.
  Mladick ear r.
  Steffanoff ear r.
  Tagliacozzi nasal r.
  Tanzer auricle r.
  Wookey pharyngoe-
    sophageal r.
reduction
  r. mammaplasty
Reese
  operation
region
  dorsal lip r.
  facial r.'s
  infraorbital r.
  mental r.
  mylohyoid r.
  orbital r.
  pterygomaxillary r.
  retromaxillary r.
  subauricular r.
  submandibular r.
  submaxillary r.
  submental r.
  zygomatic r.
Regnoli
  operation

relaxing incision
repair
    Rose-Thompson r.
resection
    mandibular r.
    maxillary r.
    submucosal r.
    submucous r. (SMR)
    submucous r. and rhinoplasty (SMRR)
    submucous r. of nasal septum
    submucous r. of vocal cord
retrenchment
retroauricular
retrusion
    mandibular r.
Reverdin
    graft
    operation
revision
    W-plasty r.
    Z-plasty r.
rhinectomy
    total r.
rhinocanthectomy
rhinocheiloplasty
rhinokyphectomy
rhinokyphosis
rhinoplasty
    augmentation r.
    submucous resection and r. (SMRR)
    Tagliacozzi r.
rhinotomy
    lateral r.
rhytidectomy
rhytidosis
Riggs disease
Riolan muscle
Risdon
    extraoral incision
"riti–" Phonetic for words beginning rhyti–.
RLN—recurrent laryngeal nerve
root canal
Rose [eponym]
    operation
    position

Rosenburg
    operation
Rosenmüller
    fossa
Rose-Thompson
    operation
    repair
rostrum (rostrums, rostra)
    r. of sphenoid
rotationplasty
RSTL—relaxed skin tension line
rule
    r. of nines
sac
    lacrimal s.
Savin
    operation
Sayoc
    operation
scale
    Lund-Browder burn s.
scapha
scarify
Scarpa
    foramina
Schimek
    operation
Schuchardt-Pfeifer
    operation
Schwartze
    mastoidectomy
"scopes" See under full name.
    microgonioscope
sculpt
section
    semithin s.
    trigeminal root s.
    ultrathin s.
Seddon nerve graft
Sédillot
    operation
"sefal–" Phonetic for words beginning cephal–.
segmental
    s. mastectomy
septa (plural of septum)
septal
    s. resection

septonasal
septoplasty
septostomy
septotomy
septum (septa)
    deviated nasal s.
    dorsal median s.
    s. mobile nasi, mobile s. of
      nose
    nasal s., s. nasi
    orbital s., s. orbitale
Serre
    operation
serrefine
    Blair s.
"serviko–" Phonetic for words
    beginning cervico–.
"sfeno–" Phonetic for words begin-
    ning spheno–.
SG—skin graft
shelf
    palatal s.
sign
    Roux s.
Silastic
    injection
Simon
    operation
simple
    s. mastectomy (SM)
    s. mastoidectomy
sin–. See also words beginning
    cin–, syn–.
sinus (sinus, sinuses)
    paranasal s.'s
"skafa" Phonetic for scapha.
Skoog
    operation
SLN—superior laryngeal nerve
slough
"sluff" Phonetic for slough.
"sluffing" Phonetic for sloughing.
SM—simple mastectomy
SMR—submucous resection
SMRR—submucous resection and
    rhinoplasty
Snellen
    operation

Sourdille
    operation
Spaeth
    operation
sphenoethmoid, sphenoethmoidal
    s. suture
sphenofrontal
sphenoidal
sphenomalar
    s. suture
sphenomaxillary
    s. suture
spheno-orbital
    s. suture
sphenopalatine
sphenovomerine
    s. suture
sphenozygomatic
    s. suture
sphincter
    s. oris
spine
    nasal s., anterior
splint
    Brown s.
    volar s.
split-thickness
    s-t. flap
    s-t. skin graft
spot
Stahr gland
Stallard
    operation
staphylectomy
staphyloplasty
staphylorrhaphy
staphylotomy
Stark line
Steffanoff ear reconstruction
Stein
    operation
Stein-Abbe lip flap
Stein-Kazanjian lower lip flap
Stenstrom foot flap
stomatoplasty
Straith
    operation

Strömbeck
    mammaplasty
    operation
STSG—split-thickness skin graft
subcutaneous
    s. mastectomy
sublabial
    s. antrotomy
submental
    s. lipectomy
submucosal
    s. resection
submucous
    s. cleft
    s. cleft palate
    s. layer
    s. resection (SMR)
    s. resection of nasal septum
    s. resection and rhinoplasty
      (SMRR)
    s. resection of vocal cord
suction
    s. lipectomy
sulci (plural of sulcus)
sulciform
sulcus (sulci)
    s. anthelicis transversus
    infraorbital s. of maxilla
    retroauricular s.
    sphenovomerian s.
    tympanic s.
    vomeral s.
supra-auricular
surgery
    See also *method, operation,*
      procedure, and *technique.*
    ambulatory s.
    conservative s.
    cosmetic s.
    day s.
    dentofacial s.
    elective s.
    general s.
    in-and-out s.
    laser s.
    major s.
    maxillofacial s.
    Mohs s.

surgery (continued)
    oral and maxillofacial s.
    plastic s.
    radical s.
    rapid in-and-out (RIO) s.
    reconstructive s.
    transsexual s.
surgical procedure
    See *operation, procedure,*
      and *technique.*
suture [material]
    See in *General Surgical*
      Terms.
suture [technique]
    See in *General Surgical*
      Terms.
syn–. See also words beginning
  cin–, sin–.
syndrome
    See also in medical specialty
      sections.
    Larsen s.
    temporomandibular dysfunc-
      tion s.
    temporomandibular joint
      (TMJ) s.
Szymanowski
    operation
Tagliacozzi
    flap
    nasal reconstruction
    rhinoplasty
Tanner-Vanderput
    graft
Tansley
    operation
Tanzer
    auricle reconstruction
    operation
tarsal
tarsoplasty
tarsorrhaphy
tarsus
    t. inferior palpebrae
    t. superior palpebrae
tattoo
TBSA—total body surface area

Teale
    operation
technique
    See also *method, operation, procedure,* and *surgery.*
    Begg light-wire differential force t.
    Mohs t.
tectonic
temporal
temporomalar
    t. suture
temporomandibular
temporozygomatic
    t. suture
Tennison
    operation
Tennison-Randall
    operation
tenoplastic
tenoplasty
"tere–" Phonetic for words beginning pteri–, ptery–.
Terry line
Tessier
    craniofacial cleft
    operation
Textor
    operation
TGAR—total graft area rejected
thelectomy
theleplasty
Thiersch
    graft
    graft operation
Thiersch-Duplay
    operation
Thompson
    dermatoplasty
TM—temporomandibular
TMJ—temporomandibular joint
TMJ syndrome
tongue
    adherent t.
    bifid t.
    cleft t.
    double t.
    split t.

tongue (continued)
    stippled t.
tori (plural of torus)
torus (tori)
    t. frontalis
    t. levatorius
    t. mandibulae
    t. mandibularis
    t. occipitalis
    palatine t.
    t. palatinus
    supraorbital t.
"tosis" Phonetic for ptosis.
total
    t. mastectomy
    t. rhinectomy
traction
    elastic t.
    intermaxillary t.
    intraoral elastic t.
    maxillomandibular t.
tragus
Trainor-Nida
    operation
TRAM—transverse rectus abdominis myocutaneous (flap)
transplant
    autogenous t.
    homogenous t.
transseptal
    t. alveolectomy
transverse
    t. palatine suture
    t. suture of Krause
Treacher Collins
    syndrome
Treacher Collins-Franceschetti
    syndrome
Tripier
    operation
Truc
    operation
tunica (tunicae)
    t. conjunctiva palpebrarum
tunicate
turbinate
tympanomastoid
    t. suture

ulcer
  Meleney chronic undermining u.
Ulloa
  operation
Ullrich-Feichtiger
  syndrome
ulotomy
unciform
unciforme ["un-si-for-mee"]
uncinate
unit
  See also in *General Medical Terms* and *Laboratory, Pathology, and Chemistry Terms*.
  burn u.
"unsi–" Phonetic for words beginning unci–.
UPP, UPPP—uvulopalatopharyngoplasty
uraniscochasma
uraniscoplasty
uraniscorrhaphy
uranoplastic
uranoplasty
uranorrhaphy
uranoschisis
uranoschism
uranostaphyloplasty
uranostaphylorrhaphy
uranostaphyloschisis
uranosteoplasty
uvula (uvulae)
  u. palatina
  palatine u.
uvular
uvularis
uvulectomy
uvulopalatopharyngoplasty (UPPP)
uvulotomy
Van Lint
  akinesia
van Millingen
  graft
  operation
vault
  cartilaginous v.

Veau
  operation
Veau-Axhausen
  operation
velopharyngeal
velopharynx
velum (vela)
  Baker v.
  v. palati
  palatine v.
  v. palatinum
Verhoeff
  operation
vermilion
  v. border
vermilionectomy
Verwey
  operation
vestibuloplasty
Vogel
  operation
vomer
vomeronasal
von Burow
  See also *Burow.*
  operation
von Haller. See *Haller.*
V-Y operation
V-Y plasty
Wardill
  palatoplasty
Wardill-Kilner
  operation
webbing
  skin w.
Webster
  line
Wharton
  duct
Wheeler
  operation
Wicherkiewicz
  operation
Wiener
  operation
Wies
  operation

Willy Meyer
   incision
   radical mastectomy
Wolfe
   graft
   operation
Wolfe-Krause
   graft
Wookey
   neck flap
   pharyngoesophageal recon-
      struction
Worth
   operation
W-plasty revision
Wright
   operation
W-Y operation
xenotransplantation
"yulo–" Phonetic for words beginning ulo–.
"zeno–" Phonetic for words beginning xeno–.

zigzag
   z. laceration
zigzagplasty
Zimany flap
zone
   vermilion z.
   vermilion transitional z.
zoograft
zoografting
zooplasty
Zovickian
   flap
Z-plasty
   incision
   operation
   revision
zygomatic
zygomaticofrontal
   z. suture
zygomaticomaxillary
   z. suture
zygomaticotemporal

Psychiatry

AA—Alcoholics Anonymous
AAA—acute anxiety attack
AACP—American Academy of
    Child Psychiatry
AAMD—age-associated memory
    disorder
        American Association on
        Mental Deficiency
AAO3, AAOx3—awake, alert, and
    oriented times three [to time,
    place, and person]
abalienated
abalienation
        a. mentis
abandonment
ability
        primary mental a.
        verbal a.
ablution
ablutomania
abreaction
absentia
absinthism
abstinence
abstract
abstraction
absurdity (absurdities)
abulia
        cyclic a.
abulic
abuse
        alcohol a.
        chemical a.
        child a.
        drug a.
        elder a.
        ethanol a.
        inhalant a.
        laxative a.
        mixed drug a.
        physical a.

abuse (continued)
        polydrug a.
        polypharmacy a.
        polysubstance a.
        psychoactive substance a.
        sexual a.
        spousal a., spouse a.
        substance a.
acalculia
acatamathesia
acataphasia
acathexis
accident prone
acclimate, acclimated
acclimation
acclimatize
accomplice
ACDF—adult child of dysfunction-
    al family
acenesthesia
acheiria
achievement
        a. scores
ACLF—adult congregate living
    facility
aconative
acoria
acousma
acousmatagnosis
acousmatamnesia
acousticophobia
acquisition
acquisitus
acrimony
acromania
acrophobia
act
        compulsive a.
        forced a.
        imperious a.
        impulsive a.

acting out
action
　　compulsive a.
activity
　　blocking a.
　　a.'s of daily living (ADL,
　　　ADLs)
aculalia
adaptability
adaptation
　　social a.
ADD—attention deficit disorder
ADDH—a. deficit disorder with
　　hyperactivity
addict
addiction
　　alcohol a.
　　drug a.
　　polysurgical a.
addictologist
addictology
ADDU—alcohol and drug depen-
　　dency unit
ADHD—attention deficit hyperac-
　　tivity disorder
adiadochokinesia
adiadochokinesis
adiaphoria
adipsia
adipsous
adjustment
　　a. disorder
ADL, ADLs—activities of daily liv-
　　ing
Adler
　　theory
adlerian psychoanalysis, psychology
"ad-oy-o-manea" Phonetic for
　　aidoiomania.
ADTP—alcohol dependency treat-
　　ment program
adversive
advocate
　　patient a.
aerodromophobia
aeroneurosis
aerophobia
"a-feem-ee-a" Phonetic for aphemia.

"af-e-fobea" Phonetic for aphephobia.
affect [noun: state of mind]
　　apathetic a.
　　bland a.
　　blunted a.
　　congruent a.
　　constricted a.
　　depressed a., depressive a.
　　euphoric a.
　　flat a.
　　impaired a.
　　inappropriate a.
　　labile a.
　　restricted a.
affection
affective
affectivity
affectomotor
"a-fo-ne-a" Phonetic for aphonia.
AFS—Alzheimer fugue state
afterglow
age
　　achievement a.
　　a. of consent
　　developmental a.
　　emotional a.
　　functional a.
　　mental a.
　　physical a., physiologic a.
agenesia
aggression
　　covert a.
　　displaced a.
　　healthy a.
aggressive
　　a. behavior
　　a. manner
agitated
agitation
agitographia
agitolalia
agitophasia
agony
agrammaphasia
agrammatica
agrammatism
agrammatologia

agraphia
    a. amnemonica
    jargon a.
agraphic
agromania
agyria
"ah-dee-fa-rahns" Phonetic for
    indifference.
aichmophobia
aidoiomania
ailurophobia
akathisia
    psychic a.
akinesthesia
"ak-mo-fobea" Phonetic for aich-
    mophobia.
alalia
    a. cophica
    developmental a.
    a. organica
    a. physiologica
    a. prolongata
alalic
Al-Anon
alcohol
    a. intoxication
alcoholemia
alcoholic
    a. psychosis
Alcoholics Anonymous (AA)
alcoholism
alcoholomania
alcoholophilia
alexithymia
algophilia
algophily
algophobia
algopsychalia
alienation
alienism
alienist
alliance
    National A. for the Mentally
      Ill (NAMI)
    therapeutic a.
    working a.
alliteration
alloeroticism

allolalia
alloplastic
alloplasty
allopsychic
allotropic
allotropy
allowance
allude, alluded
alteregoism
"al-uro-fil-ea" Phonetic for ail-
    urophilia.
"alurofobea" Phonetic for ailuro-
    phobia.
Alzheimer
    dementia
    disease
    primary degenerative
      dementia
    syndrome
amathophobia
amaxophobia
ambiguity
    lexical a.
    role a.
    sexual identity a.
    structural a.
ambisexual
ambivalence
ambivalent
ambiversion
ambivert
amenomania
American Psychiatric Association
    (APA)
amerisia
amerism
ameristic
ametamorphosis
aminoketones [a class of drugs]
amnemonic
amnesia
    affective a.
    anterograde a.
    auditory a.
    Broca a.
    concussion a.
    elective a.

amnesia (continued)
    graphokinetic a.
    hysterical a.
    immunologic a.
    incomplete a.
    infantile a.
    Korsakoff a.
    lacunar a.
    localized a.
    mimokinetic a.
    olfactory a.
    patchy a.
    postconcussion a.
    posthypnotic a.
    psychogenic a.
    retroactive a.
    retrograde a.
    systematic a.
    tactile a.
    transient global a.
amnesiac
amnesic
amnestic
amok, amuck
amoral
amoralia
amuck, amok
amychophobia
anabolic steroids [a class of drugs]
anaclitic
analysand
analysis
analysor
analytic, analytical
anamnesis
    associative a.
anancastic
anarithmia
anemophobia
anergy
anger
angina
    hysterical a.
anginal
anginophobia
angioneurotic
angophrasia

angor
    a. animi
    a. ocularis
"angzietas" Phonetic for anxietas.
anhedonia
anima
    a. mundi
animus
anomia
anorexia
    hysterical a.
    a. nervosa
anorexigenic
anthropokinetics
anthropomorphic
anthropomorphism
anthropopathy
anthropophobia
antianxiety
antidepressants [a class of drugs]
antihallucinatory
antisocial
antisocialism
Anton
    symptom
    syndrome
anxietas
    a. presenilis
    a. tibiarum
anxiety
    existential a.
    free-floating a.
    neurotic a.
    signal a.
APA— American Psychiatric Association
    American Psychological Association
apandria
apastia
apastic
apathetic
apathy
APE—acute psychotic episode
APGAR—adaptability, partnership, growth, affection, resolve [questionnaire]

aphasia
    ageusic a.
    amnemonic a.
    amnesic a.
    amnestic a.
    anosmic a.
    apractic a.
    association a.
    associative a.
    Broca a.
    color name a.
    crossed a.
    efferent motor a.
    finger a.
    gestural a.
    global a.
    kinetic motor a.
    monoglot a.
    musical a.
    paroxysmal a.
    puerperal a.
    pure motor a.
    visual a.
    Wernicke a.
aphephobia
aphonia
    hysterical a.
    a. paralytica
    a. paranoica
    spastic a.
apiphobia
apocarteresis
appearance
apperception
apperceptive
appersonification
apprehension
    a. test
aprophoria
aprosexia
apsychia
aquaphobia
arachnephobia
arachnophobia
arithmomania
arrested
articulate

ASCH—American Society of Clinical Hypnosis
asemasia
as-if personality
asphyxia
    autoerotic a.
    sexual a.
assault
    felonious a.
assaultive
assessment
    psychological a.
association
    controlled a. test
    individual practice a.
astereognosis
asthenophobia
astraphobia
astrapophobia
ataractic
ataraxia
ataxophobia
ATC—addictions treatment center
attention
    a. deficit disorder (ADD)
    a. deficit disorder with hyperactivity (ADDH)
    a. deficit hyperactivity disorder (ADHD)
attitude
    pugilistic a.
audition
    thought a.
auditory
    a. hallucinations
aula
autism
autistic
autoerotic
autoeroticism
autoerotism
autognosis
autognostic
automatism
    alcohol a.
    epileptic a.
    postepileptic a.
    postictal a.

automatism (continued)
vigil ambulatory a.
automysophobia
autonomy
autophobia
autopunition
autotopagnosia
aversive
avoidance
a. behavior
phobic a.
azaspirones [a class of drugs]
Baker
Act
"Baker-acted" Slang for "admitted
under the Baker Act."
barbiturates [a class of drugs]
bare, bared
basophobia
basophobiac
Batten
disease
Beard
disease
syndrome
behavior
adaptive b.
attachment b.
displacement b.
impulsive b.
behaviorism
Bell
delirium
mania
belle indifférence, la belle indifférence
belonephobia
Bender
Gestalt test
Visual-Motor Gestalt test
Bennett
Differential Aptitude Test
benzisoxazoles [a class of drugs]
benzodiazepines [a class of drugs]
Bernheim
therapy
beseech, beseeched
bestiality

betacism
Bianchi
syndrome
bibliotherapy
bind
bipolar double b.
unipolar double b.
Binet
test
Binet-Simon test
binge
bingeing and purging
bipolar
b. affective psychosis
b. disorder
b. double bind
b. psychosis
birth
b. order
bisexuality
bizarre
b. behavior
block
affect b.
blocking
thought
board
alphabet b.
body rocking
bouffée ["boo-fay"]
b. délirante ("day-lee-rahnt")
boundary
ego b.
bradylalia
bradylexia
bradylogia
bradyphasia
bradyphrasia
bradyphrenia
bradypsychia
brainwashing
bredouillement
"breh-dwe-maw" Phonetic for bredouillement.
bromomania
brontophobia
bruxomania

bulimia
    b. nervosa
burn-out
butyrophenones [a class of drugs]
CA—chronological age
cacergasia
cacesthenic
cacesthesia
cachexia
    psychogenic c.
cachinnation
cacodemonomania
cacolalia
cafard
callomania
camisole
cancerphobia
cannabinoid
cannabinol
cannabis
cannabism
Cannon-Bard theory
capacity
    mental c.
    testamentary c.
Capgras
    phenomenon
    symptom
    syndrome
carcinophobia
cardiophobia
"carfol–" Phonetic for words beginning carphol–.
carnal
carnophobia
carphologia
carphology
castration
catalepsy
cataleptic
cataleptiform
cataleptoid
cataphasia
cataphrenia
cataplectic
cataplexie
    c. du réveil
cataplexis

cataplexy
catathymic
catatonia
catatonic
cathectic
cathexis
cathisophobia
Cattel Infant Intelligence Scale
causation
    legal c.
cautionary
CDE—chlordiazepoxide (Librium)
CDI—Children's Depression Inventory
CDR—clinical dementia rating
CDU—chemical dependency unit
censor
    freudian c.
    psychic c.
censorship
centration
cerea flexibilitas
CES-D—Center for Epidemiological Studies of Depression
CES-D scale
CH—conversion hysteria
character
chemopsychiatry
cheromania
Cheyne-Stokes
    psychosis
choreomania
CHP—child psychiatry
chromophobia
CIL—center for independent living
cin–. See also words beginning sin–, syn–.
circuitous
circumstantiality
CIT—crisis intervention therapy
Citelli syndrome
clairaudience
clairsentience
clairvoyance
classification
    See also *index.*
    multiaxial c. (axes I–V)
claustrophilia

claustrophobia
Clérambault-Kandinsky
    complex
    syndrome
clitoromania
Clonopin [now: Klonopin]
CMHC—community mental health
    center
CMS—Clyde Mood Scale
CO—court order
coconscious
COE—court-ordered examination
cognition
cognitive
cognizant
coitophobia
commitment
compensatory
competent
    mentally c.
competitive
    c. behavior
complex
    castration c.
    Electra c.
    inferiority c.
    Oedipus c.
compulsion
compulsive
COMS—chronic organic mental
    syndrome
conation
conative
concept
conception
concretism
condensation
conditioning
    avoidance c.
    reinforcement c.
confabulation
confidentiality
conflict
confusion
congruence
congruent
    affect was c. with mood
    mood c. psychosis

conscience
consensus
constellation
    c. of symptoms
constitution
    ideo-obsessional c.
    psychopathic c.
content
    latent c.
    manifest c.
conversion
    c. disorder
    hysterical c.
    c. reaction
coprolagnia
coprolalomania
coprophagia
coprophagy
coprophilia
coprophiliac
coprophobia
corticectomy
Cotard syndrome
counterphobia
countertransference
CPI—constitutional psychopathic
    inferiority
CPS—clinical performance score
CPZ—chlorpromazine
CR—conversion reaction
crank amphetamine
CRC—crisis resolution center
criminosis
crisis (crises)
cryptesthesia
cryptomnesia
cryptomnesic
CSA—criminal sexual assault
cunnilingus
curiosity
curious
cynophobia
cytheromania
DaCosta syndrome
"daleer" Phonetic for délire.
"dazhah aproova" Phonetic for déjà
    éprouvé.
"dazhah fa" Phonetic for déjà fait.

"dazhah ontondoo" Phonetic for
déjà entendu.
"dazhah ponsa" Phonetic for déjà
pensé.
"dazhah rakonta" Phonetic for déjà
raconté.
"dazhah vakoo" Phonetic for déjà
vécu.
"dazhah voo" Phonetic for déjà vu.
"dazhah vooloo" Phonetic for déjà
voulu.
decision
    Durham d.
deem, deemed
defecalgesiophobia
defense mechanism
defiance
defiant
dehumanization
déjà entendu
déjà éprouvé
déjà fait
déjà pensé
déjà raconté
déjà vécu
déjà voulu
déjà vu
dejection
delinquency
delinquent
    juvenile d.
délire
    d. aigue
    d. alcoolique
    d. ambitieux
    d. à quatre
    d. chronique
    d. crapuleau
    d. d'embléé
    d. d'énormité
    d. de toucher
    d. ecmnesique
    d. en partie double
    d. de négation
    d. de négation généralise
    d. onirique
    d. terminal
    d. tremblant

délire (continued)
    d. vésanique
deliria (plural of delirium)
deliriant
delirifacient
delirium (deliria)
    acute d.
    Bell d.
    collapse d.
    febrile d.
    d. grandiosum
    d. grave
    low d.
    d. mussitans
    oneiric d.
    organic d.
    postcardiotomy d.
    d. schizophrenoides
    senile d.
    d. sine delirio
    substance-induced d.
    substance intoxication d.
    substance withdrawal d.
    toxic d.
    traumatic d.
    d. tremens (DTs)
de lunatico inquirendo
delusion
delusional
demented
dementia
    alcoholic d.
    Alzheimer d.
    arteriosclerotic d.
    Binswanger d.
    boxer's d.
    catatonic d.
    chronic d.
    epileptic d.
    hebephrenic d.
    hydrocephalic d.
    d. infantilis
    d. myoclonica
    myxedematous d.
    paralytic d.
    d. paralytica
    d. paranoides
    paretic d.

dementia (continued)
    post-traumatic d.
    d. praecocissima
    d. praecox
    d. praesenilis
    presenile d.
    progressive d.
    d. pugilistica
    semantic d.
    senile d.
    static d.
    terminal d.
    toxic d.
demonomania
demonophobia
dependence
    emotional d.
    physical d., physiologic d.
    polysubstance d.
    psychoactive substance d.
    psychological d.
    substance d.
dependency
dependent
depersonalization
depraved
depressants [a class of drugs]
depressed
depression
    agitated d.
    postpartum d.
    reactive d.
depressive
derealization
dereism
dereistic
despair
despairing
desperate [hopeless, despairing]
desperation
deter
deterioration
determinism
    psychic d.
deterrent
development
developmental
    d. milestones

dibenzodiazepines [a class of drugs]
dibenzothiazepines [a class of drugs]
dibenzoxazepines [a class of drugs]
dihydroindolones [a class of drugs]
dinomania
diplopiaphobia
dipsomania
dipsosis
dire
    d. consequences
    d. straits
dis–. See also words beginning dys–.
disciplinary
discord
discordance
discordant
discrimination
disease
    See also *syndrome.*
    Alzheimer d.
    Morel-Kraepelin d.
    psychosomatic d.
    Wernicke d.
"disfemia" Phonetic for dysphemia.
"disfor–" Phonetic for words begin-
    ning dysphor–.
disorder
    affective d.
    aggressive behavior d.
    alcoholic brain d.'s
    anxiety d.
    appetite d.
    attention deficit d. (ADD)
    attention deficit hyperactivi-
      ty d. (ADHD)
    attention deficit d. with
      hyperactivity (ADDH)
    bipolar d.
    character impulse d.
    conversion d.
    cyclothymic d.
    dissociative d.
    dysthymic d.
    epileptoid personality d.
    extrapyramidal d.
    gnostic d.'s
    habit d.
    hyperkinetic impulse d.

disorder (continued)
    impulse d.
    neurotic depressive d.
    obsessive-compulsive d.
      (OCD)
    panic d.
    paranoid d.
    personality d.
    post-traumatic personality d.
    post-traumatic stress d.
    psychosexual d.
    schizophrenic d.
    somatization d.
    somatoform d.
    somatoform pain d.
    stress d.
    thought d.
    transient situational person-
      ality d.
disparate [distinct, different]
dissipate
dissociation
dissociative
    d. disorder
    d. identity disorder
    d. trance disorder
distractibility
distraught
divagation
DMPE—3,4-dimethoxyphenyleth-
    ylamine
domatophobia
Don Juanism
DP—dementia praecox
dramatism
dramatization
drapetomania
dream
    clairvoyant d.
    d. interpretation
    veridical d.
dromomania
dromophobia
DT, DTs—delirium tremens
dys–. See also words beginning dis–.
dysbulia, dysboulia
dysbulic
dysergasia

dysergastic
dyslogia
dysmorphophobia
dysphemia
dysphoretic
dysphoria
    gender d.
dysphoriant
dysphoric
dysprosody
dyssocial
dyssymbolia
dysthymia
dysthymic
dystrophoneurosis
Ebbinghaus test
ecdemomania
echoing
    thought e.
echolalia
echomimia
echopathy
echophotony
echophrasia
ecmnesia
ecomania
ecophobia
ecphoria
ecphorize
ECS—electroconvulsive shock
ecstasy
"edipus" Phonetic for Oedipus.
"ee-day" Phonetic for idée.
effect [noun: result, outcome]
        See *reaction* and *phenome-*
          non.
ego
    body e.
ego-alien
egocentric
egodystonic
ego-ideal
egoism
egomania
egosyntonic
egotism
egotistic, egotistical
egotropic

eidetic
      e. image, e. imagery
ejaculation
      premature e.
"eko–" Phonetic for words begin-
      ning echo–.
elaboration
elation
Electra complex
electroconvulsive
electronarcosis
electroplexy
electroshock
electrosleep
electrotherapist
elicit
ellipsis
emasculate
emasculation
embarrass
embarrassment
embololalia
embolophrasia
emotion
emotional
empathize
empathy
encopresis
engender, engendered
engram
enomania
enosimania
entropy
enuresis [urinary incontinence, bed-
      wetting]
episode
epithet
EPS—extrapyramidal signs
      extrapyramidal symptoms
equinophobia
erectile
eremophobia
erethism
erethizophrenia
ergasia
ergasiomania
ergasiophobia
ergomania

ergomaniac
erotic
eroticomania
erotism
      anal e.
      genital e.
      muscle e.
      oral e.
erotogenesis
erotogenic
erotographomania
erotomania
erotomaniac
erotopath
erotopathy
erotophobia
erratic
erythrophobia
eschew
EST—electric shock therapy
ETOH, EtOH—ethyl alcohol
euphoretics, euphoriants, euphora-
      gens [a class of drugs]
euphoria
euphoriant
euphoric
euphorigenic
euthymic
excitability
excitable
exhibitionism
exhilarant
exhilarated
existential
existentialism
expediency
expedient
extrapsychic
extrapyramidal
extrovert
exuberance
facility
            adult congregate living f.
            (ACLF)
"fago–" Phonetic for words begin-
      ning phago–.
"fal–" Phonetic for words beginning
      phal–.

Family APGAR Questionnaire
"fan–" Phonetic for words beginning phan–.
fantasy
feeblemindedness
fellatio
felony
"fenil–" Phonetic for words beginning phenyl–.
"feno–" Phonetic for words beginning pheno–.
"fenomenon" Phonetic for phenomenon.
fetish
fetishism
5150 hold
fixation
    freudian f.
"fizeo–" Phonetic for words beginning physio–.
flagellantism
flaunt [show off]
"flegmatik" Phonetic for phlegmatic.
flexibilitas
    cerea f.
flight
    f. of ideas
floccillation
flout [scorn]
"fobia" Phonetic for phobia.
"fobic" Phonetic for phobic.
folie
    f. á deux
    f. circulaire
    f. communiquée
    f. des grandeurs
    f. du doute
    f. du pourquoi
    f. gémellaire
    f. imitative
    f. imposée
    f. induite
    f. musculaire
    f. raisonnante
forego
formation
    compromise f.
    reaction f.

formative
formboard
formication
formulation
    American Law Institute f.
free association
frenetic, frenetical
frenzy, frenzied
Freud
    cathartic method
    theory
freudian
frigidity
frustration
FT—family therapy
fugue
    dissociative f.
    psychogenic f.
    f. state
functional
GA—Gamblers Anonymous
gamophobia
Ganser
    symptom
    syndrome
garrulous
gelasmus
geophagia
geophagism
gephyrophobia
geriopsychosis
gestalt [also: Gestalt]
    Bender G. test
    g. psychology
    g. theory
    g. therapy
gestaltism
gibberish
Gjessing syndrome
glassy
globus (globi)
    g. hystericus
glossolalia
glossomantia
glossophobia
Goldstein
    classification

Gowers
        attack
        syndrome
GPA—grade-point average
grandiosity
grass [street slang for marijuana]
gratification
Griffith classification
guardian ad litem
Guilford-Zimmerman
        personality test
gynecomania
gynephobia
GZ—Guilford-Zimmerman
GZ personality test
habit
        position h.
        tongue h.
habitual
habituation
habromania
hallucination
        auditory h.
        autoscopic h.
        blank h.
        depressive h.
        epileptic h.
        gustatory h.
        haptic h.
        hypnagogic h.
        lilliputian h.
        microptic h.
        olfactory h.
        h. of perception
        psychomotor h.
        reflex h.
        stump h.
        tactile h.
        visual h.
hallucinative
hallucinatory
hallucinogen
hallucinogenesis
hallucinogenetic
hallucinogenic
hallucinosis
        acute alcoholic h.
        drug-induced h.

hallucinosis (continued)
        ethanolic h.
hallucinotic
Halstead-Reitan
        battery
        test
haphephobia
harassment
haut-mal
hebephrenia
hebetude
heboidophrenia
hedonia
hedonic
hedonism
hedonophobia
hemophobia
hermaphrodite
hermaphroditic
hermaphroditismus
heroin
herpetophobia
heterosexual
heterosexuality
heterosuggestion
"hipnahgojik" Phonetic for hypna-
        gogic.
"hipno–" Phonetic for words begin-
        ning hypno–.
"hipo–" Phonetic for words begin-
        ning hypo–.
history
        incongruous h.
histrionic
histrionism
holergasia
holergastic
holism
holistic
homicidal
homicide
homicidomania
homilophobia
homosexual
homosexuality
        ego-dystonic h.
        latent h.
        unconscious h.

hostility
hot line, hotline
hydrargyromania
hydrodipsomania
hydrophobia
hyperactive
hyperactivity
hyperarousal
hypercatharsis
hypercathartic
hyperdipsia
hyperfunction
hyperfunctioning
hypergnosis
hyperhedonia
hyperhidrosis
    emotional h.
    volar h.
Hypericum
    H. perforatum
hyperirritability
hyperlithemia
hypermania
hypermimia
hypermnesia
hypermnesic
hyperphonia
hyperphrasia
hyperphrenia
hyperpragic
hyperpraxia
hyperprosexia
hyperprosody
hypersensibility
hypersensitive
hyperserotonemia
hypersexuality
hyperstimulation
hyperthymergasia
hyperthymia
hyperthymic
hyperventilation
    hysterical h.
hypervigilance
hypnagogic
hypnagogue
hypnoanalysis
hypnogenic

hypnoid
hypnoidal
hypnology
hypnonarcosis
hypnopompic
hypnosis
hypnotherapy
hypnotics [a class of drugs]
hypnotism
hypnotist
hypnotization
hypnotize
hypoactivity
hypochondria
hypochondriac
hypochondriacal
hypochondriasis
hypodipsia
hypodipsic
hypomania
hypomaniac
hypomanic
hypomelancholia
hypomimia
hypomnesis
hyponoia
hypophonia
hypophrenia
hypophrenosis
hypoprosody
hyposexuality
hyposomnia
hypothalamotomy
hypothesis (hypotheses)
    permissive h. of affective
      disorders
hypothymia
hypothymic
hypothymism
hypovigility
hysteria
    anxiety h.
    combat h.
    conversion h.
    degenerative h.
    dissociative h.
    epidemic h.
    fixation h.

hysteria (continued)
- h. libidinosa
- major h.
- h.-malingering
- masked h.
- monosymptomatic h.
- reflex h.
- retention h.
- traumatic h.

hysteric, hysterical
hystericism
hysteriform
hysteroerotic
hysterogenic
hysteroid
hysteropsychosis
id
idea
- autochthonous i.
- complex of i.'s
- concatenated i.'s
- dominant i.
- fixed i.
- flight of i.'s
- overproductive i.'s
- overvalued i.
- i.'s of reference, referential i.'s
- ruminative i.

ideal
- ego i.

idealization
ideation
- homicidal i.
- incoherent i.
- paranoid i.
- suicidal i.

ideational
idée
- i. fixe ["feeks"]

identification
- projective i.

identity
- See also *identity disorder.*
- body i.
- core gender i.
- i. crisis
- i. diffusion
- ego i.

identity (continued)
- family i.
- gender i.
- i. integration
- sense of personal i.
- sexual i.

identity disorder
- i.d. of childhood
- dissociative i.d.
- psychosexual i.d.
- sexual and gender i.d.

ideodynamism
ideogenetic
"idetik" Phonetic for eidetic.
idioglossia
idioglottic
idiohypnotism
idiolalia
idioneurosis
idiophrenic
idiopsychologic
idiosyncrasy
idiosyncratic
idiot
- i.-savant

idiotropic
idolomania
illusion
- i. or delusions

illusional
image
- body i.
- conceptual i.
- eidetic i., visual
- eidetic i., auditory
- idealized i.
- percept i.
- personal i.
- primary memory i.
- primary mental i.
- unconscious i.

imagery
- eidetic i.
- guided i.
- guided affective i.
- hypnagogic i.
- hypnopompic i.
- spontaneous i.

imago (imagoes, imagines)
imitate
impotence
    psychic i.
impoverishment
    personality i.
    i. in thinking
impression
imprinting
impulse
    i. control disorder
    irresistible i.
impulsion
    wandering i.
inadequacy
inadequate
incest
incoherent
incompetence
incompetent
incongruent
incongruous
    i. history
incorrigible
incubus
independent
index (indexes, indices)
    See also *classification.*
    i. of mental deterioration
indifference
    i. reaction
    sexual i.
indifférence ["an-dee-fa-rahns"]
    belle i., la belle i.
indifferent
Indoklon therapy
indolones [a class of drugs]
inebriation
infantile
ingenious
inhibition
inhibitor
    monoamine oxidase i.'s
      (MAOIs) [a class of drugs]
    selective serotonin reuptake
      i.'s (SSRIs) [a class of
      drugs]

insane
    criminally i.
insanity
    adolescent i.
    affective i.
    alcoholic i.
    alternating i.
    anticipatory i.
    choreic i.
    circular i.
    climactetic i.
    collective i.
    communicated i.
    compound i.
    compulsive i.
    consecutive i.
    criminal i.
    cyclic i.
    double i.
    doubting i.
    emotional i.
    hereditary i.
    homicidal i.
    homochronous i.
    hysterical i.
    idiophrenic i.
    imposed i.
    impulsive i.
    induced i.
    manic-depressive i.
    partial i.
    perceptional i.
    periodic i.
    polyneuritic i.
    primary i.
    puerperal i.
    recurrent i.
    senile i.
    simultaneous i.
    toxic i.
insanoid
insertion
    thought i.
insight
    i. fair
    i. and judgment
insomnia
insomniac

insomnic
instinct
    death i.
    ego i.
    herd i.
instinctive
insultus
    i. hystericus
integration
    nervous i.
    structural i.
intellect
intellectualization
intelligence
    i. quotient (IQ)
intercede
intercourse
interpretation
interval
    lucid i.
intoxication
    alcohol i.
    substance i.
    water i.
intrapsychic
introjection
introspection
introspective
introversion
introvert
inversion
    sexual i.
invert
involutional
IPRT—interpersonal reaction test
IQ—intelligence quotient
irascibility
irritability
irritable
irritation
irritative
isolation
    sensory i.
ITPA—Illinois Test of Psycholin-
    guistic Abilities
jamais vu
Janet
    disease

Janet (continued)
    test
jargonaphasia
"jefirofobea" Phonetic for gephyro-
    phobia.
"jibberish" Phonetic for gibberish.
judgment
Jung
    method
jungian
"kahk–," "kak–" Phonetic for words
    beginning cac–, cach–.
Kahlbaum
    catatonic stupor
    syndrome
Kanner syndrome
katzenjammer [a hangover or
    depression]
kathisophobia
kenophobia
keraunoneurosis
"keromanea" Phonetic for cheroma-
    nia.
kinesioneurosis
Kleine-Levin
    syndrome
kleptolagnia
kleptomania
kleptomaniac
kleptophobia
Korsakoff (Korsakov)
    amnesia
    disease
    psychosis
    syndrome
Kraepelin classification
krauomania
Kretschmer types
Kussmaul
    aphasia
Labbé
    neurocirculatory syndrome
la belle indifférence
labialism
labile
    l. affect
    l. mood

lability
    emotional l.
laloneurosis
    spasmodic l.
lalopathy
lalophobia
lalorrhea
lambdacism
lambdacismus
lapsus
    l. calami
    l. linguae
    l. memoriae
lassitude
law
    Meyer l.
lesbian
lesbianism
lethargy
    hysterical l.
letheomania
lethologica
lethonomia
liaison
libidines (plural of libido)
libidinous
libido (libidines)
    bisexual l.
    ego l.
    object l.
licentious
lithium (Li)
lobotomy
logagnosia
logomania
logoneurosis
logorrhea
    jargonaphasic l.
logospasm
loquacious
LSD—lysergic acid diethylamide
lucid
lucidity
lugubrious
lunacy
lunatic
lunatism
lysergic acid diethylamide (LSD)

lyssophobia
MA—mental age
macropsia
Magnan
    movement
maieusiomania
maieusiophobia
maladjustment
malingerer
malingering
mania
    acute hallucinatory m.
    akinetic m.
    alcoholic m.
    m. á potu
    Bell m.
    dancing m.
    delirious m.
    doubting m.
    epileptic m.
    hysterical m.
    m. mitis
    periodical m.
    puerperal m.
    Ray m.
    reasoning m.
    religious m.
    transitory m.
    unproductive m.
maniac
maniacal
maniaphobia
manic
manic-depressive
mannerism
MAO—monoamine oxidase
MAOI, MAOIs—monoamine oxidase
    inhibitor(s) [a class of drugs]
marihuana, marijuana
marital
masochism
masochist
masochistic
McNaughten (pref: M'Naghten)
MCQ—multiple choice question
MD—manic depressive
    maternal deprivation
MDA—methylenedioxyamphetamine

MDMA—methylenedioxymetham-
    phetamine
mechanism
        coping m.
        defense m.
        mental m.
        neutralizing m.
        somatic m.
mediate
mediation
mediator
medicine
        behavioral m.
"meelu" Phonetic for milieu.
megalomania
megalomaniac
melancholia
        affective m.
        m. agitata
        agitated m.
        m. attonita
        flatuous m.
        m. hypochondriaca
        involution m.
        involutional m.
        m. religiosa
        m. simplex
        stuporous m.
        m. with delirium
melancholiac
melancholic
melomania
"melyuh" Phonetic for milieu.
memory
        affect m.
        anterograde m.
        m. probe
mental
mentality
mentation
mercurial
mesmerism
metapsychology
method
        See also *technique.*
        Freud cathartic m.
        introspective m.
        Jung m.

method (continued)
        Pavlov m.
metonymy
MH—mental health
micrographia
micromania
milieu
        m. therapy
Minnesota Multiphasic Personality
        Inventory (MMPI)
misanthropy
mischievous
miso–. See also words beginning
        myso–.
misocainia
misogamy
misogyn
misogyny
misologia
misoneism
misopedia
Mitchell
        treatment
"mitho–" Phonetic for words begin-
        ning mytho–.
MMPI—Minnesota Multiphasic
        Personality Inventory
M'Naghten
        rule
        test
monoamine oxidase (MAO)
monoamine oxidase inhibitors
        (MAOIs) [a class of drugs]
monogamous
monogamy
monomania
monomoria
monophasia
monosyllabic
Morel
        disease
Morel-Kraepelin disease
Morgagni
        syndrome
moria
Morita therapy
moron
moronity

morphinomania
MR—mental retardation
MS—mental status
MSRPP—Multidimensional Scale
    for Rating Psychiatric Patients
MT—music therapy
Münchausen
        by proxy syndrome
        syndrome
musicotherapy
mute
mutilate
mutism
        akinetic m.
        hysterical m.
myso–. See also words beginning
    miso–.
mysophilia
mysophobia
mysophobic
mythomania
mythophobia
NAMI—National Alliance for the
    Mentally Ill
narcism [an incorrect short form of
    narcissism]
narcissism
narcissistic
narcoanalysis
narcodiagnosis
narcohypnosis
narcolepsy
narcoleptic
narcomania
narcose
narcotic
narcotize
ND—neurotic depression
NEC—not elsewhere classified, not
    elsewhere classifiable
necromania
necromimesis
necrophilia
necrophilic
necrophilism
necrophilous
necrophobia
necrosadism

negativism
neolalia
neolalism
neologism
neomimism
neomnesis
neophasia
    polyglot n.
neophilism
neophobia
nervous
    n. breakdown
Neumann
    syndrome
neurodermatitis
neurolinguistic programming (NLP)
neuropsychiatrist
neuropsychiatry
neuropsychology
neuropsychopathy
neuropsychopharmacology
neurosis (neuroses)
    accident n.
    actual n.
    anankastic n.
    anxiety n.
    artificial n.
    association n.
    cardiac n.
    character n.
    combat n.
    compensation n.
    compulsion n.
    conversion n.
    craft n.
    defense n.
    depersonalization n.
    depressive n.
    expectation n.
    experimental n.
    fatigue n.
    fixation n.
    fright n.
    gastric n.
    homosexual n.
    housewife's n.
    hypochondriacal n.
    hysterical n.

neurosis (neuroses) (continued)
    intestinal n.
    neurasthenic n.
    obsessional n.
    obsessive-compulsive n.
    occupational n.
    organ n.
    pension n.
    phobic n.
    phobic anxiety-depersonalization n.
    prison n.
    professional n.
    pseudoschizophrenic n.
    rectal n.
    regression n.
    sexual n.
    sphenopalatine ganglion n.
    substitution n.
    torsion n.
    transference n.
    traumatic n.
    true n.
    vagabond n.
    vegetative n.
    war n.
neurotic
nihilism
    therapeutic n.
"nimfo–" Phonetic for words beginning nympho–.
NIMH—National Institute of Mental Health
NLP—Neurolinguistic Programming
noctiphobia
non compos mentis
nonplused, nonplussed
non sequitur
NOS—not otherwise specified
nosomania
nosophobia
nostomania
novel (atypical) antipsychotics [a class of drugs]
noxa (noxae)
NP—neuropsychiatric
nudophobia
nyctophobia

nympholepsy
nymphomania
nymphomaniac
obsession
obsessive
obsessive-compulsive
OCD—obsessive-compulsive disorder
OD—overdose
odontophobia
oedipism
Oedipus complex
oligergasia
oligergastic
oligomania
oligophrenia
oligophrenic
oligopsychia
oligoria
"omahl" Phonetic for haut-mal.
omnipotence of thought
onanism
oneiric
oneirism
oneiroanalysis
oneirodynia
oneirogenic
oneirogmus
oneirophrenia
oneiroscopy
"onik–" Phonetic for words beginning onych–.
oniomania
"onir–" Phonetic for words beginning oneir–.
onomatomania
onomatophobia
onomatopoiesis
onychophagy
onychotillomania
operation
    See in *General Surgical Terms.*
opiate
opioid
opium
opsomania

order
    birth o.
oreximania
organic
    o. brain syndrome (OBS)
orientation
    reality o.
oriented
    alert and o. (AO)
    o. to time, place, and person
      (OTPP)
    o. to time, place, person, and
      situation [or circumstance]
    o. times three, o. x3
orthopsychiatry
osmophobia
osteophagia
overcompensation
overdetermination
overdose (OD)
overlay
    emotional o.
    psychogenic o.
overprotection
    maternal o.
overt
overtone
    psychic o.
palilalia
panel
    urine drug p. (UDP)
panic
    acute homosexual p., homo-
      sexual p.
    p. attack
panophobia
panphobia
pantophobia
pantophobic
paradoxic, paradoxical
paragrammatism
paragraphia
paralalia
    p. literalis
paralogia
    thematic p.
paralogism

paralysis (paralyses)
    functional p.
    general p. of the insane
    histrionic p.
    hysterical p.
    psychic gaze p.
paranoia
    alcoholic p.
    amorous p.
    p. hallucinatoria
    heboid p.
    litigious p.
    p. originaria
    querulous p.
    p. simplex
paranoiac
paranoic
paranoid
paranoidism
paranomia
paranormal
paranosic
paranosis
parapathia
paraphasia
    central p.
    literal p.
    verbal p.
paraphasic
paraphasis
paraphemia
paraphernalia
paraphia
paraphilia
paraphiliac
paraphobia
paraphora
paraphrasia
paraphrenia
    p. confabulans
    p. expansiva
    involutional p.
    late p.
    p. phantastica
    p. systematica
paraphrenic
parapsychology
parapsychosis

parareaction
parasomnia
parataxic
    p. distortion
parergasia
parergastic
parorexia
parried
parry
parthenophobia
passive-aggressive
pathergasia
pathophobia
paucity
    p. of speech
Pavlov method
pavor
    p. diurnus
    p. nocturnus
PB—phenobarbital
PCP—phencyclidine
    phenylcyclohexyl piperidine
      [now: phencyclidine]
PD—psychotic depression
peccatiphobia
pederasty
pedophilia
pedophilic
pedophobia
pellagra
peotillomania
perception
perceptual
persecuted
persecutory
perseverate
perseveration
persona
personality
    affective p.
    affective p. disorder
    aggressive p.
    alternating p.
    amoral p.
    anankastic p.
    antisocial p.
    antisocial p. disorder
    as-if p.

personality (continued)
    asthenic p.
    avoidant p. disorder
    borderline p. disorder
    compulsive p.
    cycloid p.
    cycloid p. disorder
    cyclothymic p.
    cyclothymic p. disorder
    dependent p. disorder
    disordered p.
    dissociative p.
    double p.
    dual p.
    dyssocial p.
    epileptoid p. disorder
    explosive p.
    histrionic p. disorder
    hysterical p.
    inadequate p.
    kolytic p.
    multiple p.
    narcissistic p. disorder
    obsessive p.
    obsessive-compulsive p.
    obsessive-compulsive p. dis-
      order
    paranoid p.
    paranoid p. disorder
    passive p.
    passive-aggressive p.
    passive-dependent p.
    psychopathic p.
    sadistic p. disorder
    schizoid p.
    schizoid p. disorder
    schizothymic p.
    schizotypal p. disorder
    seclusive p.
    seclusive p., shut-in p.
    self-defeating p. disorder
    shut-in p.
    sociopathic p.
    split p.
    split-off p.
perversion
    sexual p.
pervert

pessimism
PET—positron emission tomography [scan]
PFQ—personality factor questionnaire
phagomania
phagophobia
phallic
phaneromania
phantasm
phantasmatomoria
phantasmoscopia
"phantasy" Phonetic for fantasy.
pharmacomania
pharmacophilia
pharmacophobia
pharmacopsychosis
phengophobia
phenomenon (phenomena)
    break-off p.
    Frégoli p.
    psi p.
    tip-of-the-tongue p.
phenothiazines [a class of drugs]
phenylbutylpiperadines [a class of drugs]
phlegmatic
phobia
    school p.
    simple p.
    social p.
    street p.
phobic
phobophobia
phonatory
phonophobia
photaugiaphobia
phren
phrenology
phthisiomania
phthisiophobia
physiognomy
physiognosis
pica
"pikno–" Phonetic for words beginning pykno–.
Pinel system

"pira–" Phonetic for words beginning pyra–.
polygamy
polypharmaceutic
polypharmacy
polyphobia
poriomania
pornographomania
Porteus maze test
postpartum
    p. depression
potency
potomania
precocious
precocity
precognition
preconscious
predilection
predisposition
pregenital
prejudice
principal [primary, main]
principle [rule]
probe
    memory p.
projection
prosody
proteinphobia
PRP—Psychotic Reaction Profile
pseudodelirium
pseudodementia
    hysterical p.
pseudologia
    p. fantastica
pseudomania
psy, psych—psychiatry, psychiatric
psychalgia
psychalgic
psychalia
psychanopsia
psychataxia
psyche
psychedelic
psychiatric
psychiatrist
psychiatry
psychic
psychoactive

psychoanaleptic
psychoanalysis
    adlerian p.
    classic p.
    jungian p.
psychoanalyst
psychoanalytic
psychoanalyze
psychoauditory
psychobiological
psychobiology
psychocatharsis
psychochemistry
psychochrome
psychochromesthesia
psychodiagnosis
psychodiagnostics
psychodrama
psychodynamics
    adaptational p.
psychodysleptic
psychogenesis
psychogenia
psychogenic
psychogeriatrics
psychognosis
psychogogic
psychogram
psychograph
psychokinesia
psychokinesis
psychokym, psychokyme
psycholagny
psycholepsy
psycholeptic
psycholinguistics
psychologic, psychological
psychologist
psychology
    abnormal p.
    analytic p., analytical p.
    animal p.
    applied p.
    behavioristic p.
    child p.
    clinical p.
    cognitive p.
    community p.

psychology (continued)
    comparative p.
    counseling p.
    criminal p.
    depth p.
    developmental p.
    dynamic p.
    environmental p.
    experimental p.
    gestalt p. [also: Gestalt]
    humanistic p.
    individual p.
    industrial p.
    infant p.
    Janet p.
    physiologic p.
    social p.
psychometer
psychometric
psychometry
psychoneurosis (psychoneuroses)
    See also *neurosis*.
    defense p.
    p. maidica
    obsessive-compulsive p.
    paranoid p.
psychoparesis
psychopath
    sexual p.
psychopathia
    p. martialis
    p. sexualis
psychopathic
psychopathology
psychopathosis
psychopathy
psychopharmacology
psychoplegia
psychoplegic
psychopneumatology
psychoreaction
psychorhythmia
psychorrhea
psychorrhexis
psychosedation
psychosedative
psychosensorial
psychosensory

psychoses (plural of psychosis)
psychosexual
psychosexuality
psychosis (psychoses)
   affective p.
   alcoholic polyneuritic p.
   alcoholic p.'s
   alternating p.
   p. of association
   atypical p.
   bipolar p.
   bipolar affective p.
   brief reactive p.
   bromide p.
   buffoonery p.
   Cheyne-Stokes p.
   chronic epileptic p.
   circular p.
   climacteric p.
   depressive p.
   drug p.
   functional p.
   gestational p.
   housewife's p.
   hysterical p.
   idiophrenic p.
   induced p.
   involutional p.
   Korsakoff p.
   manic p.
   manic-depressive p.
   organic p.
   paranoiac p.
   paranoid p.
   periodic p.
   polyneuritic p.
   p. polyneuritica
   postpartum p.
   prison p.
   puerperal p.
   reactive p.
   reactive-depressive p.
   schizoaffective p.
   schizophrenic p.
   schizophreniform p.
   senile p.
   situational p.
   symbiogenic p.

psychosis (psychoses) (continued)
   symbiotic p.
   symbiotic infantile p.
   tardive p.
   toxic p.
   unipolar p.
   Wernicke-Korsakoff p.
   windigo p.
   zoophil p.
psychosocial
psychosomatic
psychosomimetic
psychostimulant
psychosurgery
psychosyndrome
psychosynthesis
psychotechnics
psychotherapeutics
psychotherapy
   brief p.
   contractual p.
   directive p.
   dynamic p.
   existential p.
   family p.
   group p.
   hypnotic p.
   personologic p.
   psychoanalytic p.
   suggestive p.
   supportive p.
   transactional p.
psychotic
psychotogenic
psychotomimetic
psychotropic
psychrophobia
PTA—post-traumatic amnesia
puerile
puerilism
purge
purging
   bingeing and p.
pyrazolopyrimidines [a class of
   drugs]
pyrolagnia
pyromania
pyrophobia

querulous
radiophobia
"rahpor" Phonetic for rapport.
rapport
rational
rationalization
Ray mania
reaction
    acute situational r., acute
      stress r.
    adjustment r.
    alarm r. (AR)
    anniversary r.
    anxiety r.
    associative r.
    crisis r.
    defense r.
    dissociative r.
    fight-or-flight r.
    r. formation
    hyperkinetic r. of childhood
    manic-depressive r.
    psychosomatic r.
    psychotic depressive r.
    rage r.
    stress r.
reality testing
recalcitrant
    r. patient
recidivism
recidivist
redintegration
regression
    atavistic r.
Reitan-Indiana aphasic screening test
rejoinder
repertoire
repetition
repression
resistance
    drug r.
    multidrug r., multiple drug. r.
retardate
    ineducable r.
retardation
    cultural-familial mental r.
    psychomotor r.
    psychosocial r.

Rett
    syndrome
rivalry
Rorschach test
rumination
    obsessive r.
ruminative
SAD—seasonal affective disorder
sadism
    anal s.
    oral s.
sadist
sadistic
sadomasochistic
"sahn-frwa" Phonetic for sang-froid.
sang-froid ["sahn-frwa"]
sanguine
sardonic
SAT—Scholastic Aptitude Test
satiate, satiated
satyriasis
satyromania
SB—Stanford-Binet (test)
scale
    Brazelton behavioral s.
    Columbia Mental Maturity S.
    Minnesota preschool s.
    Stanford-Binet intelligence s.
    Vineland social maturity s.
    Wechsler Adult Intelligence
      S. (WAIS)
    Wechsler Intelligence S. for
      Children (WISC)
    Zung depression s.
scan
    See also in *Radiology,*
      Nuclear Medicine, and
      Other Imaging section.
    PET (positron emission
      tomography) s.
scansion
schizoid
schizophasia
schizophrenia
    acute s.
    ambulatory s.
    atypical s.
    borderline s.

schizophrenia (continued)
    catatonic s.
    childhood s.
    disorganized s.
    hebephrenic s.
    iatrogenic s.
    latent s.
    nuclear s.
    paranoid s.
    paraphrenic s.
    prepsychotic s.
    process s.
    prodromal s.
    pseudoneurotic s.
    pseudopsychopathic s.
    reactive s.
    residual s.
    schizoaffective s.
    simple s.
    undifferentiated s.
schizophreniac
schizophrenic
schizophreniform
scopophobia
scotoma (scotomata)
    mental s.
scotomization
scotophobia
screen
    urine drug s. (UDS)
scribomania
scurrile
scurrilous
SD—standard deviation
SDM—standard deviation of the mean
SDS—Self-Rating Depression Scale
sedate
sedation
sedatives [a class of drugs]
    general s.
    nervous s.
selective serotonin reuptake inhibitors (SSRIs) [a class of drugs]
self
    idealized s.
    true s.
self-absorption

self-consciousness
self-esteem
self-hypnosis
self-image
serotonin
sexual
    s. masochism
    s. sadism
shell shock
shock
    culture s.
    shell s.
SI—self-inflicted
sibling
sign
    See also *phenomenon* and *test.*
    echo s.
    Magnan s.
"sike–" Phonetic for words beginning psych–.
sin–. See also words beginning cin–, syn–.
sitomania
sitophobia
SIW—self-inflicted wound
Sjögren-Larsson
    syndrome
"skizo–" Phonetic for words beginning schizo–.
sleeplessness
sleeptalking
sleepwalking
sociology
sociopath
sodomy
somatization
somatophrenia
somatopsychosis
somnambulism
somniloquism
sophomania
sophomore
space
    personal s.
spot
    hypnogenetic s.
    mental blind s.

SSRIs—selective serotonin reuptake inhibitors [a class of drugs]
stammering
Stanford-Binet
    test
stasiphobia
status
    mental s.
stereotypy
Stewart-Morel
    syndrome
stigma (stigmas, stigmata)
stigmatic
stigmatism
stigmatization
stigmatophilia
stimulants [a class of drugs]
stress
    post-traumatic s.
"strikninomanea" Phonetic for strychninomania.
strychninomania
stupor
    depressive s.
    melancholic s.
stuporous
stuttering
subjective
sublimate
sublimation
submania
substitution
"sudo–" Phonetic for words beginning pseudo–.
suicidal
    s. ideation
suicide
superego
surprise
surrogate
symbiosis
symbol
    phallic s.
symbolism
symbolization
symbolophobia
sympathy

symptom
    See also in *General Medical Terms.*
    abstinence s.'s
    conversion s.
    factitious s.
    induced s.
    Magnan s.
    negative s.
    withdrawal s.'s
syn–. See also words beginning cin–, sin–.
syndrome
    See also *disease.*
    acquired immunodeficiency s. (AIDS)
    alcohol withdrawal s.
    Alice in Wonderland s.
    Alzheimer s.
    amnesic s.
    amnestic s.
    amnestic-confabulatory s.
    battered child s.
    Briquet s.
    Capgras s.
    Cotard s.
    delayed stress s.
    depersonalization s.
    deposed child s.
    depressive s.
    emotional deprivation s.
    empty nest s.
    extrapyramidal s.
    Ganser s.
    Gélineau s.
    gender dysphoria s.
    Gilles de la Tourette s.
    Gowers s.
    Kanner s.
    manic s.
    maternal deprivation s. (MDS)
    Morgagni s.
    Morgagni-Stewart-Morel s.
    Münchausen s.
    Neumann s.
    phobic anxiety-depersonalization s.

syndrome (continued)
>   postcardiotomy psychosis s.
>   Rett s.
>   Stewart-Morel s.
>   Tourette s.
>   Wernicke s.
>   Wernicke-Korsakoff s.
>   withdrawal s.

syphilomania
syphilophobia
syphilopsychosis
Sz—schizophrenia
tachyphrasia
tachyphrenia
taedium
>   t. vitae

taphephobia
tardive
>   t. dyskinesia (TD)

TAT—thematic apperception test
TD—tardive dyskinesia
technique
>   See also *method.*
>   play t.

telepathy
test
>   See also in *Laboratory,
>   Pathology, and Chemistry
>   Terms.*
>   Ammons Full-Range Picture
>   Vocabulary t.
>   Apgar t.
>   aptitude t.'s
>   Army General Classification
>   t.
>   association t.
>   Bender Gestalt t.
>   Bender Visual-Motor Gestalt
>   t.
>   Binet t.
>   Binet-Simon t.
>   Children's Apperception t.
>   (CAT)
>   Denver Developmental
>   Screening t.
>   draw-a-bicycle t.
>   draw-a-family t.
>   draw-a-person t.

test (continued)
>   Ebbinghaus t.
>   free association t.
>   Goodenough draw-a-man t.,
>   Goodenough draw-a-per-
>   son t.
>   Goodenough-Harris drawing
>   t.
>   Halstead-Reitan t.
>   house-tree-person (HTP) t.
>   incomplete sentences t.
>   inkblot t.
>   intelligence t. (IQ)
>   irresistible impulse t.
>   Minnesota Multiphasic Per-
>   sonality Inventory
>   (MMPI) t.
>   Porteus maze t.
>   projective human figure
>   drawing t.
>   proverbs t.
>   psychological t.
>   Rorschach ink blot t.
>   Rosenzweig picture frustra-
>   tion t.
>   Stanford-Binet t.
>   thematic apperception t.
>   (TAT)
>   WAIS (Wechsler Adult
>   Intelligence Scale) t.
>   Wechsler Adult Intelligence
>   Scale (WAIS) t.
>   Wechsler Intelligence Scale
>   for Children (WISC) t.
>   Wittenborn Psychiatric Rat-
>   ing Scale t.
>   word association t.
>   Ziehen t.
>   Zung depression scale t.

testing
>   reality t.

tetracyclics [a class of drugs]
thanatophobia
THC—tetrahydrocannabinol
theory
>   Adler t.
>   behavior t.
>   Freud t.

theory (continued)
    gestalt t. [also: Gestalt]
    Meyer t.
therapy
    art t.
    aversion t.
    behavior t.
    carbon dioxide t.
    client-centered t.
    cognitive t.
    combined t.
    conditioning t.
    convulsive shock t.
    couples t.
    drug t.
    electric convulsive t., electroconvulsive t. (ECT)
    electric shock t., electroshock t. (EST)
    family t.
    gestalt t. [also: Gestalt]
    group t.
    Indoklon convulsive t.
    lithium t.
    marriage t.
    milieu t.
    Morita t.
    orthomolecular t.
    play t.
    primal t.
    psychoanalytic t.
    relaxation t.
    sex t.
    shock t.
    sleep t.
    social t.
    suggestion t.
    supportive t.
thienobenzodiazepines [a class of drugs]
thioxanthenes [a class of drugs]
"thisio–" Phonetic for words beginning phthisio–.
thought insertion
thymergastic
"tizeo–" Phonetic for words beginning phthisio–.

TMAS—Taylor Manifest Anxiety Scale
tocophobia
topectomy
tortured
    t. expression
toxicophobia
toxiphrenia
track
    needle t.'s
tragedy
trance
    alcoholic t.
    hypnotic t.
    induced t.
    somnambulistic t.
transference
    counter t. (also: countertransference)
transsexual
transsexualism
transvestism
trauma (traumas, traumata)
    psychic t.
traumatic
traumatism
traumatize
treatment
    electroconvulsive t. (ECT), electroshock t.
    shock t.
trichologia
trichomania
trichotillomania
tricyclic
tricyclics [a class of drugs]
tristimania
type
    basic personality t.
    personality t.
    schizoid t.
typhomania
typical antipsychotics [a class of drugs]
"u–" Phonetic for words beginning eu–.
UDP—urine drug panel
UDS—urine drug screen

"ufor–" Phonetic for words beginning euphor–.

ululation

uncompensated

unit

> See also in *General Medical Terms* and *Laboratory, Pathology, and Chemistry Terms*.
>
> alcohol and drug dependency u. (ADDU)
>
> detoxification (detox) u.
>
> psychiatric u.

"unoia" Phonetic for eunoia.

urine

> u. drug panel (UDP)
>
> u. drug screen (UDS)

urolagnia

urophobia

uteromania

VDRS—Verdun Depression Rating Scale

vegetative

verbigeration

verbomania

vicious

"vitselzookt" Phonetic for witzelsucht.

Vogt-Spielmeyer

> disease

volatile

voyeurism

VS—verbal scale (IQ)

VTSRS—Verdun Target Symptom Rating Scale

vulnerability

vulnerable

Wechsler

> Adult Intelligence Scale (WAIS)
>
> Intelligence Scale for Children (WISC)

Wernicke-Korsakoff

> psychosis
>
> syndrome

WISC—Wechsler Intelligence Scale for Children

withdrawal

> w. symptoms
>
> w. syndrome
>
> thought w.

Wittenborn Psychiatric Rating Scale

> test

witzelsucht

WPRS—Wittenborn Psychiatric Rating Scale

xenophobia

Yerkes-Bridges test

"yoo–" Phonetic for words beginning eu–.

zelotypia

"zeno–" Phonetic for words beginning xeno–.

Ziehen

> test

zoomania

zoophobia

Pulmonary Medicine

a—[as a subscript] symbol for arterial blood
A—[as a subscript] symbol for alveolar gas
A-a, $(A-a)O_2$, $P(A-a)O_2$—alveolar-arterial [oxygen gradient]
AB—asthmatic bronchitis
A/B—apnea-bradycardia
A&B—apnea and bradycardia
ABA—allergic bronchopulmonary aspergillosis
ABC—airway-breathing-circulation [protocol]
    apnea, bradycardia, cyanosis
ABG, ABGs—arterial blood gas(es)
Abrahams sign
abscess
    caseous a.
    cheesy a.
    chronic a.
    embolic a.
    emphysematous a.
    fungal a.
    lung a.
    metastatic a.
    metastatic tuberculous a.
    miliary a.
    nocardial a.
    pneumococcic a.
    pulmonary a.
    streptococcal a.
    strumous a.
    tuberculous a.
abuse
    tobacco a.
acapnial
acapnic
acarbia
ACC—alveolar cell carcinoma
accessory
    a. muscles of respiration

acidosis
    carbon dioxide a.
    compensated a.
    hypercapnic a.
    lactic a.
    non-anion gap a.
    nonrespiratory a.
    respiratory a.
acidotic
acini (plural of acinus)
acinic
aciniform
acinitis
acinose [adj.]
acinotubular
acinous [adj.]
acinus (acini)
    pulmonary a.
acoustic
    a. reflection method
acromicria
actinomycosis
    pulmonary a.
action
adenocarcinoma
    alveolar a.
    bronchioalveolar a.
    bronchiolar a.
    bronchioloalveolar a.
    bronchoalveolar a.
    bronchogenic a.
    a. of lung
adenoma
    bronchial a.
    chondromatous a.
adenomatosis
    pulmonary a.
adenopathy
    hilar a.
    tracheobronchial a.

adhesion
>a. of pleura

adiaspiromycosis

adjuvant

adrenal cortical steroids, adrenocortical steroids [a class of drugs]

adrenaline

adrenergic
>a. agonists [a class of drugs]

Adson
>maneuver
>procedure
>test

adventitious
>a. sounds

AE—air entry

AEA—allergic extrinsic alveolitis

aeremia

aerocele

aerodermectasia

aeroembolism

aeroemphysema

aeroionotherapy

aeroporotomy

aerosol

aerosolization

AFRD—acute febrile respiratory disease

afterdamp

AIDS—acquired immunodeficiency syndrome

AILD—angioimmunoblastic lymphadenopathy with dysproteinemia

air
>alveolar a.
>ambient a.
>a. bronchogram
>a. bronchogram sign
>a. curtain
>a. embolism
>a. hunger
>residual a.
>tidal a.
>a. tube
>vitiated a.

airflow obstruction disease (AOD)

air space disease

airway
>anatomical a.
>artificial a.
>a. closure
>a. conductance
>conducting a.
>endotracheal a.
>a. epithelium
>esophageal obturator a.
>a. heat loss
>a. hyperactivity
>lower a.
>a. narrowing
>nasopharyngeal a.
>oropharyngeal a.
>a. osmolarity
>a. permeability
>a. reactivity
>a. receptors
>a. resistance
>respiratory a.
>a. tone

albuminoptysis

albuminoreaction

alkalosis
>acapnial a.
>carbon dioxide a.
>compensated a.
>metabolic a.
>respiratory a.

alkalotic

alkaluria

allergic
>a. bronchopulmonary aspergillosis

allergy
>bronchial a.
>delayed a.
>immediate a.
>pollen a.

Allis
>inhaler

alpha chain disease

aluminosis

alveobronchiolitis

alveolate

alveoli (genitive and plural of alveolus)

alveolitis
    allergic a.
    cryptogenic fibrosing a.
    diffuse sclerosing a.
    extrinsic allergic a.
    fibrosing a.
    a. with honeycombing
alveolobronchogram
alveolocapillary
alveolus (alveoli)
    pulmonary a.
    alveoli pulmonis
    alveoli pulmonum
Ambu bag
amebiasis
    pulmonary a.
"amp" Slang for ampicillin.
"amp and gent" Slang for ampicillin
    and gentamicin.
amphoric
amphoricity
anaerobiosis
anapnoic
anapnotherapy
Andral
    decubitus
    sign
anesthesia
    See in *General Surgical
        Terms.*
aneurysm
    mycotic a.
angina
    a. diphtheritica
angioimmunoblastic
    a. lymphadenopathy
    a. lymphadenopathy with
        dysproteinemia (AILD)
anomaly
    Freund a.
anoxiate
antagonist
    histamine H_1 a.'s [a class of
        drugs]
    leukotriene receptor a.'s [a
        class of drugs]
anthracosilicosis

anthracosis
    a. linguae
anthracotic
anthropotoxin
antiasthma
antibody (antibodies)
    See also in *Laboratory,
        Pathology, and Chemistry
        Terms.*
    monoclonal a.
antimony (Sb)
    a. pneumoconiosis
α_1-antitrypsin [alpha-1-]
antituberculous agents [a class of
    drugs]
antitussives [a class of drugs]
AP—anteroposterior [x-ray]
A&P—auscultation and percussion
APE—acute pulmonary edema
apex (apices, apexes)
    a. pulmonis, a. pulmonalis
apical
apices (plural of apex)
apicolysis
apnea
    chemoreceptor a.
    deglutition a.
    hypersomnia sleep a.
    induced a.
    initial a.
    late a.
    a. neonatorum
    obstructive sleep a.
    postanesthesia a.
    traumatic a.
apneumatosis
apneumia
apneusis
apparatus
    Fell-O'Dwyer a.
    inhalation therapy a.
    suspensory a. of pleura
appearance
arch
    aortic a.
arcus
    a. costarum

ARD—acute respiratory disease
    acute respiratory distress
ARDS—acute respiratory distress
    syndrome
    adult respiratory distress
        syndrome
area (areae, areas)
    apical a.
    asthmagenic a.
    Krönig a.
    pulmonary a.
ARF—acute respiratory failure
argon (Ar)
Arloing-Courmont test
Arneth
        syndrome
arterial
    a. blood gas (ABG)
    a. oxygen saturation
arteriogram
artery
    pulmonary a.
    subclavian a.
arytenoid
asbestos
asbestosis
aspergillosis
    pulmonary a.
asphyxia
asphyxiation
aspiration
    a. pneumonia
assay
    D-dimer a.
Assmann
    focus
    infiltrate
    tuberculous infiltrate
asthma
    allergic a.
    alveolar a.
    bronchial a.
    carder's a.
    cotton dust a.
    emphysematous a.
    essential a.
    grinder's a.
    intrinsic a.

asthma (continued)
    Millar a. [stridorous laryn-
        gismus]
    miller's a. [occupational a.
        of millers]
    miner's a.
    occupational a.
    potter's a.
atelectasis
    absorption a.
    compression a.
    congenital a.
    congestion a.
    discoid a.
    lobar a.
    lobular a.
    obstructive a.
    platelike a.
    postnatal asphyxia a.
    primary a.
    relaxation a.
    resorption a.
    rounded a.
    secondary a.
    segmental a.
atelectatic
atmograph
atmotherapy
atresia
atrium (atria)
    pulmonary a.
atrophy
    senile a. of lung
attack
    apnea a.
    Stokes-Adams a.
aura
    a. asthmatica
Austin Flint
    cavernous respiration
Ayerza
    disease
    syndrome
azygos
    a. vein
BABYbird
    respirator

Baccelli
  sign
bacille Calmette-Guérin (BCG) vac-
    cine
bacillus (bacilli)
    See in *Laboratory, Patholo-
      gy, and Chemistry Terms.*
Bacillus
    See in *Laboratory, Patholo-
      gy, and Chemistry Terms.*
bacterium (bacteria)
    See specific bacteria in *Lab-
      oratory, Pathology, and
      Chemistry Terms.*
bag
    Ambu b.
bagassosis
BAL—bronchoalveolar lavage
Balme cough
Bamberger-Marie
    disease
    syndrome
bandage
    See in *General Surgical
      Terms.*
Bard
    syndrome
baritosis
barotrauma
    pulmonary b.
base
    b. excess
bathypnea
bauxite
    b. pneumoconiosis
Bayle
    granulations
BB—blue bloater [emphysema]
BCG (bacille Calmette-Guérin) vac-
    cine
Beatty-Bright friction sound
Bethea
    method
    sign
bibasilar
    b. rales
bicarbonate

Biermer
    change
    sign
bifurcatio
    b. tracheae
bilharziosis, bilharziasis
bimodal therapy
biomarker
biopsy
    brush b.
    fine-needle b.
    fine-needle aspiration b.
    lung b.
    needle b.
    scalene lymph node b.
    transbronchial lung b.
    wedge b.
Biot
    breathing
    breathing sign
    respiration
    sign
Biox
BiPAP—bilateral positive airway
    pressure
biphasic
Bird
    respirator
    sign
bituminosis
black lung disease
Blalock-Taussig
    shunt
blast
    bechic b.
    b. chest
    b. effect
    lung b.
blastoma
    pulmonary b.
BLB—Boothby-Lovelace-Bulbulian
BLB mask
bleb
    subpleural b.
blennothorax
bloater
    blue b. [emphysema]

blood flow study
    pulmonary b.f.s.
blow-by oxygen
blue
    b. bloater [emphysema]
Blumenau
    test
body (bodies)
    creola b.
    psittacosis inclusion b.
Bohr
    equation
    isopleth method
BOOP—bronchiolitis obliterans
    organizing pneumonia
Boothby
    mask
"boo-zhe" Phonetic for bougie.
borderline
Bornholm
    disease
Bouchut
    respiration
brachytherapy
    interstitial b.
    intracavitary application b.
    remote afterloading b.
bradypnea
Bragg-Paul pulsator
breath
breath-holding
breathiness
breathing
    apneustic b.
    ataxic b.
    autonomous b.
    Biot b.
    bronchial b.
    Cheyne-Stokes b.
    continuous positive-pressure
      b. (CPPB)
    diaphragmatic b.
    frog b.
    glossopharyngeal b.
    intermittent positive-pres-
      sure b. (IPPB)
    Kussmaul b.
    labored b.

breathing (continued)
    shallow b.
    suppressed b.
    vesicular b.
breathless
breathlessness
Brehmer
    method
    treatment
Bretonneau
    angina
    disease
Brock
    syndrome
bronchadenitis
bronchi (plural of bronchus)
bronchia (plural of bronchium)
bronchial
    b. adenoma
    b. brushing
    b. challenge test
    b. circulation
    b. lavage
    b. obstruction
    b. reactivity
    b. stenosis
    b. tube
bronchiectasis
    capillary b.
    chemical b.
    cylindrical b.
    cystic b.
    follicular b.
    pseudocylindrical b.
    saccular b.
bronchiectatic
bronchiloquy
bronchiocele
bronchiocrisis
bronchiolar
    b. lavage
    b. stenoses
bronchiole
    alveolar b.
    lobular b.
    respiratory b.
    terminal b.
bronchiolectasis

bronchioli (plural of bronchiolus)
bronchiolitis
    acute obliterating b.
    b. exudativa
    b. fibrosa obliterans
    vesicular b.
    viral b.
bronchiolus (bronchioli)
    bronchioli respiratorii
bronchitic
bronchitis
    acute laryngotracheal b.
    acute suppurative b.
    arachidic b.
    asthmatic b.
    b. obliterans
    Castellani b.
    catarrhal b.
    cheesy b.
    chronic b.
    chronic obstructive b.
    croupous b.
    epidemic capillary b.
    exudative b.
    fibrinous b.
    hemorrhagic b.
    infectious asthmatic b.
    mechanical b.
    membranous b.
    phthinoid b.
    plastic b.
    polypoid b.
    productive b.
    pseudomembranous b.
    putrid b.
    secondary b.
    staphylococcal b.
    streptococcal b.
    suffocative b.
    vanadium b.
    vesicular b.
bronchium (bronchia)
bronchoadenitis
bronchoalveolar
    b. lavage
bronchoalveolitis
bronchoaspergillosis
bronchoblastomycosis

bronchoblennorrhea
bronchocandidiasis
bronchocavernous
bronchocavitary
bronchocele
bronchocentric
    b. granulomatosis
bronchoconstriction
bronchoconstrictor
bronchodilatation
bronchoegophony
bronchoesophageal
    b. fistula
bronchoesophagology
bronchoesophagoscopy
bronchofibroscopy
bronchogram
bronchography
    Cope-method b.
    percutaneous transtracheal b.
broncholith
broncholithiasis
bronchologic
bronchology
bronchomalacia
bronchomoniliasis
bronchomotor
bronchomucotropic
bronchomycosis
bronchonocardiosis
bronchopancreatic
    b. fistula
bronchopathy
bronchophony
    pectoriloquous b.
    sniffling b.
    whispered b.
bronchoplasty
bronchoplegia
bronchopleural
bronchopleuropneumonia
bronchopneumonia
    inhalation b.
    postoperative b.
bronchopneumonic
bronchopneumonitis
bronchopneumopathy

bronchopulmonary
    b. aspergillosis
    b. dysplasia
    b. lavage
    b. markings
bronchoradiography
bronchorrhagia
bronchorrhaphy
bronchorrhea
bronchoscopic
bronchoscopy
    fiberoptic b.
    nonfiberoptic b.
bronchosinusitis
bronchospasm
bronchospirochetosis
bronchospirography
bronchospirometer
bronchospirometry
    differential b.
bronchostaxis
bronchostenosis
bronchostomy
bronchotetany
bronchotomy
bronchotracheal
bronchovesicular
bronchus (bronchi)
    apical b.
    cardiac b.
    dorsal b.
    eparterial b.
    esophageal b.
    extrapulmonary b.
    hyparterial b.
    intermediate b.
    intrapulmonary b.
    left superior ventral b.
    lingular b.
    b. lingularis
    lobar b.
    b. lobares
    lower lobe b.
    main bronchi, right and left
    main stem b.
    middle lobe b.
    primary bronchi, right and left
    b. principalis dexter

bronchus (bronchi) (continued)
    b. principalis sinister
    right ventral b.
    segmental b.
    bronchi segmentales
    b. segmentalis basalis
    stem b.
    subapical b.
    tracheal b.
    upper lobe b.
"brongk–" Phonetic for words
    beginning bronch–.
"broo-ee" Phonetic for bruit.
brown lung disease
"bru-ee" Phonetic for bruit.
bruit
    b. de bois ["duh bwah"]
    b. de craquement ["duh
      krak-maw"]
    b. de cuir neuf ["duh kwer
      nuf"]
    b. de frolement ["duh frol-
      maw"]
    b. de grelot ["duh gruh-lo"]
    b. de pot fêlé [" duh po fe-
      lay"]
    b. d'airain ["da-ra"]
brush
    b. biopsy
brushing
    bronchial b.
"brwe" Phonetic for bruit.
B/S—breath sounds
BSE—bilateral, symmetrical, and
    equal
Buhl
    desquamative pneumonia
    disease
bulla (bullae)
    emphysematous b.
bullate
bullation
bullectomy
Burghart
    sign
    symptom
burn
    respiratory b.

BV—bronchovesicular
byssinosis
cadmiosis
calcicosilicosis
calcicosis
calcification
    eggshell c.
    pulmonary c.
Calmette
    vaccine
CA (cardiac-apnea) monitor
canal
    pleuropericardial c.
    pleuroperitoneal c.
cancer
    See also *carcinoma*.
    See also in *Oncology and
       Hematology* section.
    asbestos c.
    smoker's c.
candidiasis
    bronchial c.
    pulmonary c.
CAO—chronic airway obstruction
capacity
    forced vital c. (FVC)
    maximum lung c.
    oxygen c.
    timed vital c.
capillary (capillaries)
    arteriolar c.
Caplan
    nodules
    syndrome
capnea monitor
capneic
Capps
    reflex
    sign
carcinoembryonic antigen (CEA)
carcinoid
    bronchial c.
carcinoma (carcinomas, carcinomata)
    See also *cancer*.
    See also in *Oncology and
       Hematology* section.
    alveolar cell c.
    anaplastic c.

carcinoma (carcinomas, carcinomata)
    (continued)
       bronchiolar c.
       bronchogenic c.
       epidermoid c.
       squamous cell c.
carcinomatosis
    c. pleurae
cardia
    incompetent c.
cardiorespiratory
    arrest
carina
    c. of trachea
Carswell grapes
cartilage
    cricoid c.
Castellani
    bronchitis
    disease
caval
cavernoscopy
cavernostomy
cavitary
    c. lesion
CB—chronic bronchitis
CBA—chronic bronchitis with asth-
    ma
CDILD—chronic diffuse interstitial
    lung disease
cell
    See also in *Laboratory,
       Pathology, and Chemistry
       Terms*.
    ciliated c.
    clonogenic c.
    dust c.
    endocrine c.
    Langhans c.
    metaplastic c.
    mucous c.
    stem c.
centrilobular
ceramidase deficiency
CF—cystic fibrosis
CF antibody titer
CG—choking gas (phosgene)
chalicosis

change
> Biermer c.
> Gerhardt c. of sound

chest
> AP (anteroposterior) c. x-ray
> barrel c.
> emphysematous c.
> flail c.
> funnel c.
> PA (posteroanterior) and lateral c. x-ray
> pendelluft c.
> pterygoid c.

Cheyne-Stokes
> asthma
> breathing
> respiration

cholesterohydrothorax
chondroadenoma
chondroma
> c. of lung

chylaqueous
chylomediastinum
chylopleura
chylopneumothorax
chylorrhea
chylothorax
cin–. See also words beginning sin–, syn–.
cinebronchogram
cinebronchography
circadian
> c. rhythm

Clark
> electrode

classification
> International Labor Organization (ILO) C. of Pneumoconioses

clavipectoral
CLD—chronic lung disease
CMA—chronic metabolic acidosis
CMV—continuous mechanical ventilation
CNPAP—continuous nasal positive airway pressure
CO_2 [CO2]—carbon dioxide

COAD—chronic obstructive airway disease
coagulopathy
cobaltosis
cogwheel
> c. breathing

coin lesion
COLD—chronic obstructive lung disease
collapse
> c. of lung

collapsed lung
collapsotherapy
Collins
> respirometer-spirometer

concomitant
> c. metabolic acidosis

congested
congestion
> pleuropulmonary c.
> rebound c.

congestive
> c. heart failure (CHF)

coniosporosis
coniotoxicosis
COPD—chronic obstructive pulmonary disease
Cope-method bronchography
cor
> c. pulmonale

core vesicles
corporis (genitive of corpus)
corpus (corpora)
> corpora amylacea

Corrigan
> pneumonia
> respiration

corticosteroids [a class of drugs]
costal
> c. margin

costectomy
costopleural
costopneumopexy
costoversion thoracoplasty
costovertebral
cough
> aneurysmal c.
> Balme c.

cough (continued)
    barking c.
    brassy c.
    compression c.
    dry c.
    extrapulmonary c.
    habit c.
    hacking c.
    mechanical c.
    Morton c.
    nonproductive c.
    paroxysmal c.
    privet c.
    productive c.
    psychogenic c.
    reflex c.
    c. response
    smoker's c.
    Sydenham c.
    tea taster's c.
    c. threshold
    trigeminal c.
    weaver's c.
    wet c.
    whooping c.
    winter c.
CPAP—continuous positive airway
    pressure
CPE—chronic pulmonary emphyse-
    ma
CPPB—continuous positive-pres-
    sure breathing
CPT—chest physiotherapy
Craig
    test
CRD—chronic respiratory disease
crepitant
cricoid
cricopharyngeus
cricotracheotomy
croupy
crura (plural of crus)
cruris (genitive of crus)
crus (crura)
cryptococcosis
    pulmonary c.
cryptoempyema
cryptogenic

crystal
    Leyden c.'s
CSR—Cheyne-Stokes respiration
CTAP—clear to auscultation and
    percussion
culmen (culmina)
    c. of left lung
culture
    sputum c.
    tracheal aspirate c.
cupula (cupulae)
    c. of pleura
    c. pleurae
    c. pleuralis
Curschmann
    spirals
curse
    Ondine's c.
CV—closing volume
cyanosis
    pulmonary c.
cyst
    bronchogenic c.
    dermoid c.
    enteric c.
    neurenteric c.
    pericardial c.
    thymic c.
cystic
    c. fibrosis
cytogenic
D'Amato sign
Daniel
    operation
Darling
    disease
D_{co} [DCO]—diffusing capacity for
    carbon monoxide
Debove
    membrane
debris
    inflammatory cell d.
decarbonization
décollement
decortication
    d. of lung
deficiency
    α_1-antitrypsin d. [alpha-1-]

degeneration
    trabecular d.
Delmege sign
Delorme
    operation
demulcents [a class of drugs]
de Mussy
    point
    sign
Denny-Brown syndrome
density
    conglomerate d.
Desnos
    disease
    pneumonia
diaphragmatic
    d. excursion
    d. pacing
    d. paralysis
diatomite
    d. disease
    d. fibrosis
Dieulafoy
    disease
    erosion
    triad
diffusion
    d. components
    d. limitation
dimer
    D-d.
DIP—desquamative interstitial
    pneumonia
dis–. See also words beginning dys–.
discission
    d. of pleura
discrete
    d. area of consolidation
    d. area of effusion
    d. lesion
    d. nodule
disease
    See also *syndrome.*
    airflow obstruction d. (AOD)
    air space d.
    alpha chain d.
    Ayerza d.
    bird breeder's d.

disease (continued)
    black lung d.
    Bornholm d.
    brown lung d.
    Daae d.
    Darling d.
    Desnos d.
    diatomite d.
    elevator d.
    Fabry d.
    Gaucher d.
    grinder's d.
    Hamman d.
    hard metal d.
    HIB (*Haemophilus influen-*
        zae type b) d.
    Hodgkin d.
    hyaline membrane d.
    interstitial d. (ID)
    Isambert d.
    Kartagener d.
    legionnaires' d.
    Löffler d.
    Lucas-Champonnièred.
    Marie-Bamberger d.
    Newcastle d.
    pigeon breeder's d.
    Pompe d.
    pulmonary embolic d.
    Ritter d.
    Shaver d.
    silo filler's d.
    Sylvest d.
    Takayasu d.
    Whipple d.
    Woillez d.
    woolsorter's d.
D_L [DL]—diffusing capacity of lung
D_LCO [DLCO]—diffusing capacity
    of lung for carbon monoxide
DOE—dyspnea on exertion
Douglas
    bag spirometer
drainage
    water-seal d.
dressing
    See in *General Surgical*
        Terms.

Drinker respirator
Duchenne
 muscular dystrophy
Duchenne-type muscular dystrophy
Duguet siphon
dys–. See also words beginning dis–.
dysplasia
 bronchopulmonary d.
dyspnea
 exertional d.
 expiratory d.
 inspiratory d.
 nocturnal d.
 nonexpansional d.
 orthostatic d.
 paroxysmal d.
 paroxysmal nocturnal d.
  (PND)
 Traube d.
dystrophy
 Duchenne d.
 Duchenne muscular d.
 Duchenne-type muscular d.
 myotonic d.
EAA—extrinsic allergic alveolitis
EAHF—eczema, asthma, hay fever
Eaton agent pneumonia
Eaton-Lambert syndrome
EBBS—equal bilateral breath sounds
echophony
edema
 alveolar e.
 interstitial e.
 pulmonary e.
 subpleural e.
 vernal e
effect [noun: result, outcome]
 See also *phenomenon, reflex,*
  sign, and *test.*
 blast e.
 Haldane e.
 horse-race e.
effusion
 pleural e.
egophony
E/I—expiration-inspiration ratio
electrode
 Clark e.

electrophrenic
elevator
 e. disease
Ellis sign
Eloesser
 flap
 operation
embarrass
embarrassment
 respiratory e.
emboliform
embolism
 See also *embolus.*
 air e.
 hematogenous e.
 paradoxical e.
 plasmodium e.
 pulmonary e.
 venous e.
embolization
embolus (emboli)
 See also *embolism.*
 platelet e.
 pulmonary e.
 shower of emboli
emphysema
 alveolar e.
 atrophic e.
 bullous e.
 centrilobular e.
 compensatory e.
 cystic e.
 diffuse e.
 false e.
 focal-dust e.
 gangrenous e.
 generalized e.
 glass blower's e.
 hypertrophic e.
 hypoplastic e.
 idiopathic unilobar e.
 interlobular e.
 interstitial e.
 Jenner e.
 lobar e.
 loculated e.
 mediastinal e.
 obstructive e.

emphysema (continued)
    panacinar e.
    panlobular e.
    paracicatricial e.
    paraseptal e.
    pulmonary e.
    senile e.
    small-lunged e.
    subfascial e.
    surgical e.
    traumatic e.
    unilateral e.
    vesicular e.
emphysematous
empyema
    e. benignum
    interlobar e.
    metapneumonic e.
    pneumococcal e.
    putrid e.
    sacculated e.
    streptococcal e.
    synpneumonic e.
    thoracic e.
    tuberculous e.
empyemic
endobronchitis
endorphin
endothelialization
endothelioid
endothelium (endothelia)
endotracheal (ET)
    e. intubation
endotracheitis
epinephrine
epipleural
episplenitis
epithelia (plural of epithelium)
epitheliitis
epithelium (epithelia)
equation
    Henderson-Hasselbalch e.
Equen magnet
ERV—expiratory reserve volume
Escherich test
esophagism
    hiatal e.

esophagitis
    reflux e.
esophagolaryngectomy
esophagospasm
Estlander
    operation
eupnea
eupneic
eventration
    diaphragmatic e.
excavatum
    pectus e.
expansion
expectorants [a class of drugs]
expectorate
expectoration
    rusty e.
expiration
expiratory
exsufflation
exsufflator
extratracheal
extravascular
Fabry
    disease
"fago–" Phonetic for words beginning phago–.
"farin–" Phonetic for words beginning pharyn–.
"farinks" Phonetic for pharynx.
farmer's lung
Fauvel granules
faveolate
FEF—forced expiratory flow
"fenomenon" Phonetic for phenomenon.
FET—forced expiratory time
FETS—forced expiratory time in seconds
FEV—forced expiratory volume
FEV_1 [FEV1]—forced expiratory volume in one second
fever
    zinc fume f.
fiberoptic
    f. bronchoscopy
fiberscopic
fibrocystic

fibroleiomyomatosis
fibroma
    f. of lung
    periapical f.
fibromatogenic
fibromatoid
fibromatosis
fibromatous
fibroplasia
    retrolental f.
fibrosing
fibrosis
    cystic f. (CF)
    diatomite f.
    diffuse interstitial pulmo-
       nary f.
    idiopathic f.
    interstitial f.
    mediastinal f.
    pulmonary f.
fibrothorax
fibrotic
field
    clear lung f.'s
    Krönig f.
    lung f.'s
FIF—forced inspiratory flow
fine-needle
    f-n. aspiration biopsy
    f-n. biopsy
FiO_2 [FiO2]—fractional concentra-
    tion of inspired oxygen
fissura (fissurae)
fissure
    f. of lung
fistula (fistulas, fistulae)
    alveolar f.
    bronchobiliary f.
    bronchocutaneous f.
    bronchoesophageal f.
    bronchopleural f.
    esophagobronchial f.
    mediastinobronchial f.
    pleurobronchial f.
    pleurocutaneous f.
    pulmonary arteriovenous f.
    tracheal f.
    tracheoesophageal f.

flail chest
flap
    Eloesser f.
flattening
    f. of diaphragm
"flebo–" Phonetic for words begin-
    ning phlebo–.
Fleischner
    disease
    lines
"flem" Phonetic for phlegm.
flow
    effective pulmonary blood f.
    maximal midexpiratory f.
    peak expiratory f.
fluctuation
flutter
    mediastinal f.
focus (foci)
    Assmann f.
    Ghon f.
    Simon foci
"fool" Phonetic for Pfuhl.
Forlanini
    treatment
FRC—functional reserve capacity
    functional residual capacity
fremitus
    bronchial f.
    pleural f.
    rhonchal f.
    tactile f.
    tussive f.
    vocal f.
"fren–" Phonetic for words begin-
    ning phren–.
"freng-kuhl" Phonetic for Fränkel.
Freund
    anomaly
Friedländer
    bacillus pneumonia
    disease
    pneumonia
Friedrich
    operation
fuller's earth
    f.e. pneumoconiosis

fungus (fungi)
　　See specific fungi in *Laboratory, Pathology, and Chemistry Terms.*
furrow
　　Schmorl f.
FVC—forced vital capacity
Gaffky
　　scale
　　table
gallium (Ga)
　　g. scan
gangrene
　　g. of lung
gastrocamera
　　Olympus model GTF-A g.
gastroesophageal
　　g. reflux
Gaucher
　　disease
Gerhardt
　　change of sound
　　sign
Ghon
　　complex
　　focus
　　lesion
　　tubercle
Gibson rule
gland
　　Philip g.'s
glanders
　　g. of lung
glass blower's emphysema
glomectomy
glossopharyngeal
　　g. breathing
　　g. nerve
glottis (glottides)
glucocorticoids [a class of drugs]
Goldstein
　　hematemesis
　　hemoptysis
Gowers
　　attack
　　syndrome
granule
　　Fauvel g.

granuloma
　　eosinophilic g.
　　Wegener g.
granulomatosis
　　beryllium g.
　　lymphomatoid g.
　　pulmonary g.
　　sarcoid g.
　　Wegener g.
grape
　　Carswell g.'s
graphite
　　g. pneumoconiosis
graphitosis
grinder's disease
Guéneau de Mussy point
Haemophilus
hamartoma
　　h. of lung
　　intrapulmonary h.
Hamburger test
Hamman
　　disease
　　murmur
　　sign
　　syndrome
Hamman-Rich
　　disease
　　syndrome
hard metal disease
Hare syndrome
hay fever
HC—hyaline cast(s)
HCO_3 [HCO3]—bicarbonate
heaves
Heberden
　　asthma
Hecht
　　phenomenon
　　pneumonia
helium (He)
　　h. dilution method
　　h. equilibration time
　　h. washout
hematite
　　h. pneumoconiosis
hemibody

hemophilus
    See in *Laboratory, Pathology, and Chemistry Terms.*
hemoptysis
    endemic h.
    Goldstein h.
    Manson h.
    parasitic h.
hemorrhage
hemorrhagic
hemosiderosis
    idiopathic pulmonary h.
Henderson-Hasselbalch equation
HEPA—high-efficiency particulate air [filter]
hepaticopulmonary
    h. fistula
Hering-Breuer reflex
Herlitz
    disease
    syndrome
hernia
    diaphragmatic h.
    hiatal h., hiatus h.
    h. of lung
herpes
    h. zoster
hiatal, hiatus
    h. hernia
hiatus
    esophageal h.
HIB—*Haemophilus influenzae* type b
HIB disease
HIB polysaccharide vaccine
hilum (hila)
    h. of lung
    h. pulmonis
hilus (hili). See *hilum.*
"hipo–" Phonetic for words beginning hypo–.
Hirtz rales
histamine
    h. challenge
histiocytosis
    pulmonary h.
    h. X
Hitzenberg test

Hodgkin
    disease
Hoover sign
horse-race effect
hyaline membrane disease
hydropneumothorax
hydrops
    h. of pleura
hydrothorax
    chylous h.
hyparterial
    h. bronchi
hyperbaric
    h. chamber
hyperbicarbonatemia
hyperbradykininemia
hypercapnia
    permissive h.
hypercapnic
hyperchloremic
hyperchloruria
hypercyanotic
hyperinflation
hyperlucency
hyperlucent
hypernitremia
hyperoxemia
hyperoxic
hyperphonesis
hyperplasia
hyperplastic
hyperpnea
hyperpneic
hyperreactive
    h. airways
hyperresonance
hyperresonant
hyperresponsive
hyperresponsiveness
    airway h.
hypertension
    pulmonary h.
hyperventilation
    central neurogenic h.
hypocapnia
hypocapnic
hypoplasia
hypopnea

hypopneic
hypoventilation
    alveolar h.
    central h.
    chronic alveolar h.
    primary alveolar h.
hypoxemia
hypoxemic
hypoxia
hypoxic
    h. insult
idiopathic
I/E—inspiratory-expiratory [ratio]
IFR—inspiratory flow rate
ILD—interstitial lung disease
imaging
    See in *Radiology, Nuclear*
    Medicine, and Other
    Imaging section.
immunoglobulin (Ig)
    i. A (IgA)
    i. D (IgD)
    i. E (IgE)
    i. G (IgG)
    i. M (IgM)
    secretory i. A
immunohistochemistry
impaction
    mucoid i.
impressio (impressiones)
    i. cardiaca pulmonis
impression
IMV—intermittent mandatory ven-
    tilation
infection
    lower respiratory tract i.
        (LRTI)
    upper respiratory i. (URI)
    upper respiratory tract i.
        (URTI)
infiltrate
    Assmann tuberculous i.
influenza
    i. A
    i. B
    i. C
    clinical i.

influenza (continued)
    i. virus (A–C) [also: influen-
        zavirus]
influenzal
infrapulmonic
INH—isonicotinic acid hydrazide
    (isoniazid)
inhalant
    antifoaming i.
inhaler
inhibitor
    leukotriene receptor i.'s [a
        class of drugs]
INPV—intermittent negative-pres-
    sure assisted ventilation
inspiratory
    i. dyspnea
    i.-expiratory (I/E) phase ratio
    i. flow
    forced i. flow (FIF)
    i. flow rate (IFR)
    i.-inhibitory reflex
    maximum i. flow (MIF)
    maximum i. pressure (MIP)
    i. pause time
    peak i. flow (PIF)
    post-tussive i. rhonchi
    i. pressure
    i. rales
    i. reserve capacity (IRC)
    i. reserve volume (IRV)
    i. rhonchi
    i. spasm
    i. stridor
    i. triggering pressure
    i. triggering volume
insufficiency
    basilar i.
    post-traumatic pulmonary i.
    pulmonary i.
insufflation
    endotracheal i.
insult
    hypoxic i.
    respiratory i.
interlobar
intermedius
interstitial disease (ID)

intrabronchial
intracavitary
intrapleural
intrapulmonary
intubation
    endotracheal i.
ions
IPH—idiopathic pulmonary hemo-
    siderosis
IPPB—intermittent positive-pres-
    sure breathing
IPPO—intermittent positive-pres-
    sure inflation with oxygen
IPPR—intermittent positive-pres-
    sure respiration
IPPV—intermittent positive-pres-
    sure ventilation
IRC—inspiratory reserve capacity
IRV—inspiratory reserve volume
Isambert disease
"is-mus" Phonetic for isthmus.
iso—isoproterenol
isolation
    pulmonary i.
isotope
    radioactive i.
isovolume
    i. pressure
isthmi (plural of isthmus)
isthmic
isthmus (isthmi)
    Krönig i.
IV—intravenous
Jackson
    operation
Jenner emphysema
joint
    See in *Orthopedics and*
        Sports Medicine section.
judicious
Jürgensen sign
kaolin
    k. pneumoconiosis
kaolinosis
Kartagener
    disease
    syndrome
    triad

Katayama
    disease
    syndrome
Kaufman pneumonia
Kohn pores
"krico–" Phonetic for words begin-
    ning crico–.
Krogh
    apparatus
    spirometer
Krönig
    area
    field
    isthmus
    percussion
    steps
"krus" Phonetic for crus.
Kussmaul
    breathing
    respiration
    sign
Kussmaul-Kien respiration
Kveim
    test
labored breathing
Labrador lung
Laënnec
    catarrh
    pearls
    sign
"lahringo–" Phonetic for words
    beginning laryngo–.
laparothoracoscopy
"laringo–" Phonetic for words
    beginning laryngo–.
"larinjeal" Phonetic for laryngeal.
"larinks" Phonetic for larynx.
laryngopharyngitis
laryngopharynx
laryngospasm
laryngotracheal
laryngotracheitis
laryngotracheobronchitis
laryngotracheobronchoscopy
laryngotracheoscopy
laryngotracheotomy
lateral
    l. thoracoplasty

Lautier test
law
    See also *rule.*
    Laplace l.
legionella (legionellae)
    l. pneumonia
legionnaires'
    l. disease
    l. pneumonia
Legroux remission
leiomyoma (leiomyomas, leiomyomata)
Leitner syndrome
Leredde syndrome
lesion
    cavitary pulmonary l.
    coin l.
    Ghon primary l.
    precancerous l.
    target l.
leukotriene receptor antagonists (LTRAs) [a class of drugs]
leukotriene receptor inhibitors [a class of drugs]
Leyden
    crystals
light
    l. microscopy (LM)
line
    Kerley A l.'s
    Kerley B l.'s
Lingnières test
linguatuliasis
lingula (lingulae)
    l. of left lung
    l. pulmonis sinistri
lingular
    l. infiltrates
lingulectomy
LIP—lymphocytic interstitial pneumonitis
LLL—left lower lobe
lobar
    l. atelectasis
    l. pneumonia
lobe
    inferior l. of left lung
    inferior l. of right lung

lobe (continued)
    left lower l. (LLL)
    left upper l. (LUL)
    lower l. of lung
    middle l. of right lung
    pulmonary l.'s
    right lower l. (RLL)
    right upper l. (RUL)
    l.'s of lung
    superior l. of left lung
    superior l. of right lung
    upper l. of lung
lobi (plural of lobus)
lobitis
lobostomy
lobus (lobi)
locular
loculate
loculated
    l. pleural effusion
loculation
Löffler
    disease
    eosinophilia
    pneumonia
    syndrome
Louisiana pneumonia
Löwenstein
    medium
LRT—lower respiratory tract
LTB—laryngotracheobronchitis
LTRAs—leukotriene receptor antagonists [a class of drugs]
Lucas-Champonnière disease
LUL—left upper lobe
lung
    arc welder's l.
    artificial l.
    bird breeder's l.
    bird fancier's l.
    black l.
    book l., book-l.
    brown l.
    cardiac l.
    coal miner's l.
    l. collapse, collapsed l.
    collier's l.
    drowned l.

lung (continued)
    eosinophilic l.
    farmer's l.
    fibroid l.
    fluid l.
    harvester's l.
    honeycomb l.
    hyperlucent l.
    iron l.
    Labrador l.
    l. transplantation
    l. markings
    mason's l.
    miner's l.
    mushroom worker's l.
    pigeon breeder's l.
    polycystic l.
    postperfusion l.
    l. root
    shock l.
    silo filler's l.
    thresher's l.
    traumatic wet l.
    trench l.
    vanishing l.
    welder's l.
    wet l.
    white l.
Lyell
    disease
lymphangiectasis
    congenital pulmonary l.
lymphangiomyomatosis
    pulmonary l.
MAC—*Mycobacterium avium* complex
Macleod
    syndrome
macroglobulinemia
    Waldenström m.
macrophage
    alveolar m.
macule
    See also *spot.*
    coal m.
magnet
    Equen m.
main bronchi, main stem bronchus

malformation
Malpighi
    vesicles
maneuver
    See also *method.*
    Müller m.
Manson
    hemoptysis
Marfan
    sign
    syndrome
Marie-Bamberger disease
mask
    nonrebreathing m.
    partial rebreathing m.
Maugeri syndrome
MCT—mean circulation time
mechanism
    wave speed m.
mediastina (plural of mediastinum)
mediastinal
    m. crunch
mediastinoscopic
mediastinoscopy
mediastinum (mediastina)
    anterior m.
    m. anterius
    inferior m.
    m. inferius
    m. medium
    middle m.
    posterior m.
    m. posterius
    superior m.
    m. superius
medicothorax
medium (media, mediums)
    Löwenstein m.
MEF—maximal expiratory flow
MEFR—maximum expiratory flow rate
MEFV—maximum expiratory flow volume
melanoptysis
melioidosis
    pulmonary m.
membranate

membrane
> Debove m.
> hyaline m.
> pulmonary hyaline m.

Mendelson syndrome

mercury (Hg)
> millimeters of m. (mm Hg)

metastasis (metastases)

method
> See also *maneuver.*
> acoustic reflection m.
> Bohr isopleth m.

mica

micaceous

micatosis

microemboli (plural of microembolus)

microembolization

microembolus (microemboli)
> showers of microemboli

microlith

microlithiasis
> m. alveolaris pulmonum
> pulmonary alveolar m.

micronize, micronized

microthrombi (plural of microthrombus)

microthrombosis

microthrombus (microthrombi)

midthorax

MIFR—maximal inspiratory flow rate

migratory
> m. pneumonia

millimeter(s) (mm)
> m.'s of mercury (mm Hg)
> m.'s of water (mm H_2O)

minute [small]

minute gun cough

MIP—maximum inspiratory pressure

mist
> ultrasonic m.

mixed dust
> m.d. pneumoconiosis

MMEF—maximal midexpiratory flow

MMEFR—maximal midexpiratory flow rate

MMF—maximal midexpiratory flow

MMFR—maximal midexpiratory flow rate

mm Hg—millimeters of mercury

mm H_2O [mm H2O]—millimeters of water

mm pp—millimeters partial pressure

molimen (molimina)

Monaldi
> operation

monitor
> apnea m.

Morgagni-Adams-Stokes syndrome

Morton
> cough

Mounier-Kuhn syndrome

MSV—maximal sustained ventilation

MSVC—maximal sustained ventilatory capacity

mucociliary

mucoid

mucous [adj.]
> m. hypersecretion
> m. plug
> m. plugging

mucoviscidosis

mucus [noun]

Mueller
> See *Müller.*

Müller
> maneuver
> test

multilobar

murmur
> cardiopulmonary m.
> cardiorespiratory m.
> respiratory m.

muscle
> See also in *Orthopedics and Sports Medicine* section.
> accessory m.'s of respiration
> diaphragmatic m.
> inspiratory m.
> Reisseisen m.'s
> serratus m., inferior posterior
> serratus m., superior posterior
> strap m.'s

musculus (musculi)
    See in *Orthopedics and*
       Sports Medicine section.
mushroom worker's
    disease
    syndrome
MVV—maximum voluntary venti-
    lation
myasthenia
    m. gravis
    m. gravis pseudoparalytica
myasthenic
mycoplasmal
    m. pneumonia
"my-nute" Phonetic for minute
    [small].
Nathan test
nebulizer
    DeVilbiss n.
necrosis (necroses)
    embolic n.
necrotic
NEEP—negative end-expiratory
    pressure
nerve
    phrenic n.
"neu–" Phonetic for words begin-
    ning pneu–.
neuritic
neuritis
    influenzal n.
neuroendocrine
neuron-specific enolase
neurophysin
neurosecretory
"new–" Phonetic for words begin-
    ning pneu–.
Newcastle
    disease
nidus (nidi)
NO—nitric oxide
nocardial
nodal
node
    bronchopulmonary lymph n.
    mediastinal lymph n.
    pulmonary lymph n.
    tracheobronchial lymph n.

nodular
nodularity
nodulated
nodulation
nodule
    pulmonary n.'s
non-anion gap acidosis
nonfiberoptic bronchoscopy
noninvasive
"noo–" Phonetic for words begin-
    ning pneu–.
"nu–" Phonetic for words beginning
    pneu–.
"nur–" Phonetic for words begin-
    ning neur–.
O_2 [O2]—oxygen
obstructive
    o. sleep apnea (OSA)
O_2 cap [O2 cap]—oxygen capacity
oleothorax
operation
    See also in *General Surgical*
       Terms.
    Daniel o.
    Delorme o.
    Eloesser o.
    Estlander o.
    Friedrich o.
    Glenn o.
    Jackson o.
    Jacobaeus o.
    Monaldi o.
    Overholt o.
    Potts-Smith-Gibson o.
    Ransohoff o.
    Schede o.
    Semb o.
    Tuffier o.
    Wilms o.
orthodeoxia
orthopnea
    three-pillow o.
    two-pillow o.
OSA—obstructive sleep apnea
OSAS—obstructive sleep apnea
    syndrome
oscillation

osteoarthropathy
    hypertrophic pulmonary o.
    pulmonary o.
osteoplastica
    tracheopathia o.
Overholt
    operation
overinflation
    nonobstructive pulmonary o.
    obstructive pulmonary o.
overventilation
oximeter
    ear o.
    finger o.
    pulse o.
    whole blood o.
oximetry
    finger o.
    pulse o.
oxyetherotherapy
oxygen (O)
    blow-by o.
    molecular o. (O_2) [O2])
    nasal o.
    o. therapy
    T-piece o.
oxygenation
    apneic o.
ozone
PA—posteroanterior [x-ray]
P&A—percussion and auscultation
$PaCO_2$ [PaCO2]—arterial carbon
    dioxide partial pressure
$PACO_2$ [PACO2]—alveolar carbon
    dioxide partial pressure
palliative
PAM—pulmonary alveolar
    microlithiasis
panbronchiolitis
Pancoast
    syndrome
    tumor
PaO_2 [PaO2]—arterial partial pres-
    sure of oxygen (arterial pO_2)
PAO_2 [PAO2]—alveolar partial pres-
    sure of oxygen (alveolar pO_2)
PAP—positive airway pressure
    primary atypical pneumonia

PAP— (continued)
    pulmonary alveolar pro-
      teinosis
paracentesis
    p. of the chest
    p. pulmonis
    p. thoracis
parainfluenza
parapleuritis
parasite
    See specific parasites in
      Laboratory, Pathology,
      and Chemistry Terms.
paroxysmal
    p. nocturnal dyspnea (PND)
pars (partes)
PASA—*p*-aminosalicylic acid [p-,
    para-]
PAS-C—*p*-aminosalicylic acid,
    crystallized [p-, para-]
patchy
    p. infiltrates
pathogen
    See specific pathogens in
      Laboratory, Pathology,
      and Chemistry Terms.
pCO_2 [pCO2]—carbon dioxide
    pressure
PCP—*Pneumocystis carinii* pneu-
    monia
PD—postural drainage
    pulmonary disease
PE—pleural effusion
    pulmonary edema
    pulmonary embolism
peak
    p. expiratory flow rate
      (PEFR)
    p. flow gauge
    p. flow meter
pearl
    Laënnec p.
pectoriloquy
pectorophony
pectus
    p. carinatum
    p. excavatum
    p. gallinatum

pectus (continued)
    p. recurvatum
pediculus (pediculi) [anatomy]
    p. pulmonis
PEEP—positive end-expiratory
    pressure
PEF—peak expiratory flow
PEFR—peak expiratory flow rate
pen—penicillin
pendelluft
    p. chest
    p. respiration
PEPP—positive expiratory pressure
    plateau
percussion
    Krönig p.
    respiratory p.
percutaneous
    p. transtracheal bronchogra-
       phy
peribronchial
    p. cuffing
peribronchiolar
peribronchiolitis
peribronchitis
pericarditis
    tuberculous p.
perihilar
peripheral
    p. airway resistance
    p. edema
peripneumonia
    p. notha
Peyrot thorax
PFR—peak flow rate
PFT—pulmonary function test
Pfuhl
    sign
Pfuhl-Jaffe sign
PG—prostaglandin
$PGF_{2\alpha}$ [PGF2-alpha]—prostaglan-
    din $F_{2\alpha}$ [F2-alpha]
pH—hydrogen ion concentration
phagocyte
    alveolar p.
pharyngoesophageal
pharyngospasm
pharyngostenosis

pharyngotomy
phenomenon (phenomena)
    See also *effect, reflex, sign,*
      and *test.*
    first-set p.
    Friedreich p.
    Raynaud p.
    second-set p.
    Williams p.
Philip glands
phlebothrombosis
phlegm
photofluorogram
photofluorography
phrenic nerve
phrenitis
phrenoplegia
phthisis
    aneurysmal p.
    bacillary p.
    collier's p.
    diabetic p.
    essential p.
    fibroid p.
    flax dresser's p.
    grinder's p.
    miner's p.
    p. nodosa
    nonbacillary p.
    potter's p.
    pulmonary p.
    stonecutter's p.
PICU—pulmonary intensive care unit
PIE—pulmonary infiltration and
    eosinophilia
    pulmonary interstitial
      emphysema
PIF—peak inspiratory flow
PIFR—peak inspiratory flow rate
pigeon breeder's disease
pink puffer [emphysema]
piriform
pituitary
    p. fossa
    p. snuff
planigram
planimetric

plaque
    talc p.'s
platelike
    p. atelectasis
pleura (pleurae)
    cervical p.
    costal p.
    p. costalis
    diaphragmatic p.
    p. diaphragmatica
    mediastinal p.
    p. mediastinalis
    parietal p.
    p. parietalis
    pericardiac p.
    p. pericardiaca
    pericardial p.
    p. pulmonalis
    pulmonary p.
    visceral p.
    p. visceralis
pleuracentesis
pleuracotomy
pleural
    p. cavity
    p. effusion
    p. mesothelioma
    p. pressure
    p. shock
    p. space
pleuralgic
pleurectomy
pleurisy
    acute p.
    adhesive p.
    basal p.
    benign dry p.
    blocked p.
    cholesterol p.
    chronic p.
    chyliform p.
    chyloid p.
    chylous p.
    circumscribed p.
    costal p.
    diaphragmatic p.
    diffuse p.
    double p.

pleurisy (continued)
    dry p.
    p. with effusion
    encysted p.
    exudative p.
    fibrinous p.
    hemorrhagic p.
    ichorous p.
    indurative p.
    interlobular p.
    latent p.
    mediastinal p.
    metapneumonic p.
    plastic p.
    primary p.
    proliferating p.
    pulmonary p.
    pulsating p.
    purulent p.
    sacculated p.
    secondary p.
    serofibrinous p.
    serous p.
    single p.
    suppurative p.
    typhoid p.
    visceral p.
    wet p.
pleurobronchitis
pleurocele
pleurocentesis
pleuroclysis
pleurodynia
    epidemic p.
pleurogenous
pleurography
pleurohepatitis
pleurolith
pleurolysis
pleuroparietopexy
pleuroperitoneal
pleuroperitoneum
pleuropneumonia
pleuropneumonolysis
pleurorrhea
pleuroscopy
pleurothoracopleurectomy
pleurotomy

pleurotyphoid
pleurovisceral
plexus (plexus, plexuses)
    brachial p.
    esophageal p.
    mediastinal p.
    p. aorticus thoracicus
    p. pulmonalis
    subpleural mediastinal p.
plication
    fundal p.
plombage
    extraperiosteal p.
PN—pneumonia
PND—paroxysmal nocturnal dyspnea
pneogram
pneograph
pneometer
pneumal
pneumatocele
pneumatodyspnea
pneumatometer
pneumatometry
pneumatophore
pneumatosis
    p. pulmonum
pneumectomy
pneumoalveolography
pneumoangiography
pneumobronchotomy
pneumobulbar
pneumocentesis
pneumochirurgia
pneumochysis
pneumococcal
pneumococcic
pneumoconiosis (pneumoconioses)
    antimony p.
    asbestos p.
    bauxite p.
    coal worker's p., p. of coal
      workers
    collagenous p.
    complicated p.
    diatomaceous earth p.
    fuller's earth p.
    graphite p.
    hard metal p.

pneumoconiosis (pneumoconioses)
    (continued)
    hematite p.
    kaolin p.
    mica p.
    mixed dust p.
    noncollagenous p.
    polyvinyl chloride p.
    rheumatoid p.
    p. siderotica
    talc p.
    titanium dioxide p.
pneumoerysipelas
pneumogram
pneumohemia
pneumohemothorax
pneumohydrothorax
pneumolith
pneumolithiasis
pneumomalacia
pneumomediastinogram
pneumomediastinography
pneumomediastinum
pneumomelanosis
pneumomycosis
pneumonectasis
pneumonectomy
pneumonedema
pneumonemia
pneumonere
pneumonia
    abortive p.
    acute p.
    adenoviral p.
    p. alba
    alcoholic p.
    amebic p.
    anthrax p.
    apex p.
    apical p.
    p. apostematosa
    aspiration p.
    atypical p.
    bacterial p.
    bilious p.
    bronchial p.
    brooder's p.
    Buhl desquamative p.

pneumonia (continued)
   caseous p.
   catarrhal p.
   central p.
   cheesy p.
   chemical p.
   chlamydial p.
   chronic p.
   chronic eosinophilic p.
   chronic fibrous p.
   cold agglutinin p.
   congenital p.
   congenital aspiration p.
   contusion p.
   core p.
   Corrigan p.
   croupous p.
   deglutition p.
   Desnos p.
   desquamative p.
   desquamative interstitial p.
   diffuse lymphoid interstitial p.
   p. dissecans
   double p.
   Eaton agent p.
   embolic p.
   ephemeral p.
   fibrinous p.
   fibrous p.
   fibrous p., chronic
   Friedländer p.
   Friedländer bacillus p.
   gangrenous p.
   giant cell p.
   gram-negative p.
   Hecht p.
   hypostatic p.
   indurative p.
   influenzal p.
   influenza virus p.
   inhalation p.
   p. interlobularis purulenta
   interstitial p.
   interstitial plasma cell p.
   intrauterine p.
   Kaufman p.
   Klebsiella p.
   Legionella pneumophila p.

pneumonia (continued)
   legionnaires' p.
   lingular p.
   lipid p.
   lipoid p.
   lobar p.
   lobular p.
   Löffler p.
   Louisiana p.
   lymphoid interstitial p.
   massive p.
   metastatic p.
   migratory p.
   mycoplasmal p.
   neonatal p.
   obstructive p.
   oil aspiration p.
   organizing p.
   p. alba
   p. apostematosa
   parenchymatous p.
   p. dissecans
   p. interlobularis purulenta
   Pittsburgh p.
   plague p.
   plasma cell p.
   pleuritic p.
   pleurogenetic p.
   pleurogenic p.
   pneumococcal p.
   pneumocystis p.
   Pneumocystis carinii p. (PCP)
   primary atypical p.
   purulent p.
   rheumatic p.
   Riesman p.
   secondary p.
   septic p.
   staphylococcal p.
   Stoll p.
   streptococcal p.
   superficial p.
   suppurative p.
   terminal p.
   toxemic p.
   transplantation p.
   traumatic p.
   tuberculous p.

pneumonia (continued)
    tularemic p.
    typhoid p.
    unresolved p.
    vagus p.
    varicella p.
    viral p.
    wandering p.
    white p.
    woolsorter's p.
pneumonic
pneumonitis
    acute interstitial p.
    aspiration p.
    chemical p.
    cholesterol p.
    desquamative interstitial p.
    eosinophilic p.
    granulomatous p.
    hypersensitivity p.
    interstitial p.
    irradiation p. and fibrosis
    kerosene p.
    lipid p. and fibrosis
    lymphocytic interstitial p.
    lymphoid interstitial p.
    malarial p.
    oil p. and fibrosis
    pneumocystis p.
    rheumatic p.
    uremic p.
pneumonocentesis
pneumonochirurgia
pneumonocirrhosis
pneumonocyte
    granular p.
    membranous p.
pneumonograph
pneumonography
pneumonolipoidosis
pneumonolysis
pneumonomelanosis
pneumonomoniliasis
pneumonopathy
    eosinophilic p.
pneumonopexy
pneumonophthisis
pneumonoresection

pneumonorrhaphy
pneumonosis
pneumonotherapy
pneumonotomy
pneumoparesis
pneumopexy
pneumopleuritis
pneumopleuroparietopexy
pneumopyothorax
pneumoresection
pneumorrhagia
pneumosepticemia
pneumoserothorax
pneumosilicosis
pneumotachograph
pneumotachometer
pneumotachygraph
pneumotaxic center
pneumotherapy
pneumothorax
    clicking p.
    closed p.
    diagnostic p.
    extrapleural p.
    open p.
    pressure p.
    spontaneous p.
    tension p.
    traumatic p.
    valvular p.
pneumotoxin
pneumotropic
pneumotropism
pneumotyphoid
pneumotyphus
Pneumovax
    P. 23
PNPB—positive-negative–pressure breathing
pO_2 [pO2]—partial pressure of oxygen
poison
    corrosive p.
pollution
polyarteritis
    p. nodosa
polyvinyl chloride (PVC) pneumoconiosis

Pompe disease
"poo-drahzh" Phonetic for poudrage.
pore
    Kohn p.
porta (portae)
    p. of lung
    p. pulmonis
position
    See in *General Surgical Terms.*
postpneumonic
post-tussis
post-tussive
Pottenger sign
Potts-Smith-Gibson
    operation
poudrage
    pleural p.
    talc p.
PP—pink puffer [emphysema]
PPB—positive-pressure breathing
PPD—purified protein derivative (of tuberculin)
PPD-S—purified protein derivative–standard
PPV—positive-pressure ventilation
pressure
    inspiratory p.
    inspiratory triggering p.
pretracheal
principle [rule]
    See *law* and *rule.*
procedure
profundoplasty
prostaglandin (PG)
    See also in *Laboratory, Pathology, and Chemistry Terms.*
    p. $F_{2\alpha}$ [F2-alpha] ($PGF_{2\alpha}$)
    p. $F_{2\alpha}$ tromethamine [F2-alpha]
proteinosis
    pulmonary alveolar p.
prune juice sputum
pseudobronchiectasis
psittacosis
PT—pneumothorax
PTE—pulmonary thromboembolism

puffer
    chubby p. syndrome
    pink p. [emphysema]
pulmo (pulmones)
    p. dexter
    p. sinister
pulmogram
pulmolith
pulmometer
pulmometry
pulmonary
    p. abscess
    p. alveolus
    p. amyloidosis
    p. anthrax
    p. arborization
    p. ascariasis
    p. aspergillosis
    p. atresia
    p. blastomycosis
    p. candidiasis
    p. congestion
    p. cryptococcosis
    p. diffusion
    p. edema
    p. ejection clicks
    p. embolic disease
    p. embolism
    p. eosinophilia
    p. fibrosis
    p. function
    p. function test (PFT)
    p. hemosiderosis
    p. histoplasmosis
    p. hypertension
    p. infarction
    p. lymphangiectasia
    p. mucormycosis
    p. neoplasm
    p. nodulosis
    p. perfusion
    p. sarcoidosis
    p. sequestration
    p. sulcus
    p. suppuration
    p. surfactant
    p. telangiectasia
    p. thromboembolism

pulmonary (continued)
    p. thromboses
    p. toilet
    p. valve
    p. vascular markings
    p. vasculature
    p. veno-occlusive disease
    p. venules
pulmonectomy
pulmones (plural of pulmo)
pulmonis
pulmonitis
pulmonohepatic
pulmonologist
pulmonology
pulmonoperitoneal
pulsator
    Bragg-Paul p.
purpura
    lung p. with nephritis
    thrombotic thrombocytopenic p.
purulent
puruloid
PVC—polyvinyl chloride
PVC pneumoconiosis
Px—pneumothorax
pyopneumothorax
pyothorax
PZA—pyrazinamide
radiation
    interstitial r.
    r. pneumonia
    r. pneumonitis
    r. fibrosis
radices (plural of radix)
radiciform
radicis (genitive of radix)
radiocurability
radiogram
radionuclide
radiosensitivity
radix (radices)
    r. pulmonis
radon (Rn)
rale
    amphoric r.'s
    atelectatic r.'s

rale (continued)
    bibasilar r.'s
    border r.'s
    bronchial r.'s
    bubbling r.'s
    cavernous r.'s
    cellophane r.'s
    clicking r.'s
    collapse r.'s
    consonating r.'s
    crackling r.'s
    crepitant r.'s
    r. de retour
    dry r.'s
    extrathoracic r.'s
    gurgling r.'s
    guttural r.'s
    Hirtz r.'s
    r. indux
    inspiratory r.'s
    laryngeal r.'s
    marginal r.'s
    metallic r.'s
    moist r.'s
    mucous r.'s
    r. muqueux
    pleural r.'s
    r. redux
    sibilant r.'s
    Skoda r.'s
    sonorous r.'s
    subcrepitant r.'s
    tracheal r.'s
    Velcro r.'s
    vesicular r.'s
    whistling r.'s
Ramond
    point
    sign
ramus (rami)
Ransohoff
    operation
ratio
    expiratory exchange r.
    inspiratory-expiratory (I/E) phase time r.
    respiratory exchange r.
    ventilation-perfusion (V/Q) r.

Raymond
    See *Ramond.*
RDS—respiratory distress syndrome
receptor
    histamine H_1 r. [H1]
    histamine H_2 r. [H2]
recessus (recessus)
    r. pleurales
reflex
    See also *effect, phenomenon, sign,* and *test.*
    diving r.
    Hering-Breuer r.
    inspiratory-inhibitory r.
regurgitation
    esophageal r.
Reid index
remission
    Legroux r.
reoxygenation
repair
    Belsey r.
resistance
    airway r.
    pulmonary r.
    total pulmonary r.
resonance
    amphoric r.
    bandbox r.
    bell-metal r.
    cavernous r.
    cough r.
    cracked-pot r.
    hydatid r.
    shoulder-strap r.
    skodaic r.
    vesicular r.
    vesiculotympanic r.
    vocal r. (VR)
    whispering r.
    wooden r.
resonant
respiration
    abdominal r.
    absent r.
    accelerated r.
    aerobic r.
    amphoric r.

respiration (continued)
    anaerobic r.
    artificial r.
    asthmoid r.
    Austin Flint r.
    Biot r.
    Bouchut r.
    bronchial r.
    bronchocavernous r.
    bronchovesicular r.
    cavernous r.
    Cheyne-Stokes r.
    cogwheel r.
    collateral r.
    controlled diaphragmatic r.
    Corrigan r.
    costal r.
    diaphragmatic r.
    divided r.
    electrophrenic r.
    external r.
    forced r.
    granular r.
    harsh r.
    indefinite r.
    intermittent positive-pressure r. (IPPR)
    jerky r.
    Kussmaul r.
    Kussmaul-Kien r.
    labored r.
    mouth-to-mouth r.
    paradoxical r.
    pendelluft r.
    periodic r.
    puerile r.
    rude r.
    Seitz metamorphosing r.
    slow r.
    spontaneous r.'s
    stertorous r.
    supplementary r.
    suppressed r.
    thoracic r.
    tidal r.
    tubular r.
    vesicular r.
    vesiculocavernous r.

respiration (continued)
    vicarious r.
respiratory
    r. acidosis
    r. arrest
    r. bronchiolitis
    r. center drive
    r. distress
    r. distress syndrome (RDS)
    r. insufficiency
    r. paralysis
    r. rate
    r. syncytial virus (RSV)
    r. system
    r. tract
    r. tract mucosa
respirometer
    Wright r.
rete (retia)
retial
reticulonodular
retraction
retrosternal
RHLN—right hilar lymph node
rhonchal, rhonchial
rhonchus (rhonchi)
    audible rhonchi
    bibasilar rhonchi
    bilateral rhonchi
    coarse rhonchi
    diffuse rhonchi
    expiratory rhonchi
    faint rhonchi
    few rhonchi
    harsh rhonchi
    high-pitched rhonchi
    humming rhonchi
    inspiratory rhonchi
    low-pitched rhonchi
    marked rhonchi
    musical rhonchi
    occasional rhonchi
    post-tussive inspiratory
      rhonchi
    rare rhonchi
    scattered rhonchi
    sibilant rhonchi
    sonorous rhonchi

rhonchus (rhonchi) (continued)
    upper respiratory rhonchi
    whistling rhonchi
RI—respiratory illness
rib spreader
    Tuffier r.s.
Riesman
    pneumonia
ring
    vascular r.
Ritter
    disease
Riviere sign
RLC—residual lung capacity
RLL—right lower lobe
RML—right middle lobe
"rongk–" Phonetic for words begin-
    ning rhonch–.
Roussel sign
Rp—pulmonary resistance
RR—respiratory rate
RS—respiratory syncytial
RSV—respiratory syncytial virus
rub
    friction r.
    pleural r.
    pleuritic r.
    pleuropericardial r.
rubiginose, rubiginous
RUL—right upper lobe
rule
    See also *law.*
    Gibson r.
RURTI—recurrent upper respiratory
    tract infection
rusty
    r. expectoration
    r. sputum
RV—residual volume
    respiratory volume
SA—Stokes-Adams
SA attack
sacculated
saccule
sacculi (genitive and plural of sac-
    culus)
sacculiform

sacculus (sacculi)
    sacculi alveolares
SAD—small airways disease
Saethre-Chotzen syndrome
sarcoidosis
sarcoma (sarcomas, sarcomata)
        See in *Oncology and Hema-
            tology* section.
SBT—single-breath test
scan
        See also in *Radiology,
            Nuclear Medicine, and
            Other Imaging* section.
    perfusion s.
    perfusion lung s.
    ventilation s.
    ventilation-perfusion (V/Q) s.
scanning
    radionuclide s.
    ventilation-perfusion (V/Q) s.
Schede
    operation
schistosis
schistosomiasis
    pulmonary s.
Schmorl
    furrow
scimitar
    s. shadow
    s. sign
    s. syndrome
scintigraphy
    ventilation s.
scleroderma
    pulmonary s.
sclerosis
    diffuse systemic s.
    multiple s. (MS)
sedatives [a class of drugs]
    respiratory s.
segment
    bronchopulmonary s.
segmenta (plural of segmentum)
segmental
segmentum (segmenta)
        segmenta bronchopulmonalia
Seitz metamorphosing respiration

Semb
    operation
septa (plural of septum)
septi (genitive of septum)
septum (septa)
    aorticopulmonary s.
    bronchial s., s. bronchiale
sequestra (plural of sequestrum)
sequestral
sequestration
    bronchopulmonary s.
    pulmonary s.
sequestrum (sequestra)
    primary s.
    secondary s.
    tertiary s.
sequoiosis
serositis (serositides)
    adhesive s.
    multiple serositides
serpiginous
serum (serums, sera)
    antipneumococcus s.
Shaver disease
Shibley sign
shower
    s. of emboli
siderosilicosis
siderosis
    pulmonary s.
sign
        See also *effect, phenomenon,
            reflex,* and *test.*
    Abraham s.
    auscultatory s.'s
    Baccelli s.
    Bethea s.
    Biot s.
    Bird s.
    Brunati s.
    Cegka s.
    D'Amato s.
    Delmege s.
    d'Espine s.
    Ellis s.
    Eustace Smith s.
    Ewart s.
    Friedreich s.

sign (continued)
 Grancher s.
 Grocco s.
 Hamman s.
 Hoover s.
 Jürgensen s.
 Karplus s.
 Kellock s.
 Kussmaul s.
 Laënnec s.
 patent bronchus s.
 Pfuhl s.
 Pfuhl-Jaffe s.
 Pins s.
 Pottenger s.
 Ramond s.
 Riviere s.
 Roussel s.
 Schepelmann s.
 scimitar s.
 Shibley s.
 Skoda s.
 Smith s.
 spinal s.
 Sternberg s.
 vein s.
 Weill s.
 Westermark s.
 Williams s.
 Williamson s.
silica
silicatosis
silicosiderosis
silicosis
 infective s.
silicotuberculosis
silo filler's disease
SIMV—synchronized intermittent
 mandatory ventilation
sin—. See also words beginning
 cin—, syn—.
sinobronchitis
sinus (sinus, sinuses)
 costomediastinal s. of pleura
 pleural s.
 pleuroperitoneal s.
 s.'s of pulmonary trunk

siphon
 Duguet s.
"sitakosis" Phonetic for psittacosis.
situs (situs)
 s. inversus
 s. inversus viscerum
 s. perversus
 s. transversus
"sklero—" Phonetic for words beginning sclero—.
Skoda
 rale
 sign
 tympany
skodaic
 s. resonance
 s. tympany
sleep apnea
 obstructive s.a. (OSA)
 s.a. syndrome
smear
 bronchoscopic s.
Smith
 sign
snoring
SOB—shortness of breath
solanine
solanism
solitary nodule
sonorous
sound
 auscultatory s.'s
 bandbox s.
 Beatty-Bright friction s.
 bottle s.
 bronchial breath s.'s
 cavernous voice s.
 cracked-pot s.
 eddy s.'s
 friction s.
 hippocratic s.
 Korotkoff s.
 metallic s.
 percussion s.
 pericardial friction s.
 physiologic s.'s
 post-tussis suction s.
 respiratory s.

sound (continued)
    to-and-fro s.
    vesicular breath s.'s
    xiphisternal crunching s.
space
    alveolar dead s.
    anatomical dead s.
    dead s.
    dead s., anatomical
    interpleural s.
    physiologic dead s.
    pleural s.
    respiratory dead s.
    third s.
    Traube s.
spasm
    bronchial s.
    inspiratory s.
    respiratory s.
spasmodic
spectrum (spectra)
    broad-s. antibiotic
Spens
    syndrome
SPH—secondary pulmonary hemo-
    siderosis
sphingolipid
Spinhaler
spiral
    Curschmann s.'s
spirochetosis
    bronchopulmonary s.
spirograph
spirography
spirometer
    Benedict-Roth s.
    Collins respirometer-s.
    Douglas bag s.
    Krogh apparatus s.
    Tissot s.
    Venturi meter s.
    Wright respirometer-s.
spirometry
    bronchoscopic s.
    Tri-Flow incentive s.
spirophore
splenization
    hypostatic s.

splenopneumonia
splinting
spot
    See also *macule.*
    milky s.
sputum
    s. aeroginosum
    albuminoid s.
    s. coctum
    s. crudum
    s. cruentum
    egg yolk s.
    globular s.
    green s.
    icteric s.
    moss-agate s.
    mucoid s.
    nummular s.
    prune juice s.
    rusty s.
squama (squamae)
    s. alveolaris
squamous cell
standstill
    respiratory s.
stannosis
status
    s. asthmaticus
stenosis (stenoses)
    bronchial s.
    infundibular pulmonary s.
stenotracheal
step
    Krönig s.'s
stereoscopy
Sternberg sign
sternoclavicular
sternocostal
sternomastoid
Stokes
    syndrome
Stokes-Adams
    attack
    disease
    syndrome
Stoll pneumonia
streptococcal groups A, B, G

stridor
  congenital laryngeal s.
  expiratory s.
  inspiratory s.
  laryngeal s.
  s. serraticus
study
  cytological s.
  enzyme s.
subpleural
substernal
succussion
  hippocratic s.
suctioning
  endotracheal-bronchial s.
"sudo–" Phonetic for words beginning pseudo–.
suffocation
sulcate
sulci (plural of sulcus)
sulciform
sulcus (sulci)
  costal s., inferior
  pulmonary s. of thorax
  subclavian s. of lung
superior
  s. vena cava (SVC)
suppression
suture [material]
  See in *General Surgical
    Terms.*
suture [technique]
  See in *General Surgical
    Terms.*
Swyer-James
  syndrome
Swyer-James-Macleod
  syndrome
Sydenham
  cough
Sylvest
  disease
sympathomimetics [a class of drugs]
symptom
  Burghart s.
syn–. See also words beginning
  cin–, sin–.

syndrome
  See also *disease.*
  acute respiratory distress s.
    (ARDS)
  adult respiratory distress s.
    (ARDS)
  Arneth s.
  Ayerza s.
  Bard s.
  Bársony-Polgár s.
  Behçet s.
  Brock s.
  Caplan s.
  chubby puffer s.
  Eaton-Lambert s.
  Eisenmenger s.
  Goodpasture s.
  Guillain-Barré s.
  Hamman-Rich s.
  hemopleuropneumonic s.
  Hermansky-Pudlak s.
  hyperlucent lung s.
  hyperventilation s.
  immotile cilia s.
  Kartagener s.
  Leitner s.
  Leredde s.
  Löffler s.
  Macleod s.
  Marfan s.
  Maugeri s.
  Meigs s.
  Mendelson s.
  middle lobe s.
  Mounier-Kuhn s.
  Naffziger s.
  Pancoast s.
  pulmonary infiltration with
    eosinophilia (PIE) s.
  respiratory distress s. (RDS)
  respiratory distress s. (RDS)
    of newborn
  scimitar s.
  sleep apnea s.
  Stevens-Johnson s.
  Trousseau s.
  Wegener s.
  Williams-Campbell s.

syndrome (continued)
    Wilson-Mikity s.
    Young s.
syphilis
system
    respiratory s.
tabacosis
Takayasu
    syndrome
talc
    t. pneumoconiosis
talcosis
talcum
TB—tracheobronchitis
    tuberculosis
TBT—tracheobronchial toilet
TDI—toluene-diisocyanate
technique
    See *maneuver* and *method.*
tela (telae)
    t. submucosa bronchiorum
telangiectasia
    pulmonary t.
telangiectasis (telangiectases)
telar
tenting
    t. of hemidiaphragm
test
    See also *effect, phenomenon,*
      reflex, and *sign.*
    See also in *Laboratory,*
      Pathology, and Chemistry
      Terms.
    Adson t.
    Allen t.
    Arloing-Courmont t.
    Blumenau t.
    Casoni t.
    coccidioidin t.
    Craig t.
    D-dimer t.
    Escherich t.
    Hamburger t.
    Heaf t.
    histoplasmin skin t.
    Hitzenberg t.
    intracutaneous tuberculin t.
    Kveim t.

test (continued)
    Lautier t.
    Lignières t.
    Mantoux t.
    Mantoux skin t.
    match t.
    Müller t.
    Nathan t.
    patch t.
    PPD (purified protein deriv-
      ative) t.
    pulmonary function t. (PFT)
    sweat t.
    tine t., tine tuberculin t.
      (Rosenthal)
    tuberculin t.
    tuberculin patch t.
    tuberculin t., Sterneedle
    tuberculin titer t.
    tuberculosis t.
    Valsalva t.
    ventilation t.
    Visov t.
    Vollmer t.
    Weinberg t.
    Youman-Parlett t.
Teutleben ligament
TF—tactile fremitus
therapy
    aerosol t.
    gene t.
    humidification t.
    inhalation t.
    liquid air t.
    oxygen t.
    respiratory t.
    sclerosing t.
third-spacing
"thi-sis" Phonetic for phthisis.
thoracal
thoracalgia
thoracectomy
thoracentesis
thoraces (plural of thorax)
thoracicoabdominal
thoracoabdominal
thoracobronchotomy
thoracocautery

thoracocentesis
thoracocyllosis
thoracocyrtosis
thoracodorsal
thoracodynia
thoracogastroschisis
thoracograph
thoracolaparotomy
thoracolysis
    t. praecordiaca
thoracometer
thoracometry
thoracomyodynia
thoracopathy
thoracoplasty
    costoversion t.
    lateral t.
thoracopneumograph
thoracopneumoplasty
thoracoschisis
thoracoscopy
thoracostenosis
thorax (thoraces)
    amazon t.
    barrel-shaped t.
    cholesterol t.
    Peyrot t.
    pyriform t.
three-pillow orthopnea
thrombi (plural of thrombus)
thrombocytic
thrombose, thrombosed
thrombosis
    See also *thrombus.*
    See also in *Cardiology* section.
    marantic t., marasmic t.
thrombus (thrombi)
    See also *thrombosis.*
    marantic t., marasmic t.
    parietal t.
thymus
tidal volume (TV)
time (T)
    expiratory pause t.
    forced expiratory t. (FET)
    forced expiratory t. in seconds (FETS)

time (T) (continued)
    inspiratory pause t.
    mean circulating t.
    pulmonary circulation t.
tine test
"ti-sis" Phonetic for phthisis.
titanium (Ti)
    t. dioxide
titanium dioxide
    t.d. pneumoconiosis
TLC—total lung capacity
toilet
    pulmonary t.
trachea (tracheae)
    cervical t.
tracheaectasy
tracheal
    t. length
    t. mucus
    t. mucus velocity
    t. stenosis
trachealgia
tracheitis
tracheobronchial
tracheobronchitis
tracheobronchomegaly
tracheobronchoscopy
tracheocele
tracheofissure
tracheofistulization
tracheogenic
tracheolaryngeal
tracheomalacia
tracheopathia
    t. osteoplastica
tracheopharyngeal
tracheophony
tracheoplasty
tracheopyosis
tracheorrhagia
tracheorrhaphy
tracheoschisis
tracheoscopy
tracheostenosis
tracheostoma
tracheostomize
tracheotomize

tract
    respiratory t.
    upper respiratory t.
transdiaphragmatic
transplantation
    lung t.
transpulmonary
transthoracic
transthoracotomy
transtracheal
    percutaneous t. bronchography
Traube
    dyspnea
    space
trauma (traumas, traumata)
traumatopnea
treatment
    Forlanini t.
tree
    bronchial t.
    tracheobronchial t.
triad
    Kartagener t.
Trousseau
    syndrome
truncal
truncate
truncus (trunci)
    t. pulmonalis
    t. bronchomediastinalis dexter
TS—thoracic surgery
tube
    air t.
    bronchial t.
tubercle
    Ghon t.
    scalene t.
tubercular
tuberculate, tuberculated
tuberculation
tuberculitis
tuberculization
tuberculocidal
tuberculocide
tuberculoid

tuberculoma
tuberculosis (TB)
    active t.
    acute miliary t.
    adult t.
    aerogenic t.
    anthracotic t.
    avian t.
    bronchogenic t.
    bronchopneumonic t.
    cestodic t.
    exudative t.
    hilus t.
    inhalation t.
    t. of lungs
    t. miliaris disseminata
    miliary t.
    pulmonary t.
    tracheobronchial t.
tuberculostatic
tuberculotic
tuberculous
tuberosis
tuberous
    t. sclerosis
Tuffier
    operation
    rib spreader
tumor
    alveolar cell t.
    amyloid t.
    epidermoid t.
    oat cell t.
    Pancoast t.
    sulcus t.
    teratoid t.
    thymic t.
tunic
    fibrous t. of liver
    mucous t.
tunica (tunicae)
    t. mucosa
    t. muscularis
tunicate
TV—tidal volume
TVC—timed vital capacity
two-pillow orthopnea

tympany
> bell t.
> Skoda t.
> skodaic t.

"ty-sis" Phonetic for phthisis.

"u–" Phonetic for words beginning
    eu–.

ulcera (plural of ulcus)

ulcerative
> u. colitis

ulcus (ulcera)

underwater
> u. seal drainage

unit
> See also in *General Medical
> Terms* and *Laboratory,
> Pathology, and Chemistry
> Terms.*
> lung u.
> respiratory care u. (RCU)
> terminal airway u., terminal
> respiratory u.

"up-nee-a" Phonetic for eupnea.

UR—upper respiratory [tract]

URD—upper respiratory disease

URI—upper respiratory infection

URTI—upper respiratory tract
    infection

USN—ultrasonic nebulizer

V_a—arterial ventilation

V_A—alveolar ventilation

vaccine
> BCG (bacille Calmette-
> Guérin) v.

Valsalva
> maneuver
> test

valva (valvae)
> v. pulmonaria

vapor (vapores, vapors)

vaporization

vaporize

vaporizer
> Copper Kettle v.
> Fluotec v.

variation

VC—ventilatory capacity
> vital capacity

vein
> azygos v.
> brachial v.
> cephalic v.
> innominate v.
> thymic v.

Velcro
> rales

vena cava (venae cavae)

vent
> pulmonic alveolar v.'s

Ventaire

ventilation
> alveolar v.
> intermittent mandatory v.
> (IMV)
> v.-perfusion (V/Q) ratio
> v.-perfusion (V/Q) scan
> v. scintigraphy
> synchronized intermittent
> mandatory v.

ventilatory

Venti-mask

Venturi
> mask
> meter spirometer

venturimeter

vesicle [noun: blister, small sac]
> Malpighi v.'s
> pulmonary v.'s

vesiculobronchial

VF—vocal fremitus

vibration

villus (villi)
> pleural villi, villi pleurales

viral
> v. bronchopneumonia

virus
> See also in *Laboratory,
> Pathology, and Chemistry
> Terms.*
> Coxsackie v. [now: coxsack-
> ievirus]
> enteric cytopathogenic
> human orphan (ECHO) v.
> [now: echovirus]
> influenza v.
> parinfluenza v.

virus (continued)
    pneumonitis v.
    respiratory syncytial v. (RSV)
    RS (respiratory syncytial) v.
visceropleural
Visov test
visualization
    laryngoscopic v.
V_{max} [V-max]
voix
    v. de Polichinelle
volume
    inspiratory reserve v. (IRV)
    inspiratory triggering v.
von Leyden. See *Leyden.*
V/Q—ventilation-perfusion
V/Q
    distribution
    imbalance
    nonuniformity
    ratio
    scan
VRI—viral respiratory infection
VT—tidal volume
"vwah" Phonetic for voix.
Waldenström
    disease
    macroglobulinemia
    syndrome
washing
    bronchial w.'s
wave-speed mechanism
wedge
    w. resection
    w. angiogram
    w. pressure
Wegener
    granulomatosis
    syndrome
Weill
    sign

Weinberg test
Weingarten syndrome
welder's lung
Westermark sign
Whipple
    disease
Whitmore
    disease
    fever
    melioidosis
whooping cough
Williams
    sign
Williams-Campbell syndrome
Williamson
    sign
Wilms
    operation
Wilson-Mikity syndrome
windpipe
Woillez disease
wool worker's
    w.w. pneumonia
Wright
    respirometer-spirometer
xanthines, xanthine derivatives [a
    class of drugs]
xerotrachea
X histiocytosis
xiphisternal
xiphocostal
"yoo–" Phonetic for words begin-
    ning eu–.
"yoop-nee-a" Phonetic for eupnea.
Youman-Parlett test
Young
    syndrome
"zifo–" Phonetic for words begin-
    ning xipho–.
zinc fume fever

Radiology, Nuclear Medicine, and Other Imaging

AAL—anterior axillary line
AAS—acute abdominal series
abdominal
    a. aortography
aberrancy
abnormality (abnormalities)
ABR—American Board of Radiology
abscess
    atheromatous a.
abscissa
absorbance
absorbed fraction
absorbency
absorber
absorptiometry
    dual photon a.
    photon a.
absorption
    bone a.
    broad-beam a.
    a. coefficient
    x-ray a.
absorptive
absorptivity
abundance
ACAT—automated computerized
    axial tomography
ACBE—air contrast barium enema
accelerated
accelerator
    linear a.
acetabular
    a. rim
acetabulum (acetabula)
acetrizoate sodium
acetylated
acetylation
acetylator

ACG—angiocardiogram
    angiocardiography
    apexcardiogram
acinar-like
acoustic
    a. reflection method
acquisition time
actinium (Ac)
activity
    specific a.
Acuson
    128 apparatus
    computed sonography
    128 Doppler ultrasound
    echocardiographic equipment
    imager
    linear array transducer
    transvaginal sonography
    ultrasound system
    V5M multiplane trans-
      esophageal echocardio-
      graphic (TEE) transducer
adduction
adenographic
adenography
adumbration
afterglow
AFV—amniotic fluid volume
agent
    contrast a.
aggregated
air
    a. arthrography
    a. bronchogram
    a. bronchogram sign
    a. crescent sign
    a. cushion sign
    a. dome sign
    a. embolism

air (continued)
 a. encephalography
 a. insufflation
 a. monitor
 a. myelography
 a. pyelography
airflow obstruction disease (AOD)
air space disease
Åkerlund
 deformity
ALARA—as low as reasonably
 achievable
Albert
 position
albumin
 iodinated I 125 serum a.
 iodinated I 131 serum a.
 iodinated serum a.
 macroaggregated a. (MAA)
algebraic reconstruction technique
algorithm
alignment
 Cooley-Tukey a.
allowed beta transition
alpha
 a. chamber
 a. decay
 a. particles
 a. radiation
 a. ray
 a. threshold
alumina
alveolate
alveoli (genitive and plural of alveolus)
alveolobronchogram
alveologram
alveolus (alveoli)
 pulmonary a.
 alveoli pulmonis
American Board of Radiology (ABR)
American College of Radiology
 (ACR)
American Institute of Ultrasound in
 Medicine (AIUM)
American Registry of Diagnostic
 Medical Sonographers
 (ARDMS)

American Roentgen Ray Society
 (ARRS)
American Society of Radiologic
 Technologists (ASRT)
americium (Am)
amniogram
amniography
A-mod—amplitude modulation
A-mode ultrasonography
ampere (A)
amphoteric
amplification
 gas a.
 image a.
amplifier
 buffer a.
 linear a.
 nuclear pulse a.
 pulse a.
 voltage a.
amplitude
 a. image
 a. modulation
ampulla (ampullae)
 a. of Vater
analog [electronic]
 a. computations
 a. photo
 a. rate meter
analysis
 activation a.
 basic volume image a.
 correlation a.
 isotope dilution a.
 least-squares a.
 neutron activation a.
 quantitative a.
 regression a.
 saturation a.
analyzer
 multichannel a.'s
 pulse-height a.
aneurysm
 posterior inferior communicating artery (PICA) a.
angiocardiography (ACG)
 gas a.
 intravenous a.

angiocardiography (ACG) (continued)
    radionuclide a.
    rapid biplane a.
    retrograde a.
    right-sided a.
    selective a.
    venous a.
Angio-Conray contrast medium
angiogram
    fluorescein a.
    renal a.
angiography
    aortic arch a.
    biliary a.
    carotid a.
    cerebral a.
    coronary a. (CA)
    digital subtraction a. (DSA)
    emission a.
    fluorescein a.
    four-vessel a.
    intravenous renal a.
    magnetic resonance a. (MRA)
    multigated a.
    orbital a.
    peripheral a.
    pulmonary a.
    radionuclide a.
    renal a.
    spinal cord a.
    subtraction a.
    vertebral a.
    visceral a.
angiolymphangioma
angioscintigraphy
angle
    antegonial a.
    a. board
    cardiophrenic a.
    costosternal a.
    QRST a.
    subcarinal a.
Angström
    law
    unit
angular
    a. frequency

angular (continued)
    a. momentum
angulator
annihilation
    a. photons
    a. radiation
anodal
anode
    rotating a.
    stationary a.
anomalous
anomaly
antegonial
    a. angle
    a. notch
antegrade
    percutaneous a. pyelography
    percutaneous a. urography
    a. pyelography
anterior
    a. palatine suture
    a. thalamotomy
anteroposterior (AP) view
anticoincidence circuit
antineutrino
antiparticle
antiproton
aorta (aortae)
    root of a.
aortic
    a. arch
    a. arch angiography
    a. knob
aortogram
    flush a.
    transbrachial arch a.
    translumbar a.
aortography
    abdominal a.
    catheter a.
    intravenous a.
    lumbar a.
    retrograde a.
    selective visceral a.
    thoracic a.
    translumbar a.
    venous a.
    visceral a.

AP—anteroposterior [x-ray]
aperture
    coded-image a.
apical
aponeurosis (aponeuroses)
apophyseal
apophysis (apophyses)
    See also *process, prominence, protuberance,* and *swelling.*
    calcaneal a.
apparatus
    electro-oculogram a.
    stereotaxic a.
appearance
    applecore-like a.
    ball-in-hand a.
    beaded a.
    beaked a.
    beaten-brass a.
    bone-within-bone a.
    bubble-like a.
    candle drippings a.
    cobblestone a.
    cobblestone-like a.
    coiled-spring a.
    cotton ball a.
    cotton-wool a.
    double-bubble a.
    drumstick a.
    frayed-string a.
    ground-glass a.
    hair-on-end a., hair-standing-on-end a.
    hammered-brass a.
    hot-cross-bun a.
    inverse comma a.
    jail bars a.
    kernel-of-corn a., kernel-of-popcorn a.
    lacelike a.
    leafless-tree a.
    light bulb a.
    moth-eaten a.
    onion peel a., onion skin a.
    pancake a.
    panda a.
    picture frame a.
    popcorn-like a.

appearance (continued)
    pruned-tree a.
    punched-out a.
    railroad track a.
    reticulogranular a.
    rugger jersey a.
    saber-shin a.
    sandwich a.
    scottie dog a.
    shell-of-bone a.
    soap-bubble a.
    spadelike a.
    string-of-beads a.
    sunburst a.
    sun-ray a., sunray a.
    Swiss Alps a.
    trefoil a.
    trilayer a.
    weblike a.
    wineglass a.
    wormy a.
appendiculoradiography
appendoroentgenography
applecore-like appearance
applicator
    beam-therapy a.
apron
    lead-rubber a.
arachnoid
arborization
    cervical mucus a.
arboroid
Arcelin views
arch
    anastomotic a.
area (areae, areas)
    areae gastricae
    mitral valve a.
    pulmonary valve a.
    tricuspid valve a.
argon (Ar)
arm
    scanning a.
arsenic (As)
arteriogram
    coronary a.
    femoral a.
    pruned-tree a.

arteriogram (continued)
    subclavian a.
    wedge a.
arteriography
    axillary a.
    brachiocephalic a.
    carotid a.
    catheter a.
    celiac a.
    cerebral a.
    cine coronary a.
    completion a.
    coronary a.
    digital subtraction a. (DSA)
    femoral a.
    mesenteric a.
    operative a.
    peripheral a.
    pulmonary a.
    renal a.
    selective a.
    spinal a.
    vertebral a.
    visceral a.
arteriosus
    patent ductus a.
arteritis (arteritides)
arthritis (arthritides)
arthritis arthrogram
arthrogram
    double-contrast a.
arthrography
    air a.
    double-contrast a.
    opaque a.
arthroscintigram
arthroscintigraphy
articulare
articulation
artifact
    aliasing a.
artifactitious
asbestos
asbestosis
ascending
    a. pyelography
    a. urography
    a. venography

as low as reasonably achievable
    (ALARA)
ASRT—American Society of Radi-
    ologic Technologists
assay
    erythropoietin a.
    radiometric a.
Assmann
    tuberculous infiltrate
astatine (At)
asymmetry
atelectasis
    discoid a.
    lobar a.
    lobular a.
    obstructive a.
    platelike a.
    rounded a.
    segmental a.
atelectatic
atlas [C1 vertebra]
atom
    Na a.
    a. smasher
    tagged a.
atomic
    a. energy
    a. mass unit
    a. number
    a. spectrum
    a. weight (at. wt.)
atomization
attenuate, attenuated
attenuation
    a. coefficient
attenuator
Auger
    effect
    electron
autocorrelation function
autofluoroscope
    digital a.
autogenous
autoradiograph
autotomogram
autotomography
autotransformer formula

avalanche
    Townsend a.
average
    a. life
    time-weighted a.
Avogadro
    constant
    hypothesis
    law
    number
    postulate
axial
    a. transverse tomography
axillary
    a. arteriography
axis [C2 vertebra]
axis (axes)
    anteroposterior (AP) a.
    celiac a.
    craniocaudal a.
    horizontal a.
    longitudinal a.
    normal a.
    T a.
    vertical a.
    X a.
    Y a.
azygos
    a. vein
Ba—barium
background
    b. activity
    b. count
    b. erase
    b. radiation
backscatter
    b. factor
    b. peak
Ball [eponym]
    method
balloon
    b. catheterization
    b. tamponade
ballooning
    b. mitral cusp
balsa wood block
banana
    b. sign

band
barium (Ba)
    b. enema
    b. meal
    b. sulfate
    b. swallow
    b. titanate
    b. vaginography
barn
barrel
    b. chest
barreling distortion
baseline
    b. film
basial
basialis
basket cells
Baumann angle
Bayle
    granulations
BE—barium enema
bead chain cystography
beading
    b. of ribs
beam
    b. barrier
    broad b.
    b. CT scanner
    electron b.
    b. flattening filter
    b. monitor
    narrow b.
    neutron b.
    b. quality comparison
    b. splitter
    b. therapy
    useful b.
    x-ray b.
beamsplitter
beam therapy
    b.t. applicator
Béclard
    sign
becquerel (Bq)
Bergman sign
Bergonie-Tribondeau law
berkelium (Bk)
beryllium (Be)

beta
    b. decay
    b. emitter
    b. particle
    b. radiation
    b. ray
    b. transition
betatron
bevatron
biaxial
biliary
    b. angiography
bimolecular
binding energy
bioassay
    erythropoietin b.
biological half-life
biomedical
    b. radiography
bioroentgenography
biplane angiocardiography, rapid
bitewing, bite-wing, bite wing
bleb
    subpleural b.
Bloch
    scale
block
    alveolar-capillary b.
    balsa wood b.
blockage
blood-brain barrier
blood flow study
    cerebral b.f.s.
    pulmonary b.f.s.
blood pool
    b.p. imaging
    b.p. scan
blood volume measurements
blow-in fracture
blow-out fracture
blurting
blush
    angiographic b.
body section
    b.s. radiography
    b.s. roentgenography
Böhler
    calcaneal angle

Bohr
    atom
    equation
    magneton
    radius
    theory
Bolton
    plane
    point
    triangle
Bolton-nasion
    line
    plane
bombardment
bone
    b. age
    b. scan
    b. seeker
    trabecular b.
bonelet
bone marrow
    b.m. scanning
bony
    b. island
    b. suture
border
    anterior b.
    interosseous b.
    lateral b.
    medial b.
    peripheral b.
borderline
boron (B)
bosselation
BPD—biparietal diameter
Bq—becquerel(s)
brachial
brachiocephalic
    b. arteriography
brachytherapy
    interstitial b.
    intracavitary application b.
    remote afterloading b.
Bragg
    curve
    peak
brain
    b. scan

brain (continued)
    b. scanning
brain stem
braking radiation
branch
branching
    b. decay
    b. fraction
    b. ratio
breeder reactor
bregma
bregmatic
bremsstrahlung
broad-beam scattering
Broadbent-Bolton plane
bromine (Br)
bronchi (plural of bronchus)
bronchogram
bronchographic
bronchography
    Cope-method b.
    percutaneous transtracheal b.
bronchopulmonary
    b. markings
bronchoradiography
bronchoscopy
bronchus (bronchi)
    See in *Pulmonary Medicine*
      section.
BRW—Brown-Roberts-Wells
BRW CT stereotaxic guide
BSF—backscatter factor
    basal skull fracture
bubble
    b. ventriculography
bubble-like
Bucky
    diaphragm
    grid
    rays
bulla (bullae)
    emphysematous b.
bunamiodyl
Bureau of Radiological Health
burst
BV—bronchovesicular
C1 through C7—cervical vertebrae
    1–7

CA—coronary angiography
CACG—cineangiocardiogram
CAD—computer-assisted design
cadmium (Cd)
calcific
    c. shadows
calcification
    aortic c.
    coronary c.
    eggshell c.
    intracranial c.
    myocardial c.
    parentheses-like c.'s
    periarticular c.
    pericardial c.
    pulmonary c.
    valvular c.
calcium (Ca)
    c. (with scandium Sc 47)
    c. ion(s)
    ipodate c.
calculation
calculi (plural of calculus)
calculogram
calculography
calculus (calculi)
    alternating c.
    branched c.
    calcareous renal c.
    coral c.
    cystic c.
    cystine c.
    decubitus c.
    dendritic c.
    encysted c.
    fibrin c.
    gonecystic c.
    hemp seed c.
    indigo c.
    matrix c.
    mulberry c.
    nephritic c.
    noncalcareous renal c.
    oxalate c.
    prostatic c.
    renal c.
    salivary c.
    spermatic c.

calculus (calculi) (continued)
    staghorn c.
    struvite c.
    urate c.
    ureteral c.
    urethral c.
    uric acid c.
    urinary c.
    urostealith c.
    vesical c.
    vesicoprostatic c.
    xanthic c.
Caldwell
    position
    protection
Caldwell-Moloy method
calibrate
calibration
    E-dial c.
calibrator
    digital isotope c.
    dose c.
    radioisotope c.
caliectasis
californium (Cf)
calix (calices)
    major calices
    minor calices
    calices renales majores
    calices renales minores
CAM—computer-assisted myelography
camera
    Anger c.
    cine c.
    electron diffraction c.
    gamma c.
    Isocon c.
    Medx c.
    Multicrystal c.
    Orthicon c.
    pinhole c.
    positron c.
    positron scintillation c.
    radioisotope c.
    radionuclide c.
    scintillation c.
    video display c.

Camp-Gianturco method
cancelli (plural of cancellus)
cancellous [adj.]
cancellus (cancelli)
cancer
    See in *Oncology and Hematology* section.
candle-guttering
capacitance
capacitive reactance
capture
    cross-section c.
    gamma ray c.
carbon (C)
    c. dioxide
carcinoma (carcinomas, carcinomata)
    See in *Oncology and Hematology* section.
cardiac
    c. catheterization
    c. output
    c. shunt detection
    c. ventriculography
cardioangiography
    retrograde c.
cardiographic
cardiography
    M-mode c.
    radionuclide c.
    ultrasonic c.
cardiokymographic
cardiokymography
cardiophrenic
cardioscan
cardiothymic silhouette
cardiotocograph
cardiotocography
cardiotopometry
carina
carotid
    c. angiography
    c. compression tonography
carrier
    c.-free radioisotope
Carr-Purcell-Meiboom-Gill
    sequence [in MRI]
CAT—computerized axial tomography

catenary system
catheter
    c. aortography
    c. arteriography
    c.-induced thrombosis
catheterization
    balloon c.
    cardiac c.
    Seldinger c.
cathode
    hot-c. tube
    c.-ray tube (CRT)
caudad [adv.]
caudal [adj.]
caudalis
caudalward
caudate
cavitary
    c. lesion
cavogram
cavography
CBD—common bile duct
CBF—cerebral blood flow
CCT—cranial computed tomography
CDR—computed digital radiography
CECT—contrast-enhanced comput-
    ed tomography
celiac
    c. arteriography
cell
    See also in *Laboratory,*
      Pathology, and Chemistry
      Terms.
    tagged red c.'s
    tanned red c.'s
centrilobular
cephalogram
cephalomegaly
cephalometric
cephalometry
    radiographic c.
    ultrasonic c.
cephalopelvic
    c. disproportion
cephalopelvimetry
cerebral
    c. angiography
    c. arteriography

cerebral (continued)
    c. gammography
    c. pneumography
    c. sinusography
    c. ventriculography
Cerenkov
    counter
    radiation production
cerium (Ce)
cesium (Cs)
    c.with barium 137m
CG—Cardio-Green
chain
    c. cystourethrography
chamber
    cardiac c.'s
    ionization c.
    multiwire proportional c.
    pocket c.
    spark c.
    Wilson c.
Chance fracture
Chaoul
    tube
characteristic
Chassard-Lapiné projection
Chausse
    III projection (third projec-
      tion of Chausse)
    view
chelate
chelating agents [a class of drugs]
chemistry (chemistries)
    radiation c.
chemotoxic
Cherenkov. See *Cerenkov.*
chest
    AP (anteroposterior) c. x-ray
    barrel c.
    flail c.
    funnel c.
    PA (posteroanterior) and lat-
      eral c. x-ray
CHI—closed head injury
chlorine (Cl)
cholangiogram
    endoscopic retrograde c.
    intraoperative c.

cholangiogram (continued)
    intravenous c.
    operative c.
    percutaneous transhepatic c.
    retrograde c.
    transhepatic c.
    T-tube c.
cholangiographic
cholangiography
    cystic duct c.
    delayed operative c.
    direct percutaneous transhe-
      patic c.
    endoscopic c.
    endoscopic retrograde c.
      (ERC)
    fine-needle transhepatic c.
      (FNTC)
    intraoperative c.
    intravenous c. (IVC)
    operative c.
    percutaneous hepatobiliary c.
    percutaneous transhepatic c.
      (PTC)
    postoperative c.
    transabdominal c.
    transhepatic c. (TC)
    T-tube c.
cholangiopancreatography
    endoscopic retrograde c.
      (ERCP)
cholangiotomogram
Cholebrine contrast medium
cholecystocholangiogram
cholecystocholangiography
cholecystogram
cholecystographic
cholecystography
    intravenous c.
    oral c.
    post–fatty meal c.
cholecystokinin-pancreozymin
cholecystosonography
choledochogram
choledochograph
choledochography
cholegraphy
cholescintigram

cholescintigraphy
    radionuclide c.
Cholografin contrast medium
Cholovue contrast medium
chromatid-type aberration
chromatoelectrophoretic
chromatogram
chromatographic
chromium (Cr)
    c. Cr 51 serum albumin
chromoscopy
    c. time
chromosome
Ci—curie(s)
cicatrices (plural of cicatrix)
cicatricial
cicatrix (cicatrices)
cin–. See also words beginning
    sin–, syn–.
cine
    c. camera
    c. coronary arteriography
    c. CT scan
    c. study
cineangiograph
cinebronchogram
cinebronchography
cinedensigraphy
cinefluorography
cinefluoroscopy
cinematography
cinematoradiography
cinemicrography
cinephlebography
cineroentgenofluorography
cineroentgenography
cineurography
circle of confusion
circuit
    anticoincidence c.
    coincidence c.
    magnetic c.
    phototube output c.
circuitry
circular
    c. tomography
circumflex
    c. artery

cistern
    basal c.
    cerebellomedullary c.
    chiasmatic c.
    interpeduncular c.
    subarachnoidal c.
    c. of Sylvius
    terminal c
cisterna (cisternae)
cisternogram
cisternographic
cisternography
    metrizamide c.
    oxygen c.
    radionuclide c.
cisternomyelography
CIXU—constant infusion excretory
    urogram
classification
    International Labor Organi-
        zation (ILO) C. of Pneu-
        moconioses
    Salter-Harris c. of epiphy-
        seal plate injuries
    Wiberg c. of patellar types
clay shoveler's fracture
clinodactyly
    factitious c.
    traumatic c.
clinoids
cloud chamber
Clysodrast contrast medium
^{60}Co—radioactive cobalt [cobalt Co
    60]
coarse
    c. markings
coarsening
cobalt (Co)
    c. 57
    c. 58
    c. 60
    radioactive c.
Cobb method
coccygeal
Code and Carlson
    radiograph
coded-aperture imaging
Codman triangle

coefficient
    linear absorption c.
    mass absorption c.
    partition c.
coeur en sabot
coffin
coil
        See also *helix* and *spiral*.
    c. array
    birdcage c.
    breast c.
    butterfly c.
    crossed c.
    Gianturco c.
    Golay c.
    Helmholtz c.
coincidence
    c. circuit
    c. counting
    c. detection
    c. loss
    c. sum peak
coin lesion
coinlike
Colcher-Sussman method
cold
    c. lesion
    c. spot
collecting
    c. system
collimate
collimation
collimator
    automatic c.
    converging c.
    diverging c.
    focusing c.
    multihole c.
    parallel-hole c.
    pin-hole c.
    single-hole c.
    thick-septa c.
    thin-septa c.
colon
    ascending c.
    descending c.
    sigmoid c.
    transverse c.

colorimetric
colorimetrically
combined transmission-emission
    scintiphoto
comminuted
comparison view
compartmental analysis
completion arteriography
complex
    chlormerodrin-cysteine c.
Compton
    effect
    photon
    scatter
    scattering
computed
    cranial c. tomography (CCT)
    emission c. tomography
        (ECT)
    c. myelogram
    c. myelography
    quantitative c. tomography
    c. tomography (CT)
computer
    c.-assisted design (CAD)
computerized
    c. axial tomography (CAT)
    dynamic c. tomography
    c. fluoroscopy
    c. radiography
concentric
    c. pantomography
concept
    ring of bone c.
concomitant
    c. chemotherapy
    c. radiation therapy
concretion
conductivity
    thermal c.
coned-down view
Conray contrast medium
constant
    permeability c.
    Planck c.
contrast
    c. laryngography
    positive c. encephalography

contrast (continued)
    c. radiography
    c. studies
    c. ventriculography
contrast medium (contrast media)
    See also *medium.*
    Abrodil
    Acetrizoate
    acetrizoic acid
    amidotrizoic acid
    Amipaque
    Angio-Conray
    Angiografin
    Angiovist
    barium sulfate
    benzoic acid
    Biligrafin
    Biligram
    Biliodyl
    Bilivistan
    Bilopaque
    Biloptin
    bismuth
    Bracco
    brominized oil
    bunamiodyl
    calcium
    Cardiografin
    cerium
    Cholebrine
    Cholografin
    Cholovue
    Clysodrast
    Conray
    Conray 30
    Conray 43
    Conray 325
    Conray 400
    Cystografin
    Cystokon
    diaginol
    diatrizoate
    diatrizoic acid
    diodine
    diodone
    Diodrast
    Dionosil
    diprotrizoate

contrast medium (contrast media) (continued)

Duografin
Duroliopaque
dysprosium
Endobile
Endografin
Ethiodane
ethiodized oil
Ethiodol
ethyliodophenylundecyl
gadolinium
Gastrografin
glucagon
Hexabrix
Hippuran
Hypaque
hyperosmolar c.m. (HOCM)
Hytrast
Intropaque
iobenzamic acid
iobutoic acid
iocarmate meglumine
iocarmic acid
iocetamate
iocetamic acid
iodamic acid
iodamide
iodatol
iodecol
iodide
iodipamide
iodized oil
iodoalphionic acid
iodohippurate I 131
iodomethamate
iodophendylate
iodophthalein
iodopyracet
iodoxamate
iodoxamic acid
iodoxyl
ioglicate
ioglicic acid
ioglucol
ioglucomide
ioglunide
ioglycamic acid

contrast medium (contrast media) (continued)

ioglycamide
iogulamide
iohexol
iomide
ionic c.m.
Iopamidol
iopanoate
iopanoic acid
iophendylate
iophenoxic acid
ioprocemic acid
iopromide
iopronic acid
iopydol
iopydone
iosefamate
iosefamic acid
ioseric acid
iosulamide
iosumetic acid
iotasul
ioteric acid
iothalamate
iothalamic acid
iotrol
iotroxamide
iotroxic acid
ioxaglate
ioxaglic acid
ioxithalamate
ioxithalamic acid
iozomic acid
ipodate
ipodic acid
Isopaque
Isovue
Kinevac
Lipiodol
Liquipake
low-osmolar c.m. (LOCM)
magnesium
Magnevist
manganese chloride
meglumine
methiodal
methylglucamine

contrast medium (contrast media)
   (continued)
      metrizamide
      metrizoate
      metrizoic acid
      Micropaque
      Microtrast
      Monophen
      Myodil
      Neo-Iopax
      Niopam
      nonionic c.m.
      Novopaque
      Nyegaard
      Omnipaque
      Orabilex
      Oragrafin
      Oravue
      Osbil
      Pantopaque
      phenobutiodyl
      phentetiothalein
      potassium bromide
      Praestholm
      Priodax
      Propyliodone
      Raybar 75
      Rayvist
      Renografin
      Reno-M-30
      Reno-M-60
      Reno-M-Dip
      Renovist
      Renovue
      Retro-Conray
      Salpix
      sincalide
      Sinografin
      Skiodan
      Skiodan Acacia
      sodium
      sodium iodohippurate I 131
      Solu-Biloptin
      Solutrast
      Steripaque-BR
      Steripaque-V
      tantalum-178
      Telebrix

contrast medium (contrast media)
   (continued)
      Telepaque
      Teridax
      tetrabromophenolphthalein
      tetraiodophenolphthalein
      Thixokon
      thorium dioxide
      thorium tartrate
      Thorotrast
      triiodobenzoic acid
      Triosil
      Tyropanoate
      tyropanoic acid
      Umbradil
      Urografin
      Uromiro
      Uropac
      Urovision
      Vasiodone
contrecoup
conversion coefficient
convolutional
coolant
Cooley-Tukey algorithm
Coolidge
      x-ray tube
Cope-method bronchography
copper (Cu)
coprecipitation
Corbin technique
CORLA—clusters of radiolucent
   areas
coronal
      c. suture
coronary
      c. angiography (CA)
      c. arteriography
      cine c. arteriography
corresponding ray
cosmotron
costotransverse
costovertebral
      c. angle (CVA)
Cotton fracture
cotton-wool
      c.-w. appearance
coulomb force

count density
counter
> boron c.
> Cherenkov c.
> Geiger-Müller c.
> proportional c.
> radiation c.
> scintillation c.
> whole-body c.

counting rate meter
count rate
CPD—cephalopelvic disproportion
⁵¹Cr—radioactive chromium
> [chromium Cr 51]

⁵¹Cr-heated RBC
craniad [adv.]
cranial [adj.]
> c. computed tomography
> (CCT)
> c. sutures

craniograph
craniography
crater
> ulcer c.

critical mass
Crookes
> tube

cross-fire
> c-f. radiation therapy
> c-f. treatment

cross-sectional echocardiography
cruciform
crura (plural of crus)
crural
cruris (genitive of crus)
crus (crura)
> c. commune
> diaphragmatic crura

cryomagnet
cryptoscope
cryptoscopy
CSC—blow-on-blow (Fr. coup sur coup)
CT—cardiothoracic
> computed tomography

CT body scanner
CT scan
CTR—cardiothoracic ratio

CUG—cystourethrogram
culprit
> c. lesion

curie(s) (Ci)
curie-hour
curietherapy
curium (Cm)
current
> alternating c.
> direct c.
> eddy c.
> pulsating c.
> saturation c.
> single-phase c.
> three-phase c.
> unidirectional c.

curve
> Bragg c.

cut
> tomegraphic c.

Cutie Pie
CV—conjugata vera
CVO—conjugate diameter of pelvic inlet (L. conjugata vera obstetrica)
CX, CXr—chest x-ray
Cyber 170/720
Cybex ergometer
cycle
> Krebs c.
> pentose c.

cycle-length window
cyclotron
cyst
> Tornwaldt (Thornwaldt) c.

cysteine
cystic
> c. duct cholangiography

Cysto-Conray
Cystografin
Cystografin contrast medium
cystogram
> triple-voiding c.

cystography
> bead chain c.
> radionuclide c.
> retrograde c.
> triple-voiding c.

cystoid
Cystokon contrast medium
cystometrogram
cystometrography
cystopyelogram
cystopyelography
cystoradiography
cystoscopic
    c. urography
cystoureterogram
cystoureterography
cystourethrogram
    micturition c.
    retrograde c.
    voiding c.
cystourethrography
    chain c.
    expression c.
    isotope voiding c. (IVCU)
    micturating c.
    micturition c.
    radionuclide voiding c.
    retrograde c.
    voiding c. (VCUG)
dacryocystography
data (plural of datum)
    ferrokinetic d.
datacamera
datum (data)
daughter nuclide
DBC—dye-binding capacity
dead time
de Broglie wavelength
decade scaler
decay
    alpha d.
    beta d.
    branching d.
    d. constant
    exponential d.
    isometric d.
    d. mode
    nuclear d.
    positron d.
    d. product
    radioactive d.
    d. scheme
decontamination

decussation
de-excitation
defect
    filling d.
    napkin-ring d.
defibrillation
definition
deflation
deflection
deformity
    cloverleaf d.
    Erlenmeyer flask d.
    valgus d.
    varus d.
delayed
    d. operative cholangiography
delimitation
delineation
delta
    d. ray
demarcation
    no line of d.
    shell-like d.
demineralization
demyelinization
denatured
densitometer
densitometry
    quantitative CT d.
density
    background d.
    calcific d.
    inherent d.
    ionization d.
densography
dentate
    d. suture
denticulate
    d. suture
6-deoxy-1-galactose
descending
    d. urography
    d. venography
detection
    beta d.
detector
    collimation scintillation d.
    crystalline phosphor d.

detector (continued)
    dielectric track d.
    quadrature d.
    radiation d.
    semiconductor d.
    tissue-equivalent d.
    x-ray d.
deuterium
deuteron
DEXA—dual energy x-ray absorptiometry [scan]
dextrogram
DI—diagnostic imaging
diagrammatic radiography
diaphragm
    Potter-Bucky d.
diaphysis (diaphyses)
    proximal d.
diapositive
diatrizoate meglumine
diatrizoate sodium
diethylenetriaminepentaacetic acid (DTPA) [now: pentetic acid]
digital
    d. autofluoroscope
    d. fluoroscopy
    d. radiography
    d. subtraction angiography (DSA)
    d. subtraction arteriography (DSA)
digitize
diisofluorophosphate
diisopropyliminodiacetic acid (DISIDA)
dimer
    ionic d.
    nonionic d.
dimerization
Dimer X
Diodrast contrast medium
Dionosil contrast medium
dioxide
diphenyloxazole
diphosphonate
diploë
diplogram
dipolar

dipole
diprotrizoate
direct
    d. percutaneous transhepatic cholangiography
    d. vision spectroscope
dis–. See also words beginning dys–.
discharge
    d. tube
discrete
    d. area of consolidation
    d. area of effusion
    d. disease
    d. focal stenosis
    d. lesion
    d. masses
    d. narrowing
    d. nodule
    d. plaque
discriminator
disease
    See also in medical specialty sections.
    airflow obstruction d. (AOD)
    air space d.
    interstitial d. (ID)
    moyamoya d.
DISIDA—diisopropyliminodiacetic acid
disintegration rate
disk
    Note: Some specialists and references prefer disc.
    cartilaginous d.
    Engelmann d.
    floppy d.
    herniated d.
    intervertebral d.
    protruded d.
    ruptured d.
diskogram
dislocation
    Kienböck d.
distended
distortion
    pin-cushion d.
distribution
    depth dose d.

distribution (continued)
    gaussian d.
    maxwellian d.
    Poisson d.
    spatial dose d.
diverticula (plural of diverticulum)
diverticulae [incorrect spelling/pro-
    nunciation of diverticula]
diverticuli [incorrect spelling/pro-
    nunciation of diverticula]
diverticulogram
diverticulum (diverticula)
    Meckel d.
    Zenker d.
Doerner-Hoskins
    distribution law
dominance
Doppler
    echocardiography
    effect
    interrogation
    phenomenon
    principle
    study
    ultrasonography
    ultrasound
dorsomedial
    d. thalamotomy
dose
    absorbed d.
    cumulative d.
    depth d.
    doubling d.
    erythema d.
    d. estimate
    exit d.
    genetically significant d.
    integral d.
    lethal d.
    maximum permissible d.
    mean d.
    nominal single d.
    organ tolerance d.
    d. reciprocity theorem
    threshold erythema d.
    tissue tolerance d.
    tumor lethal d.

dosimeter
    pencil d.
    pocket d.
    thermoluminescent d.
    ultraviolet fluorescent d.
    Victoreen d.
dosimetric
dosimetry
    pion d.
dot
    See also *spot.*
    d. scan
Dotter
    tube
double-bubble appearance
double-contrast
    d.-c. arthrography
    d.-c. barium enema
    d.-c. radiography
    d.-c. roentgenography
doughnut sign
DPG—displacement placentogram
drip
    d. infusion pyelography
    d. infusion urography
    d. pyelography
DSA—digital subtraction angiogra-
    phy
    digital subtraction arteriog-
       raphy
DTPA—diethylenetriaminepenta-
    acetic acid [now: pentetic acid]
duct
    common bile d.
    cystic d.
    hepatic d.
    pancreatic d.
ductography
    peroral retrograde pancreati-
       cobiliary d.
duodenal
    d. bulb
    d. loop
    d. papilla
duodenogram
duodenography
    hypotonic d.
Duografin contrast medium

dura mater
. Duret
    hemorrhage
    lesion
Duroliopaque contrast medium
Duverney fracture
DXA—dual x-ray absorptiometry
D-xylose
dye
    halogenated phenolphthalein
      d.
    rose bengal d.
dynamic
    d. computed tomography
Dynapix
dyne
dynode
dys–. See also words beginning dis–.
dysprosium (Dy)
ECAT—emission computerized
    axial tomography
eccentric
    e. pantomography
ECG—electrocardiogram
    electrocardiography
echo
    e. planar imaging
    e. ranging
    e. texture
    e. time (TE)
echocardiography
    cross-sectional e.
    Doppler e.
    M-mode e.
    real-time e.
    two-dimensional e. (TDE)
echoencephalogram
echoencephalograph
    midline e.
echoencephalography
echogenic
echogenicity
echogram
echographia
echoic
echoing
echolaminography

echolucent
echo-planar imaging
echo-ranging
echo time (TE)
ECT—emission computed tomogra-
    phy
edema
    cerebral e.
edge
    Compton e.
    e. packing
E-dial calibration
EEG—electroencephalogram
    electroencephalography
EF—ejection fraction
effect [noun: result, outcome]
    See also *phenomenon* and
      sign.
    Auger e.
    Compton e.
    Doppler e.
    heel e.
    isotope e.
    mass e.
    photoelectric e.
    photonuclear e.
    radiographic e.
    scalar e.
    Wolff-Chaikoff e.
effective
    e. half-life
    e. renal plasma flow
Eindhoven
    magnet
einsteinium (Es)
ejection fraction (EF)
EKG [pref: ECG]—electrocardio-
    gram
    electrocardiography
"eko–" Phonetic for words begin-
    ning echo–.
elastic collision
electrocardiogram (ECG)
electrocardiography (ECG)
electrodiagnosis
electrodiagnostic
electrodiagnostics

electroencephalogram (EEG)
    brain death protocol e.
    flat e.
    isoelectric e.
electroencephalography (EEG)
electrogastrograph
electrogram
    See also *electroencephalogram.*
    atrial e.
    coronary sinus (CS) e.
    esophageal e.
    high right atrial (HRA) e.
    His bundle e. (HBE)
    intra-atrial e.
    intracardiac e.
    right ventricular e.
    right ventricular apical e.
    sinus node e.
electrography
electrohysterogram
electrohysterography
electrokymogram (EKY)
electrokymograph
electromagnet
electromagnetic
    e. induction
    e. radiation
electromagnetism
electrometer
    dynamic-condenser e.
    vibrating-reed e.
electron
    Auger e.
    e. beam therapy
    bound e.
    e. capture
    Compton e.
    e. multiplier tube
    e. radiography
    secondary e.
    e. volt(s)
electron-dense
electronics
electron neutrino
electrostatic
element
    daughter e.

element (continued)
    parent e.
elimination
    pyelography by e.
elliptic, elliptical
Elon
elutriation
Embden-Meyerhof glycolytic pathway
embolism
    See also *embolus.*
    air e.
    cerebral e.
    coronary e.
    pulmonary e.
    venous e.
embolus (emboli)
    See also *embolism.*
    pantaloon e.
    pulmonary e.
EMI—Electric and Musical Industries (brain scanner)
    electromagnetic interference
EMI scan
emission
    e. angiography
    beta e.
    e. computed tomography (ECT)
    filament e.
    photoelectric e.
    positron e. tomography (PET)
    positron e. transverse tomography
    radionuclide e. tomography
    e. renography
    single photon e. computed tomography (SPECT)
    thermonic e.
    e. tomography
emitter
emulsion
    nuclear e.
encephaloarteriography
encephalogram
encephalography
    air e.
    fractional e.

encephalography (continued)
    gamma e.
    positive contrast e.
encephalometry
Endobile contrast medium
endodiascopy
endoergic reaction
Endografin contrast medium
endoscopic
    e. cholangiography
    e. retrograde cholangiogra-
      phy (ERC)
    e. retrograde cholangiopan-
      creatography (ERCP)
    e. ultrasonography
enema
    air contrast barium e.
    barium e.
    cleansing e.
    Hypaque e.
    opaque e.
energy
    atomic e.
    binding e.
    chemical potential e.
    electrical potential e.
    electromagnetic e.
    e. frequency
    kinetic e.
    mechanical potential e.
    nuclear e.
    photon e.
    potential e.
    quadrant e.
    radiant e.
    e. resolution
    e. spectrum
    thermal e.
    e. wavelength
    x-ray e.
enterocleisis [closure, occlusion]
enteroclysis [injection, introduction]
enteropathy
    exudative e.
ependymoma
epididymography
epididymovesiculography
epidurography

"epifisis" Phonetic for epiphysis.
"epifizee–" Phonetic for words
    beginning epiphyse–.
epiphyseal
epiphysis (epiphyses)
equation
    Bohr e.
equilibrium
    radioactive e.
    secular e.
    transient e.
equivalence
    mass energy e.
erbium (Er)
ERC—endoscopic retrograde
    cholangiography
ERCP—endoscopic retrograde
    cholangiopancreatography
ergometer
    Cybex e.
Erlenmeyer
    flask
    flasklike deformity
erythropoietin
esophagospasm
esophagraphy
ESR—electron spin resonance
Ethiodane contrast medium
ethiodized oil
Ethiodol contrast medium
ethmoidolacrimal
    e. suture
ethmoidomaxillary
    e. suture
EU—excretory urogram
Euler number
europium (Eu)
eversion examination
    double-contrast e.e.
excavatum
    pectus e.
excretion
    e. pyelography
    e. urography
excretory
    e. cystogram
    e. urogram
    e. urography

expiration
exponential
expression
    e. cystourethrography
extension
extradural
    e. venography
extrapolate
extravasation
    e. of contrast
    e. of dye
exuberant
    e. tumor
E-zero offset
fabella (fabellae)
faceted
faceting
factitious
factor
    backscatter f.
    geometry f.
    intrinsic f.
false suture
fasciagram
fasciagraphy
fascicle
fasciculation
fast Fourier transformation
fatty meal
faveolate
fCi—femtocurie(s)
FDG—2-fluoro-2-deoxyglucose
Feist-Mankin position
femoral
    f. arteriography
    f. head
    f. neck
    f. shaft
femtocurie(s) (fCi)
"fenil–" Phonetic for words beginning phenyl–.
"fenomenon" Phonetic for phenomenon.
Ferguson
    method
fermium (Fm)
ferromagnetic relaxation
ferrous citrate Fe 59

fetogram
fetography
fiberscopic
fibroma
    calcified f.
    f. of lung
fibromatogenic
fibromatoid
fibromatosis
fibromatous
fibronuclear
fibrosis
Fick
    law
    position
    principle
field
    clear lung f.'s
    lung f.'s
filling defect
film
    f. badge
    comparison f.
    f. density calibration
    lateral decubitus f.
    plain f.
    prone f.
    sequential f.
    serial f.
filter
    inherent f.
    Thoreau f.
fine-needle
    f.-n. transhepatic cholangiography
fission
fistula (fistulas, fistulae)
fistulogram
fistulography
fixer
fixing time
flail chest
flank stripe
flash
FLASH—fast low-angle shot
flask
    Erlenmeyer f.-like deformity

flat
      f. suture
flat plate
      f.p. of abdomen
flattening
      f. of diaphragm
"flebo–" Phonetic for words begin-
      ning phlebo–.
Fleischner
      lines
flocculent
flood source
floppy disk
"flor–" Phonetic for words begin-
      ning fluor–.
flowmeter
      Doppler f.
      pulsed Doppler f.
fluid
      peritoneal f.
fluorescence
      f. microscope
      f. microscopy
fluorescent
      f. phosphor
      f. ray
      f. scan
      f. screen
fluorine (F)
      f. F 18
2-fluoro-2-deoxyglucose (FDG)
      [fluorodeoxyglucose]
fluorography
      digital f.
fluorometer
fluorometry
fluoronephelometer
fluororoentgenography
fluoroscopic
fluoroscopy
      digital f.
      image-amplified f.
"flur–" Phonetic for words begin-
      ning fluor–.
fluxes
FNTC—fine-needle transhepatic
      cholangiography

focal
      f. plane tomography
      f. spot
      f. zone
focus (foci)
      Ghon f.
      Simon foci
foramen (foramina)
      f. lacerum
      f. magnum
      obturator f.
      f. ovale
      f. spinosum
foraminal
foreign body (FB)
      retained f.b. (RFB)
formation
      Gothic arch f.
formatter
formula
      See also *law* and *method*.
      autotransformer f.
      configurational f.
      projection f.
Forssell
      sinus
fossa (fossae)
Fourier
      direct transformation imaging
      discrete transformation
      multislice modified KWE
            direct imaging
      transformation reconstruction
      transformation zeugmatogra-
            phy
      two-dimensional imaging
      two-dimensional projection
            reconstruction
four-valve-tube rectification
four-vessel angiography
Fowler
      position
fraction
      penetration f.
      scatter f.
fractional
      f. encephalography

fracture

    acute on chronic f.
    apophyseal f.
    articular f.
    avulsion f.
    Barton f.
    basal neck f.
    Bennett f.
    bimalleolar f.
    blow-out f.
    boxer f.
    bucket-handle f.
    bumper f.
    bursting f.
    butterfly f.
    buttonhole f.
    chip f.
    chisel f.
    clay shoveler's f.
    cleavage f.
    closed f.
    Colles f.
    comminuted f.
    compound f.
    compound skull f.
    compression f.
    condylar f.
    congenital f.
    cortical f.
    Cotton f.
    crush f.
    dentate f.
    depressed f.
    de Quervain f.
    diacondylar f.
    displaced f.
    Dupuytren f.
    Duverney f.
    dyscrasic f.
    epiphyseal f.
    extracapsular f.
    Galeazzi f.
    Gosselin f.
    greenstick f.
    Guérin f.
    hairline f.
    hangman's f.
    impacted f.

fracture (continued)

    intercondylar f.
    intertrochanteric f.
    intra-articular f.
    intracapsular f.
    intraperiosteal f.
    Jefferson f.
    lead pipe f.
    Le Fort f. (I–III)
    linear f.
    Lisfranc f.
    longitudinal f.
    malar f.
    mallet f.
    march f.
    midfacial f.
    Monteggia f.
    Moore f.
    nasal f.
    nasomaxillary f.
    neoplastic f.
    oblique f.
    occult f.
    open f.
    pathologic f.
    pertrochanteric f.
    pillion f.
    Pott f.
    reverse Colles f.
    segmental f.
    shaft f.
    Shepherd f.
    silver fork f.
    Skillern f.
    Smith f.
    spiral f.
    splintered f.
    spontaneous f.
    sprinter f.
    stellate f.
    Stieda f.
    strain f.
    stress f.
    subcapital f.
    subperiosteal f.
    subtrochanteric f.
    supracondylar f.
    surgical neck f.

fracture (continued)
    temporal bone f.
    tibial plateau f.
    torsion f.
    transcervical f.
    transcondylar f.
    transverse f.
    trimalleolar f.
    tuft f.
    ununited f.
    Wagstaffe f.
    willow f.
    zygomaticomaxillary f.
fracture-dislocation
    Monteggia f-d.
    posterior f-d.
frames
francium (Fr)
Frank
    lead system
free peritoneal air
Fresnel
    zone
    zone plate
frogleg, froglegged
    f. position
    f. projection
    f. view
frontal
    f. suture
frontoethmoidal
    f. suture
frontolacrimal
    f. suture
frontomalar
    f. suture
frontomaxillary
    f. suture
frontonasal
    f. suture
frontoparietal
    f. suture
frontosphenoid
    f. suture
frontozygomatic
    f. suture
fucose

fulcrum
    f. full width at half-maximum
fx—fracture
Ga—gallium
^{57}Ga citrate [gallium Ga 57 citrate]
gadolinium (Gd)
    g. Gd 159 hydroxycitrate
galactography
gallium (Ga)
    radioactive g. (gallium Ga 67)
    g. scan
    g. scanning
    g. titrate Ga 67
    g. uptake
galvanometer
gamma
    g.-aminobutyrate
    g. camera
    g. cascade
    g. emitter
    g. encephalography
    g. film
    g. heating
    g. radiation
    g. radiography
    g. rays
    g. scanning
    g. well counter
gamma ray
    g.r. counter
    g.r. level indicator
    g.r. scanner
    g.r. spectra
    g.r. spectrometer
gammography
    cerebral g.
gammopathy
    monoclonal g.
gas
    g. angiocardiography
    g. mediastinography
gastric
    g. parietography
Gastrografin contrast medium
gated
    g. blood pool imaging
    g. CT scanner
    g. imaging

gated (continued)
    g. system
gauge
    x-ray thickness g.
gaussian distribution
GB—gallbladder
GBS—gallbladder series
GE—General Electric
GE scan
Geiger
    counter
Geiger-Müller
    counter
    survey meter
    tube
General Electric CT/T7 scanner
generator
    direct current g.
    electric g.
    electrostatic g.
    molybdenum-technetium g.
    polyphase g.
    12-pulse 3-phase g.
    radionuclide g.
    resonance g.
    supervoltage g.
    technetium-99m g.
    three-phase g.
    Triphasix g.
    Van de Graaff g.
    x-ray g.
geographic, geographical
geometrical efficiency
geometry factor
germanium (Ge)
Ghon
    complex
    focus
    lesion
Girout method
glandulography
globulus (globuli)
    globuli ossei
glow
    cathode g.
    g. modular tube
goitrogen

gold (Au)
    g. Au 198
gonion gradient
    g.g. coil
    g.g. magnetic field
Gosselin fracture
graininess
GRASS—gradient recalled acquisition in a steady state
GRASS pulse sequence
gray
    scale ultrasonography
Greulich and Pyle
    bone age staging
grid
    Bucky g.
    focused g.
    oscillating g.
    Potter-Bucky g.
ground state
Gy—gray(s)
gynecography
gynogram
gynography
gyromagnetic
gyromagnetic ratio
H—Hounsfield [unit]
hafnium (Hf)
hair-on-end appearance
half-life
    biological h.
    effective h.
    physical h.
half-thickness
half-time of exchange
half-value layer
Hampton
    line
    maneuver
    view
hangman's fracture
Harrison
    curve
    groove
haustra coli
haustration
heavy particle therapy

HED—Haut-Einheits-Dosis [unit of x-ray dosage]
helicine
helicoid
helium (He)
helix (helices, helixes)
 See also *coil* and *spiral*.
 h. multihead nuclear imaging system
hemidiaphragms
hemorrhage
 cerebellar h.
 Duret h.
 epidural h.
 intracerebral h.
 intracranial h.
 intradural h.
 intraparenchymal h.
 intraventricular h.
 meningeal h.
 neonatal subdural h.
 pontine h.
 subarachnoid h.
 subdural h.
 subgaleal h.
 thalamic h.
hepatic
 h. flexure
hepatobiliary
 percutaneous h. cholangiography
hepatogram
 emission h.
hepatography
hepatolienography
hepatophlebography
hepatosplenography
Heublein method
Hexabrix contrast medium
Hg meralluride
HIDA—hepatoiminodiacetic acid [scan]
high-osmolar contrast medium (HOCM)
Hippuran contrast medium
historadiography
HOCM—high-osmolar contrast medium

holmium (Ho)
holography
homogeneity
homogeneous
homogeneously
honeycomb
 h. lung
hot
 h. area
 h. caudate lobe
 h. contrast material
 h. lesion on scan
 h. nose sign
 h. spot artifact
 h. spot imaging
 h. spot on scan
 h. thyroid nodule
hot-cross-bun
 h. appearance
 h. skull
Hounsfield unit (H)
hourglass chest
H&R—hysterectomy and radiation [therapy]
HSG—hysterosalpingogram
H-shaped vertebra
Huygens (Huyghens)
 eyepiece
 ocular
 principle
hyaline
 h. arteriosclerosis
 h. cartilage
 h. membrane disease
hybrid
hydrogen (H)
 h. atom
 radioactive h.
hydronephrosis
hydroquinone
hydroxycitrate
Hypaque [contrast medium]
 enema
 swallow
hypercycloidal tomography
hyperechoic
hyperfractionation
hyperinflation

hyperlucency
hyperlucent
hyperstereoroentgenography
hypoechoic
hypoplasia
hypotonic
    h. duodenography
hypoventilation
hysterogram
hysterograph
hysterography
hysterometry
hysterosalpingogram
hysterosalpingography
hysterotubography
Hytrast contrast medium
^{131}I—radioactive iodine [iodine I 131]
IHSA—iodinated human serum
    albumin
ilium (ilia) [hip bone]
ill-defined
image
    See also *imaging* and *scan.*
    acoustic i.
    i. aliasing
    i. amplifier
    i. analysis
    calculated i.
    i. chains
    i. contrast
    i. converter
    fluoroscopic i.
    i.-forming system
    gated i.
    i. intensification
    i. intensifier system
    i. intensifier tube
    inversion recovery i.
    i. noise
    nuclear magnetic resonance i.
    i. orthicon tube
    parametric i.
    phantom i.
    pulse echo i.
    i. quality
    radiographic i.
    i. reconstruction
    i. reformation

image (continued)
    renal i.
    i. resolution
    saturation recovery i.
    scout i.
    i. sharpness
    i. slice thickness
    spin echo i.
    static renal i.
    x-ray i.
image-amplified fluoroscopy
imaging
    See also *image* and *scan.*
    acoustic i.
    adrenal i.
    blood pool i.
    cardiac blood pool i.
    coded-aperture i.
    color flow Doppler i.
    diagnostic i.
    digital vascular i.
    digital vascular i. (DVI)
    direct Fourier transformation
      i.
    dynamic i.
    dynamic volume i.
    echo-planar i.
    electrostatic i.
    flow i.
    Fourier i.
    gated cardiac blood pool i.
    gated magnetic resonance i.
    gray-scale i.
    heavy ion i.
    hot spot i.
    infarct-avid i.
    iosotope colloid i.
    isotope hepatobiliary i.
    longitudinal section i.
    lymph node i.
    magnetic resonance i. (MRI)
    microwave i.
    multigated i.
    multiplanar i.
    multiple-gated blood pool i.
    multiple line scan i.
    multiple spin echo total vol-
      ume i.

imaging (continued)
    multislice modified KWE direct Fourier i.
    myocardial infarct i.
    myocardial perfusion i.
    nuclear i.
    nuclear magnetic resonance i.
    perfusion i.
    planar i.
    planar spin i.
    projection reconstruction i.
    pulse echo i.
    pyrophosphate i.
    quantitative brain i.
    radionuclide i.
    reconstructive i.
    reticuloendothelial i.
    rotating-frame i.
    selective excitation projection reconstruction i.
    sensitive plane projection reconstruction i.
    sequential first pass i.
    sequential plane i.
    single-slice modified KWE direct Fourier i.
    spin-echo i.
    spin-warp i.
    static i.
    stop-action i.
    technetium Tc 99m pyrophosphate i.
    thallium-201 i.
    three-dimensional i.
    three-dimensional echo planar i.
    three-dimensional Fourier i.
    three-dimensional KWE direct Fourier i.
    three-dimensional projection reconstruction i.
    transverse section i.
    two-dimensional i.
    two-dimensional Fourier i.
    two-dimensional Fourier transformation i.
    two-dimensional KWE direct Fourier i.

imaging (continued)
    two-dimensional modified KWE direct Fourier i.
    ultrasound i.
    ventilation perfusion i.
    volume i.
immobilization device
    Pigg-O-Stat i.d.
impedance
    i. venography
In—indium
^{111}In chloride [indium In 111 chloride]
^{111}In-labeled IgG [indium I 111 IgG]
^{113m}In transferrin [indium In 113m transferrin]
indirect
    i. placentography
indiscernible
indiscrete
indistinct
inductance
induction
industrial monitoring
infiltrate
    Assmann tuberculous i.
infraorbital
    i. suture
infusion
    drip i. pyelography
    i. nephrotomography
    i. pyelography
injection
    perinephric air i.
    transduodenal fiberscopic duct i.
insoluble
insufflation
    perirenal i.
    retroperitoneal gas i.
insulinase
insulin-iodine
intensification factor
interaction
intercartilaginous rim
interface
intermaxillary
    i. suture

internal conversion
internasal
    i. suture
International Commission on Radi-
    ological Protection (ICRP)
interpalatine
    i. suture
interparietal
    i. suture
interrogation
interspace
interstitial disease (ID)
intertrochanteric
intracavitary
intraoperative
    i. cholangiography
intraosseous
    i. venography
intravenous
    i. angiocardiography
    i. aortography
    i. cholangiography (IVC)
    i. cholecystography
    i. pyelography (IVP)
    i. urography (IVU)
intrinsic
Intropaque contrast medium
inverse square law
iodinated
    i. I 125 fibrinogen
    i. I 125 serum albumin
    i. I 131 aggregated albumin
      (human)
    i. I 131 serum albumin
      (human)
    i. contrast media
iodination
iodine (I)
    i. I 123
    i. I 125
    i. I 131
    i. PVP bond
    radioactive i. (iodine I 131)
iodipamide
iodoalphionic acid
iodohippurate sodium
iodomethamate
iodophthalein sodium

iodopyracet
iodoventriculography
ion
    amphoteric dipolar i.
ionic contrast medium
ionization
ionograph
ionography
Iopamidol contrast medium
iophendylate
iophenoxic acid
iopydol
iopydone
iothalamate
ipodate calcium
IRA-400 resin
iridium (Ir)
iron (Fe)
    i. hydroxide
    radioactive i.
irradiate
irradiated
irradiation
    intracavitary i.
irrigoradioscopy
ischium
island
    bone i.
    cartilage i.'s
isobar
isobaric transition
Isocon camera
isomer
isomeric
    i. decay
    i. transition
Isopaque contrast medium
isotone
isotope
    i. bone scan
    i. colloid imaging
    i. effect
    i. hepatobiliary imaging
      radioactive i.
    i. nephrography
    i. study
    i. ventriculography

isotope (continued)
   i. voiding cystourethrogra-
      phy (IVCU)
isotopic
Isovue contrast medium
IVC—intravenous cholangiogram
IVCU—isotope voiding cys-
   tourethrography
IVCV—inferior venacavography
IVH—intraventricular hemorrhage
IVP—intravenous pyelogram
IVU—intravenous urography
Jaquet apparatus
Johnson
   position
joint
   See also in *Orthopedics and*
    Sports Medicine section.
   j. mice
jugal
   j. suture
junction
   myoneural j.
   rectosigmoid j.
K-capture
kCi—kilocurie(s)
Kerley
   A lines
   B lines
"ker on sa-bo" Phonetic for coeur
   en sabot.
ketone bodies
keV, kev—kilo electron volt(s)
kidney washout
Kienböck
   dislocation
   unit
Kienböck-Adamson
   points
kilocalorie (kcal, Cal)
kilocurie(s) (kCi)
kilohertz (kHz)
kilomegacycle
kilovolt (kV)
kilovolts peak (kVp)
kineradiography
kinetic energy
kinetoscopy

Kinevac contrast medium
"kol–" Phonetic for words beginning chol–.
"kon-tre-koo" Phonetic for contrecoup.
K radiation
Krebs cycle
"krus" Phonetic for crus.
krypton (Kr)
   k. Kr 81m
   k. Kr 85
K-shell
KUB—kidney, ureter, bladder [x-ray]
kVp—kilovolts peak
kymograph
kymography
   roentgen k. (RKY)
kymoscopy
L1 through L5—lumbar vertebrae
   1–5
lacelike
lacrimoconchal
   l. suture
lacrimoethmoidal
   l. suture
lacrimomaxillary
   l. suture
lacrimoturbinal
   l. suture
lacunar
   l. infarct
LAD—left anterior descending
   [coronary artery]
LAG—lymphangiogram
lambda
lambdoid, lambdoidal
   l. suture
laminagram
laminagraph
laminagraphy
lamination
laminogram
laminography
lamp
   Wood l.
lanthanum (La)
Larsen
   disease

laryngogram
laryngography
    contrast l.
laryngopharyngography
laser beam
lateral
    l. pyelography
laterality
lattitude
Lauenstein and Hickey projection
law
    See also *principle*.
    Angström l.
    Doerner-Hoskins distribu-
       tion l.
    Fick l.
    Fick first l. of diffusion
    l. of inertia
    inverse square l.
    Ohm l.
    l. of reciprocity
    l. of thermodynamics
Law [eponym]
    position
    views
lawrencium (Lw)
layer
LDA—left descending artery
lead ["leed"]
    chest l.
    intracardiac l.
    pacemaker l., pacing l.
lead (Pb) ["led"]
    radioactive l.
lens
    Thorpe plastic l.
lepton
lesion
    annular l.
    apple core l.
    bird's nest l.
    bull's eye l.
    butterfly l.
    capsular drop l.
    caviar l.
    cavitary pulmonary l.
    central l.

lesion (continued)
    coin l.
    cold l.
    destructive l.
    diffuse l.
    doughnut l.
    dumbbell l.
    Duret l.
    ellipsoid l.
    focal l.
    frondy l.
    Ghon primary l.
    gross l.
    hot l.
    indiscriminate l.
    jet l.
    local l.
    local glomerular l.
    mass l.
    napkin-ring l.
    partial l.
    primary l.
    ring-like l.
    ring-wall l.
    sessile l.
    space-occupying l.
    space-occupying intracranial
       l.
    structural l.
    swan-neck tubular l.
    systemic l.
    target l.
    total l.
    tumor-like l.
    wedge-shaped l.
    wire-loop l.
levoangiocardiogram
levocardiogram
levogram
licorice powder
lienography
limb
    l. venography
limbal
    l. suture
limbous
    l. suture

line
  acanthomeatal l.
  auricular l.
  canthomeatal l.
  Correra l.
  glabelloalveolar l.
  glabellomeatal l.
  Granger l.
  Hampton l.
  Harris l.'s
  infraorbital l.
  infraorbitomeatal l.
  interorbital l.
  interpupillary l.
  Kerley A l.'s
  Kerley B l.'s
  McGregor l.
  pubococcygeal l.
  Reid base l.
  Shenton l.
  Skinner l.
  suture l.
  Trümmerfeld l.
linear
  l. accelerator
  l. attenuation
  l. compartmental system
  l. energy transfer
  l. focus
  l. tomography
lingular
  l. infiltrates
Lipiodol contrast medium
lipping
LIQ—lower inner quadrant
Liquipake contrast medium
list mode lithium
lithium (Li)
LLQ—left lower quadrant
LMR—localized magnetic resonance
lobar
  l. atelectasis
  l. pneumonia
lobe
  inferior l. of left lung
  inferior l. of right lung
  left lower l. (LLL)
  left upper l. (LUL)

lobe (continued)
  l. of liver, left
  l. of liver, right
  lower l. of lung
  middle l. of right lung
  right lower l. (RLL)
  right upper l. (RUL)
  superior l. of left lung
  superior l. of right lung
  upper l. of lung
lobular
localization
locular
loculated
  l. pleural effusion
longitudinal
  l. section tomography
  l. suture
  l. suture of palate
loopogram
loose bodies
Looser
  transformation zones
lopamidol
LOQ—lower outer quadrant
lordotic
  anteroposterior l. projection
  apical l. projection
low-osmolar contrast media (LOCM)
LRQ—lower right quadrant
LS—lumbosacral
LSB—left sternal border
lucent
LUL—left upper lobe
lumbar
  l. aortography
lumen (lumina)
lung
  l. collapse, collapsed l.
  fibroid l.
  honeycomb l.
  hyperlucent l.
  l. markings
  polycystic l.
  postperfusion l.
  l. root
LUQ—left upper quadrant
lutetium (Lu)

lymph
    thyroidal l. node scintigraphy
lymphangiogram
lymphangiography
    pedal l.
lymphangiotomy
lymphography
μ—micro- [prefix; alphabetized as
    m]
mA—milliampere(s)
Macleod
    syndrome
macroaggregated
    m. albumin (MAA)
macroangiography
macromolecules
macroradiography
macroscopic
macula (maculae)
macule
magenblase
magic numbers
magnet
    beam-bending m.
    cryostable m.
    Eindhoven m.
    permanent m.
    resistive m.
    superconducting m.
    superconductive m.
    Walker m.
magnetic
    m. circuit
    m. dipole
    m. disk
    m. domain
    m. field
    m. field strength
    m. flux
    m. focal plane
    m. force
    m. gradient
    m. induction
    m. lines of force
    m. material
    m. moment
    nuclear m. resonance (NMR)
    m. nuclei

magnetic (continued)
    m. permeability
    m. pole
    m. recording
    m. resonance angiography
      (MRA)
    m. resonance imaging (MRI)
    m. resonance spectroscopy
    m. retentivity
magnetization
Magnevist contrast medium
magnification
mAh, mA-h—milliampere-hour
main bronchi, main stem bronchus
malomaxillary
    m. suture
malum coxae senilis
mAm, mA-m—milliampere-minute
mammillary
    m. suture
mammogram
mammography
mandible
maneuver
    See also *method* and *tech-*
      nique.
    Hampton m.
manganese (Mn)
mannitol
maplike
mAs, mA-s—milliampere-second
mass
    atomic m.
    m. effect
    intraluminal m.
    relativistic m.
mastoid
    m. suture
MAVIS—mobile artery and vein
    imaging system
maxicamera
maxwellian distribution
Mayer
    position
    view
mC—millicoulomb(s)
McGregor line
μCi [microCi]—microcurie(s)

mCi—millicurie(s)
MCi—megacurie(s)
mCi-hr—millicurie-hour
μCi-hr [microCi-hr]—microcurie-
    hour
MCT—mean circulation time
mean
        m. deviation
        m. free path
        m. gonad dose
        m. life
measurement
Meckel
        diverticulum
        scan
media (plural of medium)
median
        m. palatine suture
mediastinal
        m. crunch
mediastinogram
mediastinography
        gas m.
        opaque m.
mediastinoscopy
medicine
        nuclear m.
medium (media, mediums)
        See also *contrast medium.*
        contrast medium
        meglumine diatrizoate m.
        metrizamide m.
        radiolucent m.
        radiopaque m.
Medx
        M. camera
        M. scanner
megavoltage
mendelevium (Md)
mercurihydroxypropane
mercury (Hg)
mesenteric
        m. arteriography
meson
metallic
metastable state
metastasis (metastases)

method
        See also *maneuver* and *tech-
            nique.*
        Ball m.
        Caldwell-Moloy m.
        Camp-Gianturco m.
        Cobb m.
        Colcher-Sussman m.
        Dooley, Caldwell, and Glass
            m.
        Ferguson m.
        Girout m.
        Heublein m.
        Monte Carlo m.
        Ottonello m.
        parallax m.
        Parama m.
        Pfeiffer-Comberg m.
        Sommer-Foegella m.
        Sweet m.
        Wolf m.
        Zimmer m.
methylcellulose gel
metopic
        m. suture
metric
        m. system
metrizamide
        m.-assisted computed
            tomography
        m. cisternography
metrizoate sodium
metrizoic acid
metrosalpingography
metrotubography
mets—metastases
MFB—metallic foreign body
mGy—milligray(s)
micaceous
mice
        joint m.
microaneurysm
microangiogram
microangiography
microangioscopy
microcalcification
microcalculus (microcalculi)
microcinematography

microcurie(s) (μCi, microCi)
microcurie-hour (μCi-hr, microCi-hr)
microdosimetry
microemboli (plural of microembolus)
microembolization
microembolus (microemboli)
    showers of microemboli
microfarad (μf)
microfracture
microinfarct
microlesion
microlith
microlithiasis
    m. alveolaris pulmonum
    pulmonary alveolar m.
micrometastasis
micron (micrometer)
micronodular
Micropaque contrast medium
microradiogram
microradiography
microroentgen (μR, microR)
microscope
    fluorescence m.
    projection x-ray m.
    x-ray m.
microscopy
    fluorescence m.
Microtrast contrast medium
microtron
micturating
    m. cystourethrography
micturition
    m. cystourethrography
middle
    m. palatine suture
"miel–" Phonetic for words beginning myel–.
Miller
    position
milliamperage
milliampere(s) (mA)
milliampere-hour (mAh, mA-h)
milliampere-minute (mAm, mA-m)
milliampere-second (mAs, mA-s)
millicoulomb(s) (mC)

millicurie(s) (mCi)
    m. destroyed (mCiδ) [mCi-delta]
    m.-hour (mCi-hr)
millicurie-hour (mCi-hr)
milligray(s) (mGy)
millirad(s) (mrad)
milliroentgen(s) (mR)
minification
minometer
minuscule
MIRD—medical internal radiation dose
MLD—median lethal dose
MLSI—multiple line scan imaging
M-mode
    M-m. cardiography
    M-m. echocardiogram
    M-m. echocardiography
    M-m. scanning
MMR—mobile mass x-ray
mode
    M-m.
modulation
    amplitude m.
    brightness m.
    image m.
    object m.
    m. transfer function
molar volume
molecular
    m. vibrations
molybdenum (Mo)
monitor
    beam m.
    radiation m.
monitoring
Monophen contrast medium
Monte Carlo method
mosaic
Mossbauer spectrometer
mottled
MPD—maximum permissible dose
mR—milliroentgen(s)
MRA—magnetic resonance angiography
mrad—millirad(s)
mrem—millirem(s)

MRI—magnetic resonance imaging
MTT—mean transit time
mucosal
    m. relief radiography
    m. relief roentgenography
MUGA—multiple gated acquisition [scan]
multangular
multicrystal camera
multigated
    m. angiography
    m. imaging
multilocular
multiplanar
    m. imaging
    m. scanning
multiple-nuclide
multiscalar
muscle
    See in *Orthopedics and Sports Medicine* section.
musculus (musculi)
    See in medical specialty sections.
myelocisternoencephalography
myelocystography
myelogram
myelography
    air m.
    computed m.
    computer-assisted m. (CAM)
    opaque m.
    oxygen m.
myocardial
    m. perfusion scintigraphy
Myodil contrast medium
Na atoms
NAD—no active disease
    no appreciable disease
nanocurie(s) (nCi)
nanogram(s) (ng)
napkin-ring
    n.r. annular stenosis
    n.r. annular tumor
    n.r. carcinoma
    n.r. defect
    n.r. lesion
    n.r. trachea

narrow-beam half-thickness
nasal
    n. suture
nasioiniac
nasion
nasofrontal
    n. suture
nasomaxillary
    n. suture
nasopharyngography
National Radiological Commission (NRC)
National Radiological Protection Board (NRPB)
nCi—nanocurie(s)
Ne—neon
necrosis (necroses)
    radiation n.
    radium n.
necrotic
NED—no evidence of disease
negatron
    n. emission
neodymium (Nd)
    n.:yttrium-aluminum-garnet (Nd:YAG) laser
Neo-Iopax contrast medium
neon (Ne)
    n. particle protocol
neostigmine
    n. methylsulfate
nephrography
    isotope n.
nephropyelography
nephrosonography
nephrostogram
nephrotomogram
nephrotomography
    infusion n.
nephrourography
neptunium (Np)
NER—no evidence of recurrence
NERD—no evidence of recurrent disease
"neu–" Phonetic for words beginning pneu–.
neuroangiographic
neurodiagnosis

neuroimaging
neuroradiology
neuroroentgenography
neurotomography
neutrino
neutron
    epithermal n.
    fast n.
    intermediate n.
    n. number
    n. radiography
    slow n.
    thermal n.
"new–" Phonetic for words beginning pneu–.
ng—nanogram(s)
Ni—nickel
nickel (Ni)
    n. carbonyl
niobium (Nb)
Niopam contrast medium
nitrogen (N)
NM—nuclear medicine
NMR—nuclear magnetic resonance
nobelium (No)
node
    lymph n.
    mesenteric n.
nodular
nodularity
nodulated
nodulation
nodule
    cold n.
    hot n.
    pulmonary n.'s
nomogram
nonfunctioning
    n. gallbladder
    n. heart valve
    n. kidney
nonhomogeneous
noninvasive
nonionic contrast media [a class of drugs]
nonlinearity
nonopaque
nonperforating

nonseptate
nonspecific
nonunion
nonvisualization
"noo–" Phonetic for words beginning pneu–.
normalized plateau slope
notch
    antegonial n.
notching
noticeable
Novopaque contrast medium
NRC—Nuclear Regulatory Commission
NSC—no significant change
NSD—no significant disease
"nu–" Phonetic for words beginning pneu–.
nuchal
nuchofrontal
nuclear
    n. angiography
    n. cardiology
    n. decay
    n. disintegration
    n. emulsion
    n. energy
    n. fission
    n. force
    n. fusion
    n. imaging
    n. magnetic moment
    n. magnetic resonance imaging (NMRI)
    n. medicine
    n. particle
    n. probe
    n. radiation
    n. reaction
    n. reactor
    n. relaxation
    n. scanner
    n. scanning
    n. scintigraphy
    n. signal
    n. spin
    n. structure

nuclear magnetic resonance (NMR)
    n.m.r. Fourier transformation
    n.m.r. image
    n.m.r. imaging
    n.m.r. phantom
    pulsed n.m.r.
    n.m.r. relaxation rate
      enhancement
    n.m.r. scanning sequence
    n.m.r. signal intensity
    n.m.r. spectra
    n.m.r. spectral parameters
    n.m.r. spectroscopy
    n.m.r. spectrometer
    n.m.r. spin warp method
    n.m.r. tomography
Nuclear Regulatory Commission
    (NRC)
nuclease
nuclei (genitive and plural of nucleus)
nucleide
nucleiform
nucleography
nucleoid
nucleoliform
nucleon
    n. number
nucleonics
nucleoprotein
nucleoreticulum
nucleotherapy
nuclide
number
    atomic n.
    Avogadro n.
    body atomic n.
    effective atomic n.
    Euler n.
    mass n.
    nucleon n.
    n. profile
Nyegaard contrast medium
obliquity
obliteration
obturator foramen
occipital
    o. suture

occipitomastoid
    o. suture
occipitoparietal
    o. suture
occipitosphenoidal
    o. suture
OCG—oral cholecystogram
odontoid
OIH—orthoiodohippurate
oligodendroglioma
Olshevsky
    tube
OM—obtuse marginal (coronary
    artery)
omentoportography
Omnipaque contrast medium
oncology
    radiation o.
opacified
opaque
    o. arthrography
    o. mediastinography
    o. myelography
operating voltage
operative
    o. arteriography
    o. cholangiography
    delayed o. cholangiography
OPG/CPA—oculoplethysmogra-
    phy/carotid phonoangiography
optimal
Orabilex contrast medium
Oragrafin contrast medium
oral
    o. cholecystography
    o. urography
Oravue contrast medium
orbital
    o. angiography
orbitography
ordography
organ
    rudimentary o.
orientation
    sagittal o.
    transverse o.
Orthicon camera
orthodiagram

orthodiagraph
orthodiagraphy
orthodiascopy
orthoiodohippurate
orthopantograph
orthopantomograph
orthopantomography
orthoroentgenography
orthoskiagraph
orthovoltage
os (ossa) [bone]
     See in *Orthopedics and*
        Sports Medicine section.
Osbil contrast medium
oscillating Bucky
osteal [bony, osseous]
osteite
osteitic
osteomyelography
osteoporosis
osteoporotic
osteoradionecrosis
osteosarcomatous
ostia (plural of ostium)
ostial [pertaining to opening, aperture, orifice]
ostium (ostia)
OTD—organ tolerance dose
Ottonello method
OURQ—outer upper right quadrant
overexposure
overinflation
overlap shadow
overriding
overvoltage
Owen
     view
oxidation
oxygen (O)
     o. cisternography
     o. myelography
moyamoya disease
^{32}P—radioactive phosphorus [phosphorus P 32]
PA—posteroanterior [x-ray]
packing fraction
pair production

palatine
     anterior p. suture
     median p. suture
     middle p. suture
     posterior p. suture
     transverse p. suture
palatoethmoidal
     p. suture
palatograph
palatography
palatomaxillary
     p. suture
palatomyograph
palladium (Pd)
palliative
palmitate
panagraphy
pancake
     p. appearance
     p. compression
pancreaticobiliary
     peroral retrograde p. ductography
pancreatogram
pancreatography
     endoscopic retrograde p.
pangynecography
panography
pan-oral radiography
panoramic
     p. radiography
     p. tomography
Panorex
pantomographic
pantomography
     concentric p.
     eccentric p.
Pantopaque contrast medium
para-aminohippuric acid
parafascicular
     p. thalamotomy (PFT)
parallax method
parallel
Parama method
parametric image
parent nuclide
parietal
     p. suture

parietography
  gastric p.
parietomastoid
  p. suture
parieto-occipital
  p.-o. suture
parietotemporal
  p. suture
particle
  viral p.
parturition
pastille radiometer
patchy
  p. infiltrates
patent
  p. ductus arteriosus (PDA)
pathologic, pathological
pathway
  Embden-Meyerhof glycolyt-
    ic p.
pattern
  alveolar p.
  broken bough p.
  butterfly p.
  convolutional p.
  corkscrew p.
  cystic p.
  fingerprint p.
  hair brush p.
  hanging-fruit p.
  haustral p.
  herring-bone p.
  honeycomb p.
  mimosa p.
  rugal p.
  signet ring p.
  solid p.
  start test p.
  three-dimensional physio-
    logic flow p.
Pauli
  exclusion principle
PAWP—pulmonary artery wedge
  pressure
pCi—picocurie(s)
PDA—patent ductus arteriosus
  posterior descending artery

peak
  Bragg p.
  kilovolts p. (kVp)
pectus
  p. carinatum
  p. excavatum
  p. recurvatum
pedal
  p. lymphangiography
PEG—pneumoencephalogram
peizoelectric
pelves (plural of pelvis)
pelvicephalography
pelvicephalometry
pelvimetry
pelviography
pelvioradiography
pelvioscopy
pelviradiography
pelviroentgenography
pelvis (pelves)
  See in *Orthopedics and
    Sports Medicine* section.
pemphigus
penetration
  radiographic p.
penetrology
penetrometer
pentetic acid (DTPA, diethylenetriaminepentaacetic acid)
pentose cycle
penumbra
percutaneous
  p. antegrade pyelography
  p. antegrade urography
  direct p. transhepatic
    cholangiography
  p. hepatobiliary cholangiog-
    raphy
  p. transhepatic cholangiog-
    raphy (PTC)
  p. transhepatic portography
  p. transtracheal bronchogra-
    phy
perfusion
  p. scintigraphy
perfusion study

peribronchial
    p. cuffing
perihilar
perinephric
peripheral
    p. angiography
    p. arteriography
    p. venography
peritoneography
permeability constant
peroral
    p. retrograde pancreaticobil-
       iary ductography
perpendicular
pertechnetate
PET—positron emission tomogra-
    phy [scan]
petrobasilar
    p. suture
petrosphenobasilar
    p. suture
petrosphenooccipital
    p. suture of Gruber
petrosquamosal
    p. suture
petrous tips
PETT—positron emission transaxial
    tomography
    positron emission transverse
       tomography
Pfeiffer-Comberg method
PFT—parafascicular thalamotomy
phalanx (phalanges)
    See in *Orthopedics and*
       Sports Medicine section.
phantom
    flood p.
pharmacoradiology
pharyngoesophagraphy
pharyngography
phenoltetrachlorophthalein
phenomenon (phenomena)
    See also *effect* and *sign*.
    Doppler p.
    interference p.
    irradiation p.
    vacuum p.
phentetiothalein

phenyldiphenyloxadiazole
phenyloxazolyl
phlebogram
phlebograph
phlebography
phonoangiography
    oculoplethysmography/carot
      id p. (OPG/CPA)
phosphate
phosphor
phosphorated
phosphorescence
phosphorus P 32 diisofluorophos-
    phate
phosphorus (P) [noun]
    labeled p.
    radioactive p.
Phospho-Soda
photocathode
photodisintegration
photodisplay unit
photoelectric
    p. absorption
    p. effect
    p. interaction
photoelectron
photoflow
photofluorogram
photofluorographic
photofluorography
photomicrograph
photomultiplier tube (PMT)
photon
    Compton p.
    degraded p.
photoneutron
photonuclear
    p. effect
    p. reaction
photopeak
photorecording
photoroentgenography
photoscanner
phototimer
phototube output circuit
PICA—posterior inferior communi-
    cating artery
PICA aneurysm

picocurie(s) (pCi)
picture-frame–like
Pigg-O-Stat immobilization device
pile
ping-pong fracture
pinhole collimator
pion beam
PIPIDA—para-isopropyliminodi-
    acetic acid technetium 99m
    hepatobiliary
PIPIDA
        hepatobiliary scan
        scan
Pirie transoral projection
piriform
pisiform
pitchblende
placentography
        indirect p.
planar
        p. spin imaging
Planck
        constant
        quantum theory
plane
        coronal p.
        cross-sectional p.
        horizontal p.
        median p.
        median-sagittal p.
        midsagittal p.
        sagittal p.
        p.'s of reference
        p. suture
        transverse p.
planigram
planigraphy
plaque
        talc p.'s
plateau
platelets
platelike
        p. atelectasis
platinum (Pt)
plesiosectional tomography
plethysmograph
        body p.
        digital p.

plethysmograph (continued)
        finger p.
pleura (pleurae)
pleural
        p. effusion
pleurography
pluridirectional tomography
plutonium (Pu)
pneumarthrogram
pneumarthrography
pneumatocele
        p. cranii
        extracranial p.
        intracranial p.
        parotid p.
pneumatogram
pneumatograph
pneumencephalography
pneumoalveolography
pneumoangiogram
pneumoangiography
pneumoarthrogram
pneumoarthrography
pneumocardiograph
pneumocardiography
pneumocystography
pneumocystotomography
pneumoencephalogram
pneumoencephalography (PEG)
        cerebral p.
        fractional p.
pneumoencephalomyelogram
pneumoencephalomyelography
pneumofasciogram
pneumogram
pneumography
        cerebral p.
        retroperitoneal p.
pneumogynogram
pneumomediastinogram
pneumomediastinography
pneumomyelography
pneumonia
        See in *Pulmonary Medicine*
        section.
pneumonitis
        See in *Pulmonary Medicine*
        section.

pneumonograph
pneumonography
pneumoperitoneal
pneumoperitoneography
pneumoperitoneum
    diagnostic p.
    transabdominal p.
pneumopreperitoneum
pneumopyelogram
pneumopyelography
pneumorachicentesis
pneumorachis
pneumoradiography
    retroperitoneal p.
pneumoretroperitoneum
pneumoroentgenogram
pneumoroentgenography
pneumothorax
    diagnostic p.
pneumotomography
pneumoventriculogram
pneumoventriculography
pocket chamber
point
    p. Ba
    Kienböck-Adamson p.'s
Poisson distribution
Poisson-Pearson formula
poker spine
polarization
polonium (Po)
polycycloidal tomography
polymer
polytomogram
polytomography
polyvinylpyrrolidone
popcorn-like
porous
portacamera
portal
    p. portography
    p. venography
portography
    percutaneous transhepatic p.
    portal p.
    splenic p.
    umbilical p.
portophlebography

portosplenography
portovenography
portwine marks
position
    See also in *General Surgical*
      Terms.
    abduction p.
    adduction p.
    Albers-Schönberg p.
    AP (anteroposterior) p.
    Béclére p.
    Benassi p.
    Blackett-Healy p.
    Broden p.
    brow-down p.
    brow-up p.
    Caldwell p.
    Camp-Coventry p.
    Cleaves p.
    cross-table lateral p.
    decubitus p.
    erect p.
    eversion p.
    extension p.
    Feist-Mankin p.
    Fick p.
    Fleischner p.
    flexion p.
    Friedman p.
    frogleg p., froglegged p.
    Gaynor-Hart p.
    Grashey p.
    Haas p.
    Hickey p.
    inlet p.
    inversion p.
    Isherwood p.
    Johnson p.
    Kurzbauer p.
    Laquerrière-Pierquin p.
    Larkin p.
    lateral p.
    Law p.
    Lawrence p.
    Leonard-George p.
    Lewis p.
    Lilienfeld p.
    Lindblom p.

position (continued)
>   Lorenz p.
>   Löw-Beer p.
>   Mayer p.
>   Meese p.
>   Miller p.
>   Nölke p.
>   oblique p.
>   PA (posteroanterior) p.
>   Pawlow p.
>   Pearson p.
>   prone p.
>   recumbent p.
>   reverse Waters p.
>   Schüller p.
>   semierect p.
>   semi-Fowler p.
>   semirecumbent p.
>   Settegast p.
>   Staunig p.
>   Stecher p.
>   Stenver p.
>   supine p.
>   Tarrant p.
>   Taylor p.
>   Titterington p.
>   Towne p.
>   Trendelenburg p.
>   Twining p.
>   Waters p.
>   Waters p., reverse
>   Wigby-Taylor p.
>   Zanelli p.
positive
>   p. contrast encephalography
positrocephalogram
positron
>   p.-coincidence
>   p. decay
>   p. emission tomography (PET)
>   p. emission transaxial tomography (PETT)
>   p. emission transverse tomography (PETT)
positronium
posterior
>   p. palatine suture

posteroanterior (PA) view
post–fatty meal cholecystography
postirradiation
postmastectomy
postoperative
>   p. cholangiography
postrelease radiography
postvoid radiography
potassium (K)
>   p. perchlorate
potential
>   p. difference
>   p. gradient
Potter-Bucky
>   diaphragm
>   grid
Praestholm contrast medium
praseodymium (Pr)
preamplifier
predetector
premaxillary
>   p. suture
presentation
>   See *position.*
>   See in *Obstetrics & Gyne-cology* section.
principal [primary, main]
principle [rule]
>   See also *law.*
>   Fick p.
>   Pauli exclusion p.
Priodax contrast medium
probe
>   fiberoptic p.
>   scintillation p.
process
>   See also *apophysis, promi-nence,* and *protuberance.*
>   acromion p.
>   articular p.
>   bremsstrahlung p.
>   capitular p.
>   condyloid p.
>   coracoid p.
>   intercondylar p.
>   mastoid p.
>   maxillary p.
>   neutron absorption p.

process (continued)
> odontoid p.
> olecranon p.
> spinous p.
> styloid p.
> superior articulating p.
> transverse p.
> xiphoid p.

processor
> array p.

projection
> See also *view.*
> anteroposterior (AP) p.
> anteroposterior lordotic p.
> apical lordotic p.
> axial p.
> axillary p.
> ball-catcher p.
> basilar p.
> basovertical p.
> biplane p.
> blow-out view p.
> Caldwell p.
> Chassard-Lapiné p.
> Chausse III p., third p. of
>   Chausse
> cone-down p.
> craniocaudad p.
> cross-sectional transverse p.
> dorsoplantar p.
> erect fluoro spot p.
> flexion, extension p.
> p. formula
> frontal p.
> half-axial p.
> Heinig p.
> Hermodsson p.
> Hughston p.
> inferior-superior p.
> inferior-superior tangential p.
> inferosuperior axial p.
> intraoral p.
> L5−S1 p.
> lateral oblique axial p.
> lateral transcranial p.
> lateral transfacial p.
> lateromedial oblique p.
> Lauenstein and Hickey p.

projection (continued)
> Laurin p.
> left anterior oblique (LAO) p.
> left posterior oblique (LPO)
>   p.
> lumbosacral p.
> medial oblique axial p.
> mediolateral p.
> Merchant p.
> mortise p.
> navicular p.
> notch p.
> nuchofrontal p.
> oblique p.
> oblique lateral p.
> open-mouth p.
> parieto-orbital p.
> pillar p.
> Pirie transoral p.
> plantodorsal p.
> posteroanterior (PA) p.
> posteroanterior lordotic p.
> recumbent lateral p.
> right anterior oblique (RAO)
>   p.
> right posterior oblique
>   (RPO) p.
> Runström p.
> scaphoid p.
> Schüller p.
> semiaxial p.
> semiaxial anteroposterior p.
> semiaxial transcranial p.
> Settegast p.
> skyline p.
> Stenver p.
> stereo right lateral p.
> stress p.
> Stryker notch p.
> submentovertex p.
> submentovertical axial p.
> sunrise p.
> superoinferior p.
> swimmer's p.
> tangential p.
> Templeton and Zim carpal
>   tunnel p.

projection (continued)
    Towne p.
    transtabular AP p.
    transtabular PA p.
    transthoracic p.
    tunnel p.
    verticosubmental p.
    Waters p.
    West Point p.
    p. x-ray microscope
promethium (Pm)
prominence
    See also *apophysis, process,*
        protuberance and *swelling.*
    styloid p.
pronate
propagation
proportional counter
propyliodone
prostatography
protactinium (Pa)
proton
    p. beam (Bragg peak)
    p. spectroscopy
protuberance
    See also *apophysis, process,*
        prominence, and *swelling.*
    external occipital p.
proximal
proximally
pruned hilum
pruned-tree
    p.-t. appearance
    p.-t. arteriogram
psoas
    p. shadow
PT—pneumothorax
PTC—percutaneous transhepatic
   cholangiography
ptosis
pubic
    inferior p. ramus
    p. rami
    superior p. ramus
    p. symphysis
pubis (genitive of pubes; used alone
   for os pubis)

pulmonary
    p. angiography
    p. arborization
    p. arteriography
    p. pedicle
    p. vascular markings
    p. vasculature
pulse-height analyzer
punctate
PVC—polyvinyl chloride
    postvoiding cystogram
"pwah-son" Phonetic for Poisson.
Px—pneumothorax
pyelofluoroscopy
pyelogram
    dragon p.
    hydrated p.
    infusion p.
    intravenous p.
    retrograde p.
pyelography
    air p.
    antegrade p.
    ascending p.
    drip p.
    drip infusion p.
    p. by elimination
    excretion p.
    infusion p.
    intravenous p. (IVP)
    lateral p.
    percutaneous antegrade p.
    respiration p.
    retrograde p.
    washout p.
pyeloscopy
pyeloureterography
pyloric
    p. string sign
pyrogen
quantification
quantitative
    q. computed tomography
quantum (quanta)
    q. theory
quenching
R—roentgen
rabbit

rachitic
rad—radiation adsorbed dose
radian (rad.)
radiant energy
radiate
radiation
    α r. [alpha]
    r. absorbed dose (rad)
    annihilation r.
    β r. [beta]
    background r.
    backscattered r.
    braking r.
    bremsstrahlung r.
    r. burn
    Cerenkov r. production
    characteristic r.
    r. colitis
    cosmic r.
    r. counter
    cyclotron r.
    r. dermatitis
    r. detector
    direct r.
    dose equivalent r.
    electromagnetic r.
    r. energy
    r. enteropathy
    r. erythema
    r. exposure
    fractionated r.
    γ r. [gamma]
    r. gastritis
    r. of Gratiolet
    r. hepatitis
    heterogeneous r.
    homogeneous r.
    Huldshinsky r.
    hysterectomy and r. (H&R)
    infrared r.
    r. injury
    r. intensity
    interstitial r.
    ionization r.
    ionizing r.
    r. leakage
    man-made environmental r.
    Maxwell theory of r.

radiation (continued)
    r. monitor
    monochromatic r.
    monoenergetic r.
    natural r.
    r. necrosis
    nonionizing r.
    nuclear r.
    occupational r.
    optic r.
    r. osteitis
    r. pericarditis
    photon theory of r.
    r. physics
    r. pneumonia
    r. pneumonitis
    primary r.
    r. protection
    protracted r.
    recoil r.
    remnant r.
    r. fibrosis
    r. myelitis
    Rollier r.
    r. oncology
    scattered r.
    r. sickness
    specific r.
    spontaneous r.
    supervoltage r.
    r. syndrome
    terrestrial r.
    r. therapy
    thermal r.
    ultraviolet r.
    useful-beam r.
    r. warning symbol
    white r.
    r. window
radiation production
    Cerenkov r.p.
radii (genitive and plural of radius)
radioactive
    r. brain scan
    r. decay
    r. disintegration
    r. effluents
    r. element

radioactive (continued)
    r. equilibrium
    r. fallout
    r. gallium
    r. gases
    r. half-life
    r. isotope
    r. nuclide
    r. series
    r. source
    r. thorium
radioactivity
    artificial r., induced r.
    natural r.
radioactor
radioanaphylaxis
radioautograph
radiobe
radiobioassay
radiobiological
radiobiologist
radiobiology
radiocalcium
radiocarbon
radiocardiogram
radiocardiography
radiochemical purity
radiochemistry
radiochemotherapy
radiochemy
radiocholecystography
radiochroism
radiochromatography
radiocinematograph
radiocolloid
radiode
radiodensity
radiodermatography
radiodiagnosis
radiodiagnostics
radiodiaphane
radioelectrocardiogram
radioelectrocardiograph
radioelectrocardiography
radioelement
radioencephalogram
radioencephalography
radiofluorine

radio frequency, radiofrequency
radiogallium
radiogenic
radiogold
radiogram
radiograph
    bite-wing r.
    cephalometric r.
    Code and Carlson r.
    extraoral r.
    intraoral r.
    lateral oblique jaw r.
    lateral ramus r.
    lateral skull r.
    maxillary sinus r.
    occlusal r.
    panoramic r.
    periapical r.
    submental vertex r.
    survey r.
    Towne projection r.
    Waters view r.
radiographic
    r. density
    r. effect
radiography
    biomedical r.
    body section r.
    computed digital r. (CDR)
    contrast r.
    digital r.
    double-contrast r.
    electron r.
    gamma r.
    mucosal relief r.
    neutron r.
    pan-oral r.
    panoramic r.
    postrelease r.
    postvoid r.
    sectional r.
    selective r.
    serial r.
    spot film r.
    stereoscopic r.
radiohepatographic
radioimmunity
radioimmunodiffusion

radioimmunoelectrophoresis
radioinduction
radioiron
radioisotope
    carrier-free r.
radiokymography
radiolabeled
radiolead
radiologic, radiological
radiologist
radiology
    dental r., oral r.
    nuclear r.
radiolucency
radiolucent
radiometallography
radiometer
    pastille r.
    photographic r.
radiometric
    r. analysis
radiomicrometer
radiomimetic
radion
radionitrogen
radionuclide
    See also *contrast medium.*
    r. angiocardiography
    r. angiography
    r. cardiography
    r. cholescintigraphy
    r. cisternography
    r. cystography
    r. emission tomography
    metastable r.
    parent r.
    r. scanning
    r. venography
    r. ventriculography
    r. voiding cystourethrography
radiopacity
radioparency
radioparent
radiopathology
radiopelvimetry
radiopharmaceutic, radiopharma-
    ceutical
radiophosphorus

radiophotography
radiophylaxis
radiopotassium
radiopotentiation
radiopulmonography
radioreceptor
radioscopy
radiosensitivity
radiosodium
radiospirometry
radiostereoscopy
radiostrontium
radiosulfur
radiotellurium
radiotherapeutics
radiotherapy
    arc r.
    computerized r.
    contact r.
    fast neutron r.
    interstitial r.
    intracavitary r.
    supervoltage r.
    whole-body r.
radiothorium
radiotomy
radiotransparency
radiotransparent
radius (radii)
    Bohr r.
radon (Rn)
RAI—radioactive iodine
RAIU—radioactive iodine uptake
ramus (rami)
range
rapid biplane angiocardiography
rate meter
ratio
    cardiothoracic r.
    gyromagnetic r.
    ^{131}I conversion r. [131-I]
    radioactive iodide conver-
        sion r.
    target-to-nontarget r.
    ventilation-perfusion (V/Q) r.
ray
    α r.'s [alpha]
    β r.'s [beta]

ray (continued)
    cathode r.'s
    central r.
    cosmic r.'s
    δ-r.'s [delta]
    fluorescent r.'s
    γ r.'s [gamma]
    grenz r.'s
    infrared r.'s
    parallel r.'s
    roentgen r.'s
    secondary r.
    vertical r.
Raybar 75 contrast medium
Rayopak
Rayvist contrast medium
RC—retrograde cystogram
RCA—radionuclide cerebral
    angiogram
reaction
    biomolecular r.
    thermonuclear r.
reactor
    nuclear r.
real-time
    r.-t. echocardiography
recanalization
recess
    azygoesophageal r.
    epitympanic r.
recovery time
recumbency
redundancy
reformat
refractory
    r. pain
region
    Broca r.
    limbic r.
region of interest
Reid baseline
relativistic mass
rem—roentgen-equivalent-man
renal
    r. angiography
    r. arteriography
    intravenous r. angiography
renocystogram

Renografin contrast medium
renogram
    isotope r.
renography
    emission r.
Reno-M-60 contrast medium
Reno-M-Dip contrast medium
Renovist contrast medium
Renovue contrast medium
"rentgen" Phonetic for roentgen.
REP—roentgen equivalent–physical
repetition time (TR)
resin
resistance
    acquired radiation r.
resistive magnet
resolution
    spatial r.
resonance
    r. capture
    electron paramagnetic r.
      (EPR)
    electron spin r. (ESR)
    nuclear magnetic r. (NMR)
    proton magnetic r. (PMR)
resonant
respiration
    r. pyelography
reticulation
reticulonodular
retrocecal
retrococcygeal
Retro-Conray contrast medium
retrograde
    r. angiocardiography
    r. aortography
    r. cardioangiography
    r. cystography
    r. cystourethrography
    endoscopic r. pancreatogra-
      phy
    peroral r. pancreaticobiliary
      ductography
    r. pyelography
    r. urography
retroperitoneal
    r. pneumography
    r. pneumoradiography

RFB—retained foreign body
RFS—renal function study
rhabdoid
    r. suture
rhenium (Re)
rhizolysis
rhizotomy
RHLN—right hilar lymph node
rhm—roentgen(s) (per) hour (at one) meter
rhodium (Rh)
rhythmeur
ribosyl
ribothymidine
ribulose
right-sided angiocardiography
ring
    Cannon r.
    r. of bone
    periosteal bone r.
ripple voltage
RISA—radioactive iodinated serum albumin
RIU—radioactive iodine uptake
RKY—roentgen kymography
RLL—right lower lobe
RLQ—right lower quadrant
R-meter
RML—right middle lobe
RO, R/O—rule out
roentgen (R)
    r.-equivalent-man (rem)
    r. kymography (RKY)
    r.'s per second (R/s)
    r. tube
roentgenogram
roentgenography
    body section r.
    double-contrast r.
    magnification r.
    mucosal relief r.
    sectional r.
    selective r.
    spot film r.
roentgenologic, roentgenological
roentgenologist
roentgenology

roentgentherapy
    intraoral r.
    intravaginal r.
rotating
    r. anode tube
rotational tomography
rotography
roto-tomography
RP—retrograde pyelogram
R/s—roentgen(s) per second
RT—radiation therapy, radiotherapy
RU—retrograde urogram
    roentgen unit
rubidium (Rb)
rudimentary
rugal pattern
rugate
rugose, rugous
RUL—right upper lobe
rule
    See *law* and *principle.*
runoff
Runström
    projection
    view
RUQ—right upper quadrant
ruthenium (Ru)
rutherford (Rd)
S1 through S5—sacral vertebrae 1–5
sacculation
sagittal
    s. suture
SAH—subarachnoid hemorrhage
salpingogram
salpingography
Salpix contrast medium
Salyrgan
samarium (Sm)
sarcoma (sarcomas, sarcomata)
    See in *Oncology and Hematology* section.
sarcomatoid
satellite lesion
saturation current
SBFT—small bowel follow-through [x-ray]
scalar
    s. coupling

scalar (continued)
    s. effect
scale
    Bloch s.
scaler
    s. counter
scalloped
scalloping
scan
    A s.
    adrenal s.
    B s.
    blood pool s.
    bone s.
    bone marrow s.
    brain s.
    C s.
    capillary blockade perfusion
       s.
    cardiac s.
    CAT (computerized axial
       tomography) s.
    C-mode s.
    compound s.
    CT (computed tomography) s.
    DISIDA (disopropylimin-
       odiacetic acid) s.
    dynamic CT s.
    EMI s.
    gallium s.
    gamma s.
    hepatobiliary s.
    HIDA (hepatoiminodiacetic
       acid) s.
    isotope bone s.
    kidney s.
    krypton s.
    liver s.
    liver-spleen s.
    mechanical compound s.
    Meckel s.
    medronate s.
    MUGA (multiple gated
       acquisition) s.
    multiple gated blood pool s.
    multislice full line s.
    nongated CT s.
    nucleotide s.

scan (continued)
    perfusion s.
    perfusion lung s.
    PET (positron emission
       tomography) s.
    PIPIDA s.
    PIPIDA hepatobiliary s.
    PYP (pyrophosphate) s.
    radioactive s.
    radionuclide s.
    RAI (radioactive iodine) s.
    renal s.
    RISA (radioactive iodinated
       serum albumin) s.
    salivary gland s.
    sector s.
    selective excitation line s.
    single sweep s.
    SPECT (single photon emis-
       sion computed tomogra-
       phy) s.
    spleen s.
    ^{99m}Tc-labeled macroaggre-
       gated albumin (MAA) s.
    technetium s.
    thallium 201 s.
    thallium myocardial s.
    thyroid s.
    ventilation s.
    ventilation-perfusion (V/Q) s.
scandium (Sc)
scanner
    CT body s.
    General Electric CT/T7 800 s.
    Medx s.
    neurodiagnostic s.
    nuclear s.
    radioisotope s.
    rectilinear s.
    tomographic multiplane s.
    whole-body s.
scanning
    A-mode (amplitude modula-
       tion) s.
    B-mode (brightness modula-
       tion) s.
    bone marrow s.
    brain s.

scanning (continued)
    cine CT s.
    compound s.
    contiguous s.
    full line s.
    gallium s.
    gamma s.
    infarct s.
    lacrimal s.
    line s.
    linear s.
    M-mode (time-motion) s.
    multiplanar s.
    nuclear s.
    nucleotide s.
    perfusion s.
    point s.
    radioisotope s.
    radionuclide s.
    real-time s.
    renal s.
    rotate-rotate s.
    rotate-stationary s.
    sector s.
    sensitive point s.
    s. sequence
    single-pass s.
    s. spot
    three-phase bone s.
    transverse s.
    ventilation-perfusion (V/Q) s.
    water path s.
    whole-body s.
scanography
    slit s.
    spot s.
scatter
    Compton s.
scattering
    Compton s.
    ultrasound s.
scimitar
    s. shadow
    s. sign
    s. syndrome
scintiangiography
scintigraphic

scintigraphy
    myocardial perfusion s.
    nuclear s.
    perfusion s.
    thallium perfusion s.
    thyroidal lymph node s.
    ventilation s.
scintillation
    s. camera
    s. scan
scintiphotography
scintiphotosplenoportography
scintiscan
scintiscanner
scintiview
"scopes" See under full name.
    autofluoroscope
    electroscope
    endodiascope
    fluoroscope
    kinescope
    kinetoscope
    kymoscope
    microscope
    orthodiascope
    photofluoroscope
    radioscope
    roentgenoscope
    sonofluoroscope
    spectroscope
    stereoscope
    thermoscope
screen
    s. craze artifact
screening
    chest s.
    s. mammography
scybala (plural of scybalum)
scybalous
scybalum (scybala)
SD—skin dose
^{75}Se—radioactive selenium [selenium Se 75]
second (s, sec.)
    milliampere s. (mAs)
section
    coronal s.
    cross s.

section (continued)
    frontal s.
sectional
    s. radiography
    s. roentgenography
"sefal–" Phonetic for words begin-
    ning cephal–.
Seidlitz
    powder test
Seldinger
    catheterization
selective
    s. arteriography
    s. radiography
    s. roentgenography
    s. venography
self-absorption
self-quenched counter tube
self-scattering
sella (sellae)
    s. turcica
semi-Fowler position
senograph
senography
sensitivity
    plane s.
    point s.
sensitometer
    electroluminescent s.
sensitometry
Sephadex
sequential
sequestra (plural of sequestrum)
sequestral
sequestration
sequestrum (sequestra)
serial
    s. radiography
serialoangiocardiography
serialogram
serialograph
series
    gastrointestinal s.
    small-bowel s.
serpiginous
serrated
    s. suture

shadow
    acoustic s.
    bat's wing s.
    heart s.
    overlap s.
    psoas s.
    sound s.
shadowgram
shadowgraph
shadowgraphy
shaggy
shape
    baseball bat s.
    cricket bat s.
Shepherd fracture
shield
    lead gonad s.
shielding
sialadenitis
sialadenography
sialoangiography
sialogram
sialography
"sibah–" Phonetic for words begin-
    ning scyba–.
side effect
sigmoidoscopy
sign
    See also *effect* and *phenom-*
      enon.
    air bronchogram s.
    air crescent s.
    air-cushion s.
    air dome s.
    banana s.
    Bergman s.
    bowler hat s.
    Carman s.
    Carman-Kirklin s.
    Carman-Kirklin meniscus s.
    coiled spring s.
    coin s.
    Cole s.
    colon cutoff s.
    crescent s.
    double-bubble s.
    doughnut s.
    E s.

sign (continued)
    fat pad s.
    floating-tooth s.
    flush-tank s.
    Granger s.
    Griesinger s.
    halo s.
    Haudek s.
    Hawkins s.
    Hefke-Turner s.
    Hennings s.
    Horner s.
    Hueter fracture s.
    Kantor string s.
    Keen s.
    Klemm s.
    Laugier s.
    lemon s.
    meniscus s.
    Mercedes-Benz s.
    Mexican hat s.
    moulage s.
    niche s.
    obturator s.
    patent bronchus s.
    pyloric string s.
    Quant s.
    reversed three s.
    rim s.
    scimitar s.
    silhouette s.
    Spalding s.
    Stierlin s.
    string s.
    string-of-beads s.
    twin peak s.
    Wegner s.
    Weill s.
    Westermark s.
    Wimberger s.
signature
    tumor s.
signet-ring pattern
silhouette
    cardiac s.
silicon (Si)
"sil-oo-et" Phonetic for silhouette.

silver (Ag)
    s. iodide
"simphysis" Phonetic for symphysis.
sin–. See also words beginning
    cin–, syn–.
Sinografin contrast medium
sinogram
sinography
"sinti–" Phonetic for words begin-
    ning scinti–.
sinus (sinus, sinuses)
    costophrenic s.
    Forssell s.
    frontal s., s. frontalis
    sphenoid s.
sinusography
    cerebral s.
sinusoidal
sinusoidalization
situs (situs)
    s. inversus
    s. inversus viscerum
    s. perversus
    s. transversus
skeletal
skiagram
skiagraph
skiagraphy
"skibah–" Phonetic for words
    beginning scyba–.
Skillern
    fracture
Skiodan contrast medium
skip
    s. areas
    s. tomography
skull
    hot-cross-bun s.
    maplike s.
    natiform s.
    sutures of s.
    West-Engstler s.
    West lacuna s.
slice
    CT s.
    s. geometry
    s. selection

slit
    s. scanography
slug
sodium (Na)
    s. bromide
    s. chromate Cr 51
    s. diatrizoate
    s. iodide I 123 (I 125, I 131)
    s. iodipamide
    s. iodohippurate I 131
    s. iodomethamate
    s. iothalamate I 125
    s. ipodate
    s. methiodal
    s. pertechnetate Tc 99m
    s. phosphate P 32
    radioactive s.
    s. radioiodide
    s. rose bengal I 131
    s. [^{99mTc}] pertechnetate [Tc
      99m]
    thallium-activated s. iodide
    s. thorium tartrate
    s. tyropanoate
solarization
solenoid
solid-state physics
solitary nodule
solubilize
Solu-Biloptin contrast medium
solution
    hundredth-normal s.
    hypertonic s.
    molal s.
Solutrast contrast medium
Sommer-Foegella method
sonar
sonarography
sonofluoroscopy
sonogram
sonography
    Acuson computed s.
    Acuson transvaginal s.
space
    Crookes s.
    retroperitoneal s.
    subarachnoid s.
spadelike

spallation
spatial
    s. vectorcardiography
specific activity
speckled
SPECT—single photon emission
    computed tomography
spectra (plural of spectrum)
spectral
spectrometer
    beta-ray s.
    gamma-ray s.
    mass s.
    Mossbauer s.
    scintillation s.
spectrometry
    pulse height s.
spectrophotofluorometer
spectrophotometer
    absorption s.
spectroscope
    direct vision s.
spectroscopic
spectroscopy
    magnetic resonance s.
    nuclear magnetic resonance s.
spectrum (spectra)
    chromatic s.
    color s.
    continuous s.
    continuous x-ray s.
    electromagnetic s.
    excitation s.
    thermal s.
    x-ray s.
SPECT scan
SPGR—spoiled GRASS [gradient
    recalled acquisition in a steady
    state]
sphenoethmoid, sphenoethmoidal
    s. suture
sphenofrontal
    s. suture
sphenomalar
    s. suture
sphenomaxillary
    s. suture

spheno-occipital
    s. suture
spheno-orbital
    s. suture
sphenoparietal
    s. suture
sphenopetrosal
    s. suture
sphenosquamous
    s. suture
sphenotemporal
    s. suture
sphenovomerine
    s. suture
sphenozygomatic
    s. suture
sphere
spherical
spinal
    s. arteriography
spinal cord
    s.c. angiography
spindling
spine
    anterior inferior iliac s.
    anterior superior iliac s.
    bamboo s.
    basilar s.
    cervical s.
    cleft s.
    ischial s.
    s. of ischium
    kissing s.'s
    lumbar s.
    lumbosacral (LS) s.
    posterior inferior iliac s.
    posterior superior iliac s.
    s. of pubic bone
    railway s.
    sacral s.
    thoracic s.
    s. of tibia
    tibial s.
    trochanteric s., greater
    trochanteric s., lesser
    s. of vertebra
    vertebral s.
spin-lattice relaxation time

spinogram
spintherometer
spintometer
spiral
    See also *coil* and *helix.*
    s. computed tomography (CT)
    s. fracture
    s. volumetric CT
splenic
    s. flexure
    s. portography
    s. venography
splenography
splenoportal venography
splenoportogram
splinting
spoiled GRASS [gradient recalled
    acquisition in a steady state]
    (SPGR)
spot
    See also *dot.*
    focal s.
    hot s.
    pelvic s.
    s. scanography
spot film
    s.f. device
    s.f. radiography
    s.f. roentgenography
    s.f. study
squamomastoid
    s. suture
squamoparietal
    s. suture
squamosphenoid
    s. suture
squamous
    s. suture
    s. suture of cranium
SSD—source-skin distance
staging
    Greulich and Pyle bone age s.
star test pattern
stenion
stenosis (stenoses)
Stenver
    position
    view

stercoraceous
stercoroma
stercorous
stercus (stercora)
stereocinefluorography
stereoencephalotomy
stereofluoroscopy
stereogram
stereograph
stereography
stereometry
stereomicroradiography
stereoradiogram
stereoradiograph
stereoradiography
stereoroentgenography
stereoroentgenometry
stereosalpingography
stereoscopic
    s. radiography
    s. zonography
stereoscopy
stereoskiagraphy
stereotactic
stereotaxis
Steripaque-BR contrast medium
Steripaque-V contrast medium
straggling
strata (plural of stratum)
stratiform
stratigram
stratigraphy
stratum (strata)
streak
    fatty s.
stress
    s. film
    s. thallium-201
string sign
stripe
    endometrial s. [on sonogram
      of uterus]
strontium (Sr)
    s. Sr 85 nitrate
    s. Sr 87m
    s. Sr 90
    radioactive s.
    s. with yttrium 90

study
    air contrast s.
    barium meal s.
    blood flow s.
    cine s.
    double-contrast s.
    dual-contrast s.
    horizontal beam s.
    iodized oil s.
    lumbar, flexion, and exten-
      sion s.
    motility s.
    perfusion s.
    perirenal air s.
    phonation s.
    quantitative regional lung
      function s.
    retrococcygeal air s.
    retroperitoneal air s.
    single-contrast s.
    spot film s.
    tracer s.
    ventilation s.
    videotape s.
    washout s.
subareolar
subluxation
subpleural
subtle
subtraction
    s. angiography
    second order s.
    s. venography
succinic semialdehyde
sulci (plural of sulcus)
sulciform
sulcus (sulci)
    s. of optic chiasm
    sigmoid s.
sulfur (S)
    colloidal s.
    radioactive s.
superimposed
superimposition
superior
    s. ramus
supinate
supination

supine
suppuration
surgery
    stereotactic s., stereotaxic s.
"sut-el" Phonetic for subtle.
suture [anatomy]
    anterior palatine s.
    bony s.
    coronal s.
    cranial s.'s
    dentate s.
    denticulate s.
    ethmoidolacrimal s.
    ethmoidomaxillary s.
    false s.
    flat s.
    frontal s.
    frontoethmoidal s.
    frontolacrimal s.
    frontomalar s.
    frontomaxillary s.
    frontonasal s.
    frontoparietal s.
    frontosphenoid s.
    frontozygomatic s.
    incisive s.
    infraorbital s.
    intermaxillary s.
    internasal s.
    interpalatine s.
    interparietal s.
    jugal s.
    lacrimoconchal s.
    lacrimoethmoidal s.
    lacrimomaxillary s.
    lacrimoturbinal s.
    lambdoid s., lambdoidal s.
    limbal s.
    limbous s.
    longitudinal s.
    longitudinal s. of palate
    malomaxillary s.
    mammillary s.
    mastoid s.
    median palatine s.
    metopic s.
    middle palatine s.
    nasal s.

suture [anatomy] (continued)
    nasofrontal s.
    nasomaxillary s.
    occipital s.
    occipitomastoid s.
    occipitoparietal s.
    occipitosphenoidal s.
    palatine s., anterior
    palatine s., median
    palatine s., middle
    palatine s., posterior
    palatine s., transverse
    palatoethmoidal s.
    palatomaxillary s.
    parietal s.
    parietomastoid s.
    parieto-occipital s.
    parietotemporal s.
    petrobasilar s.
    petrosphenobasilar s.
    petrospheno-occipital s. of
      Gruber
    petrosquamosal s.
    plane s.
    posterior palatine s.
    premaxillary s.
    rhabdoid s.
    sagittal s.
    serrated s.
    s.'s of skull
    sphenoethmoidal s.
    sphenofrontal s.
    sphenomalar s.
    sphenomaxillary s.
    spheno-occipital s.
    spheno-orbital s.
    sphenoparietal s.
    sphenopetrosal s.
    sphenosquamous s.
    sphenotemporal s.
    sphenovomerine s.
    sphenozygomatic s.
    squamomastoid s.
    squamoparietal s.
    squamosphenoid s.
    squamous s.
    squamous s. of cranium
    temporal s.

suture [anatomy] (continued)
  temporomalar s.
  temporozygomatic s.
  transverse s. of Krause
  transverse palatine s.
  true s.
  zygomaticofrontal s.
  zygomaticomaxillary s.
  zygomaticosphenoid s.
  zygomaticotemporal s.
swallow
  barium s.
  Hypaque s.
Sweet method
swelling
  See also *apophysis, process, prominence,* and *protuberance.*
  brain s.
  bulbar s.'s
swimmer's
  s. projection
  s. view
Swiss Alps appearance
Swyer-James
  syndrome
Swyer-James-Macleod
  syndrome
Sylvius cistern (cistern of Sylvius)
symmetric, symmetrical
sympexion (sympexia)
symphyseal
symphysis (symphyses)
  s. ossium pubis
  pubic s.
  s. pubica, s. pubis
symptom
  See also in *General Medical Terms.*
  crossbar s. of Fränkel
syn–. See also words beginning cin–, sin–.
synchrotron
syndrome
  See also in medical specialty sections.
  scimitar s.
synoviorthesis

system
  catenary s.
  linear s.
  mammillary s.
  metric s.
  three-compartment s.
  three-phase s.
  two-compartment s.
T—tesla
T1 through T12—thoracic vertebrae 1–12
tagged atom
tagging
tamponade
tanned red cells (TRCs)
tannic acid
tantalum (Ta)
  t. 182
  t. bronchogram
target
tautography
Taylor position
TBSA—total body surface area
Tc—technetium
⁹⁹ᵐTc-labeled 2,6-dimethylacetanilide iminodiacetic acid [Tc 99m]
⁹⁹ᵐTc-labeled pyridoxylideneglutamate (PYG) [Tc 99m]
⁹⁹ᵐTc lidofenin [Tc 99m]
TC—transhepatic cholangiography
TD—transverse diameter
TECA—technetium albumin [study]
technetium (Tc)
  t. diphosphonate
  t. Tc 99m acetanilidoiminodiacetic acid
  t. Tc 99m aggregated albumin kit
  t. Tc 99m albumin
  t. Tc 99m albumin microspheres kit
  t. Tc 99m antimony
  t. Tc 99m blood pool study
  t. Tc 99m colloid
  t. Tc 99m diethylenetriamine penta-acetic acid
  t. Tc 99m 2,3-dimercaptosuccinic acid

technetium (Tc) (continued)
- t. Tc 99m etidronate sodium kit
- t. Tc 99m ferric hydroxide
- t. Tc 99m generator
- t. Tc 99m glucoheptonate
- t. Tc 99m HAM perfusion scan
- t. Tc 99m imidodiphosphonate
- t. Tc 99m iminodiacetic acid
- t. Tc 99m macroaggregates
- t. Tc 99m medronate sodium kit
- t. Tc 99m methylene diphosphonate
- t. Tc 99m microspheres
- t. Tc 99m pentetate sodium kit
- t. Tc 99m pertechnetate
- t. Tc 99m phosphate uptake
- t. Tc 99m phytate
- t. Tc 99m pyridoxylidene glutamate
- t. Tc 99m pyrophosphate
- t. Tc 99m radiopharmaceutical
- t. Tc 99m serum albumin kit
- t. Tc 99m stannous pyrophosphate/polyphosphate kit
- t. Tc 99m sulfur colloid

technetium albumin (TECA) study
technetium-sulfur colloid
technique
    See also *maneuver* and *method.*
- autoradiographic t.
- cerebral flow image t.
- chromatographic-fluorometric t.
- Corbin t.
- drip infusion t.
- pulse echo t.
- supervoltage t.
- Welin t.

TEE—transesophageal echocardiogram
Telebrix contrast medium

telecobalt
telefluoroscopy
telemetry
teleoroentgenogram
teleoroentgenography
Telepaque contrast medium
teleradiography
teleroentgenogram
teleroentgenography
teleroentgentherapy
teletherapy
tellurium (Te)
Templeton and Zim carpal tunnel projection
temporal
- t. suture
temporomalar
- t. suture
temporozygomatic
- t. suture
tenting
- t. of hemidiaphragm
terbium (Tb)
Teridax contrast medium
termination
tesla
test
- chlormerodrin accumulation t.
- fat absorption t.
- gallbladder function t.
- gastrointestinal blood loss t.
- gastrointestinal protein loss t.
- positive washout t.
- radioactive renogram t.
- radioimmunoprecipitation t.
- radioiodine t.
- radioisotope renogram t.
- Seidlitz powder t.
- sniff t.
- string t.
- tanned red cell (TRC) t.
- triiodothyronine red cell uptake t.
- triiodothyronine resin t.
- ultrasound t.
- washout t.
thalamectomy

thalamotomy
    anterior t.
    dorsomedial t.
    parafascicular t. (PFT)
thallium (Tl)
    t. 201 imaging
    t. myocardial scan
    t. perfusion scintigraphy
    t. stress testing
thallous chloride Tl 201
theorem
    Bayes t.
theory
    Planck quantum t.
therapy
    beam t.
    Chaoul t.
    contact radiation t.
    deep roentgen ray t.
    electron beam t.
    endocrine ablative t.
    gamma-ray t.
    grid t.
    high-voltage roentgen t.
    interstitial radiation t.
    interstitial radium t.
    megavolt t., megavoltage t.
    radionuclide t.
    radium t.
    radium beam t.
    rotation t.
    x-ray t.
    zone t.
thermal neutrons
thermograph
thermography
thermoluminescent
thermonuclear
thermovision
thiosemicarbazide
Thixokon contrast medium
Thoms
    method
thoracic
    t. aortography
Thoreau filter
thorium (Th)
    t. dioxide

Thorotrast contrast medium
Thorpe
    plastic lens
three-phase system
threshold
thrombi (plural of thrombus)
thrombosis
    See in *Cardiology* section.
thrombus (thrombi)
    See in *Cardiology* section.
thulium (Tm)
    t. thumb-printing
thymidine
thyratron
thyroidal lymph node scintigraphy
Thyrx timer
time (T)
    acquisition t.
    arm-lung t.
    chromoscopy t.
    circulation t.
    colonic transit t.
    echo t. (TE)
    t. of flight
    longitudinal relaxation t.
    mean circulating t.
    real-t.
    recovery t.
    repetition t. (TR)
    rise t.
    spin-lattice relaxation t.
    spin-spin relaxation t.
    T_1 relaxation t. [T1]
    T_2 relaxation t. [T2]
    thermal relaxation t.
    transit t.
    transverse relaxation t.
time-activity curve
timer
    Thyrx t.
tin (Sn)
    t. with indium 113m
titanium (Ti)
    t. dioxide
Tl—thallium
TLA—translumbar aortogram
TNI—total nodal irradiation

tomography
    axial transverse t.
    circular t.
    computed t. (CT)
    computerized axial t. (CAT)
    contrast-enhanced computed
      t. (CECT)
    cranial computed t. (CCT)
    dynamic computed t.
    emission t.
    emission computed t. (ECT)
    emission computerized axial
      t. (ECAT)
    focal plane t.
    hypercycloidal t.
    linear t.
    longitudinal section t.
    metrizamide-assisted com-
      puted t.
    nuclear magnetic resonance t.
    panoramic t.
    plesiosectional t.
    pluridirectional t.
    polycycloidal t.
    positron emission t. (PET)
    positron emission transaxial
      t. (PETT)
    positron emission transverse
      t. (PETT)
    quantitative computed t.
    radionuclide emission t.
    rotational t.
    simultaneous multifilm t.
    single photon emission com-
      puted t. (SPECT)
    skip t.
    transversal t.
    ultrasonic t.
    wide-angle t.
tomolaryngography
tomoscopy
tonography
    carotid compression t.
topographic, topographical
tortuous
Towne
    position
    projection ratiograph

Towne (continued)
    view
Townsend avalanche
tracer
tracheobronchoscopy
transabdominal
    t. cholangiography
transducer
    sector t.
transferrin
transformation
    fast Fourier f.
transformer
    filament t.
    high-voltage t.
    ratio t.
    step-down t.
    step-up t.
transhepatic
    t. cholangiography (TC)
    direct percutaneous t.
      cholangiography
    fine-needle t. cholangiogra-
      phy (FNTC)
    percutaneous t. cholangiog-
      raphy (PTC)
    percutaneous t. portography
transition
translumbar aortography
transmutation
transtracheal
    percutaneous t. bronchogra-
      phy
transversal tomography
transverse
    axial t. tomography
    t. colon
    t. magnetization
    t. palatine suture
    t. suture of Krause
trauma (traumas, traumata)
TRC—tanned red cell(s)
tree
    tracheobronchial t.
Treitz
    ligament
Trendelenburg
    position

triangle
    Codman t.
triangular
triangulation
trichloroacetic acid
triolein (glyceral trioleate) I 131
Triosil contrast medium
Triphasix generator
triple-voiding cystography
tritium
triton
trochanter
    greater t.
    lesser t.
true suture
TSD—target skin distance
TT—transit time
T tube, T-tube
    T-t. cholangiogram
    T-t. cholangiography
tube
    cathode-ray t. (CRT)
    Chaoul t.
    Coolidge x-ray t.
    Crookes t.
    discharge t.
    Dotter t.
    electron multiplier t.
    Geiger-Müller t.
    glow modular t.
    hot-cathode t.
    image intensifier t.
    image orthicon t.
    Olshevsky t.
    photomultiplier t. (PMT)
    roentgen t.
    rotating anode t.
    valve t.
    x-ray t.
tuber (tubers, tubera)
tubercle
tubercula (plural of tuberculum)
tuberculate, tuberculated
tuberculation
tuberculoid
tuberculosis (TB)
tuberculum (tubercula)
tuberosis

tuberositas (tuberositates)
tungsten (W)
TVC—triple voiding cystogram
T_1-weighted [T1-]
T_2-weighted [T2-]
two-dimensional
    t.-d. echocardiography (TDE)
tympanography
UGI—upper gastrointestinal
UGI
    study
    tract
UIQ—upper inner quadrant
ULQ—upper left quadrant
ultrasonic
    u. cardiography
    u. tomography
ultrasonogram
ultrasonograph
ultrasonographic
ultrasonography
    A-mode u.
    Doppler u.
    endoscopic u.
    gray-scale u.
ultrasound
    Doppler u.
    real-time u.
umbilical
    u. portography
Umbradil contrast medium
undulating
unit
    Angström u.
    Behnken u. (R)
    cobalt 60 beam therapy u.
    electromagnetic u.'s
    Hampson u.
    Hounsfield (H) u.
    Kienböck u. (X)
    quantum u.
    X u.
    x-ray u.
unsaturated
    u. compounds
UOQ—upper outer quadrant
upper GI series
uranium (U)

ureterocystography
ureterogram
ureterography
ureteropyelography
urethrocystogram
urethrocystography
urethrocystometry
urethrogram
        excretory u.
urethrography
Urografin contrast medium
urogram
        drip infusion u.
urography
        ascending u.
        cystoscopic u.
        descending u.
        drip infusion u.
        excretion u.
        excretory u.
        intravenous u. (IVU)
        oral u.
        percutaneous antegrade u.
        retrograde u.
urokymography
Uromiro contrast medium
Uropac contrast medium
uroradiology
Uroselectan
Urovision contrast medium
URQ—upper right quadrant
US—ultrasonography
        ultrasound
uterine
        u. venography
uterography
uterosalpingogram
uterosalpingography
uterotubography
vaginogram
vaginography
        barium v.
valve
        v. tube
vanadium (V)
Van de Graaff
        generator

Vascoray
vascular
        v. groove
vasculitic
Vasidone contrast medium
vasiform
vasoepididymography
vasography
Vater
        ampulla (ampulla of Vater)
VCG—vectorcardiogram
        vectorcardiography
VCU, VCUG—voiding cystoure-
        throgram
vectocardiogram
vectocardiography
vectorcardiography (VCG)
        spatial v.
Velpeau axillary view
venacavogram
venacavography
        inferior v. (IVCV)
venogram
        renal v.
venography
        ascending v.
        descending v.
        extradural v.
        impedance v.
        intraosseous v.
        limb v.
        peripheral v.
        portal v.
        radionuclide v.
        selective v.
        splenic v.
        splenoportal v.
        subtraction v.
        uterine v.
        vertebral v.
venous
        v. angiocardiography
        v. aortography
ventilation
        v.-perfusion (V/Q) scan
        v. scintigraphy
ventriculogram

ventriculography
   bubble v.
   cardiac v.
   cerebral v.
   contrast v.
   isotope v.
   radionuclide v.
vermography
vertebra (vertebrae)
       See also in *Orthopedics and
       Sports Medicine* section.
   abdominal vertebrae
   basilar v.
   butterfly v.
   caudal vertebrae, caudate
       vertebrae
   cervical v. (C1–C7)
   cleft v.
   vertebrae coccygeae, coc-
       cygeal vertebrae
   codfish v.
   vertebrae colli
   cranial v.
   v. dentata
   dorsal vertebrae
   false vertebrae
   hourglass v.
   H-shaped v.
   ivory v.
   vertebrae lumbales
   lumbar vertebrae (L1–L5)
   v. magnum
   movable v.
   odontoid v.
   picture frame v.
   v. plana
   primitive v.
   v. prominens, prominent v.
   sacral v., vertebrae sacrales
       (S1–S5)
   vertebrae spuriae
   sternal v.
   tail v.
   terminal v., great
   thoracic vertebrae (T1–T12)
   vertebrae thoracicae
   vertebrae thoracales
   toothed v.

vertebra (vertebrae) (continued)
       tricuspid v.
       true vertebrae
       v. vera
vertebral
       v. angiography
       v. arteriography
       v. venography
vesiculogram
       seminal v.
vesiculography
vibex (vibices)
Victoreen dosimeter
videodensitometric
videodensitometry
videometry
view
       See also *projection*.
       ball catcher's v.
       Chausse v.
       comparison v.
       coned-down v.
       decubitus v.
       dorsal v.
       frog-leg v.
       Hampton v.
       kyphotic v.
       lateral v.
       lateral decubitus v.
       Law v.
       lordotic v.
       Mayer v.
       normal anteroposterior v.
       oblique v.
       overcouch v.
       panoramic v.
       pantomographic v.
       plantar v.
       posterior v.
       profile ray v.
       recumbent v.
       Runström v.
       scottie dog v.
       scout v.
       skyline v.
       Stenver v.
       stereoscopic v.
       stress v.

view (continued)
    submentovertical v.
    superoinferior v.
    swimmer's v.
    tangential v.
    Towne v.
    Velpeau axillary v.
    Waters v.
visceral
    v. angiography
    v. aortography
    v. arteriography
    selective v. aortography
viscerography
visualization
    double-contrast v.
voiding
    v. cystourethrography
      (VCUG)
    isotope v. cystourethrogra-
      phy (IVCU)
    radionuclide v. cys-
      tourethrography
voltage
volume
    atomic v.
    v. imaging
    molar v.
voxel [*vol*ume *el*ement]
V/Q—ventilation-perfusion
V/Q
    scan
W—wehnelt [unit of x-ray penetrat-
    ing ability]
Wagstaffe fracture
Walker magnet
washout
    w. pyelography
Waters [eponym]
    projection
    view
wave
    electromagnetic w.'s
waveform
wavelength
    Compton w.
    de Broglie w.

WBR—whole-body radiation [ther-
    apy]
WD—well-differentiated
weight
    atomic w. (at. wt.)
Weill
    sign
Welin technique
Westmark sign
whole-body counting
wide-angle tomography
Wilson
    chamber
WNL—within normal limits
Wolf
    method
wolfram [tungsten]
X—Kienböck unit of x-ray dosage
X axis
XC—excretory cystogram
xenon (Xe)
    x. Xe 127
    x. Xe 133
xerogram
xerography
xeromammography
xeroradiogram
xeroradiograph
xerosialography
xerotomography
x-ray
    x-r. microscope
    projection x-r. microscope
    x-r. tube
XU—excretory urogram
Y axis
ytterbium (Yb)
    y. pentetate sodium
yttrium (Y)
zeugmatography
    Fourier transformation z.
Zimmer method
zinc (Zn)
zirconium (Zr)
    z. with niobium 95
zone
    Fresnel z.
    Looser transformation z.'s

zone (continued)
    umbau z.'s
zone plate
    Fresnel z.p.
zonogram
zonography
    stereoscopic z.
zwitterion

zygomaticofrontal
    z. suture
zygomaticomaxillary
    z. suture
zygomaticosphenoid
    z. suture
zygomaticotemporal
    z. suture

Urology and Nephrology

abdominal
 a. nephrectomy
 a. nephrotomy
abdominogenital
abdominoscrotal
abdominovesical
aberratio
 a. testis
ability
 impaired urinary concentrat-
  ing a.
ablation
abscess
 chronic a.
 kidney a.
 lacunar a.
 parafrenal a.
 paranephric a.
 pelvic a.
 pelvirectal a.
 perinephric a.
 perirenal a.
 periurethral a.
 perivesical a.
 prostatic a.
 renal a.
 retrovesical a.
 spermatic a.
 urethral a.
 urinary a.
 urinous a.
absence
 enuretic a.
accelerator
 serum thrombotic a.
access
 hemodialysis vascular a.
acetonemic
acetonuria
acetylsulfadiazine
acetylsulfaguanidine

acetylsulfathiazole
achromaturia
acidosis
 bicarbonate wastage renal
  tubular a.
 carbon dioxide a.
 hyperchloremic renal a.
 renal tubular a. (types 1, 2, 4)
 uremic a.
aciduric
acini (plural of acinus)
acinic
aciniform
acinitis
acinose [adj.]
acinotubular
acinous [adj.]
acinus (acini)
 a. renalis [malpighii]
 a. renis [malpighii]
aconuresis
acraturesis
acrobystia
acrobystiolith
acrobystitis
acrolein
acroposthitis
action
acuminatum (acuminata, acuminatae)
 condyloma acuminatum,
  condylomata acuminata
 verruca acuminata, verrucae
  acuminatae
acystia
acystinervia
acystineuria
Adamantiades-Behçet
 syndrome
Addis
 method

Addison
    crisis
    disease
addisonian
    a. syndrome
addisonism
adenine phosphoribosyl transferase
    (APRT) deficiency
adenitis
    syphilitic inguinal a.
adenocarcinoma
    acinar a.
    acinic cell a.
    acinous a.
    ductal a. of prostate
    a. of infantile testis
    a. of kidney
    renal a.
    testicular a. of infancy
    urachal a.
adenoma
    adrenocortical a.
    cortical a.
    feminizing a.
    mesonephric a.
    renal cortical a.
    a. substantiae corticalis
        suprarenalis
    testicular a.
    tubular a. of Pick
    tubulovillous a.
adenomyosarcoma
adenosarcoma
    embryonal a.
adhesion
    preputial a.
adiposis
    a. orchalis
    a. orchia
    a. orchica
adiposogenital dystrophy
adiposuria
adrenal
    a. adenoma
    a. cortex
    a. crisis
    a. gland
    a. hyperplasia

adrenal (continued)
    a. hypoplasia
    a. insufficiency
    Marchand a.
    a. medulla
    a. steroids
    a. virilism
adrenalinuria
adrenoceptive
adrenocorticohyperplasia
adrenogenital
    a. syndrome
adrenoreceptor
adrenostatic
adrenotoxin
adrenotropic
adrenotropin
adrenotropism
aerocystography
aerocystoscopy
aerourethroscopy
agalactosuria
agenesis
    renal a.
agenitalism
agenosomia
agenosomus
aglomerular
AGN—acute glomerulonephritis
agonad
agonadal
agonadism
AHC—acute hemorrhagic cystitis
air
    a. pyelography
Albarran
    disease
    gland
    test
    tubules
albiduria
Albright
    solution
    syndrome
albuginea
    a. penis
    a. testis
    albugineotomy

albugineous
albuginitis
albuminaturia
albuminorrhea
albuminuria
> adventitious a.
> globular a.
> nephrogenous a.
> postrenal a.
> renal a.
> residual a.

albuminuric
> a. retinitis

Alcock
> canal

alcoholuria
aldosterone
> a. adenoma
> a. suppression test

aldosteronoma
aldosteronopenia
aldosteronuria
Aldrich-Mees
> lines

Aldridge
> operation

Alexander-Adams
> operation

aleydigism
alginuresis
alkaptonuric
Allemann
> syndrome

allotransplantation
alpha
> a.-galactosidase A
> a.-keto acid dehydrogenase

amebiasis
> a. of bladder

aminoaciduria
> imidazole a.
> overflow a.
> renal a.
> transport a.

aminoglutethimide
β-aminoisobutyricaciduria [beta-]
δ-aminolevulinic acid (ALA) [delta-]

ampulla (ampullae)
> a. ductus deferentis
> Henle a.
> a. of vas deferens

Amussat
> valvula

amyloidosis
> kidney a.
> renal a.

anastomosis (anastomoses)
> See also *operation* and *procedure.*
> pyeloileocutaneous a.
> transuretero-ureteral a.

anatrophic
> a. nephrotomy

Andrews operation
androgen
> a. ablation
> adrenal a.
> a. deprivation
> a. precursors
> a. suppression

androgenic
androgenization
androgenized
androgenous
androgens [a class of drugs]
anesthesia
> See in *General Surgical Terms.*

aneurysmatic
angiogram
> renal a.

angiography
> intravenous renal a.
> renal a.

angiokeratoma
> a. corporis diffusum
> a. corporis diffusum universale
> diffuse a.
> a. of Fordyce
> scrotal a., a. of scrotum

angiomyolipoma
angioplasty
> percutaneous transluminal renal a. (PTRA)

angle
   costovertebral a.
anischuria
ankylurethria
annulus (annuli) [compare: anulus]
   a. urethralis
anogenital
anomaly
anoperineal
anorchia
anorchid
anorchidic
anorchidism
anorchis
anorchism
anorgasmy
anovesical
ANS—acute nephritic syndrome
antegrade
   percutaneous a. pyelography
   percutaneous a. urography
   a. pyelography
anterior
   a. nephrectomy
antiandrogen
antibody (antibodies)
   See also in *Laboratory,*
      Pathology, and Chemistry
      Terms.
   cytophilic a.
   cytotoxic a.
   monoclonal a.
antidiuretic
   a. hormone
antidiuretics [a class of drugs]
antigen (Ag)
   See also in *Laboratory,*
      Pathology, and Chemistry
      Terms.
   A a.
   B a.
   cryptic T a.
   factor VIII a.
   O a.
   P54 a.
   T a.
   Thomsen-Friedenreich a.
   transplantation a.

antigenic
   a. modulation
anti–glomerular basement membrane
   (anti-GBM) antibody disease
antilithics [a class of drugs]
anulus (anuli) [compare: annulus]
anuresis [urinary retention, anuria]
anuretic
anuria
   angioneurotic a.
   calculous a.
   compression a.
   obstructive a.
   postrenal a.
   prerenal a.
   renal a.
   suppressive a.
anuric
A&P—anterior and posterior [repair]
APD—ambulatory peritoneal dialysis
apex (apices, apexes)
   a. of bladder
   a. prostatae, a. of prostate
      gland
   a. vesicae, a. vesicalis
APKD—adult polycystic kidney
   disease
aplasia
   gonadal a.
APN—acute pyelonephritis
aponeurosis (aponeuroses)
   Denonvilliers a.
   perineal a.
   superficial perineal a.
apoplexy
   urethral a.
appearance
   cobblestone a.
   cobblestone-like a.
   ground-glass a.
   stack-of-coins a.
   string-of-beads a.
   tadpole-like a.
   toxic a.
arch
   cortical a.'s of kidney
arcuate
arcuation

ardor
    a. urinae
area (areae, areas)
    genital a.'s
ARF—acute renal failure
Arnold and Gunning method
arteriogram
arteriography
    renal a.
arteriole
    glomerular a.
    glomerular a., afferent
    glomerular a., efferent
    Isaacs-Ludwig a.
    postglomerular a.
    preglomerular a.
    renal a.
artery
    arcuate a.
    cremasteric a.
    dorsal a.
    gluteal a.
    helicine a.
    hypogastric a.
    iliac a.
    interlobar a.
    interlobular a.
    pudendal a.
    renal a.
    spermatic a.
    vesical a.
arthritis (arthritides)
    urethral a.
ascending
    a. pyelography
    a. urography
ascites
    dialysis a.
    nephrogenic a.
Ask-Upmark
    kidney
    syndrome
aspermatism
aspermatogenesis
aspermia
aspiration
assay
    estrogen receptor a. (ERA)

asthenospermia
atonia
atonic
atonicity
atony
atresia
    meatal a.
atrophy
    renal a.
    testicular a.
AUA—American Urological Association
autonephrectomy
azoospermatism
azoospermia
azotemia
    extrarenal a.
    prerenal a.
azotemic
    a. ostcodystrophy
azoturia
azoturic
bacille Calmette-Guérin (BCG) vaccine
bacillus (bacilli)
    See in *Laboratory, Pathology, and Chemistry Terms.*
Bacillus
    See in *Laboratory, Pathology, and Chemistry Terms.*
backflow
    pyelolymphatic b.
    pyelorenal b.
    pyelosinus b.
    pyelotubular b.
    pyelovenous b.
bacterium (bacteria)
    See specific bacteria in *Laboratory, Pathology, and Chemistry Terms.*
bacteriuria
bacteriuric
"bah-fon" Phonetic for bas-fond.
balanic
balanitis
    b. circinata
    b. circumscripta plasmacellularis

balanitis (continued)
    b. diabetica
    Follmann b.
    b. gangraenosa
    gangrenous b.
    b. xerotica obliterans
balanoblennorrhea
balanocele
balanoplasty
balanoposthitis
balanoposthomycosis
balanopreputial
balanorrhagia
balanus
Balkan
    B. nephritis
    B. nephropathy
ballotable
ballottement
    kidney b.
Bamberger
    hematogenic albuminuria
band
    See also *line* and *frenulum.*
    genitomesenteric b.
bandage
    See *dressing.*
    See also in *General Surgical*
       Terms.
baruria
base
    b. of bladder
    b. of renal pyramid
basement membrane
bas-fond
basket
    Buerhenne stone b. technique
basketing
basket procedure
Bates
    operation
BCG (bacille Calmette-Guérin) vac-
    cine
bead chain cystography
beading
Belfield
    operation

Bell
    muscle
Bellini
    ducts
    ligaments
    tubules
Bence Jones
    albumin
    albumosuria
    cylinders
    globulin
    protein
    protein method
    proteinuria
    urine
bend
    iliac b. of ureter
Benedict and Franke method
Benedict and Osterberg method
Bengt-Johanson repair
Bennett
    operation
Bergenhem
    operation
Berger
    See also *Buerger.*
    disease
    focal glomerulonephritis
Bergman sign
Bertin
    column
Bertrand method
beta
    b.-aminoisobutyricaciduria
    b.-galactosidase
Bevan
    operation
Bevan-Rochet
    operation
Bigelow
    litholapaxy
    operation
bilateral
    b. lithotomy
bilharzial
biliuria
biomodulation

biopsy
>   brush b.
>   fine-needle aspiration b.
>   renal b.
>   transperineal b.
>   transrectal b.
>   transurethral b.

Bittorf reaction

Björk-Shiley
>   heart valve

bladder
>   atonic b.
>   autonomic b.
>   dome of b.
>   encysted b.
>   fasciculated b.
>   hypertonic b.
>   hypotonic b.
>   ileocecal b.
>   irritable b.
>   nervous b.
>   neurogenic b.
>   sacculated b.
>   stammering b.
>   trabeculated b.
>   transurethral resection of b.
>   (TURB)
>   urinary b.

blennuria

Boari
>   operation

body (bodies)
>   compressible cavernous b.
>   b. of epididymis
>   falciform b.
>   b. of Highmore
>   juxtaglomerular b.
>   malpighian b.'s of kidney
>   penile b.
>   b. of pubis
>   Savage perineal b.
>   wolffian b.

Boettcher. See *Böttcher.*

boggy
>   b. prostate

"boo-shahr(z)" Phonetic for
>   Bouchard.

"boo-ton-year" Phonetic for bouton-
>   nière.

"boo-zhe" Phonetic for bougie.

Böttcher (Boettcher)
>   crystals

Bottini
>   operation

Bouchard
>   coefficient

boutonnière

Bowen
>   disease

Bowman
>   capsule
>   disks
>   space
>   theory

BPH—benign prostatic hyperplasia
>   benign prostatic hypertrophy

brachytherapy
>   interstitial b.
>   intracavitary application b.
>   remote afterloading b.

Brackin
>   ureterointestinal anastomosis
>   technique

bradyspermatism

bradyuria

branched-chain α-keto acid dehy-
>   drogenase [alpha-]

Brescia-Cimino fistula

Brewer
>   infarcts
>   point

Bricker
>   operation

bridle

Bright
>   disease

brightic

brightism

Brödel white line

"broo-ee" Phonetic for bruit.

Browne
>   operation

bruit
>   See in *Cardiology* and *Pul-
>   monary Medicine* sections.*

Brunn (von Brunn)
    epithelial nests
    nests
brush
    b. biopsy
"brwe" Phonetic for bruit.
BT—bladder tumor
bubo
    chancroidal b.
    Frei b.
    gonorrheal b.
    indolent b.
    nonvenereal b.
    pestilential b.
    strumous b.
    venereal b.
Buck
    fascia
Buerhenne
    stone basket technique
bulb
    b. of corpus cavernosum
bulbitis
bulbocavernosus
bulbourethral
bulbus
    b. penis
    b. urethrae
BUN—blood urea nitrogen
Burnett
    syndrome
Burow
    vein
Buschke-Löwenstein tumor
butterfly
    b. rash
button
    Biskra b.
Bywaters
    syndrome
Cacchi-Ricci
    syndrome
cachexia
    urinary c.
cadaveric
calculi (plural of calculus)
calculosis
calculous [adj.]

calculus (calculi)
    alternating c.
    branched c.
    calcareous renal c.
    coral c.
    cystic c.
    cystine c.
    decubitus c.
    dendritic c.
    encysted c.
    fibrin c.
    gonecystic c.
    hemp seed c.
    indigo c.
    matrix c.
    mulberry c.
    nephritic c.
    noncalcareous renal c.
    oxalate c.
    prostatic c.
    renal c.
    salivary c.
    spermatic c.
    staghorn c.
    struvite c.
    urate c.
    ureteral c.
    urethral c.
    uric acid c.
    urinary c.
    urostealith c.
    vesical c.
    vesicoprostatic c.
    xanthic c.
caliber
calibrate
calibration
calibrator
caliceal
calicectasis
calicectomy
calicine
caliectasis
calix (calices)
    major calices
    minor calices
    calices renales majores
    calices renales minores

Calmette
    vaccine
Camey
    ileocystoplasty
Campbell
    procedure
Camper
    angle
    chiasm
    fascia
    ligament
    plane
canal
    vesicourethral c.
canaliculus (canaliculi)
    apical c.
cancer
    See also *carcinoma.*
    See also in *Oncology and*
      Hematology section.
    testicular c.
cannulate
cannulation, cannulization [intro-
  duction of a cannula]
CAPD—continuous ambulatory
  peritoneal dialysis
capillarectasia
capillaritis
capillaropathy
capillary (capillaries)
    peritubular c.
capistration
capita (plural of caput)
capsula (capsulae)
    c. adiposa renis
    c. fibrosa renis
    c. glomeruli
capsular
capsulation
capsule
    adipose c.
    Bowman c.
    fibrous c. of corpora caver-
      nosa penis
    Gerota c.
    glomerular c.
    c. of glomerulus
    müllerian c.

capsule (continued)
    pelvioprostatic c.
    perinephric c.
    suprarenal c.
capsulectomy
capsuloma
capsuloplasty
capsulorrhaphy
capsulotomy
caput (capita)
    c. gallinaginis
carbohydraturia
carbonuria
carbunculoid
Carcassonne
    ligament
    perineal ligament
carcinoembryonic antigen (CEA)
carcinoma (carcinomas, carcinomata)
    See also *cancer.*
    See also in *Oncology and*
      Hematology section.
    embryonal c.
    embryonal c. of testis
    epibulbar c.
    granular cell c.
    c. in situ
    renal cell c.
    c. scroti
    seminal c.
    squamous cell c.
    transitional cell c.
    verrucous c.
carnosinuria
caruncle
    morgagnian c.
    urethral c.
caruncular
cast
    blood c.
    epithelial c.
    fat c.
    granular c.
    wax c., waxy c.
castrate
castration
    radiologic c.
catecholaminergic

catecholamines
Cathelin segregator
catheterization
    retrourethral c.
    suprapubic c.
catheterize
cauda (caudae)
    c. epididymidis
cava (plural of cavum)
CAVH—continuous arteriovenous
    hemofiltration
cavography
cavum (cava)
    c. pelvis
    c. retzii
    c. vesicouterinum
CBI—continuous bladder irrigation
CC, C_{cr}—creatinine clearance
CCPD—continuous cycled peri-
    toneal dialysis
C_{cr}, CC—creatinine clearance
C&D—cystoscopy and dilatation
cecal
    c. cystoplasty
Cecil
    operation
    repair
cecocystoplasty
cell
    See also in *Laboratory,*
      Pathology, and Chemistry
      Terms.
    Leydig c.
    renal c.
    Sertoli c.
    signet c.
    suppressor c.
cellule
centrilobular
ceramidase deficiency
cervicalgia
cervicalis
cervicectomy
cervices (plural of cervix)
cervicitis
cervicocolpitis
cervicodynia
cervicoplasty

cervicovaginal
cervicovaginitis
cervicovesical
cervix (cervices)
CG—chronic glomerulonephritis
CGN—chronic glomerulonephritis
chain
    c. cystourethrography
challenge
    fluid c.
chancre
    Nisbet c.
chancroid
chancroidal
chancrous
chemolysis
cholecystopyelostomy
chondroitinuria
chondrosarcoma
chondrosarcomatosis
chondrosarcomatous
chorda (chordae)
    c. gubernaculum
    c. spermatica
chordal
chordee
chorditis
choriocarcinoma
chorioepithelioma
chromaffinoma
chromosomal
    c. markers
chromoureteroscopy
chylocele
    parasitic c.
chyloderma
chyluria
cin–. See also words beginning
    sin–, syn–.
cinefluorography
cineurography
circuitous
circumcise
circumferential
Civiale
    operation
CIXU—constant infusion excretory
    urogram

Cl—chloride
Clark
    operation
classification
    Jewett c. of bladder carcinoma (stages 0, A–D)
    Jewett and Strong c. of bladder carcinoma (stages 0, A–D)
    Marshall-Jewett-Strong c.
clean-catch urine specimen
cloaca (cloacae)
    congenital c.
    persistent c.
cloacal
CMGN—chronic membranous glomerulonephritis
coarse
    c. gravel
    c. material
cocarcinogen
Cock
    operation
colic
    renal c.
colicky pain
colicystopyelitis
colitis (colitides)
    uremic c.
colla (plural of collum)
collecting
    c. system
    c. tubes
Colles fascia
colliculectomy
colliculi (plural of colliculus)
colliculitis
colliculus (colliculi)
    bulbar c.
    seminal c.
    c. seminalis
collum (colla)
    c. glandis penis
    c. vesicae felleae
colony count
colovesical
    c. fistula
colpocystourethropexy

column
    Bertin c.
    c. of Sertoli
columna (columnae)
    columnae bertini
    columnae renales
competent
    c. bladder
computed
    c. tomography (CT)
computerized
    c. axial tomography (CAT)
concrement
condyloma (condylomata)
    flat c.
    giant c.
    c. latum, condylomata lata
    pointed c.
condylomatosis
congestion
    renal c.
continence
continent
"coo-day" Phonetic for coudé.
Cooke-Apert-Gallais syndrome
cooler
    Eissner prostatic c.
Cooper
    fascia
    irritable testis
copulation
copulatory
Corbus
    disease
cord
    genital c.
    gubernacular c.
    nephrogenic c.
    spermatic c.
corditis
corona (coronae)
    c. glandis penis
    c. of glans penis
coronal
corporis (genitive of corpus)
corpus (corpora)
    corpora amylacea
    corpora cavernosa

corpus (corpora) (continued)
    c. epididymidis
    c. Highmore
    c. penis
    c. spongiosum penis
    c. Wolffi
cortex (cortices)
    aberrant suprarenal c.
    adrenal c.
    fetal adrenal c.
    c. glandulae suprarenalis
    renal c.
      c. renis
cortiadrenal
cortices (plural of cortex)
corticis (genitive of cortex)
Cortrosyn stimulation test [trademark for cosyntropin]
costovertebral
    c. angle (CVA)
    c. angle tenderness (CVAT)
cosyntropin stimulation test
counterirritation
Cowper gland
CP—chronic pyelonephritis
CPD—congenital polycystic disease
CPN—chronic pyelonephritis
crab louse
CRD—chronic renal disease
Creevy
    evacuator
cremaster
    internal c. of Henle
CRF—chronic renal failure
CRI—chronic renal insufficiency
crisis (crises)
    Dietl c.
crista (cristae)
    c. urethralis masculinae
    c. urethralis virilis
cristal
cristate
crossover, cross-over
    c. vasectomy
crura (plural of crus)
cruris (genitive of crus)
crus (crura)
    c. penis

cryogenic
cryopreservation
crypt
    c.'s of Haller
    c.'s of Littre
    c. of Morgagni
cryptorchid
cryptorchidectomy
cryptorchidism
cryptorchidopexy
crystalloid
crystalluridrosis
CUG—cystourethrogram
Culp
    ureteropelvioplasty
Culp-DeWeerd
    ureteropelvioplasty
cuneiform
cunnilingus
cutaneous
    c. ureterostomy
    c. vesicostomy
CVA—costovertebral angle
CVAT—costovertebral angle tenderness
CVRD—cardiovascular renal disease
CVS—clean-voided specimen
cylinders
    Bence Jones c.
cylindruria
Cys-Cys—cystine
cyst
    adrenal c.
    dermoid c.
    epidermoid c.
    medullary c.
    pyelogenic c.
    renal c.
    retroperitoneal c.
    testicular c.
    wolffian c.
cystalgia
cystathionine γ-lyase [gamma-]
cystatrophia
cystauchenitis
cystauxe
cystectasia
cystectasy

cystectomy
cysteine
cystelcosis
cystendesis
cysterethism
cysthypersarcosis
cystidoceliotomy
cystidotrachelotomy
cystistaxis
cystitis
    allergic c.
    amicrobic c.
    bacterial c.
    catarrhal c.
    chemical c.
    c. colli
    croupous c.
    cystic c.
    c. cystica
    diphtheritic c.
    c. emphysematosa
    eosinophilic c.
    exfoliative c.
    c. follicularis
    gangrenous c.
    glandular c.
    c. glandularis
    hemorrhagic c.
    incrusted c.
    interstitial c.
    mechanical c.
    panmural c.
    papillary c.
    c. papillomatosa
    c. senilis feminarum
    subacute c.
    submucous c.
cysto—cystoscopy
cystocele
cystochrome
cystochromoscopy
cystocolostomy
cystodynia
cystoenterocele
cystoepiplocele
cystoepithelioma
cystofibroma

cystogram
    air c.
    excretory c.
    gravity c.
    postvoiding c.
    voiding c.
cystography
    bead chain c.
    radionuclide c.
    retrograde c.
    triple-voiding c.
cystolith
cystolithectomy
cystolithiasis
cystolithic
cystolithotomy
cystometer
    Lewis c.
cystometric
cystometrogram
cystometrography
cystometry
    flow c.
cystonephrosis
cystoneuralgia
cystoparalysis
cystopexy
cystophotography
cystophthisis
cystoplasty
    cecal c.
cystoplegia
cystoproctostomy
cystoprostatectomy
cystoptosis
cystopyelitis
cystopyelogram
cystopyelography
cystopyelonephritis
cystoradiography
cystorectocele
cystorectostomy
cystorrhagia
cystorrhaphy
cystorrhea
cystosarcoma
    c. phyllodes
cystoschisis

cystoscirrhus
cystosclerosis
cystoscopic
    c. urography
cystoscopy
    c. and dilatation (C&D)
cystospasm
cystospermitis
cystostaxis
cystostomy
cystotomy
    suprapubic c.
cystotrachelotomy
cystoureteritis
cystoureterocele
cystoureterogram
cystoureterography
cystoureteropyelitis
cystoureteropyelonephritis
cystourethrectomy
cystourethritis
cystourethrocele
cystourethrogram
cystourethrography
    chain c.
    expression c.
    isotope voiding c. (IVCU)
    micturating c.
    micturition c.
    radionuclide voiding c.
    retrograde c.
    voiding c. (VCUG)
cystourethropexy
cystous
cytometry
    flow c.
cytophilic
cytophotometry
Danubian endemic familial
    nephropathy
dartoic
dartoid
dartos
Daseler zone
Davat
    operation
Davis
    sound

Debré-de Toni-Fanconi
    syndrome
debris
    clots and d.
    purulent d.
    stonelike d.
decapsulation
decortication
    renal d.
deferentectomy
Defer method
del Castillo syndrome
delta
    d.-aminolevulinic acid (ALA)
demasculinization
Deming
    operation
Demme method
Denis Browne
    operation
    technique
Denonvilliers
    aponeurosis
    fascia
descending
    d. urography
descensus
    d. testis
de Toni-Debré-Fanconi
    syndrome
de Toni-Fanconi
    syndrome
de Toni-Fanconi-Debré
    syndrome
detrusor
    d. urinae
diabetes
    d. insipidus
    d. mellitus
dialysance
dialysate
dialysis
    peritoneal d.
    renal d.
dialyze, dialyzed
dialyzer
diaphragm
    urogenital d.

Dietl crisis
"diff" Slang for differential.
differential
dis–. See also words beginning dys–.
discrete
    d. masses
    d. narrowing
    d. nodule
    d. organ enlargement
disease
    See also *syndrome.*
    Addison d.
    anti–glomerular basement
      membrane (anti-GBM)
      antibody d.
    Bowen d.
    Bright d.
    Corbus d.
    Ducrey d.
    Durand-Nicholas-Favre d.
    Ebstein d.
    end-stage renal d. (ESRD)
    extramammary Paget d.
    Fournier d.
    Harley d.
    Hartnup d.
    Hodgkin d.
    hypertensive renal d.
    Klebs d.
    Kyrle d.
    Lignac d.
    Lignac-Fanconi d.
    Marion d.
    medullary cystic d.
    Munk d.
    Paget d.
    Paget d. of penis
    Peyronie d.
    polycystic d.
    Potter d.
    Reiter d.
    renal artery d.
    renal cystic d.
    Stühmer (Stuehmer) d.
    Wilkins d.
dislodger
    stone d.

Dittel
    operation
    sound
diuresis (diureses)
    alcohol d.
    osmotic d.
    tubular d.
    water d.
diuretic
    d. effect
diuretics [a class of drugs]
    hydragogue d.
    loop d.
    osmotic d.
    potassium-sparing d.
    refrigerant d.
diuria
diversion
    ileal conduit d.
    ileocecal cutaneous d.
    jejunal cutaneous urinary d.
    Leadbetter ileal loop d.
diverticula (plural of diverticulum)
diverticulae [incorrect spelling/pro-
    nunciation of diverticula]
diverticular
diverticulectomy
    vesical d.
diverticuli [incorrect spelling/pro-
    nunciation of diverticula]
diverticulum (diverticula)
    d. ampullae ductus deferentis
    bladder d.
    calyceal d.
    ureteric d.
    urethral d.
    vesical d.
DLE—disseminated lupus erythe-
    matosus
Doppler
    operation
dorsa (plural of dorsum)
dorsi (genitive of dorsum)
dorsum (dorsa)
    d. penis, d. of penis
    d. of testis
Douglas
    pouch

Doyen
    operation
dressing
    See also in *General Surgical
      Terms.*
dribbling
drip
    d. infusion pyelography
    d. infusion urography
    d. pyelography
Ducrey
    disease
duct
    Bellini d.
    ejaculatory d.
    Leydig d.
    mesonephric d.
    d. of Wolff
    wolffian d.
ductal
ductulus (ductuli)
    d. aberrans superior
    ductuli aberrantes
    ductuli prostatica
ductus (ductus)
    d. aberrans
    d. deferens
    d. ejaculatorius
    d. epididymidis
    d. excretorius glandulae bul-
      bourethrales
    d. excretorius vesiculae sem-
      inalis
    d. glandulae bulbourethralis
    d. mesonephricus
    d. Muelleri
    d. paraurethrales
    d. prostatica
    d. spermaticus
    d. wolffi
Duplay
    operation
Dupuytren
    hydrocele
Durand-Nicholas-Favre
    disease
dynamoscopy
dys–. See also words beginning dis–.

dysgenesis
    gonadal d.
dysgenitalism
dysgonesis
dystrophy
    oculocerebrorenal d.
dysuresia
dysuria
    psychic d.
    spastic d.
dysuriac
dysuric
dyszoospermia
Ebstein
    disease
ectopia
    e. testis
    e. vesicae
Edebohls
    operation
    position
edema
    nephritic e.
effect [noun: result, outcome]
    See *phenomenon, reaction,
      reflex, sign,* and *test.*
    diuretic e.
    estrogen e., estrogenic e.
efferent
efflux
    e. of clear urine
Eissner prostatic cooler
ejaculate
ejaculatio
    e. deficiens
    e. praecox
    e. retardata
ejaculation
    premature e.
ejaculum
electrocystography
electrode
    ball-tip e.
    bayonet-tip e.
    Bugbee e.
    Collings e.
    conical-tip e.
    Hamm e.

electrode (continued)
    McCarthy e.
    Neil-Moore e.
electrodialysis
electrodialyzer
electroendosmosis
electrolithotrity
electromyography (EMG)
    ureteral e.
electroureterogram
electroureterography
elephantiasis
    e. scroti
elimination
    pyelography by e.
Ellik evacuator
emasculate
emasculation
embolism
embolus (emboli)
    renal cholesterol e.
embryonal
emission
endometrioid
endometriosis
    e. vesicae
endopelvic
endothelia (plural of endothelium)
endothelialization
endothelium (endothelia)
endourethral
end-stage renal disease (ESRD)
enorchia
enterovesical
    e. fistula
enucleator
    Young e.
enuresis [urinary incontinence, bed-
    wetting]
    diurnal e.
    nocturnal e.
enuretic
enzyme
    degradative e.
epicystitis
epicystotomy
epididymal
epididymectomy

epididymis
epididymitis
    spermatogenic e.
epididymodeferentectomy
epididymodeferential
epididymography
epididymo-orchitis
epididymotomy
epididymovasectomy
epididymovasostomy
epididymovesiculography
epinephrectomy
epinephritis
epinephroma
epinephros
epispadiac
epispadial
epispadias
    balanitic e.
    penile e.
    penopubic e.
epistaxis
    Gull renal e.
epithelia (plural of epithelium)
epitheliitis
epithelium (epithelia)
    surface e.
    visceral e.
EPL—extracorporeal piezoelectric
    lithotriptor
Epstein
    disease
    nephrosis
    syndrome
ER—estrogen receptor
ERA—estrogen receptor assay
erectile
erection
erythematosus
    disseminated lupus e. (DLE)
erythrocyturia
erythroplasia
    e. of Queyrat
    Zoon e.
Esbach method
estrogen
    e. effect

ESWL—extracorporeal shock wave
    lithotripsy
EU—excretory urogram
evacuator
    Creevy e.
    Ellik e.
    McCarthy e.
    Toomey e.
Everett-TeLinde
    operation
excavatio (excavationes)
    e. rectovesicalis
    e. vesicouterina
excavation
    rectovesical e.
    vesicouterine e.
excretion
    e. pyelography
    e. urography
excretory
    e. cystogram
    e. urogram
    e. urography
exercise
    Kegel e.'s
exophytic
expression
    e. cystourethrography
exstrophy
    e. of bladder
external
    e. urethrotomy
extracorporeal shock wave lithotrip-
    sy (ESWL)
extragonadal
extramammary Paget disease
extravasation
    pyelosinus e.
extremitas (extremitates)
extremity
    inferior e. of kidney
    inferior e. of testis
    superior e. of kidney
    superior e. of testis
exudative
"fal–" Phonetic for words beginning
    phal–.

fallopian
    f. arch
Fanconi
    syndrome
Fanconi-Albertini-Zellweger syn-
    drome
fascia (fasciae)
    Buck f.
    Camper f.
    cervical visceral f.
    Colles f.
    cremasteric f.
    f. cremasterica
    dartos f. of scrotum
    deep cervical f.
    deep f. of penis
    Denonvilliers f.
    Gerota f.
    inferior f.
    investing f.
    f. lata, fasciae latae
    f. penis profunda
    f. penis superficialis
    perirenal f.
    f. propria cooperi
    f. of prostate
    pubic f.
    pubovesicocervical f.
    rectovesical f.
    renal f.
    f. renalis
    Scarpa f.
    f. spermatica externa
    f. spermatica interna
    spermatic f., external
    spermatic f., internal
    subserous f.
    superficial f. of urogenital
        trigone
    f. transversalis
    f. of urogenital trigone
Feleki instrument
feminization
    testicular f.
feminize, feminizing
femoral
    f. triangle

"fenil–" Phonetic for words beginning phenyl–.
"fenomenon" Phonetic for phenomenon.
Fenwick-Hunner ulcer
"feo–" Phonetic for words beginning pheo–.
Ferrein
    tubes
    tubules
fetoprotein
α-fetoprotein (AFP) [alpha-]
fetoprotein
    α-f. [alpha-]
"fi–" Phonetic for words beginning
phi–.
fibroma
    f. of testis
fibromatogenic
fibromatoid
fibromatosis
fibromatous
fibromectomy
fibrosis
    retroperitoneal f.
Fiessinger-Leroy-Reiter
    syndrome
filling defect
filtrate
filtration
fine-needle
    f-n. aspiration biopsy
Fishberg method
fistula (fistulas, fistulae)
    Brescia-Cimino f.
    congenital urethrorectal f.
    enterovesical f.
    radiocephalic f.
    urinary f.
    uterovesical f.
    vesicoabdominal f.
    vesicocolonic f.
    vesicointestinal f.
    vesicorectal f.
    vesicoumbilical f.
    vesicovaginal f.
fistulization

FJN—familial juvenile nephroph-
thisis
"flegmon" Phonetic for phlegmon.
fluctuation
fluid
    See also *liquor.*
    seminal f.
    straw-colored f.
fluoresceinuria
"foke-mahn" Phonetic for Volkmann.
Foley
    ureteropelvioplasty
    Y-plasty
    Y-type ureteropelvioplasty
    Y-V ureteropelvioplasty
Folin
    filtrate
    gravimetric method
    method
Folin and Bell
    method
Folin, Benedict, and Myers
    method
Folin and Berglund
    method
Folin and Denis
    method
Folin and Farmer
    method
Folin and Flander
    method
Folin and Hart
    method
Folin and Macallum
    method
Folin, McEllroy, and Peck
    method
Folin and Wright
    method
Folin and Youngburg
    method
Follmann balanitis
foreskin
    redundant f.
Formad kidney
formula
    Van Slyke f.
Foroblique

fossa (fossae)
    intrabulbar f.
    f. ischioanalis
    lateral f. of preputial space
    f. of male urethra
    f. of Morgagni navicular
    f. navicularis urethrae
    f. ovalis
    paravesical f.
    f. subinguinalis
Fournier
    disease
    gangrene
    sign
    syphiloma
Franco
    operation
Frank
    operation
frena (plural of frenum)
frenal
frenectomy
frenoplasty
frenulum (frenula)
    See also *band.*
    f. of prepuce of penis
    f. preputii penis
frenum (frena)
    See *band* and *frenulum.*
frequency
Freyer
    operation
friable
Fröhlich (Froehlich)
    syndrome
frond
fulguration
Fuller
    operation
functional
    f. anastomosis
fundic
fundiform
fundus (fundus)
    f. of bladder
    f. of urinary bladder
    f. vesicae urinariae

fungating
    f. growth
fungus (fungi)
    See also specific fungi in
       Laboratory, Pathology,
       and Chemistry Terms.
    f. testis
funicular
funiculate
funiculi (genitive and plural of
    funiculus)
funiculitis
funiculoepididymitis
funiculopexy
funiculus (funiculi)
    f. spermaticus
galactoma
α-galactosidase A [alpha-]
β-galactosidase [beta-]
galactosuria
galacturia
gamete
gametic
gametocidal
gametocide
gametocyst
ganglioneuroblastoma
Gasser
    syndrome
GBM—glomerular basement mem-
    brane
GC—gonococcus
    granular cast
genitalia [grammatically plural; no
    singular form]
genitocrural
genitofemoral
genitoinfectious
genitoplasty
genitorectal
Gerhardt
    test for urobilin in urine
germinomatous
Gerota
    capsule
    fascia
    method
GFR—glomerular filtration rate

Gibbon
  hydrocele
Gilbert-Behçet
  syndrome
Gilbert-Dreyfus
  syndrome
Giraldes
  organ
gland
  adrenal g.
  Albarran g.
  bulbourethral g.
  Cowper g.
  Home g.
  Littre g.
  mucous g. of urethra
  paraurethral g.
  preputial g.
  prostate g.
  Skene g.
  suprarenal g.
  urethral g.'s of male urethra
glandula (glandulae)
glandular
  g. cystitis
  g. metaplasia
glandule
glandulous [adj.]
glans
  g. penis
Gleason
  grading score
  score on prostate carcinoma
gleet
Glenn
  technique
glischruria
globi (plural of globus)
globulinuria
globus (globi)
  g. major epididymidis
  g. minor epididymidis
glomerular
  g. insufficiency
  g. proteinuria
  g. sclerosis
glomeruli (plural of glomerulus)
glomerulocapillary

glomerulonephritis
  anti–glomerular basement
    membrane (anti-GBM)
    antibody g.
glomerulonephropathy
glomerulopathy
glomerulosclerosis
glomerulose
glomerulus (glomeruli)
  malpighian glomeruli
  renal glomeruli, glomeruli
    renis
  Ruysch glomeruli
GN—glomerulonephritis
Goldblatt
  hypertension
  kidney
  phenomenon
gonad
gonadal
gonadectomize
gonadectomy
gonadial
gonadoblastic
gonadopathy
gonadotherapy
gonadotropism
gonaduct
gonangiectomy
gonecyst
gonecystis
gonecystitis
gonecystolith
gonecystopyosis
gonocele
gonococci
gononephrotome
gonophore
gonorrhea
Goodpasture
  syndrome
Gordon
  syndrome
gorget
  Teale g.
Gorlin-Chaudhry-Moss
  syndrome

graft
    Thiersch g.
granuloma
    g. inguinale
granulomatous
    g. prostatitis
granulosa
    g.-theca cell tumor
gravity
    specific g.
Grawitz
    cachexia
    tumor
GU—genitourinary
    gonococcal urethritis
gubernacula (plural of gubernaculum)
gubernacular
gubernaculum (gubernacula)
    chorda g.
    Hunter g.
    g. testis
Gull
    renal epistaxis
GUS—genitourinary system
Guyon
    sign
    sound
gynandroblastoma
gynoblastoma
Hagner
    operation
Hallé
    point
hamartoma
    renal h.
hanging
    h. panniculus
Harley disease
Hartnup
    disease
    syndrome
Heintz method
Heitz-Boyer procedure
Heller-Nelson
    syndrome
hematocele
    scrotal h.

hematoma
    perinephric h.
hematonephrosis
hematoscheocele
hematospermatocele
hematospermia
hematuria
    angioneurotic h.
    endemic h.
    essential h.
    microscopic h.
    renal h.
    urethral h.
    vesical h.
hemaurochrome
hemihypertrophy
heminephrectomy
heminephroureterectomy
hemipyonephrosis
hemiscrotectomy
hemispherium (hemispheria)
    h. bulbi urethrae
hemodialysis
    sequential ultrafiltration h.
    simultaneous h. and
        hemofiltration
hemofiltration
    simultaneous hemodialysis
        and h.
hemoglobinuria
    intermittent h.
hemorrhage
    glomerular h.
hemorrhagic
    h. cystitis
hemospermia
Hendrickson lithotrite
Henle
    ampulla
    internal cremaster
    loop
    sphincter
    tubules
hermaphrodism
hermaphrodite
hermaphroditic
hermaphroditism
hermaphroditismus

hernia
   parastomal h.
herpes
   genital h.
   h. praeputialis
   h. progenitalis
Hess
   operation
Hesselbach
   triangle
Heyd syndrome
high
   h. lithotomy
Highmore
   body
   corpus
hilum (hila)
   h. of adrenal gland
   h. glandulae suprarenalis
   h. of kidney
   renal h.
   h. renale
   h. renalis
   h. of suprarenal gland
hilus (hili). See *hilum.*
hind-kidney
Hinman reflux
"hipo–" Phonetic for words beginning hypo–.
Hippel-Lindau. See *von Hippel-Lindau.*
Hodgkin
   disease
Home
   gland
   lobe
homotransplant
horseshoe
Houston
   muscle
Huggins
   operation
Hughes reflex
Hunner
   stricture
   ulcer
Hunter
   gubernaculum

hunterian
   h. chancre
hydatid
   h. of Morgagni
   sessile h.
hydatidocele
hydatiduria
hydrocele
   bilocular h.
   chylous h.
   communicating h.
   Dupuytren h.
   encysted h.
   funicular h.
   Gibbon h.
   Maunoir h.
   noncommunicating h.
   scrotal h.
   spermatic h.
   h. of testis
hydrocelectomy
hydrohematonephrosis
hydronephrosis
hydronephrotic
hydroperinephrosis
hydropigenous
hydropyonephrosis
hydrosarcocele
hydroscheocele
hydrostatic
hydroureter
hydroureteronephrosis
hydroureterosis
hydrouria
hyperacidaminuria
hyperallantoinuria
hyperammonuria
hyperandrogenism
hyperazotemia
hyperazoturia
hypercalciuria
   absorptive h.
   idiopathic h.
   renal h.
   resorptive h.
   secondary h.
hyperdiuresis
hypereccrisia

hypereccritic
hyperechoic
hyperexcretory
hyperfiltration
hypergenitalism
hypergonadism
hypergonadotropic
hypergranulation
    juxtaglomerular cell h.
hyperleydigism
hyperlithic
hyperlithuria
hypernatremia
hypernatremic
hypernephritis
hypernephroid
hypernephroma
hyperorchidism
hyperosmolality
hyperosmolarity
hyperosmotic
hyperoxaluria
    enteric h.
    primary h. (type I, type II)
    secondary h.
hyperpipecolatemia
hyperplasia
    adrenal cortical h., adreno-
      cortical h.
    benign prostatic h. (BPH)
    congenital adrenal h. (CAH)
    congenital adrenocortical h.
    cystic prostatic h.
    Leydig cell h.
    lipoid adrenal h.
    nodular adrenal h.
    nodular adrenocortical h.
hyperplastic
    h. polyp
hyperposia
hyperreninemia
hyperreninemic
hypersthenuria
hypersuprarenalism
hypertension
    adrenal h.
    essential h.
    Goldblatt h.

hypertension (continued)
    renal h.
    secondary h.
hypertensive
    h. renal disease
hypertestosteronism
hypertrophy
    benign prostatic h. (BPH)
    prostatic h.
hyperuresis
hyperuricemia
hyperuricemic
hyperuricuria
hypoadrenocorticism
    pituitary h.
    secondary h.
hypoaldosteronemia
hypoaldosteronism
    hyporeninemic h.
    isolated h.
hypoaldosteronuria
hypoandrogenism
hypocalcinuria
hypoeccrisia
hypoeccritic
hypogenitalism
hypogonadal
hypogonadism
    familial hypogonadotropic h.
    pituitary h.
    h. with anosmia
hypogonadotropic
hypoleydigism
hyponatremia
hyponatremic
hyponatruria
hypo-orchidism
hypo-osmolality
hypoperfusion
hypophosphatasia
hypophosphatemia
    hereditary h.
    renal h.
    X-linked h.
hypophosphatemic
hypophosphaturia
hypoplasia
    oligonephronic h.

hypospadiac
hypospadias
 balanic h., balanitic h.
 glandular h.
 penile h.
 penoscrotal h.
 perineal h.
 pseudovaginal h.
hypostasis
hypostatic
hyposuprarenalism
hypothalamic
 h. suppression
hypotonia
hypotonic
hypouremia
hypouresis
hypouricuria
hypourocrinia
hysterocystic
hysterocystocleisis
hysterocystopexy
IADH—inappropriate antidiuretic
 hormone
ileal [pertaining to ileum (bowel)]
 i. conduit diversion
ileocecal
 i. cutaneous diversion
ileocystoplasty
 Camey i.
 LeDuc-Camey i.
ileocystostomy
iliac [hip bone]
iliocostal
iliohypogastric
ilioinguinal
imaging
 See in *Radiology, Nuclear*
 Medicine, and Other
 Imaging section.
immunohistochemistry
immunosuppressants [a class of
 drugs]
immunosurveillance
immunotherapy
implant
 Silastic i.

implantation
 radioactive isotope i.
impotence
 functional i.
 organic i.
 orgastic i.
 paretic i.
 psychic i.
 secondary i.
 symptomatic i.
impotentia
 i. coeundi
 i. erigendi
incision
 pyelotomy i.
inclusion
incontinence
 overflow i.
 paradoxical i.
 paralytic i.
 stress i.
 urinary i.
 i. of urine
incontinent
incontinentia
 i. urinae
indoxyl
indoxyluria
induration
 penile i.
infarct
 bilirubin i
 Brewer i.
 uric acid i.
infarction
 renal i.
infection
 urinary tract i. (UTI)
inferior vena cava (IVC)
infiltrating
infrarenal
infravesical
infundibula (plural of infundibulum)
infundibuliform
infundibulopelvic
infundibulum (infundibula)
 i. of kidney
 i. of urinary bladder

infusion
> drip i. pyelography
> i. nephrotomography
> i. pyelography

inguinoscrotal

inoperable

insertion
> cystoradium i.

insipidus
> diabetes i.

instrument
> Feleki i.

insufficiency
> capsular i.
> renal i.

integument

intercourse

interlobar

interlobular

internal
> i. urethrotomy

interposition
> i. operation

interureteral

interureteric

intrarenal

intratesticular

intratubular

intraureteral

intraurethral

intravenous
> i. pyelography (IVP)
> i. urography (IVU)

intravesical

intumescence

intumescent

inversion
> i. of bladder

involution

I&O—intake and output

Isaacs-Ludwig arteriole

ischemia
> renal i.

ischiopubic

island
> Wolff i.

"is-mus" Phonetic for isthmus.

isotope
> i. nephrography
> i. voiding cystourethrography (IVCU)

Israel
> operation

isthmectomy

isthmi (plural of isthmus)

isthmic

isthmus (isthmi)
> i. prostatae
> i. urethrae

isuria

IV—intravenous

IVCU—isotope voiding cystourethrography

IVP—intravenous pyelogram

IVU—intravenous urography

Jaffe
> test

Jaksch (von Jaksch)
> test

jejunal
> j. cutaneous urinary diversion

Jewett
> bladder carcinoma classification
> sound

Jewett-Strong system

JG—juxtaglomerular

Johanson-Blizzard syndrome

joint
> See in *Orthopedics and Sports Medicine* section.

Joseph
> syndrome

judicious

junction
> ureteropelvic j.
> ureterovesical j.

juxtavesical

"kahk–," "kak–" Phonetic for words beginning cac–, cach–.

KB—ketone body

Kegel exercises

Kelly
> operation
> sign

Kelly-Deming
    operation
Kelly-Stoeckel
    operation
keratoderma
    k. blennorrhagica
keratosis (keratoses)
    k. blennorrhagica
α-keto acid dehydrogenase [alpha-]
ketone bodies
kidney
    amyloid k.
    arteriosclerotic k.
    artificial k.
    atrophic k.
    cake k.
    cicatricial k.
    cirrhotic k.
    coarsely granular k.
    congenital double k.
    congested k.
    contracted k.
    crush k.
    cyanotic k.
    cystic k.
    disk k.
    doughnut k.
    dump k.
    dystopic k.
    ectopic k.
    fatty k.
    finely granular k.
    flea-bitten k.
    floating k.
    Formad k.
    fused k.
    Goldblatt k.
    gouty k.
    granular k.
    hind k.
    horseshoe k.
    hypermobile k.
    hypoplastic k.
    infarcted k.
    lardaceous k.
    large red k.
    lump k.
    medullary sponge k.

kidney (continued)
    mortar k.
    multilobar k.
    mural k.
    myelin k.
    palpable k.
    pelvic k.
    polycystic k.
    primordial k.
    k. punch
    putty k.
    Rokitansky k.
    Rose-Bradford k.
    sacciform k.
    sclerotic k.
    sigmoid k.
    single k.
    soapy k.
    solitary k.
    sponge k.
    k. stone
    supernumerary k.
    unilateral fused k.
    unilobar k.
    wandering k.
    waxy k.
Kimmelstiel-Wilson
    disease
    syndrome
Klebs disease
KLS—kidneys, liver, spleen
Kocher
    maneuver
Kock
    pouch
    reservoir
"koo-day" Phonetic for coudé
"kor–" Phonetic for words begin-
    ning cor– and chor–.
Korean hemorrhagic
    nephrosonephritis
kraurosis
    penile k.
Krause
    ligament
"krus" Phonetic for crus.
KUB—kidney, ureter, bladder [x-ray]

KW—Kimmelstiel-Wilson [syndrome]
"kyl–" Phonetic for words beginning chyl–.
Kyrle
    disease
labia (plural of labium)
labial
labium (labia)
    See also *margin.*
    l. urethrae
labyrinth
    cortical l.
    Ludwig l.'s
    renal l.
    Santorini l.
lactaciduria
lacuna (lacunae)
    great l. of urethra
    l. magna
    lacunae of Morgagni
    l. of muscles
    lacunae of urethra, urethral
        lacunae
    urethral lacunae of Morgagni
lacunar
lacunula (lacunulae)
lacunule
lamina (laminae)
laminar
Lancereaux
    nephritis
laparocystectomy
laparonephrectomy
laparoscopy
Lashmet and Newburgh
    method
lateral
    l. lithotomy
    l. pyelography
Launois-Cléret
    syndrome
law
    Bell l.
layer
    submucous l. of bladder
LCM—left costal margin
LD—living donor

Leadbetter
    ileal loop diversion
    maneuver
Leadbetter-Politano
    ureterovesicoplasty
LeDuc-Camey
    ileocystoplasty
Le Fort
    sound
leiomyoma (leiomyomas, leiomyomata)
    l. of seminal vesicles
lesion
    Armanni-Ebstein l.
    Baehr-Löhlein l.
    Ebstein l.
    Kimmelstiel-Wilson l.
    local glomerular l.
    Löhlein-Baehr l.
    precancerous l.
    wire-loop l.
leukemia
    testicular l.
leukoplakia
    l. of penis
levator (levatores)
    l. ani
Lewis
    cystometer
Leydig
    cells
    duct
leydigarche
libidinal
libido (libidines)
libidogen
lice (plural of louse)
lichen
    l. planus
Lichtheim
ligament
    fallopian l.
    lateral false l.
    lateral puboprostatic l.
    medial puboprostatic l.
    middle umbilical l.
    pubic l. of Cowper
    pubovesical l.

ligament (continued)
    round l.
Lightwood
    syndrome
Lignac
    disease
    syndrome
Lignac-Fanconi
    disease
    syndrome
limbus (limbi)
Lindau-von Hippel. See *von Hippel-Lindau.*
line
    See also *band.*
    Aldrich-Mees l.'s
    Brödel white l.
    Mees l.'s
    Sergent white adrenal l.
linea (lineae)
    l. alba
    l. nigra
liquid
    See *fluid* and *liquor.*
liquor (liquors, liquores)
    See also *fluid.*
    l. prostaticus
    l. seminis
lithangiuria
lithectasy
lithiasis
lithocenosis
lithoclysmia
lithocystotomy
lithodialysis
lithokonion
litholabe
litholapaxy
litholysis
litholyte
litholytics [a class of drugs]
lithometer
lithomyl
lithonephria
lithonephritis
lithonephrotomy
lithophone

lithotomy
    bilateral l.
    high l.
    lateral l.
    marian l.
    median l.
    mediolateral l.
    perineal l.
    prerectal l.
    rectal l.
    rectovesical l.
    suprapubic l.
    vaginal l.
    vesicovaginal l.
lithotriptic
lithotriptoscopy
    extracorporeal shock wave l.
    (ESWL)
lithotrity
lithous
lithoxiduria
lithuresis
lithureteria
lithuria
Littre glands
LK—left kidney
Lloyd sign
LN—lipoid nephrosis
    lupus nephritis
lobe
    Home l.
    lateral l.'s of prostate gland
    median l. of prostate
    renal l.'s
    l.'s of prostate
lobectomy
lobi (plural of lobus)
lobulated
lobulation
lobule
    cortical l.'s of kidney
    glomerular l.
    l. of testis
lobuli (plural of lobulus)
lobulization
lobulose
lobulus (lobuli)
    lobuli testis

lobus (lobi)
Löhlein nephritis
loop
    Cordonnier ureteroileal l.
    l. diuretics [a class of drugs]
    Henle l., l. of Henle
louse (lice)
    crab l.
    pubic l.
Löwe
    disease
    syndrome
Lowsley
    lithotrite
    operation
    tractor
Luder-Sheldon syndrome
lumbar
    l. nephrectomy
lumen (lumina)
lupus
    drug-induced l.
    l. nephritis
    systemic l. erythematosus
        (SLE)
luteinizing hormone (LH)
luxation
Luy segregator
lymphogranuloma
    l. inguinale
    venereal l.
    l. venereum
lymphoma
    testicular l.
lymphopathia
    l. venereum
macrogenitosomia
macula (maculae)
    m. densa
macular
Mainz pouch urinary reservoir
Makkas
    operation
malacoplakia
    m. vesicae
Malassez
    disease

Malpighi
    pyramids
malpighian
    m. bodies
malrotation
maneuver
    See also *method* and *technique.*
    Kocher m.
    Leadbetter m.
Marchiafava-Micheli
    disease
    syndrome
margin
    See also *labium.*
    convex m. of testis
    m. of kidney, lateral
    m. of kidney, medial
margo (margines)
marian
    m. lithotomy
Marion disease
Marshall
    test
Marshall-Jewett-Strong classification
Marshall-Marchetti
    operation
Marshall-Marchetti-Birch
    operation
Marshall-Marchetti-Krantz (MMK)
    operation
Marshall and Tanner pubertal staging
marsupial
marsupium (marsupia)
Martin
    operation
Martius
    operation
Martius-Harris
    operation
Matson
    operation
Maunoir hydrocele
Mays
    operation
MB—methylene blue
MBAS—methylene blue active substance

MBD—methylene blue dye
McCarthy
    electrode
    evacuator
McGill
    operation
meatal
meati [incorrect word for plural of
    meatus]
meatoplasty
    Stacke m.
meatorrhaphy
meatoscopy
    ureteral m.
meatotomy
    ureteral m.
meatus (meatus)
    fish-mouth m.
    m. of urethra
    m. urinarius
    urinary m.
mechanism
    suspensory m.
median
    m. bar of prostate
    m. lithotomy
mediastinum (mediastina)
    m. testis
mediolateral
    m. lithotomy
medorrhea
medulla (medullae)
    adrenal m.
    m. glandulae suprarenalis
    m. of kidney
    m. nephrica
    m. renalis
    m. renis
    suprarenal m.
    m. of suprarenal gland
medullary
medullary cystic disease
medullated
medullation
medullectomy
medulliadrenal
medulloadrenal
medulloid

medullosuprarenoma
megabladder
megalocystis
megalopenis
megaloureter
megalourethra
melasma
    m. addisonii
    m. suprarenale
mellitus
    diabetes m.
membrana (membranae)
membranate
membrane
    glomerular m.
    Toldt m.
membranolysis
membranous
    m. urethra
membrum (membra)
    m. virile
Mercier
    bar
    operation
mesangium
mesenchyma
mesenchymal
mesenchymoma
    benign m.
    malignant m.
mesoblastic
mesonephric
mesonephroi (plural of mesonephros)
mesonephroma
mesonephron
mesonephros (mesonephroi)
    caudal m.
    cranial m.
    genital m.
metanephros (metanephroi)
metastasis (metastases)
method
    See also *maneuver* and *technique.*
    acid hematin m.
    Addis m.
    Arnold and Gunning m.
    Bence Jones protein m.

method (continued)
  Benedict and Franke m.
  Benedict and Osterberg m.
  Bertrand m.
  Defer m.
  Demme m.
  Esbach m.
  Fishberg m.
  Folin m.
  Folin and Bell m.
  Folin, Benedict, and Myers
    m.
  Folin and Berglund m.
  Folin and Denis m.
  Folin and Farmer m.
  Folin and Flander m.
  Folin gravimetric m.
  Folin and Hart m.
  Folin and Macallum m.
  Folin, McEllroy, and Peck m.
  Folin and Wright m.
  Folin and Youngburg m.
  Heintz m.
  Lashmet and Newburgh m.
  Naunyn-Minkowski m.
  Osborne and Folin m.
  Permutit m.
  Power and Wilder m.
  Shohl and Pedley m.
  Sjöqvist m.
  Sumner m.
  Volhard and Fahr m.
MGN—membranous glomeru-
  lonephritis
microalbuminuria
microcalculus (microcalculi)
microcalix
microgenitalism
microlith
microlithiasis
  pulmonary alveolar m.
micro-orchidism
microphallus
microrchidia
microvillus (microvilli)
miction
micturate

micturating
  m. cystourethrography
micturition
  m. cystourethrography
migration
  retrograde m.
"mik" Slang for Mikulicz.
mika operation
Miller
  syndrome
minute [small]
MM—Marshall-Marchetti
MM operation
MMK—Marshall-Marchetti-Krantz
  [operation]
molluscum
  m. contagiosum
mononephrous
monorchidic
monorchism
morcellement
  m. operation
Morgagni
  caruncle
  fossa of M.
  fovea
  hydatid
  lacunae
  sinus
Morris syndrome
"mor-sel-maw" Phonetic for morcellement.
motility
  altered sperm m.
MPGN—membranoproliferative
  glomerulonephritis
MSK—medullary sponge kidney
MT—malignant teratoma
MTI—malignant teratoma, intermediate
MTT—malignant teratoma, trophoblastic
Muckle-Wells
  syndrome
Muelleri
  ductus M.
müllerian
  m. capsule

multicentric
Munk disease
muscle
> See also in *Orthopedics and Sports Medicine* section.
> Bell m.
> Braune m.
> bulbocavernous m.
> cremaster m.
> dartos m. of scrotum
> detrusor m. of bladder
> erector m. of penis
> external oblique m.
> Guthrie m.
> Houston m.
> iliopsoas m.
> interfoveolar m.
> internal oblique m.
> interspinal m.'s of loins
> ischiocavernous m.
> Jarjavay m.
> latissimus dorsi m.
> levator ani m.
> levator m. of prostate
> oblique m. of abdomen (external, internal)
> obturator m. (external, internal)
> organic m.
> m.'s of pelvic diaphragm
> perineal m.'s, m.'s of perineum
> psoas m. (greater, smaller)
> pubicoperitoneal m.
> pubococcygeal m.
> puboprostatic m.
> puborectal m.
> pubovaginal m.
> pubovesical m.
> pyramidal m.
> rectourethral m.
> rectovesical m.
> rectus m.
> Riolan m.
> Santorini m.'s, circular
> Sebileau m.
> sphincter m. of membranous urethra

muscle (continued)
> sphincter m. of urethra
> sphincter m. of urinary bladder
> transverse m. of abdomen
> transverse perineal m. (deep, superficial)
> transverse m. of perineum (deep, superficial)
> m.'s of urogenital diaphragm
> visceral m.
> Wilson m.
musculus (musculi)
> See also *muscle.*
> See also in *Orthopedics and Sports Medicine* section.
> m. bulbocavernosus
> m. bulbospongiosus
> m. cremaster
> m. pubococcygeus
> m. puborectalis
> m. pubovesicalis
> m. rectus abdominis
> m. transversus abdominis
myelolipoma
"my-nute" Phonetic for minute [small].
myosarcoma
myxocystitis
Narath
> operation
National Prostatic Cancer Treatment Group (NPCTG)
Naunyn-Minkowski method
nebula (nebulae)
necrosis (necroses)
> acute tubular n.
> bilateral renal cortical n.
> cortical n.
> fibrinoid n.
> glomerular n.
> laminar cortical n.
> nephrotoxic tubule n.
> renal coagulation n.
> n. of renal papillae, renal papillary n.
> tubular n.
necrospermia

necrospermic
necrotic
necrozoospermia
"nefrosis" Phonetic for nephrosis.
Nélaton
    sphincter
neoadjuvant
neobladder
neocystostomy
    ureteral n.
    ureteroileal n.
neoplasm
    adrenal n.
    vascular n.
neoplastic
neostigmine
    n. methylsulfate
neostomy
neovagina
nephradenoma
nephralgia
    idiopathic n.
nephralgic
nephrapostasis
nephrasthenia
nephratonia
nephratony
nephrauxe
nephrectasia
nephrectasis
nephrectasy
nephrectomize
nephrectomy
    abdominal n.
    anterior n.
    lumbar n.
    paraperitoneal n.
    posterior n.
    radical n.
    simple n.
    transthoracic n.
nephredema
nephrelcosis
nephremia
nephremphraxis
nephria
nephric
nephridium

nephrism
nephritis (nephritides)
    acute n.
    acute focal n.
    acute interstitial n.
    acute serum sickness n.
    albuminous n.
    allergic n.
    anaphylactoid purpura n.
    anti–glomerular basement
        membrane (anti-GBM)
        antibody n.
    arteriosclerotic n.
    azotemic n.
    bacterial n.
    Balkan n.
    capsular n.
    n. caseosa, caseous n.
    catarrhal n.
    cheesy n.
    chloroazotemic n.
    chronic n.
    chronic interstitial n.
    clostridial n.
    congenital n.
    croupous n.
    degenerative n.
    desquamative n.
    diffuse n.
    diffuse suppurative n.
    n. dolorosa
    dropsical n.
    embolic n.
    epidemic n.
    exudative n.
    familial hemorrhagic n.
    fibrolipomatous n.
    fibrous n.
    focal n.
    focal embolic n.
    glomerular n.
    glomerulocapsular n.
    n. gravidarum
    hemorrhagic n.
    hereditary n.
    Heymann n.
    hydremic n.
    hydropigenous n.

nephritis (nephritides) (continued)
hypogenetic n.
idiopathic n.
indurative n.
interstitial n.
interstitial granulomatous n.
interstitial nonsuppurative n.
interstitial scarlatinal n.
interstitial syphilitic n.
Lancereaux n.
latent n.
leptospiral n.
lipomatous n.
Löhlein n.
lupus n.
Masugi n.
n. mitis
nephrotoxic serum n.
parenchymatous n.
parenchymatous n., chronic
phenacetin n.
pneumococcus n.
post-streptococcal n.
potassium-losing n.
n. of pregnancy
productive n.
radiation n.
n. repens
salt-losing n.
saturnine n.
scarlatinal n.
Schönlein-Henoch purpura n.
shunt n.
Steblay n.
subacute n.
suppurative n.
suppurative n., acute
suppurative n., chronic
suppurative cortical n.
syphilitic n.
tartrate n.
transfusion n.
trench n.
tubal n., tubular n.
tuberculous n.
tubulointerstitial n.
vascular n.
Volhard n.

nephritis (nephritides) (continued)
war n.
water-losing n.
nephritogenic
nephroabdominal
nephroangiosclerosis
nephroblastomatosis
nephrocapsectomy
nephrocardiac
nephrocele
nephrocolic
nephrocolopexy
nephrocoloptosis
nephrocystanastomosis
nephroerysipelas
nephrogastric
nephrogenic
nephrogenous
nephrography
isotope n.
nephrohemia
nephrohydrosis
nephrohypertrophy
nephroid
nephrolith
nephrolithotomy
nephrologist
nephrology
nephrolysis
nephrolytic
nephroma
embryonal n.
mesoblastic n.
nephromalacia
nephromegaly
nephron
nephroncus
nephronophthisis
familial juvenile n.
nephro-omentopexy
nephroparalysis
nephropathia
n. epidermica
nephropathic
nephropathy
acute hypokalemic n.
acute urate n.
amphotericin B n.

nephropathy (continued)
    analgesic n.
    Balkan n.
    bismuth n.
    cadmium n.
    carbon tetrachloride n.
    chronic hypokalemic n.
    chronic urate n.
    copper n.
    Danubian endemic familial n.
    diabetic n.
    dropsical n.
    epidemic n.
    familial n.
    gold n.
    gouty n.
    human immunodeficiency
       virus–associated n. [HIV-]
    hypazoturic n.
    hypercalcemic n.
    hypochloruric n.
    hypokalemic n.
    IgA n.
    iodide n.
    iron n.
    kaliopenic n.
    kanamycin n.
    lead n.
    malarial n.
    membranous n.
    mesangial n.
    obstructive n.
    oxalate n.
    phenacetin n.
    polymyxin n.
    n. of potassium depletion
    reflux n.
    salt-losing n.
    silver n.
    streptomycin n.
    sulfonamide n.
    tetracycline n.
    toxic n.
    tubular n.
    urate n.
    vascular n.
nephropexy
nephrophagiasis

nephrophthisis
nephropoietic
nephropoietin
nephroptosia
nephroptosis
nephropyelitis
nephropyelography
nephropyelolithotomy
nephropyeloplasty
nephropyosis
nephrorosein
nephrorrhagia
nephrorrhaphy
nephroscleria
nephrosclerosis
    arteriolar n.
    benign n.
    hyaline arteriolar n.
    hyperplastic arteriolar n.
    intercapillary n.
    malignant n.
    senile n.
nephrosclerotic
nephroscopy
nephrosis (nephroses)
    acute n.
    amyloid n.
    cholemic n.
    chronic n.
    congenital n.
    Epstein n.
    glycogen n.
    Haymann n.
    hydropic n.
    hypokalemic n.
    infectious avian n.
    larval n.
    lipid n.
    lipoid n.
    lower nephron n.
    mercurial n.
    necrotizing n.
    osmotic n.
    pure n.
    toxic n.
    vacuolar n.
nephrosonephritis
    hemorrhagic n.

nephrosonephritis (continued)
  Korean hemorrhagic n.
nephrosonography
nephrospasis
nephrosplenopexy
nephrostogram
nephrostolithotomy
  percutaneous n. (PCNL)
nephrotic
nephrotome
nephrotomogram
nephrotomography
  infusion n.
nephrotomy
  abdominal n.
  anatrophic n.
  lumbar n.
nephrotoxic
nephrotoxicity
nephrotoxin
nephrotresis
nephrotropic
nephrotuberculosis
nephrotyphoid
nephrotyphus
nephroureterectomy
nephroureterocystectomy
nephrourography
nephrozymase
nephrozymosis
nerve
      cavernous n.'s of penis
      dorsal n. of penis
      ilioinguinal n.
      scrotal n.'s, anterior
      scrotal n.'s, posterior
nerve block
      dorsal penile n.b. (DPNB)
nest
      Brunn n.
      von Brunn n.
net
      See *plexus* and *rete.*
network
      See *plexus* and *rete.*
neuroendocrine
neurogenic
      n. bladder

neuronephric
NGU—nongonococcal urethritis
nil
      n. disease
Nisbet
      chancre
nitrite
nitrosamine
nocturnal
      n. enuresis
      n. penile tumescence (NPT)
nodular
nodularity
nodulated
nodulation
nonfunctioning
      n. kidney
Nonnenbruch
      syndrome
nonoliguric
nonopaque
nonseminomatous
nonvisualization
Nourse
      syringe
NPCTG—National Prostatic Cancer
      Treatment Group
NPT—nocturnal penile tumescence
NSU—nonspecific urethritis
NTN—nephrotoxic nephritis
Nussbaum
      experiment
obstructive
      o. uropathy
obturator
      Alcock-Timberlake o.
      Timberlake o.
occlusion
      o. of renal artery
oligohydruria
oligonecrospermia
oligophosphaturia
oligospermatic
oligospermatism
oligozoospermatism
oligozoospermia
Ombrédanne
      operation

operation

  See also *maneuver, method,*
    procedure, surgery, and
    technique.
  Aldridge o.
  Alexander-Adams o.
  Andrews o.
  Bates o.
  Belfield o.
  Bennett o.
  Bergenhem o.
  Bevan o.
  Bevan-Rochet o.
  Bigelow o.
  Boari o.
  Bottini o.
  Bricker o.
  Browne o.
  Cecil o
  Civiale o.
  Clark o.
  Cock o.
  Davat o.
  Deming o.
  Denis Browne o.
  Dittel o.
  Doppler o.
  Doyen o.
  Duplay o.
  Edebohls o.
  Everett-TeLinde o.
  Franco o.
  Frank o.
  Freyer o.
  Fuller o.
  Hagner o.
  Hess o.
  Huggins o.
  interposition o.
  Israel o.
  Kelly o.
  Kelly-Deming o.
  Kelly-Stoeckel o.
  Lowsley o.
  Makkas o.
  Marian o.
  Marshall-Marchetti o.
  Marshall-Marchetti-Birch o.

operation (continued)
  Marshall-Marchetti-Krantz
    (MMK) o.
  Martin o.
  Martius o.
  Martius-Harris o.
  Matson o.
  Mays o.
  McGill o.
  Mercier o.
  mika o.
  morcellement o.
  Narath o.
  Ombrédanne o.
  Petersen o.
  Rigaud o.
  sling o.
  Spivack o.
  Stanischeff o.
  Steinach o.
  Torek o.
  Tuffier o.
  Turner-Warwick o.
  van Hook o.
  Vidal o.
  Vogel o.
  Volkmann o.
  Voronoff o.
  Wheelhouse o.
  White o.
  Wood o.
  Young o.
oral
  o. urography
orchialgia
orchichorea
orchidalgia
orchidectomy
orchidic
orchiditis
orchidocelioplasty
orchidoepididymectomy
orchidoncus
orchidopathy
orchidopexy
orchidoplasty
orchidoptosis
orchidorrhaphy

orchidotherapy
orchidotomy
orchiencephaloma
orchiepididymitis
orchilytic
orchiocatabasis
orchiocele
orchiococcus
orchiodynia
orchiomyeloma
orchioncus
orchioneuralgia
orchiopathy
orchiopexy
orchioplasty
orchiorrhaphy
orchioscheocele
orchioscirrhus
orchiotomy
orchis
orchitic
orchitis
    metastatic o.
    mumps o.
    o. parotidea
    spermatogenic granuloma-
       tous o.
    traumatic o.
    o. variolosa
orchitolytic
orchotomy
organ
    o. of Giraldes
orgasm
orifice
    o. of male urethra
    o. of ureter
    ureteral o.
    o. of urethra
    vesicourethral o.
orificia (plural of orificium)
orificial
orificium (orificia)
    o. urethrae externum
      muliebris
    o. urethrae externum virilis
    o. urethrae internum
"orkitis" Phonetic for orchitis.

Osborne and Folin
    method
oscheal
oscheitis
oscheocele
oscheohydrocele
oscheolith
oscheoma
oscheoncus
oscheoplasty
oscillation
osmolality
    urine o.
osmotherapy
osmotic diuretics [a class of drugs]
osteodystrophy
    azotemic o.
    renal o.
osteomalacia
    renal tubular o.
osteosarcoma
ostia (plural of ostium)
ostial [pertaining to opening, aper-
    ture, orifice]
ostium (ostia)
    o. urethrae externum femini-
      nae
    o. urethrae externum mas-
      culinae
    o. urethrae internum
ostomy. See specific procedure.
    neostomy
    ureterostomy
    vesicostomy
Otis
    sound
ovarium (ovaria)
    o. masculinum
Paget
    disease
    disease of penis
pagetoid
panendoscopy
panniculalgia
panniculus (panniculi)
    p. adiposus
    hanging p.
PAP—prostatic acid phosphatase

papilla (papillae)
 renal papillae, papillae renales
 urethral p.
papillate
papillation
papilliferous
papilliform
papillitis
 necrotizing p., necrotizing
  renal p.
papilloma
 p. of bladder
 hirsutoid p.'s of penis
 p. of renal pelvis
 squamous cell p.
 p. venereum
papule
 moist p., mucous p.
 pearly penile p.
papulosis
 bowenoid p.
para
 p.-aminohippuric acid (PAH,
  PAHA) synthetase
paradidymal
paradidymis
paragenitalis
paraglobulinuria
paralysis (paralyses)
 Brown-Séquard p.
paranephric
paranephritis
 lipomatous p.
paranephroma
paranephros
paraperitoneal
 p. nephrectomy
paraphimosis
paraprostatitis
pararenal
parasite
 See specific parasites in
  Laboratory, Pathology,
  and Chemistry Terms.
paratesticular
paraureteric [beside or near the
 ureter]
paraurethra

paraurethral
paraurethritis
paravesical
parenchyma
 p. of kidney
 p. testis
pars (partes)
particulate
pathogen
 See specific pathogens in
  Laboratory, Pathology,
  and Chemistry Terms.
pattern
 rugal p.
PBPI—penile-brachial pressure index
PCNL—percutaneous nephrostolithotomy
pelves (plural of pelvis)
pelvicaliceal, pelvicalyceal
pelvilithotomy
pelvioileoneocystostomy
pelviolithotomy
pelvioneocystostomy
pelvioneostomy
pelvioperitonitis
pelvioplasty
pelvioradiography
pelvioscopy
pelviostomy
pelviotomy
pelviperitonitis
pelviradiography
pelvirectal
pelviroentgenography
pelvis (pelves)
 See also in *Orthopedics and*
  Sports Medicine section.
 bifid p.
 bony p.
 extrarenal p.
 pseudospider p.
 renal p., p. renalis
 spider p.
 split p.
 p. of ureter
pelviureteral
pelviureteroradiography
penectomy

penial
penile
 p. body
 p.-brachial pressure index (PBPI)
 dorsal p. nerve block (DPNB)
 p. epispadias
 p. hypospadias
 p. induration
 p. kraurosis
 nocturnal p. tumescence (NPT)
 pearly p. papule
 p. reflex
 p. root
 p. tumescence
 p. urethra
penis
 p. captivus
 chordeic p.
 cleft p.
 clubbed p.
 concealed p.
 double p.
 p. palmatus
 p. plastica
 webbed p.
penischisis
penitis
penoscrotal
peotomy
percutaneous
 p. antegrade pyelography
 p. antegrade urography
 p. nephrostolithotomy (PCNL)
 p. transluminal renal angioplasty (PTRA)
periarteritis
 p. gummosa
 p. nodosa
pericystitis
perididymis
perididymitis
perineal
 p. body
 p. lithotomy
 p. pad

perineal (continued)
 p. prostatectomy
 p. sensation
perineoscrotal
perineostomy
perinephric
perinephritic
perinephritis
perinephrium
perineum
 anterior p.
 posterior p.
 watering-can p.
perineural
periorchitis
 p. adhaesiva
 p. purulenta
periorchium
peripenial
periprostatic
periprostatis
perirenal
perispermatitis
 p. serosa
peritoneal
 p. cavity, greater
 p. cavity, lesser
 p. dialysis
peritoneum
periureteral [around or encircling the ureter]
periureteric
periureteritis
periurethral
periurethritis
perivesical
perivesicular
perivesiculitis
Permutit method
Petersen
 operation
Peyronie disease
PG—prostaglandin
PGE$_2$ [PGE2]—prostaglandin E$_2$
PH—prostatic hypertrophy
phallalgia
phallanastrophe
phallaneurysm

phallectomy
phallic
phallitis
phallocampsis
phallocrypsis
phallodynia
phalloncus
phalloplasty
    reconstructive p.
phallorrhagia
phallorrhea
phallotomy
phallus
phenomenon (phenomena)
    See also *reaction, reflex,*
        sign, and *test.*
    first-set p.
    Schramm p.
    second-set p.
phenylketonuria (PKU)
    p. II
    p. III
    atypical p.
    maternal p.
phimosiectomy
phimosis
phimotic
phlegmon
photoradiation
photoscan
Picchini
    syndrome
"pielo–" Phonetic for words begin-
    ning pyelo–.
Piersol point
pile
    prostatic p.
pilimiction
"pilitis" Phonetic for pyelitis.
"pio–" Phonetic for words begin-
    ning pyo–.
Pitres sign
plaque
    Randall p.'s
plexus (plexus, plexuses)
    See also *rete.*
    p. cavernosus penis
    cavernous p. of penis

plexus (plexus, plexuses) (continued)
    hypogastric p.
    pampiniform p.
    p. pampiniformis
    pelvic p.
    prostatic p.
    prostaticovesical p.
    p. prostaticus
    renal p.
    p. renalis
    sacral p.
    Santorini p.
    spermatic p.
    p. spermaticus
    suprarenal p.
    p. suprarenalis
    testicular p.
    p. testicularis
    ureteric p.
    p. uretericus
    p. venosus prostaticus
    vesical p.
    p. vesicale
    p. vesicalis
    vesicoprostatic p.
plica (plicae)
    p. pubovesicalis
    p. vesicalis transversa
ploidy
PN—pyelonephritis
pneumatocele
    scrotal p.
pneumokidney
pneumopyelography
pole
    caudal p. of testis
    cranial p. of testis
    inferior p. of kidney
    inferior p. of testis
    pelvic p.
    upper p. of kidney
    upper p. of testis
polychloruria
polycystic disease
polydipsia
polyorchidism
polyorchis

polyp
> inflammatory p.
> neoplastic p.
> non-neoplastic p.
> pedunculated p.
> sessile p.

polyspermia
polyspermism
polyspermy
polyuria
porotomy
porphyrinuria
porphyruria
porta (portae)
> p. renis

position
> See in *General Surgical Terms.*
> semi-Fowler p.

posterior
> p. nephrectomy

postglomerular
posthetomy
posthioplasty
posthitis
postholith
postirradiation
postvoid radiography
potassium-sparing diuretics [a class of drugs]

Potter
> disease

pouch
> p. of Douglas
> Koch p.
> obturator p.
> paravesical p.
> perineal p., deep
> perineal p., superficial
> rectovesical p.
> uterovesical p.
> vesicouterine p.

Power and Wilder method
PPTT—prepubertal testicular tumor
Prehn sign
preperitoneal
prepubertal

prepuce
> p. of penis

preputial
preputiotomy
preputium
> p. clitoridis
> p. penis

prerectal
> p. lithotomy

prerenal
> p. azotemia

preurethritis
prevesical
> retropubic p. prostatectomy

priapism
> secondary p.

priapitis
priapus
principal [primary, main]
principle [rule]
procedure
> See also *maneuver, method, operation,* and *technique.*
> Campbell p.
> Heitz-Boyer p.

proctocystocele
proctocystoplasty
proctocystotomy
proctoelytroplasty
profound
> p. hematuria

progenital
pronephros
prostaglandin (PG)
> See also in *Laboratory, Pathology, and Chemistry Terms.*
> p. E_2 [E2] (PGE_2)

prostata
prostatalgia
prostatauxe
prostate
> funnel-neck p.

prostatectomy
> perineal p.
> radical p.
> radical retropubic p.
> retropubic prevesical p.

prostatectomy (continued)
    suprapubic p. (SPP)
    suprapubic transvesical p.
    transurethral p.
prostatelcosis
prostateria
prostatic
    benign p. hyperplasia (BPH)
    benign p. hypertrophy (BPH)
prostaticovesical
prostaticovesiculectomy
prostatism
    vesical p.
prostatisme
    p. sans prostate
prostatitic
prostatitis
    granulomatous p.
    tuberculous p.
prostatocystitis
prostatocystotomy
prostatography
prostatolith
prostatolithotomy
prostatomegaly
prostatometer
prostatomy
prostatomyomectomy
prostatorrhea
prostatotomy
prostatotoxin
prostatovesiculectomy
prostatovesiculitis
proteinuria
    adventitious p.
    Bence Jones p.
    cardiac p.
    colliquative p.
    cyclic p.
    emulsion p.
    enterogenic p.
    febrile p.
    globular p.
    gouty p.
    hematogenous p.
    intrinsic p.
    nephrogenous p.
    palpatory p.

proteinuria (continued)
    postrenal p.
    residual p.
proteinuric
pruritus
    p. scroti
    uremic p.
pseudohermaphrodite
pseudohermaphroditism
pseudohydronephrosis
pseudosarcoid
PSGN—poststreptococcal glomeru-
    lonephritis
psoas
    p. muscle
ptosis
    p. of kidney
    renal p.
PTRA—percutaneous transluminal
    renal angioplasty
puberty
    delayed p.
    precocious p.
pubes (pubes)
pubic
    inferior p. ligament
    p. lice
    p. ligament of Cowper
    p. region
    superior p. ligament
    p. symphysis
pubis
    symphysis p.
puboprostatic
pubovesical
pubovesicalis
pudenda (plural of pudendum)
pudendal
pudendum (pudenda)
punch
    kidney p.
    Murphy kidney p.
    Turkel p.
puncture
    suprapubic p.
purpura
    lung p. with nephritis
purulent

puruloid
pustule
PV—postvoiding
PVC—postvoiding cystogram
pyelectasia
pyelectasis
pyelic
pyelitic
pyelitis
    calculous p.
    p. cystica
    defloration p.
    encrusted p.
    p. glandularis
    p. granulosa
    p. gravidarum
    hematogenous p.
    hemorrhagic p.
    suppurative p.
    urogenous p.
pyelocaliectasis
pyelocystanastomosis
pyelocystitis
pyelocystostomosis
pyelofluoroscopy
pyelogram
    dragon p.
    hydrated p.
    infusion p.
    intravenous p.
    retrograde p.
pyelograph
pyelography
    air p.
    antegrade p.
    ascending p.
    drip p.
    drip infusion p.
    p. by elimination
    excretion p.
    infusion p.
    intravenous p. (IVP)
    lateral p.
    percutaneous antegrade p.
    respiration p.
    retrograde p.
    washout p.
pyeloileocutaneous

pyelointerstitial
pyelolithotomy
pyelometer
pyelometry
pyelonephritis
    acute p.
    acute nonobstructive p.
    ascending p.
    asymptomatic p.
    calculous p.
    chronic p.
    chronic bacterial p.
    hematogenous p.
    p. of pregnancy
    xanthogranulomatous p.
pyelopathy
pyeloplasty
pyeloplication
pyeloscopy
pyelostomy
pyelotomy
    p. incision
pyelotubular
pyeloureteral
pyeloureterectasis
pyeloureteritis cystica
pyeloureterogram
pyeloureterography
pyeloureterolysis
pyeloureteroplasty
pyelovenous
pyocalix
pyocele
pyohydronephrosis
pyonephritis
pyonephrolithiasis
pyonephrosis
pyonephrotic
pyospermia
pyoureter
pyovesiculosis
pyramid
    p. of kidney
    renal p.
    p.'s of Malpighi
pyramis (pyramides)
    pyramides Malpighii

pyuria
> abacterial p.

RA—renal artery

"rabdo–" Phonetic for words begin-
> ning rhabdo–.

radical [adj.]
> r. nephrectomy
> r. prostatectomy
> r. retropubic prostatectomy

radices (plural of radix)

radiciform

radicis (genitive of radix)

radioenzymatic

radiography
> postvoid r.

radionuclide
> r. cystography
> r. voiding cystourethrography

radix (radices)
> r. penis

"ra-fee" Phonetic for raphe.

Ralks
> adapter

ramus (rami)

Randall
> plaques

raphe (raphae)
> median r. of perineum
> r. penis
> perineal r., r. perinealis, r.
> > perinei, r. of perineum
> r. scroti, r. of scrotum

raphes (genitive of raphe)

RAS—renal artery stenosis

RBC—red blood cell(s)

RC—retrograde cystogram

reabsorption

reaction
> See also *phenomenon, reflex,*
> > *sign,* and *test.*
> Bittorf r.

receptor
> volume r.'s

recessus (recessus)

reconstructive
> r. phalloplasty

rectal
> r. lithotomy

rectocystotomy

rectourethral

rectovesical
> r. lithotomy

rectovestibular

rectum

reflex
> See also *phenomenon, reac-
> tion, sign,* and *test.*
> See also in *Neurology and
> Pain Management* section.
> bulbospongiosus r.
> dartos r.
> micturition r.
> penile r., penis r.
> scrotal r.
> sexual r.
> urinary r.'s
> virile r.

reflux
> Hinman r.
> intrarenal r.
> r. nephropathy
> pyelorenal r.
> pyelotubular r.
> urethrovesiculodifferential r.
> vesicoureteral r. (VUR)
> vesicoureteric r.

region
> genitourinary r.
> inguinal r.
> ischiorectal r.
> pelvic r.
> perineal r.
> pubic r.
> suprapubic r.
> urogenital r.

regurgitation
> vesicoureteral r.

Reiter
> disease
> syndrome

rejection

Reliquet lithotrite

ren
> r. mobilis
> r. unguliformis

renal
- r. agenesis
- r. angiography
- r. arteriography
- r. artery
- r. blastema
- r. calculi
- r. cell carcinoma
- r. cortex
- r. cortical necrosis
- r. cyst
- r. dysgenesis
- r. dysplasia
- r. ectopia
- r. failure
- r. fascia
- r. hyperplasia
- r. insufficiency
- intravenous r. angiography
- r. lithiasis
- r. medulla
- r. osteodystrophy
- r. papillae
- r. parenchyma
- r. pedicle
- r. pelvis
- percutaneous transluminal r. angioplasty (PTRA)
- r. plexus
- r. pouch
- r. rickets
- r. sinus
- r. toxicity
- r. transplant
- r. transplantation
- r. tubular acidosis
- r. tubular necrosis
- r. tubule
- r. vein
- r. vein thrombosis
- r. venogram

renes
renicapsule
renicardiac
reniculus (reniculi)
reninoma
renipelvic
reniportal

renipuncture
renocortical
renogastric
renogram
- isotope r.
renointestinal
renoprival
renopulmonary
renotrophic
renotropic
repair
- Bengt-Johanson r.
- Cecil r.
resection
- transurethral r. (TUR)
- transurethral r. of bladder (TURB)
- transurethral r. of prostate (TURP)
respiration
- r. pyelography
rete (retia)
- See also *plexus*.
- r. testis
retia (plural of rete)
retial
retraction
retrograde
- r. cystography
- r. cystourethrography
- r. ejaculation
- r. pyelography
- r. urography
retroperitoneal
retropubic
- r. prevesical prostatectomy
- radical r. prostatectomy
retrourethral
- r. catheterization
retrovesical
Retzius
- space
RFS—renal function study
rhabdoid
rhabdomyomatous
rhabdosarcoma
- renal r.

ridge
  interureteric r.
Rigaud
  operation
RigiScan
  device
  measurement
  penile tumescence monitor
rima (rimae)
  r. pudendi
  r. vulvae
rimal
RK—right kidney
RLD—related living donor
Roche sign
Rokitansky
  kidney
root
  penile r.
Rose-Bradford kidney
RP—retrograde pyelogram
RPG—retrograde pyelogram
RPGN—rapidly progressive
  glomerulonephritis
RTA—renal tubular acidosis
RU—retrograde urogram
ruga (rugae)
  r. of urinary bladder
rugal pattern
rugate
runoff
Ruysch
  glomeruli
RVR—renal vascular resistance
RVRA—renal vein renin activity
  renal vein renin assay
RVRC—renal vein renin concentration
RVT—renal vein thrombosis
Santorini plexus
sarcocele
sarcoma (sarcomas, sarcomata)
  See also in *Oncology and
    Hematology* section.
  botryoid s., s. botryoides
  clear cell s.
  embryonal s.
  s. of testis

sarcomatous
Savage perineal body
scan
  See also in *Radiology,
    Nuclear Medicine, and
    Other Imaging* section.
  adrenal s.
  gallium s.
  kidney s.
  renal s.
scanning
  gallium s.
scapus (scapi)
  s. penis
Scardino
  ureteropelvioplasty
Scardino-Prince
  ureteropelvioplasty
Scarpa
  fascia
  sheath
  triangle
Schachowa
  spiral tubes
schistosomiasis
  urinary s.
  vesical s.
Schramm phenomenon
schwannoma
Schweizer-Foley
  Y-plasty
sclerosis
  focal glomerular s.
  glomerular s.
  renal arteriolar s.
  systemic s. of kidney
score
  Gleason grading s.
scrotal
  s. fat necrosis
  s. hemangioma
  s. lymphangioma
  s. panniculitis
scrotectomy
scrotitis
scrotocele
scrotoplasty

scrotum
    s. lapillosum
    lymph s.
    watering-can s.
sediment
    urinary s.
segmenta (plural of segmentum)
segmental
segmentum (segmenta)
segregator
    Cathelin s.
    Harris s.
    Luy s.
semen
semenuria
semi-Fowler position
seminal
    s. vesiculotomy
semination
seminiferous
seminologist
seminology
seminoma
seminomatous
seminome
seminuria
septa (plural of septum)
septi (genitive of septum)
septulum (septula)
    septula testis
septum (septa)
    s. bulbi urethrae
    cloacal s.
    s. glandis penis, s. of glans
      penis
    s. pectiniforme
    s. penis
    rectovesical s.
    s. renis
    scrotal s., s. of scrotum
    septa of testis
    urorectal s.
Sergent white adrenal line
Sertoli
    cell
    column
    tumor
Sertoli cell–only syndrome

serum (serums, sera)
    s. acid phosphatase
    s. alkaline phosphatase
    s. blocking factor
    s. urate level
    s. urea nitrogen (SUN)
    s. uric acid
serumuria
"serviko–" Phonetic for words
    beginning cervico–.
shaft
    s. of penis
"shangker" Phonetic for chancre.
"shangkroid" Phonetic for chancroid.
sheath
    bulbar s.
    fascial s. of prostate
    s. of prostate
    Scarpa s.
shelf
    rectal s.
Shohl and Pedley method
shower
    uric acid s.
shunt
    dialysis s.
"shwah-no-mah" Phonetic for
    schwannoma.
siderosis
    urinary s.
"sifilis" Phonetic for syphilis.
"sifilo–" Phonetic for words begin-
    ning syphilo–.
sigmoid
    s. conduit
sigmoidovesical
sign
    See also *phenomenon, reac-*
      tion, reflex, and *test.*
    Bergman s.
    Brodie s.
    flush-tank s.
    Gilbert s.
    Guyon s.
    Kelly s.
    ligature s.
    Lloyd s.
    Pitres s.

sign (continued)
    Prehn s.
    Roche s.
    Rommelaere s.
    string s.
    Sumner s.
    Thornton s.
"simphysis" Phonetic for symphysis.
simple
    s. nephrectomy
sin–. See also words beginning
    cin–, syn–.
sinus (sinus, sinuses)
    s. epididymidis, s. of epi-
      didymis
    Guérin s.
    s. of kidney
    mucous s.'s of male urethra
    prostatic s.
    renal s.
    urogenital s.
Sipple syndrome
situs (situs)
    s. inversus
    s. inversus viscerum
    s. perversus
    s. transversus
Sjöqvist
    method
Skene
    gland
"skis–" Phonetic for words begin-
    ning schis–.
"sklero–" Phonetic for words begin-
    ning sclero–.
SLE—systemic lupus erythematosus
sling
    s. operation
smegma
    s. praeputii
Smith-Lemli-Opitz
    syndrome
"so-as" Phonetic for psoas.
"so-is" Phonetic for psoas.
solution
    See *fluid* and *liquor.*
sore
    venereal s.

space
    Bowman s.
    capsular s.
    Colles s.
    intravesical s.
    perineal s., deep
    perineal s., superficial
    preperitoneal s.
    preputial s.
    prevesical s.
    retroperitoneal s.
    Retzius s., s. of Retzius
    suprapubic s.
    urogenital s.
specific gravity
sperm
    muzzled s.
spermacrasia
spermagglutination
spermalist
spermatemphraxis
spermatic
spermaticide
spermatid
spermatin
spermatism
spermatitis
spermatoblast
spermatocele
spermatocelectomy
spermatocidal
spermatocyst
spermatocystectomy
spermatocystitis
spermatocystotomy
spermatocytal
spermatocyte
spermatocytic
spermatocytogenesis
spermatogenesis
spermatogenic
spermatogenous
spermatogeny
spermatogone
spermatogonium
spermatoid
spermatology
spermatolysin

spermatolysis
spermatolytic
spermatomere
spermatomerite
spermatopathia
spermatopoietic
spermatorrhea
spermatoschesis
spermatovum
spermatozoa
spermatozoal
spermatozoon
spermaturia
spermectomy
spermia
spermiation
spermicidal
spermicide
spermiduct
spermiocyte
spermiogenesis
spermioteleosis
spermioteleotic
spermium
spermoblast
spermoculture
spermolith
spermoloropexy
spermolytic
spermoneuralgia
spermophlebectasia
spermoplasm
spermosphere
spermotoxic
spermotoxin
sp gr—specific gravity
sphincter
    Henle s.
    inguinal s.
    Nélaton s.
    s. urethrae
    s. vesicae
sphincteric
sphincterismus
sphincteritis
Spivack
    operation
splenonephroptosis

sponge
    medullary s. kidney
SPP—suprapubic prostatectomy
squamous
    s. metaplasia
SRFS—split renal function study
stain
    Ziehl-Neelsen s.
Stanischeff
    operation
stasis
    urinary s.
Steinach
    operation
stellate
stenosis (stenoses)
    meatal s.
    posterior s. of urethra
    renal artery s.
stent
    double-J silicone s.
    Gibbon ureteral s.
    pigtail s.
stereocilium (stereocilia)
sterile, sterilely
sterility
    absolute s.
    male s.
    primary s.
    relative s.
    secondary s.
sterilization
sterilize
stigma (stigmas, stigmata)
    syphilitic s.'s
stigmatic
stigmatism
stigmatization
stoma
    Turnbull loop s.
stone
    bladder s.
    cystine s.
    kidney s.
    s. searcher
strangulation
    s. of bladder
stranguria

strangury
strata (plural of stratum)
stratiform
stratum (strata)
    submucous s. of bladder
streak
    See *band* and *line.*
stria (striae)
    See *band* and *line.*
stricture
    Hunner s.
string sign
stromal
Stühmer (Stuehmer)
    disease
stuttering
    urinary s.
submucous
    s. cystitis
    s. layer of bladder
    s. ulcer
subscapular
suburethral
succus (succi)
    s. prostaticus
"sudo–" Phonetic for words beginning pseudo–.
sulci (plural of sulcus)
sulciform
sulcus (sulci)
summit
    s. of bladder
Sumner
    method
suprahilar
suprapubic
    s. catheterization
    s. cystotomy
    s. lithotomy
    s. prostatectomy (SPP)
    s. transvesical prostatectomy
suprarenal
suprarenalectomy
suprarenalism
suprarenalopathy
suprarene
suprarenoma

surgery
    See also *maneuver, method, operation, procedure,* and *technique.*
    transsexual s.
surgical procedure
    See *operation, procedure,* and *technique.*
suspensory
suture [material]
    See in *General Surgical Terms.*
suture [technique]
swelling
    genital s.
    scrotal s.
symphyseal
symphysis (symphyses)
    s. ossium pubis
    pubic s.
    s. pubica, s. pubis
symptom
    See also in *General Medical Terms.*
    incarceration s.
syn–. See also words beginning cin–, sin–.
syndrome
    See also *disease.*
    acute nephritic s.
    adrenogenital s.
    Allemann s.
    androgenital s.
    Bartter s.
    Bywaters s.
    Cacchi-Ricci s.
    compression s.
    Conn s.
    Cooke-Apert-Gallais s.
    crush s.
    Cushing s.
    Cushing s. medicamentosus
    Debré-de Toni-Fanconi s.
    del Castillo s.
    de Toni-Debré-Fanconi s.
    de Toni-Fanconi s.
    de Toni-Fanconi-Debré s.
    Epstein s.

syndrome (continued)
  Fanconi s.
  Fiessinger-Leroy-Reiter s.
  Gasser s.
  gasserian s.
  Gilbert s.
  Gilbert-Behçet s.
  Gilbert-Dreyfus s.
  Goodpasture s.
  Gordon s.
  Gorlin-Chaudhry-Moss s.
  gynecomastia-aspermato-
    genesis s.
  Hartnup s.
  Heller-Nelson s.
  hemolytic-uremic s.
  hepatorenal s.
  Heyd s.
  Hippel-Lindau s.
  Kimmelstiel-Wilson s.
  Klinefelter s.
  Labbé s.
  Launois-Cléret s.
  Leriche s.
  Lightwood s.
  Lignac s.
  Lignac-Fanconi s.
  Luder-Sheldon s.
  male Turner s.
  Marañon s.
  megacystis-megaureter s.
  Miller s.
  Muckle-Wells s.
  nephrotic s.
  Nonnenbruch s.
  Reifenstein s.
  Rovsing s.
  rudimentary testis s.
  Schmidt s.
  Sertoli-cell-only s.
  Sipple s.
  suprarenogenic s.
  Thorn s.
  Turner s.
  Turner s., male
  Waterhouse-Friderichsen s.
synorchidism
synorchism

synoscheos
syphilis
syphilitic
syringe
  Nourse s.
  Toomey s.
system
  Jewett-Strong s.
systemic
  s. lupus erythematosus (SLE)
TAR—thrombocytopenia–absent
  radius [syndrome]
technique
  See also *maneuver* and
    method.
  Denis Browne t.
  Glenn t.
Teilum tumor
tela (telae)
  t. subserosa vesicae urinariae
telar
tenesmus
  vesical t.
teratoblastoma
teratocarcinoma
teratoma (teratomas, teratomata)
  adult t.
  anaplastic malignant t.
  benign cystic t.
  cystic t.
  differentiated t.
  immature t.
  malignant t.
  mature t.
  solid t.
  tropoblastic malignant t.
  undifferentiated malignant t.
teratomatous
teratospermia
test
  See also *phenomenon, reac-
    tion, reflex,* and *sign.*
  See also in *Laboratory,
    Pathology, and Chemistry
    Terms.*
  Albarran t.
  aldosterone suppression t.
  blood urea nitrogen (BUN) t.

test (continued)
    clonidine suppression t.
    Coombs t.
    creatinine clearance t.
    FTA-ABS (fluorescent tre-
        ponemal antibody absorp-
        tion) t.
    glucose t.
    immunodiffusion t.
    ketone body t.
    kidney function t.
    Lange t. (for acetone in urine)
    leukocyte adherence inhibi-
        tion t.
    Marshall t.
    methylene blue t.
    nitrites t.
    nitrogen retention t.
    pH t.
    proteinuria t.
    radioisotope renal excretion t.
    radioisotope renogram t.
    renal function t. (RFT)
    renin stimulation t.
    rhubarb t.
    saline suppression t.
    semen analysis t.
    serologic t. for syphilis (STS)
    serum creatinine t.
    specific gravity t.
    specific red cell adherence t.
    split renal function t.
    Sulkowitch t.
    Trousseau t.
    tubular reabsorption of
        phosphate t.
    ultrasound t.
    urine chloride t.
    urine concentration t.
    VDRL (Venereal Disease
        Research Laboratories) t.
        [abbreviation not expand-
        ed]
    Watson-Schwartz t.
testes (plural of testis)
testicle
    retained t.
    undescended t.

testicular
testiculi (plural of testiculus)
testiculoma
testiculus (testiculi)
testis (testes)
    abdominal t.
    Cooper irritable t.
    ectopic t.
    femoral t.
    inguinal t.
    inverted t.
    t. muliebris
    obstructed t.
    perineal t.
    pulpy t.
    t. redux
    retained t.
    undescended t.
testitis
testitoxicosis
testoid
testopathy
testosterone
    t. cypionate
    t. propionate
therapy
    immunosuppressive t.
    replacement t.
thiazides [a class of drugs]
Thiersch graft
Thiersch-Duplay
    urethroplasty
Thompson
    lithotrite
Thomsen-Friedenreich
    antigen
thoracoabdominal
Thorn salt-depletion syndrome
Thornton sign
thrombi (plural of thrombus)
thrombosis
    See also in *Cardiology* sec-
        tion.
    renal vein t.
thrombus (thrombi)
    See *thrombosis*.
    See also in *Cardiology* sec-
        tion.

Tm—maximal tubular excretory
     capacity of kidneys
TNM—tumor, nodes, metastases
     [tumor staging system]
Toldt
     membrane
"tolt" Phonetic for Toldt.
tomography
     computed t. (CT)
     computerized axial t. (CAT)
Toomey
     evacuator
     syringe
Torek
     operation
tori (plural of torus)
torsion
tortuous
     t. ureter
torus (tori)
     t. uretericus
tour de maître
trabecula (trabeculae)
     trabeculae of corpora caver-
          nosa of penis
     trabeculae corporis spon-
          giosi penis
     trabeculae corporum caver-
          nosorum penis
     trabeculae of corpus spon-
          giosum of penis
trabecularism
trabeculate
trabeculation
     t. of bladder dome
tract
     genitourinary (GU) t.
     urinary t.
     urogenital t.
tractor
     Lowsley t.
transabdominal
transcutaneous
transitional
transluminal
     percutaneous t. renal angio-
          plasty (PTRA)
transperineal

transplantation
     kidney t.
     renal t.
transrectal
transsexual
transthoracic
     t. nephrectomy
transureteroureterostomy
transurethral
     t. prostatectomy
     t. resection (TUR)
     t. resection of bladder
          (TURB)
     t. resection of prostate
          (TURP)
transverse
transversourethralis
transversus
transvesical
     suprapubic t. prostatectomy
transvestism
transvestite
trauma (traumas, traumata)
Trendelenburg
     position
triangle
     Hesselbach t.
     Scarpa t.
trigonal
trigone
     urogenital t.
trigonitis
trigonotome
trigonum (trigona)
     t. urogenitale
     t. vesicae, t. vesicae (Lieu-
          taudi)
triple-voiding cystography
TSPAP—total serum prostatic acid
     phosphatase
tube
     collecting t.'s
     Ferrein t.'s
     Schachowa spiral t.'s
tuberculocele
tuberculosis (TB)
     adrenal t.
     genital t.

tuberculosis (TB) (continued)
  genitourinary t.
  t. of kidney and bladder
  renal t.
tubular
  t. necrosis
  t. stenosis
tubule
  Albarran t.
  Bellini t.
  Henle t.'s
  mesonephric t.
  metanephric t.
  renal t.
  seminiferous t.
  testicular t.
  urine-collecting t.
  uriniferous t.
  uriniparous t.
tubuli (plural of tubulus)
tubulitis
tubulointerstitial
tubulopathy
tubulorrhexis
tubulosaccular
tubulous [adj.]
tubulus (tubuli)
Tuffier
  operation
  retractor
tuft
  malpighian t.
  renal t.
tumescence
  nocturnal penile t. (NPT)
  penile t.
tumescent
tumor
  Brenner t.
  Buschke-Löwenstein t.
  cystic t.
  germ cell t.
  granulosa-theca cell t.
  Grawitz t.
  juxtaglomerular t.
  luteinized granulosa-theca
    cell t.
  rhabdoid t.

tumor (continued)
  Teilum t.
  thrombus t.
  Wilms t.
  yolk sac t.
tunic
  fibrous t. of liver
  mucous t.
  muscular t.
  proper t.
  t.'s of spermatic cord
tunica (tunicae)
  t. adventitia
  t. albuginea
  t. albuginea testis
  t. dartos
  t. fibrosa
  t. mucosa
  t. muscularis
  t. propria
  t. serosa
  t. spongiosa urethrae femini-
    nae
  tunicae testis
  t. vasculosa
tunicate
TUR—transurethral resection
TURB—transurethral resection of
    bladder
Turkel
  punch
Turnbull loop stoma
Turner-Warwick
  operation
  urethroplasty
TURP—transurethral resection of
    prostate
TVC—triple voiding cystogram
UA—urinalysis
UC—urethral catheterization
UD—urethral discharge
UG—urogenital
ulcer
  decubitus u.
  Hunner u.
  submucous u.
ulcera (plural of ulcus)

ulcus (ulcera)
    u. penetrans
    u. simplex vesicae
ultrasonogram
    renal u.
undescended testis
unit
    See also in *General Medical*
       Terms and *Laboratory,*
       Pathology, and Chemistry
       Terms.
    international adrogen u.
    international u. of male hor-
       mone
UP—ureteropelvic
U/P—urine-plasma [ratio]
UPJ—ureteropelvic junction
urachal
urachovesical
urachus
uracrasia
uracratia
uragogue
uraturia
urea nitrogen (UN)
uremia
    azotemic u.
    extrarenal u.
    prerenal u.
    retention u.
uremic medullary cystic disease
ureter
    aberrant u.
    circumcaval u.
    double u.
    ectopic u.
    postcaval u.
    retrocaval u.
    retroiliac u.
ureteral
    u. electromyography
    u. meatoscopy
    u. neocystostomy
    u. reflux
    u. stent
ureteralgia
ureterectasia
ureterectasis

ureterectomy
ureteric
    u. ridge
ureteritis
    u. cystica
    u. glandularis
ureterocele
    ectopic u.
ureterocelectomy
ureterocervical
ureterocolostomy
ureterocutaneostomy
ureterocutaneous
ureterocystanastomosis
ureterocystography
ureterocystoneostomy
ureterocystostomy
ureterodialysis
ureteroduodenal
ureteroenteric
ureteroenteroanastomosis
ureteroenterostomy
ureterogram
ureterography
ureteroheminephrectomy
ureteroileal
    u. neocystostomy
ureteroileostomy
ureterointestinal
ureterolith
ureterolithiasis
ureterolithotomy
ureterolysis
ureteromeatotomy
ureteroneocystostomy
ureteroneopyelostomy
ureteronephrectomy
ureteropathy
ureteropelvic
ureteropelvioneostomy
ureteropelvioplasty
    Culp u.
    Culp-DeWeerd u.
    Foley u.
    Foley Y-type u.
    Foley Y-V u.
    Scardino u.
    Scardino-Prince u.

ureterophlegma
ureteroplasty
ureteroproctostomy
ureteropyelitis
ureteropyelography
ureteropyeloneostomy
ureteropyelonephritis
ureteropyelonephrostomy
ureteropyeloplasty
ureteropyelostomy
ureteropyosis
ureterorectal
ureterorectoneostomy
ureterorectostomy
ureterorenoscopy
ureterorrhagia
ureterorrhaphy
ureteroscopy
ureterosigmoid
ureterosigmoidostomy
ureterostegnosis
ureterostenoma
ureterostenosis
ureterostoma
ureterostomosis
ureterostomy
    cutaneous u.
ureterotomy
ureterotrigonoenterostomy
ureterotrigonosigmoidostomy
ureteroureteral
ureteroureterostomy
ureterouterine
ureterovaginal
ureterovesical
ureterovesicoplasty
    Leadbetter-Politano u.
ureterovesicostomy
urethra
    female u.
    u. feminina
    male u.
    u. masculina
    u. muliebris
    penile u.
    u. virilis
urethralgia
urethratresia

urethrectomy
urethremphraxis
urethreurynter
urethrism
urethritis
    u. cystica
    u. glandularis
    gonorrheal u.
    gouty u.
    u. granulosa
    nonspecific u.
    u. orificii externi
    u. petrificans
    polypoid u.
    prophylactic u.
    specific u.
    u. venerea
urethroblennorrhea
urethrobulbar
urethrocele
urethrocystitis
urethrocystocele
urethrocystogram
urethrocystography
urethrocystometry
urethrocystopexy
urethrocystoscopy
urethrodynia
urethrogram
urethrograph
urethrography
urethrometer
urethrometry
urethropenile
urethroperineal
urethroperineoscrotal
urethropexy
urethrophraxis
urethrophyma
urethroplasty
    Thiersch-Duplay u.
    Turner-Warwick u.
urethroprostatic
urethrorectal
urethrorrhagia
urethrorrhaphy
urethrorrhea
urethroscopic

urethroscopy
urethroscrotal
urethrospasm
urethrostaxis
urethrostenosis
urethrostomy
urethrotomy
    external u.
    internal u.
urethrotrigonitis
urethrovaginal
urethrovesical
uretic
uricaciduria
uricometer
uricosuria
urina
    u. chyli
    u. cibi
    u. cruenta
    u. galactodes
    u. jumentosa
    u. potus
    u. sanguinus
    u. spastica
urinable
urinacidometer
urinal
urinary
    u. bladder
    u. diversion
    u. fistula
    u. frequency
    u. incontinence
    u. meatus
    u. retention
    u. sphincter
    u. tract
urinate
urination
    precipitant u.
    stuttering u.
urine
    anemic u.
    Bence Jones u.
    black u.
    chylous u.
    clean-catch u. specimen

urine (continued)
    crude u.
    u. cytology
    diabetic u.
    dyspeptic u.
    febrile u.
    gouty u.
    milky u.
    nebulous u.
    nervous u.
    residual u.
    straw-colored u.
    voided u.
urinemia
urine urea nitrogen (UUN)
uriniferous
uriniparous
urinocryoscopy
urinogenital
urinogenous
urinoglucosometer
urinologist
urinology
urinoma
urinometer
urinometry
urinosexual
urinous
urobilinogenuria
urobilinuria
urocele
urochezia
urochrome
urochromogen
uroclepsia
urocrisia
urocrisis
urocriterion
urocyanogen
urocyst
urocystic
urocystis
urocystitis
urodeum
urodialysis
urodochium
urodynamic
urodynamics

urodynia
uroedema
uroerythrin
uroflavin
uroflometer
urofuscin
urofuscohematin
urogenital
    u. trigone
urogenous
uroglaucin
urogram
    excretory u.
    intravenous u.
urography
    ascending u.
    cystoscopic u.
    descending u.
    excretion u.
    excretory u.
    intravenous u. (IVU)
    oral u.
    percutaneous antegrade u.
    retrograde u.
urohematin
urohematonephrosis
urohematoporphyrin
urohypertensin
urokinetic
urokymography
urolith
urolithiasis
urolithic
urolithology
urolithotomy
urologic, urological
urologist
urology
urolutein
uromancy
uromantia
uromelanin
urometer
uromucoid
uroncus
uronephrosis
uronology
urononcometry

uronophile
uronoscopy
uropathogen
uropathy
    obstructive u.
uropenia
uropepsinogen
urophanic
urophein
urophosphometer
uroplania
uropoiesis
uropoietic
uroporphyria
uroporphyrinogen
uropsammus
uropterin
uropyonephrosis
uropyoureter
uroradiology
urorhythmography
urorrhagia
urorrhea
urorrhodin
urorrhodinogen
urorubin
urorubinogen
urorubrohematin
urosaccharometry
uroscheocele
uroschesis
uroscopic
uroscopy
urosemiology
urosepsin
urosepsis
uroseptic
urosis
urospectrin
urostalagmometry
urostealith
urothelial
urothelium
urotherapy
urotoxia
urotoxic
urotoxicity
urotoxin

uroureter
uroxanthin
uterus (uteri)
    u. masculinus
UTI—urinary tract infection
utricle
    prostatic u.
    urethral u.
utricular
utriculi
utriculitis
utriculosaccular
utriculus
    u. masculinus
    u. prostaticus
    u. vestibuli
U-tube
UV—ureterovesical
    urethrovesical
    urine volume
UVA—urethrovesical angle
UVJ—ureterovesical junction
    urethrovesical junction
uvula (uvulae)
    u. of bladder
    Lieutaud u.
    u. vesicae
uvular
uvularis
vaccine
    BCG (bacille Calmette-
      Guérin) v.
vagina (vaginae)
    v. masculina
vaginal
    v. lithotomy
vaginalitis
    plastic v.
vaginate
valve
    anterior urethral v.'s
    posterior urethral v.'s
    ureteral v.
    urethral v.'s
valvula (valvulae)
    v. fossae navicularis
    v. prostatica
valvule

valvulectomy
van Buren
    disease
van Hook
    operation
variation
varicocelectomy
vas (vasa)
    v. aberrans
    v. afferens glomeruli
    vasa afferentia
    v. deferens
    v. efferens glomeruli
    v. epididymidis
vasalgia
vasculitic
vasculum (vascula)
    v. aberrans
vasectomized
vasectomy
    crossover v.
vasiform
vasitis
    v. nodosa
vasodilators [a class of drugs]
vasoepididymography
vasoepididymostomy
vasoligation
vaso-orchidostomy
vasopuncture
vasoresection
vasorrhaphy
vasosection
vasostomy
vasotomy
vasovasostomy
vasovesiculectomy
vasovesiculitis
VCU, VCUG—voiding cystourethrogram
vein
    arcuate v.
    interlobar v.
venacavography
venae cavernosae penis
venereal
    v. disease (VD)

venogram
　　renal v.
venter (ventres)
ventrocystorrhaphy
venula (venulae)
　　venulae rectae renis
　　venulae stellatae renis
venular
venule
　　stellate v. of kidney
　　straight v. of kidney
verruca (verrucae)
　　v. acuminata, verrucae
　　　acuminatae
verrucous
vertebra (vertebrae)
　　picture frame v.
vertebral
vertex (vertices)
　　v. of urinary bladder
　　v. vesicae urinariae
verumontanitis
verumontanum
vesica (vesicae)
　　v. prostatica
　　v. urinaria
vesical [adj.: pertaining to the bladder]
　　v. compliance
　　v. diverticulectomy
　　v. exstrophy
　　v. external sphincter dyssynergia (VSD)
　　v. fibrosis
　　v. fistula
　　v. neck
vesicle [noun: blister, small sac]
　　prostatic v.
　　seminal v.
　　spermatic v.
　　spermatic v., false
vesicoabdominal
vesicocavernous
vesicocele
vesicocervical
vesicoclysis
vesicocolonic
vesicoenteric

vesicofixation
vesicointestinal
vesicoperineal
vesicoprostatic
vesicopubic
vesicopustule
vesicorectal
vesicorectostomy
vesicorenal
vesicosigmoid
vesicosigmoidostomy
vesicospinal
vesicostomy
　　cutaneous v.
vesicotomy
vesicoumbilical
vesicourachal
vesicoureteral
　　v. reflux (VUR)
　　v. regurgitation
vesicoureteric
vesicourethral
vesicouterine
vesicouterovaginal
vesicovaginal
　　v. lithotomy
vesicovaginorectal
vesicula (vesiculae)
　　v. prostatica
　　v. seminalis
vesiculectomy
vesiculiform
vesiculitis
vesiculocavernous
vesiculogram
vesiculography
vesiculoprostatitis
vesiculotomy
　　seminal v.
vesiculotubular
vessel
　　internal spermatic v.
　　pudendal v.
vestibulourethral
vestige
vestigial
vestigium (vestigia)
　　v. processus vaginalis

Vidal
    operation
vinculum (vincula)
    See *band* and *frenulum.*
virilizing
virus
    See specific viruses in *Laboratory, Pathology, and Chemistry Terms.*
visceralgia
visceroptosis
VMA—vanillylmandelic acid
Vogel
    operation
void
voiding
    v. cystourethrography (VCUG)
    isotope v. cystourethrography (IVCU)
    radionuclide v. cystourethrography
Voillemier point
Volhard
    nephritis
Volhard and Fahr
    method
Volkmann
    operation
von Brunn. See *Brunn.*
von Hippel-Lindau
    disease
    syndrome
von Jaksch. See *Jaksch.*
von Rokitansky. See *Rokitansky.*
Voronoff
    operation
VSD—vesical external sphincter dyssynergia
Walther
    sound
washout
    w. pyelography
waste
    nitrogenous w.

WBC/hpf—white blood cell(s) per high-power field
Weinstein syndrome
Wheelhouse
    operation
White [eponym]
    operation
Wilkins disease
Wilks
    disease
Wilms tumor
Wilson
    muscle
Wolff
    corpus (corpus of Wolff)
    duct (duct of Wolff)
wolffian
    w. body
    w. cyst
    w. duct
Wood [eponym]
    operation
xanthogranuloma
    juvenile x.
XC—excretory cystogram
XU—excretory urogram
YAG laser therapy
yolk sac tumor
Young
    enucleator
    operation
    tractor
Youssef syndrome
Y-plasty
    Foley Y-p.
    Schweizer-Foley Y-p.
"zheel-bare" Phonetic for Gilbert [Nicolas Augustin Gilbert].
zone
    Daseler z.
    glomerular z.
    nephrogenic z.
Zoon erythroplasia
zoospermia
Zylytol

Sloane's
Medical
Word
Book

Part Three

Guide to Terminology

Abbreviations

a—[as a subscript] symbol for arterial blood
A—adenine
    adenosine
    [as a subscript] symbol for alveolar gas
    amplitude of accommodation
    artery
    atropine
    before (L. ante)
    start of anesthesia
    water (L. aqua)
A_{1c} [A1C]—hemoglobin A_{1c} [glycosylated hemoglobin]
A_2 [A2]—aortic second sound
aa—arteries
AA—Alcoholics Anonymous
    amino acid
    aminoacyl
    ascending aorta
A&A—aid and attendance
A-a, $(A-a)O_2$, $P(A-a)O_2$—alveolar-arterial [oxygen gradient]
AAA—abdominal aortic aneurysm
    acquired aplastic anemia
    acute anxiety attack
    amalgam
AABB—American Association of Blood Banks
AAC—antibiotic-associated colitis
AACN—American Association of Colleges of Nursing
    American Association of Critical-Care Nurses
AACP—American Academy of Child Psychiatry
AAD—American Academy of Dermatology
    antibiotic-associated diarrhea
AADP—American Academy of Denture Prosthetics

AADR—American Academy of Dental Radiology
AADS—American Association of Dental Schools
AAE—active assistive exercise
    American Association of Endodontists
AAFP—American Academy of Family Practice
    American Association of Family Physicians
AAGP—American Academy of General Practice
AAI—acute adrenal insufficiency
    American Association of Immunologists
    arm-ankle index
AAID—American Academy of Implant Dentistry
AAL—anterior axillary line
AAMA—American Association of Medical Assistants
AAMD—age-associated memory disorder
    American Association on Mental Deficiency
AAMT—American Association for Medical Transcription
AAN—American Academy of Neurology
AANA—American Association of Nurse Anesthetists
AAO—American Academy of Ophthalmology
    American Academy of Otolaryngology
    American Association of Orthodontists
AAO3, AAOx3—awake, alert, and oriented times three [to time, place, and person]

AAOS—American Academy of Orthopaedic Surgeons

AAP—acute apical periodontitis
American Academy of Pediatrics
American Academy of Pedodontics
American Academy of Periodontology
American Association of Pathologists

AAPA—American Academy of Physician Assistants

AAPB—American Association of Pathologists and Bacteriologists

AAPMC—antibiotic-associated pseudomembranous colitis

AAPMR—American Academy of Physical Medicine and Rehabilitation

AART—American Association of Respiratory Therapy

AAS—acute abdominal series
aortic arch syndrome

AAT—auditory apperception test

AAV—adeno-associated virus

Ab, ab—abortion

Ab—antibody

AB—Ace bandage
apex beat
asthmatic bronchitis
axiobuccal

A/B—apnea-bradycardia

A&B—apnea and bradycardia

ABA—allergic bronchopulmonary aspergillosis

ABC—Adriamycin, bleomycin, cisplatin
airway-breathing-circulation [protocol]
apnea, bradycardia, cyanosis
applesauce, bananas, cereal [diet]
aspiration biopsy cytology
axiobuccocervical

ABD, Abd, abd—abdomen, abdominal

ABE—acute bacterial endocarditis

ABEP—auditory brain stem evoked potential

ABF—aortobifemoral [bypass]

ABG—axiobuccogingival

ABG, ABGs—arterial blood gas(es)

ABI—ankle-brachial index

ABL—axiobuccolingual

ABLB—alternate binaural loudness balance (test)

ABMT—autologous bone marrow transplantation

ABN, Abn, abn—abnormal, abnormality

ABP—arterial blood pressure

ABR—absolute bed rest
American Board of Radiology
auditory brain stem response

abs—absolute

ABS—acute brain syndrome

abst, abstr—abstract

ABV—Adriamycin, bleomycin, vinblastine

ac—acute

a.c.—before meals (L. ante cibum)

AC—acromioclavicular
air conduction
alternating current
anterior chamber
anterior colporrhaphy
anticoagulant
anticomplement
anti-inflammatory corticoid
axiocervical

Ac—actinium

ACA—adenocarcinoma
anterior cerebral artery

ACAT—automated computerized axial tomography

ACBE—air contrast barium enema

ACBG—aortocoronary bypass graft

ACBGS—aortocoronary bypass graft surgery

ACBS—aortocoronary bypass surgery

ACC—adenoid cystic carcinoma
alveolar cell carcinoma
ambulatory care center

ACC— (continued)
　American College of Cardi-
　　ology
　anodal closure contraction
ACCP—American College of Chest
　Physicians
ACD—absolute cardiac dullness
　adult celiac disease
　allergic contact dermatitis
　anterior chest discomfort
　anticonvulsant drug
ACDF—adult child of dysfunction-
　al family
　anterior cervical diskectomy
　　and fusion
ACE—angiotensin-converting
　enzyme
ACEIs—ACE inhibitors [a class of
　drugs]
ACEP—American College of
　Emergency Physicians
ACF—acid-fast culture
　acute care facility
ACG—American College of Gas-
　troenterology
　angiocardiogram
　angiocardiography
　angle closure glaucoma
　apexcardiogram
AChRab—acetylcholine receptor
　antibody
ACL—anterior cruciate ligament
ACLF—adult congregate living
　facility
ACLS—advanced cardiac life support
ACNM—American College of
　Nurse-Midwives
ACOG—American College of
　Obstetricians and Gynecologists
ACOS—American College of
　Osteopathic Surgeons
ACP—aspirin, caffeine, phenacetin
ACPS—acrocephalopolysyndactyly
ACRM—American College of
　Rehabilitation Medicine
ACS—American Cancer Society
　American College of Sur-
　　geons

ACS— (continued)
　anodal closing sound
ACSM—American College of
　Sports Medicine
ACT—activated coagulation time
ACTH—adrenocorticotropic hor-
　mone
ACTH-RF—ACTH-releasing factor
ACVD—acute cardiovascular disease
　arteriosclerotic cardiovascu-
　　lar disease
　autoimmune collagen vascu-
　　lar disease
AD—admitting diagnosis
　advance directive
　axiodistal
　right ear (L. auris dextra)
ADA—American Dental Association
　American Diabetes Associa-
　　tion
　American Dietetic Associa-
　　tion
　anterior descending artery
ADAA—American Dental Assis-
　tants Association
ADC—anodal duration contraction
　axiodistocervical
ADD—attention deficit disorder
ADDU—alcohol and drug depen-
　dency unit
ADE—acute disseminated
　encephalitis
ADEM—acute disseminated
　encephalomyelitis
ADG—atrial diastolic gallop
　axiodistogingival
ADH—antidiuretic hormone
ADHA—American Dental Hygien-
　ists Association
ADHD—attention deficit hyperac-
　tivity disorder
adhib—to be administered (L.
　adhibendus)
ADI—axiodistoincisal
ADL, ADLs—activities of daily liv-
　ing
ad lib—as desired, at pleasure (L.
　ad libitum)

adm, admit—admission
admov—let there be added (L. admove)
ADO—axiodisto-occlusal
ADR—absence of deep reflexes
    adverse drug reaction
ADS—anonymous donor sperm
    antibody-deficient syndrome
    antidiuretic substance
ADT—any desired thing (placebo)
ADTP—alcohol dependency treatment program
AdV—adenovirus
AE—above-elbow
    air entry
AEA—above-elbow amputation
    allergic extrinsic alveolitis
AED—antiepileptic drug
    automatic external defibrillator
AEq—age equivalent
AER—albumin excretion rate
    auditory evoked response
AF—acid-fast
    amniotic fluid
    Asian female
    atrial fibrillation
Af—atrial flutter
AFB—acid-fast bacilli
AFBG—aortofemoral bypass graft
AFO—ankle-foot orthosis
AFP—alpha-fetoprotein
    atrial filling pressure
AFRD—acute febrile respiratory disease
AFS—acid-fast smear
    Alzheimer fugue state
    American Fertility Society
AFV—amniotic fluid volume
AG—anion gap
    antiglobulin
    axiogingival
Ag—antigen
AGA—acute gonococcal arthritis
    American Gastroenterological Association
    appropriate for gestational age
AGC—absolute granulocyte count

AGE—acute gastroenteritis
    angle of greatest extension
AGF—angle of greatest flexion
AGG—agammaglobulinemia
AGH—amenorrhea-galactorrhea hypothyroidism
AGL—acute granulocytic leukemia
AGN—acute glomerulonephritis
AGS—adrenogenital syndrome
    American Geriatric Society
AH—abdominal hysterectomy
Ah—hypermetropic astigmatism
A&H—amenorrhea and hirsutism
AHA—acquired hemolytic anemia
    American Heart Association
    American Hospital Association
    autoimmune hemolytic anemia
AHC—acute hemorrhagic cystitis
AHD—arteriosclerotic heart disease
    atherosclerotic heart disease
    autoimmune hemolytic disease
AHIMA—American Health Information Management Association
AHP—Assistant House Physician
AHS—Assistant House Surgeon
AI—artificial insemination
    axioincisal
AICD—automatic implantable cardioverter-defibrillator
AID—acute infectious disease
    artificial insemination by donor
AIDS—acquired immunodeficiency syndrome
AIH—artificial insemination by husband
AILD—angioimmunoblastic lymphadenopathy with dysproteinemia
AK—above-knee, above-the-knee
AKA—above-knee amputation
A/kg—ampere per kilogram
AL—axiolingual
ALA—alpha-lipoic acid
    aminolevulinic acid

ALARA—as low as reasonably achievable
ALS—advanced life support
    antilymphocyte serum
am—meter-angle
a.m.—before noon (L. ante meridiem)
AM—Asian male
    myopic astigmatism
AMA—against medical advice
    American Medical Association
    antimitochondrial antibody
Amb, amb—ambulate, ambulation, ambulatory
AMBL—acute myeloblastic leukemia
AMH—automated medical history
AMI—acute myocardial infarction
A-mod—amplitude modulation
AML—acute myelogenous leukemia
AMP—adenosine monophosphate
    average mean pressure
AMPPE—acute multifocal placoid pigment epitheliopathy
AMRA—American Medical Record Association [now: AHIMA]
AMRL—Aerospace Medical Research Laboratories
amt—amount
ANA—antinuclear antibody
ANC—absolute neutrophil count
anes—anesthesia
    anesthesiology
ANS—acute nephritic syndrome
ant—anterior
ante—before
ANUG—acute necrotizing ulcerative gingivitis
AOA—American Optometric Association
    American Osteopathic Association
AOB—alcohol on breath
AOTA—American Occupational Therapy Association
AP—action potential
    alkaline phosphatase

AP— (continued)
    angina pectoris
    antepartum
    anteroposterior [x-ray]
    aortic pressure
    apical pulse
    attending physician
    axiopulpal
A&P—anterior and posterior [repair]
    auscultation and percussion
APA—acute pain attack
    aldosterone-producing adenoma
    American Podiatric Association
    American Psychiatric Association
    American Psychological Association
APACHE—acute physiology and chronic health evaluation
APB—atrial premature beat
APC—acetylsalicylic acid, phenacetin, caffeine
    adenomatous polyposis coli
    aspirin, phenacetin, caffeine
    atrial premature contraction
APC-C—aspirin, phenacetin, caffeine with codeine
APD—abdominal postoperative dehiscence
    action potential duration
    ambulatory peritoneal dialysis
    anteroposterior diameter
    atrial premature depolarization
APE—acute psychotic episode
    acute pulmonary edema
    aminophylline, phenobarbital, ephedrine
APGAR—adaptability, partnership, growth, affection, resolve [questionnaire]
APH—adenohypophysial hormone
    antepartum hemorrhage
    anterior pituitary hormone
APHA—American Public Health Association

APKD—adult polycystic kidney disease
APN—acute pyelonephritis
apo—apolipoprotein
APPG—aqueous procaine penicillin G
APR—abdominoperineal resection
  anterior pituitary reaction
APRT—adenine phosphoribosyl transferase
APTT, aPTT—activated partial thromboplastin time
APUD—amine precursor uptake decarboxylase
AQS—additional qualifying symptoms
Ar—argon
AR—artificial respiration
AIIRAs—angiotensin II receptor antagonists [a class of drugs]
ARC—abnormal retinal correspondence
  American Red Cross
ARD—acute respiratory disease
  acute respiratory distress
  anorectal dressing
  arthritis and rheumatic disease
ARDMS—American Registry of Diagnostic Medical Sonographers
ARDS—acute respiratory distress syndrome
  adult respiratory distress syndrome
ARF—acute renal failure
  acute respiratory failure
Arg—arginine
ARL—average remaining lifetime
ARM—artificial rupture of membranes
ARP—at-risk period
ARSB—arylsulfatase B
ART—automated reagin test
ARVD—Association for Research in Vision and Ophthalmology
AS—androsterone sulfate
  antistreptolysin
  aortic stenosis

AS— (continued)
  arteriosclerosis
  left ear (L. auris sinistra)
ASA—American Society of Anesthesiologists
  American Surgical Association
ASAL—argininosuccinic acid lyase
ASAS—American Society of Abdominal Surgeons
  argininosuccinic acid synthetase
ASCH—American Society of Clinical Hypnosis
ASCI—American Society for Clinical Investigation
ASCLT—American Society of Clinical Laboratory Technicians
ASCO—American Society of Clinical Oncology
  American Society of Contemporary Ophthalmology
ASCP—American Society of Clinical Pathologists
ASF—aniline, sulfur, formaldehyde
ASGE—American Society for Gastrointestinal Endoscopy
ASH—American Society of Hematology
AsH—hyperopic astigmatism
ASHA—American Speech and Hearing Association
ASIM—American Society of Internal Medicine
ASL—argininosuccinic lyase
Asn—asparagine
ASRT—American Society of Radiologic Technologists
ASS—argininosuccinic synthetase
ATA—alimentary toxic aleukia
ATC—addictions treatment center
ATG—antithymocyte globulin
ATL—antitension line
atm—atmosphere(s)
ATP—adenosine triphosphate
ATPase—adenosine triphosphatase
ATS—American Thoracic Society
att—attending

ATT—arginine tolerance test
AU—antitoxin unit
       arbitrary unit(s)
       each ear (L. auris utraque)
          [not: auris uterque]
Au—gold
AUA—American Urological Asso-
       ciation
AUG—acute ulcerative gingivitis
AUL—acute undifferentiated leuke-
       mia
AV—aortic valve
AV, A-V—arteriovenous
          atrioventricular
AVM—arteriovenous malformation
AVN—atrioventricular node
AVR—aortic valve replacement
A&W—alive and well
AWI—anterior wall infarction
AZT—azidothymidine [now:
       zidovudine]
b—born
Ba—barium
BA—betamethasone acetate
BA, B.A.—Bachelor of Arts
BAC—buccoaxiocervical
BAL—bronchoalveolar lavage
BAT—blunt abdominal trauma
BB—blood bank
       blue bloater [emphysema]
       both bones
       breakthrough bleeding
       breast biopsy
       buffer base
BBA—born before arrival [of doc-
       tor or midwife]
BBB—blood buffer base
BBT—basal body temperature
BC—birth control
       buccocervical
BCAA—branched-chain amino acid
BCF—basophil chemotactic factor
BCNU—bis-chloroethyl-nitrosourea
BCP, BCPs—birth control pills
BD—buccodistal
BDE—bile duct exploration
BE—barium enema
Be—beryllium

BF—bouillon filtrate (tuberculin)
BG—bone graft
       buccogingival
BHAPs—bisheteroarylpiperazines
       [a class of drugs]
BI—burn index
Bi—bismuth
b.i.d.—twice a day (L. bis in die)
BiPAP—bilateral positive airway
       pressure
BL—baseline
       blood loss
       borderline
       buccolingual
BLB—Boothby-Lovelace-Bulbulian
BLN—bronchial lymph nodes
BLS—basic life support
BM—body mass
       bone marrow
       bowel movement
       buccomesial
BMET—basic metabolic panel
       [also: profile]
BMG—benign monoclonal gam-
       mopathy
BMP—basic metabolic panel [also:
       profile]
BMR—basal metabolic rate
BO—bucco-occlusal
BOM—bilateral otitis media
BOOP—bronchiolitis obliterans
       organizing pneumonia
BP—bathroom privileges
       birthplace
       blood pressure
       bypass
BPD—biparietal diameter
BPH—benign prostatic hyperplasia
       benign prostatic hypertrophy
bpm—beats per minute
Bq—becquerel(s)
BR—bathroom
       bed rest, bedrest
Br—breath
       bridge
BRAT—bananas, rice cereal, apple-
       sauce, toast [diet]
BRM—biuret-reactive material

BRP—bathroom privileges
    bilirubin production
BRW—Brown-Roberts-Wells
BS—Babinski sign
    blood sugar
    bowel sounds
    breaking strength
B/S—breath sounds
BS, B.S.—Bachelor of Science
BSA—bismuth-sulfite agar
    body surface area
BSB—body surface burned
BSE—bilateral, symmetrical, and
    equal
    breast self-examination
BSER—brain stem evoked response
BSF—backscatter factor
    basal skull fracture
BSI—bound serum iron
BSN—bowel sounds normal
BSO—bilateral salpingo-oophorec-
    tomy
BSR—basal skin resistance
BSS—balanced salt solution
    black silk suture
    buffered saline solution
BSV—binocular single vision
BT—bladder tumor
    brain tumor
BTB—breakthrough bleeding
BTE—behind the ear
BTL—bilateral tubal ligation
BTR—Bezold-type reflex
BTU—British thermal unit
BU—base (of prism) up
    Bodansky unit
    burn unit
BUDR—bromodeoxyuridine [now:
    broxuridine]
BUE—both upper extremities
BUN—blood urea nitrogen
BUO—bleeding of undetermined
    origin
BUS—Bartholin, urethral, Skene
    [glands]
BV—biologic value
    blood vessel
    blood volume

BV— (continued)
    bronchovesicular
BVA—best corrected visual acuity
BVH—biventricular hypertrophy
BVI—blood vessel invasion
BW—biological warfare
    birthweight
Bx—biopsy
$\bar{c}$—with (L. cum)
c—calorie
    cup
    homeopathic symbol for
        centesimal scale of poten-
        cies ($1/100^c$)
C—calculus
    carbohydrate
    Caucasian
    Celsius
    centigrade
    certified
    cervical
    chest
    clearance rate
    clonus
    closure
    color sense
    contraction
    contracture
    correct
    hundred
C.—Clostridium
    Cryptococcus
°C—degree Celsius
    degree centigrade [pref:
        degree Celsius]
C1 through C7—cervical vertebrae
    1–7
C1–C9—complement components
    1–9 (C1q, C1r, C1s to C9q,
    C9r, C9s)
CA—cardiac-apnea
    cardiac arrest
    cardiac arrhythmia
    carotid artery
    cervicoaxial
    cholic acid
    chronological age
    cold agglutinin

CA— (continued)
    corneal abrasion
    coronary angiography
    coronary arrest
    coronary artery
    corpora amylacea
    croup-associated [virus]
Ca—calcium
Ca, CA—cancer
    carcinoma
CAB—coronary artery bypass
CABG—coronary artery bypass graft
CACC—cathodal closure contraction
CACG—cineangiocardiogram
CAD—cadaver
    computer-assisted design
    computer-assisted diagnosis
    coronary artery disease
CADTe—cathodal-duration tetanus
CAF—continuous atrial fibrillation
    coronary arteriovenous fistula
    cyclophosphamide, Adria-
      mycin, fluorouracil
CAG—chronic atrophic gastritis
CAH—chronic active hepatitis
    congenital adrenal hyperpla-
      sia
CAHC—chronic active hepatitis
    with cirrhosis
CAHD—coronary arteriosclerotic
    heart disease
    coronary atherosclerotic
      heart disease
CAI—computer-assisted instruction
CAL—computer-assisted learning
Cal, Kcal—kilocalorie
C_{alb}—albumin clearance
CALLA—common acute lym-
    phoblastic leukemia antigen
C_{am}—amylase clearance
CAM—Caucasian adult male
    chorioallantoic membrane
    computer-assisted myelogra-
      phy
    contralateral axillary metas-
      tasis
CAMP—computer-assisted menu
    planning

cAMP, cyclic AMP—cyclic adeno-
    sine monophosphate
CAO—chronic airway obstruction
cap.—capsule (L. capsula)
CAP—catabolite activator protein
    College of American Pathol-
      ogists
CAPD—continuous ambulatory
    peritoneal dialysis
CAPS—caffeine, alcohol, pepper,
    spicy foods
CAS—chronic alcohol syndrome
CAST—Cardiac Arrhythmia Sup-
    pression Trial
    color allergy screening test
CAT—computerized axial tomogra-
    phy
cath—cathartic
CAV—congenital absence of vagina
    congenital adrenal virilism
    croup-associated virus
    cyclophosphamide, Adria-
      mycin, vincristine
CAVB—complete atrioventricular
    block
CAVH—continuous arteriovenous
    hemofiltration
CB—chronic bronchitis
C&B—crown and bridge
CBA—chronic bronchitis with asth-
    ma
CBBB—complete bundle branch
    block
CBC—complete blood count
CBD—common bile duct
CBF—cerebral blood flow
    coronary blood flow
CBG—corticosteroid-binding glob-
    ulin
    cortisol-binding globulin
CBI—continuous bladder irrigation
CBP—complete breech presentation
CBS—capillary blood sugar
    chronic brain syndrome
CBV—catheter balloon valvuloplasty
    central blood volume
    circulating blood volume
    corrected blood volume

CBW—chemical and biological warfare

cc, cm³ [cm3], cu cm—cubic centimeter(s)

CC—cardiac cycle
cervical collar
chest compression
circulatory collapse
clinical course
closing capacity
commission certified
cord compression
costochondral
cradle cap
critical care
critical condition
current complaints

CC, C_{cr}—creatinine clearance

CC, C/C—chief complaint

CCA—circumflex coronary artery
common carotid artery
congenital contractural arachnodactyly

CCAT—conglutinating complement absorption test

CCC—cathodal-closing contraction
cathodal closure contraction
chronic calculous cholecystitis
consecutive case conference

CCCl—cathodal-closure clonus

CCF—carotid cavernous fistula
cephalin-cholesterol flocculation
compound comminuted fracture
congestive cardiac failure

CCK—cholecystokinin

CCN—coronary care nursing

CCP—chronic calcifying pancreatitis

CCPD—continuous cycled peritoneal dialysis

C_{cr}, CC—creatinine clearance

CCS—casualty clearing station

CCT—composite cyclic therapy
cranial computed tomography

CCTe—cathodal-closure tetanus

CCU—coronary care unit
critical care unit

CCW—counterclockwise

CD—cadaver donor
cardiac disease
cardiac dullness
caudal
common duct
conjugata diagonalis, conjugate diameter (diagonal conjugate diameter of pelvic inlet)
consanguineous donor
curative dose
cystic duct

C/D, C/d—cigarettes per day

CD_{50} [CD50]—median curative dose

C&D—cystoscopy and dilatation

CDC—calculated date of confinement
Centers for Disease Control and Prevention
chenodeoxycholate

CDCA—chenodeoxycholic acid

CDD—certificate of disability for discharge

CDE—chlordiazepoxide (Librium)
common duct exploration

CDH—chronic daily headache
congenital diaphragmatic hernia
congenital dislocation of the hip

CDI—Children's Depression Inventory

CDILD—chronic diffuse interstitial lung disease

CDP—comprehensive discharge planning
cytidine diphosphate

CDR—clinical dementia rating
computed digital radiography
cup-to-disk ratio

CDSS—clinical decision support system

CDU—chemical dependency unit

CE—cardiac enlargement
cerebral edema

CE— (continued)
    cholesterol esters
    contractile element
CEA—carcinoembryonic antigen
    carotid endarterectomy
CECT—contrast-enhanced computed tomography
CEG—chronic erosive gastritis
cent—centimeter
CEOM—chronic exudative otitis media
CEP—cortical evoked potential
    counterelectrophoresis
CER—central episiotomy and repair
CERA—cortical evoked response audiometry
Cert—certified
CES—central excitatory state
    clitoral engorgement syndrome
CESD—cholesteryl ester storage disease
CES-D—Center for Epidemiological Studies of Depression
cf—compare (L. confer)
CF—carbolfuchsin
    cardiac failure
    carrier-free
    Caucasian female
    chemotactic factor
    Christmas factor
    citrovorum factor
    complement fixation, complement-fixing
    contractile force
    count fingers
    cystic fibrosis
CFA—common femoral artery
    complement-fixing antibody
    complete Freund adjuvant
    craniofacial abnormality
CFF—critical flicker fusion test
    critical fusion frequency
CFIDS—chronic fatigue immune deficiency syndrome
CFP—chronic false-positive
    cystic fibrosis of pancreas
CFS—chronic fatigue syndrome

CFT—clinical full-time
    complement fixation test
cfu—colony-forming unit(s)
CG—Cardio-Green
    choking gas (phosgene)
    chorionic gonadotropin
    chronic glomerulonephritis
    colloidal gold
CGI—clinical global impression
CGL—chronic granulocytic leukemia
c̄ gl—correction with glasses
cGMP, 3′,5′-GMP—cyclic guanosine monophosphate
CGN—chronic glomerulonephritis
CG/OQ—cerebral glucose oxygen quotient
CGP—choline glycerophosphatide
    chorionic growth hormone prolactin
    circulating granulocyte pool
CGRP—calcitonin gene-related peptide
CGS—catgut suture
CGS, c.g.s.—centimeter-gram-second
CGT—chorionic gonadotropin
CGTT—cortisone glucose tolerance test
CH—case history
    community health
    convalescent hospital
    conversion hysteria
    crown-heel (length)
CHA—congenital hypoplastic anemia
    chronic hemolytic anemia
CHB—complete heart block
CHC—community health center
CHD—childhood disease
    congenital heart disease
CHE—cholinesterase
chem—chemistry [panel, profile]
CHF—congestive heart failure
CHH—cartilage-hair hypoplasia
CHI—closed head injury
CHL—chloramphenicol
CHO—carbohydrate (diet order)
chol—cholesterol
Chol est—cholesterol esters

CHOP—cyclophosphamide, hydroxydaunomycin, Oncovin, prednisone
CHP—child psychiatry
    comprehensive health planning
chr—chronic
Chr.—Chromobacterium
CHS—cholinesterase
    compression hip screw
CI—cardiac index
    cardiac insufficiency
    cerebral infarction
    clinical investigator
    colloidal iron
    complete iridectomy
    coronary insufficiency
    crystalline insulin
Ci—curie(s)
CIBD—chronic inflammatory bowel disease
CICE—combined intracapsular cataract extraction
CICU—cardiac intensive care unit
    coronary intensive care unit
CID—combined immunodeficiency disease
    cytomegalic inclusion disease
CIDS—cellular immune deficiency syndrome
    continuous insulin delivery system
CIE, CIEP—counterimmunoelectrophoresis
cig—cigarettes
CIHD—chronic ischemic heart disease
CIL—center for independent living
C_{in}—insulin clearance
CIN—cervical intraepithelial neoplasia
CIOH—chronic idiopathic orthostatic hypotension
CIPN—chronic idiopathic peripheral neuropathy
circ—circulation
    circumcision

CIS—carcinoma in situ
    central inhibitory state
CIT—crisis intervention therapy
CIXU—constant infusion excretory urogram
CJD—Creutzfeldt-Jakob disease
ck—check
CK—creatine kinase
CL—chest and left arm (ECG lead)
    Clostridium
Cl—chloride
    chlorine
CLAS—congenital localized absence of skin
CLD—chronic lung disease
CLL—chronic lymphocytic leukemia
CLO—cod liver oil
cm—centimeter
cm^2 [cm2], sq cm—square centimeter
cm^3 [cm3], cc, cu cm—cubic centimeter(s)
CM—capreomycin
    chloroquine-mepacrine
    cochlear microphonic [potential]
    costal margin
CMA—Certified Medical Assistant
    chronic metabolic acidosis
CMB—carbolic methylene blue
CMC—carpometacarpal (joint)
    critical micellar concentration
CME—continuing medical education
    cystoid macular edema
CMET—comprehensive metabolic panel [also: profile]
CMF—chondromyxoid fibroma
    cyclophosphamide, methotrexate, 5-fluorouracil
CMGN—chronic membranous glomerulonephritis
CMHC—community mental health center
cm H_2O [cm H2O]—centimeter(s) of water
CMI—cell-mediated immunity
    cellular-mediated immune [response]

CMI— (continued)
    cytomegalic inclusion
c/min—cycle(s) per minute
CML—cell-mediated lympholysis
    chronic myelocytic leukemia
    chronic myelogenous leuke-
        mia
    chronic myeloid leukemia
CMM—cutaneous malignant mela-
    noma
CMN—cystic medial necrosis
CMN-AA—cystic medial necrosis
    of the ascending aorta
CMO—cardiac minute output
    comfort measures only
C-MOPP—cyclophosphamide,
    mechlorethamine, Oncovin,
    procarbazine, prednisone
CMP—complete metabolic panel
    [also: profile]
    comprehensive metabolic
        panel [also: profile]
    cytidine monophosphate
CMR—carpometacarpal ratio
    cerebral metabolic rate
    crude mortality ratio
CMRG—cerebral metabolic rate of
    glucose
CMRO—cerebral metabolic rate of
    oxygen
CMS—Clyde Mood Scale
CMT—Certified Massage Therapist
    Certified Medical Transcrip-
        tionist
    Charcot-Marie-Tooth [atro-
        phy, disease, syndrome]
CMV—continuous mechanical ven-
    tilation
    cytomegalovirus
CN—clinical nursing
    cranial nerve
    cyanogen
CNA—Certified Nurse Anesthetist
CND—cause not determined
    congenital neuromuscular
        disorder
CNE—chronic nervous exhaustion
CNH—community nursing home

CNL—cardiolipin natural lecithin
CNM—Certified Nurse-Midwife
CNPAP—continuous nasal positive
    airway pressure
CNS—central nervous system
CNSD—chronic nonspecific diarrhea
CNV—conduction nerve velocity
co—contraction [syndrome]
c/o—complains of
CO—carbon monoxide
    cardiac output
    castor oil
    cervicoaxial
    coenzyme
    corneal opacity
    coronary occlusion
    court order
CO_2 [CO2]—carbon dioxide
Co—cobalt
^{60}Co—radioactive cobalt [cobalt Co
    60]
CoA—coenzyme A
COAD—chronic obstructive airway
    disease
coag—coagulation
COAG—chronic open-angle glau-
    coma
COC—cathodal-opening clonus
    cathodal-opening contraction
    combination-type oral con-
        traceptive
COCl—cathodal-opening clonus
COD—cause of death
    condition on discharge
COE—court-ordered examination
COG—closed angle glaucoma
COGTT—cortisone-primed oral
    glucose tolerance test
COHb—carboxyhemoglobin
COLD—chronic obstructive lung
    disease
coll—eyewash (L. collyrium)
collyr—eyewash (L. collyrium)
comp—complaint
    complication
COMS—chronic organic mental
    syndrome

COMT—catechol-*O*-methyl transferase
ConA—concanavalin A
COP—cyclophosphamide, Oncovin, prednisone
COPD—chronic obstructive pulmonary disease
COR—conditioned orientation response
CORA—conditioned orientation reflex audiometry
CORLA—clusters of radiolucent areas
COT—critical off-time
COTe—cathodal-opening tetanus
CP—cerebral palsy
    chemically pure
    chest pain
    chloropurine
    chloroquine and primaquine
    chronic pyelonephritis
    closing pressure
    cochlear potential
    combination product
    combining power
    coproporphyrin
    cor pulmonale
C/P—cholesterol-phospholipid ratio
C&P—compensation and pension
C_{pah}—para-aminohippurate clearance
CPAP—continuous positive airway pressure
CPB—cardiopulmonary bypass
CPBS—cardiopulmonary bypass surgery
CPC—cetylpyridinium chloride
    chronic passive congestion
    clinicopathologic conference
CP&C—cast post and core
CPD—calcium pyrophosphate dihydrate (crystals)
    cephalopelvic disproportion
    citrate-phosphate-dextrose
    congenital polycystic disease
CPE—cardiogenic pulmonary edema
    chronic pulmonary emphysema

CPE— (continued)
    compensation, pension, and education
CPEO—chronic progressive external ophthalmoplegia
CPI—congenital pain indifference
    constitutional psychopathic inferiority
    coronary prognostic index
CPID—chronic pelvic inflammatory disease
CPK—creatine phosphokinase [now: creatine kinase (CK)]
cpm—counts per minute
CPM—central pontine myelinolysis
    continuous passive motion
CPN—chronic pyelonephritis
CPPB—continuous positive-pressure breathing
CPPD—calcium pyrophosphate dihydrate (crystals)
CPR—cardiopulmonary resuscitation
    cerebral-cortex perfusion rate
    cortisol production rate
c.p.s., cps—cycles per second (Hz)
CPS—carbamoyl phosphate synthetase
    clinical performance score
    cumulative probability of success
CPT—chest physiotherapy
CPZ—chlorpromazine
CQ—chloroquine-quinine
    circadian quotient
CR—calculus removed
    chest and right arm (ECG lead)
    colon resection
    complete remission
    conditioned reflex
    conditioned response
    conversion reaction
    corneal reflex
    crown-rump (length)
CR1, CR2, CR3, CR4—complement receptors 1, 2, 3, 4
^{51}Cr—radioactive chromium [chromium Cr 51]

CRAO—central retinal artery occlusion

CRBBB—complete right bundle branch block

CRC—crisis resolution center

CRD—chronic renal disease
chronic respiratory disease
crown-rump distance

creat—creatinine

CREST—calcinosis cutis, Raynaud phenomenon, esophageal dysfunction/hypermotility, sclerodactyly, telangiectasia [syndrome]

CRF—cardiac risk factor(s)
chronic renal failure
corticotropin-releasing factor

CRH—corticotropin-releasing hormone

CRI—cardiac risk index
chronic renal insufficiency

CRL—crown-rump length

CRM—cross-reacting material

CRNA—Certified Registered Nurse Anesthetist

CROS—contralateral routing of signals

CRP—C-reactive protein

CRS—Chinese restaurant syndrome
colorectal surgery

CRU—clinical research unit

CRV—central retinal vein

CRVO—central retinal vein occlusion

CS—Central Service
Central Supply
cesarean section
chondroitin sulfate
conditioned stimulus
conscious
coronary sinus
corticosteroid
current strength
cycloserine

C&S—conjunctiva and sclera
culture and sensitivity

CSA—chondroitin sulfate A
criminal sexual assault

CSC—blow-on-blow (Fr. coup sur coup)

C-section—cesarean section

CSF—cerebrospinal fluid
colony-stimulating factor

CSH—chronic subdural hematoma
cortical stromal hyperplasia

CSIU—cardiac surgery intermediate unit

CSL—cardiolipin synthetic lecithin

CSLR—crossed straight leg raising [test]

CSM—corn-soy milk

CSMT—capillary refill, sensation, motor function, temperature

CSN—carotid sinus nerve

CSR—Cheyne-Stokes respiration
corrected sedimentation rate
cortisol secretion rate

CSS—carotid sinus stimulation

CT—cardiothoracic
carotid tracing
carpal tunnel
cerebral thrombosis
chlorothiazide
circulation time
clotting time
coagulation time
collecting tubule
computed tomography
connective tissue
contraction time
coronary thrombosis
corrected transposition
corrective therapy
cover test
crest time
cytotechnologist

CTAB—cetyltrimethylammonium bromide [now: cetrimonium bromide (CTBA)]

CTAP—clear to auscultation and percussion

CTC—chlortetracycline

CTD—carpal tunnel decompression
congenital thymic dysplasia

CTH—ceramide trihexoside

CTL—cytotoxic T lymphocyte

CTR—cardiothoracic ratio
CTS—carpal tunnel syndrome
CTx—chemotherapy
CTZ—chemoreceptor trigger zone
    chlorothiazide
cu—cubic
C_u—urea clearance
CU—convalescent unit
cu cm, cm^3 [cm3], cc—cubic cen-
    timeter(s)
CUG—cystourethrogram
cu mm, mm^3 [mm3]—cubic mil-
    limeter(s)
CUSA—Cavitron ultrasonic aspirator
CV—cardiovascular
    central venous
    cerebrovascular
    closing volume
    color vision
    conjugata vera
    conversational voice
    corpuscular volume
    cresyl violet, cresylecht violet
CVA—cardiovascular accident
    cerebrovascular accident
    costovertebral angle
CVAT—costovertebral angle tender-
    ness
CVB—chorionic villus biopsy
CVC—central venous catheter
CVD—cardiovascular disease
    cerebrovascular disease
    collagen vascular disease
CVF—central visual field
CVH—combined ventricular hyper-
    trophy
    common variable hypogam-
      maglobulinemia
CVI—cerebrovascular insufficiency
    common variable immuno-
      deficiency
CVIU—cardiovascular intermediate
    unit
CVO—central vein occlusion
    conjugate diameter of pelvic
      inlet (L. conjugata vera
      obstetrica)

CVOD—cerebrovascular occlusive
    disease
CVP—central venous pressure
    cyclophosphamide, vincris-
      tine, prednisone
CVR—cardiovascular-respiratory
    [system]
    cerebrovascular resistance
CVRD—cardiovascular renal disease
CVS—cardiovascular surgery
    cardiovascular system
    clean-voided specimen
cw—clockwise
CW—cardiac work
    case work
    chemical warfare
    chest wall
    children's ward
    continuous wave
CWP—childbirth without pain
CWS—cotton-wool spot
cx—cervix
    convex
CX, CXr—chest x-ray
Cx—cancel
CxMT—cervical motion tenderness
Cy—cyanogen
cyclic AMP, cAMP—cyclic adeno-
    sine monophosphate
cyclic GMP, cGMP—cyclic guano-
    sine monophosphate
cyclo—cyclophosphamide
    cyclopropane
Cys—cysteine
Cys-Cys—cystine
cysto—cystoscopy
CZI—crystalline zinc insulin
d—dextro- [prefix]
d—diameter
    dose (L. dosis)
    give (L. da)
    right (L. dexter)
d.—day (L. die)
D—daughter
    dead
    deciduous
    density
    dermatology

D— (continued)
    deuterium
    deuteron
    died
    diopter
    diplomate
    distal
    divorced
    dorsal
    duration
    mean dose
    vitamin D unit
DA—degenerative arthritis
    dental assistant
    developmental age
    direct agglutination
    disaggregated
    dopamine
    ductus arteriosus
Da—dalton
dA—deoxyadenosine
DAB—dimethylaminoazobenzene
DAD—delayed after-depolarization
dADP—deoxyadenosine disphos-
    phate
DAF—decay antibody-accelerating
    factor
DAG—diacylglycerol
DAH—disordered action of the heart
DALA—δ-aminolevulinic acid
    [delta-]
DAM—degraded amyloid
    diacetyl monoxime
dAMP—deoxyadenosine mono-
    phosphate
DAN—diabetic autonomic neuropa-
    thy
DAO—diamine oxidase
DAP—dihydroxyacetone phosphate
    direct agglutination pregnan-
    cy (test)
DAPT—direct agglutination preg-
    nancy test
Dapt—Daptazole
DAT—differential agglutination titer
    diphtheria antitoxin
    direct antiglobulin test
dATP—deoxyadenosine triphosphate

db—disability
DB—date of birth
    dextran blue
    distobuccal
dB, db—decibel
DBA—dibenzanthracene
DBC—dye-binding capacity
DBCL—dilute blood clot lysis
    (method)
DBM—demineralized bone matrix
    dibromomannitol
DBO—distobucco-occlusal
DBP—diastolic blood pressure
    distobuccopulpal
DC—daily census
    deoxycholate
    diagnostic code
    diphenylarsine cyanide
    direct current
    discharge
    discontinue
    distocervical
DC, D.C.—Doctor of Chiropractic
D&C—dilatation and curettage
    dilation and curettage
DCA—deoxycholate-citrate agar
    deoxycholic acid
    desoxycorticosterone acetate
DCC—double concave
dCDP—deoxycitidine diphosphate
DCF—direct centrifugal flotation
DCG—disodium cromoglycate
DCHFB—dichlorohexafluorobutane
DCI—dichloroisoproterenol
dCMP—deoxycitidine monophos-
    phate
D_{co} [DCO]—diffusing capacity for
    carbon monoxide
DCTMA—desoxycorticosterone tri-
    methylacetate
dCTP—deoxycitidine triphosphate
DCTPA—desoxycorticosterone
    triphenylacetate
DCx—double convex
DD—died of the disease
    differential diagnosis
    disk diameter

D&D—Drake and Drake [medical reference books]
DDAVP—desmopressin acetate [trademarked name]
DDC—diethyldithiocarbamic acid
direct display console
DDC, ddC—dideoxycytidine
DDD—degenerative disk disease
dichlorodiphenyl-dichloroethane
DDH—dissociated double hyper-tropia
DDP, cis-DDP—cisplatin
DDS, D.D.S.—Doctor of Dental Surgery
DDT—dichlorodiphenyl-trichloro-ethane
DDx—differential diagnosis
discharge diagnosis
DE—dream elements
duration of ejection
D&E—dilatation and evacuation
dilation and evacuation
DEAE—diethylaminoethanol
diethylaminoethyl
DEAE-D—diethylaminoethyl dextran
DEBA—diethylbarbituric acid
dec—deceased
deciduous
decoct
decoction
decrease
DEC—dendritic epidermal cell
decr—decrease
decub—lying down (L. decubitus)
DEF, def—decayed, extracted, filled
def—deficiency
deg—degree
del—delivery
Dem—Demerol (meperidine)
dep—dependent(s)
derm—dermatology
DES—diethylstilbestrol
diffuse esophageal spasm
dest—distilled (L. destilla)
DET—diethyltryptamine
DEXA—dual energy x-ray absorp-tiometry [scan]

DF—decapacitation factor
deficiency factor
degree of freedom
desferrioxamine
diabetic father
discriminant function
disseminated foci
DFA—direct fluorescent antibody [test]
DFDT—difluorodiphenyl-trichloro-ethane
DFO—deferoxamine
DFP—diisopropyl fluorophosphate
DFU—dead fetus in utero
dideoxyfluorouridine
dg—decigram
DG—deoxyglucose
diastolic gallop
diglyceride
distogingival
DG, Dx—diagnosis
DH—delayed hypersensitivity
DHA—dihydroxyacetone
DHAP—dihydroxyacetone phosphate
DHE—dihydroergotamine
DHEA—dehydroepiandrosterone
DHEAS—dehydroepiandrosterone sulfate
DHFR—dihydrofolate reductase
DHIA—dehydroisoandrosterone
DHL—diffuse histiocytic lymphoma
DHT—dihydrotachysterol
dihydrotestosterone
DI—diagnostic imaging
diag—diagnosis
DIC—diffuse intravascular coagula-tion
disseminated intravascular coagulation
DID—dead of intercurrent disease
DIE—died in Emergency Room
DIM—divalent ion metabolism
DIMOAD—diabetes insipidus, dia-betes mellitus, optic atrophy, deafness [syndrome]
DIP—desquamative interstitial pneumonia
diisopropyl phosphate

DIP— (continued)
    distal interphalangeal
DIPJ—distal interphalangeal joint
dis—disease
disc—discontinue
disch—discharge
DISI—dorsiflexion intercalated segment instability
DISIDA—diisopropyliminodiacetic acid
disp—dispensatory
    dispense
dist—distill
DIT—diet-induced thermogenesis
    diiodotyrosine
div—divide
DJD—degenerative joint disease
DK—decay
    dog kidney
DKA—diabetic ketoacidosis
dL, dl—deciliter
DL—danger list
    difference limen
    distolingual
    Donath-Landsteiner (test)
D_L [DL]—diffusing capacity of lung
DLA—distolabial
DLAI—distolabioincisal
$D_L CO$ [DLCO]—diffusing capacity of lung for carbon monoxide
DLE—disseminated lupus erythematosus
DLI—distolinguoincisal
DLO—distolinguo-occlusal
DLP—distolinguopulpal
DM—diabetic mother
    diastolic murmur
    dopamine
DMA—dimethyladenosine
DMAB—dimethylamino-benzaldehyde
DMARD—disease-modifying antirheumatic drug
DMBA—dimethylbenzanthracene
DMCT—demethylchlortetracycline
DMD, D.M.D.—Doctor of Dental Medicine

DMF—decayed, missing, or filled (teeth)
DMM—dimethylmyleran
DMN—dimethylnitrosamine
DMO—dimethyloxazolidinedione
DMPA—depomedroxyprogesterone acetate
DMPE—3,4-dimethoxyphenylethylamine
DMPP—dimethylphenyl-piperazinium
DMS—dimethylsulfoxide
DMSO—dimethylsulfoxide
DMT—dimethyltryptamine
DN—dicrotic notch
D/N—dextrose-nitrogen [ratio]
D&N—distance and near [vision]
DNA—deoxyribonucleic acid
DNase—deoxyribonuclease
DNB—dinitrobenzene
DNC—dinitrocarbanilide
DND—died a natural death
DNFB—dinitrofluorobenzene
DNP—deoxyribonucleoprotein
DNPH—dinitrophenylhydrazine
DNPM—dinitrophenylmorphine
DNR—do not resuscitate
DNT—did not test
DO—diamine oxidase
    disto-occlusal
DO, D.O.—Doctor of Osteopathy
DOA—dead on arrival
DOB—date of birth
DOC—deoxycholate
    deoxycorticosterone
    died of other causes
DOCA—deoxycorticosterone acetate
DOCs—deoxycorticoids
DOD—date of death
    dead of disease
DOE—dyspnea on exertion
DOM—deaminated-O-methyl metabolite
    dimethoxymethyl amphetamine
DOMA—dihydroxymandelic acid
DON—diazo-oxonorleucine
DOPA—dihydroxyphenylalanine

DOPAC—dihydroxyphenylacetic acid
DP—dementia praecox
    diastolic pressure
    directional preponderance
    disability pension
    distopulpal
DPA—dipropylacetate
DPC—delayed primary closure
DPDL—diffuse poorly differentiated lymphoma
DPG—diphosphoglycerate
    displacement placentogram
DPGM—diphosphoglyceromutase
DPGP—diphosphoglycerate phosphatase
DPH—diphenylhydantoin
DPI—disposable personal income
DPL—distopulpolingual
dpm—disintegrations per minute
DPM, D.P.M.—Doctor of Podiatric Medicine
DPN—diphosphopyridine nucleotide
DPO—dimethoxyphenyl penicillin
DPS—dimethylpolysiloxane
DPT—diphtheria, pertussis, tetanus
    dipropyltryptamine
DPVNS—diffuse pigmented villonodular synovitis
DQ—developmental quotient
DR—diabetic retinopathy
dr—drachm
    drain
Dr.—doctor
DRF—dose-reduction factor
DRGs—diagnosis related groups
DRI—Discharge Readiness Inventory
DS—dead space
    dextrose-saline
    dry swallow
DSA—digital subtraction angiography
    digital subtraction arteriography
DSAP—disseminated superficial actinic porokeratosis
DSC, DSCG—disodium cromoglycate

DSM—dextrose solution mixture
DT—diphtheria [vaccine] and tetanus toxoids [vaccine]
    distance test
    duration tetany
    dye test
dT—diphtheria [booster] and tetanus toxoids [vaccine]
DT, DTs—delirium tremens
DTBC—D-tubocurarine
DTBN—di-*tert*-butyl nitroxide
DTC—D-tubocurarine
dTDP—deoxythymidine diphosphate
DTH—delayed-type hypersensitivity
DTIC—dacarbazine
D time—dream time
DTM—dermatophyte test medium
DTMP—deoxythymidine monophosphate
DTN—diphtheria toxin normal
DTNB—dithiobisnitrobenzoic acid
DTP—diphtheria and tetanus (toxoids) pertussis (vaccine)
    distal tingling on pressure
DTPA—diethylenetriaminepentaacetic acid [now: pentetic acid]
DTRs—deep tendon reflexes
dTTP—deoxythymidine triphosphate
DTZ—diatrizoate
DU—deoxyuridine
    diagnosis undetermined
    dog unit
DUB—dysfunctional uterine bleeding
DUMP—deoxyuridine monophosphate
duod—duodenum
DUSN—diffuse unilateral subacute neuroretinitis
DV—dependent variable
    dilute volume
    double vision
D&V—diarrhea and vomiting
DVA—distance visual acuity
DVD—dissociated vertical deviation
    dissociated vertical divergence
DVT—deep vein thrombosis
    deep venous thrombosis

DW—distilled water
    dry weight
D/W—dextrose in water
D5W, D$_5$W, D5/W—5% dextrose in water
Dx, DG—diagnosis
DX—dextran
DXA—dual x-ray absorptiometry
DXD—discontinued
DXM—dexamethasone
DXT—deep x-ray therapy
Dy—dysprosium
DZ—dizygous (twins)
E—electric charge
    electromotive force
    electron emmetropia
    energy
    epinephrine
    erythrocyte
    esophoria
    esotropia
    experimenter
    eye
E.—Entamoeba
    Escherichia
ea—each
EA—educational age
    erythrocyte antibody
    ethacrynic acid
E&A—evaluate and advise
EAA—extrinsic allergic alveolitis
EAb, EAB—elective abortion
EAC—Ehrlich ascites carcinoma
    erythrocyte antibody complement
    external auditory canal
EACA—epsilon-aminocaproic acid
EACD—extrinsic allergic contact dermatitis
EAHF—eczema, asthma, hay fever
EAM—external auditory meatus
EAP—epiallopregnanolone
EAST—external rotation and abduction stress test
EB—elementary body
    epidermolysis bullosa
    Epstein-Barr [virus]
    escape beat

EB— (continued)
    estradiol benzoate
EBF—elastic band fixation [of fracture]
    erythroblastosis fetalis
EBI—emetine bismuth iodide
EBL—estimated blood loss
EBNA—Epstein-Barr nuclear antigen [test]
EBV—Epstein-Barr virus
EC—ejection click
    electron capture
    enteric-coated (aspirin, tablets)
    entrance complaint
    Escherichia coli
    exaltation-contraction
    extracapsular
    extracellular
    eyes closed
EC, ECA—ethacrynic acid
ECAT—emission computerized axial tomography
ECBV—effective circulating blood volume
ECC—edema, clubbing, cyanosis
    endocervical curettage
    extracapsular cataract
    extracorporeal circulation
ECCE—extracapsular cataract extraction
ECD—endothelial corneal dystrophy
ECE—endocervical ecchymosis
ECF—eosinophil chemotactic factor
    epicanthic fold
    extended care facility
ECFA—eosinophil chemotactic factor of anaphylaxis
ECG—electrocardiogram
    electrocardiography
ECHO—enteric cytopathogenic human orphan [now: echovirus]
ECIB—extracorporeal irradiation of blood
ECIL—extracorporeal irradiation of lymph
ECM—erythema chronicum migrans
    extracellular material

E. coli—Escherichia coli
ECS—electroconvulsive shock
ECT—emission computed tomography
ECV—extracellular volume
ECW—extracellular water
ED—effective dose
 epileptiform discharge
 erythema dose
ED_{50} [ED50]—median effective dose
EDB—ethylene dibromide
EDC—estimated date of confinement
 expected date of confinement
EDD—expected date of delivery
EDP—electronic data processing
 end-diastolic pressure
EDR—electrodermal response
EDTA—edetic acid
 ethylenediaminetetra-acetic acid
 ethylenediaminetetra-acetate
EDV—end-diastolic volume
EE—end-to-end
 eye and ear
EEA—electroencephalic audiometry
EEC—enteropathogenic *Escherichia coli*
EEE—eastern equine encephalomyelitis
EEG—electroencephalogram
 electroencephalography
EEME—ethinylestradiol methyl ether
EENT—eyes, ears, nose, and throat
EER—electroencephalic response
EF—ectopic focus
 ejection fraction
 encephalitogenic factor
EFA—extrafamily adoptees
EFA, EFAs—essential fatty acid(s)
EFC—endogenous fecal calcium
EFE—endocardial fibroelastosis
e.g.—for example (L. exempli gratia)
EG—esophagogastrectomy
EGA—estimated gestational age
EGF—epidermal growth factor
EGG—electrogastrogram
EGM—electrogram

EGOT—erythrocyte glutamic-oxaloacetic transaminase
EH—essential hypertension
EHBF—estimated hepatic blood flow
 extrahepatic blood flow
EHC—enterohepatic circulation
 essential hypercholesterolemia
EHDP— ethane hydroxydiphosphate
EHF—exophthalmos-hyperthyroid factor
EHL—endogenous hyperlipidemia
EHO—extrahepatic obstruction
EHP—excessive heat production
E/I—expiration-inspiration ratio
EID—electroimmunodiffusion
 emergency infusion device
EIEC—enteroinvasive *Escherichia coli*
EIP—extensor indicis proprius
EIT—erythrocyte iron turnover
EK—erythrokinase
EKC—epidemic keratoconjunctivitis
EKG [pref: ECG]—electrocardiogram
 electrocardiography
EKY—electrokymogram
el—elixir
ELAM—endothelial leukocyte adhesion molecule
elb—elbow
ELITT—endometrial laser intrauterine thermotherapy
elix—elixir
ELT—euglobulin lysis time
EM—ejection murmur
 erythrocyte mass
Em—emanation
 emmetropia
EM, EMC—electron microscopy
EMB—embryology
 eosin methylene blue
 ethambutol
 ethambutol-myambutol
EMC—encephalomyocarditis
EMD—electromechanical dissociation

EMF—electromagnetic flowmeter
electromotive force
endomyocardial fibrosis
erythrocyte maturation factor
EMG—electromyogram
electromyography
exophthalmos, macroglossia,
gigantism
EMI—Electric and Musical Industries (brain scanner)
electromagnetic interference
EMIT—enzyme-multiplied immunoassay technique
emp—a plaster (L. emplastrum)
EMS—emergency medical service
EMT—emergency medical technician
emul—emulsion
EN—enema
erythema nodosum
ENG—electronystagmogram
electronystagmography
ENL—erythema nodosum leprosum
ENT—ear, nose, and throat
EO—eosinophil
ethylene oxide
eyes open
eod—entry on duty
EOG—electro-oculogram
electro-olfactogram
EOM—extraocular movement(s)
extraocular muscle(s)
EOMI—extraocular muscles intact
eos—eosinophils
EP—ectopic pregnancy
erythrocyte protoporphyrin
EPA—eicosapentaenoic acid
EPC—epilepsia partialis continua
EPEC—enteropathogenic *Escherichia coli*
EPF—exophthalmos-producing factor
epith—epithelium
EPL—extracorporeal piezoelectric
lithotriptor
EPP—end-plate potential
erythropoietic protoporphyria
EPR—electron paramagnetic reso-
nance

EPR— (continued)
electrophrenic respiration
estradiol production rate
EPS—electrophysiology study
exophthalmos-producing
substance
expressed prostatic secretions
extrapyramidal signs
extrapyramidal symptoms
EPSP—excitatory postsynaptic
potential
EPTE—existed prior to enlistment
EPTS—existed prior to service
eq—equivalent
ER—ejection rate
emergency room
endoplasmic reticulum
estrogen receptor
evoked response
external resistance
Er—erbium
ERA—electric response audiometry
evoked response audiometry
ERC—endoscopic retrograde
cholangiography
ERCP—endoscopic retrograde
cholangiopancreatography
ERG—electroretinogram
ERP—effective refractory period
equine rhinopneumonitis
estrogen receptor protein
ERV—expiratory reserve volume
ES—end-to-side
Expectation Score
Es—einsteinium
ESB—electrical stimulation to brain
ESC—electromechanical slope
computer
Esch.—*Escherichia*
ESD—electronic summation device
ESF—erythropoietic-stimulating
factor
ESL—end-systolic length
ESM—ejection-systolic murmur
eso—esophagoscopy
esophagus
ESP—end-systolic pressure

ESP— (continued)
    eosinophil stimulation pro-
      motor
    extrasensory perception
ESR—electron spin resonance
    erythrocyte sedimentation rate
ess—essential
ESS—erythrocyte-sensitizing sub-
    stance
ess neg—essentially negative
est—estimated
EST—electric shock therapy
ESU—electrostatic unit
ESV—end-systolic volume
ESWL—extracorporeal shock wave
    lithotripsy
ET—ejection time
    endotracheal
    esotropia
    etiology
Et—ethyl
ETA—ethionamide
ETAF—epithelial thymic-activating
    factor
et al.—and others (L. et alii)
ETEC—enterotoxic *Escherichia coli*
ETH—elixir of terpin hydrate
ETH/C—elixir of terpin hydrate
    with codeine
etiol—etiology
ETKM—every test known to man
ETM—erythromycin
ETOH, EtOH—ethyl alcohol
ETOX—ethylene oxide
ETP—entire treatment period
ETT—extrathyroidal thyroxine
ETV—educational television
EU—Ehrlich unit(s)
    enzyme unit(s)
    excretory urogram
Eu—europium
EUA—examination under anesthesia
ev—electron-volt
EV—extravascular
eval—evaluation
EVG—endovascular graft
EVLW—extravascular lung water

ew—elsewhere
EW—Emergency Ward
EWB—estrogen withdrawal bleeding
EWL—egg-white lysozyme
ex—excision
    exophthalmos
exam—examination
exc—excision
exp, expir—expiration
    expired
ext—exterior
    external
    extract
F—Fahrenheit
    fat
    father
    fellow
    female
    field of vision
    filaria
    fluorine
    formula
    fusiformis
F, Fr—French [catheter gauge]
FA—far advanced
    fatty acid(s)
    femoral artery
    field ambulance
    first aid
    fluorescence assay
    fluorescent antibody
    forearm
    free acid
Fab—fragment, antigen-binding
Facb—fragment, antigen-and-com-
    plement-binding
FACD—Fellow of the American
    College of Dentists
FACOG—Fellow of the American
    College of Obstetricians and
    Gynecologists
FACP—Fellow of the American
    College of Physicians
FACS—Fellow of the American
    College of Surgeons
    fluorescence-activated cell
      sorter

FACSM—Fellow of the American College of Sports Medicine
FAD—flavin adenine dinucleotide
FADF—fluorescent antibody dark-field [examination]
FAE—follicle-associated epithelium
fam doc—family doctor
FAN—fuchsin, amido black, naphthol yellow
FAP—familial adenomatous polyposis
FAT—fluorescent antibody test
FB—fingerbreadth
 foreign body
FBP—femoral blood pressure
 fibrinogen breakdown product
FBS—fasting blood sugar
 fetal bovine serum
FC—finger clubbing
 finger counting
FCA—ferritin-conjugated antibodies
 Freund complete adjuvant
fCi—femtocurie(s)
FD—fatal dose
 focal distance
 foot drape
 freeze-dried
FD_{50} [FD50]—median fatal dose
F&D—fixed and dilated
FDA—Food and Drug Administration
FDE—final drug evaluation
FDG—2-fluoro-2-deoxyglucose
FDP—fibrin degradation product
 flexor digitorum profundus
 frontodextra posterior
 fructose 1,6-diphosphate
FDS—flexor digitorum superficialis
Fe—iron
FEC—free erythrocyte coproporphyrin
FECG—fetal electrocardiogram
FECP—free erythrocyte coproporphyria
FEF—forced expiratory flow
FEKG—fetal electrocardiogram
fem—female

FEP, FEPP—free erythrocyte protoporphyrin
FER—familial exudative retinopathy
FES—forced expiratory spirogram
FET—forced expiratory time
FETS—forced expiratory time in seconds
FEV—familial exudative vitreoretinopathy
 forced expiratory volume
FEV_1 [FEV1]—forced expiratory volume in one second
FF—fat-free
 father factor
 fecal frequency
 filtration fraction
 finger-to-finger
 flat feet
 force fluids
 forearm flow
 foster father
FFA—free fatty acid(s)
FFDW—fat-free dry weight
FFF—flicker, fusion, frequency (test)
FFM—fat-free mass
FFP—fresh frozen plasma
FFT—flicker fusion threshold
FFWW—fat-free wet weight
FG—fibrinogen
FGF—father's grandfather
 fresh gas flow
FGM—father's grandmother
FH—family history
 fetal head
 fetal heart
FHR—fetal heart rate
FHS—fetal heart sound(s)
FHT—fetal heart tone(s)
FI—fibrinogen forced inspiration
FIA—fluoroimmunoassay
 Freund incomplete adjuvant
FID—flame ionization detector
 free induction decay
FIF—forced inspiratory flow
fig—figure
FIGE—field inversion gel electrophoresis
FIGLU—formiminoglutamic acid

FIGO—Federation of International Gynecology and Obstetrics

FiO₂ [FiO2]—fractional concentration of inspired oxygen

fist—fistula

FITC—fluorescein isothiocyanate

FJN—familial juvenile nephrophthisis

fl.—fluid

FLA—left frontoanterior (L. frontolaeva anterior)

FLASH—fast low-angle shot

filt—filter

flor—flowers

fl. oz.—fluid ounce(s)

FLP—left frontoposterior (L. frontolaeva posterior)

FLSA—follicular lymphosarcoma

FLT—left frontotransverse (L. frontolaeva transversa)

Fl up—flare-up

FM—flowmeter

FME—full-mouth extraction

FMG—foreign medical graduate

FMN—flavin mononucleotide

FMR—fetal-to-maternal ratio

FMS—fat-mobilizing substance
full-mouth series

FN—false-negative
finger-to-nose

FNTC—fine-needle transhepatic cholangiography

FO—fronto-occipital

FOAVF—failure of all vital forces

FOD—free of disease

f.p.—foot-pound

FP—false-positive
family practice
freezing point
frontoparietal
frozen plasma

FPC—familial polyposis coli
fish protein concentrate

FPM—filter paper microscopic (test)

FPP—familial paroxysmal polyserositis

fps—frames per second

Fr—francium

Fr, F—French [catheter gauge]

FR—Fisher-Race (notation)
flocculation reaction
flow rate

F&R—force and rhythm (of pulse)

frag—fragility
fragment

FRC—functional reserve capacity
functional residual capacity

FRF—follicle-stimulating hormone-releasing factor

frict—friction

FROM—full range of motion

FRP—functional refractory period

FRS—furosemide

FS—full scale (IQ)
function study

FSD—focal skin distance

FSF—fibrin-stabilizing factor

FSH—follicle-stimulating hormone

FSH/LH-RH—follicle-stimulating hormone and luteinizing hormone–releasing hormone

FSH-RF—follicle-stimulating hormone–releasing factor

FSH-RH—follicle-stimulating hormone–releasing hormone

FSPs—fibrin split products

FSR—fusiform skin revision

FSW—field service worker

ft.—foot

FT—false transmitter
family therapy
fibrous tissue
free thyroxine
full term

FTA—fluorescent treponemal antibody

FTA-AB, FTA-ABS—fluorescent treponemal antibody absorption test

FTLB—full-term live birth

FTND—full-term normal delivery

FTT—failure to thrive

FU—fecal urobilinogen
fluorouracil
follow-up

FUDR, FUdR—5-fluorouracil deoxyribonucleoside [now: floxuridine]

FUO—fever of undetermined origin
fever of unknown origin

FUR—fluorouracil riboside

FV—fluid volume

FVC—forced vital capacity

FVL—femoral vein ligation

FW—Felix-Weil (reaction)
Folin and Wu (method)
fragment wound

FWHM—full width at half-maximum

FWR—Felix-Weil reaction

fx—fracture

FYI—for your information

FZ—focal zone

g—gram(s)

G—gauge
gingival
glucose
gonidial (colony)
good
gravida
Greek

GA—Gamblers Anonymous
gastric analysis
general anesthesia
gestational age
gingivoaxial
glucuronic acid
gut-associated

Ga—gallium

GABA—γ-aminobutyric acid [gamma-]

GAG—glycosaminoglycan

gal—gallon

GALT—gastrointestinal-associated lymphoid tissue
gut-associated lymphoid tissue

galv—galvanic

GAPD, GAPDH—glyceraldehyde phosphate dehydrogenase

garg—gargle

GB—gallbladder

GBA—ganglionic-blocking agent
gingivobuccoaxial

GBH—graphite-benzalkonium-heparin

GBM—glomerular basement membrane

GBS—gallbladder series

GC—gas chromatography
glucocorticoid
gonococcus
granular cast
guanine cytosine

GCA—giant cell arteritis

g-cal—gram-calorie

g-cm—gram-centimeter

GCS—general clinical service
Glasgow Coma Scale

GCSF—granulocyte colony-stimulating factor

GDA—germine diacetate

GDH—glycerophosphate dehydrogenase

GDS—Gradual Dosage Schedule

GE—gastroenterology
gastroenterostomy
General Electric

G/E—granulocyte-erythroid [ratio]

gen—general

GER—gastroesophageal reflux

GERD—gastroesophageal reflux disease

GERL—Golgi endoplasmic reticulum lysosomes

GET—gastric emptying time
general endotracheal

GET½—gastric emptying half-time

GF—germ-free
gluten-free
grandfather

GFD—gluten-free diet

GFR—glomerular filtration rate

GG—gamma globulin

GGA—general gonadotropic activity

GGT—gamma-glutamyl transferase

GGTP—gamma-glutamyl transpeptidase

GH—growth hormone

GHD—growth hormone deficiency

GH-IH—growth hormone-inhibiting hormone

GH-RF—growth hormone–releasing factor
GH-RH—growth hormone–releasing hormone
GH-RIH—growth hormone release–inhibiting hormone
GHz—gigahertz
GI—gastrointestinal
    globin insulin
GIK—glucose, insulin, and potassium
GIM—gonadotropin inhibitory material
GIP—gastric inhibitory polypeptide
    gastrointestinal polyposis
GIS—gas in stomach
    gastrointestinal system
GIT—gastrointestinal tract
GITT—glucose-insulin tolerance test
GK—glycerol kinase
GL—greatest length
GLA—gingivolinguoaxial
GLC—gas-liquid chromatography
GLI—glucagon-like immunoreactivity
glob—globulin
GLP—group living program
glu, gluc—glucose
g-m—gram-meter
GM—gastric mucosa
    general medicine
    geometric mean
    grandmother
    grand multiparity
GMA—glyceryl methacrylate
GMC—general medical council
GM-CSF—granulocyte-macrophage colony-stimulating factor
GMK—green monkey kidney
GMP—guanosine monophosphate
3′,5′-GMP, cGMP—cyclic guanosine monophosphate
GM&S—general medical and surgical
GMT—geometric mean titer
GMW—gram-molecular weight
GN—glomerulonephritis
    gram-negative

G/N—glucose-nitrogen [ratio]
GNB—gram-negative bacilli
GNID—gram-negative intracellular diplococci
Gn-RH—gonadotropin-releasing hormone
GOK—God only knows
GOT—glutamic-oxaloacetic transaminase
gp—group (muscle)
GP—general paresis
    general practice
    general practitioner
    glycoprotein
    guinea pig
    gutta-percha
GPA—grade-point average
GPAIS—guinea pig anti-insulin serum
GPC—giant papillary conjunctivitis
G6PD, G6PDH—glucose-6-phosphate dehydrogenase
GPI—general paralysis of the insane
    gingival periodontal index
    glucose phosphate isomerase
GPT—glutamic-pyruvic transaminase
GPUT—galactose phosphate uridyl transferase
gr.—grain(s)
GR—gastric resection
    glutathione reductase
GRA—gonadotropin-releasing agent
grad—gradually, by degrees
GRAS—generally recognized as safe
GRASS—gradient recalled acquisition in a steady state
GRF—gonadotropin-releasing factor
    growth hormone–releasing factor
GRH—growth hormone–releasing hormone
GRP—gastrin-releasing peptide
GS—general surgery
G/S—glucose and saline
GSA—guanidinosuccinic acid
GSC—gas-solid chromatography
    gravity-settling culture
GSD—genetically significant dose

GSE—gluten-sensitive enteropathy
GSH—glutathione (reduced)
    growth-stimulating hormone
GSR—galvanic skin response
    generalized Shwartzman
    reaction
GSSG—glutathione (oxidized)
GSSR—generalized Sanarelli-
    Shwartzman reaction
GSW—gunshot wound
gt.—drop (L. gutta)
GT—gingiva, treatment of
    glucose tolerance
    glutamyl transpeptidase
G&T—gowns and towels
GTH—gonadotropic hormone
GTN—gestational trophoblastic
    neoplasia
    glyceryl trinitrate
GTP—glutamyl transpeptidase
    guanosine triphosphate
gtt.—drops (L. guttae)
GTT—glucose tolerance test
GU—genitourinary
    gonococcal urethritis
GUS—genitourinary system
GV—gentian violet
GVH—graft-versus-host
GVHD—graft-versus-host disease
GVHR—graft-versus-host reaction
GW—group work
Gy—gray(s)
gyn, GYN—gynecology
Gy/s—gray(s) per second
GZ—Guilford-Zimmerman
H—height
    high
    Holzknecht [unit]
    horizontal
    hormone
    Hounsfield [unit]
    hour
    hydrogen
    hydrogen ion
    hypermetropia
    hyperphoria
    hypo
H.—*Haemophilus*

HA—headache
    height age
    hemadsorbent
    hemagglutinating antibody
    high anxiety
    hospital admission
    hyaluronic acid
    hydroxyapatite
HAD—hemadsorption
HAE—hereditary angioneurotic
    edema
HAHTG—horse antihuman thymus
    globulin
HAI—hemagglutination inhibition
    hemagglutinin inhibition
hal—halothane
HANE—hereditary angioneurotic
    edema
HAP—heredopathia atactica
    polyneuritiformis
    histamine phosphate acid
HAPA—hemagglutinating antipeni-
    cillin antibody
HASHD—hypertensive arterioscle-
    rotic heart disease
HAT—hypoxanthine-aminopterin-
    thymidine (medium)
HAV—hepatitis A virus
HB—heart block
    hepatitis B
    housebound
Hb, Hgb—hemoglobin
HBB—hydroxybenzyl benzimidazole
HBD, HBDH—hydroxybutyrate
    dehydrogenase
HBF—hepatic blood flow
HBI—high-serum-bound iron
HBLV—human B lymphotropic virus
HBO—hyperbaric oxygen
HBP—high blood pressure
HBV—hepatitis B virus
HBW—high birthweight
HC—head compression
    hepatic catalase
    hospital course
    house call
    hyaline cast(s)
    hydroxycorticoid

HCA—hypothalamic chronic anovulation

HCC—hepatocellular carcinoma hydroxycholecalciferol

hCG—human chorionic gonadotropin

HCH—hexachlorocyclohexane

HCL—hard contact lenses

HCl—hydrochloride

HCO$_3$ [HCO3]—bicarbonate

HCP—hepatocatalase peroxidase hereditary coproporphyria

hCS, hCSM—human chorionic somatomammotropin

HCT—homocytotrophic

Hct, hct—hematocrit

HCTZ—hydrochlorothiazide

HCU—homocystinuria

HD—hearing distance high dosage

HDC—histidine decarboxylase

HDCV—human diploid cell (rabies) vaccine

HDI—hexamethylene diisocyanate

HDL—high-density lipoprotein

HDLW—distance at which a watch is heard by the left ear

HDP—hydroxydimethylpyrimidine

HDRW—distance at which a watch is heard by the right ear

HE—hereditary elliptocytosis human enteric

H&E—hematoxylin and eosin [stain]

HEAT—human erythrocyte agglutination test

HEC—hydroxyergocalciferol

HED—Haut-Einheits-Dosis [unit of x-ray dosage]

HEENT—head, eyes, ears, nose, and throat

HEK—human embryo kidney (cell culture)

HEL—human embryo lung (cell culture)

HEMA—hydroxyethyl methacrylate

HEPA—high-efficiency particulate air [filter]

HES—hydroxyethyl starch

HET—helium equilibration time

HETE—hydroxy-eicosatetraenoic acid

HETP—hexaethyltetraphosphate

HF—Hageman factor heart failure high flow high frequency

HFI—hereditary fructose intolerance

HFP—hexafluoropropylene

Hg—mercury

Hgb, Hb—hemoglobin

HGF—hyperglycemic-glycogenolytic factor

hGG—human gamma globulin

hGH—human growth hormone

HGPRT—hypoxanthine-guanine phosphoribosyl transferase

HH—hydroxyhexamide

HHb—hypohemoglobin, reduced hemoglobin, un-ionized hemoglobin

HHS—Department of Health and Human Services

HHT—hereditary hemorrhagic telangiectasia

HI—hemagglutination inhibition high impulsiveness hydroxyindole

HIA—hemagglutination-inhibition antibody

5-HIAA—hydroxyindoleacetic acid

HIB—*Haemophilus influenzae* type b

HIDA—hepatoiminodiacetic acid [scan]

HIHA—high impulsiveness, high anxiety

HILA—high impulsiveness, low anxiety

history past medical h. (PMH)

HIT—hemagglutination-inhibition test hypertrophic infiltrative tendinitis

HIV—human immunodeficiency virus

HJ—Howell-Jolly

HJB—Howell-Jolly bodies

HK—heat-killed
heel-to-knee
hexokinase
HKLM—heat-killed *Listeria mono-cytogenes*
HL—hearing level
hearing loss
histocompatibility locus
hypermetropia, latent
H&L—heart and lungs
HLDH—heat-stable lactate dehy-drogenase
hLH—human luteinizing hormone
H-L-K—heart, liver, kidney
HLR—heart-lung resuscitator
hLT—human lymphocyte transfor-mation
hlth—health
HLV—herpes-like virus
HM—human milk
hydatidiform mole
manifest hyperopia
HME—heat and moisture exchanger
HMF—hydroxymethylfurfural
hMG—human menopausal gonado-tropin
HMG—hydroxymethylglutaryl
HMK—high-molecular-weight kininogen
HML—human milk lysozyme
HMO—health maintenance organi-zation
HMP—hexose monophosphate
hexose monophosphate pathway
hot moist pack
HMPG—hydroxymethoxy-phenyl-glycol
HMPS—hexose monophosphate shunt
HMSAS—hypertrophic muscular subaortic stenosis
HMSN—hereditary motor and sen-sory neuropathy
HN—hereditary nephritis
hilar node
nitrogen mustard, mechlor-ethamine

HNP—herniated nucleus pulposus
hnRNA—heterogeneous nuclear RNA
HO—high oxygen
h/o, H/O—history of
H_2O [H2O]—water
H_2O_2 [H2O2]—hydrogen peroxide
HOA—hypertrophic osteoarthroscopy
HOC—hydroxycorticoid
HOCM—high-osmolar contrast medium
hypertrophic obstructive car-diomyopathy
HOOD—hereditary osteo-onycho-dysplasia
HOP—high oxygen pressure
hosp—hospital
hp—haptoglobin
HP—high protein
house physician
human pituitary
H&P—history and physical
HPA—hypothalamic-pituitary-adre-nal (axis)
HPAA—hydroxyphenylacetic acid
HPE—history and physical exami-nation
hpf—high-power field
HPF—heparin-precipitable fraction
hPFSH—human pituitary follicles-stimulating hormone
hPG—human pituitary gonadotropin
HPI—history of present illness
hPL—human placental lactogen
HPLC—high-performance liquid chromatography
high-pressure liquid chro-matography
HPO—high-pressure oxygen
HPP—hereditary pyropoikilocytosis
hydroxypyrazolopyrimidine
HPPA—hydroxyphenylpyruvic acid
HPPH—hydroxyphenyl-phenylhy-dantoin
HPS—hematoxylin-phloxine-saffron
hypertrophic pyloric stenosis
HPT—hyperparathyroidism

HPV—*Haemophilus pertussis* vaccine
    human papillomavirus
HPVG—hepatic portal venous gas
HR—heart rate
    hospital record
    hospital report
H&R—hysterectomy and radiation [therapy]
hr—hour
HRA—health risk appraisal
HRF—histamine-releasing factor
HRIG—human rabies immune globulin
HRR—Hardy-Rand-Ritter (plates)
HRS—Hamilton Rating Scale
h.s.—at bedtime (L. hora somni)
HS—heat stable
    heme synthetase
    hereditary spherocytosis
    herpes simplex
    horse serum
    house surgeon
HSA—human serum albumin
HSG—hysterosalpingogram
HSV—herpes simplex virus
ht—heart
    height
HT—hemagglutination titer
    histologic technician
    hydroxytryptamine
    hypermetropia, total
HT, htn—hypertension
HT—hypothalamus
Ht—total hyperopia
HTA—hydroxytryptamine
HTLV—human T-cell lymphotrophic virus [now: HIV]
HTOH—hydroxytryptophol
HTP—hydroxytryptophan
HTV—herpes-type virus
HU—hemagglutinating unit
    Hounsfield unit
    hydroxyurea
    hyperemia unit
HuIFN—human interferon
HUS—hyaluronidase unit for semen

HV—hepatic vein
    herpesvirus
    hospital visit
    hyperventilation
H&V—hemigastrectomy and vagotomy
HVA—homovanillic acid
HVE—high-voltage electrophoresis
HVH—herpesvirus hominis
HVL—half-value layer
HVM—high-velocity missile
HVSD—hydrogen-detected ventricular septal defect
Hx—history
Hy—hypermetropia
    hysteria
hypo—hypodermic (injection)
    under
hys—hysteria
HZ—herpes zoster
Hz—hertz
HZV—herpes zoster virus
I—inactive, optically
    incisor, deciduous
    incisor, permanent
    intensity of magnetism
    iodine
^{131}I—radioactive iodine [iodine I 131]
IA—internal auditory
    intra-aortic
    intra-arterial
IABP—intra-aortic balloon pump
IAC—internal auditory canal
IADH—inappropriate antidiuretic hormone
IAHA—immune adherence hemagglutination assay
IAM—internal auditory meatus
IAS—interatrial septum
    intra-amniotic saline
IASD—interatrial septal defect
IASP—International Association for the Study of Pain
IAT—invasive activity test
    iodine-azide test
IB—immune body
IBB—intestinal brush border
IBC—iron-binding capacity

IBF—immunoglobulin-binding factor
IBU—international benzoate unit
IC—immune complex
    inspiratory capacity
    intensive care
    intercostal
    intermediate care
    intermittent claudication
    internal conversion
    intracavitary
    intracellular
    intracerebral
    intracranial
    intracutaneous
    irritable colon
    isovolumic contraction
I/C—incomplete
ICA—internal carotid artery
    intracranial aneurysm
ICAM-1—intercellular adhesion
    molecule-1
ICAO—internal carotid artery
    occlusion
ICC—Indian childhood cirrhosis
    intensive coronary care
ICCU—intensive coronary care unit
ICD—International Classification of
    Diseases
    intrauterine contraceptive
      device
    ischemic coronary disease
ICD, ICDH—isocitric dehydrogenase
ICE—iridocorneal-endothelial [syn-
    drome]
ICF—intermediate care facility
ICG—indocyanine green
ICLH—Imperial College, London
    Hospital
ICM—intercostal margin
ICP—intracranial pressure
ICS—intercostal space
ICT—inflammation of connective
    tissue
    isovolumic contraction time
ICU—intensive care unit
ICW—intracellular water
id—the same (L. idem)

ID—identification
    immunodeficiency
    infant death(s)
    Infectious Disease [service]
    infectious disease(s)
    infective dose
    inside diameter
    internal diameter
    intradermal
ID_{50} [ID50]—median infective dose
I&D—incision and drainage
    irrigation and débridement
IDA—image display and analysis
IDD—insulin-dependent diabetes
IDDM—insulin-dependent diabetes
    mellitus
IDI—induction-delivery interval
IDL—intermediate-density lipopro-
    tein
IDM—infant of diabetic mother
IDP—initial dose period
IDR—intradermal reaction
IDS—immunity deficiency state
    inhibitor of DNA synthesis
IDU—idoxuridine
    iododeoxyuridine
IDVC—indwelling venous catheter
I/E—inspiratory-expiratory [ratio]
IEF—isoelectric focusing
IEL—intraepithelial lymphocytes
IEM—immune electron microscopy
    inborn error of metabolism
IEMG—integrated electromyogram
IEOP—immunoelectro-osmophoresis
IEP—immunoelectrophoresis
    isoelectric point
    isoelectric precipitation
IF—immunofluorescence
    initiation factor
    interferon
    interstitial fluid
    intrinsic factor
IFA—immunofluorescence assay
    indirect fluorescent antibody
IFC—intrinsic factor concentrate
IFN—interferon
IFR—inspiratory flow rate

IFRA—indirect fluorescent rabies antibody (test)
IG—immune globulin
    intragastric
Ig—immunoglobulin [IgA, IgD, IgE, IgG, IgM]
IGDM—infant of gestational diabetic mother
IGF-1—insulin-like growth factor-1
IGT—impaired glucose tolerance
IGV—intrathoracic gas volume
IH—idiopathic hyperprolactinemia
    infectious hepatitis
    inner half
IHA—indirect hemagglutination
IHC—idiopathic hypercalciuria
    immunohistochemistry
IHO—idiopathic hypertrophic osteoarthropathy
IHR—intrinsic heart rate
IHSA—iodinated human serum albumin
IHSS—idiopathic hypertrophic subaortic stenosis
IIF—indirect immunofluorescence
IJP—internal jugular [vein] pressure
IJV—internal jugular vein
IL—interleukin [IL-1, IL-2, IL-3]
IL-2R—interleukin-2 receptor
ILA—insulin-like activity
ILB, ILBW—infant of low birthweight
ILD—interstitial lung disease
    ischemic leg disease
    ischemic limb disease
IM—infectious mononucleosis
    internal medicine
    intramedullary
    intramuscular
    intramuscularly
IMA—internal mammary artery
IMAA—iodinated macroaggregated albumin
IMB—intermenstrual bleeding
IMBC—indirect maximum breathing capacity
IMC—irregular menstrual cycle

IMH—idiopathic myocardial hypertrophy
IMHP—1-iodomercuri-2-hydroxypropane
IMI—intramuscular injection
imp—impression
    improved
    inosine monophosphate
IMPA—incisal mandibular plane angle
IMR—infant mortality rate
IMRAD—introduction, methods, results, discussion
IMS—incurred in military service
IMV—intermittent mandatory ventilation
In—indium
in.—inch
IN—intranasal
inc—increase
    incurred
incr—increase
ind—independence
INDM—infant of nondiabetic mother
INE—infantile necrotizing encephalomyelopathy
inf—inferior
    infusion
info—information
INH—isonicotine hydrazine inhibitor
    isonicotinic acid hydrazide (isoniazid)
inj—inject
inl—inlay
INO—internuclear ophthalmoplegia
inoc—inoculate
INPV—intermittent negative-pressure assisted ventilation
int—intermediate
    intermittent
    internal
int med—internal medicine
IO—internal os
    intestinal obstruction
    intraocular
I&O—in and out (surgery)
    intake and output
IOL—intraocular lens

IOP—intraocular pressure
IOU—intensive therapy observation unit
IP—incisioproximal
    incubation period
    instantaneous pressure
    interphalangeal
    intraperitoneal
    isoelectric point
I-para—primipara
IPC—isopropyl chlorophenyl
IPG—impedance plethysmography
IPH—idiopathic pulmonary hemosiderosis
IPL—intrapleural
IPP—intermittent positive pressure
IPPB—intermittent positive-pressure breathing
IPPI—interruption of pregnancy for psychiatric indication
IPPO—intermittent positive-pressure inflation with oxygen
IPPR—intermittent positive-pressure respiration
IPPV—intermittent positive-pressure ventilation
IPRT—interpersonal reaction test
IPS—initial prognostic score
IPSP—inhibitory postsynaptic potential
IPU—inpatient unit
IPV—inactivated poliovirus vaccine
IQ—intelligence quotient
IR—immunoreactive
    internal resistance
IRC—inspiratory reserve capacity
IRG—immunoreactive glucagon
IRHCS—immunoradioassayable human chorionic somatomammotropin
IRhGH—immunoreactive human growth hormone
IRI—immunoreactive insulin
IRMA—intraretinal microvascular abnormalities
irr—irradiation
IRS—infrared spectrophotometry
IRV—inspiratory reserve volume

is—in place (L. in situ)
IS—immune serum
    intercostal space
    interspace
    intraspinal
ISA—intrinsic sympathomimetic activity
ISD, ISDN—isosorbide dinitrate
ISG—immune serum globulin
ISH—icteric serum hepatitis
iso—isoproterenol
ISP—interspace
IST—insulin sensitivity test
ISW—interstitial water
IT—implantation test
    inhalation test
    inhalation therapy
    intradermal test
    intrathecal
    intratracheal
    intratumoral
    isomeric transition
ITC—imidazolyl-thioguanine chemotherapy
ITE—in the ear [hearing aid]
ITLC—instant thin-layer chromatography
ITP—idiopathic thrombocytopenic purpura
ITPA—Illinois Test of Psycholinguistic Abilities
ITT—insulin tolerance test
ITU—intensive therapy unit
IU—immunizing unit
    international unit(s)
    intrauterine
IUCD—intrauterine contraceptive device
IUD—intrauterine death
    intrauterine device
IUGR—intrauterine growth rate
    intrauterine growth retardation
IUM—intrauterine fetally malnourished
IUT—intrauterine transfusion
IV—interventricular
    intervertebral

IV— (continued)
    intravascular
    intravenous
    intraventricular
    invasive
IVC—inferior vena cava
    intravenous cholangiogram
IVCC—intravascular consumption
    coagulopathy
IVCD—intraventricular conduction
    defect
IVCP—inferior vena cava pressure
IVCU—isotope voiding cys-
    tourethrography
IVCV—inferior venacavography
IVD—intervertebral disk
IVGTT—intravenous glucose toler-
    ance test
IVH—intraventricular hemorrhage
IVM—intravascular mass
IVP—intravenous pyelogram
    intraventricular pressure
IVS—interventricular septum
IVSD—interventricular septal defect
IVT—intravenous transfusion
IVTTT—intravenous tolbutamide
    tolerance test
IVU—intravenous urography
IWL—insensible water loss
IWMI—inferior wall myocardial
    infarction
J—joule
    journal
JA—juvenile arthritis
JCA—juvenile chronic arthritis
JCAHO—Joint Commission on
    Accreditation of Healthcare
    Organizations
jej—jejunum
JG—juxtaglomerular
JND—just noticeable difference
JRA—juvenile rheumatoid arthritis
jt—joint
JV—jugular vein
    jugular venous
JVP—jugular venous pressure
    jugular venous pulse
JXG—juvenile xanthogranuloma

K—absolute zero
    cathode
    electrostatic capacity
    Kell blood system
    Kelvin
    potassium
KA—ketoacidosis
    King-Armstrong (units)
KAU—King-Armstrong units
kb—kilobase
KB—ketone body
KBr—potassium bromide
kc—kilocycle
KC—cathodal closing
Kcal, Cal—kilocalorie
KCC—cathodal-closing contraction
KCG—kinetocardiogram
kCi—kilocurie(s)
KCl—potassium chloride
kcps—kilocycles per second
KCT—cathodal-closing tetanus
KD—cathodal duration
KDT—cathodal-duration tetanus
KE—kinetic energy key
keV, kev—kilo electron volt(s)
KFAB—kidney-fixing antibody
kg—kilogram(s)
kg-cal—kilogram-calorie
KGS—ketogenic steroid
kHz—kilohertz
KIU—kallikrein-inhibiting unit
KLH—keyhole limpet hemocyanin
KLS—kidneys, liver, spleen
km—kilometer(s)
KM—kanamycin
KMnO—potassium permanganate
KMV—killed measles virus vaccine
KOC—cathodal-opening contraction
KP—keratitic precipitates
    keratitis punctata
KPTT—kaolin partial thromboplas-
    tin time
KRB—Krebs-Ringer bicarbonate
    buffer
KRP—Kolmer test with Reiter pro-
    tein
    Krebs-Ringer phosphate

KS—ketosteroid
    Kveim-Siltzbach (test)
KSC—cathodal-closing contraction
KST—cathodal-closing tetanus
KU—Karmen units
KUB—kidney, ureter, bladder [x-ray]
kv, kV—kilovolt
KV—kanamycin and vancomycin
    killed vaccine
    killed virus
KVO—keep vein open [IV line]
kVp—kilovolts peak
KW—Keith-Wagener [retinopathy]
    Kimmelstiel-Wilson [syn-
       drome]
    Kugelberg-Welander [syn-
       drome]
kW—kilowatt(s)
KWB—Keith, Wagener, Barker
    [classification, groups 1–4]
kWh, kW-hr—kilowatt-hour
l—lethal (L. letha)
    pound (L. libra)
ʟ—levo- [prefix]
L—coefficient of induction
    Latin
    left
    length
    leucine
    ligament
    light sense
    liter(s)
    low
    lower
    lumbar
L.—Lactobacillus
    Leishmania
L1 through L5—lumbar vertebrae
    1–5
LA—lactic acid
    latex agglutination (test)
    left arm
    left atrial
    left atrium
    leucine aminopeptidase
    linguoaxial
    local anesthesia
    low anxiety

L&A—light and accommodation
LAA—leukocyte ascorbic acid
lab—laboratory
LAD—left anterior descending
    [coronary artery]
    leukocyte adhesion deficiency
LADA—left anterior descending
    artery
LAE—left atrial enlargement
LAF—laminar air flow
LAG—labiogingival
    lymphangiogram
LAH—lactalbumin hydrolysate
    left atrial hypertrophy
LAI—labioincisal
LAIT—latex agglutination-inhibi-
    tion test
LAL—limulus amebocyte lysate
LAO—left anterior oblique [projec-
    tion]
LAP—left atrial pressure
    leucine aminopeptidase (test)
    leukocyte alkaline phos-
      phatase
    lyophilized anterior pituitary
LAR—left arm recumbent
LAS—linear alkylate sulfonate
LASER—light amplification by
    stimulated emission of radia-
    tion [now: laser]
LASIK—laser-assisted in situ kera-
    tomileusis
    laser-assisted intrastromal
      keratomileusis
lat—lateral
LATS—long-acting thyroid stimula-
    tor
LATS-p—LATS protector
LAV—lymphadenopathy-associated
    virus
LB—live birth(s)
lb.—pound (L. libra)
LBB—left bundle branch
LBBB—left bundle branch block
LBCD—left border of cardiac dull-
    ness
LBF—*Lactobacillus bulgaricus* fac-
    tor

LBI—low serum-bound iron
LBM—lean body mass
LBNP—lower-body negative pressure
LBW—low birthweight
LBWI—low-birthweight infant
LBWR—lung-body weight ratio
LC—lethal concentration
    lipid cytosomes
    living children
LCA—left circumflex coronary artery
    left carotid artery
    lithocholic acid
LCAT—lecithin-cholesterol-acyl-transferase
LCD—liquor carbonis detergens
LCF, LCx—left circumflex [coronary artery]
LCFA—long-chain fatty acid
LCL—Levinthal-Coles-Lillie (bodies)
    lymphocytic lymphosarcoma
LCM—left costal margin
    lymphatic choriomeningitis
    lymphocytic choriomeningitis
LCT—liquid crystal thermogram
    liquid crystal thermography
    long-chain triglyceride
LD—left deltoid
    lethal dose
    light difference
    linguodistal
    living donor
    low dosage
    lymphocyte-defined
L-D—Leishman-Donovan (bodies)
L/D—light-dark [ratio]
LD_{50} [LD50]—median lethal dose
LDA—left descending artery
    left dorsoanterior [position]
    linear displacement analysis
LDD—light-dark discrimination
LDDS—local dentist
LDH—lactate dehydrogenase
LDL—loudness discomfort level
    low-density lipoprotein
LDLP—low-density lipoprotein
LDP—left dorsoposterior

LE—left eye
    leukoerythrogenetic
    lower extremity
LED—lupus erythematosus disseminatus
LES—local excitatory state
LET—linear energy transfer
LF—laryngofissure
    limit flocculation
LFA—left femoral artery
    left frontoanterior [position]
LFD—lactose-free diet
    least fatal dose
LFN—lactoferrin
LFP—left frontoposterior [position]
LFT—latex flocculation test
    left frontotransverse [position]
    liver function test
lg—large
LG—laryngectomy
    left gluteal
    linguogingival
LGB—lateral geniculate body
LGN—lateral geniculate nucleus
LGV—lymphogranuloma venereum
LH—lower half
    luteinizing hormone
LHL—left hepatic lobe
LHRF—luteinizing hormone–releasing factor
LHRH—luteinizing hormone–releasing hormone
LI—linguoincisal
    low impulsiveness
LIA—leukemia-associated inhibitory activity
LIAFI—late infantile amaurotic familial idiocy
LIBC—latent iron-binding capacity
LIF—left iliac fossa
    leukocyte inhibitory factor
lig—ligament
LIHA—low impulsiveness, high anxiety
LILA—low impulsiveness, low anxiety
LIP—lymphocytic interstitial pneumonitis

liq—liquid
    liquor
LIQ—lower inner quadrant
LIS—lobular in situ
LK—left kidney
LKP—lamellar keratoplasty
LL—left leg
    left lower
    left lung
    lower lobe
    lysolecithin
LLC—long leg cast
LLE—left lower extremity
LLF—Laki-Lorand factor
LLL—left lower lobe
LLM—localized leukocyte mobilization
LLQ—left lower quadrant
LLS—lazy leukocyte syndrome
LM—light microscopy
    light minimum
    linguomesial
LMA—left mentoanterior [position]
LMD—local medical doctor
    low-molecular-weight dextran
LMDX—low-molecular-weight dextran
LMF—lymphocyte mitogenic factor
LMK—low-molecular-weight kininogen
LMP—last menstrual period
    left mentoposterior [position]
LMR—localized magnetic resonance
LMT—Licensed Massage Therapist
    left mentotransverse [position]
LMW—low molecular weight
LMWD—low-molecular-weight dextran
LN—lipoid nephrosis
    lupus nephritis
    lymph node
L/N—letter-numerical (system)
LNMP—last normal menstrual period
LNPF—lymph node permeability factor
LO—linguo-occlusal

LOA—leave of absence
    left occipitoanterior [position]
LOD—line of duty
LOM—limitation of motion
    loss of motion
LOP—left occipitoposterior [position]
LOQ—lower outer quadrant
LOT—left occipitotransverse [position]
LOWBI—low-birthweight infant
LP—latency period
    leukocyte-poor
    light perception
    linguopulpal
    lipoprotein
    low protein
    lumbar puncture
    lymphoid plasma
L/P— lactate-pyruvate [ratio]
LPA—left pulmonary artery
LPE—lipoprotein electrophoresis
LPF—leukocytosis-promoting factor
    localized plaque formation
    low-power field
    lymphocytosis-promoting factor
LPH—lipotropic hormone
LPL—lipoprotein lipase
lpm—liter(s) per minute
LPN—licensed practical nurse
LPO—left posterior oblique [projection]
    light perception only
LPS—lipopolysaccharide
LPV—left pulmonary vein
LR—laboratory references
    lactated Ringer
    light reaction
L/R—left-to-right [ratio]
L&R—left and right
LRF—luteinizing hormone–releasing factor
LRH—luteinizing hormone–releasing hormone
LRQ—lower right quadrant
LRS—lactated Ringer solution
LRT—lower respiratory tract

LS—left side
    legally separated
    liver and spleen
    lumbosacral
    lymphosarcoma
LSA—left sacroanterior [position]
    lymphosarcoma
LSB—left sternal border
LScA—left scapuloanterior [position]
LScP—left scapuloposterior [position]
LSCS—lower segment cesarean section
LSD—lysergic acid diethylamide
LSH—lutein-stimulating hormone
LSM—late systolic murmur
LSP—left sacroposterior [position]
LST—left sacrotransverse [position]
LSV—left subclavian vein
lt—left
LT—left thigh
    leukotriene
    levothyroxine
    long-term
    lymphotoxin
LTB—laryngotracheobronchitis
LTB_4—leukotriene B_4
LTF—lymphocyte-transforming factor
LTH—lactogenic hormone
    luteotropic hormone
lt lat—left lateral
LTPP—lipothiamide pyrophosphate
LTRAs—leukotriene receptor antagonists [a class of drugs]
LU—left upper
L&U—lower and upper
LUE—left upper extremity
LUL—left upper lobe
LUQ—left upper quadrant
LV—left ventricle
    leukemia virus
    live virus
LVAD—left ventricular assist device
LVDP—left ventricular diastolic pressure
LVE—left ventricular enlargement

LVEDP—left ventricular end-diastolic pressure
LVEDV—left ventricular end-diastolic volume
LVEF—left ventricular ejection fraction
LVET—left ventricular ejection time
LVF—left ventricular failure
    low-voltage fast
    low-voltage foci
LVH—left ventricular hypertrophy
LVN—licensed vocational nurse
LVP—left ventricular pressure
    lysine-vasopressin
LVS—left ventricular strain
LVSP—left ventricular systolic pressure
LVSV—left ventricular stroke volume
LVSW—left ventricular stroke work
LVW—left ventricular work
LW—lacerating wound
    Lee-White (method)
L&W, L/W—living and well
LX—local irradiation
lymphs—lymphocytes
lzm—lysozyme
μ—mu (Greek letter)
    mean
    micro- [prefix; alphabetized as m]
m—median
    meter
    milli
    minim
    molar, deciduous
M—male
    married
    mega
    mesial
    minute
    mix
    molar, permanent
    month
    mother
    multipara
    murmur
    muscle

M— (continued)
 myopia
 strength of pole
 thousand (L. mil., milli)
M_1—mitral first sound
M_2—mitral second sound
ma—meter-angle
mA—milliampere(s)
μA [microA]—microampere(s)
MA—mandelic acid
 mean arterial [blood pressure]
 medical audit
 mental age
 Miller-Abbott (tube)
 moderately advanced
MA, M.A.—Master of Arts
MAA—macroaggregated albumin
MABP—mean arterial blood pressure
mac—macerate
MAC—maximum allowable concentration
 membrane attack complex
 minimum alveolar concen-
 tration
 Mycobacterium avium complex
MACC—methotrexate, Adriamycin,
 cyclophosphamide, CCNU
 (lomustine)
MAF—macrophage-activating factor
MAFH—macroaggregated ferrous
 hydroxide
mAh, mA-h—milliampere-hour
MAI—*Mycobacterium avium-intracellulare*
mAm, mA-m—milliampere-minute
M+Am—myopia plus astigmatism
MAM—methylazomethanol
man—manipulate
manip—manipulation
MAO—maximal acid output
 monoamine oxidase
MAOI, MAOIs—monoamine oxidase
 inhibitor(s) [a class of drugs]
MAP—mean aortic pressure
 mean arterial pressure
 methylacetoxyprogesterone
 methylaminopurine

MAP— (continued)
 muscle action potential
mAs, mA-s—milliampere-second
MASER—microwave amplification
 by stimulated emission of radiation [now: maser]
MASH—Mobile Army Surgical
 Hospital
MAST—military antishock trousers
 multiple antigen stimulation
 test
MAVIS—mobile artery and vein
 imaging system
max—maximum
mb, mbar—millibar(s)
MB—mesiobuccal
 methylene blue
MBA—methylbovine albumin
MBAS—methylene blue active substance
MBC—maximal breathing capacity
 minimal bactericidal concentration
MBD—methylene blue dye
 minimal brain damage
 minimal brain dysfunction
MBF—myocardial blood flow
MBFLB—monaural bifrequency
 loudness balance
MBL—minimal bactericidal level
MBO—mesiobucco-occlusal
MBP—mean blood pressure
 mesiobuccopulpal
 myelin basic protein
MBSA—methylated bovine serum
 albumin
MC—maximum concentration
 metacarpal
 mineralocorticoid
 myocarditis
MC, MTC—mytomycin C
Mc—megacycle
 megacycle(s)
mC—millicoulomb(s)
MCA—methylcholanthrene
 middle cerebral artery
MCBR—minimum concentration of
 bilirubin

MCC—minimum complete-killing concentration
mean corpuscular [hemoglobin] concentration
MCCU—mobile coronary care unit
MCD—mean corpuscular diameter
MCF—macrophage chemotactic factor
MCFA—medium-chain fatty acid(s)
mcg, μg—microgram(s)
MCH—mean corpuscular hemoglobin
MCHC—mean corpuscular hemoglobin concentration
MCHg—mean corpuscular hemoglobin
μCi [microCi]—microcurie(s)
mCi—millicurie(s)
MCi—megacurie(s)
mCi-hr—millicurie-hour
μCi-hr [microCi-hr]—microcurie-hour
MCL—midclavicular line
midcostal line
most comfortable loudness level
MCMI—Millon clinical multiaxial inventory
MCP—metacarpophalangeal
mitotic-control protein
mc p s—megacycles per second
MCQ—multiple choice question
MCR—message competition ratio
metabolic clearance rate
M-CSF—macrophage colony-stimulating factor
MCT—mean circulation time
mean corpuscular thickness
medium-chain triglyceride [oil]
medullary carcinoma of thyroid
MCV—mean clinical value
mean corpuscular volume
MD—malic dehydrogenase
manic depressive
Mantoux diameter
maternal deprivation

MD— (continued)
medium dosage
movement disorder
muscular dystrophy
myocardial damage
MD, M.D.—medical doctor (L. Medicinae Doctor)
Md—mendelevium
MDA—methylenedioxyamphetamine
motor discriminative acuity
right mentoanterior (L. mentodextra anterior) [position]
MDC—minimum detectable concentration
MDD—mean daily dose
MDF—mean dominant frequency
myocardial depressant factor
MDH—malic dehydrogenase
MDM—minor determinant mixture
MDMA—methylenedioxymethamphetamine
MDP—muramyl dipeptide
right mentoposterior (L. mentodextra posterior) [position]
MDR—minimum daily requirement
MDT—median detection threshold
right mentotransverse (L. mentodextra transversa) [position]
MDTR—mean diameter-thickness ratio
MDY—month, date, year
ME—medical education
medical examiner
mercaptoethanol
middle ear
Me—methyl
M/E—myeloid-erythroid [ratio]
MEA—mercaptoethylamine
multiple endocrine adenomatosis
med—median
medical
medicine
MED—minimal effective dose
minimal erythema dose

MEDAC—multiple endocrine deficiency–autoimmune candidiasis
meds—medications
medicines
MEF—maximal expiratory flow
MEFR—maximum expiratory flow
rate
MEFV—maximum expiratory flow
volume
meg—megakaryocyte
MEG—magnetoencephalograph
mercaptoethylguanidine
MEM—minimum essential medium
MEN—multiple endocrine neoplasia
mep—meperidine
MEP—motor evoked potential
multimodality evoked potential
MEPP—miniature end-plate potential
mEq—milliequivalent(s)
MER—mean ejection rate
methanol extraction residue
methanol-extruded residue
mets—metastases
mev—millielectron volts
MeV, Mev—megaelectron volt(s)
mf—microfilaria
μF [microF]—microfarad(s)
MF—medium frequency
microscopic factor
mycosis fungoides
myelin figures
M&F—mother and father
M/F—male-female [ratio]
MFB—metallic foreign body
MFD—midforceps delivery
minimum fatal dose
MFP—monofluorophosphate
MFR—mucus flow rate
MFWs—multiple fragment wounds
μg, mcg—microgram(s)
mg—milligram(s)
mg%—milligrams percent
MG—mesiogingival
methyl glucoside
muscle group
myasthenia gravis
Mg—magnesium

MGF—mother's grandfather
MGGH—methylglyoxal guanylhy-
drazone
mgh—milligram-hour
mg/L—milligrams per liter
MGM—mother's grandmother
MGN—membranous glomeru-
lonephritis
MGP—marginal granulocyte pool
MGR—modified gain ratio
mgtis—meningitis
mGy—milligray(s)
MH—mammotropic hormone
marital history
medical history
mental health
MHA—methemalbumin
microhemagglutination assay
mixed hemadsorption
MHB—maximum hospital benefit
methemoglobin
MHC—major histocompatibility
complex
MHD—mean hemolytic dose
minimum hemolytic dose
MHN—massive hepatic necrosis
MHP—1-mercuri-2-hydroxypropane
MHPG—methoxyhydroxy-phenyl-
glycol
MHR—maximal heart rate
mHz—milliherz
MHz—megahertz
MI—mercaptoimidazole
mitral incompetence
mitral insufficiency
myocardial infarction
MIC—Maternity and Infant Care
minimum inhibitory concentration
MICU—medical intensive care unit
mobile intensive care unit
MID—maximum inhibiting dilution
mesioincisodistal
mesioincisodistal minimum
minimal inhibiting dose
minimum infective dose
midnoc—midnight

MIF—macrophage-inhibiting factor
 migration inhibitory factor
 mixed immunofluorescence
 müllerian inhibitory factor
MIFR—maximal inspiratory flow
 rate
mIg—membrane immunoglobulin
MIH—migratory inhibitory hormone
MILIS—Multicenter Investigation
 for the Limitation of Infarct Size
min—minim
 minimal
 minute
MIO—minimum identifiable odor
MIP—maximum inspiratory pressure
MIRD—medical internal radiation
 dose
MIRU—myocardial infarction
 research unit
MIT—monoiodotyrosine
mixt—mixture
mJ—millijoule(s)
mkat—millikatal(s)
MKS—meter-kilogram-second
MKV—killed-measles vaccine
μL, μl—microliter(s)
mL, ml—milliliter(s)
ML—mesiolingual
 middle lobe
 midline
M/L—monocyte-lymphocyte [ratio]
MLA—left mentoanterior (L. men-
 tolaeva anterior) [position]
 mesiolabial
 monocytic leukemia, acute
MLAI—mesiolabioincisal
MLAP—mean left atrial pressure
MLC—minimum lethal concentration
 mixed leukocyte culture
 multilamellar cytosome
 myelomonocytic leukemia,
 chronic
MLD—median lethal dose
 metachromatic
 minimum lethal dose
MLF—medial longitudinal fasciculus
MLI—mesiolinguoincisal
MLN—mesenteric lymph node

MLNS—mucocutaneous lymph
 node syndrome
MLO—mesiolinguo-occlusal
MLP—left mentoposterior (L. men-
 tolaeva posterior) [position]
 mesiolinguopulpal
MLR—mixed lymphocyte reaction
MLS—mean lifespan
 myelomonocytic leukemia,
 subacute
MLSI—multiple line scan imaging
MLT—left mentotransverse (L. men-
 tolaeva transverse) [position]
MLV—Moloney leukemogenic virus
 mouse leukemia virus
μm—micromicron
mμ—millimicron
μM [microM]—micromolar(s)
mm—millimeter(s)
 muscles
mm^2 [mm2], sq mm—square mil-
 limeter(s)
mm^3 [mm3], cu mm—cubic mil-
 limeter(s)
mM—millimolar
MM—malignant melanoma
 Marshall-Marchetti
 medial malleolus
 mucous membrane
 multiple myeloma
 muscularis mucosa
 myeloid metaplasia
M&M—milk and molasses
MMA—methylmalonic acid
mμc—millimicrocurie [now:
 nanocurie]
$\mu\mu$c—micromicrocurie [now: pico-
 curie]
MMC—minimum medullary concentration
MMD—minimum morbidostatic
 dose
MMEF—maximal midexpiratory
 flow
MMEFR—maximal midexpiratory
 flow rate
MMF—maximal midexpiratory flow

MMFR—maximal midexpiratory
flow rate

mμg—millimicrogram [now:
nanogram]

μμg—micromicrogram [now:
picogram]

mm Hg—millimeters of mercury

mm H₂O [mm H2O]—millimeters
of water

MMK—Marshall-Marchetti-Krantz
[operation]

μmm—micromillimeter(s)

MMM—myeloid metaplasia with
myelofibrosis
myelosclerosis with myeloid
metaplasia

mmol—millimole(s)

mmol/L—millimoles per liter

MMP—matrix metalloproteinase

MMPI—Minnesota Multiphasic
Personality Inventory

mm pp—millimeters partial pressure

MMPR—methylmercaptopurine
riboside

MMR—mass miniature radiography
measles, mumps, rubella
[vaccine]
mobile mass x-ray
myocardial metabolic rate

mN—millinormal

Mn—manganese

MN—midnight
multinodular
myoneural

M/N, M&N—morning and night

MNCV—motor nerve conduction
velocity

MNU—methylnitrosourea

mo—month

MO—medical officer
mesio-occlusal
mineral oil

Mo—molybdenum

mod—moderate

MOD—mesio-occlusodistal

MODY—maturity-onset diabetes of
the young

mol—mole(s)

molc—molar concentration

mol wt—molecular weight

MOM—milk of magnesia

MOMA—methoxyhydroxymandel-
ic acid

monos—monocytes

MOPP—nitrogen mustard, Oncovin, prednisone, procarbazine

MOPV—monovalent oral poliovirus vaccine

mOs—milliosmolal

mOsm—milliosmole(s)

MOTT—mycobacteria other than
tubercle (bacilli) [nontubercu-
lous mycobacteria]

MP—mean pressure
melting point
menstrual period
mercaptopurine
mesiopulpal
metacarpophalangeal
monophosphate
mucopolysaccharide
multiparous

MPA—main pulmonary artery
medroxyprogesterone acetate
methylprednisolone acetate

MPAP—mean pulmonary arterial
pressure

MPC—marine protein concentrate
maximum permissible con-
centration
meperidine, promethazine,
chlorpromazine
minimum mycoplasmacidal
concentration

MPD—maximum permissible dose

MPEH—methylphenyl-ethylhydan-
toin

MPGN—membranoproliferative
glomerulonephritis

MPHR—maximum predicted heart
rate

MPJ—metacarpophalangeal joint

MPL—mesiopulpolingual

MPLA—mesiopulpolabial

MPN—most probable number

MPO—myeloperoxidase

MPP—mercaptopyrazidopyrimidine

MPS—mononuclear phagocyte system
    mucopolysaccharidosis

MPSS—methylprednisolone sodium succinate

MR—megaroentgen(s)
    mental retardation
    metabolic rate
    methyl red
    mitral reflux
    mitral regurgitation
    mortality rate
    mortality ratio
    muscle relaxant

mR—milliroentgen(s)

MRA—magnetic resonance angiography

mrad—millirad(s)

MRAP—mean right atrial pressure

MRC—Medical Reserve Corps

MRD—minimum reacting dose

mrem—millirem(s)

MRF—melanocyte-stimulating hormone–releasing factor
    mesencephalic reticular formation

MRFIT—Multiple-Risk Factor Intervention Trial

MRI—magnetic resonance imaging

MRSA—methicillin-resistant *Staphylococcus aureus*

MRT—median recognition threshold
    milk-ring test

MRVP—mean right ventricular pressure

ms, msec—millisecond(s)

μs—microsecond(s)

ms, mss—manuscript(s)

MS—mental status
    mitral stenosis
    morphine sulfate
    mucosubstance
    multiple sclerosis
    musculoskeletal

MSER—mean systolic ejection rate

MSG—monosodium glutamate

MSH—medical self-help
    melanocyte-stimulating hormone
    melanophore-stimulating hormone

MSH-IF—melanocyte-stimulating hormone–inhibiting factor

MSH-RF—melanocyte-stimulating hormone–releasing factor

MSK—medullary sponge kidney

MSL—midsternal line

MSN—mildly subnormal

MSRPP—Multidimensional Scale for Rating Psychiatric Patients

MSS—mental status schedule

MSU—monosodium urate

MSV—maximal sustained ventilation
    Moloney sarcoma virus
    murine sarcoma virus

MSVC—maximal sustained ventilatory capacity

MT—empty
    malignant teratoma
    massage therapist
    maximal therapy
    medical technologist
    medical transcriptionist
    membrana tympani
    metatarsal
    methyltyrosine
    more than
    music therapy

MTC—mytomycin C

MTD—maximum tolerated dose

MTDT—modified tone decay test

MTF—maximum terminal flow
    modulation transfer function

MTHF—methyltetrahydrofolic acid

MTI—malignant teratoma, intermediate
    minimum time interval

MTP—metatarsophalangeal

MTR—Meinicke turbidity reaction

MTT—malignant teratoma, trophoblastic
    marrow transit time
    mean transit time
    monotetrazolium

MTV—mammary tumor virus
MTX—methotrexate
μU [microU]—microunit(s)
mU—milliunit(s)
MU—Mache unit
    Montevideo unit
    mouse unit(s)
muc—mucilage
MUP—motor unit potential
MUST—medical unit, self-con-
    tained, transportable
μV [microV]—microvolt(s)
mV—millivolt(s)
MV—megavolt(s)
    minute volume
    mitral valve
    mixed venous
MVP—mean platelet volume
    mitral valve prolapse
MVR—massive vitreous retraction
MVV—maximum voluntary venti-
    lation
mw—microwave
mW—milliwatt(s)
μW [microW]—microwatt(s)
MW—megawatt(s)
    molecular weight
My—myopia
MyG—myasthenia gravis
MZ—monozygotic
n—nano- [prefix]
    nerve
N—nasal
    neurology
    nitrogen
    normal
    size of sample
    unit of neutron dosage
N.—Neisseria
    Nocardia
Na—sodium
NA—neutralizing antibody
    Nomina Anatomica [former
      system of anatomical
      classification; now: Ter-
      minologia Anatomica]
    noradrenaline
    not admitted

NA— (continued)
    numerical aperture
N/A, NA—not applicable
    not available
NAA—no apparent abnormalities
NaBr—sodium bromide
NaCl—sodium chloride
NAD—nicotinamide adenine dinu-
    cleotide
    no active disease
    no acute distress
    no apparent distress
    no appreciable disease
    nothing abnormal detected
NADH—nicotinamide adenine
    dinucleotide [reduced form]
NADP—nicotinamide adenine
    dinucleotide phosphate
NADPH—nicotinamide adenine
    dinucleotide phosphate
    [reduced form]
NAMI—National Alliance for the
    Mentally Ill
NANA—N-acetylneuraminic acid
NAPA—N-acetyl-p-aminophenol
NB—newborn
    nitrous oxide–barbiturate
NBM—nothing by mouth
NBO—nonbed occupancy
NBS—normal blood serum
NBT—nitroblue tetrazolium
NBTE—nonbacterial thrombotic
    endocarditis
NBW—normal birthweight
NC—no casualty
    no change
    noise criterion
    noncontributory
    not cultured
N/C—no complaints
NCA—neurocirculatory asthenia
    nonspecific cross-reacting
      antigen
NCD—not considered disabling
NCF—neutrophil chemotactic factor
nCi—nanocurie(s)
NCI—National Cancer Institute

NCRPM—National Council on Radiation Protection and Measurements
NCV—nerve conduction velocity
noncholera vibrios
ND—neonatal death
neurotic depression
no data
no disease
nondisabling
normal delivery
not detectable
not detected
not determined
not done
NDA—National Dental Association
no data available
no demonstrable antibodies
NDGA—nordihydroguaiaretic acid
NDMA—nitrosodimethylaniline
NDP—net dietary protein
Ne—neon
NE—nerve ending
neurologic examination
no effect
nonelastic
norepinephrine
not evaluated
not examined
NEC—necrotizing enterocolitis
not elsewhere classified, not elsewhere classifiable
NED—no evidence of disease
NEEP—negative end-expiratory pressure
NEFA—nonesterified fatty acid(s)
NEG—negative
NEM—N-ethylmaleimide
NER—no evidence of recurrence
NERD—no evidence of recurrent disease
neur—neurology
neuro—neurologic
NF—National Formulary
none found
normal flow
not found
NFTD—normal full-term delivery

ng—nanogram(s)
NG—nasogastric
NGF—nerve growth factor
NGU—nongonococcal urethritis
NHA—nonspecific hepatocellular abnormality
NHC—neonatal hypocalcemia
NHLI—National Heart and Lung Institute
NHMRC—National Health and Medical Research Council
NHS—normal human serum
NI—no information
not identified
not isolated
Ni—nickel
NIA—no information available
NIAID—National Institute of Allergy and Infectious Diseases
NIAMD—National Institute of Arthritis and Metabolic Diseases
NICHHD—National Institute of Child Health and Human Development
NICU—neonatal intensive care unit
neurological intensive care unit
NIDD—non–insulin-dependent diabetes
NIDDM—non–insulin-dependent diabetes mellitus
NIDR—National Institute of Dental Research
NIH—National Institutes of Health
NIMH—National Institute of Mental Health
NINDB—National Institute of Neurologic Diseases and Blindness
NIOSH—National Institute of Occupational Safety and Health
NK—natural killer
not known
NKA—no known allergies
NKDA—no known drug allergies
NKH—nonketotic hyperosmotic
nl—nanoliter(s)
NLA—neuroleptanalgesia

NLP—Neurolinguistic Programming
no light perception
NLT—normal lymphocyte transfer test
nm—nanometer(s)
NM—neuromuscular
not measurable
not measured
not mentioned
nuclear medicine
NMA—National Medical Association
NMG—no Marcus Gunn [phenomenon]
NMN—nicotinamide mononucleotide
NMP—normal menstrual period
NMR—nuclear magnetic resonance
nn—nerves
N:N—[indicates presence of] the azo group
NND—neonatal death
NNM—Nicolle-Novy-MacNeal (medium)
NO—nitric oxide
No.—number
N/O—none obtained
non-REM—non–rapid eye movement
non rep—do not repeat (L. non repetatur)
NOS—not otherwise specified
NP—nasopharyngeal
nasopharynx
neuropathology
neuropsychiatric
normal plasma
not performed
nucleoprotein
nurse practiner
nursing procedure
NPA—National Perinatal Association
NPB—nodal premature beat
NPC—near point of convergence
NPCTG—National Prostatic Cancer Treatment Group
NPDL—nodular, poorly differentiated lymphocytes

NPH—neutral protamine Hagedorn (insulin)
normal-pressure hydrocephalus
NPN—nonprotein nitrogen
n.p.o., NPO—nothing by mouth (L. nil per os)
NPT—neoprecipitin test
nocturnal penile tumescence
NPU—net protein utilization
nr—do not repeat (L. non repetatur)
NR—nonreactive
no radiation
no response
normal not readable
not recorded
not resolved
NRC—National Radiological Commission
National Research Council
normal retinal correspondence
Nuclear Regulatory Commission
NRD—nonrenal death
NREM—non–rapid eye movement
NRPB—National Radiological Protection Board
NRS—normal reference serum
NS—nervous system
neurologic survey
neurosurgery
nonspecific
nonsymptomatic
normal saline
no sample
no specimen
not significant
not sufficient
ns, nsec—nanosecond(s)
NSA—no serious abnormality
no significant abnormality
NSAIA—nonsteroidal anti-inflammatory agent
NSAID, NSAIDs—nonsteroidal anti-inflammatory drug(s) [a class of drugs]
NSC—no significant change
not service-connected

NSCD—nonservice-connected disability

NSD—nominal single dose
normal spontaneous delivery
no significant defect
no significant difference
no significant disease

NSE—neuron-specific enolase

nsec, ns—nanosecond(s)

nsg—nursing

NSHD—nodular sclerosing Hodgkin disease

NSILA—nonsuppressible insulin-like activity

NSM—neurosecretory material

NSND—nonsymptomatic, nondisabling

NSQ—not sufficient quantity

NSR—normal sinus rhythm

NSS—normal saline solution

NST—nonstress test

NSU—nonspecific urethritis

NSVD—normal spontaneous vaginal delivery

NT—nasotracheal
neutralization test
neutralizing nontypable
not tested

NTAB—nephrotoxic antibody

NTG—nontoxic goiter

NTN—nephrotoxic nephritis

NTP—normal temperature and pressure

nU—nanounit(s)

NUD—non-ulcer dyspepsia

NV—negative variation

Nv—naked vision

N&V—nausea and vomiting

NVA—near visual acuity

nvCJD—new variant Creutzfeldt-Jakob disease

NVD—nausea, vomiting, diarrhea
Newcastle virus disease

NWB—nonweightbearing, non-weightbearing, non–weight-bearing, no weightbearing

NYD—not yet diagnosed

o—ortho- [prefix]

0 [zero]—suture size

O—eye (L. oculus)
none
nonmotile organism
obstetrics
occiput
opening
oral
orderly
respirations [anesthesia chart]

O_2 [O2]—oxygen

O_3 [O3]—ozone

OA—occipital artery
occiput anterior
osteoarthritis
oxalic acid

OAAD—ovarian ascorbic acid depletion

OAF—osteoclast-activating factor

OAP—osteoarthropathy

OAR—other administrative reasons

OAV—oculoauriculovertebral (dysplasia)

OB—objective benefit
obstetrics

OBG, OB-GYN—obstetrics and gynecology

obl—oblique

OBS—obstetrics service
organic brain syndrome

OC—occlusocervical
office call
on call
oral contraceptive
original claim

OCA—oral contraceptive agent

O_2 cap [O2 cap]—oxygen capacity

occ—occasional

OCD—obsessive-compulsive disorder

OCG—oral cholecystogram

OCR—optical character recognition

OCT—ornithine carbamyl transferase
oxytocin challenge test

OCV—ordinary conversational voice

OD—optical density
outside diameter
overdose

OD— (continued)
    right eye (L. oculus dexter)
OD, O.D.—Doctor of Optometry
ODA—right occipitoanterior (L. occipitodextra anterior) [position]
ODD—oculodentodigital
ODN—ophthalmodynamometry
ODP—right occipitoposterior (L. occipitodextra posterior) [position]
ODT—right occipitotransverse (L. occipitodextra transversa) [position]
O&E—observation and examination
OER—oxygen enhancement ratio
OF—Ovenstone factor
OFC—occipitofrontal circumference
OFD—oral-facial-digital
    orofaciodigital
Off—official
OG, O&G—obstetrics and gynecology
OGS—oxogenic steroid
OGTT—oral glucose tolerance test
OH—occupational history
OH, OHCS—hydroxycorticosteroids
OHP—oxygen under high pressure
OI—osteogenesis imperfecta
OIF—oil immersion field
OIH—orthoiodohippurate
OJ—orange juice
OKN—opticokinetic nystagmus
OL—left eye (L. oculus laevus)
OLA—left occipitoanterior (L. occipitolaeva anterior) [position]
OLH—ovine lactogenic hormone
OLP—left occipitoposterior (L. occipitolaeva posterior) [position]
OLT—left occipitotransverse (L. occipitolaeva transversa) [position]
OM—obtuse marginal (coronary artery)
    otitis media
    outer membrane
OMI—old myocardial infarction

OMPA—octamethyl-pyrophosphoramide
    otitis media, purulent, acute
OMT—osteopathic manipulative therapy
OOB—out of bed
OP—opening pressure
    operation
    osmotic pressure
OP, OPT—outpatient
O&P—ova and parasites
OPC—outpatient clinic
OPD—outpatient department
OPG—oxypolygelatin
OPG/CPA—oculoplethysmography/carotid phonoangiography
oph, ophth—ophthalmology
OPK—optokinetic
OPS—outpatient service
OPT—outpatient treatment
OPT, OP—outpatient
OPV—oral poliovirus vaccine
OR—operating room
ORD—optical rotatory dispersion
ORF—open reading frame
ORIF—open reduction and internal fixation
ORS—orthopedic surgery
orth, ortho—orthopedics
OS—left eye (L. oculus sinister)
    opening snap
    oral surgery
OSA—obstructive sleep apnea
OSAS—obstructive sleep apnea syndrome
OSHA—Occupational Safety and Health Administration
OSM—oxygen saturation meter
OST—object sorting test
OT—occlusion time
    occupational therapy
    old tuberculin
    orotracheal
    otolaryngology
OTC—ornithine transcarbamylase
    over-the-counter
    oxytetracycline
OTD—organ tolerance dose

oto, otol—otology
oto, otolar—otolaryngology
OTR—Ovarian Tumor Registry
OU—each eye (L. oculus uterque)
OURQ—outer upper right quadrant
ov—egg (L. ovum)
OV—office visit
OVD—occlusal vertical dimension
OW—out of wedlock
O/W—oil in water
    oil-water [ratio]
ox—oxymel
oz.—ounce
p—after (L. post)
    pico- [prefix]
    probability
p—para- [prefix]
P—para
    partial
    pharmacopeia
    phosphate
    phosphorus
    plasma
    position
    postpartum
    premolar
    presbyopia
    pressure
    primipara
    properdin
    protein
    psychiatry
    pulse
    pupil
P.—*Pasteurella*
    Plasmodium
    Proteus
P1—parental generation
^{32}P—radioactive phosphorus [phosphorus P 32]
P_1—pulmonic first sound
P_2—pulmonic second sound
pa—yearly (L. per annum)
PA—paralysis agitans
    pathology
    phakic-aphakic
    posteroanterior [x-ray]
    primary amenorrhea

PA— (continued)
    pulmonary artery
    pulpoaxial
PA, P.A.—physician's assistant
Pa—pascal(s)
P&A—percussion and auscultation
PAB—*p*-aminobenzoate [p-, para-]
PABA—*p*-aminobenzoic acid [p-, para-]
PAC—papular acrodermatitis of childhood
    pericarditis, arthropathy, camptodactyly (syndrome)
    phenacetin, aspirin, caffeine
    premature atrial contraction
$PaCO_2$ [PaCO2]—arterial carbon dioxide partial pressure
$PACO_2$ [PACO2]—alveolar carbon dioxide partial pressure
PAF—platelet-activating factor
    pulmonary arteriovenous fistula
PAFD—percutaneous abscess and fluid drainage
PAFIB—paroxysmal atrial fibrillation
PAH—pulmonary artery hypertension
PAH, PAHA—*p*-aminohippuric acid [p-, para-]
PAIDS—pediatric AIDS
PAL—posterior axillary line
PALS—periarterial lymphoid sheath
PAM—crystalline penicillin G in 2% aluminum monostearate
    phenylalanine mustard
    pralidoxime
    pulmonary alveolar macrophage(s)
    pulmonary alveolar microlithiasis
    pyridine aldoxime methiodide
PAN—periodic alternating nystagmus
    peroxyacetyl nitrate
    polyarteritis nodosa
PANS—puromycin aminonucleoside
PAO—peak acid output
PaO_2 [PaO2]—arterial partial pressure of oxygen (arterial pO_2)

PAO$_2$ [PAO2]—alveolar partial pressure of oxygen (alveolar pO$_2$)

PAOD—peripheral arterial occlusive disease
 peripheral arteriosclerotic occlusive disease

Pap—Papanicolaou

PAP—peroxidase-antiperoxidase
 positive airway pressure
 primary atypical pneumonia
 prostatic acid phosphatase
 pulmonary alveolar proteinosis
 pulmonary artery pressure

PAPP—para-aminopropiophenone

PAPS—phosphoadenosyl-phosphosulfate

PAPVC—partial anomalous pulmonary venous connection

PAPVR—partial anomalous pulmonary venous return

PAR—postanesthesia room
 pulmonary arteriolar resistance

PAS—*p*-aminosalicylic [p-, para-]
 periodic acid–Schiff
 peripheral anterior synechia
 pulmonary artery stenosis

PASA—*p*-aminosalicylic acid [p-, para-]

PAS-C—*p*-aminosalicylic acid, crystallized [p-, para-]

PASG—pneumatic antishock garment

PASM—periodic acid-silver methenamine

Past.—*Pasteurella*

PAT—paroxysmal atrial tachycardia
 prism adaptation test
 prism adaption test

path—pathology

PAWP—pulmonary artery wedge pressure

PB—phenobarbital
 phonetically balanced
 pressure breathing

Pb—barometric pressure
 lead

PBA—pulpobuccoaxial

PBC—prebed care
 primary biliary cirrhosis

PBC, PcB—point of basal convergence

PBE—perlsucht bacillen emulsion

PBF—pulmonary blood flow

PBG—porphobilinogen

PBI—protein-bound iodine

PBL—peripheral blood lymphocytes

PBN—paralytic brachial neuritis

PBO—penicillin in beeswax
 placebo

PBPI—penile-brachial pressure index

PBS—phosphate-buffered saline

PBT$_4$—protein-bound thyroxine

PBV—predicted blood volume
 pulmonary blood volume

PBZ—pyribenzamine

p.c.—after meals (L. post cibum)

PC—pentose cycle
 phosphate cycle
 phosphatidyl choline
 phosphocreatine
 phosphocreatinine
 platelet concentrate
 platelet count
 portacaval
 pubococcygeus
 pulmonic closure

PCA—passive cutaneous anaphylaxis
 patient-controlled analgesia

PCB—paracervical block
 polychlorinated biphenyl

PcB, PBC—point of basal convergence

PCc—periscopic concave

PCD—phosphate-citrate-dextrose
 posterior corneal deposits

PCE—pseudocholinesterase

PCG—phonocardiogram

PCH—paroxysmal cold hemoglobinuria

pCi—picocurie(s)

PCI—pneumatosis cystoides intestinalis

PCM—protein-calorie malnutrition

PCN—penicillin

PCNL—percutaneous nephrostolithotomy
PCO—polycystic ovary
pCO₂ [pCO2]—carbon dioxide
pressure
PCP—parachlorophenol
phencyclidine
phenylcyclohexyl piperidine
[now: phencyclidine]
Pneumocystis carinii pneumonia
PCPA—parachlorophenylalanine
PCR—polymerase chain reaction
pcs—preconscious
PCS—portacaval shunt
PCT—plasmacrit
porphyria cutanea tarda
portacaval transposition
PCV—packed cell volume
polycythemia vera
PCV-M—polycythemia vera with
myeloid metaplasia
PCW—pulmonary capillary wedge
(pressure)
PCx—periscopic convex
PD—papilla diameter
Parkinson disease
patent ductus
pediatrics
phosphate dehydrogenase
plasma defect
poorly differentiated
postural drainage
potential difference
pressor dose
prism diopter
progression of disease
psychotic depression
pulmonary disease
pulpodistal
pupillary distance
PDA—patent ductus arteriosus
pediatric allergy
posterior descending artery
PDAB—para-dimethyl-aminoben-
zaldehyde
PDC—pediatric cardiology
PDD—pyridoxine-deficient diet

PDGF—platelet-derived growth
factor
PDH—packaged disaster hospital
phosphate dehydrogenase
PDI—periodontal disease index
pdl—pudendal
PDLL—poorly differentiated lymphocytic lymphoma
PDP—piperidino-pyrimidine
PDR—*Physicians' Desk Reference*
proliferative diabetic retinopathy
PE—pharyngoesophageal
phenylephrine
phosphatidylethanolamine
physical evaluation
physical examination
pleural effusion
polyethylene
potential energy
probable error
pulmonary edema
pulmonary embolism
PEBG—phenethylbiguanide
ped, peds—pediatrics
PEEP—positive end-expiratory
pressure
PEF—peak expiratory flow
PEFR—peak expiratory flow rate
PEG—percutaneous endoscopic
gastrostomy
pneumoencephalogram
polyethylene glycol
pen—penicillin
pent—pentothal
PEO—progressive external ophthalmoplegia
PEP—preejection period
PEPP—positive expiratory pressure
plateau
PER—protein efficiency ratio
PERL—pupils equal, react to light
PERLA—pupils equal, react to
light and accommodation
perpad—perineal pad
PERRLA—pupils equal, round, react
to light and accommodation

PET—positron emission tomography [scan]
    pre-eclamptic toxemia
PETN—pentaerythritol tetranitrate
PETT—positron emission transaxial tomography
    positron emission transverse tomography
PF—personality factor
    picture-frustration (study)
    platelet factor
P/F—pass-fail system
PFGE—pulsed field gradient gel electrophoresis
PFIB—perfluoroisobutylene
PFK—phosphofructokinase
PFQ—personality factor questionnaire
PFR—peak flow rate
PFT—parafascicular thalamotomy
    pulmonary function test
PFU—plaque-forming unit(s)
pg—picogram(s)
PG—plasma triglyceride
    pregnant
    prostaglandin
    pyoderma gangrenosum
PGA—pteroylglutamic acid
PGD—phosphogluconate dehydrogenase
    phosphoglyceraldehyde dehydrogenase
PGD_2 [PGD2]—prostaglandin D_2
PGDH—phosphogluconate dehydrogenase
PGDR—plasma glucose disappearance rate
PGE_1 [PGE1]—prostaglandin E_1
PGE_2 [PGE2]—prostaglandin E_2
$PGF_{2\alpha}$ [PGF2-alpha]—prostaglandin $F_{2\alpha}$ [F2-alpha]
PGG_2 [PGG2]—prostaglandin G_2
PGH—pituitary growth hormone
PGH_2 [PGH2]—prostaglandin H_2
PGI—phosphoglucoisomerase
    potassium, glucose, and insulin

PGI_2 [PGI2]—prostaglandin I_2 [prostacyclin]
PGK—phosphoglycerate kinase
PGL—persistent generalized lymphadenopathy
PGM—paternal grandmother
PGP—postgamma proteinuria
PGTR—plasma glucose tolerance rate
pH—hydrogen ion concentration
PH—past history
    personal history
    pharmacopeia
    prostatic hypertrophy
    public health
    pulmonary hypertension
Ph—phenyl
PHA—phytohemagglutinin
phar., pharm.—pharmaceutical
phar, pharm—pharmacy
Phar.D., Pharm.D.—Doctor of Pharmacy (L. Pharmaciae Doctor)
PHBB—propylhydroxybenzyl benzimidazole
PHC—posthospital care
PhD, Ph.D.—Doctor of Philosophy
PHI—phosphohexoisomerase
PHK—platelet phosphohexokinase
PHLA—postheparin lipolytic activity
PHM—posterior hyaloid membrane
PHP—primary hyperparathyroidism
    pseudohypoparathyroidism
phys—physiology
PI—pacing impulse
    performance intensity
    periodontal index
    peripheral iridectomy
    phosphatidylinositol
    pre-induction (examination)
    present illness
    protamine insulin
    pulmonary incompetence
    pulmonary infarction
PIA—plasma insulin activity
PICA—posterior inferior cerebellar artery
    posterior inferior communicating artery

PICU—pediatric intensive care unit
  pulmonary intensive care unit
PID—pelvic inflammatory disease
  plasma-iron disappearance
PIDT—plasma-iron disappearance
  time
PIE—pulmonary infiltration and
  eosinophilia
  pulmonary interstitial
  emphysema
PIF—peak inspiratory flow
  prolactin-inhibiting factor
  proliferation-inhibitory factor
PIFR—peak inspiratory flow rate
PIH—prolactin-inhibiting hormone
PII—plasma inorganic iodine
PIP—proximal interphalangeal
PIPJ—proximal interphalangeal joint
PIT—plasma iron transport rate
  plasma iron turnover
PITR—plasma iron turnover rate
PK—Prausnitz-Kustner (reaction)
  psychokinesis
  pyruvate kinase
PKP—penetrating keratoplasty
PKU—phenylketonuria
PKV—killed poliomyelitis vaccine
PL—light perception
  phospholipid
  placebo
  placental lactogen
  pulpolingual
PLA—pulpolabial
  pulpolinguoaxial
PLD—platelet defect
PLED—periodic lateralized epilep-
  tiform discharge
pls—please
PLS—prostaglandin-like substance
PLT—primed, lymphocyte typing
PLV—live poliomyelitis vaccine
  panleukopenia virus
  phenylalanine-lysine-vaso-
  pressin
PM—after death (L. post mortem)
  pacemaker
  physical medicine
  polymorph (white blood cell)

PM— (continued)
  postmortem
  presystolic murmur
  preventive medicine
  pulpomesial
p.m., PM—after noon (L. post
  meridian)
  afternoon, evening, nighttime
PMA—papillary, marginal, attached
  [prevalence of gingivitis]
  phorbol myristate acetate
  progressive muscular atrophy
PMB—para-hydroxymercuribenzoate
  polymorphonuclear basophil
  (leukocyte)
  postmenopausal bleeding
PMC—percutaneous mitral commissurotomy
  pseudomembranous colitis
PMD—progressive muscular dystrophy
PME—polymorphonuclear
  eosinophil (leukocyte)
PMH—past medical history
PMI—point of maximal impulse
  point of maximal intensity
PML—polymorphous light eruption
  progressive multifocal
  leukoencephalopathy
PMMA—polymethyl methacrylate
  [usually not expanded]
PMN—polymorphonuclear neutrophil (leukocyte)
PMP—past menstrual period
  previous menstrual period
PMR—perinatal mortality rate
  physical medicine and rehabilitation
  polymyalgia rheumatica
  proportionate morbidity ratio
PMS—phenazine methosulfate
  postmitochondrial supernatant
  pregnant mare's serum
  premenstrual syndrome
PMT—Porteus maze test
  premenstrual tension
PN—perceived noise
  percussion note

PN— (continued)
    periarteritis nodosa
    peripheral nerve
    peripheral neuropathy
    pneumonia
    polyneuritis
    pyelonephritis
PNa—plasma sodium
PND—paroxysmal nocturnal dyspnea
    postnasal drip, postnasal
      drainage
PNH—paroxysmal nocturnal hemo-
    globinuria
PNI—Prognostic Nutritional Index
    psychoneuroimmunology
PNP—para-nitrophenol
    purine nucleoside phospho-
      rylase
PNPB—positive-negative–pressure
    breathing
PNPP—para-nitrophenylphosphate
PNS—partial nonprogressing stroke
    peripheral nervous system
PNU—protein nitrogen unit
p.o.—by mouth (L. per os)
pO_2 [pO2]—partial pressure of oxy-
    gen
PO—parieto-occipital
    period of onset
    phone order
POA—pancreatic oncofetal antigen
    point of application
POB—phenoxybenzamine
    place of birth
POC—point of care
    postoperative care
    postoperative course
POD—place of death
    postoperative day
PODx—preoperative diagnosis
polio—poliomyelitis
poly—polymorphonuclear leukocyte
POMC—pro-opiomelanocortin
POMP—prednisone, Oncovin,
    methotrexate, 6-mercaptopurine
POMR—problem-oriented medical
    record

POP—plasma oncotic pressure
    plaster of Paris
POR—problem-oriented record
pos—positive
pos pr—positive pressure
poss—possible
post—posterior
postop—postoperative
pot—potassium
p.p.—after meals (L. post prandium)
PP—partial pressure
    pellagra preventive
    permanent partial
    pink puffer [emphysema]
    pinpoint
    postpartum
    postprandial
    private practice
    prothrombin-proconvertin
    protoporphyrin
    proximal phalanx
    pulse pressure
    pyrophosphate
PPA—phenylpyruvic acid
ppb—parts per billion
PPB—platelet-poor blood
    positive-pressure breathing
PPBS—postprandial blood sugar
PPC—progressive patient care
PPCA—proserum prothrombin con-
    version accelerator
PPCF—plasmin prothrombin-con-
    verting factor
PPD—paraphenylenediamine
    phenyldiphenyloxadiazole
    purified protein derivative
    (of tuberculin)
PPD-S—purified protein deriva-
    tive–standard
ppg—picopicogram(s)
PPH—postpartum hemorrhage
    primary pulmonary hyper-
    tension
    protocollagen proline
    hydroxylase
PPHP—pseudopseudo-
    hypoparathyroidism

PPLO—pleuropneumonia-like organism
ppm—parts per million
PPNG—penicillinase-producing *Neisseria gonorrhoeae*
PPO—preferred provider organization
PPP—pentose phosphate pathway
PPR—Price precipitation reaction
PPT—plant protease test
Ppt, ppt—precipitate
PPTT—prepubertal testicular tumor
PPV—positive-pressure ventilation
PQ—permeability quotient
 pyrimethamine-quinine
p.r.—through the rectum (L. per rectum)
Pr—presbyopia
 prism
PR—partial remission
 peer review
 peripheral resistance
 pregnancy rate
 production rate
 professional relations
 prosthion
 protein
 public relations
 pulse rate
PRA—plasma renin activity
PRBV—placental residual blood volume
PRCs—packed red cells
PRD—postradiation dysplasia
pre—preliminary
preg—pregnant
preop—preoperative
prep—prepare
PRF—prolactin-releasing factor
PRFM—prolonged rupture of fetal membranes
PRH—prolactin-releasing hormone
PRI—phosphoribose isomerase
primip—primipara [woman bearing first child]
PRIST—paper radioimmunosorbent test
PRL—prolactin

PRM—phosphoribomutase
 preventive medicine
p.r.n., prn, PRN—as necessary (L. pro re nata)
pro—prothrombin
proct—proctology
prog—prognosis
PROM—premature rupture of membranes
 prolonged rupture of membranes
prot—protein
prox—proximal
PRP—panretinal photocoagulation
 pityriasis rubra pilaris
 platelet-rich plasma
 progesterone receptor proteins
 Psychotic Reaction Profile
PRPP—phosphoribosyl-pyrophosphate
PRRE—pupils round, regular, and equal
PRT—phosphoribosyltransferase
PRU—peripheral resistance unit
ps—per second
PS—performing scale (IQ)
 periodic syndrome
 physical status
 plastic surgery
 population sample
 Porter-Silber (chromogen)
 prescription
 psychiatric
 pulmonary stenosis
 pyloric stenosis
P/S—polyunsaturated-saturated fatty acid [ratio]
Ps.—*Pseudomonas*
PSA—polyethylene sulfonic acid
PSC—Porter-Silber chromogen
 primary sclerosing cholangitis
PSD—peptone-starch-dextrose
PSG—peak systolic gradient
 presystolic gallop
PSGN—poststreptococcal glomerulonephritis
PSH—past surgical history
psi—pounds per square inch

PSP—periodic short pulse
  phenolsulfonphthalein
  positive spike pattern
  progressive supranuclear
    palsy
PSRO—Professional Standards
  Review Organization
PSS—physiologic saline solution
  progressive systemic sclerosis
PST—penicillin, streptomycin,
  tetracycline
psy, psych—psychiatry, psychiatric
  psychology
pt—patient
  pint
PT—parathyroid
  paroxysmal tachycardia
  permanent and total
  pharmacy and therapeutics
  physical therapist
  physical therapy
  physical training
  pneumothorax
  prothrombin time
PTA—persistent truncus arteriosus
  phosphotungstic acid
  post-traumatic amnesia
  prior to admission
  prior to arrival
PTAH—phosphotungstic acid
  hematoxylin
PTAV—percutaneous transluminal
  atrial valvuloplasty
PTB—patellar tendon–bearing
  prior to birth
PTBD—percutaneous transhepatic
  biliary drainage
PTC—percutaneous transhepatic
  cholangiography
  phenothiocarbazine
  phenylthiocarbamide
PTCA—percutaneous transluminal
  coronary angioplasty
PTD—permanent and total disability
PTE—parathyroid extract
  pulmonary thromboembolism
PTF—plasma thromboplastin facto

PTFE—polytetrafluoroethylene
  [See *Teflon* in *General Surgi-
  cal Terms.*]
PTH—parathyroid hormone
  post-transfusion hepatitis
PTHS—parathyroid hormone secre-
  tion [rate]
PTI—persistent tolerant infection
PTM—post-transfusion mononucle-
  osis
PTMA—phenyltrimethylammonium
PTMV—percutaneous transluminal
  mitral valvuloplasty
PTP—post-tetanic potentiation
  prior to program
PTR—peripheral total resistance
PTRA—percutaneous transluminal
  renal angioplasty
PTSA—para-toluenesulfonic acid
PTT—particle transport time
  partial thromboplastin time
PTU—propylthiouracil
PTX—parathyroidectomy
PU—pregnancy urine
PUD—peptic ulcer disease
PUE—pyrexia of unknown etiology
PUFA—polyunsaturated fatty acid(s)
pul, pulm—pulmonary
PUO—pyrexia of unknown origin
PUVA—psoralens and ultraviolet A
PV—peripheral vascular
  peripheral vein
  peripheral vessels
  plasma volume
  polycythemia vera
  portal vein
  postvoiding
  through the vagina (L. per
    vaginam)
P&V—pyloroplasty and vagotomy
PVA—polyvinyl alcohol
PVC—polyvinyl chloride
  postvoiding cystogram
  premature ventricular con-
    traction
  pulmonary venous congestion
PVD—peripheral vascular disease
PVF—portal venous flow

PVP—penicillin V potassium
 peripheral vein plasma
 polyvinylpyrrolidone [now:
  povidone]
 portal venous pressure
PVR—peripheral vascular resistance
 pulmonary vascular resistance
PVS—premature ventricular systole
pvt—private
PVT—paroxysmal ventricular
 tachycardia
 portal vein thrombosis
PW—posterior wall
PWA—person with AIDS
PWB—partial weightbearing
 (weight-bearing)
PWC—physical work capacity
PWI—posterior wall infarction
PWM—pokeweed mitogen
Px—physical examination
 pneumothorax
 prognosis
PXE—pseudoxanthoma elasticum
PYLL—potential years of life lost
PZ—pancreozymin
PZA—pyrazinamide
PZ-CCK—pancreozymin-cholecys-
 tokinin
PZI—protamine zinc insulin
q.—every (L. quaque)
Q—coulomb (unit of electric quantity)
 query [sometimes used for
  questionable diagnosis]
q.a.m.—every morning (L. quaque
 ante meridiem)
QC—quinine-colchicine
q.d.—every day (L. quaque die)
q.h.—every hour (L. quaque hora)
q.2h.—every two hours
q.3h.—every three hours
q.4h.—every four hours
q.h.s.—every hour of sleep
q.i.d.—four times a day (L. quater
 in die)
q.n.s.—quantity not sufficient (L.
 quantum non satis)
QO_2, qO_2—oxygen quotient

q.o.d.—every other day [coined
 expression, not Latin]
QP—Quanti-Pirquet reaction
q.p.m.—every night (L. quaque post
 meridiem)
QRZ—wheal reaction time
q.s.—sufficient quantity, enough (L.
 quantum satis)
q.s. ad—to a sufficient quantity
qt—quiet
qt.—quart
quant—quantity
q.v.—which see (L. quod vide)
R—Behnken unit
 Rankine (scale)
 Réaumur (scale)
 rectal
 regression coefficient
 remote
 resistance
 respiration
 right
 Rinne test
 roentgen
 rough (colony)
R.—*Rickettsia*
RA—airway resistance
 renal artery
 rheumatoid arthritis
 right arm
 right atrial
 right atrium
rad—radial
 radiation adsorbed dose
 root (L. radix)
RAD—right axis deviation
RAE—right atrial enlargement
RAF—rheumatoid arthritis factor
RAH—right atrial hypertrophy
RAI—radioactive iodine
RAIU—radioactive iodine uptake
RAO—right anterior oblique [pro-
 jection]
RAP—rheumatoid arthritis precipitin
 right atrial pressure
RAR—right arm recumbent
RARLS—rabbit antirat lymphocyte
 serum

RAS—renal artery stenosis
    reticular-activating system
RAST—radioallergosorbent test
RATx—radiation therapy
RB—rating board
RBB—right bundle branch
RBBB—right bundle branch block
RBC—red blood cell(s)
    red blood cell count
    red blood [cell] count
RBC IT—red blood cell iron turnover
RBCV—red blood cell volume
RBE—relative biologic(al) effec-
    tiveness
RBF—renal blood flow
RBL—Reid base line
RBP—resting blood pressure
RC—retrograde cystogram
RCA—radionuclide cerebral
    angiogram
    red cell aplasia
    right coronary artery
RCBV—regional cerebral blood
    volume
RCD—relative cardiac dullness
RCF—relative centrifugal force
RCM—right costal margin
RCR—respiratory control ratio
RCU—red cell utilization
    respiratory care unit
RCV—red cell volume
rd—rutherford
RD—reaction of degeneration
    resistance determinant
    retinal detachment
    right deltoid
RDA—recommended daily
    allowance
    recommended dietary
      allowance
    right dorsoanterior [position]
RDDA—recommended daily die-
    tary allowance
RDI—rupture-delivery interval
RDP—right dorsoposterior [position]
RDS—respiratory distress syndrome
RDW—red blood cell distribution
    width index

RE—radium emanation
    regional enteritis
    resting energy
    reticuloendothelial
    right eye
R&E—research and education
rect—rectified
REE—resting energy expenditure
REF—renal erythropoietic factor
REG—radioencephalogram
rehab—rehabilitation
rem—removal
    roentgen-equivalent-man
REM—rapid eye movement
REP—roentgen equivalent–physical
RER—rough endoplasmic reticulum
res—research
res, resp—respectively
    respiratory
RES—reticuloendothelial system
RF—radio frequency [also:
    radiofrequency]
    Reitland-Franklin (unit)
    relative fluorescence
    releasing factor
RFA—right femoral artery
    right frontoanterior [position]
RFB—retained foreign body
RFLA—rheumatoid factor–like
    activity
RFLP—restriction fragment length
    polymorphism
RFP—right frontoposterior [position]
RFS—renal function study
RFT—right frontotransverse [posi-
    tion]
    rod-and-frame test
RFW—rapid-filling wave
RG—right gluteal
RGP—rigid gas-permeable (contact
    lens)
rh—rheumatic
RH—relative humidity
    releasing hormone
Rh—Rhesus
RHD—relative hepatic dullness
rheum—rheumatic
RHL—right hepatic lobe

RHLN—right hilar lymph node
rhm—roentgen(s) (per) hour (at one) meter
Rh neg—Rhesus factor–negative
Rh pos—Rhesus factor–positive
RI—recession index
    regional ileitis
    respiratory illness
RIA—radioimmunoassay
RID—radial immunodiffusion
RIF—right iliac fossa
RIFA—radioiodinated fatty acid(s)
RIH—right inguinal hernia
RIHSA—radioactive iodinated human serum albumin
RIMA—right internal mammary anastomosis
    right internal mammary artery
RIND—reversible ischemic neurologic disability
RINE—reversible ischemic neurologic event
RIP—radioimmunoprecipitation
    rapid infusion pump
RIPA—radioimmunoprecipitation assay
RISA—radioactive iodinated serum albumin
RIST—radioimmunosorbent test
RITC—rhodamine isothiocyanate
RIU—radioactive iodine uptake
RK—radial keratotomy
    right kidney
RKY—roentgen kymography
RL—right leg
    right lung
R-L—right-to-left
RLC—residual lung capacity
RLD—related living donor
RLE—right lower extremity
RLF—retrolental fibroplasia
RLL—right lower lobe
RLN—recurrent laryngeal nerve
RLP—radiation-leukemia-protection
RLQ—right lower quadrant
RLS—Ringer lactated solution
RM—radical mastectomy
    respiratory movement

RMA—right mentoanterior [position]
RMK—Rhesus monkey kidney
RML—right middle lobe
RMP—rapidly miscible pool
    right mentoposterior [position]
RMS—root-mean-square
RMT—retromolar trigone
    right mentotransverse [position]
RMV—respiratory minute volume
RN, R.N.—registered nurse
RNA—ribonucleic acid
RNAse, RNase—ribonuclease
RND—radical neck dissection
RNP—ribonucleoprotein
RO—Ritter-Oleson [technique]
RO, R/O—rule out
ROA—right occipitoanterior [position]
roent—roentgenology
ROM—range of motion
    rupture of membranes
ROMI—rule out myocardial infarction
ROP—right occipitoposterior [position]
ROS—review of systems
rot—rotating
ROT—right occipitotransverse [position]
RP—reactive protein
    refractory period
    resting pressure
    rest pain
    retinitis pigmentosa
    retrograde pyelogram
Rp—pulmonary resistance
RPA—right pulmonary artery
RPCF, RPCFT—Reiter protein complement fixation test
RPE—retinal pigment epithelium
RPF—renal plasma flow
RPG—retrograde pyelogram
RPGN—rapidly progressive glomerulonephritis
RPh, R.Ph.—Registered Pharmacist
rpm—revolutions per minute

RPO—right posterior oblique [projection]
RPR—rapid plasma reagin (test)
RPR-CT—rapid plasma reagin circle card test
RPS—renal pressor substance
RPV—right pulmonary vein
RQ—recovery quotient
    respiratory quotient
RR—radiation response
    recovery room
    renin release
    respiratory rate
    response rate
R&R—rest and recuperation
RRA—radioreceptor assay
RR&E—round, regular, and equal
RR-HPO—rapid recompression–high-pressure oxygen
rRNA—ribosomal RNA
RRP—relative refractory period
RRR—renin-release rate
R/s—roentgen(s) per second
RS—rating schedule
    respiratory syncytial
    right side
RSA—relative specific activity
    right sacroanterior [position]
RSB—right sternal border
RSC—rested-state contraction
RScA—right scapuloanterior [position]
RScP—right scapuloposterior [position]
RSNA—Radiological Society of North America
RSP—right sacroposterior [position]
RSR—regular sinus rhythm
RST—radiosensitivity test
    rapid surfactant test
    reagin screen test
    right sacrotransverse [position]
RSTL—relaxed skin tension line
RSV—respiratory syncytial virus
    right subclavian vein
    Rous sarcoma virus
rt—right

RT—radiation therapy, radiotherapy
    reaction time
    reading test
    recreational therapy
    right thigh
    room temperature
RTA—renal tubular acidosis
RTD—routine test dilution
RTF—replication and transfer
    resistance transfer factor
rt lat—right lateral
rtn—return
RU—resistance unit
    retrograde urogram
    right upper
    roentgen unit
RUE—right upper extremity
RUL—right upper lobe
RUQ—right upper quadrant
RUR—resin-uptake ratio
RURTI—recurrent upper respiratory tract infection
RV—rat virus
    residual volume
    respiratory volume
    right ventricle
    rubella virus
RVB—red venous blood
RVD—relative vertebral density
RVE—right ventricular enlargement
RVEDP—right ventricular end-diastolic pressure
RVH—right ventricular hypertrophy
RVR—renal vascular resistance
    resistance to venous return
RVRA—renal vein renin activity
    renal vein renin assay
RVRC—renal vein renin concentration
RVS—Relative Value Schedule
    Relative Value Study
RVT—renal vein thrombosis
RW—ragweed
℞ [R_x, Rx]—prescription
    take (L. recipe)
    therapy
    treatment
s̄—without (L. sine)

s, sec.—second(s)
S_1–S_4 [S1–S4]—heart sounds (first through fourth)
S—left (L. sinister)
    second
    serum
    single
    soluble
    spherical lens
    subject
    sulfur
    supravergence
    surgery
    Svedberg (unit of sedimentation coefficient)
S.—*Salmonella*
    Schistosoma
    Spirillum
    Staphylococcus
    Streptococcus
S1 through S5—sacral vertebrae 1–5
SA—salicylic acid
    sarcoma
    secondary amenorrhea
    serum albumin
    sinoatrial
    slightly active
    specific activity
    Stokes-Adams
    sustained action
    sympathetic activity
SAA—severe aplastic anemia
SACH—solid-ankle, cushioned-heel (foot prosthesis)
SAD—seasonal affective disorder
    small airways disease
    source to axis distance
SAH—subarachnoid hemorrhage
sal—saline
SAM—sulfated acid mucopolysaccharide
    systolic anterior motion
SAP—serum alkaline phosphatase
    systemic arterial pressure
SAS—supravalvular aortic stenosis
sat—saturated
SAT—Scholastic Aptitude Test

SB—serum bilirubin
    single breath
    Stanford-Binet (test)
    sternal border
    stillbirth
SBE—subacute bacterial endocarditis
SBF—splanchnic blood flow
SBFT—small bowel follow-through [x-ray]
SBP—systemic blood pressure
    systolic blood pressure
SBT—serum bacterial titer
    single-breath test
s̄ c, s̄ gl—without correction (glasses) (L. sine correctione)
SC—sacrococcygeal
    scleral cautery
    secretory component
    self-care
    semicircular
    semiclosed
    service-connected (disability)
    sick call
    sickle cell
    single chemical
    special care
    sternoclavicular (joint)
    subclavian (vein)
    subconjunctival
    subcutaneous
    succinylcholine
    sugar-coated
    supportive care
    supraclavicular
SC, S.C.—semilunar (valve) closure
SCA—single-chain antigen-binding
SCAT—sickle cell anemia test
SCBA—self-contained breathing apparatus
SCD—service-connected disability
ScDA—right anterior scapular (L. scapulodextra anterior) [position]
ScDP—right posterior scapular (L. scapulodextra posterior) [position]
SCG—serum chemistry graft
SCH—succinylcholine

sched—schedule
schiz—schizophrenia
SCI—structured clinical interview
SCIDS—severe combined immunodeficiency syndrome
SCK—serum creatine kinase
ScLA—left anterior scapular (L.
scapulolaeva anterior) [position]
ScLP—left posterior scapular (L.
scapulolaeva posterior) [posi-
tion]
scop—scopolamine
SCP—single-celled protein
SCPK—serum creatine phosphokinase [now: serum creatine
kinase (SCK)]
scr—scruple
SCT—sex chromatin test
staphylococcal clumping test
SCU—special care unit
SD—septal defect
serum defect
skin dose
spontaneous delivery
standard deviation
streptodornase
sudden death
S/D—systolic-to-diastolic [ratio]
SDA—right anterior sacral (L.
sacrodextra anterior) [position]
Seventh Day Adventist
specific dynamic action
SDCL—symptom distress checklist
SDE—specific dynamic effect
SDH—serine dehydrase
sorbitol dehydrogenase
succinate dehydrogenase
SDM—standard deviation of the
mean
SDO—sudden-dosage onset
SDP—right posterior sacral (L.
sacrodextra posterior) [position]
SDS—Self-Rating Depression Scale
sodium dodecyl sulfate
sudden death syndrome
SDT—right transverse sacral (L.
sacrodextra transversa) [posi-
tion]

SE—sphenoethmoidal suture
standard error
Starr-Edwards (prosthesis)
^{75}Se—radioactive selenium [seleni-
um Se 75]
sec., s—second(s)
sed rate—sedimentation rate
SED—skin erythema dose
spondyloepiphyseal dysplasia
SEE—Seeing Essential English
SEG—sonoencephalogram
segs—segmented neutrophils
SEM—scanning electron microscopy
semi—half
SEP—somatosensory evoked potential
systolic ejection period
seq—sequela
sequestrum
SER—smooth endoplasmic reticulum
somatosensory evoked
response
systolic ejection rate
SERMs—selective estrogen receptor
modulators [a class of drugs]
SES—socioeconomic status
SET—systolic ejection time
sev—severe
severed
SF—shell fragment
shrapnel fragment
Svedberg flotation unit(s)
synovial fluid
SFEMG—single-fiber electromyogram
SFP—screen filtration pressure
SFS—split-function study
SFT—skinfold thickness
SFW—shell fragment wound
shrapnel fragment wound
SG—serum globulin
skin graft
specific gravity
Surgeon General
S-G—Sachs-Georgi [test]
SGA—small for gestational age
s̄ gl, s̄ c—without glasses (correc-
tion) (L. sine correctione)

SGOT—serum glutamic-oxaloacetic transaminase [now: AST]
SGP—serine glycerophosphatide
SGPT—serum glutamic-pyruvic transaminase [now: ALT]
sh—shoulder
SH—serum hepatitis
    sex hormone
    sinus histiocytosis
    social history
    sulfhydryl
    surgical history
SHB—sulfhemoglobin
SHBD—serum hydroxybutyrate dehydrogenase
SHBG—sex hormone–binding globulin
SHG—synthetic human gastrin
SHO—secondary hypertrophic osteoarthropathy
SI—International System of Units (Fr. Système International d'Unités)
    sacroiliac
    self-inflicted
    seriously ill
    serum iron
    soluble insulin
    stimulation index
Si—silicon
SICD—serum isocitric dehydrogenase
SICU—surgical intensive care unit
SID—sudden infant death
SIDS—sudden infant death syndrome
sig—let it be labeled (L. signetur)
    significant
SIg—surface immunoglobulin
SIJ—sacroiliac joint
simul—simultaneously, at the same time
SIMV—synchronized intermittent mandatory ventilation
SIRS—soluble immune response suppressor
SIW—self-inflicted wound
SJR—Shinawora-Jones-Reinhart (units)

SK—streptokinase
SKSD—streptokinase-streptodornase
sl—slight
    sublingual
SL—sensation level
    streptolysin
SLA—left anterior sacral (L. sacrolaeva anterior) [position]
SLD, SLDH—serum lactate dehydrogenase
SLE—systemic lupus erythematosus
slg—secretory immunoglobulin
SLKC—superior limbic keratoconjunctivitis
SLN—superior laryngeal nerve
SLO—streptolysin-O
SLP—left posterior sacral (L. sacrolaeva posterior)
    sacrolaeva posterior [position]
    sex-limited protein
SLR—straight leg raising
    Streptococcus lactis R
SLRT—straight leg-raising test
SLT—left transverse sacral (L. sacrolaeva transversa) [position]
sm—small
SM—simple mastectomy
    skim milk
    streptomycin
    submucous
    suction method
    symptoms
    systolic mean
    systolic murmur
SMA—sequential multiple analyzer [SMA 6/60, SMA 12/60, SMA 20/60]
    superior mesenteric artery
    supplementary motor area
SMAC ["smack"]—sequential multiple analyzer plus computer [SMAC 7, SMAC 12, SMAC 20]
SMC—somatomedin C
    special monthly compensation
SMO—slip made out

SMON—subacute myelo-opti-
coneuropathy
SMP—slow-moving protease
special monthly pension
SMR—somnolent metabolic rate
submucous resection
SMRR—submucous resection and
rhinoplasty
SN—serum-neutralizing
suprasternal notch
SNB—scalene node biopsy
SNF ["sniff"]—skilled nursing
facility
SNM—Society of Nuclear Medicine
SNS—sympathetic nervous system
SO—salpingo-oophorectomy
SOA-MCA—superficial occipital
artery to middle cerebral artery
SOAP—Subjective, Objective,
Assessment, Plan [format for
medical reports]
SOB—shortness of breath
SOC—sequential-type oral contra-
ceptive
SOD—superoxide dismutase [now:
orgotein]
SOM—secretory otitis media
serous otitis media
SOMI—sternal occipital mandibu-
lar immobilizer
SOP—standard operating procedure
sp, spp—species
SP—shunt procedure
skin potential
steady potential
summating potential
suprapubic
symphysis pubis
systolic pressure
S/P, SP—status post
SPA—suprapubic aspiration
SPAI—steroid protein activity index
SPBI—serum protein-bound iodine
SPCA—serum prothrombin conversion accelerator
SPE—serum protein electrophoresis
SPECT—single photon emission
computed tomography

SPEP—serum protein electrophoresis
SPF—specific pathogen-free
split products of fibrin
sp gr—specific gravity
SPGR—spoiled GRASS [gradient
recalled acquisition in a steady
state]
SPH—secondary pulmonary hemosiderosis
spherical
spherical lens
SPI—serum precipitable iodine
SPL—sound pressure level
SPP—suprapubic prostatectomy
spt—spirit
SPTA—spatial peak temporal average
SPWB—Saunders Pharmaceutical
Word Book
sq—square
SQ—social quotient
subcutaneous
SR—sarcoplasmic reticulum
secretion rate
sedimentation rate
sensitization response
service record
sigma reaction
sinus rhythm
skin resistance
stimulation ratio
superior rectus
systemic resistance
systems research
systems review
SRF—skin reactive factor
somatotropin-releasing factor
split renal function
SRFS—split renal function study
SRH—somatotropin-releasing hormone
SRIF—somatotropin
release–inhibiting factor
SRP—short rib polydactyly
SRR—slow rotation room
SRS—slow-reacting substance
SRS-A—slow-reacting substance of
anaphylaxis

SRT—sedimentation rate test
 speech reception test
 speech reception threshold
SS—side-to-side
 signs and symptoms
 soapsuds [enema]
 somatostatin
 subaortic stenosis
 sum of squares
 supersaturated
SSA—salicylsalicylic acid (salsalate)
 skin-sensitizing antibody
 sulfosalicylic acid (test)
SSc—systemic sclerosis
SSD—source to skin distance
 source-skin distance
SSE—soapsuds enema
SSKI—saturated solution of potassium iodide
SSN—severely subnormal
SSP—Sanarelli-Shwartzman phenomenon
SSP, SSPE—subacute sclerosing panencephalitis
s.s.s.—layer upon layer (L. sub signo veneni)
SSS—sick sinus syndrome
 specific soluble substance
SSSS—staphylococcal scalded skin syndrome
SSU—sterile supply unit
st—stage [of disease]
 straight
ST—esotropia
 skin test
 stable toxin
 standardized test
 sternothyroid
 subtalar
 subtotal
 surface tension
 survival time
STA—serum thrombotic accelerator
STA-MCA—superficial temporal artery to middle cerebral artery
staph—staphylococcus
stat, STAT—immediately (L. statim)
STC—soft tissue calcification

std—saturated
STD—skin test dose
 skin-to-tumor distance
 standard test dose
STH—somatotropic (growth) hormone
STK—streptokinase
STM—streptomycin
STP—scientifically treated petroleum
 standard temperature and pressure
STPD—standard temperature and pressure, dry (0°C, 760 mm Hg)
strep—streptococcal
 streptococci
STS—serologic test for syphilis
STSG—split-thickness skin graft
STT—serial thrombin time
STU—skin test unit
STVA—subtotal villous atrophy
SU—sensation unit
SUA—serum uric acid
subcu, subq—subcutaneous
SUD—sudden unexpected death
 sudden unexplained death
SUDS—sudden unexplained death syndrome
SUID—sudden unexplained infant death
SUN—serum urea nitrogen
sup—superficial
 superior
surg—surgery
SUS—stained urinary sediment
SUUD—sudden unexpected, unexplained death
SV—severe
 simian virus
 sinus venosus
 snake venom
 stroke volume
 subclavian vein
 supravital
SVAS—supravalvular aortic stenosis
SVC—slow vital capacity
 superior vena cava
SVCG—spatial vectorcardiogram
SVD—spontaneous vaginal delivery

SVM—syncytiovascular membrane
SVR—systemic vascular resistance
SVT—supraventricular tachycardia
SW—spiral wound
    stroke work
SWS—slow-wave sleep
Sx—symptoms
sym—symmetrical
sym, symp—symptoms
syr—syrup
Sz—schizophrenia
t—temporal
T—thorax
    temperature
    tension (intraocular)
    tesla
    time
    tumor
T.—*Taenia*
    Treponema
    Trichophyton
    Trypanosoma
T− (T minus)—decreased tension
    (T−1, T−2)
T+ (T plus)—increased tension
    (T+1, T+2)
T1 through T12—thoracic vertebrae
    1–12
T_3 [T3]—triiodothyronine [test]
T_4 [T4]—thyroxine [test]
TA—Terminologia Anatomica [current system of anatomical classification]
    therapeutic abortion
    titratable acid
    toxin-antitoxin
T&A—tonsillectomy and adenoidectomy
TA-AB—teichoic acid antibody
TA-AIDS—transfusion-associated AIDS
tab—tablet
TAB—typhoid, paratyphoid A, paratyphoid B
TADAC—therapeutic abortion, dilation, aspiration, curettage
TAF—toxoid-antitoxin floccules
    trypsin-aldehyde-fuchsin

TAH—total abdominal hysterectomy
TAL—tendo Achillis lengthening
    thymic alymphoplasia
TAM—toxoid-antitoxin mixture
TAME—toluene-sulfo-trypsin arginine methyl ester
TAMI—Thrombolysis and Angioplasty in Myocardial Infarction [trial]
TAO—thromboangiitis obliterans
    triacetyloleandomycin
TAP—tension by applanation
TAPVD—total anomalous pulmonary venous drainage
TAR—thrombocytopenia–absent radius [syndrome]
TAT—tetanus antitoxin
    thematic apperception test
    thromboplastin activation test
    total antitryptic activity
    toxin-antitoxin
    turn-around time
    tyrosine aminotransferase
TB—toluidine blue
    total base
    tracheobronchitis
    tuberculin
    tuberculosis
Tb—terbium
TBA—tertiary butylacetate
    testosterone-binding affinity
    thiobarbituric acid
TBE—tuberculin bacillin emulsion
TBF—total body fat
TBG—thyroxine-binding globulin
TBGP—total blood granulocyte pool
TBII—thyrotropin-binding inhibitory immunoglobulin
TBM—tuberculous meningitis
TBP—thyroxine-binding protein
TBPA—thyroxine-binding prealbumin
TB-RD—tuberculosis-respiratory disease
tbs., tbsp.—tablespoon(s)
TBS—tribromosalicylanilide
    triethanolamine-buffered saline

TBSA—total body surface area
TBT—tolbutamide test
    tracheobronchial toilet
TBV—total blood volume
Tc—technetium
TC—taurocholate
    temperature compensation
    tetracycline
    thermal conductivity
    tissue culture
    to contain
    total capacity
    total cholesterol
    transhepatic cholangiography
    tuberculin
    tubocurarine
TCII—transcobalamin II
TCA—tricarboxylic acid
    trichloroacetate
    trichloroacetic acid
TCAP—trimethylcetylammonium
    pentachlorophenate
TCC—trichlorocarbanilide
TCD—tissue culture dose
TCD_{50} [TCD50]—median tissue
    culture dose
TCE—trichloroethylene
TCF—total coronary flow
TCGF—T-cell growth factor
TCH—total circulating hemoglobin
TCI—to come in
    transient cerebral ischemia
TCi—tetracurie(s)
TCID—tissue culture infective dose
$TCID_{50}$ [TCID50]—median tissue
    culture infective dose
TCIE—transient cerebral ischemic
    episode
TCM—tissue culture medium
TCMI—T-cell–mediated immunity
TCP—therapeutic continuous peni-
    cillin
    tricresyl phosphate
TCPA—tetrachlorophthalic anhydride
TcR—T-cell receptor
TCSA—tetrachlorosalicylanilide
TCT—thrombin-clotting time
    thyrocalcitonin

TD—tardive dyskinesia
    tetanus-diphtheria [vaccine—
      pediatric initial dose]
    therapy discontinued
    thoracic duct
    threshold of discomfort
    threshold dose
    thymus-dependent
    tic douloureux
    time disintegration
    to deliver
    tone decay
    torsion dystonia
    total disability
    toxic dose
    transverse diameter
    treatment discontinued
Td—tetanus-diphtheria [vaccine—
    adult booster dose]
TD_{50} [TD50]—median toxic dose
TDA—TSH-displacing antibody
TDE—tetrachlorodiphenylethane
    (pesticide)
TDF—thoracic duct fistula
    thoracic duct flow
TDI—toluene-diisocyanate
    total-dose infusion
TDL—thoracic duct lymph
TDP—thoracic duct pressure
    thymidine diphosphate
TDT—tone decay test
TdT—tetanus and diphtheria toxoids
TE—threshold energy
    tissue-equivalent
    tooth extracted
    total estrogen (excretion)
    tracheoesophageal
Te—tetanus
TEA—tetraethylammonium
TEAC—tetraethylammonium chlo-
    ride
TeBG—testosterone-estradiol–bind-
    ing globulin
TECA—technetium albumin [study]
TED—threshold erythema dose
    thromboembolic disease
TEE—transesophageal echocardio-
    gram

TEE— (continued)
    tyrosine ethyl ester
TEF—tracheoesophageal fistula
TEIB—triethylene-iminobenzo-
    quinone
TEM—transmission electron
    microscopy
    triethylenemelamine
TEN—toxic epidermal necrolysis
tenac—tenaculum
TENS—transcutaneous electrical
    nerve stimulator
TEPP—tetraethyl pyrophosphate
ter—threefold
    three times
TES—trimethylaminoethane-sul-
    fonic acid
tet—tetanus
TETD—tetraethylthiuram disulfide
TF—tactile fremitus
    tetralogy of Fallot
    thymol flocculation
    tissue-damaging factor
    to follow
    total flow
    transfer factor
TFA—total fatty acid(s)
TFCC—triangular fibrocartilage
    complex
TFE—tetrafluoroethylene
TG—thioguanine
    thyroglobulin
    toxic goiter
    triglyceride
TGA—transient global amnesia
    transposition of the great
      arteries
TGAR—total graft area rejected
TGF—T-cell growth factor
    transforming growth factor
TGFA—triglyceride fatty acid(s)
TGT—thromboplastin generation test
    thromboplastin generation
    time
TGV—thoracic gas volume
    transposition of the great
      vessels
th—thoracic

TH—thyrohyoid
THA—total hydroxyapatite
THAM—trihydroxymethyl-
    aminomethane
THBR—thyroid hormone–binding
    ratio
THC—tetrahydrocannabinol
THDOC—tetrahydrodeoxycorticos-
    terone
ther—therapy
THF—humoral thymic factor
    tetrahydrofolate
THFA—tetrahydrofolic acid
THO—titrated water
THP—total hydroxyproline
TI—time interval
    transverse inlet
    tricuspid incompetence
    tricuspid insufficiency
TIA—transient ischemic attack
TIBC—total iron-binding capacity
TIC—trypsin-inhibitory capacity
t.i.d.—three times a day (L. ter in die)
TID—titrated initial dose
TIE—transient ischemic episode
TIG—tetanus immunoglobulin
TIMI—Thrombolysis in Myocardial
    Infarction [TIMI II trial]
tinct—tincture
TIPS—transjugular intrahepatic
    portosystemic shunt
TIS—tumor in situ
TIT—triiodothyronine
TIVC—thoracic inferior vena cava
TKA—transketolase activity
TKD—tokodynamometer
TKG—tokodynagraph
TL—temporal lobe
    time lapse
    time-limited
    total lipids
    tubal ligation
Tl—thallium
TLA—translumbar aortogram
TLC—tender loving care
    thin-layer chromatography
    total L-chain concentration
    total lung capacity

TLC— (continued)
  total lung compliance
TLD—thermoluminescent dosimeter
  transcutaneous lumbar
    diskectomy
  tumor lethal dose
T/LD_{100}—minimum dose causing
  death or malformation of
  100% of fetuses
TLE—thin-layer electrophoresis
TLQ—total living quotient
TLSO—thoracolumbosacral orthosis
TLV—threshold limit value
TM—temporomandibular
  time motion
  trademark
  transmetatarsal
  tympanic membrane
Tm—maximal tubular excretory
  capacity of kidneys
  transport maximum
TMAb—thyroid microsomal anti-
  body
TMAS—Taylor Manifest Anxiety
  Scale
TmG—maximal tubular reabsorp-
  tion of glucose
TMI—threatened myocardial
  infarction
  transmural infarction
TMIF—tumor-cell migration–inhi-
  bition factor
TMJ—temporomandibular joint
TML—tetramethyl lead
TMP—thymidine monophosphate
  trimethoprim
TMTD—tetramethylthiuram disulfide
TMV—tobacco mosaic virus
TN—total negatives
  true negative
Tn—normal intraocular tension
TND—term normal delivery
TNF—tumor necrosis factor
TNI—total nodal irradiation
TNM—tumor, nodes, metastases
  [tumor staging system]
TNT—trinitrotoluene
TNTC—too numerous to count

TO—telephone order
  tincture of opium (L. tinc-
    tura opii)
TOA—tubo-ovarian abscess
TOCP—triorthocresyl phosphate
tonoc—tonight
TOPS—Take Off Pounds Sensibly
  [program]
TOPV—trivalent oral poliovirus
  vaccine
TORCH—toxoplasmosis, other
  agents, rubella, cytomegalovirus, herpes simplex [syndrome]
TORP—total ossicular replacement
  prosthesis
tot prot—total protein
TP—temperature and pressure
  threshold potential
  thrombocytopenic purpura
  total positives
  total protein
  true positive
  tryptophan
TPA—tetradecanoylphorbol-13-ace-
  tate
  Treponema pallidum agglu-
    tination
t-PA, tPA, TPA—tissue plasminogen activator
TPBF—total pulmonary blood flow
TPC—thromboplastic plasma com-
  ponent
TPCF—*Treponema pallidum* complement fixation
TPG—transplacental gradient
TPH—transplacental hemorrhage
TPHA— *Treponema pallidum*
  hemagglutination assay
TPI—*Treponema pallidum* immobilization
  triose phosphate isomerase
TPM—triphenylmethane
TPN—total parenteral nutrition
  triphosphopyridine nucleotide
TPNH—reduced triphosphopyridine
  nucleotide
TPP—thiamine pyrophosphate

TPPN—total peripheral parenteral nutrition

TPR—temperature, pulse, respiration
testosterone production rate
total peripheral resistance
total pulmonary resistance

TPS—tumor polysaccharide substance

TPT—typhoid-paratyphoid

TPTZ—tripyridyltriazine

TPVR—total pulmonary vascular resistance

TQ—tourniquet

tr—tincture
trace

TR—tetrazolium reduction
therapeutic radiology
time-release
total resistance
total response
tricuspid regurgitation
tuberculin residue

TRA—transaldolase

TRAIDS—transfusion-related AIDS

TRAM—transverse rectus abdominis myocutaneous (flap)
Treatment Rating Assessment Matrix
Treatment Response Assessment Method

TRBF—total renal blood flow

TRC—tanned red cell(s)
total ridge-count

TRF—T-cell–replacing factor
thymus-replacing factor
thyrotropin-releasing factor

TRH—thyrotropin-releasing hormone

TRI—tetrazolium reduction inhibition

TRIC—trachoma-inclusion conjunctivitis

trit—triturate

TRK—transketolase

TRMC—tetramethylrhodamino-isothiocyanate

tRNA—transfer RNA

TRNG—tetracycline-resistant *Neisseria gonorrhoeae*

troch—troche (L. trochiscus)

TRP—tubular reabsorption of phosphate

TRPT—theoretical renal phosphorus threshold

TRU—turbidity-reducing unit

TS—thoracic surgery
total solids
tricuspid stenosis
triple strength
tropical sprue

TSA—technical surgical assistance
tumor-specific antigen

T_4SA [T4SA]—thyroxine-specific activity

TSB—trypticase soy broth

TSC—technetium sulfur colloid
thiosemicarbizide

TSD—target skin distance

TSE—trisodium edetate

TSF—tissue-coding factor

TSH—thyroid-stimulating hormone

TSH-RF—thyroid-stimulating hormone–releasing factor

tsp.—teaspoon(s), teaspoonful

TSP—total serum protein

TSPAP—total serum prostatic acid phosphatase

TSR—thyroid-to-serum ratio

TST—tumor skin test

TSY—trypticase soy yeast

TT—tetrazol
thrombin time
thymol turbidity
tooth, treatment of
total thyroxine
total time
transit time
transthoracic

TTC—triphenyltetrazolium chloride

TTD—tissue tolerance dose

TTH—thyrotropic hormone
tritiated thymidine

TTP—thrombotic thrombocytopenic purpura
thymidine triphosphate

TTR—transacting transcriptional regulation

TTS—temporary threshold shift
TTT—tolbutamide tolerance test
TU—thiouracil
 toxic unit
TUG—total urinary gonadotropin
TUR—transurethral resection
TURB—transurethral resection of
 bladder
TURP—transurethral resection of
 prostate
TV—tidal volume
 trial visit
TVC—timed vital capacity
 total volume capacity
 transvaginal cone
 triple voiding cystogram
TVH—total vaginal hysterectomy
TW—tap water
TWL—transepidermal water loss
Tx—traction
 treatment
Ty—type
 typhoid
U—unit
 unknown
 upper
 uracil
 uridine
 urology
UA—unaggregated
 uric acid
 urinalysis
 uterine aspiration
UAP—uterine arterial pressure
UB—ultimobranchial body
UBBC—unsaturated vitamin
 B_{12}-binding capacity
UBF—uterine blood flow
UBI—ultraviolet blood irradiation
UC—ultracentrifugal
 unchanged
 unclassifiable
 unit clerk
 urea clearance
 urethral catheterization
 uterine contraction
U&C—usual and customary

UCD, UChD—usual childhood dis-
 eases
UCG—urinary chorionic gonado-
 tropin
UCP—urinary coproporphyrin
UCS—unconditioned stimulus
 unconscious
UCTS—undifferentiated connective
 tissue syndrome
UD—urethral discharge
 uroporphyrinogen decar-
  boxylase
UDCA—ursodeoxycholic acid
UDP—uridine diphosphate
 urine drug panel
UDPG—uridine diphosphate-glucose
UDPGA—uridine diphosphoglu-
 curonic acid
UDPGT—uridine diphosphoglu-
 curonyl transferase
UDS—urine drug screen
UE—upper extremity
UFA—unesterified fatty acid(s)
UG—urogenital
UGI—upper gastrointestinal
UH—upper half
UI—uroporphyrin isomerase
UIBC—unsaturated iron-binding
 capacity
UIF—undegraded insulin factor
UIQ—upper inner quadrant
UK—unknown
 urokinase
UL—upper lobe
U&L—upper and lower
ULN—upper limit of normal
ULQ—upper left quadrant
UM—uracil mustard
umb—umbilicus
UMP—uridine monophosphate
UN—urea nitrogen
ung—ointment (L. unguentum)
uni-—one [prefix]
unk, unkn—unknown
UOQ—upper outer quadrant
UP—upright posture
 ureteropelvic
 uroporphyrin

U/P—urine-plasma [ratio]
UPG—uroporphyrinogen
UPI—uteroplacental insufficiency
UPJ—ureteropelvic junction
UPOR—usual place of residence
UPP—uterine perfusion pressure
UPP, UPPP—uvulopalatopharyngo-
    plasty
ur—urine
UR—unconditioned response
    upper respiratory [tract]
    utilization review
URD—upper respiratory disease
URF—unidentified reading frame
URI—upper respiratory infection
urol—urology
URQ—upper right quadrant
URTI—upper respiratory tract
    infection
US—ultrasonic
    ultrasonography
    ultrasound
USAN—United States Adopted
    Name
USDA—United States Department
    of Agriculture
USN—ultrasonic nebulizer
USO—unilateral salpingo-
    oophorectomy
USP—United States Pharmacopeia
USPHS—United States Public
    Health Service
USR—unheated serum reagin (test)
UTBG—unbound thyroxine–bind-
    ing globulin
UTI—urinary tract infection
UTP—uridine triphosphate
UU—urine urobilinogen
UUN—urine urea nitrogen
UV—ultraviolet
    umbilical vein
    ureterovesical
    urethrovesical
    urine volume
UVA—ultraviolet A
    urethrovesical angle
UVB—ultraviolet B
UVC—ultraviolet C

UVJ—ureterovesical junction
    urethrovesical junction
UVL—ultraviolet light
UVP—uterine venous pressure
v—see (L. vide)
    very
    volt
V—vein
    vision
    visual acuity
    voice volume
    volt(s)
    voltage
    volume
V.—Vibrio
VA—vacuum aspiration
    ventriculoatrial
    vertebral artery
VA, V.A.—Veterans Administration
    Veterans Affairs
Va—visual acuity
V_a—arterial ventilation
V_A—alveolar ventilation
vag—vagina
    vaginal
VALE—visual acuity, left eye
VAMP—vincristine, amethopterine,
    6-mercaptopurine, prednisone
var—variation
VARE—visual acuity, right eye
vasc—vascular
VASC—Verbal Auditory Screen for
    Children
VB—viable birth
VB, VBL—vinblastine
VBS—veronal-buffered saline
VC—acuity of color vision
    vena cava
    ventilatory capacity
    vital capacity
VC, VCR—vincristine
VCG—vectorcardiogram
    vectorcardiography
VCU, VCUG—voiding cystoure-
    throgram
VD—vapor density
VDA—visual discriminatory acuity

VDBR—volume of distribution of bilirubin
VDEL—Venereal Disease Experimental Laboratory
vdg—voiding
VDL—visual detection level
VDM—vasodepressor material
VDP—vincristine, daunorubicin, prednisone
VDRS—Verdun Depression Rating Scale
VDS—venereal disease–syphilis
VE—visual efficiency
    volumic ejection
VEE—vagina ectocervix and endocervix
    Venezuelan equine encephalomyelitis
VEM—vasoexcitor material
VEP—visual evoked potential
VER—visual evoked response
ves—vesicular
v.f.—visual field
VF—left leg (electrode)
    ventricular fibrillation
    ventricular fluid
    visual field
    vocal fremitus
VFP—ventricular fluid pressure
VG—ventricular gallop
VH—vaginal hysterectomy
    venous hematocrit
    ventricular hypertrophy
    viral hepatitis
    vitreous hemorrhage
VHD—valvular heart disease
VHF—visual half-field
VIA—virus-inactivating agent
vib—vibration
VIG—vaccinia-immune globulin
VIP—vasoactive intestinal polypeptide
    very important patient
    voluntary interruption of pregnancy
VIS—vaginal irrigation smear
VISC—vitreous infusion suction cutter

vit—vitamin
vit cap—vital capacity
VLDL, VLDLP—very low-density lipoprotein
VM—viomycin
    voltmeter
VMA—vanillylmandelic acid
VMR—vasomotor rhinitis
VN—virus-neutralizing
VNS—villonodular synovitis
VO—verbal order
vol—volume
VOU—vision, each eye (L. visio oculus uterque)
VP—vasopressin
    venipuncture
    venous pressure
    Voges-Proskauer [reaction]
    volume pressure [curve]
    vulnerable period
V&P—vagotomy and pyloroplasty
VPB—ventricular premature beat
VPC—ventricular premature complex
    ventricular premature contraction
    volume of packed cells
    volume per cent
VPF—vascular permeability factor
V/Q—ventilation-perfusion
VR—valve replacement
    vascular resistance
    venous return
    ventilation ratio
    vocal resonance
    vocational rehabilitation
VR&E—vocational rehabilitation and education
VRI—viral respiratory infection
vs—against (L. versus)
    vibration seconds
    voids
VS—vaccination scar
    venisection
    ventricular septum
    verbal scale (IQ)
    vital signs
    without glasses

VSD—ventricular septal defect
vesical external sphincter dyssynergia
VSS—vital signs stable
VSV—vesicular stomatitis virus
VSW—ventricular stroke work
VT—tidal volume
ventricular tachycardia
V&T—volume and tension
VTSRS—Verdun Target Symptom Rating Scale
vv.—veins (L. venae)
v/v—volume (of solute) per volume (of solvent)
VV—viper venom
VW—vessel wall
VZ—varicella-zoster
VZIG—varicella-zoster immune globulin
VZV—varicella-zoster virus
w, w/—with
W—water
watt(s)
Weber [test]
week
wehnelt [unit of x-ray penetrating ability]
weight
widowed
wife
W+—weakly positive
WAIS—Wechsler Adult Intelligence Scale
WAS—Wiskott-Aldrich syndrome
WB—weightbearing (weight-bearing)
whole blood
Willowbrook (virus)
Wb—weber(s)
WBC—white blood cell
white blood [cell] count
WBC/hpf—white blood cell(s) per high-power field
WBF—whole-blood folate
WBH—whole-blood hematocrit
WBR—whole-body radiation [therapy]

WC—water closet
whooping cough
work capacity
WCC—white cell count
WD—wallerian degeneration
well-developed
well-differentiated
with disease
W4D—Worth four-dot (test)
WDLL—well-differentiated lymphocytic lymphoma
WDWN—well-developed, well-nourished
WEE—western equine encephalomyelitis
WF—Weil-Felix (reaction)
white female
WFR—Weil-Felix reaction
WG—water gauge
WH—well-healed
WHO—World Health Organization
WIA—wounded in action
WIC—Women, Infants, and Children [a government assistance program]
WISC—Wechsler Intelligence Scale for Children
wk—weak
week
WL—waiting list
wavelength
work load
WM—white male
whole milk
WMF—white middle-aged female
WMM—white middle-aged male
WMR—work metabolic rate
WN—well-nourished
WNF—well-nourished female
WNL—within normal limits
WNM—well-nourished male
w/o, wo—without
WO—water in oil
WP—weakly positive
working point
WPRS—Wittenborn Psychiatric Rating Scale

WPW—Wolff-Parkinson-White (syndrome)
wr—wrist
WR—Wasserman reaction
 weakly reactive
WRCs—washed red cells
WRE—whole ragweed extract
ws—watts-second
WS—water swallow
wt—weight
 white
WV—whispered voice
w/v—weight (of solute) per volume (of solvent)
w/w—weight (of solute) per weight (of solvent)
x—homeopathic symbol for the decimal scale of potencies $(1/10^x)$
 times
X—Kienböck unit of x-ray dosage
 magnification
 removal of
 respirations [anesthesia chart]
 start of anesthesia
 symbol for an unknown
XC—excretory cystogram
Xe—xenon
XLA—X-linked agammaglobulinemia

XM—crossmatch
XMP—xanthosine monophosphate
XR—x-ray
XS—excess
 xiphisternum
XT—exotropia
XU—excretory urogram
 x-unit
yr.—year
YAG—yttrium-aluminum-garnet
Yb—ytterbium
yd.—yard(s)
YF—yellow fever
y/o, Y/O—year-old
 years old
YOB—year of birth
YPLL—years of potential life lost
yr—year
YS—yellow spot (of the retina)
 yolk sac
YST—yolk sac tumor
Z—atomic number
 impedance
 zero
 Zuckung (contraction)
Z/D—zero defects
Z/G, ZIG—zoster immune globulin
ZSR—zeta sedimentation rate

Anatomy Plates

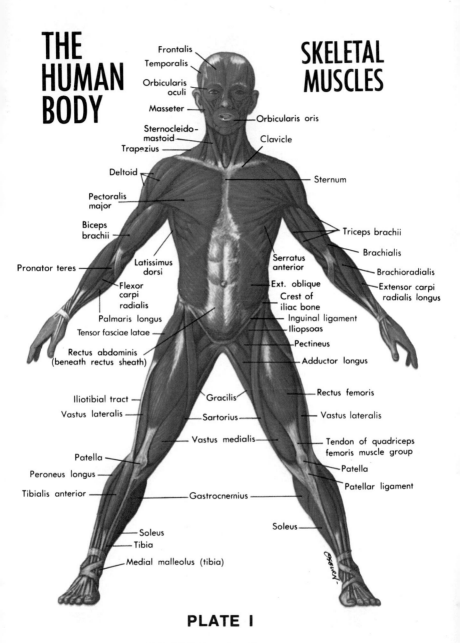

THE HUMAN BODY

SKELETAL MUSCLES

Frontalis
Temporalis
Orbicularis oculi
Masseter
Orbicularis oris
Sternocleido-mastoid
Clavicle
Trapezius
Deltoid
Sternum
Pectoralis major
Biceps brachii
Triceps brachii
Brachialis
Pronator teres
Latissimus dorsi
Serratus anterior
Brachioradialis
Flexor carpi radialis
Ext. oblique
Extensor carpi radialis longus
Crest of iliac bone
Palmaris longus
Inguinal ligament
Tensor fasciae latae
Iliopsoas
Rectus abdominis (beneath rectus sheath)
Pectineus
Adductor longus
Iliotibial tract
Gracilis
Rectus femoris
Vastus lateralis
Sartorius
Vastus lateralis
Vastus medialis
Patella
Tendon of quadriceps femoris muscle group
Peroneus longus
Patella
Tibialis anterior
Gastrocnemius
Patellar ligament
Soleus
Soleus
Tibia
Medial malleolus (tibia)

PLATE I

© by W. B. Saunders Company

BONES

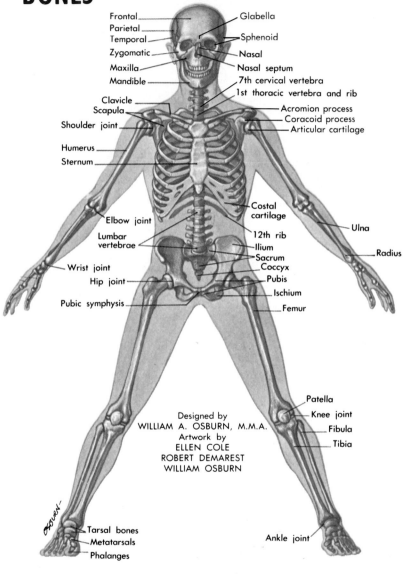

Frontal
Parietal
Temporal
Zygomatic
Maxilla
Mandible
Clavicle
Scapula
Shoulder joint
Humerus
Sternum
Elbow joint
Lumbar vertebrae
Wrist joint
Hip joint
Pubic symphysis

Glabella
Sphenoid
Nasal
Nasal septum
7th cervical vertebra
1st thoracic vertebra and rib
Acromion process
Coracoid process
Articular cartilage
Costal cartilage
Ulna
12th rib
Ilium
Sacrum
Coccyx
Radius
Pubis
Ischium
Femur

Patella
Knee joint
Fibula
Tibia

Designed by
WILLIAM A. OSBURN, M.M.A.
Artwork by
ELLEN COLE
ROBERT DEMAREST
WILLIAM OSBURN

Tarsal bones
Metatarsals
Phalanges

Ankle joint

PLATE II

DETAILS OF CIRCULATORY STRUCTURES

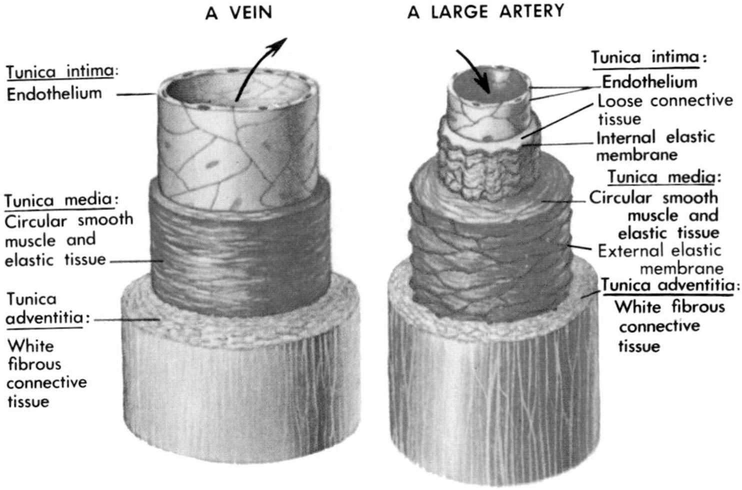

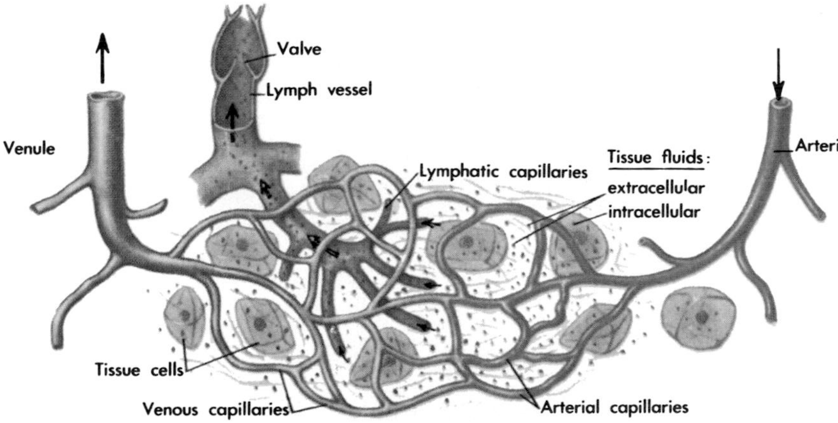

A VEIN

Tunica intima:
Endothelium

Tunica media:
Circular smooth
muscle and
elastic tissue

Tunica
adventitia:

White
fibrous
connective
tissue

A LARGE ARTERY

Tunica intima:
Endothelium
Loose connective
tissue
Internal elastic
membrane
Tunica media:
Circular smooth
muscle and
elastic tissue
External elastic
membrane
Tunica adventitia:
White fibrous
connective
tissue

Valve
Lymph vessel

Venule

Lymphatic capillaries

Tissue fluids:
extracellular
intracellular

Arteriole

Tissue cells
Venous capillaries

Arterial capillaries

A CAPILLARY BED

PLATE IX

THE BRAIN AND SPINAL NERVES

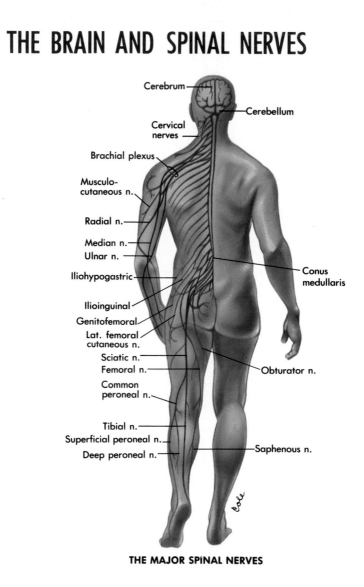

THE MAJOR SPINAL NERVES

PLATE X

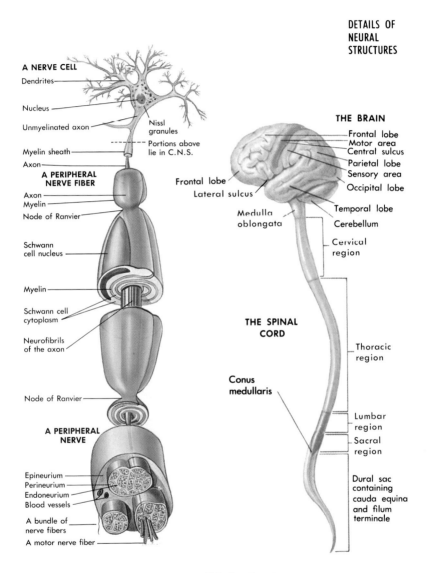

DETAILS OF
NEURAL
STRUCTURES

A NERVE CELL

Dendrites

Nucleus

Unmyelinated axon

Nissl granules

Portions above lie in C.N.S.

Myelin sheath

Axon

A PERIPHERAL NERVE FIBER

Axon
Myelin
Node of Ranvier

Schwann cell nucleus

Myelin

Schwann cell cytoplasm

Neurofibrils of the axon

Node of Ranvier

A PERIPHERAL NERVE

Epineurium
Perineurium
Endoneurium
Blood vessels

A bundle of nerve fibers

A motor nerve fiber

THE BRAIN

Frontal lobe
Motor area
Central sulcus
Parietal lobe
Sensory area
Occipital lobe

Frontal lobe
Lateral sulcus

Temporal lobe

Medulla oblongata

Cerebellum

Cervical region

THE SPINAL CORD

Conus medullaris

Thoracic region

Lumbar region

Sacral region

Dural sac containing cauda equina and filum terminale

PLATE XI

ORGANS OF SPECIAL SENSE THE EAR

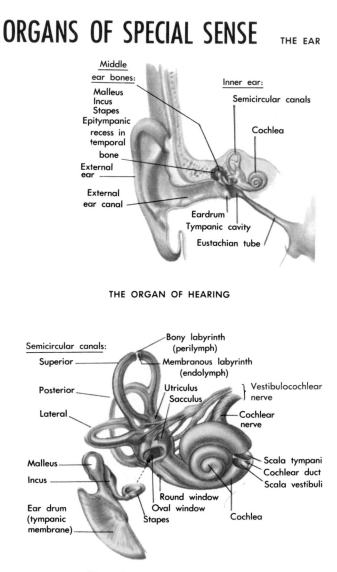

Middle
ear bones:

Malleus
Incus
Stapes
Epitympanic
recess in
temporal
bone
External
ear

External
ear canal

Inner ear:

Semicircular canals

Cochlea

Eardrum
Tympanic cavity
Eustachian tube

THE ORGAN OF HEARING

Semicircular canals:

Superior

Posterior

Lateral

Malleus

Incus

Ear drum
(tympanic
membrane)

Bony labyrinth
(perilymph)
Membranous labyrinth
(endolymph)

Utriculus
Sacculus

Vestibulocochlear
nerve

Cochlear
nerve

Scala tympani
Cochlear duct
Scala vestibuli

Round window
Oval window
Stapes

Cochlea

THE MIDDLE EAR AND INNER EAR

PLATE XII

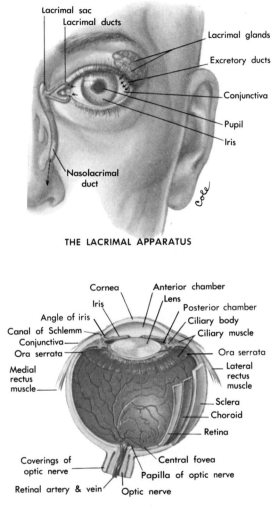

THE LACRIMAL APPARATUS

HORIZONTAL SECTION OF THE EYE

PLATE XIII

STRUCTURAL DETAILS

SKELETAL MUSCLE

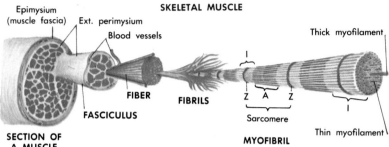

Epimysium (muscle fascia)
Ext. perimysium
Blood vessels
Thick myofilament

FIBER
FIBRILS
FASCICULUS

Z A Z
Sarcomere

Thin myofilament

SECTION OF A MUSCLE

MYOFIBRIL

BRAIN

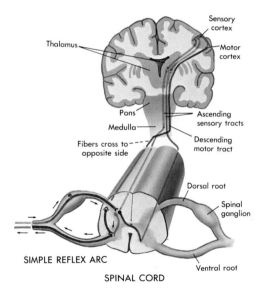

Thalamus
Sensory cortex
Motor cortex

Pons
Medulla
Fibers cross to opposite side

Ascending sensory tracts
Descending motor tract

Dorsal root
Spinal ganglion

SIMPLE REFLEX ARC

Ventral root

SPINAL CORD

PLATE XIV

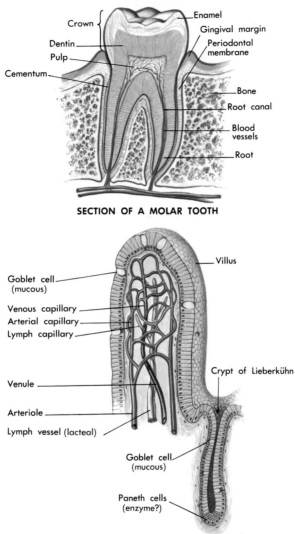

SECTION OF A MOLAR TOOTH

Crown {
Dentin
Pulp
Cementum

Enamel
Gingival margin
Periodontal membrane
Bone
Root canal
Blood vessels
Root

Goblet cell (mucous)
Venous capillary
Arterial capillary
Lymph capillary
Venule
Arteriole
Lymph vessel (lacteal)

Villus
Crypt of Lieberkühn
Goblet cell (mucous)
Paneth cells (enzyme?)
Intestinal gland

SECTIONS OF SMALL INTESTINE WALL

PLATE XV

THE PARANASAL SINUSES

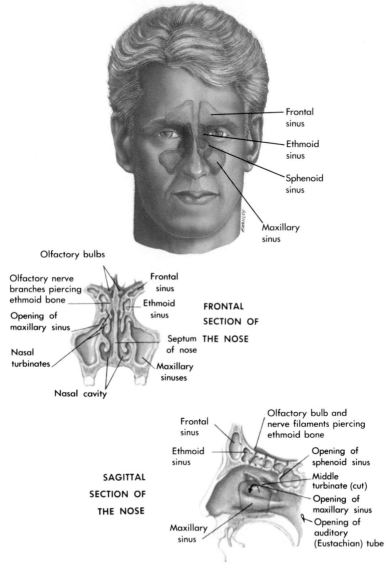

Frontal sinus

Ethmoid sinus

Sphenoid sinus

Maxillary sinus

Olfactory bulbs

Olfactory nerve branches piercing ethmoid bone

Opening of maxillary sinus

Nasal turbinates

Nasal cavity

Frontal sinus

Ethmoid sinus

Septum of nose

Maxillary sinuses

FRONTAL SECTION OF THE NOSE

SAGITTAL SECTION OF THE NOSE

Frontal sinus

Ethmoid sinus

Maxillary sinus

Olfactory bulb and nerve filaments piercing ethmoid bone

Opening of sphenoid sinus

Middle turbinate (cut)

Opening of maxillary sinus

Opening of auditory (Eustachian) tube

PLATE XVI

Combining Forms in Medical Terminology

The following is a list of combining forms encountered frequently in the vocabulary of medicine. A dash or dashes are appended to indicate whether the form usually precedes (as *ante-*) or follows (as *-agra*) the other elements of the compound or usually appears between the other elements (as *-em-*). Following each combining form, the first item of information is the Greek or Latin word, or both a Greek and a Latin word, from which it is derived. Greek words have been transliterated into Roman characters. Latin words are identified by [L.], Greek words by [Gr.]. Information necessary to an understanding of the form appears next in parentheses. Then the meaning or meanings of the words are given, followed where appropriate by reference to a synonymous combining form. Finally, an example is given to illustrate the use of the combining form in a compound English derivative.

a-	*a-* [L.] (*n* is added before words beginning with a vowel) negative prefix. Cf. in-³. *a*metria
ab-	*ab* [L.] away from. Cf. apo-, *ab*ducent
abdomin-	*abdomen, abdominis* [L.] abdomen. *abdomin*oscopy
ac-	See ad-, *ac*cretion
acet-	*acetum* [L.] vinegar. *acet*ometer
acid-	*acidus* [L.] sour. *acid*uric
acou-	*akouō* [Gr.] hear. *acou*esthesia. (Also spelled acu-)
acr-	*akron* [Gr.] extremity, peak. *acr*omegaly
act-	*ago, actus* [L.] do, drive, act. rea*ct*ion
actin-	*aktis, aktinos* [Gr.] ray, radius. Cf. radi-. *actin*ogenesis
acu-	See acou-. oste*o*acu*s*is
ad-	*ad* [L.] (*d* changes to *c, f, g, p, s,* or *t* before words beginning with those consonants) to. *ad*renal
aden-	*adēn* [Gr.] gland. Cf. gland-. *aden*oma
adip-	*adeps, adipis* [L.] fat. Cf. lip- and stear-. *adip*ocellular
aer-	*aēr* [Gr.] air. an*aer*obiosis
aesthe-	See esthe-. *aesthe*sioneurosis
af-	See ad-. *af*ferent
ag-	See ad-. *ag*glutinant

-agogue	*agōgos* [Gr.] leading, inducing. galact*agogue*
-agra	*agra* [Gr.] catching, seizure. pod*agra*
alb-	*albus* [L.] white. Cf. leuk-. *alb*ocinereous
alg-	*algos* [Gr.] pain. neur*alg*ia
all-	*allos* [Gr.] other, different. *all*ergy
alve-	*alveus* [L.] trough, channel, cavity. *alve*olar
amph-	See amphi-. *amph*eclexis
amphi-	*amphi* [Gr.] (*i* is dropped before words beginning with a vowel) both, doubly. *amphi*celous
amyl-	*amylon* [Gr.] starch. *amyl*osynthesis
an-¹	See ana-, *an*agogic
an-²	See a-. *an*omalous
ana-	*ana* [Gr.] (final *a* is dropped before words beginning with a vowel) up, positive. *ana*phoresis
ancyl-	See ankyl-, *ancyl*ostomiasis
andr-	*anēr, andros* [Gr.] man. gyn*andr*oid
angi-	*angeion* [Gr.] vessel. Cf. vas-. *angi*emphraxis
ankyl-	*ankylos* [Gr.] crooked, looped. *ankyl*odactylia. (Also spelled ancyl-)
ant-	See anti-. *ant*ophthalmic
ante-	*ante* [L.] before. *ante*flexion

anti- *anti* [Gr.] (*i* is dropped before words beginning with a vowel) against, counter. Cf. contra-. *anti*pyogenic

antr- *antron* [Gr.] cavern. *antr*odynia

ap-¹ See apo-. *ap*heter

ap-² See ad, *ap*pend

-aph- *haptō, haph-* [Gr.] touch. dys*aph*ia. (See also hapt-)

apo- *apo* [Gr.] (*o* is dropped before words beginning with a vowel) away from, detached. Cf. ab-. *apo*physis

arachn- *arachnē* [Gr.] spider. *arachn*odactyly

arch- *archē* [Gr.] beginning, origin. *arch*enteron

arter(i)- *arteria* [Gr.] windpipe, artery. *arter*iosclerosis, peri*arter*itis

arthr- *arthron* [Gr.] joint. Cf. articul-. syn*arthr*osis

articul- *articulus* [L.] joint. Cf. arthr-. dis*articul*ation

as- See ad-. *as*similation

at- See ad-. *at*trition

aur- *auris* [L.] ear. Cf. ot-. *aur*inasal

aux- *auxō* [Gr.] increase. enter*aux*e

ax- *axōn* [Gr.] or *axis* [L.] axis. *ax*ofugal

axon- *axōn* [Gr.] axis. *axon*ometer

ba- *bainō, ba-* [Gr.] go, walk, stand. hypno*ba*tia

bacill- *bacillus* [L.] small staff, rod. Cf. bacter-. actino*bacill*osis

bacter- *bactērion* [Gr.] small staff, rod. Cf. bacill-. *bacter*iophage

ball- *ballō, bol-* [Gr.] throw. *ball*istics. (See also bol-)

bar- *baros* [Gr.] weight. pedo*bar*ometer

bi-¹ *bios* [Gr.] life. Cf. vit-. aero*bi*c

bi-² *bi-* [L.] two. *bi*lobate (See also di-¹)

bil- *bilis* [L.] bile. Cf. chol-. *bil*iary

blast- *blastos* [Gr.] bud, child, a growing thing in its early stages. Cf. germ-. *blast*oma, zygo*blast*

blep- *blepō* [Gr.] look, see. hemi*ablep*sia

blephar- *blepharon* [Gr.] (from *blepō*; see blep-) eyelid. Cf. cili-. *blephar*oncus

bol- See ball-. em*bol*ism

brachi- *brachiōn* [Gr.] arm. *brachi*ocephalic

brachy- *brachys* [Gr.] short. *brachy*cephalic

brady- *bradys* [Gr.] slow. *brady*cardia

brom- *brōmos* [Gr.] stench. podo*bro*midrosis

bronch- *bronchos* [Gr.] windpipe. *bronch*oscopy

bry- *bryō* [Gr.] be full of life. em*bry*onic

bucc- *bucca* [L.] cheek. disto*bucc*al

cac- *kakos* [Gr.] bad, abnormal. Cf. mal-. *cac*odontia, arthro*cac*e. (See also dys-)

calc-¹ *calx, calcis* [L.] stone (cf. lith-), limestone, lime. *calc*ipexy

calc-² *calx, calcis* [L.] heel. *calc*aneotibial

calor- *calor* [L.] heat. Cf. therm-. *calor*imeter

cancr- *cancer, cancri* [L.] crab, cancer. Cf. carcin-. *cancr*ology (Also spelled chancr-)

capit- *caput, capitis* [L.] head. Cf. cephal-. de*capit*ator

caps- *capsa* [L.] (from *capio*; see cept-) container. en*caps*ulation

carbo(n)- *carbo, carbonis* [L.] coal, charcoal. *carbo*hydrate, *carbon*uria

carcin- *karkinos* [Gr.] crab, cancer. Cf. cancr-. *carcin*oma

cardi- *kardia* [Gr.] heart. lipo*cardi*ac

cary- See kary-. *cary*okinesis

cat- See cata-. *cat*hode

cata- *kata* [Gr.] (final *a* is dropped before words beginning with a vowel) down, negative. *cata*batic

caud- *cauda* [L.] tail. *caud*ad

cav- *cavus* [L.] hollow. Cf. coel-. con*cav*e

cec- *caecus* [L.] blind. Cf. typhl-. *cec*opexy

cel-¹ See coel-. amphi*cel*ous

cel-² See -cele. *cel*ectome

-cele *kēlē* [Gr.] tumor, hernia. gastro*cele*

cell- *cella* [L.] room, cell. Cf. cyt-. *cell*iferous

cen- *koinos* [Gr.] common. *cen*esthesia

cent- *centum* [L.] hundred. Cf. hect-. Indicates fraction in metric system.* *centi*meter, *centi*pede

cente- *kenteō* [Gr.] to puncture. Cf. punct-. entero*cente*sis

centr- *kentron* [Gr.] or *centrum* [L.] point, center. neuro*centr*al

cephal- *kephalē* [Gr.] head. Cf. capit-. en*cephal*itis

cept- *capio, -cipientis, -ceptus* [L.] take, receive. re*cept*or

cer- *kēros* [Gr.] or *cera* [L.] wax. *cer*oplasty, *cer*omel

cerat- See kerat-. a*cerat*osis

cerebr- *cerebrum* [L.] brain. *cerebr*ospinal

cervic- *cervix, cervicis* [L.] neck. Cf. trachel-. *cervic*itis

chancr- See cancr-. *chancr*iform

cheil-   *cheilos* [Gr.] lip. Cf. labi-.
     *cheil*oschisis
cheir-   *cheir* [Gr.] hand. Cf. man-.
     macro*cheir*ia (Also spelled
     chir-)
chir-   See cheir-. *chir*omegaly
chlor-   *chlōros* [Gr.] green. a*chlor*opsia
chol-   *cholē* [Gr.] bile. Cf. bil-.
     hepato*chol*angeitis
chondr-   *chondros* [Gr.] cartilage.
     *chondr*omalacia
chord-   *chordē* [Gr.] string, cord.
     peri*chord*al
chori-   *chorion* [Gr.] protective fetal
     membrane. endo*chori*on
chro-   *chrōs* [Gr.] color. poly*chro*matic
chron-   *chronos* [Gr.] time. syn*chron*ous
chy-   *cheō, chy-* [Gr.] pour. ec*chy*mosis
-cid(e)   *caedo, -cisus* [L.] cut, kill. infan-
     ti*cide*, germi*cid*al
cili-   *cilium* [L.] eyelid. Cf. blephar-.
     super*cili*ary
cine-   See kine-. auto*cine*sis
-cipient   See cept-. in*cipient*
circum-   *circum* [L.] around. Cf. peri-.
     *circum*ferential
-cis-   *caedo, -cisus* [L.] cut, kill.
     ex*cis*ion
clas-   *klaō* [Gr.] break. cranio*clas*t
clin-   *klinō* [Gr.] bend, incline, make
     lie down. *clin*ometer
clus-   *claudo, -clusus* [L.] shut.
     mal*occlus*ion
co-   See con-. *co*hesion
cocc-   *kokkos* [Gr.] seed, pill. gono*cocc*us
coel-   *koilos* [Gr.] hollow. Cf. cav-.
     *coel*enteron (Also spelled cel-)
col-[1]   See colon-. *col*ic
col-[2]   See con-. *col*lapse
colon-   *kolon* [Gr.] lower intestine. *colon*ic
colp-   *kolpos* [Gr.] hollow, vagina. Cf.
     sin-. endo*colp*itis
com-   See con-. *com*masculation
con-   *con-* [L.] (becomes co- before
     vowels or *h*; col- before *l*;
     com- before *b, m,* or *p*; cor-
     before *r*) with, together. Cf.
     syn-. *con*traction
contra-   *contra* [L.] against, counter. Cf.
     anti-. *contra*indication
copr-   *kopros* [Gr.] dung. Cf. sterco-.
     *copr*oma
cor-[1]   *korē* [Gr.] doll, little image,
     pupil. iso*cor*ia
cor-[2]   See con-. *cor*rugator
corpor-   *corpus, corporis* [L.] body. Cf.
     somat-. intra*corpor*al
cortic-   *cortex, corticis* [L.] bark, rind.
     *cortic*osterone

cost-   *costa* [L.] rib. Cf. pleur-.
     inter*cost*al
crani-   *kranion* [Gr.] or *cranium* [L.]
     skull. peri*crani*um
creat-   *kreas, kreato-* [Gr.] meat, flesh.
     *creat*orrhea
-crescent   *cresco, crescentis, cretus* [L.]
     grow. ex*crescent*
cret-[1]   *cerno, cretus* [L.] distinguish,
     separate off. Cf. crin-. dis*cret*e
cret-[2]   See -crescent. ac*cret*ion
crin-   *krinō* [Gr.] distinguish, separate
     off. Cf. cret-[1]. endo*crin*ology
crur-   *crus, cruris* [L.] shin, leg.
     brachio*crur*al
cry-   *kryos* [Gr.] cold. *cry*esthesia
crypt-   *kryptō* [Gr.] hide, conceal.
     *crypt*orchism
cult-   *colo, cultus* [L.] tend, cultivate.
     *cult*ure
cune-   *cuneus* [L.] wedge. Cf. sphen-.
     *cune*iform
cut-   *cutis* [L.] skin. Cf. derm(at)-.
     sub*cut*aneous
cyan-   *kyanos* [Gr.] blue. antho*cyan*in
cycl-   *kyklos* [Gr.] circle, cycle.
     *cycl*ophoria
cyst-   *kystis* [Gr.] bladder. Cf. vesic-.
     nephro*cyst*itis
cyt-   *kytos* [Gr.] cell. Cf. cell-.
     plasmo*cyt*oma
dacry-   *dakry* [Gr.] tear [tēr]. *dacry*ocyst
dactyl-   *daktylos* [Gr.] finger, toe. Cf.
     digit-. hexa*dactyl*ism
de-   *de* [L.] down from. *de*composition
dec-[1]   *deka* [Gr.] ten. Indicates multiple
     in metric system.* Cf. dec-[2].
     *dec*agram
dec-[2]   *decem* [L.] ten. Indicates fraction
     in metric system.* Cf. dec-[1].
     *deci*para, *deci*meter
dendr-   *dendron* [Gr.] tree. neuro*dendr*ite
dent-   *dens, dentis* [L.] tooth. Cf.
     odont-. inter*dent*al
derm(at)-   *derma, dermatos* [Gr.] skin. Cf.
     cut-. endo*derm, dermat*itis
desm-   *desmos* [Gr.] band, ligament.
     syn*desm*opexy
dextr-   *dexter, dextr-* [L.] right-hand.
     ambi*dextr*ous
di-[1]   *di-* [Gr.] two. *di*morphic. (See
     also bi-[2])
di-[2]   See dia-. *di*uresis
di-[3]   See dis-. *di*vergent
dia-   *dia* [Gr.] (*a* is dropped before
     words beginning with a
     vowel) through, apart. Cf.
     per-. *dia*gnosis
didym-   *didymos* [Gr.] twin. Cf. gemin-.
     epi*didym*al

digit- *digitus* [L.] finger, toe. Cf. dactyl-. *digit*igrade

diplo- *diploos* [Gr.] double. *diplo*myelia

dis- *dis-* [L.] (*s* may be dropped before a word beginning with a consonant) apart, away from. *dis*location

disc- *diskos* [Gr.] or *discus* [L.]disk. *disc*oplacenta

dors- *dorsum* [L.] back. ventro*dors*al

drom- *dromos* [Gr.] course. hemo*dro*mometer

-ducent See duct-. ad*ducent*

-duct *duco, ducentis, ductus* [L.] lead, conduct. ovi*duct*

dur- *durus* [L.] hard. Cf. scler-. in*dur*ation

dynam(i)- *dynamis* [Gr.] power, *dyna*moneure, neuro*dynam*ic

dys- *dys-* [Gr.] bad, improper. Cf. mal-. *dys*trophic. (See also cac-)

e- *e* [L.] out from. Cf. ec- and ex-. *e*mission

ec- *ek* [Gr.] out of. Cf. e-. *ec*centric

-ech- *echō* [Gr.] have, hold, be. syn*ech*otomy

ect- *ektos* [Gr.] outside. Cf. extra-. *ect*oplasm

ede- *oideō* [Gr.] swell. *ede*matous

ef- See ex-. *ef*florescent

-elc- *helkos* [Gr.] sore, ulcer. enter*el*cosis. (See also helc-)

electr- *ēlectron* [Gr.] amber. *electr*otherapy

em-[1] See en-. *em*bolism, *em*pathy, *em*phlysis

-em-[2] *haima* [Gr.] blood. an*em*ia. (See also hem(at)-)

en- *en* [Gr.] (*n* changes to *m* before *b, p,* or *ph*) in, on. Cf. in-[2]. *en*celitis

end- *endon* [Gr.] inside. Cf. intra-. *end*angium

enter- *enteron* [Gr.] intestine. dys*enter*y

ep- See epi-. *ep*axial

epi- *epi* [Gr.] (*i* is dropped before words beginning with a vowel) upon, after, in addition. *epi*glottis

erg- *ergon* [Gr.] work, deed. en*erg*y

erythr- *erythros* [Gr.] red. Cf. rub(r)-. *erythr*ochromia

eso- *esō* [Gr.] inside. Cf. intra-. *eso*phylactic

esthe- *aisthanomai, aisthē-* [Gr.] perceive, feel. Cf. sens-. an*esthe*sia

eu- *eu* [Gr.] good, normal. *eu*pepsia

ex- *ex* [Gr., L.] out of. Cf. e-. *ex*cretion

exo- *exō* [Gr.] outside. Cf. extra-. *exo*pathic

extra- *extra* [L.] outside of, beyond. Cf. ect-, exo-. *extra*cellular

faci- *facies* [L.] face. Cf. prosop-. brachio*faci*olingual

-facient *facio, facientis, factus, -fectus* [L.] make. Cf. poie-. cale*facient*

-fact- See facient-. arte*fact*

fasci- *fascia* [L.] band. *fasci*orrhaphy

febr- *febris* [L.] fever. Cf. pyr-. *febr*icide

-fect- See -facient. de*fect*ive

-ferent *fero, ferentis, latus* [L.] bear, carry. Cf. phor-. ef*ferent*

ferr- *ferrum* [L.] iron. *ferr*oprotein

fibr- *fibra* [L.] fiber. Cf. in-[1]. chondro*fibr*oma

fil- *filum* [L.] thread. *fil*iform

fiss- *findo, fissus* [L.] split. Cf. schis-. *fiss*ion

flagell- *flagellum* [L.] whip. *flagell*ation

flav- *flavus* [L.] yellow. Cf. xanth-. ribo*flav*in

-flect- *flecto, flexus* [L.] bend, divert. de*flect*ion

-flex- See -flect. re*flex*ometer

flu- *fluo, fluxus* [L.] flow. Cf. rhe-. *flu*id

flux- See flu-. af*flux*ion

for- *foris* [L.] door, opening. per*for*ated

-form *forma* [L.] shape. Cf. -oid. ossi*form*

fract- *frango, fractus* [L.] break. re*fract*ive

front- *frons, frontis* [L.] forehead, front. naso*front*al

-fug(e) *fugio* [L.] flee, avoid. vermi*fuge*, centri*fug*al

funct- *fungor, functus* [L.] perform, serve, function. mal*funct*ion

fund- *fundo, fusus* [L.] pour. in*fund*ibulum

fus- See fund-. dif*fus*ible

galact- *gala, galactos* [Gr.] milk. Cf. lact-. dys*galact*ia

gam- *gamos* [Gr.] marriage, reproductive union. a*gam*ont

gangli- *ganglion* [Gr.] swelling, plexus. neuro*gangli*itis

gastr- *gastēr, gastros* [Gr.] stomach. cholangio*gastr*ostomy

gelat- *gelo, gelatus* [L.] freeze, congeal. *gelat*in

gemin- *geminus* [L.] twin, double. Cf. didym-. quadri*gemin*al

gen- *gignomai, gen-, gon-* [Gr.] become, be produced, originate, or *gennaō* [Gr] produce, originate. cyto*gen*ic

germ- *germen, germinis* [L.] bud, a growing thing in its early stages. Cf. blast-. *germ*inal, ovi*germ*

gest-	*gero, gerentis, gestus* [L.] bear, carry. con*gest*ion
gland-	*glans, glandis* [L.] acorn. Cf. aden-. intra*gland*ular
-glia	*glia* [Gr.] glue. neuro*glia*
gloss-	*glōssa* [Gr.] tongue. Cf. lingu-. tricho*gloss*ia
glott-	*glōtta* [Gr.] tongue, language. *glott*ic
gluc-	See glyc(y)-. *gluc*ophenetidin
glutin-	*gluten, glutinis* [L.] glue. ag*glutin*ation
glyc(y)-	*glykys* [Gr.] sweet. *glyc*emia, *gly*cyrrhizin. (Also spelled gluc-)
gnath-	*gnathos* [Gr.] jaw. ortho*gnath*ous
gno-	*gignōsiō, gnō* [Gr.] know, discern. diag*no*sis
gon-	See gen, anphi*gon*y
grad-	*gradior* [L.] walk, take steps. retro*grad*e
-gram	*gramma* [Gr.] letter, drawing. cardio*gram*
gran-	*granum* [L.] grain, particle. lipo*gran*uloma
graph-	*graphō* [Gr.] scratch, write, record. histo*graph*y
grav-	*gravis* [L.] heavy. multi*grav*ida
gyn(ec)-	*gynē, gynaikos* [Gr.]woman, wife. andro*gyn*y, *gynec*ologic
gyr-	*gyros* [Gr.] ring, circle. *gyr*ospasm
haem(at)-	See hem(at)-. *haem*orrhagia, *haemat*oxylon
hapt-	*haptō* [Gr.] touch. *hapt*ometer
hect-	*hekt-* [Gr.] hundred. Cf. cent-. Indicates multiple in metric system.* *hect*ometer
helc-	*helkos* [Gr.] sore, ulcer. *helc*osis
hem(at)-	*haima, haimatos* [Gr.] blood. Cf. sanguin-. *hem*angioma, *hemat*ocyturia. (See also -em-)
hemi-	*hēmi-* [Gr.] half. Cf. semi-. *hemi*ageusia
hen-	*heis, henos* [Gr.] one. Cf. un-. *hen*ogenesis
hepat-	*hēpar, hēpatos* [Gr.] liver. gastro*hepat*ic
hept(a)-	*hepta* [Gr.] seven. Cf. sept-². *hepta*tomic, *hepta*valent
hered-	*heres, heredis* [L.] heir. *hered*oimmunity
hex-¹	*hex* [Gr.] six. Cf. sex-. *hex*yl-. An *a* is added in some combinations
hex-²	*echō, hex-* [Gr.] (added to *s* becomes *hex*-) have, hold, be. cac*hex*ia
hexa-	See hex-¹. *hexa*chromic
hidr-	*hidros* [Gr.] sweat. hyper*hidr*osis
hist-	*histos* [Gr.] web, tissue. *histo*dialysis
hod-	*hodos* [Gr.] road, path. *hod*oneuromere. (See also od- and -ode¹)
hom-	*homos* [Gr.] common, same. *hom*omorphic
horm-	*ormē* [Gr.] impetus, impulse. *horm*one
hydat-	*hydōr, hydatos* [Gr.] water. *hydat*ism
hydr-	*hydōr, hydr-* [Gr.] water. Cf. lymph-. anclor*hydr*ia
hyp-	See hypo-. *hyp*axial
hyper-	*hyper* [Gr.] above, beyond, extreme. Cf. super-. *hyper*trophy
hypn-	*hypnos* [Gr.] sleep. *hypn*otic
hypo-	*hypo* [Gr.] (*o* is dropped before words beginning with a vowel) under, below. Cf. sub-. *hypo*metabolism
hyster-	*hystera* [Gr.] womb. colpo*hyster*opexy
iatr-	*iatros* [Gr.] physician. ped*iatr*ics
idi-	*idios* [Gr.] peculiar, separate, distinct. *idi*osyncrasy
il-	See in-²,³. *il*linition (in, on); *il*legible (negative prefix)
ile-	See ili- [ile- is commonly used to refer to the portion of the intestines known as the ileum]. *ile*ostomy
ili-	*ilium (ileum)* [L.] lower abdomen, intestines [ili- is commonly used to refer to the flaring part of the hip bone known as the ilium]. *ili*osacral
im-	See in-²,³. *im*mersion (in, on); *im*perforation (negative prefix)
in-¹	*is, inos* [Gr.] fiber. Cf. fibr-. *in*osteatoma
in-²	*in* [L.] (*n* changes to *l, m,* or *r* before words beginning with those consonants) in, on. Cf. en-. *in*sertion
in-³	*in-* [L.] (*n* changes to *l, m,* or *r* before words beginning with those consonants) negative prefix. Cf. a-. *in*valid
infra-	*infra* [L.] beneath. *infra*orbital
insul-	*insula* [L.] island. *insul*in
inter-	*inter* [L.] among, between. *inter*carpal
intra-	*intra* [L.] inside. Cf. end-, eso-. *intra*venous
ir-	See in-²,³. *ir*radiation (in, on); *ir*reducible (negative prefix)
irid-	*iris, iridos* [Gr.] rainbow, colored circle. kerato*irid*ocyclitis
is-	*isos* [Gr.] equal. *is*otope
ischi-	*ischion* [Gr.] hip, haunch. *ischi*opubic

jact-   *iacio, iactus* [L.] throw. *jact*itation
-ject   *iacio, -iectus* [L.] throw. in*ject*ion
jejun-   *ieiunus* [L.] hungry, not partak-
     ing of food. gastro*jejuno*stomy
jug-   *iugum* [L.] yoke. con*jug*ation
junct-   *iungo, iunctus* [L.] yoke, join.
     con*junct*iva
kary-   *karyon* [Gr.] nut, kernel, nucleus.
     Cf. nucle-. mega*kary*ocyte.
     (Also spelled cary-)
kerat-   *keras, keratos* [Gr.] horn. *kera*-
     *to*lysis. (Also spelled cerat-)
kil-   *chilioi* [Gr.] one thousand. Cf.
     mill-. Indicates multiple in
     metric system.* *kilo*gram
kine-   *kineō* [Gr.] move. *kine*mato-
     graph. (Also spelled cine-)
labi-   *labium* [L.] lip. Cf. cheil-.
     gingivo*labi*al
lact-   *lac, lactis* [L.] milk. Cf. galact-.
     gluco*lact*one
lal-   *laleō* [Gr.] talk, babble. glosso*lal*ia
lapar-   *lapara* [Gr.] flank. *lapar*otomy
laryng-   *larynx, laryngos* [Gr.] windpipe.
     *laryng*endoscope
lat-   *fero, latus* [L.] bear, carry. See
     -ferent. trans*lat*ion
later-   *latus, lateris* [L.] side.
     ventro*later*al
lent-   *lens, lentis* [L.] lentil. Cf. phac-.
     *lent*iconus
lep-   *lambanō, lēp-* [Gr.] take, seize.
     cata*lep*tic
leuc-   See leuk-. *leuc*inuria
leuk-   *leukos* [Gr.] white. Cf. alb-. *leuk*-
     orrhea. (Also spelled leuc-)
lien-   *lien* [L.] spleen. Cf. splen-.
     *lien*ocele
lig-   *ligo* [L.] tie, bind. *lig*ate
lingu-   *lingua* [L.] tongue. Cf. gloss-.
     sub*lingu*al
lip-   *lipos* [Gr.] fat. Cf. adip-. glyco*lip*in
lith-   *lithos* [Gr.] stone. Cf. calc-¹.
     nephro*lith*otomy
loc-   *locus* [L.] place. Cf. top-.
     *loc*omotion
log-   *legō, log-* [Gr.] speak, give an
     account. *log*orrhea, embryo*log*y
lumb-   *lumbus* [L.] loin. dorso*lumb*ar
lute-   *luteus* [L.] yellow. Cf. xanth-.
     *lute*oma
ly-   *lyō* [Gr.] loose, dissolve. Cf.
     solut-. kerato*ly*sis
lymph-   *lympha* [Gr.] water. Cf. hydr-.
     *lymph*adenosis
macr-   *makros* [Gr.] long, large.
     *macr*omyeloblast
mal-   *malus* [L.] bad, abnormal. Cf.
     cac-, dys-. *mal*function
malac-   *malakos* [Gr.] soft. osteo*malac*ia

mamm-   *mamma* [L.] breast. Cf. mast-.
     sub*mamm*ary
man-   *manus* [L.] hand. Cf. cheir-.
     *man*iphalanx
mani-   *mania* [Gr.] mental aberration.
     *mani*graphy, klepto*mani*a
mast-   *mastos* [Gr.] breast. Cf. mamm-.
     hyper*mast*ia
medi-   *medius* [L.] middle. Cf. mes-.
     *medi*frontal
mega-   *megas* [Gr.] great, large; one mil-
     lion. Indicates multiple in
     metric system.* *mega*colon,
     *mega*dyne. (See also megal-)
megal-   *megas, megalou* [Gr.] great,
     large. acro*megal*y
mel-   *melos* [Gr.] limb, member.
     sym*mel*ia
melan-   *melas, melanos* [Gr.] black.
     hippo*melan*in
men-   *mēn* [Gr.] month. dys*men*orrhea
mening-   *mēninx, mēningos* [Gr.] mem-
     brane. encephalo*mening*itis
ment-   *mens, mentis* [L.] mind. Cf.
     phren-, psych-, thym-. de*ment*ia
mer-   *meros* [Gr.] part. poly*mer*ic
mes-   *mesos* [Gr.] middle. Cf. medi-.
     *mes*oderm
met-   See meta-. *met*allergy
meta-   *meta* [Gr.] (*a* is dropped before
     words beginning with a
     vowel) after, beyond, accom-
     panying. *meta*carpal
metr-¹   *metron* [Gr.] measure. stereo*metr*y
metr-²   *metra* [Gr.] womb. endo*metr*itis
micr-   *mikros* [Gr.] small. photo*micr*o-
     graph
mill-   *mille* [L.] one thousand. Cf. kil-.
     Indicates fraction in metric
     system. *mill*igram, *mill*ipede
miss-   See -mittent. intro*miss*ion
-mittent   *mitto, mittentis, missus* [L.] send.
     inter*mittent*
mne-   *mimnērcō, mnē-* [Gr.] remember.
     pseudo*mne*sia
mon-   *monos* [Gr.] only, sole.
     *mono*plegia
morph-   *morphē* [Gr.] form, shape.
     poly*morph*onuclear
mot-   *moveo, motus* [L.] move.
     vaso*mot*or
my-   *mys, myos* [Gr.] muscle.
     inoleio*my*oma
-myces   *mykēs, mykētos* [Gr.] fungus.
     myelo*myces*
myc(et)-   See -myces. asco*mycet*es,
     strepto*myc*in
myel-   *myelos* [Gr.] marrow. polio*myel*itis
myx-   *myxa* [Gr.] mucus. *myx*edema

narc-   *narkē* [Gr.] numbness. topo*nar*-
cosis

nas-   *nasus* [L.] nose. Cf. rhin-.
palato*nas*al

ne-   *neos* [Gr.] new, young. *ne*ocyte

necr-   *nekros* [Gr.] corpse. *necr*ocytosis

nephr-   *nephros* [Gr.] kidney. Cf. ren-.
para*nephr*ic

neur-   *neuron* [Gr.] nerve.
esthesio*neur*e

nod-   *nodus* [L.] knot *nod*osity

nom-   *nomos* [Gr.] (from *nemō*- deal
out, distribute) law, custom.
tax*onom*y

non-   *nona* [L.] nine. *non*acosane

nos-   *nosos* [Gr.] disease. *nos*ology

nucle-   *nucleus* [L.] (from *nux, nucis*
nut) kernel. Cf. kary-. *nucle*ide

nutri-   *nutrio* [L.] nourish. mal*nutri*tion

ob-   *ob* [L.] (*b* changes to *c* before
words beginning with that
consonant) against, toward,
etc. *ob*tuse

oc-   See ob-. *oc*clude

ocul-   *oculus* [L.] eye. Cf. ophthalm-.
*ocul*omotor

-od-   See -ode[1]. peri*od*ic

-ode[1]   *hodos* [Gr.] road, path. cath*ode*.
(See also hod-)

-ode[2]   See -oid. nemat*ode*

odont-   *odous, odontos* [Gr.] tooth. Cf.
dent-. orth*odont*ia

-odyn-   *odynē* [Gr.] pain, distress.
gastr*odyn*ia

-oid   *eidos* [Gr.] form. Cf. -form. hy*oid*

-ol   See ole-. cholester*ol*

ole-   *oleum* [L.] oil. *ole*oresin

olig-   *oligos* [Gr.] few, small.
*olig*ospermia

omphal-   *omphalos* [Gr.] navel.
peri*omphal*ic

onc-   *onkos* [Gr.] bulk, mass.
hemat*onc*ometry

onych-   *onyx, onychos* [Gr.] claw, nail.
an*onych*ia

oo-   *ōon* [Gr.] egg. Cf. ov-.
peri*oo*thecitis

op-   *horaō, op*- [Gr.] see. erythr*op*sia

ophthalm-   *ophthalmos* [Gr.] eye. Cf. ocul-.
ex*ophthalm*ic

or-   *os, oris* [L.] mouth. Cf.
stom(at)-. intra*or*al

orb-   *orbis* [L.] circle. sub*orb*ital

orchi-   *orchis* [Gr.] testicle. Cf. test-.
*orchi*opathy

organ-   *organon* [Gr.] implement,
instrument. *organ*oleptic

orth-   *orthos* [Gr.] straight, right,
normal. *orth*opedics

oss-   *os, ossis* [L.] bone. Cf. ost(e)-.
*oss*iphone

ost(e)-   *osteon* [Gr.] bone. Cf. oss-.
en*ost*osis, *oste*anaphysis

ot-   *ous, ōtos* [Gr.] ear. Cf. aur-.
par*ot*id

ov-   *ovum* [L.] egg. Cf. oo-. syn*ov*ia

oxy-   *oxys* [Gr.] sharp. *oxy*cephalic

pachy(n)-   *pachynō* [Gr.] thicken. *pachy*derma, myo*pachyn*sis

pag-   *pēgnymi, pag*- [Gr.] fix, make
fast. thoraco*pag*us

par-[1]   *pario* [L.] bear, give birth to.
primi*par*ous

par-[2]   See para-. *par*epigastric

para-   *para* [Gr.] (final *a* is dropped
before words beginning with a
vowel) beside, beyond.
*para*mastoid

part-   *pario, partus* [L.] bear, give birth
to. *part*urition

path-   *pathos* [Gr.] that which one under-
goes, sickness. psycho*path*ic

pec-   *pēgnymi, pēg*- [Gr.] (*pēk*- before *t*)
fix, make fast. sym*pec*tothiene.
(See also pex-)

ped-   *pais, paidos* [Gr.] child. ortho*ped*ic

pell-   *pellis* [L.] skin, hide. *pell*agra

-pellent   *pello, pellentis, pulsus* [L.] drive.
re*pellent*

pen-   *penomai* [Gr.] need, lack.
erythrocyto*pen*ia

pend-   *pendeo* [L.] hang down. ap*pend*ix

pent(a)-   *pente* [Gr.] five. Cf. quinque-.
*pent*ose, *penta*ploid

peps-   *peptō, peps*- [Gr.] digest.
brady*peps*ia

pept-   *peptō* [Gr.] digest. dys*pept*ic

per-   *per* [L.] through. Cf. dia-. *per*nasal

peri-   *peri* [Gr.] around. Cf. circum-.
*peri*phery

pet-   *peto* [L.] seek, tend toward.
centri*pet*al

pex-   *pēgnumi, pēg*- [Gr.] (added to *s*
becomes *pēx*) fix, make fast.
hepato*pex*y

pha-   *phēmi, pha*- [Gr.] say, speak.
dys*pha*sia

phac-   *phakos* [Gr.] lentil, lens. Cf.
lent-. *phac*osclerosis. (Also
spelled phak-)

phag-   *phagein* [Gr.] eat. lipo*phag*ic

phak-   See phac-. *phak*itis

phan-   See phen-. dia*phan*oscopy

pharmac-   *pharmakon* [Gr.] drug.
*pharmac*ognosy

pharyng-   *pharynx, pharyng*- [Gr.] throat.
glosso*pharyng*eal

phen-   *phainō, phan*- [Gr.] show, be
seen. phos*phen*e

pher-   *pherō, phor-* [Gr.] bear, support. peri*phery*

phil-   *phileō* [Gr.] like, have affinity for. eosino*phil*ia

phleb-   *phleps, phlebos* [Gr.] vein. peri*phleb*itis

phleg-   *phlogō, phlog-* [Gr.] burn, inflame. adeno*phleg*mon

phlog-   See phleg-. anti*phlog*istic

phob-   *phobos* [Gr.] fear, dread. claustro*phob*ia

phon-   *phōne* [Gr.] sound. echo*phon*y

phor-   See pher-. Cf. -ferent. exo*phor*ia

phos-   See phot-. *phos*phorus

phot-   *phōs, phōtos* [Gr.] light. *phot*erythrous

phrag-   *phrassō, phrag-* [Gr.] fence, wall off, stop up. Cf. sept-¹. dia*phrag*m

phrax-   *phrassō, phrag-* [Gr.] (added to *s* becomes *phrax-*) fence, wall off, stop up. em*phrax*is

phren-   *phrēn* [Gr.] mind, midriff. Cf. ment-. meta*phren*ia, meta*phren*on

phthi-   *phthinō* [Gr.] decay, waste away. *phthi*sis

phy-   *phyō* [Gr.] beget, bring forth, produce, be by nature. noso*phy*te

phyl-   *phylon* [Gr.] tribe, kind. *phyl*ogeny

-phyll   *phyllon* [Gr.] leaf. xantho*phyll*

phylac-   *phylax* [Gr.] guard. *prophylac*tic

phys(a)-   *physaō* [Gr.] blow, inflate. *physo*cele, *physa*lis

physe-   *physaō, physē-* [Gr.] blow, inflate. em*physe*ma

pil-   *pilus* [L.] hair. epi*pil*ation

pituit-   *pituita* [L.] phlegm, rheum. *pituit*ous

placent-   *placenta* [L.] (from *plakous* [Gr.]) cake. extra*placent*al

plas-   *plassō* [Gr.] mold, shape. cine*plas*ty

platy-   *platys* [Gr.] broad, flat. *platy*rrhine

pleg-   *plēssō* [Gr.] strike. di*pleg*ia

plet-   *pleo, -pletus* [L.] fill. de*plet*ion

pleur-   *pleura* [Gr.] rib, side. Cf. cost-. peri*pleur*al

plex-   *plēssō, plēg-* [Gr.] (added to *s* becomes *plēx-*) strike. apo*plex*y

plic-   *plico* [L.] fold. com*plic*ation

pne-   *pneuma, pneumatos* [Gr.] breathing. traumato*pne*a

pneum(at)-   *pneuma, pneumatos* [Gr.] breath, air. *pneum*odynamics, *pneumat*othorax

pneumo(n)-   *pneumōn* [Gr.] lung. Cf. pulmo(n)-. *pneumo*centesis, *pneumon*otomy

pod-   *pous, podos* [Gr.] foot. *pod*iatry

poie-   *poieō* [Gr.] make, produce. Cf. -facient. sarco*poie*tic

pol-   *polos* [Gr.] axis of a sphere. peri*pol*ar

poly-   *polys* [Gr.] much, many. *poly*spermia

pont-   *pons, pontis* [L.] bridge. *pont*ocerebellar

por-¹   *poros* [Gr.] passage. myelo*pore*

por-²   *poros* [Gr.] callus. *poro*cele

posit-   *pono, positus* [L.] put, place. re*positor*

post-   *post* [L.] after, behind in time or place. *post*natal, *post*oral

pre-   *prae* [L.] before in time or place. *pre*natal, *pre*vesical

press-   *premo, pressus* [L.] press. *press*oreceptive

pro-   *pro* [Gr., L.] before in time or place. *pro*gamous, *pro*cheilon, *pro*lapse

proct-   *prōktos* [Gr.] anus. entero*proct*ia

prosop-   *prosōpon* [Gr.] face. Cf. faci-. di*prosop*us

pseud-   *pseudēs* [Gr.] false. *pseud*oparaplegia

psych-   *psychē* [Gr.] soul, mind. Cf. ment-. *psycho*somatic

pto-   *piptō, ptō-* [Gr.] fall. nephro*pto*sis

pub-   *pubes, puber, puberis* [L.] adult. ischio*pub*ic. (See also puber-)

puber-   *puber* [L.] adult. *puber*ty

pulmo(n)-   *pulmo, pulmonis* [L.] lung. Cf. pneumo(n)-. *pulmo*lith, cardio*pulmon*ary

puls-   *pello, pellentis, pulsus* [L.] drive. *puls*ion

punct-   *pungo, punctus* [L.] prick, pierce. Cf. cente-. *punct*iform

pur-   *pus, puris* [L.] pus. Cf. py-. sup*pur*ation

py-   *pyon* [Gr.] pus. Cf. pur-. nephro*py*osis

pyel-   *pyelos* [Gr.] trough, basin, pelvis. nephro*pyel*itis

pyl-   *pylē* [Gr.] door, orifice. *pyl*ephlebitis

pyr-   *pyr* [Gr.] fire. Cf. febr-. galacto*pyr*a

quadr-   *quadr-* [L.] four. Cf. tetra-. *quadr*igeminal

quinque-   *quinque* [L.] five. Cf. pent(a)-. *quinque*cuspid

rachi-   *rachis* [Gr.] spine. Cf. spin-. encephalo*rachi*dian

radi-   *radius* [L.] ray. Cf. actin-. ir*radi*ation

re-   *re-* [L.] back, again. *re*traction

ren-   *renes* [L.] kidneys. Cf. nephr-. ad*ren*al

ret-	*rete* [L.] net. *ret*othelium

retro-	*retro* [L.] backward. *retro*deviation

rhag-	*rhēgnymi, rhag-* [Gr.] break, burst. hemor*rhag*ic

rhaph-	*rhaphē* [Gr.] suture. gastror*rhaph*y

rhe-	*rhaphē* [Gr.] flow. Cf. flu-. diar*rhe*al

rhex-	*rhēgnymi, rhēg-* [Gr.] (added to s becomes *rhēx*) break, burst. metror*rhex*is

rhin-	*rhis, rhinos* [Gr.] nose. Cf. nas-. basi*rhin*al

rot-	*rota* [L.] wheel. *rot*ator

rub(r)-	*ruber, rubri* [L.] red. Cf. erythr-. bili*rub*in, *rubr*ospinal

salping-	*salpinx, salpingos* [Gr.] tube, trumpet. *salping*itis

sanguin-	*sanguis, sanguinis* [L.] blood. Cf. hem(at)-. *sanguin*eous

sarc-	*sarx, sarkos* [Gr.] flesh. *sarc*oma

schis-	*schizō, schid-* [Gr.] (before *t* or added to *s* becomes *schis-*) split. Cf. fiss-. *schis*torachis, rachi*schis*is

scler-	*sklēros* [Gr.] hard. Cf. dur-. *scler*osis

scop-	*skopeō* [Gr.] look at, observe. endo*scope*

sect-	*seco, sectus* [L.] cut. Cf. tom-, *sect*ile

semi-	*semi* [L.] half. Cf. hemi-. *semi*flexion

sens-	*sentio, sensus* [L.] perceive, feel. Cf. esthe-. *sens*ory

sep-	*sepō* [Gr.] rot, decay. *sep*sis

sept-[1]	*saepio, saeptus* [L.] fence, wall off, stop up. Cf. phrag-. naso*sept*al

sept-[2]	*septem* [L.] seven. Cf. hept(a)-. *sept*an

ser-	*serum* [L.] whey, watery substance. *ser*osynovitis

sex-	*sex* [L.] six. Cf. hex-[1]. *sex*digitate

sial-	*sialon* [Gr.] saliva. poly*sial*ia

sin-	*sinus* [L.] hollow, fold. Cf. colp-. *sin*obronchitis

sit-	*sitos* [Gr.] food. para*sit*ic

solut-	*solvo, solventis, solutus* [L.] loose, dissolve, set free. Cf. ly-. dis*solut*ion

-solvent	See solut-. dis*solvent*

somat-	*sōma, somatōs* [Gr.] body. Cf. corpor-. psycho*somat*ic

-some	See somat-. dictyo*some*

spas-	*spaō, spas-* [Gr.] draw, pull. *spas*m, *spas*tic

spectr-	*spectrum* [L.] appearance, what is seen. micro*spectr*oscope

sperm(at)-	*sperma, spermatos* [Gr.] seed. *sperm*acrasia, *spermat*ozoon

spers-	*spargo, -spersus* [L.] scatter. di*spers*ion

sphen-	*sphēn* [Gr.] wedge. Cf. cune-. *sphen*oid

spher-	*sphaira* [Gr.] ball. hemi*spher*e

sphygm-	*sphygmos* [Gr.] pulsation. *sphygm*omanometer

spin-	*spina* [L.] spine. Cf. rachi-. cerebro*spin*al

spirat-	*spiro, spiratus* [L.] breathe. in*spirat*ory

splanchn-	*splanchna* [Gr.] entrails, viscera. neuro*splanchn*ic

splen-	*splēn* [Gr.] spleen. Cf. lien-. *splen*omegaly

spor-	*sporos* [Gr.] seed. *spor*ophyte, zygo*spor*e

squam-	*squama* [L.] scale. de*squam*ation

sta-	*histēmi, sta-* [Gr.] make stand, stop. genesi*sta*sis

stal-	*stellō, stal-* [Gr.] send. peri*stal*sis. (See also stol-)

staphyl-	*staphylē* [Gr.] bunch of grapes, uvula. *staphyl*ococcus, *staphyl*ectomy

stear-	*stear, steatos* [Gr.] fat. Cf. adip-. *stear*odermia

steat-	See stear-. *steat*opygous

sten-	*stenos* [Gr.] narrow, compressed. *sten*ocardia

ster-	*stereos* [Gr.] solid. chole*ster*ol

sterc-	*stercus* [L.] dung. Cf. copr-. *sterc*oporphyrin

sthen-	*sthenos* [Gr.] strength. a*sthen*ia

stol-	*stellō, stol-* [Gr.] send. dia*stol*e

stom(at)-	*stoma, stomatos* [Gr.] mouth, orifice. Cf. or-. ana*stom*osis, *stomat*ogastric

strep(h)-	*strephō, strep-* (before *t*) [Gr.] twist. Cf. tors-. *streph*osymbolia, *strep*tomycin. (See also stroph-)

strict-	*stringo, stringentis, strictus* [L.] draw tight, compress, cause pain. con*strict*ion

-stringent	See strict-. a*stringent*

stroph-	*strephō, stroph-* [Gr.] twist. ana*stroph*ic. (See also strep(h)-)

struct-	*struo, structus* [L.] pile up (against). ob*struct*ion

sub-	*sub* [L.] (*b* changes to *f* or *p* before words beginning with those consonants) under, below. Cf. hypo-. *sub*lumbar

suf-	See sub-. *suf*fusion

sup-	See sub-. *sup*pository

super-	*super* [L.] above, beyond, extreme. Cf. hyper-. *super*motility

sy-	See syn-. *sy*stole

syl- See syn-. *syl*lepsiology

sym- See syn-. *sym*biosis, *sym*metry, *sym*pathetic, *sym*physis

syn- *syn* [Gr.] (*n* disappears before *s*, changes to *l* before *l*, and changes to *m* before *b*, *m*, *p*, and *ph*) with, together. Cf. con-. myo*syn*izesis

ta- See ton-. ec*ta*sis

tac- *tassō, tag-* [Gr.] (*tak* before *t*) order, arrange. a*tac*tic

tact- *tango, tactus* [L.] touch. con*tact*

tax- *tassō, tag-* [Gr.] (added to *s* becomes *tax-*) order, arrange. a*tax*ia

tect- See teg-. pro*tect*ive

teg- *tego, tectus* [L.) cover. in*teg*ument

tel- *telos* [Gr.] end. *tel*osynapsis

tele- *tēle* [Gr.] at a distance. *tele*ceptor

tempor- *tempus, temporis* [L.] time, timely or fatal spot, temple. *tempor*omalar

ten(ont)- *tenon, tenontos* [Gr.] (from *teinō* stretch) tight stretched band. *ten*odynia, *ten*onitis, *tenont*agra

tens- *tendo, tensus* [L.] stretch. Cf. ton-. ex*tens*or

test- *testis* [L.] testicle. Cf. orchi-. *test*itis

tetra- *tetra-* [Gr.] four. Cf. quadr-. *tetra*genous

the- *tithēmi, thē-* [Gr.] put, place. syn*the*sis

thec- *thēkē* [Gr.] repository, case. *thec*ostegnosis

thel- *thēlē* [Gr.] teat, nipple. *thel*erethism

therap- *therapeia* [Gr.] treatment. hydro*therap*y

therm- *thermē* [Gr.] heat Cf. calor-. dia*therm*y

thi- *theion* [Gr.] sulfur. *thi*ogenic

thorac- *thōrax, thōrakos* [Gr.] chest. *thorac*oplasty

thromb- *thrombos* [Gr.] lump, clot. *thromb*openia

thym- *thymos* [Gr.] spirit. Cf. ment-. dys*thym*ia

thyr- *thyreos* [Gr.] shield (shaped like a door *thyra*). *thyr*oid

tme- *temnō, tmē-* [Gr.] cut. axono*tme*sis

toc- *tokos* [Gr.] childbirth. dys*toc*ia

tom- *temnō, tom-* [Gr.] cut. Cf. sect-. appendec*tom*y

ton- *teino, ton-* [Gr.] stretch, put under tension. Cf. tens-. peri*ton*eum

top- *topos* [Gr.] place. Cf. loc-. *top*esthesia

tors- *torqueo, torsus* [L.] twist. Cf. strep-. ec*tors*ion

tox- *toxicon* [Gr.] (from *toxon* bow) arrow poison, poison. *tox*emia

trache- *tracheia* [Gr.] windpipe. *trache*otomy

trachel- *trachēlos* [Gr.] neck. Cf. cervic-. *trachel*opexy

tract- *traho, tractus* [L.] draw, drag. pro*tract*ion

traumat- *trauma, traumatos* [Gr.] wound. *traumat*ic

tri- *treis, tria* [Gr.] or *tri-* [L.] three. *tri*gonid

trich- *thrix, trichos* [Gr.] hair. *trich*oid

trip- *tribō* [Gr.] rub. en*trip*sis

trop- *trepō, trop-* [Gr.] turn, react. sito*trop*ism

troph- *trepō, troph-* [Gr.] nurture. a*troph*y

tuber- *tuber* [L.] swelling, node. *tuber*cle

typ- *typos* [Gr.] (from *typto* strike) type. a*typ*ical

typh- *typhos* [Gr.] fog, stupor. adeno*typh*us

typhl- *typhlos* [Gr.] blind. Cf. cec-. *typhl*ectasis

un- *unus* [L.] one. Cf. hen-. *un*ioval

ur- *ouron* [Gr.] urine. poly*ur*ia

vacc- *vacca* [L.] cow. *vacc*ine

vagin- *vagina* [L.] sheath. in*vagin*ated

vas- *vas* [L.] vessel. Cf. angi-. *vas*cular

vers- See vert-. in*vers*ion

vert- *verto, versus* [L.] turn. di*vert*iculum

vesic- *vesica* [L.] bladder. Cf. cyst-. *vesic*ovaginal

vit- *vita* [L.] life. Cf. bi-[1]. de*vit*alize

vuls- *vello, vulsus* [L.] pull, twitch. con*vuls*ion

xanth- *xanthos* [Gr.] yellow, blond. Cf. flav-, lute-. *xanth*ophyll

-yl- *hylē* [Gr.] substance. cacod*yl*

zo- *zoē* [Gr.] life, *zōon* [Gr.] animal. micro*zo*aria

zyg- *zygon* [Gr.] yoke, union. *zyg*odactyly

zym- *zymē* [Gr.] ferment. en*zym*e

---

*It is the custom in the metric system to identify fractions of units by stems from the Latin, as centimeter, decimeter, and millimeter, and multiples of units by the similar stems from the Greek, as hectometer, decameter, and kilometer.

Compiled by Lloyd W. Daly, AM, PhD, LittD, Allen Memorial Professor of Greek Emeritus, University of Pennsylvania. Adapted from Miller, B.F., and Keane, C.B.: Encyclopedia and Dictionary of Medicine, Nursing, and Allied Health, 4th ed. Philadelphia, W.B. Saunders Company, 1987.

Rules for Forming Plurals

As with English words, many medical words form their plurals by adding **s** or **es**. Irregular plural forms are included alphabetically in the specialty sections of this book with the explanation "plural of" in parentheses. The singular form is also followed by the irregular plural form in parentheses. The rules for forming plurals of common medical terms are listed below. Examples and a few exceptions are noted. Memorizing these rules and the exceptions will improve the quality and accuracy of your work and increase your speed.

1. For singular nouns ending in **a**, retain the **a** and add **e**.

Singular	Plural
vertebr<u>a</u>	vertebr<u>ae</u>
burs<u>a</u>	burs<u>ae</u>
bull<u>a</u>	bull<u>ae</u>

2. For singular nouns ending in **um**, drop the **um** and add **a**.

Singular	Plural
	adnexa*
bacteri<u>um</u>	bacteri<u>a</u>
diverticul<u>um</u>	diverticul<u>a</u>**
ov<u>um</u>	ov<u>a</u>

Adnexa (meaning appendages) is always plural. It is sometimes incorrectly dictated as adnexae or adnexi.
**The plural of diverticulum is often incorrectly dictated and spelled as diverticulae or diverticuli.

Note: *Data*, the plural of datum (rarely used), may be singular or plural. If used in the noncounting sense as a synonym for information (more data is needed), it would take a singular verb; if used to mean a number of individual pieces of information (all the data point to . . .), it would be plural. *Medium*, the singular form of *media*, is rarely used in medical reports.

3. For singular nouns ending in **on**, drop the **on** and add **a**.

Singular	Plural
acromion	acromia
ganglion	ganglia
phenomenon	phenomena
prodromon	prodroma*
spermatozoon	spermatozoa

Prodroma is often incorrectly (even in some references) thought to be the singular form and made plural as *prodromata*. The singular form *prodromon* is rarely used, if at all. *Prodrome*, the English form, is most commonly dictated.

4. A. For singular nouns ending in **us**, drop the **us** and add **i**.

Singular	Plural
calculus	calculi
bronchus	bronchi
nucleus	nuclei

B. A few singular nouns ending in **us** form the plural by dropping the **us** and adding **era** or **ora**.

Singular	Plural
genus	genera
glomus	glomera
latus	latera
tempus	tempora
ulcus	ulcera
viscus	viscera
vulnus	vulnera

Exceptions:

Certain words ending in **us** do not change in the plural form.

Singular	Plural
meatus	meatus*
abortus	abortus**

*The plural of meatus is often incorrectly written as meati.
**Abortus* is sometimes incorrectly dictated as *aborta,* particularly in expressions such as "gravida 6, para 3, abortus 3."
The plural form of *pus* is pura. Other exceptions include sinuses and viruses.

5. A. For singular nouns ending in **sis**, drop the **is** and add **es**.

Singular	Plural
anastomos*is*	anastomos*es*
metastas*is*	metastas*es*
epiphys*is*	epiphys*es*
prosthes*is*	prosthes*es*

Exception:
Naris ends only in **is**, but the plural is nar*es*. The singular form is often incorrectly dictated as *nare,* an erroneous back-formation of *nares.*

B. For singular nouns ending in **itis** or **is** not preceded by "s," drop the **s** and add **des**.

Singular	Plural
arterit*is*	arterit*des*
arthrit*is*	arthrit*des*
epididym*is*	epididym*des*
epiglott*is*	epiglott*des*
Ir*is*	ir*des*

Note: *Pubis,* often thought to be a singular noun, is actually the genitive of *pubes* which is unchanged in the plural. *Pubis* is used alone as an alternative for *os pubis,* the pubic bone.

6. For singular nouns ending in **y**, drop the **y** and add **ies**.

Singular	Plural
cavit*y*	cavi*ties*
ovar*y*	ovar*ies*

7. For singular nouns ending in **en**, drop the **en** and add **ina**.

Singular	Plural
cerum*en*	cerum*ina*
foram*en*	foram*ina*
lum*en*	lum*ina*
velam*en*	velam*ina*

8. For singular nouns ending with **x**:
   A. If the word ends in **ax** or **ox**, drop the **x** and add **ces**.

Singular	Plural
thora*x*	thora*ces*
vo*x*	vo*ces*

8. B. If the word ends in **ix** or **ex**, drop the **ix** or **ex** and add **ices**.

Singular	Plural
ap<u>ex</u>	ap<u>ices</u>
var<u>ix</u>	var<u>ices</u>

Exceptions:

refl<u>ex</u>	refl<u>exes</u>
s<u>ex</u>	s<u>exes</u>

C. If the word ends in **nx**, drop the **x** and add **ges**.

Singular	Plural
phalan<u>x</u>	phalan<u>ges</u>
salpin<u>x</u>	salpin<u>ges</u>
menin<u>x</u>	menin<u>ges</u>

9. For singular nouns ending in **oma**, retain the **oma** and add **ta**.

Singular	Plural
carcin<u>oma</u>	carcinom<u>ata</u>*
condyl<u>oma</u>	condylom<u>ata</u>*
my<u>oma</u>	myom<u>ata</u>*

*A simple **s** ending is also correct: carcin<u>omas</u>, condyl<u>omas</u>, my<u>omas</u>.

10. For singular nouns ending in **o**, drop the **o** and add **ines**.

Singular	Plural
lentig<u>o</u>	lentig<u>ines</u>
libid<u>o</u>	libid<u>ines</u>
marg<u>o</u>	marg<u>ines</u>

Exceptions:
Some words ending in **o** form the plural by simply adding **nes**.

Singular	Plural
pulm<u>o</u>	pulmo<u>nes</u>
radiati<u>o</u>	radiatio<u>nes</u>

11. A few nouns used in medical reports are always plural. Some may appear singular in form, but the following terms all take plural verbs.

adnexa	feces
genitalia	menses
fauces	rhagades

12. A few terms used in medical reports *sound* plural but are actually singular.

agenda*	facies	measles
ascites	insignia*	mumps
herpes	lues	regalia*

*These nonmedical Latin plural forms have become singular in English and take a singular verb. They may be occasionally used in medical reports.

13. Some terms may be either singular or plural depending on their use.

biceps*	meatus	sordes
forceps**	scissors**	tongs**
pubes	series	tweezers**

*Biceps is an adjective that is sometimes used alone to mean the biceps muscle or muscles.
**These surgical instruments may be used with either a singular or plural verb, but are usually plural.

14. Other irregularly formed plurals include the following:

Singular	Plural	Singular	Plural
caput	capita	os [bone]	ossa
cavitas	cavitates	os [mouth]	ora
comes	comites	pancreas	pancreata
cuspis	cuspides	paries	parietes
dens	dentes	pars	partes
foot	feet	rete	retia
louse	lice	tooth	teeth
mesonephros	mesonephroi	venter	ventres

Sloane's
Medical
Word
Book

Appendix

Table of Elements

Name	Symbol	At. No.	At. Wt.†
Actinium	Ac	89	(227.028)
Aluminum	Al	13	26.982
Americium	Am	95	(243.061)
Antimony	Sb	51	121.760
Argon	Ar	18	39.948
Arsenic	As	33	74.922
Astatine	At	85	(209.987)
Barium	Ba	56	137.327
Berkelium	Bk	97	(247.070)
Beryllium	Be	4	9.012
Bismuth	Bi	83	208.980
Boron	B	5	10.811
Bromine	Br	35	79.904
Cadmium	Cd	48	112.411
Calcium	Ca	20	40.078
Californium	Cf	98	(251.080)
Carbon	C	6	12.011
Cerium	Ce	58	140.115
Cesium	Cs	55	132.905
Chlorine	Cl	17	35.453
Chromium	Cr	24	51.996
Cobalt	Co	27	58.933
Copper	Cu	29	63.546
Curium	Cm	96	(247.070)
Dysprosium	Dy	66	162.503
Einsteinium	Es	99	(252.087)
Element 104*	Unq	104	(261.11)
Element 105*	Unp	105	(262.114)
Element 106*	Unh	106	(263.118)
Element 107*	Uns	107	(262.12)
Element 108*	Uno	108	
Element 109*	Une	109	
Erbium	Er	68	167.26
Europium	Eu	63	151.965
Fermium	Fm	100	(257.095)
Fluorine	F	9	18.998
Francium	Fr	87	(223.020)
Gadolinium	Gd	64	157.25
Gallium	Ga	31	69.723
Germanium	Ge	32	72.61
Gold	Au	79	196.967
Hafnium	Hf	72	178.49
Helium	He	2	4.003
Holmium	Ho	67	164.930
Hydrogen	H	1	1.008
Indium	In	49	114.818

Table of Elements (continued)

Name	Symbol	At. No.	At. Wt.†
Iodine	1	53	126.904
Iridium	Ir	77	192.217
Iron	Fe	26	55.845
Krypton	Kr	36	83.80
Lanthanum	La	57	138.906
Lawrencium	Lw	103	(262.11)
Lead	Pb	82	207.2
Lithium	Li	3	6.941
Lutetium	Lu	71	174.967
Magnesium	Mg	12	24.305
Manganese	Mn	25	54.938
Mendelevium	Md	101	(258.10)
Mercury	Hg	80	200.59
Molybdenum	Mo	42	95.94
Neodymium	Nd	60	144.24
Neon	Ne	10	20.180
Neptunium	Np	93	(237.048)
Nickel	Ni	28	58.693
Niobium	Nb	41	92.906
Nitrogen	N	7	14.007
Nobelium	No	102	(259.101)
Osmium	Os	76	190.2
Oxygen	0	8	15.999
Palladium	Pd	46	106.42
Phosphorus	P	15	30.974
Platinum	Pt	78	195.08
Plutonium	Pu	94	(244.064)
Polonium	Po	84	(209.982)
Potassium	K	19	39.098
Praseodymium	Pr	59	140.908
Promethium	Pm	61	(144.913)
Protactinium	Pa	91	(231.039)
Radium	Ra	88	(226.025)
Radon	Rn	86	(222.018)
Rhenium	Re	75	186.207
Rhodium	Rh	45	102.906
Rubidium	Rb	37	85.468
Ruthenium	Ru	44	101.07
Samarium	Sm	62	150.36
Scandium	Sc	21	44.956
Selenium	Se	34	78.96
Silicon	Si	14	28.086
Silver	Ag	47	107.868
Sodium	Na	11	22.990
Strontium	Sr	38	87.62
Sulfur	S	16	32.066
Tantalum	Ta	73	180.948
Technetium	Tc	43	(97.907)
Tellurium	Te	52	127.60
Terbium	Tb	65	158.925
Thallium	Tl	81	204.383

Table of Elements (continued)

Name	Symbol	At. No.	At. Wt.†
Thorium	Th	90	232.038
Thulium	Tm	69	168.934
Tin	Sn	50	118.710
Titanium	Ti	22	47.867
Tungsten	W	74	183.84
Uranium	U	92	238.029
Vanadium	V	23	50.942
Xenon	Xe	54	131.29
Ytterbium	Yb	70	173.04
Yttrium	Y	39	88.906
Zinc	Zn	30	65.39
Zirconium	Zr	40	91.224

*Multiple, and sometimes conflicting, names have been proposed for elements 104–108. The symbols given for elements 104–109 are based on the IUPAC systematic names.

†Atomic weights are corrected to conform with the 1993 values of the International Union of Pure and Applied Chemistry, expressed to the fourth decimal point, rounded off to the nearest thousandth. The numbers in parentheses are the mass numbers of the most stable or most common isotope for certain radioactive elements.

Source: Dorland's Illustrated Medical Dictionary, 29th ed. Philadelphia, W.B. Saunders Company, 2000, p. 579.

Tables of Weights and Measures

Measures of Mass

Avoirdupois Weight

Grains	Drams	Ounces	Pounds	Grams*
1	0.0366	0.0023	0.00014	0.0647989
27.34	1	0.0625	0.0039	1.772
437.5	16	1	0.0625	28.350
7000	256	16	1	453.5924277

*Metric equivalents.

Apothecaries' Weight

Grains	Scruples	Drams	Ounces	Pounds	Grams*
1	0.05	0.0167	0.0021	0.00017	0.0647989
20	1	0.333	0.042	0.0035	1.296
60	3	1	0.125	0.0104	3.888
480	24	8	1	0.0833	31.103
5760	288	96	12	1	373.24177

*Metric equivalents.

Troy Weight

Grains	Pennyweights	Ounces	Pounds	Grams*
1	0.042	0.002	0.00017	0.0647989
24	1	0.05	0.0042	1.555
480	20	1	0.083	31.103
5760	240	12	1	373.24177

*Metric equivalents.

Metric Weight

Micro-gram	Milli-gram	Centi-gram	Deci-gram	Gram	Deka-gram	Hecto-gram	Kilo-gram	Equivalents Avoirdupois	Apothecaries
1	—	—	—	—	—	—	—	0.000015 grains	
10^3	1	—	—	—	—	—	—	0.015432 grains	
10^4	10	1	—	—	—	—	—	0.154323 grains	
10^5	10^2	10	1	—	—	—	—	1.543235 grains	
10^6	10^3	10^2	10	1	—	—	—	15.432356 grains	
10^7	10^4	10^3	10^2	10	1	—	—	5.6438 dr.	7.7162 scr.
10^8	10^5	10^4	10^3	10^2	10	1	—	3.527 oz.	3.215 oz.
10^9	10^6	10^5	10^4	10^3	10^2	10	1	2.2046 lb.	2.6792 lb.

Measures of Capacity

Apothecaries' (Wine) Measure

Minims	Fluid Drams	Fluid Ounces	Gills	Pints	Quarts	Gal- lons	Cubic Inches	Milli- liters	Cu. Centi- meters
1	0.0166	0.002	0.0005	0.00013	—	—	0.00376	0.06161	0.06161
60	1	0.125	0.0312	0.0078	0.0039	—	0.22558	3.6967	3.6967
480	8	1	0.25	0.0625	0.0312	0.0078	1.80468	29.5737	29.5737
1920	32	4	1	0.25	0.125	0.0312	7.21875	118.2948	118.2948
7680	128	16	4	1	0.5	0.125	28.875	473.179	473.179
15360	256	32	8	2	1	0.25	57.75	946.358	946.358
61440	1024	128	32	8	4	1	231	3785.434	3785.434

Metric Measure

Micro- liter	Milli- liter	Centi- liter	Deci- liter	Liter	Deka- liter	Hecto liter	Kilo- liter	Equivalents (Apothecaries' Fluid)
1	—	—	—	—	—	—	—	0.01623108 minim
10^3	1	—	—	—	—	—	—	16.23 minims
10^4	10	1	—	—	—	—	—	2.7 fluid drams
10^5	10^2	10	1	—	—	—	—	3.38 fluid ounces
10^6	10^3	10^2	10	1	—	—	—	2.113363738 pints
10^7	10^4	10^3	10^2	10	1	—	—	2.64 gallons
10^8	10^5	10^4	10^3	10^2	10	1	—	26.418 gallons
10^9	10^6	10^5	10^4	10^3	10^2	10	1	264.18 gallons

Measures of Length

Metric Measure

Micro- meter	Milli- meter	Centi- meter	Deci- meter	Meter	Deka- meter	Hecto meter	Kilo- meter	Equivalents	
1	0.001	10^{-4}	—	—	—	—	—	0.000039	inch
10^3	1	10^{-1}	—	—	—	—	—	0.03937	inch
10^4	10	1	—	—	—	—	—	0.3937	inch
10^5	10^2	10	1	—	—	—	—	3.937	inches
10^6	10^3	10^2	10	1	—	—	—	39.37	inches
10^7	10^4	10^3	10^2	10	1	—	—	10.9361	yards
10^8	10^5	10^4	10^3	10^2	10	1	—	109.3612	yards
10^9	10^6	10^5	10^4	10^3	10^2	10	1	1093.6121	yards

Unit Conversions

Measures of Mass

Avoirdupois to Metric

1 ounce	=	28.350 grams
1 pound	=	453.59 grams

Metric to Avoirdupois

1 gram	=	0.035274 ounces
1 kilogram	=	35.274 ounces
1 kilogram	=	2.2046 pounds

Apothecaries' to Metric

1 grain	=	0.065 grams
1 scruple	=	1.296 grams
1 dram	=	3.888 grams
1 ounce	=	31.103 grams

Metric to Apothecaries'

1 milligram	=	0.015432 grains
1 milligram	=	1/60 grain
1 gram	=	15.4320 grains
1 gram	=	0.2572 drams
1 gram	=	0.03215 ounces
1 kilogram	=	2.68 pounds

Liquid Measure

Apothecaries' to Metric*

1 minim	=	0.06 milliliters
1 fluid dram	=	3.70 milliliters
1 fluid ounce	=	29.57 milliliters
1 pint	=	473.18 milliliters
1 quart	=	946.36 milliliters
1 gallon	=	3785.43 milliliters

Metric* to Apothecaries'

1 milliliter	=	16.231 minim
1 milliliter	=	0.27 fluid drams
1 liter	=	33.815 fluid oz.

*A milliliter (mL) is approximately equal to a cubic centimeter.

Temperature

Conversion Formulas

$$°F = (°C \times \tfrac{9}{5}) + 32$$
$$°C = (°F - 32) \times \tfrac{5}{9}$$

Source: Miller, B.F. and Keane, C.B.: Encyclopedia and Dictionary of Medicine, Nursing, and Allied Health, 6th ed. Philadelphia, W.B. Saunders Company, 1997.